Antibiotics in Laboratory Medicine

Sixth Edition

Antibiotics in Laboratory Medicine

Sixth Edition

Daniel Amsterdam, PhD, ABMM, FAAAS, FIDSA

Professor
Departments of Microbiology & Immunology, Medicine, and Pathology
School of Medicine and Biomedical Sciences
State University of New York at Buffalo;
Chief of Service, Department of Laboratory Medicine
Erie County Medical Center
Buffalo, New York

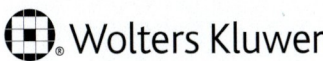 Wolters Kluwer

Philadelphia • Baltimore • New York • London
Buenos Aires • Hong Kong • Sydney • Tokyo

Acquisitions Editor: Julie Goolsby
Product Development Editors: Kristina Oberle and Andrea Vosburgh
Production Project Manager: Joan Sinclair
Design Coordinator: Terry Mallon
Manufacturing Coordinator: Beth Welsh
Prepress Vendor: Absolute Service, Inc.

6th edition

9 8 7 6 5 4 3 2 1

Printed in China.

Library of Congress Cataloging-in-Publication Data

Antibiotics in laboratory medicine / [edited by] Daniel Amsterdam. — Sixth edition.
  p. ; cm.
 Includes bibliographical references and index.
 ISBN 978-1-4511-7675-9 (alk. paper)
 I. Amsterdam, Daniel, editor.
 [DNLM: 1. Microbial Sensitivity Tests. 2. Anti-Bacterial Agents—pharmacology. 3. Drug Resistance, Microbial—physiology. QW 25.5.M6]
 QR69.A57
 615.3'29—dc23
                    2014022704

    Care has been taken to confirm the accuracy of the information presented and to describe generally accepted practices. However, the authors, editors, and publisher are not responsible for errors or omissions or for any consequences from application of the information in this book and make no warranty, expressed or implied, with respect to the currency, completeness, or accuracy of the contents of the publication. Application of this information in a particular situation remains the professional responsibility of the practitioner; the clinical treatments described and recommended may not be considered absolute and universal recommendations.
    The authors, editors, and publisher have exerted every effort to ensure that drug selection and dosage set forth in this text are in accordance with the current recommendations and practice at the time of publication. However, in view of ongoing research, changes in government regulations, and the constant flow of information relating to drug therapy and drug reactions, the reader is urged to check the package insert for each drug for any change in indications and dosage and for added warnings and precautions. This is particularly important when the recommended agent is a new or infrequently employed drug.
    Some drugs and medical devices presented in this publication have Food and Drug Administration (FDA) clearance for limited use in restricted research settings. It is the responsibility of the health care provider to ascertain the FDA status of each drug or device planned for use in his or her clinical practice.

LWW.com

For Victor Lorian, MD (deceased), my mentors and coauthors in this and other works, and as always, for my steadfast wife, Carol, and my children, Jonathan and Valerie.

Acknowledgments

As a former contributor to *Antibiotics in Laboratory Medicine*, I am pleased and honored to take on the editorial leadership of the sixth edition to carry on the vision of the founding editor, Victor Lorian, MD. Dr. Lorian's editorial direction spanned more than 30 years and this acknowledgment is a small tribute to his role. In the nascent edition, there were only antibacterial agents deliberated. Succeeding editions witnessed the expanding role of antifungal and antiviral compounds.

In addition to Dr. Lorian's vital contribution, this edition acknowledges the efforts of chapter authors from previous editions who were unable to continue in this work.

Preface

Since their discovery and introduction into the armamentarium of medicines, antibiotics have saved countless lives and contributed to the rapid advancement of modern medicine. The legacy drugs, penicillin, tetracycline, and their contemporary successors have been essential in sustaining health and dealing with human diseases. Their use to treat infections should be considered a global health resource that needs to be carefully conserved. Yet, we are confronted by the expanding scope of drug resistance and more pointedly multidrug resistance, which highlights the reliance on laboratory antimicrobial susceptibility and resistant gene testing. It has become patently clear that for many organisms once considered reliably susceptible to a number of broad-spectrum agents, unexpected resistance can occur as a result of foreign travel or multidrug courses of therapy during a hospital admission.

In recent editions of *Antibiotics in Laboratory Medicine*, which have now has spanned more than 35 years, nearly half the antibiotic era, readers have witnessed the role of newer compounds and drug classes including antifungal and antiviral agents, albeit limited the past decade, and had access to methods and approaches for determining efficacy and detailing the mechanisms of action and resistance of these compounds in vivo and in vitro.

New for this edition are the introductory "Perspectives" and the Appendix. The former deals with the outlook of antiinfective compounds; their origin and archeologic niche in nature; and their current role, development, and future application. In the Appendix are the Web addresses that readers can select for learning more about the nature of the drugs, current resistance patterns and trends, and their clinical application. Each of the intervening chapters, by new or former author(s) expanded and reworked, represent current science and laboratory practice. Several aspects of this volume are worth highlighting. In Chapter 1, Winkler et al. detail the criteria and considerations that Clinical and Laboratory Standards Institute uses in defining breakpoints, the essential divide between the classification of agents as "susceptible" or "resistant" or as we also know as "nonsusceptible." Examples and rationale are presented for changing breakpoints. In ensuing chapters, Drs. Turnidge and Bell and I expand on previously detailed information in experimentally defining susceptibility/resistance when using agar- or broth-based analytical systems. Drs. Venugopal and Hecht expertly update susceptibility of anaerobes, which, although essential, has recently become a less focused clinical challenge. Drs. Thompson and Patterson discuss and refine the testing modalities and clarified terms for defining and interpreting the activity of antifungal agents. Dr. Inderlied along with new coauthor Dr. Edward Desmond addresses the expanding role of the laboratory in evaluating the susceptibility of the mycobacteria to antimycobacterial agents. Dr. Rolain provides readers with a comprehensive review of susceptibility testing of unusual microorganisms for which there is a paucity of information. In Chapter 8, Dr. Edberg and new coauthors Drs. Latte and Sordillo update application and methods for measuring levels of antimicrobial agents in body fluids. Dr. Sundsfjord and colleagues from Norway in Chapter 9 examine the varied molecular methods that have come into use for detection of antibacterial resistance genes. In the ensuing Chapter 10, Dr. Stratton updates the molecular mechanism of action of antimicrobial agents, which is essential to understanding the MOA of drugs and designing new compounds. The chapter addressing antiviral agents (Chapter 11) discusses the several newly developed antiviral classes for HIV, cytomegalovirus, and influenza. Dr. Ostrov in collaboration with Dr. Amsterdam have reorganized and updated the chapter that addresses antiseptics and disinfectants. In Chapter 13, Drs. Frimodt-Møller and colleagues have done an extensive update on the evaluation of antimicrobial agents in experimental animal infections; new models and more than 50 new references have been added to the previously cited reference list. In the last work, Chapter 14, Dr. Bamberger and colleagues have used their vast clinical experience and knowledge and document the distribution of antimicrobial agents in extravascular compartments.

As a former (and current) contributor, I am cognizant of and in awe of my fellow authors who participated in this work and made this edition of *Antibiotics in Laboratory Medicine* scientifically sound and clinically meaningful. The sixth edition is authored by an international group of distinguished scientists and physicians, expert in their discipline, brilliant in their vision, and recognized worldwide.

Daniel Amsterdam

Contributing Authors

Paul G. Ambrose, PharmD
Associate Research Professor
Pharmacy Practice
School of Pharmacy and Pharmaceutical Services
University at Buffalo
Amherst, New York

Daniel Amsterdam, PhD, ABMM, FAAAS, FIDSA
Professor
Departments of Microbiology & Immunology, Medicine, and Pathology
School of Medicine and Biomedical Sciences
State University of New York at Buffalo;
Chief of Service, Department of Laboratory Medicine
Erie County Medical Center
Buffalo, New York

David R. Andes, MD
Professor
Departments of Medicine and Microbiology
Chief, Division of Infectious Diseases
University of Wisconsin
Madison, Wisconsin

David M. Bamberger, MD
Professor of Medicine
University of Missouri-Kansas City School of Medicine;
Chief, Section of Infectious Diseases
Truman Medical Centers
Kansas City, Missouri

Jan M. Bell, BSc (Hons), BA
SA Pathology
Women's and Children's Hospital
North Adelaide, Australia

Franklin R. Cockerill III, MD
Ann and Leo Markin Professor of Medicine and Microbiology
Department of Laboratory Medicine and Pathology
Mayo Clinic College of Medicine
Rochester, Minnesota

Edward Desmond, PhD, DABMM
Chief
Myocobacteriology and Mycology Section
Microbial Diseases Laboratory
California Department of Public Health
Richmond, California

Stephen C. Edberg, PhD, ABMM, FAAM
Professor Emeritus
Yale University;
Mount Sinai Health System
New York, New York

John W. Foxworth, PharmD
Professor of Medicine, Bioinformatics and Personalized Health
Department of Medicine, Division of Clinical Pharmacology
University of Missouri School of Medicine
Kansas City, Missouri

Niels Frimodt-Møller, Professor, MD, DMSc
Senior Consultant
Department of Clinical Microbiology
Hvidovre Hospital
Hvidovre, Denmark

Dale N. Gerding, MD
Professor
Department of Medicine
Loyola University Chicago Stritch School of Medicine
Maywood, Illinois

David W. Hecht, MD, MS, MBA
Senior Vice President of Clinical Affairs/Chief Medical Officer
Department of Medicine
Loyola University Medical Center
Maywood, Illinois
Department of Medicine
Hines VA Hospital
Hines, Illinois

Joachim Hegstad, MSc
Department of Microbiology and Infection Control
University Hospital of North Norway
Tromsø, Norway

Kristin Hegstad, PhD
Reference Centre for Detection of
    Antimicrobial Resistance
Department of Microbiology and Infection Control
University Hospital of North Norway;
Research Group for Host-Microbe Interactions
Department of Medical Biology
University of Tromsø - The Arctic
    University of Norway
Tromsø, Norway

Clark B. Inderlied, PhD
Emeritus Professor of Clinical Pathology
University of Southern California
Keck School of Medicine
Los Angeles, California

Michael A. Kallenberger, PharmD
Clinical Lead Pharmacist
Antimicrobial Stewardship
Truman Medical Centers
Kansas City, Missouri

Shelly Latte, MD
Attending Physician
Division of Infectious Diseases
Division of Hospital Medicine
St. Luke's and Roosevelt Hospital Center
Mount Sinai Health System
New York, New York

Alexander J. Lepak, MD
Assistant Professor
Department of Medicine
University of Wisconsin School of Medicine and
    Public Health
Madison, Wisconsin

Barbara E. Ostrov, MD
Vice Chair, Department of Pediatrics
Professor of Pediatrics and Medicine
Penn State Hershey Children's Hospital
Penn State Hershey Medical Center
Hershey, Pennsylvania

Thomas F. Patterson, MD, FACP
Professor of Medicine
The University of Texas Health Science Center at
    San Antonio;
Department of Medicine/Infectious Diseases
South Texas Veterans Health Care System
San Antonio, Texas

Brian S. Pepito, MD
Clinical Assistant Professor
Department of Medicine
University of South Dakota School of
    Medicine
Sioux Falls, South Dakota

Jean-Marc Rolain, PharmD, PhD
Professor
Faculté de Médecine et de Pharmacie
URMITE CNRS-IRD-INSERM
IHU Méditerranée Infection
Marseille, France

Ørjan Samuelsen, PhD
Reference Centre for Detection of
    Antimicrobial Resistance
Department of Microbiology and
    Infection Control
University Hospital of North Norway
Tromsø, Norway

Emilia Mia Sordillo, MD, PhD, FACP
Senior Attending
Departments of Medicine and Pathology and
    Laboratory Medicine
Medical Director, Microbiology and Molecular
    Diagnostics
Mount Sinai St. Luke's and
    Mount Sinai Roosevelt
Mount Sinai Health System
New York, New York

Charles William Stratton, MD
Director, Clinical Microbiology Laboratory
Vanderbilt University Medical Center
Nashville, Tennessee

Arnfinn Sundsfjord, MD, PhD
Professor
National Reference Laboratory for
  Detection of Antimicrobial Resistance
Department of Clinical Microbiology and
  Infection Control
University Hospital of North Norway;
Department of Medical Biology
Faculty of Health Sciences
University of Tromsø - The Arctic
  University of Norway
Tromsø, Norway

George R. Thompson III, MD
Assistant Professor of Medicine
Department of Medical Microbiology and
  Immunology
Department of Medicine, Division of
  Infectious Diseases
University of California Davis
Davis, California

**John D. Turnidge, MBBS, FRACP,
FRCPA, MASM**
Professor
Departments of Pediatrics, Pathology, and
  Molecular and Biomedical Sciences
University of Adelaide
Adelaide, South Australia

Anilrudh A. Venugopal, MD
Associate Professor
Department of Medicine
Loyola University Medical Center
Maywood, Illinois

Matthew A. Wikler, MD
Vice President
The Medicines Company
Parsippany, New Jersey

Contents

Color Plates

Color Plates

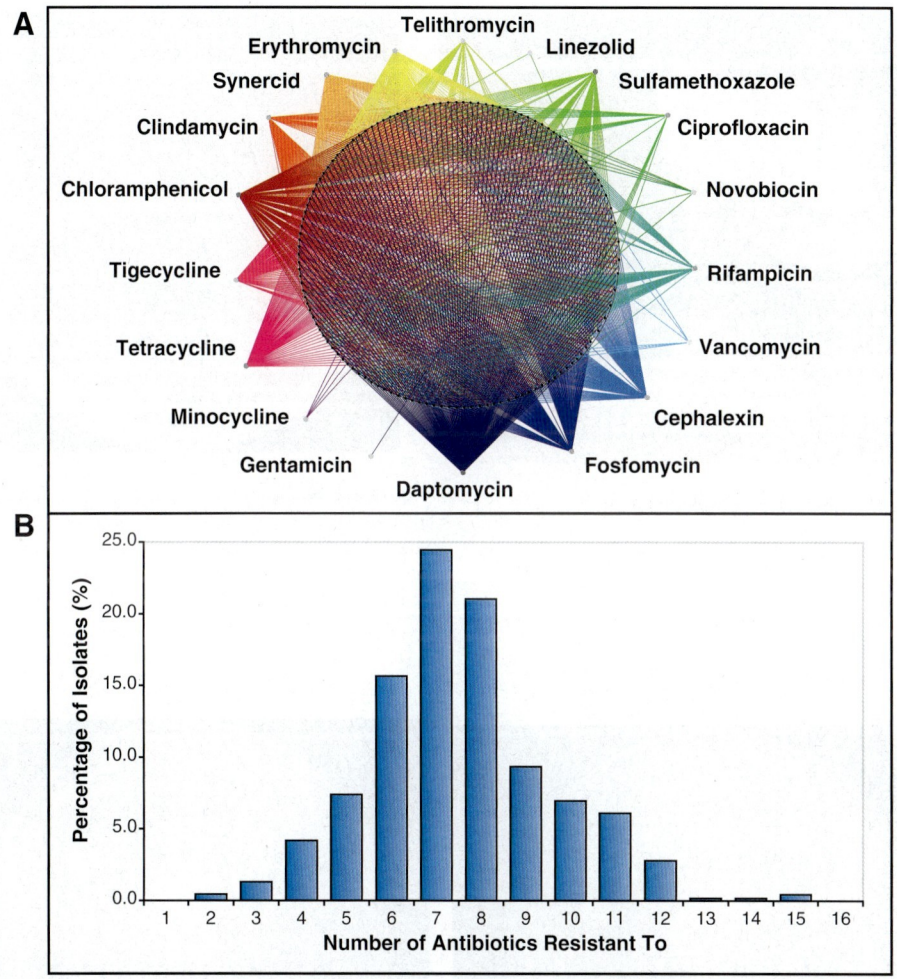

Figure 1 ■ Antibiotic resistance profiling of 480 soil-derived bacterial isolates. **A:** Schematic diagram illustrating the phenotypic density and diversity of resistance profiles. The central circle of 191 black dots represents different resistance profiles, where a line connecting the profile to the antibiotic indicates resistance. **B:** Resistance spectrum of soil isolates. Strains were individually screened from spores on solid *Streptomyces* isolation media (SIM) against 21 antibiotics at 20 mg of antibiotic per milliliter of medium (mg/mL). Resistance was defined as reproducible growth in the presence of antibiotic. (From D'Costa VM, McGrann KM, Hughes DW, et al. Sampling the antibiotic resistome. *Science* 2006;311:375.)

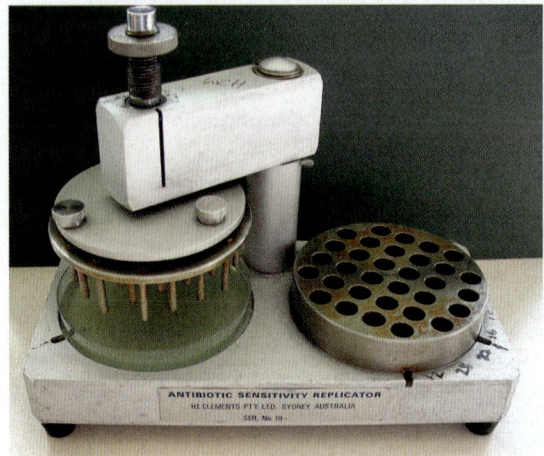

Figure 2.1 ■ Replicator for agar dilution.

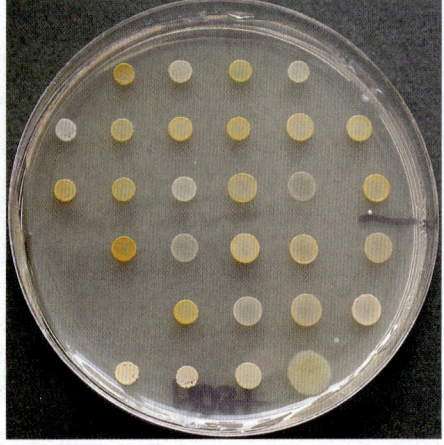

Figure 2.2 ■ Agar dilution plate after 24 hours of incubation. The medium is Mueller-Hinton agar. The strains are of *Staphylococcus aureus*. The last spot at bottom right is a control. Three strains have not grown at this concentration.

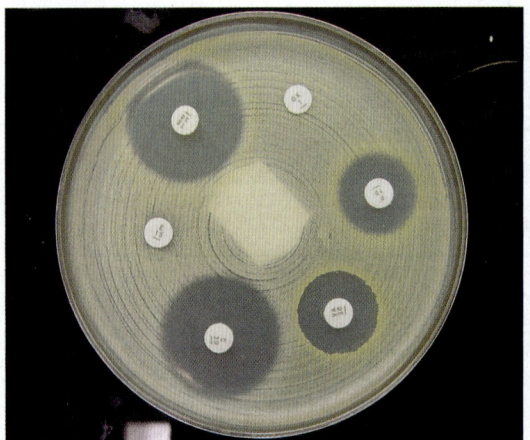

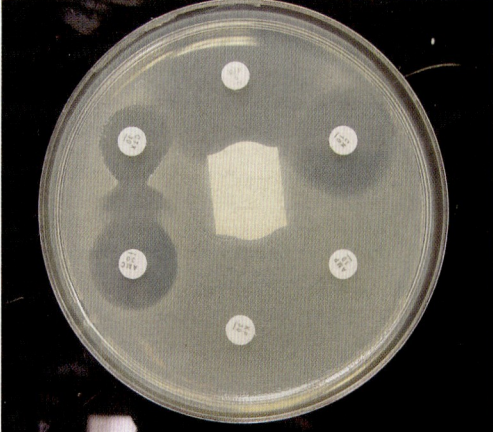

Figure 2.3 ■ Disk diffusion test: CLSI method on 90-mm plates. **A:** *Staphylococcus aureus*. **B:** *Escherichia coli*. This strain possesses an extended-spectrum β-lactamase and shows "keyhole" synergy between cefotaxime and amoxicillin-clavulanate.

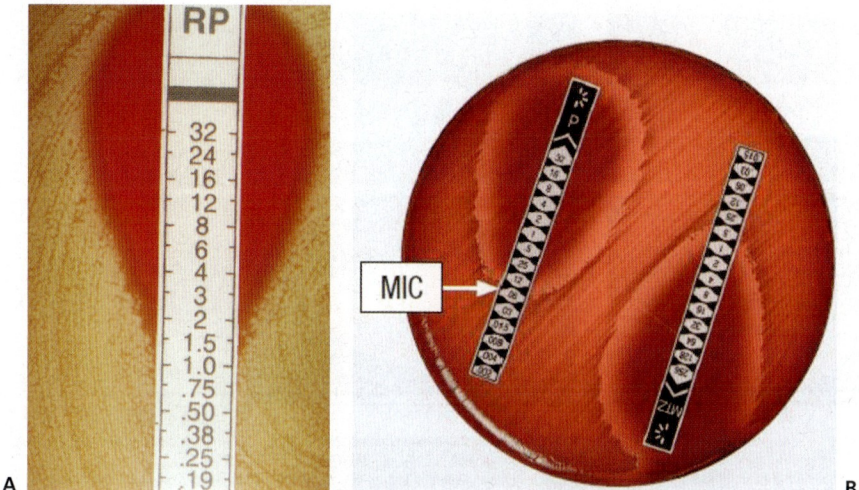

Figure 2.5 ■ **A.** Etest gradient diffusion test for *Streptococcus pneumoniae* and quinupristin/dalfopristin. **B.** M.I.C.E gradient diffusion test for *Helicobacter pylori* with penicillin and metronidazole. The MIC is where the growth of the strain meets the strip, ignoring the zone of hemolysis.

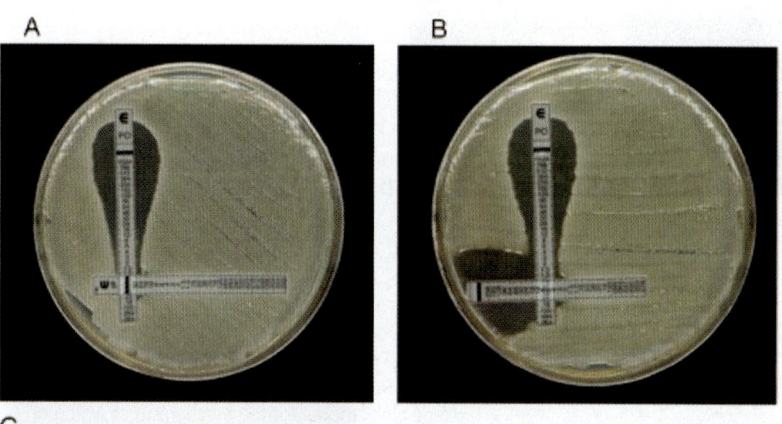

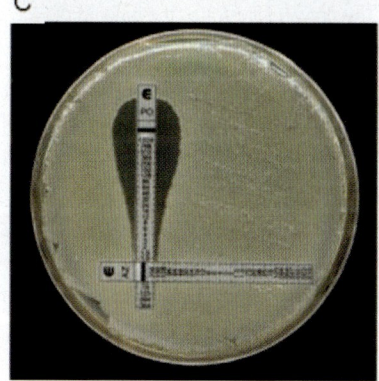

Figure 2.9 ■ Synergy study using three antimicrobial agents, one of which is incorporated into the agar. Activity of polymyxin B in combination with imipenem, rifampicin, and azithromycin versus a multidrug-resistant *A. baumannii* OXA-23 clones using the Etest method. **A:** Polymyxin and imipenem. **B:** Polymyxin and rifampicin. **C:** Polymyxin and azithromycin. (From Wareham DW, Bean DC. In-vitro activity of polymyxin B in combination with imipenem, rifampicin and azithromycin versus multidrug resistant strains of *Acinetobacter baumannii* producing Oxa-23 carbapenemase. *Ann Clin Microbiol Antimicrob* 2006;5:10.)

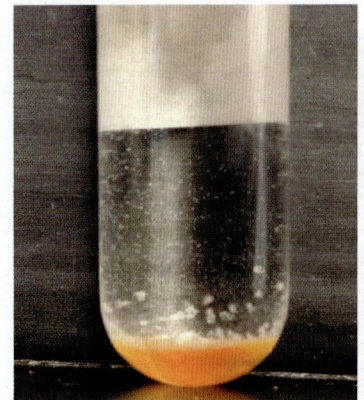
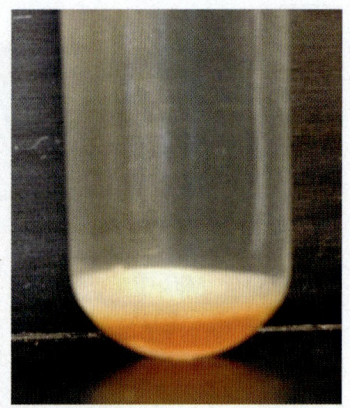

A

B

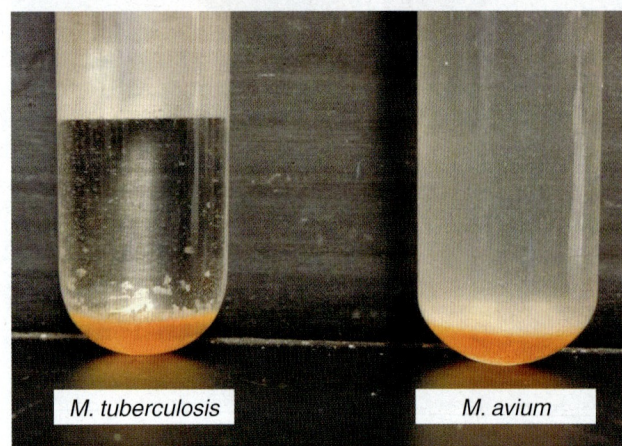

Figure 5.2 ■ Growth in MGIT 960 medium comparing *M. tuberculosis* with *M. avium* before **(A,B)** and after **(C,D)** slight swirling. *M. tuberculosis* **(A,C)**. *M. avium* **(B,D)**. (Photographs courtesy of Jane Wenger, California Department of Public Health.)

M. tuberculosis

M. avium

C

D

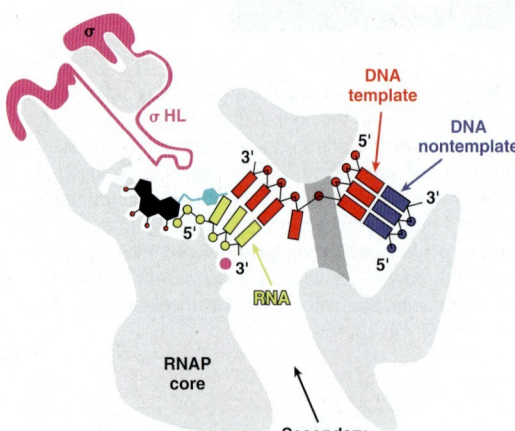

Figure 5.7 ■ Rifampin mechanism of action. The steric block model for the mechanism of action of rifamycins. The drawing illustrates the binding of rifampin sterically blocking the growing RNA chain in the transcription initiation complex of RNAP. (Adapted from Aristoff PA, Garcia GA, Kirchhoff PD, et al. Rifamycins—obstacles and opportunities. *Tuberculosis [Edinb]* 2010;90[2]:94–118; Artsimovitch I, Vassilyev DG. Is it easy to stop RNA polymerase? *Cell Cycle* 2006;5[4]:399–404.)

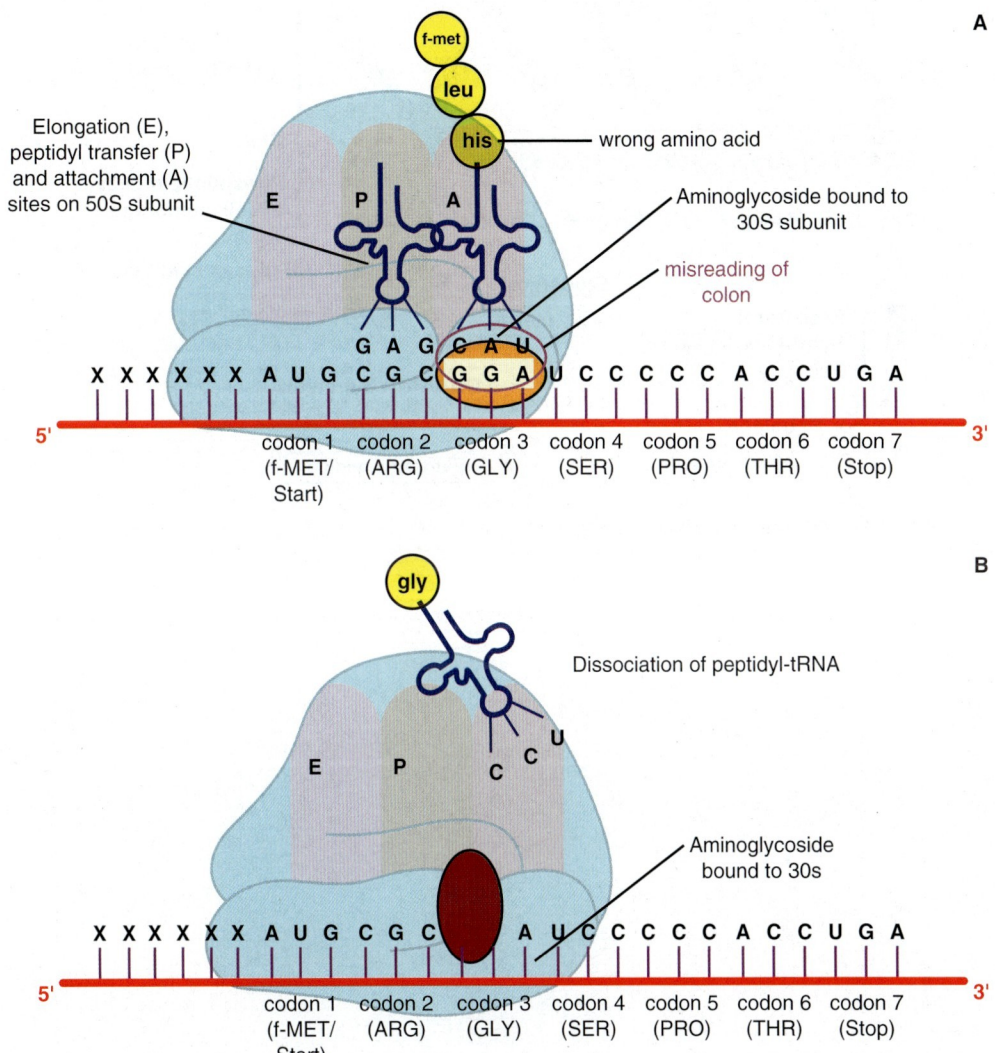

Figure 5.9 ■ Aminoglycosides prevent protein synthesis by **(A)** causing translation errors (proofreading errors) and the misreading of codons and insertion of incorrect amino acids) or **(B)** translocation errors or the dissociation of peptidyl-tRNA. Aminoglycoside resistance in *M. tuberculosis* is most commonly caused by three mutations in the rrs gene (16S rRNA): A1401G, C1402T, and G1484T. (Graphics adapted from http://pharmaxchange.info/press/2011/05 /mechanism-of-action-of-aminoglycosides/ by Akul Mehta with animation by G. Kaiser.)

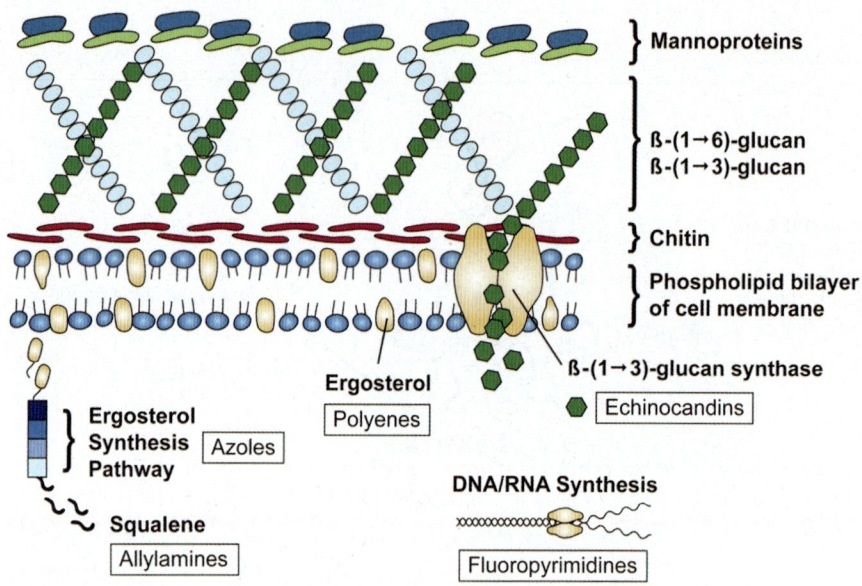

Figure 6.1 ■ Targets of systemic antifungal agents.

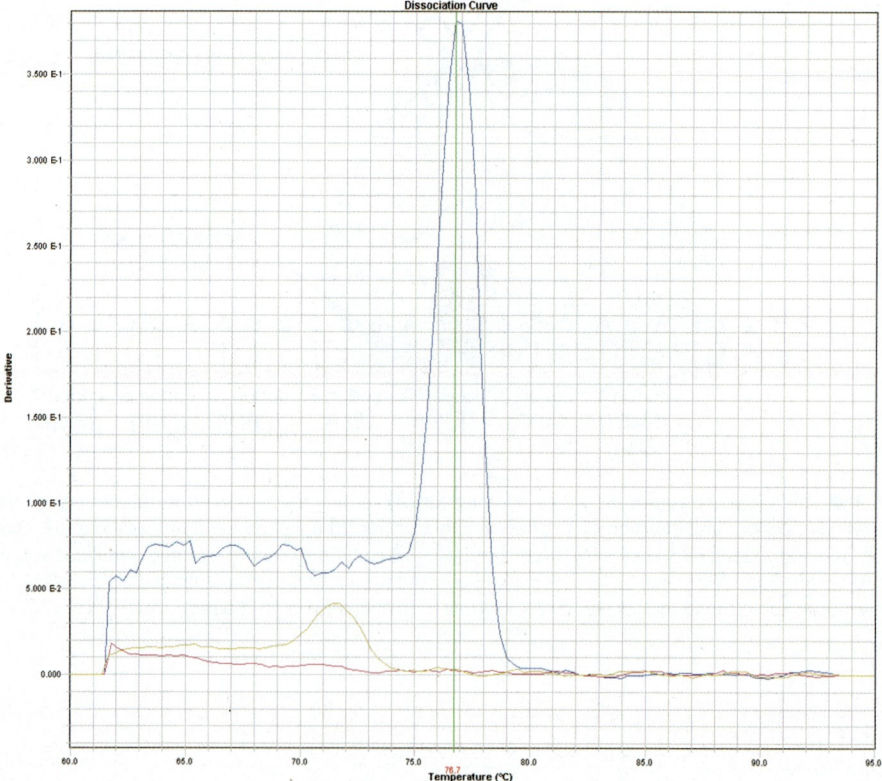

Figure 9.1 ■ SYBR Green I melt-curve analysis illustrating a positive *nuc* gene amplification with a Tm 76,7°C (*blue*), and two negative samples (*red* and *orange*). The *orange* melt-curve has an unspesific amplification most likely a primer dimer.

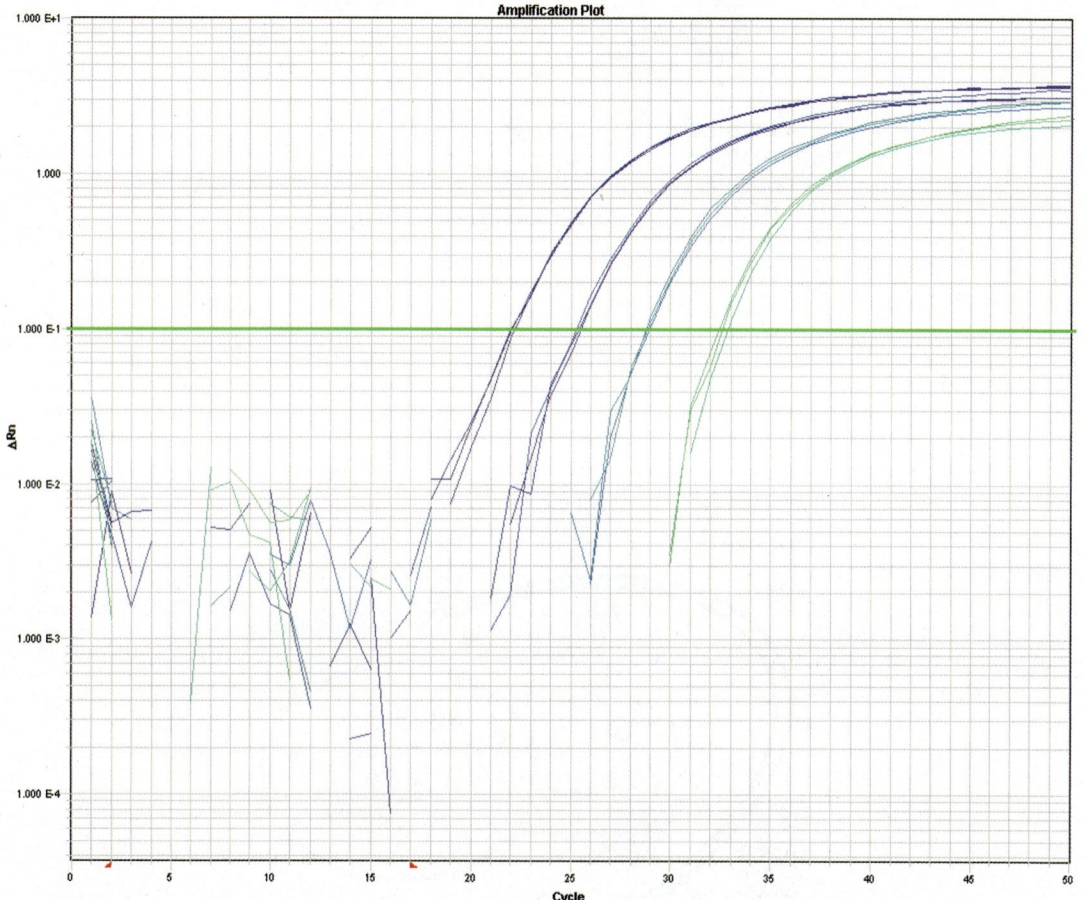

Figure 9.2 ■ Amplification plot showing four 10-fold dilutions of MRSA samples in triplicates, targeting *SCC mec* I gene. Detecion by molecular beacon probe, labeled with Fam in 5′and Dabcyl in 3′end. The *x axis* shows the number of PCR cycles, and the *y axis* shows fluorescent units in a logarithmic scale. The *green horizontal line* defines the cycle threshold value (CT-value) of each positive sample that crosses this line and is read at the *x axis*. A sample with a low CT-value has a higher starting concentration of the target compared to a sample with a higher CT-value.

PROTEASE INHIBITORS

ENTRY INHIBITORS: FUSION, CCR5, CXCR4

CD4 CELL

REVERSE TRANSCRIPTASE INHIBITORS: NUCLEOSIDE, NUCLEOTIDE, NON-NUCLEOSIDE

INTEGRASE INHIBITORS

Figure 11.1 ■ Replication cycle of HIV: sites of antiviral action.

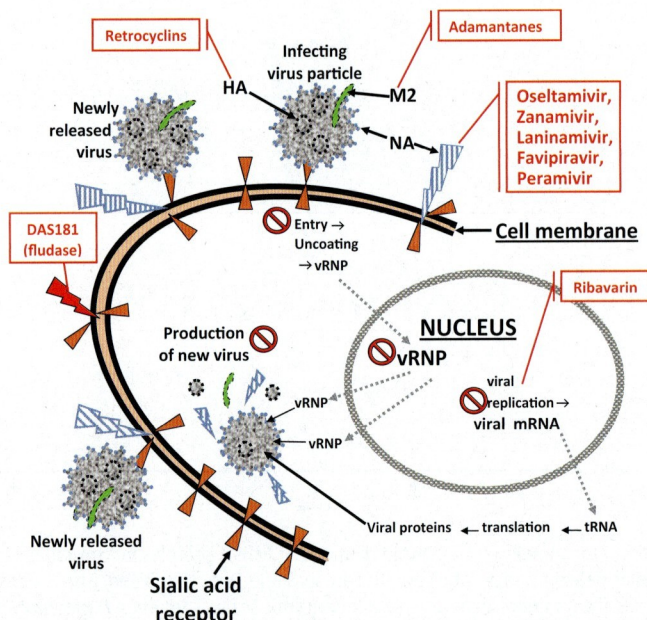

Figure 11.6 ■ Therapeutic targets for treatment of influenza A. Schematic of the life cycle of influenza A and its viral proteins. Old and new drugs targeting influenza pathways are identified in red boxes. Future targets for influenza viral/host immune response and cellular interactions are identified as red crossed circles ⊘. Influenza enters the host cell through the sialic acid receptor via neuraminidase alteration of the receptor. Then, viral RNA synthesis occurs in the infected host nucleus using RNP as a template. Viral translation occurs in host cytoplasm. New virus is produced then exported from host cells. Neuraminidase and the experimental agent DAS181 (Fludase) "cut" the sialic acid receptor at the cell membrane (sawtooth). NA, neuraminidase; HA, hemagglutinin; M2, matrix 2 protein ion channel; vRNP, viral ribonucleoproteins; viral mRNA, viral messenger RNA; tRNA, transfer RNA. (Adapted from Samji T. Influenza A: understanding the viral life cycle. *Yale J of Biol and Med* 2009;82:153–159; Centers for Disease Control and Prevention. Influenza antiviral medications: summary for clinicians. http://www.cdc.gov/flu/pdf/professionals /antiviral-summary-clinicians.pdf. Accessed December 15, 2013; Hayden FG. Newer influenza antivirals, biotherapeutics and combinations. *Influenza Other Respir Viruses* 2013;7[Suppl 1]:63–75.)

Intersection of Drug Development, Challenges of Antimicrobial Resistance, and Predicting Antimicrobial Efficacy

Daniel Amsterdam and Charles William Stratton

In 2009, the World Health Organization (WHO) referred to the problem of antibiotics and antibiotic resistance, stating, "Antibiotic Resistance – one of the three greatest threats to human health." In the 8 years since the last publication of this volume, there have been numerous and significant advances in our understanding of the effects of antimicrobial agents on the human (and animal) microbiome, the increase and recognition of new antimicrobial (i.e., antiinfective resistance mechanisms), as well as the tremendous advances in technology that have led to the detection of these multiloci mechanisms especially among the gram-negative Enterobacteriaceae. Unfortunately, progress in all these areas is dimmed by the apparent disinterest of pharmaceutical companies in the development of new, more effective compounds to combat the increasing number of drug-resistant infections. Several themes are incorporated into this perspective and limn the changing landscape of antimicrobial development and the means with associated technology for estimating efficacy in human or animal hosts. These are the constriction of the antibiotic development pipeline, origins of antibiotic resistance, developing knowledge about the human and animal microbiomes, the predictive value of antimicrobial susceptibility testing, and new technologies especially "next-generation" sequencing, which has the capability of examining the entire microbial sequence rapidly and for reasonable costs.

THE CONSTRICTED ANTIBIOTIC PIPELINE

In the United States and around the world, the incidence of drug-resistant infections and associated morbidity have increased. WHO identified the resistance of microorganisms to antimicrobial agents as one of the three greatest threats to human health. Recent reports by the Infectious Diseases Society of America (IDSA) (1) and the European Centre for Disease Prevention and Control and the European Medicines Agency (2) document that the number of candidate drugs in the developing pipeline, which are beneficial compared to existing drugs that will be capable to treat infections due to the group of pathogens termed "ESKAPE" (*Enterococcus faecium, Staphylococcus aureus, Klebsiella pneumoniae, Acinetobacter baumannii, Pseudomonas aeruginosa*, and *Enterobacter* species) are few. The aforementioned six species/groups cause the majority of US hospital infections and are not always contained by the available armamentarium of antibacterial drugs (3).

It is the IDSA's view that the antibiotic pipeline problem can be dealt with by engaging global, political, scientific, industry, economic, intellectual property, policy, medical, and philanthropic leaders to develop creative incentives that will serve to stimulate new and ongoing research and development in this area. In this regard, it has been inferred that the financial gains and advantages for major pharmaceuticals may not be particularly advantageous for the development of new antimicrobial agents because the costs for treatment regimens, and reimbursement schedules in comparison to antineoplastic, biologic respiratory, and allergy drugs. In short, the economic advantage of antimicrobial agents relative to other drug class candidates presents an economic disadvantage (4).

Despite the confluence of these negative factors, it is the IDSA's aim that the "creation of sustainable global antibacterial drug R&D enterprise" achieve in the short term 10 new, safe, and effective antibiotics by 2020. Toward this end, IDSA (5) launched a new collaboration entitled the "IDX '20" initiative, which several American and European groups and societies have endorsed. This declaration is a noble effort that no doubt will be reviewed in the next few years—or by the next publication of *Antibiotics in Laboratory Medicine*.

The development of new antimicrobial agents is one of three strategies that have been proposed to meet the challenge of multiresistant diverse microorganism types (extended-spectrum β-lactamases [ESBLs], *Klebsiella pneumoniae* carbapenemase [KPC], methicillin-resistant *Staphylococcus aureus* [MRSA], vancomycin-resistant enterococci [VRE], etc.) collectively referred to as multidrug-resistant organisms (MDROs). The other two strategies include interrupting the cross-transmission of MDROs and effective pharmacology oversight-stewardship in the treatment of these infections. This latter strategy incorporates tactics for appropriate initiation, selection, and de-escalation of antimicrobial therapy.

TRACING THE ORIGINS OF ANTIBIOTIC RESISTANCE

The marvel of antibiotic discovery, now more than 70 years old, gave rise to an era of drug innovation and discoveries that have been tempered by the emergence of resistant microorganisms (6).

Almost every chapter in this volume addresses the detection and identification of microbes that are resistant to a particular drug or class of anti-infectives. In examining the history and development of antimicrobial resistance, should this be interpreted to mean that antibiotic resistance in clinically significant bacteria is a contemporary phenomenon? Recent studies of modern human (and environmental) commensal microbial genomes suggest that these genomes possess a greater concentration of antibiotic resistance genes than had been previously recognized (7–9). A highly varied collection of genes encoding resistance to β-lactam, tetracycline, and glycopeptide antibiotics was recently found in 30,000-year-old Beningian permafrost sediments in Alaska (7). D'Costa and colleagues (7) documented through structure and function studies the complete vancomycin resistance element vanA and confirmed its similarity to modern variants. In earlier work, D'Costa et al. (10) analyzed the antibiotic resistance potential of soil microorganisms. In this study, it was alarming to discover that the frequency of high-level resistance detected in this study was to antibiotics that have served as the standard therapeutic regimens for decades. No class of antibiotic natural or synthetic was spared with respect to bacterial target. A summary of the 18 antibiotics and the extent of inactivation of the 480 strains that formed the library is noted in Figure 1. In general, without exception, investigators found that every strain in the library was resistant on average to 7 or 8 antimicrobials; two strains were resistant to 15 of the 21 drugs. Several antimicrobials, including cephalexin, the synthetic dihydrofolate reductase inhibitor trimethoprim, and the more recently developed lipopeptide daptomycin were almost universally ineffective against the library of bacterial strains. This wide dissemination of antibiotic resistance elements tempers the contemporary hypothesis for the emergence of antibiotic resistance and instead implies a natural history of resistance.

PREDICTIVE VALUE OF ANTIMICROBIAL SUSCEPTIBILITY TESTING RESULTS

This volume is dedicated to tests that estimate the interactive end point of "bug" and drug. It is noteworthy, and without alarming revelation, that diseases other than those caused by infectious agents are treated by medicating the host. In contrast, therapy for infectious disease attempts to eliminate the pathogens from the host while minimizing adverse sequelae due to host immune responses and drug side effects. The target then for drug therapy is the pathogen; however, this frequently results in collateral damage.

A wide variety of manual and automated tests are described in this volume and in particular in Chapters 2 and 3, they review the development and detail of these assays during the latter half of the last century. Results of those assays are interpreted in the form of categorical values ("S," "I," or "R") or with numerical equivalents and defined

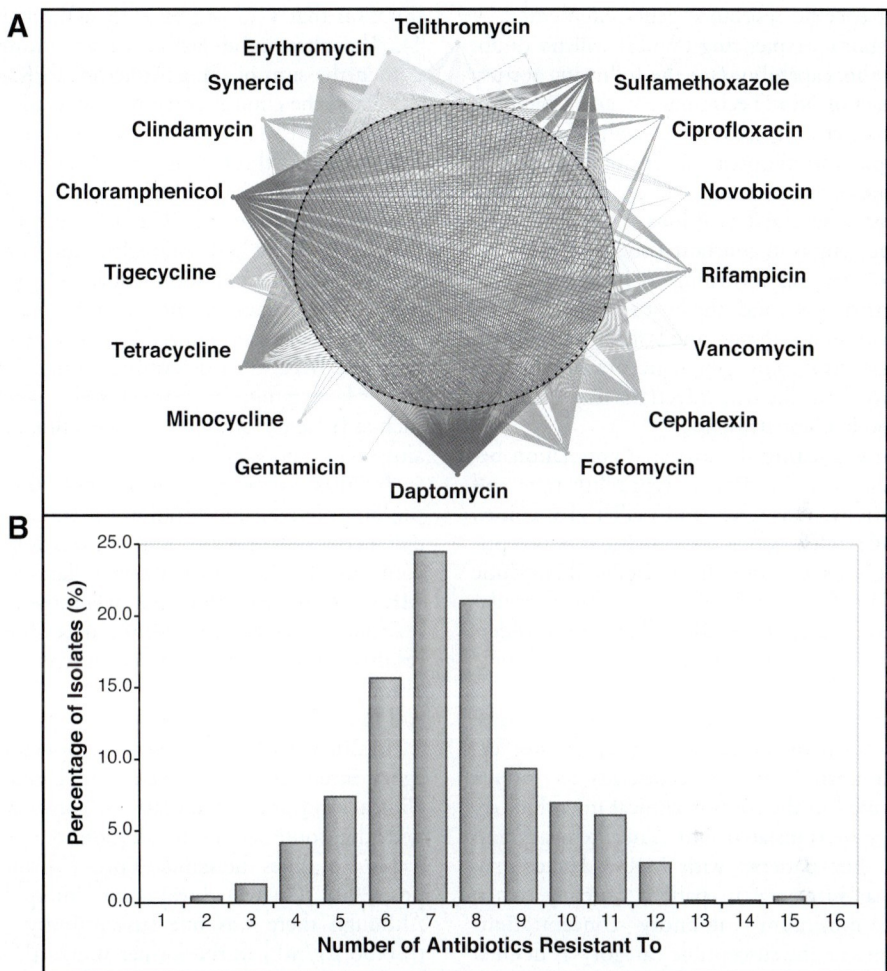

Figure 1 ■ Antibiotic resistance profiling of 480 soil-derived bacterial isolates. A: Schematic diagram illustrating the phenotypic density and diversity of resistance profiles. The central circle of 191 black dots represents different resistance profiles, where a line connecting the profile to the antibiotic indicates resistance. **B:** Resistance spectrum of soil isolates. Strains were individually screened from spores on solid *Streptomyces* isolation media (SIM) against 21 antibiotics at 20 mg of antibiotic per milliliter of medium (mg/mL). Resistance was defined as reproducible growth in the presence of antibiotic. (From D'Costa VM, McGrann KM, Hughes DW, et al. Sampling the antibiotic resistome. *Science* 2006;311:375.) (See Color Plate in the front of the book.)

by at least two major consensus groups—Clinical and Laboratory Standards Institute (CLSI) in the United States and European Committee on Antimicrobial Susceptibility Testing (EUCAST) in the European Union. In Chapter 1, Wikler and colleagues explore and discuss the reasoning/rationale for defining the "breakpoint," the dividing quantitative line between susceptibility and resistance that is the underpinning of antibacterial susceptibility tests. The question posed here

is how successful are these results in predicting a positive outcome in patients with infection.

When using mortality as an outcome indicator, several studies (11–15) executed between 1996 and 2003 demonstrated that mortality was reduced by 40% to 60% when the first antimicrobial agent administered was "susceptible." Resistance as determined by in vitro testing is considered in these studies to be an independent risk factor for therapeutic failure. The advent of molecular methods to detect specific resistance genes augmented by whole genome sequencing (WGS) will no doubt enhance this capability (see the following section on "Impact of New Technologies" and Chapter 9 by Hegstad et al.). Clearly, the standard, that is, phenotypic antimicrobial susceptibility tests that we use today fail to mimic the physiologic status of the host in several dimensions. First, in the "test tube," the drug is in constant association with the host—not varying according to its pharmacokinetic construct; second, the host's cellular and antibody entities are absent; and last, the bioburden, that is, the test system agent concentration may be at variance from the true infectious dose extant in various body compartments.

When evaluating the expected correlation between results of in vitro susceptibility tests and therapeutic response, Rex and Pfaller (16) coined the "90–60 rule," which indicated that a susceptible result is associated with a favorable therapeutic response in 90% to 95% of patients. The formulative predictions are beclouded when one considers immunocompromised patients with polymicrobic infections.

Several pertinent and directed questions can be posed to form the essential meaning of this section. Can antimicrobial susceptibility test results as performed in the routine clinical microbiology laboratory be translated into clinical efficacy and potency? For patients with MRSA bacteremia, is there a difference in patient outcome when reported minimum inhibitory concentrations (MICs) are in the susceptible category as defined by consensus organizations? Should there be a difference in categorical interpretation (S, I, or R) for pneumococcal meningitis–associated and non–meningitis-associated disease? When documented nosocomial bacteremia is caused by *P. aeruginosa*, is patient outcome associated with reduced piperacillin-tazobactam MICs?

Clearly, the response in each of the previously cited cases is the critical establishment of the breakpoint concentration by regulatory oversight groups that define the chasm between susceptible and "resistant." In Chapter 1 of this volume, Wikler and coauthors define this parameter and the necessary evidence to establish it. Simply stated, each antimicrobial agent/drug pair is dependent on the pharmacokinetic (PK) and pharmacodynamic (PD) properties of the antiinfective compound and the associated clinical outcome. Specific parameters that are pertinent to evaluating the PK/PD are the area under the curve of C_{max} (peak) and above the resulted bug–drug MIC, and the time

duration that C_{max} is greater than the MIC (Fig. 1). The pharmacodynamics of an antimicrobial is then the sum of the antimicrobial PK plus the MIC and the clinical outcome. Generally, the application of PK/PD parameters for drugs can be categorized as those drugs which are concentration-dependent; that is, higher concentrations are required in relation to MIC to kill pathogens (e.g., fluoroquinolones and aminoglycosides) and time-dependent (concentration independent) agents whose effectiveness is measured by duration of exposure above a recognized inhibitory concentration (the MIC_{90}) to determine killing. Examples of this latter group include cell wall–active agents such as β-lactam antibiotics (penicillins and cephalosporins) and vancomycin.

In 2004, Sakoulas and associates (17) redefined the interpretive concentration for successful (i.e., enhanced) outcome in the interpretation of vancomycin MIC for bloodstream isolates (BSIs) or MRSA. They determined that when the MIC was less than or equal to 0.5 µg/mL, successful therapy resulted in a 55.6% improved outcome as compared to 9.5% when MICs were 1 or 2 µg mL—still in the susceptible category.

In 2008, the CLSI revised the susceptible category interpretation for penicillin based on the clinical syndrome (meningitis vs. non-meningitis) and the route of administration of penicillin. Table 1 outlines the standard pre- ("former") and post-2008 ("new") breakpoint interpretations. Although there was one susceptibility category (≤0.06 µg/mL) in the former standard, the new standard defined three categories based on clinical syndrome and route of administration (18).

In a 2008 study of *P. aeruginosa* bacteremia patients treated with piperacillin-tazobactam, Tam et al. (19) determined that when susceptibility to piperacillin-tazobactam was 32/64 µg/mL, there was a fourfold increase in 30-day mortality (85.7% vs. 22.2%) compared to isolates with susceptibility of 16 µg/mL.

In each of the previously mentioned examples, credence for the predictive value of an MIC and the associated susceptible or resistant categorical interpretation can only prove meaningful when sufficient in vitro studies have been completed along with the necessary clinical outcome evaluations.

In efforts to integrate clinical microbiologic data, that is, antimicrobial susceptibility results and pharmacologic data, programs have been developed under the banner of "antimicrobial stewardship" that are designed to "monitor and direct antimicrobial use at a health care institution, thus

Table 1

Penicillin and *Streptococcus pneumoniae*: Comparison of Former (pre-2008) and New Penicillin Breakpoints (MIC)—Clinical and Laboratory Standards Institute, 2008

Standard	Susceptibility Category MIC (µg/mL)		
	Susceptible	**Intermediate**	**Resistant**
Former—all clinical syndromes and penicillin routes	≤0.06	0.12–1	≥2
New (by clinical syndrome and penicillin route)			
Meningitis, IV penicillin	≤0.06	—[a]	>0.12
Nonmeningitis, IV penicillin	≤2	4	≥8
Nonmeningitis, oral penicillin	≤0.06	0.12–1	≥2

[a]No intermediate category defined under new standard.
MIC, minimum inhibitory concentration; IV, intravenous.

providing a standard evidence-based approach to judicial antimicrobial use" (20,21). Outcome measures that are desired include improved patient outcome, improved safety, reduced resistance, and reduced cost (22). These measures may be difficult to assess as well as difficult to achieve. Within the frame of "antimicrobial stewardship program" (ASP), the use of clinical pharmacists and the electronic health record offer a streamlined method for implementation (23,24). Moreover, new approaches in rapid pathogen detection and identification can prove highly effective when integrated into an ASP (25).

THE HUMAN AND ANIMAL MICROBIOME

The microbiome, whether animal or human, can be defined as the aggregate genomes of their respective microbiota and the varied metabolic activities which they encode. The accumulated information has the potential to revolutionize the way we view contemporary therapeutics. During the past century, the information that has been gathered in the area of pharmacology, describing rates of absorption, distribution, metabolism, and excretion for hundreds of compounds—in our case, antibiotics—referred to today as xenobiotics (compound foreign to a living organism, which include antimicrobial agents as well as other therapeutic drugs). As yet a poorly understood component of xenobiotic metabolism is the effect-impact of the vast number (trillions, 10^7) of microorganisms that reside in the gastrointestinal tract. Although the discovery of antibiotics is decades old, spanning the past century, it appears we are

at the beginning of determining the "intended" collateral damages that antibiotics can impart on the symbiotic microorganisms living in our gastrointestinal tract (26). The gathering of the varied and numerous microbial members within our person play vital roles in the maintenance of human health by freeing nutrients and/or energy from otherwise inaccessible dietary substrates, promoting the differentiation of host cells and tissues, stimulating the immune system, and protecting the host from invasion by pathogens. The assemblage of human-associated microbial communities does not generally proceed smoothly. There are several examples where some fraction of the community is removed or killed (e.g., oral hygiene). The effect of antimicrobial agents on the gut microbiota serves as a model for disturbance in human-associated communities. It is estimated, that on any given day, 1% to 3% of people in the developed world are exposed to pharmacologic doses of antibiotics (27).

Antimicrobial therapy is intended to achieve sufficient drug concentration for a sufficient duration in a particular body compartment so that the targeted pathogen is eliminated. Even if this aim were always attained, the antibiotic will also be found at varied concentrations of several locations within the body depending on the mode of administration and PK properties. When members of the microbiota are exposed to antibiotics that affect their growth rate without killing them, there is selection for resistance. The horizontal transfer of antibiotic-resistant determinants takes place in the human gut and oral communities and their reservoir serves as the starting point/place for transfer to pathogens as well as the resident microbiota. The collateral damage to the human microbiome exerted by contemporary antimicrobials through overuse and extended spectrum has likely been the driving force behind the proliferation of MDROs and members of the ESKAPE group. Understanding the balance and fragility of the human microbiome so as to use "microbiome-sparing antimicrobial therapy," develop techniques to restore and maintain the indigenous microbiota, as well as use protective mechanisms encoded by an intact microbiome will limit the expanding scope of resistance (28).

As we decipher the heterogeneous environment of the human body/microbiome, we recognize that microorganisms encounter these environments replaced with transient chemical and nutrient gradients. Clinically, antibiotic gradients develop when a patient begins, ends, or neglects a prescribed regimen. To simulate in vivo conditions, Zhang et al. (29) constructed a microfluidic device consisting of a tiny chamber device. The investigators then determined the effect of the microenvironment generated within the chambers on bacterial populations grown in them. They found that when the test organism *Escherichia coli* is grown in a heterogeneous environment that contains a steep antibiotic concentration, ciprofloxacin in their simulated experiments, they demonstrated rapid and repeatable acquisition and fixation of ciprofloxacin mutations compared with bacteria grown in homogeneous environments. If we suppose that some parts of the human body resemble heterogeneous environments rather than the in vitro containment of a Petri dish and a flask, then the environment proposed by Zhang et al. (29) would provide a more relevant model for the development of antimicrobial resistance.

IMPACT OF NEW TECHNOLOGIES

More than 10 years have elapsed since the first polymerase chain reaction (PCR) assays for antimicrobial resistance was evaluated. For this event, the assay was directed to MRSA. Few targeted assays have followed but have included vancomycin resistance in *Enterococcus* spp and rifampin resistance in *Mycobacterium tuberculosis*. To date, there has not been a developed panel/array of molecular susceptibility testing for several common drug resistance mechanisms.

A barrier for molecular susceptibility testing has been the characterization of mutation(s) associated with the resistance phenotype and the subsequent development of tests specific for these markers. For example, mutants generated during in vitro selection of antimicrobial-resistant strains can differ from those that develop naturally in human populations and cause clinical disease (30).

By far, in the second decade of the 21st century, the greatest need and challenge in molecular assay development is the capability to detect resistance determinants among the gram-negative bacilli. In the family Enterobacteriaceae, several hundred mechanisms have been reported causing resistance to β-lactams, cephalosporins, monobactams, and/or carbapenems. Among Enterobacteriaceae, β-lactam resistance has been attributed to several mechanisms, which include ESBLs, AmpCs, metallo-β-lactamases (MBLs), and KPCs. The number of genotypically unique ESBLs total more than 200 (31).

Directed detection of the several and as yet uncovered resistance mechanism requires technology with efficient and specific methodology capable to be multiplexed beyond that of PCR platforms extant and will probably be based on microarrays, metabolite detection assays, or direct sequencing. Key to the widespread acceptance of these newer technologies will be the evidence to demonstrate the high negative predictive values and the associated sensitivity to detect low levels of gene expression.

Which technologies of those that are currently in use will prove meaningful for future development is unknown. Although real-time PCR has revolutionized clinical molecular diagnostics, permitting detection of targets in a closed system within a 45-minute to 2-hour time frame, an associated limitation is the number of fluorophores that can be used for simultaneous detection of multiple targets—usually six. For detection of a multiplicity of targets (more than six), liquid- and solid-phase microarrays may best suit this requirement. Examples of this technology would be XTAG (Luminex, Austin, TX) or BeadExpress (Illumina, San Diego, CA). Solid arrays which have been in use for several years in research laboratories as represented by Nanosphere, Inc. (Northbrook, IL) are an alternative. Other solid array systems such as GeneChip (Affymetrix, Santa Clara, CA) and BioFilmChip (Autogenomics, Vista, CA) are other alternatives.

Recent advances in nucleic acid sequencing technology have made sequencing the entire human genome—or for this discussion, the microbial code—both technically and economically feasible. In clinical medicine, WGS has been heralded to clarify molecular diagnosis and guide therapy—giving rise to the concept of personalized medicine. Several benchtop, high-throughput sequencing platforms no larger than our all-in-one printer are available for this function. Among them, the 454 GS Junior (Roche, Branford, CT), MiSeq (Illumina, San Diego, CA), and the Ion Torrent PGM (Life Technologies, Carlsbad, CA) offer modest setup and operating costs. Each instrument can generate sufficient data for a draft bacterial genome (32). It is not unlikely that given the multiple bioinformatic methods available, the capability to analyze the information encoded within the complete genome sequence for determining antimicrobial resistance would be available. In the context of this discussion, reference is made to using the decoded microbial genome to identify resistance markers that would redirect health care providers from treating patients with those drugs that would predictably become ineffective when the microbial target would produce the inactivating enzymes or processes that would render the antiinfective useless. Although the time required to accomplish this is rapid (days) compared to earlier sequencing iterations, it does not meet the clinical needs for "rapid" diagnosis. Each instrument can generate the data required for a draft bacterial genome sequence suitable for identifying and characterizing pathogens.

Deciphering DNA sequences is essential for virtually all areas of biologic investigation. The classical capillary electrophoresis (CE)–based sequencing has enabled the elucidation of genetic information in almost any organism or biologic system. In order to overcome inherent barriers in this experimental system, a fundamentally different technology was developed—next-generation sequencing (NGS). NGS is especially suited for microbial systems as it has the capability to evaluate alterations throughout the genome without prior knowledge and is therefore adaptable for unculturable microorganisms. NGS has increased the rate of data output each year since its inception in 2007 so that in 2012, 1 terabase (Tb) of data is available in a single sequencing run compared to 1 gigabase (Gb) in 2007. Associated with this exponential increase in output is a 10^5-fold decrease in the cost of determining the genome of a microorganism. In 1995, sequencing the 1.8-megabase (Mb) genome of *Haemophilus influenzae* with CE technology costed approximately $1 million and took about 1 year. Sequencing the 5-Mb genome of *E. coli* in 2012 with NGS technology can be accomplished in 1 day at a cost of about $100.

The molecular detection of resistance is an attractive concept; however, it fails to direct or recommend any specific treatment plan, antiinfective, or course of action. Genotypic resistance approaches have been used throughout the development of antiretroviral agents to monitor the treatment of HIV. But this was necessitated as the routine phenotype testing for susceptibility (or resistance) was not readily accessible to clinical laboratories because of biosafety precautions necessary when dealing with the human immunoproliferative agent—HIV. As is the case in WGS, the issue will become for microbial targets, the capability of dedicated software to interrogate the decoded microbial sequence to identify resistant markers for extant antimicrobial agents.

Recent reports have demonstrated how high-throughput genome sequencing of bacterial genomes were used to monitor disease spread and control infections in hospital settings. These investigations were associated with an outbreak of carbapenem-resistant *K. pneumonia*, which occurred at the U.S. National Institute of Health Clinical Center (33); cases of group A streptococcus (GAS; *Streptococcus pyogenes*) isolates associated with outbreaks of puerperal sepsis in Australian hospitals (32); and an outbreak of MRSA in a neonatal intensive care unit at a hospital in Cambridge, United Kingdom (34). These three studies show the future direction of clinical laboratory studies, which enable same-day diagnosis antibiotic resistance gene profiling and virulence gene detection.

A departure from traditional molecular diagnostics for targeting either DNA or RNA that encode resistance determinants would encompass the identification of proteins responsible for resistance—the field of proteomics. Advances in mass spectrometry describe matrix-associated laser desorption-time of flight (MALDI-TOF) identification of bacteria. This technique establishes the protein signature that can fingerprint the identification of clinically significant bacteria; however, direct detection of resistance determinants has not been established because several proteins can be involved in drug resistance (35).

As antibiotic resistance mechanisms among pathogenic microorganisms, especially the Enterobacteriaceae, are discerned, there is compelling need to rapidly and definitively identify them. Advanced diagnostics employing molecular methods is considered to be a key driver to improve therapeutic outcome—molecular arrays and NGS are key to providing the most promising opportunities.

REFERENCES

1. Boucher HW, Talbot GH, Bradley JS, et al. Bad bugs, no drugs: no ESKAPE! An update from the Infectious Diseases Society of America. *Clin Infect Dis* 2009;48:1–12.
2. European Centre for Disease Prevention and Control/ European Medicines Agency Joint Technical Report. The bacterial challenge: time to react. http://www.ema.europa.eu/docs/en_GB/document_library/Report/2009/11/WC500008770.pdf. Updated September 2009. Accessed May 17, 2014.
3. Rice LB. Federal funding for the study of antimicrobial resistance in nosocomial pathogens: no ESKAPE. *J Infect Dis* 2008;197:1079–1081.
4. Tillotson GS. Stimulating antibiotic development. *Lancet Infect Dis* 2010;10:2–3.
5. Infectious Diseases Society of America. The 10 × '20 initiative pursuing a global commitment to develop 10 new antibacterial drugs by 2020. *Clin Infect Dis* 2010;50:1081–1083.
6. Wright GD. The antibiotic resistome: the nexus of chemical and genetic diversity. *Nature Rev Microbiol* 2007;5:175–186.
7. D'Costa VM, King CE, Kalan L, et al. Antibiotic resistance is ancient. *Nature* 2011;477:457–461.
8. Sommer MOA, Dantas G, Church GM. Functional characterization of the antibiotic resistance reservoir in the human microflora. *Science* 2009;325:1128–1131.
9. Dantas G, Sommer MOA, Oluwasegun RD, et al. Bacteria subsisting on antibiotics. *Science* 2008;3201:100–103.
10. D'Costa VM, McGrann KM, Hughes DW, et al. Sampling the antibiotic resistome. *Science* 2006;311:374–377.
11. Garnacho-Montero J, Garcia-Garmendia JL, Barrero-Almodora A, et al. Impact of adequate empirical antibiotic therapy on the outcome of patients admitted to the intensive care unit with sepsis. *Crit Care Med* 2003;31:2742–2751.
12. Vallees J, Rello J, Ochagavia A, et al. Community-acquired bloodstream infection in critically ill adult patients: impact of shock and inappropriate antibiotic therapy on survival. *Chest* 2003;123:1615–1624.
13. Ibrahim EH, Sherman G, Ward S, et al. The influence of inadequate antimicrobial treatment of bloodstream infections on patient outcomes in the ICU. *Chest* 2000;118:145–155.
14. Rello J, Gallego M, Mariscal D, et al. The value of routine microbial investigation in ventilator-associated pneumonia. *Am J Respir Crit Care Med* 1997;156:196–200.
15. Alvarez-Lerma F. Modification of empiric antibiotic treatment in patients with pneumonia acquired in the intensive care unit. ICU-Acquired Pneumonia Study Group. *Intensive Care Med* 1996;22:387–394.
16. Rex JH, Pfaller MA. Has antifungal susceptibility testing come of age? *Clin Infect Dis* 2002;35:982–989.
17. Sakoulas G, Moise-Broder PA, Schentag J, et al. Relationship of MIC and bactericidal activity to efficacy of vancomycin for treatment of methicillin-resistant *Staphylococcus aureus* bacteremia. *J Clin Micro* 2004;42:2398–2402.
18. Centers for Disease Control and Prevention. Effects of penicillin susceptibility breakpoints for *Streptococcus pneumoniae*. United States, 2006-2007. *MMWR Morb Mortal Wkly Rep* 2008;50:1353–1355.
19. Tam VH, Gamez EA, Westan JS, et al. Outcomes of bacteremia due to *Pseudomonas aeruginosa* with reduced susceptibility to piperacillin-tazobactam: implications on the appropriateness of the resistance breakpoint. *Clin Infect Dis* 2008;46:862–867.
20. Delit TH, Owens RC, McGowan JE Jr, et al. Infectious Diseases Society of America and the Society for Healthcare Epidemiology of America guidelines for developing an institutional program to enhance antimicrobial stewardship. *Clin Infect Dis* 2007;44:159–177.
21. Tamma PD, Cosgrove SE. Antimicrobial stewardship. *Infect Dis Clin North Am* 2011;25:245–260.
22. McGowan JE. Antimicrobial stewardship—the state of the art in 2011: focus on outcome and methods. *Infect Control Hosp Epidemiol* 2012;33:331–337.
23. Salmasian H, Freedberg DE, Abrams JA, et al. An automated tool for detecting medication overuses based on the electronic health records. *Pharmacoepidemiol Drug Saf* 2013;22:183–189.
24. Linsky A, Simon SR. Medication discrepancies in integrated electronic health records. *BMJ Qual Saf* 2013;22:103–109.
25. Perez KK, Olsen RJ, Musick WL, et al. Integrating rapid pathogen identification and antimicrobial stewardship significantly decreases hospital costs. *Arch Pathol Lab Med* 2013;137:1247–1254.
26. Blaser M. Antibiotic overuse: stop the killing of beneficial bacteria. *Nature* 2011;476:393–394.
27. Goossens H, Ferech M, Vander Stichele R, et al. Outpatient antibiotic use in Europe and association with resistance: a cross-national database study. *Lancet* 2005;365:579–587.
28. Tosh PK, McDonald LC. Infection control in the multidrug-resistant era: tending the human microbiome. *Clin Infect Dis* 2012;54:707–713.
29. Zhang Q, Lambert G, Liao D, et al. Acceleration of emergence of bacterial antibiotic resistance in connected microenvironments. *Science* 2011;333(6050):1764–1767.
30. Piatek AS, Telenti A, Murray MR, et al. Genotypic analysis of *Mycobacterium tuberculosis* in two distinct populations using molecular beacons: implications for rapid susceptibility testing. *Antimicrob Agents Chemother* 2000;44:103–110.
31. Leinberger DM, Grimm V, Rubtsova M, et al. Integrated detection of extended-spectrum-beta-lactam resistance by DNA microarray-base genotyping of TEM, SHV, and CTX-M genes. *J Clin Microbiol* 2010;48:460–471.
32. Loman NJ, Misra RN, Dallman TJ, et al. Performance comparison of benchtop high-throughput sequencing platforms. *Nature Biotechnol* 2012;30(5):434–439.
33. Ben Zakour NL, Venturini C, Beatson SA, et al. Analysis of *Streptococcus pyogenes* peripheral sepsis cluster by use of whole-genome sequencing. *J Clin Microbiol* 2012;50:2224–2228.
34. Köser CU, Holden MT, Ellington MJ, et al. Rapid whole-genome sequencing for investigation of a neonatal MRSA outbreak. *N Engl J Med* 2012;366:2267–2275.
35. Carapetis JR, Steer AC, Mulholland EK, et al. The global burden of group A streptococcal disease. *Lancet Infect Dis* 2005;5:685–694.
36. Shah NH, Gharbia SE, eds. *Mass spectrometry for microbial proteomics*. New York: John Wiley and Sons, 2010.

Chapter 1

The Breakpoint

Matthew A. Wikler, Franklin R. Cockerill III, and Paul G. Ambrose

DEFINITION AND CLINICAL UTILITY OF ANTIMICROBIAL BREAKPOINTS

A breakpoint, in its simplest terms, represents the concentration of an antimicrobial agent that separates populations of microorganisms. Breakpoints are used in many ways, and so there may be more than one breakpoint for a specific antimicrobial agent–microorganism combination. It is also of interest that a breakpoint may change from time to time for a variety of reasons, as discussed later. In addition, breakpoints can vary from one country to another and from one official body to another in the same country. For example, in the United States, both the Clinical and Laboratory Standards Institute (CLSI), formerly the National Committee for Clinical Laboratory Standards (NCCLS), and the U.S. Food and Drug Administration (FDA) may provide breakpoints for the same antimicrobial agents. Additionally, breakpoints in the European Union (EU) are set by the European Committee on Antimicrobial Susceptibility Testing (EUCAST). The determination of a specific breakpoint is not a black-and-white decision, as many factors must be considered when selecting breakpoints.

To assist physicians in selecting antimicrobial agents to treat patients, clinical microbiologists categorize clinical isolates as drug susceptible, drug intermediate, or drug resistant. A result of "susceptible" assumes that an infection due to the isolate may be appropriately treated with the dosage of an antimicrobial agent recommended for that type of infection and infecting species. A result of "resistant" assumes that the isolate is not inhibited by the usually achievable concentrations of the agent with normal dosage schedules and/or falls in the range where specific microbial resistance mechanisms are likely and clinical efficacy has not been reliably attained in treatment studies. A result of "intermediate" assumes that an infection due to the isolate may be appropriately treated in body sites where the drugs are physiologically concentrated or when a high dosage of the drug can be used. The category of intermediate is also used as a "buffer zone" to prevent small, uncontrolled technical factors from causing major discrepancies in interpretations (1).

Ultimately, the purpose of breakpoints is to provide clinicians with information to assist in making decisions about antimicrobial treatments for patients with infections. Breakpoints serve many purposes, some of which are important for an individual patient, others for epidemiologic reasons. If breakpoints did not result in better patient care, then there would be little need to determine them other than as an academic exercise.

The remainder of this chapter focuses on breakpoints for bacteria, as these are currently the most advanced; however, many of the principles apply to the setting of breakpoints for other types of microorganisms (e.g., fungi).

HISTORICAL EVOLUTION AND CURRENT CRITERIA FOR ESTABLISHING BREAKPOINTS

CLSI has been providing standards for the testing of bacteria and breakpoints since 1975. Initially, breakpoints were established by examining scatterplots of the distributions of bacterial isolates versus the results of susceptibility testing conducted with antibacterial agents. Such scatterplots would frequently divide the bacterial isolates into two populations, one of which would appear to be more susceptible to the antibacterial agent being tested, the other less susceptible. The breakpoint would be the drug concentration separating the two populations. Establishing breakpoints in such a manner is probably suitable for epidemiologic purposes, as it allows one to easily determine shifts in the populations of organisms and to identify the emergence of resistant populations. From a clinical perspective, however, such an approach does not take into account the clinical implications.

In an attempt to improve the process for establishing breakpoints, CLSI has provided specific guidelines contained in a special document. The first version of this document was published in 1994 (2) and introduced the concept of looking at other types of data, including clinical data, in an attempt to correlate proposed breakpoints with what is likely to occur in the clinical setting. A revision of this document was published in 2001 (3). At the current time, so-called clinical breakpoints (antimicrobial susceptibility test interpretive categories) are determined by CLSI utilizing the following types of information: microbiologic data, animal modeling data, pharmacokinetic (PK) and pharmacodynamic (PD) modeling data, and human clinical data. These data are all considered and compared one against the other. In an ideal world, these data would all correlate with one another so that a breakpoint could be determined with certainty.

The microbiologic data considered consist of distributions of bacterial isolates and their minimum inhibitory concentrations (MICs). Numerous distributions are evaluated including those for a broad spectrum of organisms against which the antimicrobial agent is likely to be utilized and those for select populations of organisms that have specific types of resistance mechanisms. As clinical studies are conducted with a new antimicrobial agent, the susceptibility patterns observed in actual patients enrolled in studies are also reviewed. By utilizing data of this type, one can gain a sense of the various populations of organisms that exist and their relative susceptibility to the antimicrobial agent. Animal studies are quite useful in determining which pharmacokinetic-pharmacodynamic (PK-PD) measure one should be evaluating when trying to predict clinical efficacy. The three most common PK-PD measures are the duration of time the drug concentrations remain above the MIC (T>MIC), the ratio of the maximal drug concentration to the MIC (C_{max}:MIC ratio), and the ratio of the area under the concentration time curve at 24 hours to the MIC (AUC_{0-24}:MIC ratio). For most classes of antimicrobial agents, animal studies have demonstrated the ability to predict clinical efficacy by examining specific parameters (4). For example, it has been clearly demonstrated for β-lactam antibiotics that the most critical parameter predictive of clinical outcomes is the time that free drug plasma concentrations remain above the MIC of the causative organism (5–7). This is an example of a class of antibiotics where the predictive parameter is "time dependent." For cephalosporin antibiotics and *Streptococcus pneumoniae*, it appears that clinical success is likely if the free drug concentration above the MIC of the causative organism is maintained for 40% to 50% of the dosing interval, while for penicillins, the target appears to be 30% to 40% of the dosing interval (4).

The area under the drug concentration time curve (AUC) is a measure of drug exposure. Mathematically, the AUC is calculated as the integral of the drug concentration time curve. Response to drugs in vivo can usually be linked to the AUC. In some instances, the shape of the concentration time curve can affect in vivo response to a drug, and thus other measures of exposure (e.g., C_{max}, C_{min}) can also be important. Fluoroquinolone antibiotics have been demonstrated in animal models to be "concentration dependent"; that is, clinical outcomes can be predicted based on the AUC:MIC ratio and/or by the C_{max}:MIC. For the fluoroquinolones, it appears that clinical success (8,9) depends on attaining a free drug AUC:MIC ratio of around 30 for gram-positive organisms and around 100 for gram-negative organisms.

Although these general PK-PD targets tend to apply to many types of infections, one must keep in mind that levels obtained in certain tissues and body fluids may result in these targets not being predictive. For example, for drugs that are excreted by the kidneys and where active drug is concentrated in the urine, one would anticipate the ability to successfully treat organisms in the urinary tract with higher MICs. On the other hand, most drugs do not achieve high levels in the cerebrospinal fluid (CSF), and so one would anticipate that higher doses of an antimicrobial agent may be required to adequately treat an infection in that site. It would not be sufficient only to determine PK-PD targets based on responses in animal models, and so it is important that the results of clinical studies be correlated with these targets. Such work has been done for many classes of antimicrobial agents (4,8,10–14). Unfortunately, for new classes of antimicrobial agents, including LpxC inhibitors (deacetylase inhibitors of endotoxin biosynthesis), topoisomerase type-B subunit inhibitors, β-lactam–β-lactamase inhibitors, the correlations between the targets and the clinical outcomes in humans have yet to be well studied.

Once the PK-PD measure and target predicting clinical success has been identified, one can integrate this information with human PK data to estimate the probability of attaining drug exposures sufficient across a range of MIC values. One of the best ways to conduct such an analysis is by using Monte Carlo techniques (15,16). Basically, the strategy is to take (a) the PK parameters along with anticipated variability and (b) the MIC values of organisms likely to cause an infection along with the proportion of time; a specific MIC value is achieved or exceeded by in vivo concentrations of antimicrobial agent and then model patients by randomly matching up PK profiles and MICs. By using such a technique, one can easily simulate 5,000 or 10,000 patients and make predictions as to what MICs one is likely to be able to treat successfully with various dosing regimens (17,18). Ideally, this process should be accomplished in the earliest stages of drug development, as this allows one to determine the optimal dosing regimen likely to result in a successful clinical outcome while minimizing the potential for toxicity. Such PK-PD modeling can also be utilized to justify the initial breakpoint for a new antimicrobial agent prior to the availability of a large amount of clinical data (19,20).

Ultimately, the purpose of breakpoints is to provide information to the clinician for the selection of optimal antimicrobial therapy. Because of this, it is critical to evaluate clinical data from well-designed clinical studies which correlate breakpoints with clinical outcomes. Unfortunately, this is far from an exact science, as there are many factors that determine clinical outcomes other than the antimicrobial agent used. Consequently, clinical correlations are generally used to confirm susceptibility breakpoints predicted by the previously mentioned techniques and data.

For many reasons, the true limits of an antimicrobial agent are rarely tested in clinical studies conducted for the purpose of gaining regulatory approval. First, most of these studies exclude or discontinue patients whose infections are caused by organisms with an MIC above a tentative breakpoint. As a result, even if clinical studies could demonstrate a breakpoint, the probability of this happening is greatly reduced. In most cases, clinical studies can be ethically designed in a manner that would blind the investigator to susceptibility test results, allowing the decision to continue or discontinue therapy with the study drug to be determined by clinical and microbiologic responses. Clinical studies so designed are

more likely to aid in determining a clinical breakpoint. Another reason that breakpoints often fail to be determined by clinical data is that many of the newer antibiotics being developed are quite potent and only a small percentage of organisms will have MICs high enough to truly test their limits. In fact, few or no patients may be enrolled who have infections due to organisms with MICs at a sufficient level to uncover the limits of the antibiotic being evaluated.

ESTABLISHING BREAKPOINTS BY SITE OF INFECTION

It is sometimes necessary to consider the need for different breakpoints based on the site of the infection for which the antimicrobial agent is intended. For example, the ability of a drug to concentrate within the CSF is frequently quite different from the ability of the same drug to be concentrated in the urine or into tissues such as lung. As a result, it is reasonable to anticipate the requirement for a different breakpoint for the treatment of meningitis, urinary tract infections, or pneumonia.

As an example, CLSI recommends different penicillin breakpoints for *S. pneumoniae* isolated from spinal fluid as compared with respiratory secretions. Due to PK/PD and outcome data, lower (more stringent) breakpoints are provided for CSF isolates versus higher (more lenient) breakpoints for respiratory isolates (13).

ESTABLISHING BREAKPOINTS WHEN THERE ARE NO RESISTANT BACTERIAL STRAINS

As previously noted, many of the newer antimicrobial agents being developed are relatively potent and few resistant bacterial strains exist. When there is a dearth of resistant strains, it is difficult to obtain animal or clinical data to determine the true breakpoint. In these circumstances, the breakpoint is generally set at one or two 2-tube dilutions above the known susceptible population of strains for that organism. In such a situation, only a susceptible and not a resistant breakpoint is usually published, along with a notation that any strains isolated with a higher MIC should be sent to a reference laboratory to confirm the results. With time, a population of less susceptible strains will frequently emerge, and additional animal and clinical data may become available. At that point, it may become possible to establish a breakpoint reflective of the new situation.

CORRELATION BETWEEN MINIMAL INHIBITORY CONCENTRATION AND DISK ZONES

Many laboratories do not do MIC testing but rather depend on disk diffusion susceptibility testing methods. In order to meet the needs of these institutions, breakpoints are set for disk diffusion methods by correlating MIC results and disk diffusion results. Once again, various types of MIC distributions of clinical isolates of bacteria are reviewed, including distributions for a broad spectrum of organisms against which the antimicrobial agent is likely to be used and for select populations of organisms that have specific types of resistance mechanisms. Statistical methods are generally utilized to determine the best correlation between disk zones and MICs. Once the disk zone breakpoint is statistically determined, the rates of discrepant results are evaluated (i.e., where one method predicts susceptible and the other predicts resistant or intermediate). The number of discrepancies that occur within one twofold dilution of the intermediate MIC is less important than the number of discrepancies that occur at other MICs. After analysis of such discrepancies, the disk test may be adjusted to make it more predictive of the MIC test (i.e., by reducing the number of discrepancies). In some cases, it is impossible to develop a disk test that correlates with the MIC test. A recommendation is then made to not perform disk testing.

OVERRIDING THE BREAKPOINT

There are circumstances in which the breakpoint determined utilizing the standard methods is known to be inaccurate. When this occurs, the laboratory is instructed to override the results of the test and to adjust the report to the physician. For example, in recent years, gram-negative organisms that produce extended-spectrum β-lactamases (ESBLs) emerged. The standard testing methods that were used produced results indicating that the organism was susceptible to cephalosporins; however, because of the presence of an ESBL, these drugs were ineffective against such strains. As a result, CLSI developed specific testing methods to detect ESBL-producing strains. When such strains were detected using these specific methods, laboratories were instructed to override all MIC results previously interpreted as susceptible with the interpretation of resistant (21). Recently, CLSI has modified the MIC breakpoints for these drugs so that ESBL-producing strains are essentially captured. However, until these new breakpoints are adopted by laboratories, the specific ESBL tests must still be used with "overriding of results" as directed. As new mechanisms of resistance develop, it is critical that organizations and agencies that produce standardized antimicrobial susceptibility testing methods and interpretive criteria be diligent in looking for circumstances where the results of such tests are not accurate.

THE USE OF SUSCEPTIBILITY TESTS OF ONE ANTIBIOTIC TO PREDICT THE SUSCEPTIBILITY OF ANOTHER ANTIBIOTIC

Laboratories often use testing systems developed by antimicrobial susceptibility testing manufacturers. Such testing systems may contain a panel of antibiotics that do not replicate the available agents in a particular hospital or within the formulary of a particular health care system. In such a case, a laboratory may wish to use the results for one antibiotic to predict the susceptibility of an organism to another similar antibiotic. This has been a common practice, for example, with various cephalosporin antibiotics. In Table 1 of CLSI document M100 (21), there are suggestions as to when this may be possible. One must be aware that the correlations for certain types of organisms may be much better than for others within the same antibiotic class and that depending on one antimicrobial agent to predict another will invariably lead to some reporting errors.

WHY ARE THERE DIFFERENT BREAKPOINTS IN VARIOUS PARTS OF THE WORLD?

It is not uncommon to find that the clinical breakpoints for an antimicrobial agent–microorganism combination are different in different parts of the world. The reasons for this should become clear when one examines the variables involved in determining breakpoints. Breakpoints are set based on results achieved using a standardized testing method. If everyone used exactly the same testing method with adequate controls, the results would be expected to be similar. Unfortunately, testing methods are not currently standardized around the world, and thus there is the potential for different breakpoints to be established using different methods. Second, an antimicrobial agent might be used differently in different geographic areas. If it is customary to use an antimicrobial agent at a higher dose or to dose more frequently (including constant infusion) in one geographic area, the breakpoint will likely be higher in that area. Third, different microorganisms are encountered in different parts of the world. If resistant strains of bacteria are present in one geographic area but not other areas, it may be necessary to regionally adjust the breakpoints to ensure that the new resistant strains are being properly reported. There are also public health reasons why a breakpoint may vary. Public health authorities in one geographic area may want to avoid a resistance problem, deal with a resistance problem, or promote the use of certain antimicrobial agents over others. One way to impact antimicrobial use is to adjust breakpoints.

CURRENT EFFORTS TO DEVELOP STANDARDIZED METHODS AND BREAKPOINTS IN OTHER PARTS OF THE WORLD

Currently, efforts are being undertaken in various parts of the world to develop standardized methods for susceptibility testing. Ultimately, it would be ideal if one standardized testing method was accepted worldwide, as this would allow the direct comparison of results from one part of the world to another. The lack of harmonization of methods can create significant problems when evaluating epidemiologic trends. For example, suppose the goal is to examine the development of resistance for a particular organism and its spread in various parts of the world. The use of different methods makes it impossible to ascertain the true level of resistance. Even if one standardized testing method was accepted and utilized throughout the world, it is likely that there would still be different clinical breakpoints, for the reasons noted previously.

Another problem resulting from the lack of standardized methods for susceptibility testing concerns the development of new antibiotics. When conducting clinical trials and looking for correlations between outcomes and MICs or disk zones, it is necessary to use the same methods wherever the drug is tested.

The EUCAST is a standing committee of the European Society of Clinical Microbiology and Infectious Diseases (ESCMID). EUCAST was set up to standardize susceptibility testing in Europe so that comparable results and interpretations would be produced. It has both a general committee, whose membership includes representatives from all European countries, from the pharmaceutical industry, and from the in vitro media and device industries, and an ESCMID-appointed steering committee, which consists of a chair, a scientific secretary, six National Breakpoint Committee representatives, and two representatives from the general committee. Decisions are made by the steering committee after consultation with the general committee (ESCMID Web site, https://www.escmid.org). Unlike the CLSI, which develops only clinical breakpoints, EUCAST is in the process of developing both epidemiologic and clinical breakpoints. Epidemiologic breakpoints are breakpoints that differentiate the wild-type strains from strains that have developed resistance. Epidemiologic breakpoints can be extremely valuable when one wants to evaluate the emergence of resistant populations of organisms. The methods used by EUCAST (22,23) are in general agreement with those of the CLSI. EUCAST has been collecting MIC distribution data from worldwide sources for the purposes of establishing epidemiologic breakpoints. This extensive database is available on the EUCAST Web site (www.eucast.org).

WHY THE BREAKPOINTS OF CLSI AND THE FDA MAY DIFFER

At times, breakpoints contained in the FDA-approved package insert for an antimicrobial agent do not agree with the breakpoints published in CLSI documents. There are many reasons why this may occur, including differences in the interpretation of data and differences in how the two organizations function. When a new antimicrobial agent is approved by the FDA, interpretive criteria utilizing the CLSI standardized methods are approved and included in the product label. Most pharmaceutical sponsors will also submit a package of data to CLSI within a year of a new drug approval requesting breakpoints. Although there is general agreement between the FDA and CLSI, at times there are differences based on interpretation of the data. It is common for differences to occur after an antimicrobial agent has been on the market for a few years, as new resistance mechanisms become apparent requiring a reevaluation of the breakpoint. Unlike the FDA, CLSI has the ability to review breakpoints for any antimicrobial agent when there appears to be a need to do so. As a result, CLSI will make changes in single drugs or will frequently evaluate a class of drugs at the same time and make whatever adjustments seem necessary. Currently, the FDA generally considers a change in a breakpoint only when the sponsor submits a package to the FDA requesting a change. FDA staff participate in CLSI meetings as advisors and reviewers. Sponsors are encouraged to submit new data to the FDA to allow for updating the product label.

The obvious question arising from this is which breakpoints will clinical laboratories in the United States use? When there are published CLSI breakpoints, US laboratories use these breakpoints when testing organisms and providing reports to physicians. In fact, US laboratories are tested and accredited based on their compliance with CLSI methods and interpretive standards. If US laboratories use devices provided by in vitro diagnostic (IVD) manufacturers, those manufacturers must receive FDA approval at the breakpoints the FDA specifies before marketing these devices.

THE IMPORTANCE OF QUALITY CONTROL

The ability of the laboratory to follow the standardized testing methods utilized for setting breakpoints and the ability of the automated testing system to replicate the results that would be obtained utilizing the standard methods are critically important. Clearly, if such methods are not followed and well controlled, then the MIC or disk zone reported may be inaccurate, potentially resulting in a misinterpretation and inaccurate reporting to the health care provider. For this reason, care must be taken in performing these tests, and proper quality control must be implemented. In order to help the laboratory, CLSI and other organizations that produce documents outlining standardized methods provide quality control ranges for various standard bacterial strains tested against specific antibiotics. It is critical to ensure that the test performed on the quality control strains produces results that are within the accepted ranges. In addition, the laboratory must make certain that the breakpoints applied are those based on the methods that are being utilized. It is also critical that growth of the bacterial strain is sufficient for an accurate MIC or disk

zone to be obtained. That is why it is necessary to have a control well or area on the test plate where the bacterial strain can grow uninfluenced by the antimicrobial agent.

HOW TO REPORT AND USE BREAKPOINTS

Although breakpoint information is valuable when used for a specific patient, it can also have an impact on antimicrobial agent selection for a much larger group of patients. Most antimicrobial agent use is empiric; that is, a patient appears with what seems to be a bacterial infection, and the physician prescribes an antimicrobial agent without knowledge of the causative organism or its susceptibility. If the laboratory periodically collects its susceptibility testing data, summarizes such data, and distributes them to its physicians, then physicians are in a better position to prescribe antimicrobial agents likely to be successful. Most hospitals publish an antibiogram once or twice a year just for this purpose. There are numerous things one must consider when constructing antibiograms, and CLSI document M39-A3 (24) provides a guideline to help laboratories in developing them.

RESETTING BREAKPOINTS

Although epidemiologic breakpoints tend to be static, clinical breakpoints are not. There are numerous reasons why a breakpoint may need to be changed, and many of them are outlined in CLSI document M23 (3):

1. Strains less susceptible and/or more resistant to an antimicrobial agent may evolve.
2. Organisms with new mechanisms of resistance may develop.
3. New dosages or formulations of an antimicrobial agent and/or new clinical uses may require a change.
4. New clinical and/or pharmacologic data may suggest the need for reassessment.
5. Actions by and/or data from the FDA or other regulatory authorities, the Centers for Disease Control and Prevention (CDC), the College of American Pathologists, or other sources may suggest the need for reassessment.
6. Changes in CLSI-approved reference methods may have an impact on interpretive criteria and/or quality control parameters.

7. Other in vitro testing may suggest the need for reassessment.
8. Changes may also be made when public health concerns require action in situations where clinical information is limited.

As a recent example, in January 2010, CLSI changed the breakpoints for cefazolin against Enterobacteriaceae to reflect the emergence of resistance caused by ESBLs. However, after further review of common dosing regimens, MIC distributions and PK-PD data, this correction was determined to be too severe. Therefore, in January 2011, CLSI increased the MIC concentration interpretation for resistance by one twofold dilution (25).

PUBLIC HEALTH CONSIDERATIONS

The setting of breakpoints has an impact not only on individual patients but also on public health. The breakpoints will determine how antimicrobial agents will be perceived to work against specific organisms. As a result, when a physician receives an antibiogram of the susceptibility patterns of the organisms in his or her hospital and/or the local community, the physician's antimicrobial agent use patterns may be affected. Because the vast majority of bacterial infections are treated empirically, physicians depend on the antibiogram to direct their selection of initial antimicrobial therapy. If a breakpoint is changed and the change results in a commonly used antimicrobial agent no longer appearing to be efficacious, this may lead physicians to alter their prescribing habits. As a result, one class of drugs may end up being substituted for another. This shift in antimicrobial use can have an impact on future resistance patterns in the hospital and the community. For example, a previously low MIC that defined resistance for penicillin against *S. pneumoniae* for nonmeningitis infection resulted in a greater use of vancomycin. The increased use of vancomycin in hospitals appears to have led to an increase in the incidence of vancomycin-resistant enterococci. In addition, if a change in a breakpoint leads to the use of more expensive antimicrobial agents, there is an economic impact on the health care system. Clearly, there are important economic and health consequences when a breakpoint change results in the development of more problematic and difficult-to-treat organisms. These potential issues must be carefully considered when setting and/or changing breakpoints.

NEED FOR GREATER UNDERSTANDING OF BREAKPOINTS

As stated previously, the primary reason for breakpoints is to provide information to health care providers that will allow for the selection of antimicrobial agents likely to successfully treat infections. If a health care provider neither understands what the susceptibility report means nor understands the assumptions that underlie the report, then the actions taken may not be optimal for the patient. For example, if the breakpoint is set based on a specific dose of an antimicrobial agent being used, and if the physician uses a lower dose, then the actual clinical result may not be as anticipated. It is critical that efforts be made to properly communicate to health care providers what breakpoints mean and the assumptions that go into these interpretive standards. Information concerning some of the assumptions made in selecting breakpoints is contained in the documents and tables developed by CLSI and other standards-setting organizations. Unfortunately, this information rarely is communicated to physicians. If breakpoints are to be optimally utilized to maximize patient care, greater communication and education must occur. The education process could involve scientific publications that specifically discuss the decisions made by CLSI and other standards-setting organizations and the rationales for the decisions and the assumptions made. Such publications would likely be of interest primarily to microbiologists, infectious disease physicians, and hospital epidemiologists. These health care professionals should then convey the information they acquire to physicians through local educational activities.

In summary, breakpoints allow microbiology laboratories to provide valuable information to clinicians for the optimal selection of antimicrobial therapies. Epidemiologic breakpoints make it easier to detect the emergence of resistant populations of bacteria. Clinical breakpoints may vary due to differences in testing methods and in how antimicrobial agents are used in different parts of the world. Health care providers must be knowledgeable about the assumptions that go into the setting of breakpoints if they are to utilize such information to optimize patient care.

ACKNOWLEDGMENT

Ms. Tracy Dooley is thanked for her review and helpful comments for this manuscript.

REFERENCES

1. Clinical and Laboratory Standards Institute. *Methods for dilution antimicrobial susceptibility tests for bacteria that grow aerobically; approved standard—ninth edition.* Wayne, PA: Clinical and Laboratory Standards Institute, 2012. CLSI document M07-A9.
2. National Committee for Clinical Laboratory Standards. *Development of in vitro susceptibility testing criteria and quality control parameters.* Villanova, PA: National Committee for Clinical Laboratory Standards, 1994. NCCLS document M23-A.
3. Clinical and Laboratory Standards Institute. *Development of in vitro susceptibility testing criteria and quality control parameters; approved guideline—third edition.* Wayne, PA: Clinical and Laboratory Standards Institute, 2008. CLSI document M23-A3.
4. Craig WA. Pharmacodynamics of antimicrobials: general concept and applications. In: Nightingale CH, Murakawa T, Ambrose PG, eds. *Antimicrobial pharmacodynamics in theory and clinical practice.* New York: Marcel-Dekker, 2002:1–22.
5. Andes D, Craig WA. In vivo activities of amoxicillin and amoxicillin-clavulanate against *Streptococcus pneumoniae*: application to breakpoint determinations. *Antimicrob Agents Chemother* 1998:2375–2379.
6. Eagle H, Fleischman R, Musselman AD. Effect of schedule of administration on therapeutic efficacy of penicillin: importance of aggregate time penicillin remains at effective bactericidal levels. *Am J Med* 1950;9:280–299.
7. Eagle H, Fleischman R, Levy M. Continuous vs. discontinuous therapy with penicillin. *N Engl J Med* 1953; 238:481–486.
8. Ambrose PG, Grasela DM, Grasela TH, et al. Pharmacodynamics of fluoroquinolones against *Streptococcus pneumoniae* in patients with community-acquired respiratory tract infections. *Antimicrob Agents Chemother* 2001;45:2793–2797.
9. Craig WA, Andes DR. Correlation of the magnitude of the AUC24/MIC for 6 fluoroquinolones against *Streptococcus pneumoniae* with survival and bactericidal activity in an animal model. In: Program and abstracts of the 40th Interscience Conference on Antimicrobial Agents and Chemotherapy; September 2000; Toronto, Canada.
10. Bodey GP, Ketchel SJ, Rodriguez N. A randomized study of carbenicillin plus cefamandole or tobramycin in the treatment of febrile episodes in cancer patients. *Am J Med* 1979;67:608–616.
11. Forrest A, Chodosh S, Amantea MA, et al. Pharmacokinetics and pharmacodynamics of oral grepafloxacin in patients with acute exacerbation of chronic bronchitis. *J Antimicrob Chemother* 1997;40(Suppl A):45–57.
12. Forrest A, Nix DE, Ballow CH, et al. Pharmacodynamics of ciprofloxacin in seriously ill patients. *Antimicrob Agents Chemother* 1993;37:1073–1081.
13. Preston SL, Drusano GL, Berman AL, et al. Pharmacodynamics of levofloxacin: a new paradigm for early clinical trials. *JAMA* 1997;279:125–129.
14. Ambrose PG, Bhavnani SM, Rubino CM, et al. Pharmacokinetics-pharmacodynamics of antimicrobial therapy: it's not just for mice anymore. *Clin Infect Dis* 2007;44:79–86.
15. Drusano GL. Antimicrobial pharmacodynamics: critical interactions between "drug and bug." *Nat Rev Microbiol* 2004;2:289–300.
16. Dudley MN, Ambrose PG. Pharmacodynamics in the study of resistance and establishing in vitro susceptibility breakpoints: ready for primetime. *Curr Opin Microbiol* 2000;3:515–521.
17. Ambrose PG, Craig WA, Bhavnani BM, et al. Pharmacodynamic comparisons of different dosing regimens of penicillin G against penicillin-susceptible and -resistant pneumococci. In: Program and abstracts of the 42nd Interscience Conference on Antimicrobial Agents and Chemotherapy; September 27–30; San Diego, CA. Abstract A-635.
18. Dudley MN, Ambrose PG. Monte Carlo simulation and new cefotaxime, ceftriaxone, and cefepime breakpoints for *S. pneumoniae*, including strains with reduced susceptibility to penicillin. In: Program and abstracts of the 42nd Interscience Conference on Antimicrobial Agents and Chemotherapy; September 27–30; San Diego, CA. Abstract A-1263.
19. Ambrose PG, Grasela DM. The use of Monte Carlo simulation to examine the pharmacodynamic variance of drugs: fluoroquinolones against *Streptococcus pneumoniae*. *Diagn Microbiol Infect Dis* 2000;38:151–157.
20. Drusano GL, Preston SL, Hardalo C, et al. Use of preclinical data for selection of a phase II/III dose for evernimicin and identification of a preclinical MIC breakpoint. *Antimicrob Agents Chemother* 2001;45:13–22.
21. Clinical and Laboratory Standards Institute. *Performance standards for antimicrobial susceptibility testing; twenty-third informational supplement.* Wayne, PA: Clinical and Laboratory Standards Institute; 2013. CLSI document M100-S23.
22. EUCAST Definitive Document E. Def 2.1. Determination of antimicrobial susceptibility test breakpoints. *Clin Microbiol Infect* 2000;6:570–572.
23. EUCAST Definitive Document E. Def 3.1. Determination of minimum inhibitory concentrations (MICs) of antibacterial agents by agar dilution. *Clin Microbiol Infect* 2000;6:509–515.
24. Clinical and Laboratory Standards Institute. *Analysis and presentation of cumulative antimicrobial susceptibility test data; approved guideline—third edition.* Wayne, PA: Clinical and Laboratory Standards Institute; 2009. CLSI document M39-A3.
25. Turnidge JD. Cefazolin and Enterobacteriaceae: rationale for revised susceptibility testing breakpoints. *Clin Infect Dis* 2011;52:917–924.

Chapter 2

Antimicrobial Susceptibility on Solid Media

John D. Turnidge and Jan M. Bell

Susceptibility testing on solid media is a widely used alternative to the traditional broth-based testing developed originally to measure minimum inhibitory concentrations. With rare exceptions, it relies on the use of agar as the solidifying agent and the nature of agar, which permits slow diffusion of chemicals through its three-dimensional matrix. There are three formats for testing using solid media: agar dilution, disk diffusion, and gradient diffusion. Of these, the one that has proven most popular and adaptable to routine laboratory testing is disk diffusion. It has been the subject of excellent chapters in previous editions of this book (1,2). The first edition of this book (3) contains an excellent chapter on some of the basic issues with testing in agar that are not fully explored here.

Of note, this chapter addresses the use of agar in susceptibility testing of conventional bacteria of human and animal origin and does not address susceptibility testing of mycobacteria, nocardiae or other aerobic actinomycetes, mycoplasmas, yeast, or molds. Methods for testing such organisms using agar have been described, and readers are referred to the standards from the Clinical and Laboratory Standards Institute (CLSI) (4–7).

FEATURES OF SOLIDIFYING AGENTS

Solidifying agents for susceptibility testing and culture media generally need the following features to be useful: (a) water solubility, (b) ability to remain solid at incubation temperatures (≤42°C), (c) ability to liquefy at higher temperatures to permit pouring and incorporation of additives, (d) chemical inertness, (e) relative transparency, and (f) resistance to bacterial degradative enzymes.

Agar

Agar is a natural product obtained from several red seaweeds from the Rhodophyceae class and related seaweeds such as *Pterocladia*, which collectively are called agarophytes. It takes its name from the Malay word *agar-agar*, which describes these seaweeds. Agar also has wide application in the food industry as a thickening and emulsifying agent. Agar liquefies when heated to boiling and does not gel until cooled to 45°C to 50°C. After gelling, it requires reheating to near boiling to liquefy again. For the preparation of bacteriologic grade agar, *Gelidium* species are almost always used because they have the preferred lower gelling temperature of 34°C to 36°C, allowing the addition of supplements (8,9).

The principal components of agar are the polysaccharides agarose and agaropectin. Purified agarose has become one of the mainstays of solid-phase electrophoretic analysis. As a natural product, agar is subject to lot-to-lot variation. Variation occurs in the presence of sulfate ions, which affect the overall negative charge of the polysaccharides, which in turn can affect diffusion of certain chemicals. Calcium is also essential in small amounts to permit gelling. Of greater importance is brand-to-brand and lot-to-lot variation in the concentrations of divalent cations, which can affect the activity of certain antimicrobials, as discussed in the following section.

Other Solidifying Agents

A range of other gelling agents have been experimented with over the years, but none has yet displaced agar for susceptibility tests. In part, this relates not only to cost but also to the daunting

17

challenge of recalibrating end points (minimum inhibitory concentrations [MICs], zone diameters) for a very broad range of bacteria and drugs. Substances that have been examined include Separan NP10 (Dow Chemical Co, Midland, MI), a polyacrylamide that allows smaller concentrations of agar to be used; Gelrite (Merck & Co, Kelco Division, Rahway, NJ), a gellan gum formed from the fermentation products of a *Pseudomonas* species; and Neutra-Gel (Union Carbide Corp, Tuxedo, NY), a polyoxyethylene polymer that held the greatest promise when combined with a synthetic amino acid medium. Gelrite (Merck & Co, Kelco Division, Rahway, NJ) is the only one still available commercially.

FEATURES AND CHOICE OF AGAR

Since the development and promulgation of the European Committee of Antimicrobial Susceptibility Testing (EUCAST) disk diffusion methods (10), the agar main medium now used for conventional bacterial susceptibility testing is Mueller-Hinton. Sensitest and Iso-Sensitest agars are still used by minor susceptibility testing methods in Australia (11) and the United Kingdom (12). Mueller-Hinton agar has become the de facto standard agar medium in large part because it was selected for disk susceptibility testing when it was first standardized in the United States by Bauer et al. (13). Curiously, the medium was originally developed for the cultivation of *Neisseria* species. A large number of criticisms have been leveled at Mueller-Hinton over the years. Its problems include the possibility of different MIC values in broth versus the agar version, antagonism of tetracyclines, high levels of folate synthesis inhibitor antagonists, variation in performance between manufacturers due to difference in peptone sources, poor support for streptococcal species, and variable growth rates with gram-positive bacteria generally (14). Most of these problems were overcome through the intensive efforts of investigators and manufacturers toward its standardization, including intensive quality control procedures (15) and subsequently the development of "golden pound" reference lots (16). Currently, a new International Standards Organization (ISO) standard is being prepared which permits the calibration of Mueller-Hinton agar and broth based on performance rather than by comparison to a reference golden pound (17).

Iso-Sensitest agar was a common choice in some European countries until supplemented by EUCAST methods (18). Iso-Sensitest was developed by Oxoid from the original diagnostic sensitivity test agar and then Sensitest agar and is designed to minimize the amount of variable nutrients and maximize the defined components. To a lesser extent, problems have been encountered over the years in the performance of Iso-Sensitest (19). Nevertheless, it remains the basis of the British Society of Antimicrobial Chemotherapy disk diffusion test (12). Paper disk method (PDM) antibiotic sensitivity medium, long recommended (along with Iso-Sensitest) by the Swedish Reference Group on Antibiotics (20), has been withdrawn from the market.

The medium recommended for anaerobe susceptibility testing is Brucella agar or Wilkins-Chalgren (21,22). Less attention has been paid overall to the suitability of different media for anaerobes. Studies by a number of investigators have shown that supplemented Brucella agar supports the growth of a wider range of anaerobes than other media (23–25) and is now recommended as the reference medium by CLSI (22).

There are considerable differences in the formulas of different agars (Table 2.1).

FACTORS IN AGAR COMPOSITION

Antagonists of Folate Synthesis Inhibitors

Paraaminobenzoic acid (*p*-ABA) is a potent inhibitor of sulfonamides. Concentrations found in certain media such as peptone water and nutrient agar will virtually eliminate sulfonamide activity (26). Susceptibility testing agar used in any of the current published methods has minimal concentrations of *p*-ABA.

Thymidine and thymine in sufficient concentrations antagonize the dihydrofolate reductase (DHFR) inhibitors such as trimethoprim, increasing MICs and reducing zone diameters in agar diffusion tests. This nucleoside and its pyrimidine base possibly act by competing for the target enzyme. Thymidine is by far the more potent of the two, and methods to reduce or eliminate its presence in agar will restore DHFR inhibitor activity. Indeed, one common method is to use lysed horse blood, which is rich in the enzyme thymidine phosphorylase, which converts thymidine to thymine and 2-deoxyribose-1-phosphate.

Table 2.1

Formulations of Agar Media Used in Current Susceptibility Testing Methods

	Mueller-Hinton (CLSI, EUCAST)	Iso-Sensitest (BSAC)	Sensitest (CDS)	Wilkins-Chalgren (CA-SFM)	Brucella (CLSI)	GC (CLSI)
Protein source	Dehydrated beef infusion 300 g/L (or similar) Hydrolyzed casein 17.5 g/L	Hydrolyzed casein 11 g/L Peptones 3 g/L	Hydrolyzed casein 11 g/L Peptones 3 g/L	Tryptone 10 g/L Gelatin peptone 10 g/L	Peptone 10 g/L Dehydrated meat extract 5 g/L	Peptones from meat and/or casein source 15 g/L
Sugars		Glucose 2 g/L	Glucose 2 g/L	Glucose 1 g/L	Glucose 10 g/L	
Starch	1.5 g/L	1 g/L	1 g/L			1 g/L
Sodium chloride		3 g/L	3 g/L		5 g/L	5 g/L
Buffers		Sodium acetate 1 g/L Disodium hydrogen phosphate 2 g/L	Buffer salts 3.3 g/L			Dipotassium hydrogen phosphate 4 g/L Potassium dihydrogen phosphate 1 g/L
Calcium	Supplement after autoclaving	Calcium gluconate 0.1 g/L				
Magnesium	Supplement after autoclaving	Magnesium glycerophosphate 0.2 g/L				
Metal salts	Cobaltous sulfate 0.001 g/L Cupric sulfate 0.001 g/L Zinc sulfate 0.001 g/L Ferrous sulfate 0.001 g/L Manganous chloride 0.002 g/L					
Yeast extract				5 g/L		In some formulations
Vitamins		Menadione 0.001 g/L Cyanocobalamin 0.001 g/L		Thiamine 0.00002 g/L	Menadione 0.0005 g/L Haemin 0.005 g/L	
Amino acids		L-Cysteine hydrochloride 0.02 g/L L-Tryptophan 0.02 g/L Pyridoxine 0.003 g/L Pantothenate 0.003 g/L Nicotinamide 0.003 g/L Biotin 0.0003 g/L Thiamine 0.00004 g/L			L-Arginine 1 g/L Sodium pyruvate 1 g/L	
Nucleosides		Adenine 0.01 g/L Guanine 0.01 g/L Xanthine 0.01 g/L Uracil 0.01 g/L	Nucleoside bases 0.02 g/L			
Agar	17 g/L (12–18 g/L)	8 g/L	8 g/L	10 g/L	15 g/L	10 g/L
pH	7.3 ± 0.2	7.4 ± 0.2	7.4 ± 0.02	7.1 ± 0.2	7.5 ± 0.2	7.2 ± 0.2

CLSI, Clinical and Laboratory Standards Institute; EUCAST, European Committee of Antimicrobial Susceptibility Testing; BSAC, British Society for Antimicrobial Chemotherapy; CDS, calibrated dichotomous sensitivity; CA-SFM, Comité de l'Antibiogramme de la Société Française de Microbiologie; GC, gas chromatography.

Further, most bacteria, except *Enterococcus faecalis*, cannot utilize thymine as a substrate (26). Some bacterial strains require thymidine for growth and will grow poorly or not at all on susceptibility testing agar. Because such strains are naturally DHFR inhibitor resistant, no problems of testing occur when thymidine is added back into the medium.

Although Mueller-Hinton agar is purportedly low in thymidine and thymine, occasionally, problems can arise. CLSI has developed a quality control procedure to test for low thymidine content using either of two American Type Culture Collection (ATCC) strains of *E. faecalis* and trimethoprim-sulfamethoxazole disks (27). This procedure is now embraced in the new ISO standard to Mueller-Hinton lot acceptance criteria (17).

Calcium, Magnesium, Zinc, and Manganese

The principal problem with Mueller-Hinton over the years has been the variability in the concentrations of divalent cations, especially calcium (Ca^{++}) and magnesium (Mg^{++}), which can have significant effects on the activity of aminoglycosides and some other antimicrobials, particularly against *Pseudomonas aeruginosa* (28,29). For the broth, this has now been overcome during the manufacturing process, and the concentrations are adjusted to within an acceptable range specified by ISO 16782 (17). However, the addition of agar to Mueller-Hinton will alter the cation concentration in unpredictable ways, such that for some newer antimicrobial agents heavily influenced by cation concentration, such as Ca^{++} with daptomycin (30) and manganese (Mn^{++}) with tigecycline (31,32), it has not been possible to develop agar dilution or diffusion standards. The great variability in cation concentrations with different brands of Mueller-Hinton agar has recently been highlighted (31,33).

The divalent cations of Ca^{++} and Mg^{++} are well-known antagonists of aminoglycosides. The antagonism is complex and cannot simply be accounted for by the concentrations of the cations themselves (34). It appears to be affected to a large extent by other constituents such as sodium chloride and phosphate. The effects are most obvious when testing *P. aeruginosa* (35–37). The variability of concentrations in Mueller-Hinton agar in the past has been one reason that certain European countries have favored Iso-Sensitest agar, where the divalent cation concentrations are defined in the formulation. Ostensibly, agar

itself is processed to remove free cations and anions (14), but recent studies have demonstrated that there can still be a wide range of calcium and magnesium concentrations in different batches of Mueller-Hinton agar (30,31,33). In contrast to Mueller-Hinton broth, the concentration of divalent cations in Mueller-Hinton is not stipulated in the ISO 16782 standard. However, other susceptibility test media have not been subject to control of their divalent cations, and the reproducibility of aminoglycoside results with different lots has not been examined.

The concentration of Ca^{++} is critical to the interpretation of daptomycin susceptibility (30). Daptomycin activity varies greatly with Ca^{++} concentration, and specified concentrations are required in the media (usually those seen physiologically). For this reason, daptomycin has not yet been completely standardized for tests in agar, and supplementation is required for broth testing (30). Cation concentrations are also known to affect the activity of the polymyxins in susceptibility tests at least for *P. aeruginosa* and *Acinetobacter baumannii* (33,35). Calcium and magnesium concentrations can also affect the action of tetracycline against *Pseudomonas* species, although this is of little importance because tetracyclines are not considered clinically active against these species.

The concentrations of another cation, zinc (Zn^{++}), in Mueller-Hinton (38–40) agar and Iso-Sensitest agar (41) has an impact on the activity of imipenem and possibly other carbapenems, at least for common nonfermentative gram-negative. Again, the concentrations of Zn^{++} can be quite variable in different brands of Mueller-Hinton agar (32,33).

A summary of two recent publications that have examined cation concentrations in Mueller-Hinton agar is presented in Table 2.2.

Sodium Chloride

Less well known is the effect of sodium chloride concentration on the activity of aminoglycosides (42,43). As summarized by Waterworth (34), variations in NaCl can have quite significant effects: an increase in concentration from 22 to 174 mM can increase the MIC of gentamicin by as much as 32-fold. NaCl is not part of the Mueller-Hinton formulation, but the manufacture to a reference standard at least generates consistent results. NaCl is part of the Iso-Sensitest formulation, but viable amounts could also come from the hydrolyzed casein and peptones.

Table 2.2

Variations in Cation Concentration in Commercial Formulations of Mueller-Hinton Agar

Reference	Manufacturer	Cation Concentration									
		Ca	Mg	Zn	Fe	Ni	Cd	Mn	Cu	Pb	Hg
Fernández-Mazarrasa et al. (31)	Merck	12.2	8.2	0.18	0.5	0.08	0.01	11.5	0.08	0.01	bld
	Difco	13.5	7.8	0.38	0.3	0.08	0.01	0.05	bld	0.02	bld
	Oxoid	13.8	16.8	0.14	0.6	0.08	0.01	0.05	bld	0.02	bld
Girardello et al. (33)	Merck	7.5	6.2	bld	bld			19.3			
	Difco	16.1	4.9	1.1	bld			bld			
	Oxoid	20.9	13.3	bld	bld			bld			
	Himedia	25.3	31.2	bld	bld			bld			

Ca, calcium; Mg, magnesium; Zn, zinc; Fe, iron; Ni, nickel; Cd, cadmium; Mn, manganese; Cu, copper; Pb, lead; Hg, mercury; bld, below limit of detection.

pH

Major variation in the pH of the medium can result in major changes in the activity of aminoglycosides, macrolides, and tetracyclines. Aminoglycoside activity is substantially increased in alkaline conditions and substantially inhibited in acidic conditions. Similar effects are observed with macrolides. Susceptibility testing agars are manufactured to performance standards of pH, and in some testing methods, such as those of CLSI, it is recommended to confirm the pH in the cooled, prepoured state or with a surface pH meter after pouring, once the agar has been prepared from the dried powder in the routine laboratory.

The pH effect does become significant, however, when agar plates are incubated in increased concentrations of CO_2; such is recommended for streptococci and *Haemophilus* species in most methods. Rosenblatt and Schoenknecht (44) have shown an increase in pH from 7.4 to 8.4 over a period of 24 hours when Mueller-Hinton blood agar plates are incubated in 5% to 7% CO_2 in air. Carbon dioxide is absorbed onto the surface during incubation, some of which will be converted to carbonic acid initially and then carbonate ions, first decreasing and later increasing the pH at the surface (44). Acidity is known to reduce the activity of macrolides in particular (including the azalides and ketolides) (45–55) and of aminoglycosides to some extent (56,57) while increasing the activity of tetracyclines (2). In agar-based tests, this effect will result in higher MICs and smaller zones for macrolides and aminoglycosides, as the pH at the surface will be more acidic at the critical time.

Additives

Some bacterial species require the addition of specific nutrients to ensure adequate growth. The most common of these is blood, usually sheep or horse blood, at a concentration of 5%. When testing sulfonamides, horse blood is preferred, as it is low in sulfonamide antagonists.

Specific reagent additives are required for certain fastidious species or for nonfastidious species against certain antimicrobial agents, as described in Table 2.3.

Defined Growth Supplement

One important additive, noted here and in CLSI documents as *defined growth supplement*, is a complex mixture of vitamins, cofactors, and other nutrient substances. The two most recognizable and important brands are IsoVitaleX (Becton, Dickinson and Company, Sparks, MD) and Vitox (Thermo Scientific, West Palm Beach, FL). These products contain 1.1 g L-cystine, 0.03 g guanine, 3 mg thiamine HCl, 13 mg *p*-ABA, 0.001 to 0.012 g vitamin B_{12}, 0.1 g cocarboxylase, 0.25 g nicotinamide adenine dinucleotide (NAD), 1 g adenine, 10 g L-glutamine, 100 g glucose, 0.02 g ferric nitrate, and 25.9 mg cysteine HCl per liter of water. It is most commonly used at a 1% concentration to ensure the growth of the fastidious organisms, especially *Neisseria gonorrhoeae*.

Table 2.3

Specific Additives to Agars Used for Susceptibility Testing

Method	Medium	Species	Antimicrobial Agent(s)	Additive(s)
CLSI agar dilution and disk diffusion	Mueller-Hinton	*Staphylococcus* spp.	Oxacillin, nafcillin, methicillin	2% NaCl
		All relevant	Fosfomycin	25 mg/L Glucose-6-phosphate
		Streptococcus spp. *Neisseria meningitidis Campylobacter jejuni/coli Pasteurella* spp *Mannheimia haemolytica*	All relevant	5% Sheep blood
		Helicobacter pylori	All relevant	5% Aged sheep blood (≥2 weeks old)
		Haemophilus spp	All relevant	15 mg/L β-NAD 15 mg/L Bovine or porcine hematin 5 g/L Yeast extract ±0.2 IU Thymidine phosphory-lase (if testing folate antagonists) (*Haemophilus* test medium)
		Histophilus somni Actinobacillus pleuropneumoniae		10 g/L Hemoglobin 1% Defined growth supplement ("Chocolate Mueller-Hinton")
	GC base	*Neisseria gonorrhoeae*	All relevant	1% Defined growth supplement
	Brucella	Anaerobes	All relevant	5% Laked sheep blood 5 mg/L Hemin 1 mg/L Vitamin K_1
EUCAST disk diffusion	Mueller-Hinton	*Streptococcus* spp *Haemophilus* spp *Moraxella catarrhalis Listeria monocytogenes*	All relevant	5% Horse blood 20 mg/L β-NAD (Mueller-Hinton-F)
BSAC disk diffusion	Iso-Sensitest	*Streptococcus pneumoniae* β-Hemolytic *Streptococcus* spp *Moraxella catarrhalis Neisseria gonorrhoeae Neisseria meningitidis Campylobacter* spp.	All relevant	5% Horse blood
		α-Hemolytic *Streptococcus* spp *Haemophilus* spp *Pasteurella multocida Bacteroides fragilis Bacteroides thetaiotaomicron Clostridium* spp *Coryneform bacteria*	All relevant	5% Horse blood 20 mg/L β-NAD

(Continued)

Table 2.3 (Continued)

Specific Additives to Agars Used for Susceptibility Testing

Method	Medium	Species	Antimicrobial Agent(s)	Additive(s)
CDS disk diffusion	Sensitest	*Corynebacterium* spp *Enterococcus* spp *Listeria* spp *Streptococcus* spp *Erysipelothrix rhusiopathiae* *Moraxella catarrhalis* *Campylobacter* spp *Neisseria meningitidis* *Pasteurella* spp	All relevant	5% Horse blood
	Mueller-Hinton	*Haemophilus* spp	All relevant	15 mg/L β-NAD 15 mg/L Bovine or porcine hematin 5 g/L Yeast extract
	Columbia	*Helicobacter pylori* *Neisseria gonorrhoeae*	All relevant	8% "Chocolatized" horse blood
	Brucella	Anaerobes		5% Horse blood 5 mg/L Hemin 1 mg/L Vitamin K_1

CLSI, Clinical and Laboratory Standards Institute; NAD, nicotinamide adenine dinucleotide; GC, gas chromatography; EUCAST, European Committee of Antimicrobial Susceptibility Testing; BSAC, British Society for Antimicrobial Chemotherapy; CDS, calibrated dichotomous sensitivity.

PARANITROPHENYLGLYCEROL AND OTHER ANTISWARMING AGENTS

Paranitrophenylglycerol (PNPG) has been used among other techniques to prevent the swarming of *Proteus mirabilis* and *Proteus vulgaris* across agar surfaces. This is mostly a problem for agar dilution testing when multiple strains including strains of these two species are being tested on a single series of plates. As a result of the swarming, spots close to the *Proteus* species can be difficult or impossible to read. However, PNPG has been shown to affect the MIC results of a number of bacterial species and antimicrobials, especially *Pseudomonas aeruginosa* (58,59).

A second antiswarming agent, Dispersol LN, has also been evaluated and shown to affect the activity of some antimicrobials (60). The addition of PNPG or another antiswarming agent is no longer recommended routinely in any method and should only be used if there are data to show that the agent does not interfere with the MICs of that organism–antimicrobial combination. Another natural chemical, $10'(Z),13'(E)$-heptadecadienylhydroquinone, has been shown to increase susceptibility of *P. mirabilis* to polymyxin B (61).

Higher concentrations of agar (e.g., 2%) can be used to inhibit swarming. None of the three options—use of PNPG, use of Dispersol LN, or increasing the concentration of agar—is now recommended.

Strains with Special Growth Requirements

Special problems arise with strains or species with unusual growth requirements. The so-called nutritionally variant "streptococci" *Abiotrophia defectiva* (previously *Streptococcus defectivus*) and *Granulicatella adiacens* (previously *Streptococcus adiacens, Abiotrophia adiacens*) require pyridoxal for growth. Media can be supplemented with pyridoxal (0.001%) and lysed horse blood to ensure growth of the strains (63–65) and allow interpretation of MICs at least (no breakpoints have been determined).

Occasionally, mutant strains of *Staphylococcus aureus* will depend on thiamine or menadione (vitamin K_3) for growth. These often exhibit small colonies on primary isolation. The addition of thiamine (2 mg/L) and menadione (0.5 mg/L) to susceptibility testing media will allow susceptibility (MIC) tests to be performed (66).

Strains of *Escherichia coli* and other gram-negatives dependent on thymine for growth are sometimes encountered. They can be selected for during treatment with folate synthesis inhibitors (67). Strains of Enterobacteriaceae dependent for growth on thymidine, cysteine, or glutamine may be tested by adding the appropriate nutrient to the basal medium (7), although experience with this is limited due to the infrequency with which these strains are isolated.

AGAR DILUTION SUSCEPTIBILITY TESTING

Agar dilution susceptibility testing is the solid equivalent of broth dilution susceptibility testing, either in macro- or microbroth format. One advantage it offers over broth-based methods is that it allows the simultaneous testing of a large number of strains on a single agar plate, for example, 32 on a 90-mm plate using a Steers-Foltz or similar replicator (Fig. 2.1). It is therefore well suited to the rapid evaluation of new compounds or for large-scale centralized surveillance programs. The comparative disadvantages of this method are that it includes an additional variable (agar) in the medium and that, once prepared, the plates have a limited shelf life owing to degradation of the antimicrobial.

Most important, although agar dilution susceptibility testing, such as that described by CLSI

(62) and EUCAST (18), has traditionally been accepted as equivalent to broth microdilution, it is not the international (ISO) reference standard, and users of agar dilution need to be aware that there may be differences from the ISO standard for some antimicrobial agent–microorganism combinations, particularly in the light of uncontrolled cation concentrations in Mueller-Hinton agar versus Mueller-Hinton broth as specified for susceptibility testing. In the future, it will be necessary to establish equivalence to the ISO standard for new antimicrobial agents as they are developed. Methods for establishing equivalence have been described (68).

The two major published agar dilution susceptibility testing methods for common human pathogens (18,62) are essentially equivalent. In the usual approach to determining MICs on agar, the antimicrobial is incorporated into molten agar over a series of twofold dilutions, gently rotated to ensure even distribution of the antimicrobial, and then poured into Petri plates. The major elements of the test are described in the following sections.

Antimicrobial Powders

Antimicrobial powders should be obtained as "pure substance" from the manufacturer or from a reputable chemical supplier (e.g., Sigma-Aldrich Corporation). It is not appropriate to use powders found in vials for parenteral drug administration, as these may contain preservatives, surfactants,

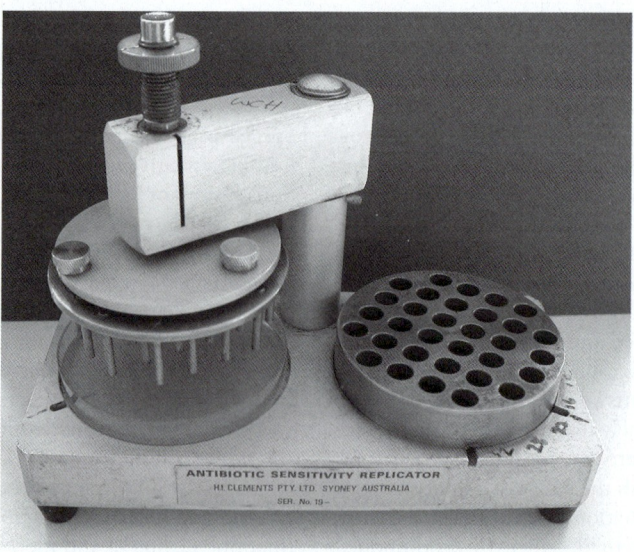

Figure 2.1 ■ Replicator for agar dilution. (See Color Plate in the front of the book.)

fillers, or other substances that could interfere with the antimicrobial activity, and their contents may vary legally by as much as 10% above or below the label amount. Each powder should come with an expiration date and an indication of its potency and (sometimes) water content. It is vital that all these data be taken into account before preparation of stock solutions. Data should also be available from the manufacturer or another reliable source on choice of solvent and solubility before preparing stock solutions. One easily accessible source is Table 5A in CLSI's M100 document, which is updated yearly (69).

Powders should be stored as recommended by the manufacturer. If no instructions for storage are available, then store powders at −20°C in a desiccator, preferably under vacuum (69). This will ensure the product retains its potency for the maximum time.

Choice of Dilution Range

Before preparing stock solutions, it is essential that an appropriate dilution range be chosen. Suggested ranges for different species or bacterial types have been published (21). A full range is generally 10 to 12 doubling dilutions. Doubling dilutions are appropriate because they provide the narrowest integer series on a logarithmic scale, and MICs for a single bug–drug combination are log-normally distributed in the wild type, that is, in the absence of a resistance mechanism. Although any series could be used, the most widely accepted doubling dilution series is that of base 2. This implies that preferably the highest concentration (the concentration at the start) should be a power of 2 (e.g., $2^7 = 128$). Following this pattern will allow comparison with the majority of published data and MICs for published quality control strains.

Preparation of Stock Solutions

Stock solutions should be prepared by weighing out the *exact amount* of powder using a balance designed for milligram amounts. Ideally, amounts less than 100 mg should not be weighed out. Alternatively, an approximate amount can be weighed out, and using the following formula, the *exact volume* can be added. The amount weighed is calculated using the formula

$$W = \frac{V \times C}{P}$$

where W = weighted amount (μg), V = volume of stock solution required (mL), C = concentration of solution required (μg/mL), and P = potency in μg/mg. Usually, a potency value is provided. If not, it will need to be calculated from the values provided in the certificate of analysis. These values are purity (as measured, e.g., by high-performance liquid chromatography [HPLC]), water content (as measured, e.g., by Karl Fischer analysis), and active fraction, which will be lower for salts than for free acids or bases.

$$\text{Potency} = \text{Purity} \times \text{Active fraction} \times (1 - \text{Water content [\%]})$$

The choice of final concentration will depend on whether the antimicrobial is being used immediately or whether it is intended for aliquoting and storage. Stock solutions for storage are best prepared as a 10-fold concentration of the highest dilution being used. Concentration choices will also be determined by the solubility of the antimicrobial. Stock solutions should be stored frozen at −20°C or lower and only thawed once before use; any unused thawed stock should be discarded.

Some antimicrobial agents require special solvents to achieve the high concentrations required in stock solutions. A comprehensive list of appropriate solvents and diluents is provided in reference 70 and is kept updated on a yearly basis as new antimicrobial agents in clinical development are added.

Preparation of Dilution Range

In order to avoid compounding minor errors in pipetting that would occur if low volumes were used or with repeated dilution, dispensing and dilution schemes such as those recommended by CLSI (69), the British Society for Antimicrobial Chemotherapy (BSAC) (21), and EUCAST (18) should be followed. These are adaptations of the original dilution scheme proposed by Ericsson and Sherris (71). An antimicrobial-free control plate should be added to any dilution series for quality control (i.e., to ensure that the selected strains are indeed viable).

Agar Selection

The description of each method identifies which agar media to use for particular bacterial groups or species. As all subsequent interpretations depend on data generated from these media, the nominated media for each method must be used. The ranges of media specified for each method are listed in Table 2.1.

Preparation of Agar Plates

Agars are generally prepared from a dehydrated base following the manufacturer's instructions with regard to amounts of base, water, and autoclaving. After autoclaving, bottles should be cooled to 45°C to 50°C by placing them in a water bath at this temperature. When the agar has reached this temperature, antimicrobial dilutions and supplements—and blood if required—are added aseptically. An additional plate should be prepared without the incorporation of antimicrobials as a plate to ensure that there is adequate growth of test and control strains on the medium.

Adequate mixing of the antibiotic in the molten agar is essential, and this is best achieved by mixing each antibiotic solution in a small decanted volume of molten agar and then mixing the result with the bottle of molten agar. If the antibiotic solution is added directly to the whole bottle of molten agar, the solution should be warmed to avoid small portions of agar solidifying around the solution as it is added. The antimicrobial solution is mixed into the molten agar by gentle swirling and inverting the bottle rather than by shaking so that frothing is avoided. Plates should be poured onto a level surface as soon as practical after mixing.

The pH of each batch of agar should be measured after preparation. An aliquot of molten agar can be poured into a beaker or cup over a suitably designed pH electrode and allowed to gel and reach room temperature. Alternatively, a surface electrode can be placed on an aliquot of agar poured into a Petri dish and allowed to reach room temperature. It is also possible to macerate a sufficient amount of set agar and submerge the tip of an electrode.

Agar plates are then poured from the cooled molten agar as soon as possible after mixing in order to minimize any impact on the antimicrobial concentration. There is no specified depth, but 20 mL of molten agar in a 90-mm plate is considered adequate. It is advisable to dry the plates, for instance, in a fan-assisted drying cabinet for 10 minutes (21) or in a 35°C to 37°C incubator inverted with the lids off (72), as moisture buildup is common if covers are placed over cooling agar in Petri dishes.

Preparation of Inoculum

Most standards offer the choice of two methods for the preparation of inocula: the "growth" method and the "direct" method. The direct method is often preferred for inocula prepared from fastidious organisms, as growth of these organisms in broth can be a little unpredictable. The solution for final suspension varies somewhat between standards and sometimes between groups or species being tested but is generally either 0.85% to 0.9% NaCl, the same type of broth used in the agar, or phosphate-buffered saline (PBS). For reference work, inocula should be prepared from subcultures in order to ensure purity.

Calibration of Turbidity

Inocula are always calibrated to a turbidity standard, usually a McFarland turbidity standard, which employs particulate suspensions of barium sulfate. McFarland 0.5 is the most common choice and can be prepared as described in various texts (62,72). Briefly, it is a 0.5-mL aliquot of 1.175% w/v $BaCl_2\cdot2H_2O$ added to 99.5 mL of 1% w/v H_2SO_4 (62). Alternative turbidity standards made from other materials such as latex particles but optically equivalent to 0.5 McFarland are available commercially (e.g., Remel Inc, Lenexa, KS). Normally, a visual comparison is made with the turbidity standard. It is important that this be done in good lighting and against a card with a white background and a contrasting black line. More recently, there has been a move to the use of a nephelometer or photometer to achieve this calibration. For instance, at a wavelength of 550 nm, a 5-mL glass tube with 2 mL of inoculum suspension with an optical density of 0.1 to 0.12 approximates a 0.5 McFarland barium sulfate standard (72). Equally, at 625 nm and a light path of 1 cm, the standard has an optical density of 0.08 to 0.10 (62).

Barium sulfate standards are affected by light and heat, and hence they should be stored between uses in a dark place at room temperature. Their turbidity should be checked in a nephelometer or photometer monthly. They also require vigorous agitation at each use.

Growth Method

Usually, two to five morphologically similar colonies are picked from a primary or subculture plate. The wire loop is used to touch each colony, and it is then immersed in about 5 mL of the recommended broth (e.g., tryptic soy broth in the CLSI method). The broth is incubated at 35°C until it equals or exceeds the correct turbidity, generally 2 to 6 hours for rapidly growing pathogens. The broth is then diluted with a suitable sterile fluid such as broth, saline, or PBS according to the instructions until 0.5 McFarland is reached.

Direct Colony Suspension Method

In this method, two to five colonies are touched or picked up and suspended directly in the fluid of choice. Clearly, the turbidity should be adjusted subsequently as for the growth method. This method is acceptable in almost all situations. Hence, it remains an option. The choice of growth versus direct method depends on laboratory workflow. Almost all standards prefer the direct suspension method for fastidious organisms such as *Haemophilus* species and *N. gonorrhoeae*.

Plate Inoculation

In almost all circumstances, it is preferable to use a replicator apparatus to inoculate the agar plates, such as a Steers replicator (see Fig. 2.1). These are expensive items but last indefinitely. They generally come with 32 to 36 pins to deliver this number of strains to a 90-mm agar plate. The size of the pins is critical to decisions about how or whether the inoculum to be used for various species is to be further diluted. Prongs of 3 mm deliver approximately 2 μL (range 1 to 3 μL) to the plate surface; prongs of 2.5 mm generally deliver around 1 μL (18), while prongs of 1 mm deliver around 10-fold less (0.1 to 0.2 μL) (73). Hence, some standards recommend dilution for some organism groups or species when using the 3-mm pins.

There is some variation between standards regarding whether further dilution of the standardized inoculum prepared as outlined earlier should be performed and how it should be performed. The commonly stated intention is that each spot on the plate should contain around 10^4 colony-forming units (CFUs). However, in preparing standardized inocula, there are considerable differences between species in the number of CFU per milliliter for a given turbidity (74).

Incubation

Temperature and Duration

Most organisms should be incubated at 35°C to 37°C. An incubator set at 36°C can generally operate within this range. The CLSI method specifies 35°C ± 2°C for all bacteria. The duration of incubation depends on the species. For rapidly growing species such as the Enterobacteriaceae, the glucose-nonfermenting gram-negative bacilli, *Enterococcus* species, and *Staphylococcus* species, overnight incubation for a minimum of 16 hours is needed. Longer incubation is recommended for fastidious species (18 to 20 hours plus), for

Staphylococcus species when testing against antistaphylococcal penicillins (24 hours), for *Campylobacter* species (24 to 48 hours depending on the standard and incubation temperature), for *Helicobacter pylori* (CLSI 3 days), and for anaerobes (42 to 48 hours).

Atmosphere

Enrichment of air with CO_2 is recommended in most standards for a variety of fastidious species, including *Streptococcus pneumoniae*, *Haemophilus influenzae*, sometimes other *Streptococcus* species, and *N. gonorrhoeae*. The concentration is usually 5%, although some standards tolerate ranges of 4% to 6%. The effect on the activity of certain drugs under these circumstances was discussed earlier.

Campylobacter species and *H. pylori* demand incubation in a microaerophilic atmosphere, identical to that recommended for primary isolation. Commercial systems are available for generating the required microaerophilic environment.

Anaerobic bacteria should obviously be incubated in the standard anaerobic environment used for primary isolation of anaerobes. Either an anaerobic chamber or jar is acceptable.

Plate Stacking

The effect of stacking plates on the incubation temperature is not widely recognized. After placement in the incubator, plates in the middle of a stack will take longer to reach the desired incubation temperature than plates at the top and bottom (75,76). This is important because the incubation temperature can have a profound effect on the generation time of bacteria, which in turn will affect the end point determination. In general, no more than five plates should be used in a stack. Even then, it can take up to 4 hours for the center plate to reach the incubator temperature (76).

Reading

Plates should be read with optimum lighting, preferably on a dark, nonreflecting surface. For instance, in Figure 2.2, growth has obviously occurred at some spots but not at others. The MIC is taken as the first concentration at which no growth occurs. Most standards recommend that the appearance of one or two colonies or a faint haze can be ignored. However, if there are one or two colonies at a number of concentrations rather than a single one above the putative MIC, then

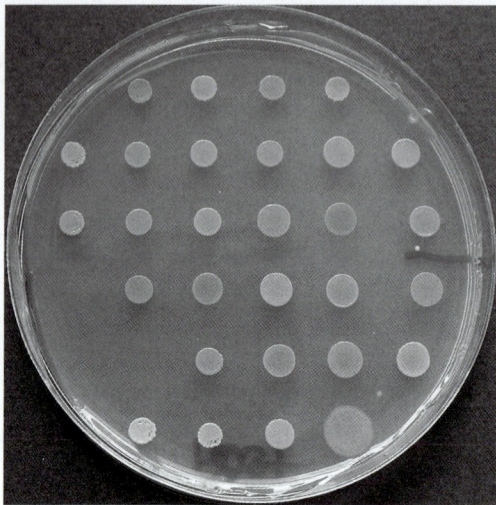

Figure 2.2 ■ Agar dilution plate after 24 hours of incubation. The medium is Mueller-Hinton agar. The strains are of *Staphylococcus aureus*. The last spot at bottom right is a control. Three strains have not grown at this concentration. (See Color Plate in the front of the book.)

the MIC is that concentration at which no colonies are seen. If this is the case, the purity of the strain should be checked, as it may be an indication of contamination. The only significant exception to these reading rules occurs in the reading of the end points for folate synthesis inhibitors, where growth can diminish gradually over a range of concentrations. CLSI recommends that the end point be read as that concentration resulting in 80% inhibition of growth (62). Other bacteriostatic drugs, such as chloramphenicol, clindamycin, tetracycline, and linezolid, can exhibit the same phenomenon to a lesser degree.

Quality Control

Quality control procedures in the performance of agar dilution are designed to ensure the reproducibility of the test and to confirm the performance of the reagents and the persons conducting the test. Most importantly, it is designed to detect errors of concentration or dilution of the antimicrobials, a not infrequent hazard in agar dilution testing. It is assumed that the laboratory is using reagents and materials from trusted suppliers who undertake quality control checks during manufacture. Using a trusted supplier does not prevent problems that may develop during shipping and handling, and hence, there is a need to have a quality control system at the laboratory level.

Quality Control Strains

The main component of quality control is the testing of reference quality control strains. The number tested varies between standards and with the type of strains being tested. Wherever possible, it is desirable to test a quality control strain of the same family, genus, and species as the strains under examination. The following ATCC reference strains have become almost universal as quality control strains for testing rapidly growing aerobic bacteria: *Escherichia coli* ATCC 25922, *Staphylococcus aureus* ATCC 29213, *P. aeruginosa* ATCC 27853, and *Enterococcus faecalis* ATCC 29212. Other strains recommended by different standards include *Escherichia coli* ATCC 35218 (CLSI for β-lactamase inhibitor combinations), *Staphylococcus aureus* Collection de l'Institut Pasteur (CIP) 6525 (Comité de l'Antibiogramme de la Société Française de Microbiologie [CA-SFM] for methicillin and oxacillin), *Haemophilus influenzae* ATCC 49217 (CLSI and BSAC), *Haemophilus influenzae* ATCC 49766 (CLSI), *Haemophilus influenzae* National Collection of Type Cultures (NCTC) 8468 (EUCAST), *N. gonorrhoeae* ATCC 49226 (CLSI and BSAC), *Streptococcus pneumoniae* ATCC 49619 (CLSI and BSAC), *Helicobacter pylori* ATCC 43504 (CLSI), *Campylobacter jejuni* ATCC 33560 (CLSI), *Bacteroides fragilis* ATCC 25285 (CLSI), *B. fragilis* NCTC 9343 (BSAC), *Bacteroides thetaiotaomicron* ATCC 29741 (CLSI), *Eubacterium lentum* ATCC 43055 (CLSI), and *Clostridium difficile* ATCC 700057. The CLSI also has special control strains for veterinary testing: *Histophilus somni* ATCC 700025 and *Actinobacillus pleuropneumoniae* ATCC 27090.

The selection of quality control strains involves a compromise between the objective of getting strains with MICs close to the center of a dilution series of a range of antimicrobials (62) and the number of strains that would be required to achieve this objective. The strains commonly recommended have also been selected for their stability over long periods of time and repeated subculture. There is nothing to prevent a laboratory from developing and using its own quality control strains.

Storage of Quality Control Strains

Stock cultures of the quality control strains should be maintained in the freezer below −20°C (ideally at −70°C) in a suitable stabilizer such as fetal calf serum, glycerol broth, or skim milk or should be freeze-dried. Some workers recommend that two sets of stock cultures be stored: one set to create working cultures and the other as emergency backup. This will guarantee that the laboratory always has unaltered quality control strains. Working cultures should be stored on agar slants at 2°C to 8°C and subcultured each week for no more than 3 successive weeks. New working cultures are generated each month from frozen or freeze-dried stock and subcultured twice before use.

Frequency of Testing and Corrective Action

Each standard provides MIC quality control ranges for these strains against some or all of the antimicrobials of interest. The recommended quality control strains are included in each test run. When these strains fall within the quality control range, the test run is valid. When one or more results are out of this range, the test run must be considered invalid and be rerun.

Use in Routine Susceptibility Testing

Agar dilution can be adapted to routine susceptibility testing. Essentially, it is a truncated method that incorporates one or two selected concentrations of antimicrobial, usually at breakpoint values (so-called breakpoint susceptibility testing). It has been advocated as an option for routine testing by some authorities in the past (77) but is slowly being supplanted by other methods. The advantages and disadvantages of this method have been described in detail by BSAC (77). When testing multiple strains of gram-negative bacteria that may include *P. mirabilis* and *P. vulgaris*, it is necessary to include an antiswarming agent, which, as discussed earlier, can affect results. The method offers specific challenges in terms of quality control because the limited number of concentrations will only detect the most gross of preparation errors in standard quality control organisms and will often fail to detect the most common error—a 10-fold error in antibiotic dilutions. To overcome this, there are a number of options available: (a) assaying antibiotic dilutions prepared from stock solutions, (b) assaying agar plugs removed from a poured agar plate (78), and (c) assaying paper disks applied for a fixed interval to the surface of a poured agar plate (79). McDermott et al. (79) provided a detailed analysis of two of these methods and recommended methods with high precision.

DISK DIFFUSION SUSCEPTIBILITY TESTING

Disk diffusion susceptibility testing has a long history, having evolved out of antibiotic diffusion from wells used for drug assay and susceptibility testing. The method in its various forms still has wide popularity owing to its ease of use and low cost compared with other methods. It has spawned many variants around the world. Unlike in dilution methods, an MIC value is not generated. Instead, in the development of the test, zone diameters must be compared with the MIC values of the same strains in order to determine which zone diameters predict which MIC values and hence which category of susceptibility.

Theoretical Aspects

All disk diffusion methods are based on the diffusion through agar of drug released from an impregnated disk. There are a large number of variables affecting this diffusion. Important features of antibiotic diffusion were worked out by Cooper and others in the 1950s (75,76,80–83). They have been clearly explained by Barry (3,84), who detailed the dynamics of zone formation and the "critical concentration," "critical time," and "critical population."

　　When an antibiotic is placed in a well cut into the agar or in a disk applied to the agar surface, the drug commences diffusion immediately and diffuses in a decreasing gradient of concentration from the edge of the well or disk. Over a number of hours, the height of this gradient deceases from very steep initially to quite shallow as the drug continues to diffuse (85). In disk susceptibility testing, disks are applied after the surface has been inoculated with bacteria. The formation of the zone edge is thus a contest between the diffusion of the drug and the growth rate of the bacterial inoculum, including any initial lag phase after incubation commences. The critical concentration is the concentration just capable of inhibiting growth, and it is also that concentration found at the zone edge at the critical time. It is similar but not identical to the MIC as measured by dilution methods. The critical time is the time it takes for the critical concentration to be reached at what ultimately becomes the zone edge. It is generally around 3 to 4 hours under standard test conditions. The critical population is the number of bacterial cells found at the critical time at the ultimate zone edge. The relationships between these parameters are as follows:

$$C_c = \frac{M}{4\pi D T_0 h}\, e^{\frac{r^2}{4DT_0}}$$

$$T_0 = L + G \log_2\left(\frac{N'}{N_0}\right)$$

where C_C = critical concentration, M = disk content, T_0 = critical time, D = diffusion coefficient of drug, h = depth of agar, r = zone radius, L = lag time, G = generation time, N'^2 = critical population at the critical time, and N_0 = number of viable cells at beginning of incubation. Although the following description is inaccurate, it is useful to simplify these relationships by imagining the zone of inhibition as a "cylinder" in which the drug is evenly distributed. The concentration of drug in this cylinder is thus the disk content (M) divided by the volume of the cylinder, namely $pd^2h/4$, where d is the zone diameter and h is the depth of the agar and therefore $d = \sqrt{4M/\pi hC}$. Thus, the zone diameter increases in proportion to the square root of the disk content and decreases in proportion to the square root of the agar depth. This defines the essential relationships between zone size, disk content, and agar depth and how variations in these affect zone diameters.

Disk Production

Disks for almost all antimicrobials can be obtained commercially. Even drugs that are still under development are likely to have disks available for use in the laboratory and clinical development programs. From time to time, it may be useful for a laboratory to manufacture its own disks. Strict standards must be adhered to if this is done. The same stipulations in drug sourcing and preparation of stocks as have been described in the section on agar dilution apply. Paper disks should be obtained that adhere to the same standards that apply to commercial manufacturers. In the United States, the standard is 740-E (Schleicher and Schuell, Keene, NH), and the paper used should be 30 ± 4 mg/cm^2 (86).

Solvents used in disk manufacture are described in a previous edition of this book (86).

Factors Influencing Zone Diameters

A large range of factors can influence the zone sizes produced. The most important are the disk content (also called *potency*, *mass*, or *strength*, namely,

the amount of drug in the disk), the disk size, the diffusion characteristics of the drug, the depth of the agar, the growth rate of the bacterium (including the initial lag phase), the density of the inoculum, and the activity of the drug against the strain being tested. Other factors such as medium composition, pH, and the effect of additives are dealt with at the beginning of this chapter.

Disk Content

The amount of drug impregnated into the disk is somewhat arbitrary. Amounts are chosen that are likely to produce zones of moderate size (15 to 35 mm) under normal conditions. Different disk methods have often selected different disk contents based on early experience with the antibiotic during development and precedents set within antibiotic classes.

Disk contents will be subject to variation during manufacture, and regulators such as the U.S. Food and Drug Administration (FDA) have set tolerances on the true amount in the disk in the range of 90% to 125% of the label. Such small errors will have a small effect on the zone diameter because it is proportional to the square root of the disk content, which means that the possible variation in the diameter ranges from about -5% to $+12\%$.

The difference in zone diameters with different disk contents has been exploited to determine critical concentrations (84). When three or more disks with a range of antibiotic contents are used, the resulting zone diameters, when squared, are directly proportional to the logarithms of the disk contents. The results can be plotted using linear regression, extrapolation of which to no zone yields the critical concentrations. These values will often be good approximations of the MICs as measured by other methods (3).

Disk Size

The extent of drug diffusion will obviously be affected by the width of the disk. Paper disks are now almost universally manufactured to be 6 mm wide. Further, the nature of the paper is subject to regulation, as different varieties of paper have been shown to affect the release characteristics of antibiotics (86). One disk method, that of Neo-Sensitabs produced by the Danish company Rosco Diagnostica A/S, Taastrup, Denmark (87,88), uses 9-mm disks made from hardened inert "chalk-like" substances. These larger disks result in larger zones for the same disk content.

Diffusion Characteristics of the Drug

The two crucial properties of the drug molecules are size and charge. In general, larger molecules diffuse more slowly, and the zones formed as a consequence are smaller. Large molecules demonstrating this include the glycopeptides such as vancomycin and teicoplanin (89). Strongly cationic molecules such as the polymyxins polymyxin B and colistin will also be inhibited in their diffusion owing to interaction with acid or sulfate groups on the agar polymer. Aminoglycosides are cationic to a lesser extent, and their diffusion is reduced slightly as a result (2).

Agar Depth

As noted, agar depth will naturally alter the size of the inhibition zone. Most methods have settled on a depth of 4 mm or a similar amount. This represents a balance between a smaller depth, which is likely to generate a reasonable zone size, and a larger depth, which is designed to reduce the zone size variation due to small variations in depth. A number of studies have demonstrated greater plate-to-plate variation in zone diameter when the agar depth is less than 3 mm (89a,89b).

Time between Inoculation and Disk Placement

The period of delay between the inoculation of the agar surface and the placement of the disks prior to incubation will have a significant effect on the ultimate zone diameter. This is a direct result of the concept of "the critical time" discussed earlier. Many bacteria are capable of initiating growth at room temperature, the temperature at which plates are usually inoculated. If the plates are preincubated at 35°C, the effect will be exaggerated. Studies examining this phenomenon have been used to elucidate the critical time (3). With two exceptions, disk diffusion methods recommend that the disks be applied within 15 minutes of plate inoculation.

Incubation Time

With rapidly growing bacteria, the zone diameter is formed within a few hours of commencing incubation (3). In theory, therefore, it is possible to read zone diameters when growth becomes visible. With further incubation—recommended for all organisms in all methods—there can be subtle changes in the zone diameter beyond the time when growth first becomes visible. These changes are the result of (a) delayed growth, (b) better visualization of partial inhibition, and/or (c) the delayed appearance of resistant variants. As zone diameter breakpoints are applied to species after specified incubation periods, it is not generally possible to use these values to determine susceptibility earlier. However, if the zone of inhibition is clearly in the resistant range, further incubation is only likely to make the zone smaller, and, therefore, it would be possible to categorize a strain as resistant when growth becomes visible. Incubation of the plate for a few hours longer than typically recommended (e.g., Enterobacteriaceae for 24 rather than 18 hours) will not usually influence the interpretation significantly. Some bacteria need longer intervals of incubation than 24 hours, such as *H. pylori* (3 days) and some strains of *Yersinia pestis* (48 hours).

A specific incubation duration of 24 hours is recommended in many methods for staphylococci when tested against the antistaphylococcal penicillins, usually represented by oxacillin or methicillin, and the glycopeptides, represented by vancomycin. In parallel with broth-based susceptibility testing methods, which can use 2% NaCl, this duration is used in order to maximize the expression of strains with heteroresistance. It must be used in consort with an incubation temperature of 35°C (and no greater). In the BSAC disk method, incubation at 30°C and the addition of 2% NaCl are also used, as these factors are known to enhance heteroresistance expression (90,91). Incubation for 24 hours is also recommended for enterococci when testing them against vancomycin in the CLSI method (27).

Incubation Temperature

Incubation temperatures are designed to optimize the growth of the organisms under test. Most human bacterial pathogens are adapted to optimum growth at 37°C. Most methods therefore recommend growth at 35°C to 37°C. Incubation at 30°C is known to enhance the expression of heteroresistance to methicillin and other antistaphylococcal penicillins (90) and has been recommended as part of the recently developed BSAC disk susceptibility test (12).

Inoculum Density

Inoculum density probably has a greater effect on the ultimate zone diameter than any other variable. As described by Barry (84), the critical population is one of the three critical parameters in determining zone size. Higher inoculum densities will result in bacterial numbers reaching the critical population sooner, at a time when the critical concentration has diffused less than with lower inoculum densities (84). In the case of very dense inocula, it is likely that no zone at all will be formed, even if the organism is susceptible. Inoculum density is particularly important when the bacteria produce inactivating enzymes such as β-lactamases, especially if the enzyme requires induction, as in the case of staphylococcal penicillinase. At low inoculum densities, the drug has the ability to kill the organism before sufficient enzyme is produced, and much larger zones will result.

In the development of different methods internationally, two approaches have been taken to the choice of inoculum density. Some methods have opted for simplicity and use inocula calibrated to a turbidity standard, almost always a McFarland 0.5 barium sulfate standard. This has been shown to result in quite different inoculum densities (in terms of CFUs per milliliter) for different species (74). Denser inocula (i.e., those with higher turbidity) are required for selected species such as *H. pylori* to ensure prompt and adequate growth (65).

Zone Edge

The features of the zone edge will be determined by the drug activity–species relationship, the resistance mechanism (if present), and occasional peculiarities of the species. Certain drug classes are notorious for producing "fuzzy" zone edges, where there is a gradual decrease in inhibition over a distance of 1 to 5 mm. This is a standard feature of sulfonamides and will be seen sometimes with DHFR inhibitors, amphenicols, and oxazolidinones. Most methods recommend that when a fuzzy zone is seen, the reader should make a judgment as to where approximately 80% inhibition occurs and define that as the zone edge. Judging 80% inhibition accurately and consistently takes practice. Studies presented at CLSI meetings have shown that linezolid zone diameters are most reproducibly read when viewed in transmitted rather than reflected light (27).

A second phenomenon, a "heaped" zone edge, is seen occasionally, but it is a normal feature of penicillinase-producing *S. aureus*. It is recommended that a heaped edge be interpreted as showing that the strain is producing penicillinase.

P. mirabilis and *P. vulgaris* typically swarm up the disk even when susceptible to the drug. When the organism is susceptible, a thin film is observed inside a more or less distinct zone of inhibition. This film should be ignored when making zone diameter interpretations.

Disk Spacing

Although inappropriate disk spacing is a common problem, it has not been studied in any systematic way. The distance between individual disks will be determined principally by the disk contents and organism growth rate. Higher disk contents and slower growth produce larger zones. If zones are large enough, ones from adjacent disks can run into each other and reduce the chance of accurately determining the zone diameter. The CLSI method, among others, specifies the distance between adjacent disks (24 mm from center to center) to minimize the chances of zone overlap. This limits to five the number of disks that can be placed on a 90- to100-mm plate, a considerable inconvenience if six to eight drugs need to be tested, as the cost of large plates is often substantially more that the cost of the common 90- or100-mm Petri plate. The EUCAST disk method has similar recommendations, namely 6 disks for a 100-mm plate and 12 disks for a 150-mm plate (10). The additional disk for the smaller plates is possible as a number of disks in the EUCAST have strengths lower than that of CLSI. All methods agree that disks should be placed to minimize the risk of zone overlap and possible misreading.

Current Disk Susceptibility Testing Methods

Currently, there are six methods published internationally and are kept up to date through constant revision and the addition of new agents (CLSI, EUCAST, BSAC, CA-SFM, calibrated dichotomous sensitivity [CDS], and Neo-Sensitabs [Rosco Diagnostica A/S, Taastrup, Denmark]). Of these, the most widely applied are the CLSI and EUCAST methods. The other methods are largely confined in their use to single countries—BSAC in the United Kingdom, CA-SFM in France, CDS in Australia, and Neo-Sensitabs in Denmark. Methodologically, there is nothing to recommend one method over another. However, the CLSI and EUCAST processes of setting MIC breakpoints and zone diameter criteria is based on the most comprehensive data set, which includes pharmacodynamic considerations and a large amount of clinical outcome data when available.

Further, these two methods are calibrated back to the now firmly established ISO reference broth microdilution method, whereas the others have not. Because zone diameter interpretive criteria are standardized for each individual method, it is not possible to either deviate from the method or use zone diameter criteria from another method unless all testing procedures and conditions are the same.

Testing of Problematic Species

Anaerobes

Two disk diffusion methods are described for anaerobes: that of the CA-SFM method (92), which uses Wilkins-Chalgren agar, and that of BSAC (12), which uses Iso-Sensitest agar supplemented with 5% horse blood and 20 mg/L of NAD. There have been several significant attempts to develop such methods in the United States (93–95), but the results have never been considered sufficiently robust for full development. In part, this relates to the prevailing view that routine testing of anaerobic bacteria is not required. Rather, it is believed that these bacteria should be tested in specific clinical circumstances or in batches to determine trends in resistance (22). BSAC has recently provided disk susceptibility testing methods for rapidly growing anaerobes on Wilkins-Chalgren agar supplemented with 5% horse blood, including interpretative criteria for a limited number of drugs (96). This effort must be considered tentative.

Campylobacter Species

After a considerable amount of work by the veterinary subcommittee of CLSI, there is now an established method for disk susceptibility testing of the principal two species (*C. jejuni* and *Campylobacter coli*) (65). The medium employed is Mueller-Hinton supplemented with 5% sheep blood. BSAC has also recently published a method using Iso-Sensitest supplemented with 5% horse blood for these two species (12). EUCAST have also recently provided a standardized disk diffusion method for these species using Mueller-Hinton-F medium (10).

Helicobacter pylori

Some authorities believe that disk susceptibility testing of *H. pylori* is not feasible (12,96). Their doubts are understandable given the slow-growing nature and special growth requirement of this species. However, CA-SFM has standardized a disk

test on Mueller-Hinton supplemented with 10% defibrinated horse blood and developed interpretive criteria for erythromycin and ciprofloxacin (92). There have also been several preliminary studies looking at the action of macrolides and other agents against this species (97–102). There is generally excellent agreement between disk and MIC results in these methods, and testing for resistance to macrolides and metronidazole by disk only requires multilaboratory comparison and quality control development to become a fully validated method, as clinical correlates are well established (100).

Quality Control

The main features of quality control in disk susceptibility testing revolve around the regular testing of quality control strains. Each methodology has a slightly different approach and range of quality control strains. Many advocate the testing of β-lactamase–producing strains of *E. coli* and *H. influenzae* as control organisms for β-lactamase inhibitor combinations. Careful attention must be paid to the storage of quality control strains (see the earlier discussion on agar dilution). Suitable detailed guidance is provided by CLSI (27). Quality control limits are defined for the common antimicrobials and relevant control strains. Ideally, quality control tests are conducted every time that the susceptibility tests are performed. The two major methods, CLSI and EUCAST, allow the shift to weekly testing if daily testing has proven satisfactory. Usually 1 in 20 or 3 in 30 results out of range can be tolerated. Better still is the option of graphing daily results on a Shewhart chart or similar quality control chart to detect obvious trends. If there is no obvious cause for out-of-range testing, the suspect combination should be tested daily for 5 days. If all the results are within the acceptable range, normal quality control procedures can be resumed. Otherwise, a detailed analysis of the source of errors should be undertaken. Sources of error include (a) incorrect measurement or transcription of zone diameters; (b) inadequately mixed, expired, or incorrectly stored turbidity standard; (c) one or more of the materials out of date or incorrectly stored; (d) incorrect incubation temperature or atmosphere; (e) malfunctioning equipment (e.g., dispensers); (f) incorrectly stored disks; (g) altered or contaminated control strain; (h) incorrectly prepared inocula; and (i) inoculum source more than 24 hours old. Judgment is required when deciding whether patient results relevant to the out-of-range quality control tests should be reported.

Reading of Zone Diameters

Manual Methods

Good lighting is essential to proper manual reading of zone diameters. Optimally, the plate is held a few centimeters above a black, nonreflecting background illuminated with reflected light. For transparent media, zones should be measured from the back of the plate; for opaque media such as those containing blood, zones are measured on the upper agar surface in reflected light. Two typical plates are shown in Figure 2.3. All methods normally recommend that zone diameters be measured and recorded. Although measurement is time consuming, there are long-term advantages, as interpretive criteria can change, and retrospective adjustment of interpretation is possible when breakpoints change (as they do from time to time when new resistance emerges). Measuring and recording zone diameters are probably less frequently practiced (103). Most zone diameters are simple to read. The important exceptions are where the zone edge is not sharp, as noted earlier. Very faint growth inside the zone can be ignored. When there are multiple discrete colonies within the zone, either the strain has resistant mutants (and should be reported as resistant) or the inoculum was mixed. Either way, these colonies should be subcultured and the test repeated from the original plate or inoculum. Care should be taken with hemolytic streptococci not to read the zone of hemolysis rather than the zone edge.

Automated Methods

Significant advances have been made in recent years in imaging and scanning technology. As a result, there are now a small range of commercial systems that can read and interpret zone diameters. These include the Oxoid Aura (Oxoid, Basingstoke, United Kingdom), the BIOMIC V3 system (Giles Scientific, Santa Barbara, CA), and the Adagio system (Bio-Rad Laboratories, Hercules, CA). These systems have been developed over a long period and have been extensively validated. They have benefited from significant advances in scanning and imaging technology as well as in computer software. Intersubject variability in reading is virtually eliminated, although all systems allow for manual override. Zone diameter breakpoints can be adjusted to whatever method is being used. When interfaced with laboratory information systems, zone-reading systems can save reporting time and reduce transcription errors.

Establishment of Interpretive Criteria

Although formulas have been devised for the relationship between the zone diameter and the MIC of the organism (discussed earlier), in practice it turns out that breakpoint zone diameter criteria cannot really be defined using such formulas. One obstacle is that zone diameters vary continuously and MICs are measured on a discontinuous (grouped) scale of twofold dilutions. An MIC measurement implies that the strain has an MIC within the range of that particular twofold dilution; for example, a measured MIC of 16 mg/L

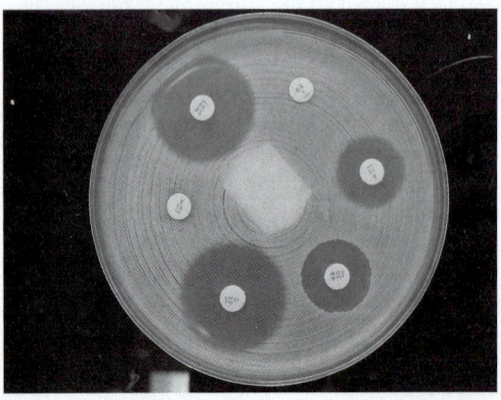
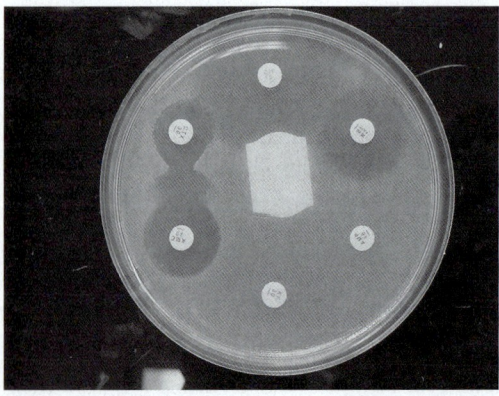

Figure 2.3 ■ **Disk diffusion test: CLSI method on 90-mm plates. A:** *Staphylococcus aureus.* **B:** *Escherichia coli.* This strain possesses an extended-spectrum β-lactamase and shows "keyhole" synergy between cefotaxime and amoxicillin-clavulanate. (See Color Plate in the front of the book.)

implies that the true MIC is somewhere between 8 mg/L and 16 mg/L. Also, as can be seen from the theoretical example in Figure 2.3, there is often a broad range (scatter) of zone diameters for strains with the same MIC. Finally, it is common for both zone diameters and MICs to have "off-scale" values (less than or equal to some number or greater than some number).

"Linear" regression has often been applied in the past to the paired MIC–zone diameter data. It is linear regression only in the sense that it uses standard linear regression methods on log-transformed MIC versus untransformed zone diameter data. However, it has little value, and its validity can be questioned. First, it is not possible to perform true linear regression if there are off-scale values. Either these data must be assigned some arbitrary value or omitted. Either way, bias is introduced into the regression as a result. Second, as the MIC data are discontinuous, there are unproven assumptions that the true MICs at each point are log-normally distributed. Third, no one has yet defined a satisfactory way of "reading out" the breakpoint zone diameters from linear regression. Instead, alternative statistical methods have been developed (and are evolving) to select zone diameter criteria given previously selected MIC breakpoint criteria.

At present, there are no internationally agreed approaches. The most popular method to date is based on that originally devised by Metzler and DeHaan (104), the so-called error rate–bound method. This is based on the minimization of "errors" (discrepancies between the zone diameter and MIC) with potential clinical impact. In the modern interpretation of MIC–zone diameter discrepancies, assuming that an intermediate category is desired, there are three types of errors: *minor*, where the MIC is intermediate (I) and the zone diameter is either susceptible (S) or resistant (R) or where the zone diameter is I and the MIC is either S or R; *major*, where the MIC is S and the zone diameter is R (i.e., the zone diameter is falsely resistant), which would deter the prescriber from choosing this drug; and *very major*, where the MIC is R and the zone diameter is S (i.e., the zone diameter is falsely susceptible), which could cause the prescriber to choose the drug to which the organism is really resistant. Minor errors will not occur if single MIC and zone diameter breakpoints are selected. Metzler and DeHaan (104) proposed that major errors should account for no more than 5% of the sample and very major errors for no more than 1%. They made no proposal for

the percentage of minor errors that could be tolerated, other than to suggest that a large intermediate range of zone diameters is "not useful." The selection of zone diameters was based simply on any one or pair of zone diameters that gave the desired percentages of major and very major errors. Metzler and DeHaan's (104) paper examined single MIC breakpoints and one or two zone diameter breakpoints. Brunden et al. (105) extended the observations to the more common modern situation of having or wishing to have two breakpoint criteria each for MICs and zone diameters. They also introduced more sophisticated iterative methods for zone diameter selection and applied a recommendation that the minor errors tolerated should be no more than 5%.

This method was developed further by CLSI, which has codified the error rate tolerances for setting zone diameter breakpoints depending on the size of the intermediate MIC range (0, 1, or 2 dilutions), compensating for both the inherent error in MIC determinations (often quoted as ±1 dilution, although this an oversimplification) and the number of strains in the different susceptibility categories (Table 2.4) (106). Even more sophisticated statistical techniques have been proposed and have been proven to work well on published data (107). Very recently, these have been implemented, along with the error rate–bound method, as an online analytics tool (108), although this has yet to be adopted by any authority.

By way of showing how these methods work, the data in Figure 2.4 would yield the following error rates using the Metzler-DeHaan method: very major, 1/132 (<1%); major, 1/132 (<1%); and minor, 3/132 (2.3%). By the CLSI method (two intermediate concentrations), the rates for those with an MIC greater than one dilution above the resistance breakpoint are as follows: very major, 0/25 (0%); and minor, 0/25 (0%). The rates for those with an MIC from the resistant to the susceptible breakpoint are as follows: very major, 1/21 (4.8%); major, 1/21 (4.8%); and minor, 1/21 (4.8%). The rates for those with an MIC less than one dilution below the susceptible breakpoint are as follows: major, 0/86 (0%); and minor, 0/86 (0%).

Rapid Disk Testing

As zone diameters for rapidly growing bacteria become visible after a few hours and after the critical time has passed (see "Theoretical Aspects" earlier in this chapter), interest has been shown in the

Table 2.4

Clinical and Laboratory Standards Institute Criteria for Tolerable Discrepancy Rates in Setting Zone Diameter Breakpoints

	Discrepancy Rates (% of MIC Category)[a]		
MIC Category	**Very Major**	**Major**	**Minor**
No intermediate range[b]			
MIC >1 dilution above resistance breakpoint	<2%	NA	<5%
MIC <1 dilution below susceptible breakpoint	NA	<2%	<5%
MIC = resistant and susceptible breakpoint	<10%	<10%	<40%
Single or two intermediate dilutions[b]			
MIC >1 dilution above resistance breakpoint	<2%	NA	<5%
MIC = 1 dilution above resistance breakpoint to 1 dilution below susceptible breakpoint	<10%	<10%	<40%
MIC <1 dilution below susceptible breakpoint	NA	<40%	<5%

[a]Percentages are the proportion of strains in that particular category, not the whole population.
[b]The resistance breakpoint is the MIC *at or above* which the strain is resistant; the susceptible breakpoint is the MIC *at or below* which the strain is susceptible.
MIC, minimum inhibitory concentration; NA, not applicable.

possibility of reading disk susceptibility results earlier than the conventional 16 to 20 hours (85,109–112). High degrees of correlation with standard testing have been shown for reading at 4 to 5 hours for Enterobacteriaceae (98.9%), gram-positive cocci (98.7%), and *Pseudomonas* species (97.9%) (2). One quarter of the strains of *P. aeruginosa* will have grown insufficiently at 5 hours and will require longer incubation times (85). In the single study of

Salmonella typhi, results of reading at 8 hours were 100% concordant with test results after conventional incubation (112).

In order to achieve good correlation with standard disk testing, conditions for the test need to be modified. Plates should be prewarmed to 37°C prior to inoculation; the inoculum should be adjusted to McFarland 1.0 (not 0.5); 5% blood should be added for testing all gram-positive

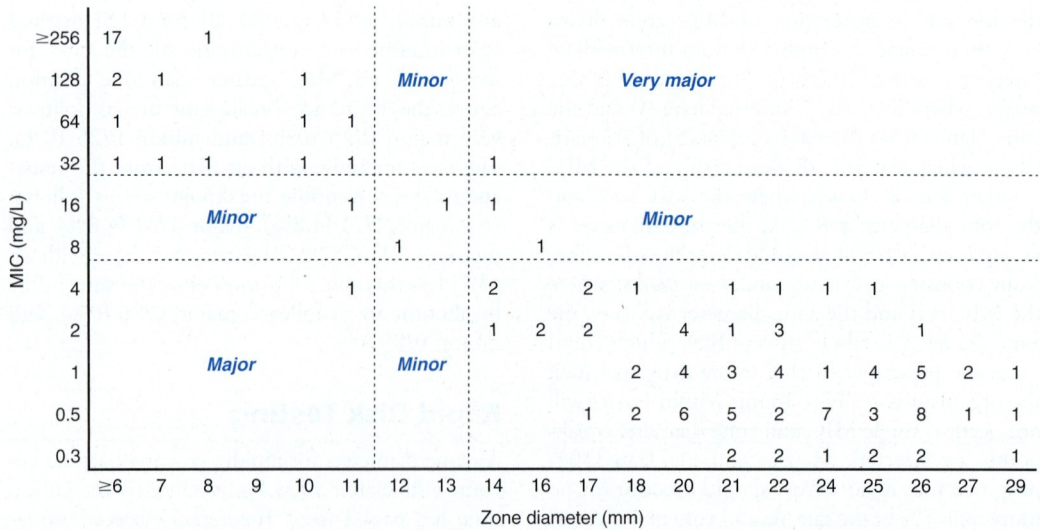

Figure 2.4 ■ **Relationship between zone diameters and MICs.** MIC, minimum inhibitory concentration.

cocci to maximize growth rates; and strains classified as intermediate but with zones close to the susceptible borderline should be reclassified as susceptible (2).

Rapid reading has not become popular despite its good performance, and it is not currently offered as an alternative by any standard-setting organization. This relates partly to workflow in the laboratory; unless plates can be set up early in the day, it is often not possible to generate the results in sufficient time for the clinician to make use of them on the same day.

Direct Disk Testing

Direct susceptibility testing involves the use of the specimen as the source of the inoculum. Few specimens are suitable for direct testing because the organism being tested in the specimen may be mixed with other pathogens and contaminants. Considerable error can occur when mixed strains are present in the disk test (113).

Studies on direct testing have been conducted principally on urine and positive blood cultures, although direct testing is feasible on a wider range of specimens, especially those obtained from sterile body sites such as cerebrospinal fluid. A single study on testing wound exudates gave unreliable results (114). The results of all such tests must be considered preliminary, and tests should be repeated by a standardized method once the organism or organisms have been isolated. The benefit of direct testing is that it can generate a preliminary result a day sooner and guide the clinician in choosing an antibiotic earlier in treatment. It is of greatest value when the clinical circumstances are urgent and/or life-threatening. In the one prospective study that compared rapid testing with conventional testing, significant benefits were seen for patient care and outcomes in the group whose results were generated rapidly (115).

Urine

The possibility of direct antimicrobial susceptibility testing of potentially infected urine was recognized many years ago (116). A number of prospective studies have been conducted examining the accuracy of direct disk diffusion testing (117–131). With few exceptions, direct susceptibility testing shows a high degree of accuracy (94% to 98% agreement with conventional testing), provided strict criteria are followed for the selection of results that can be interpreted. Problems encountered that might prevent interpretation include (a)

low bacterial concentrations despite true urinary infection, (b) inaccuracies due to the nonstandardized inoculum, and (c) mixed cultures (128).

The studies in which CLSI methods were used have provided the best examples of how direct testing of urine should be undertaken (127–129,131). Specimens for direct testing should be selected using microscopy criteria indicating probable urinary tract infection: an elevated white cell count (8 to 10 cells/mm^3) and an absence or a paucity of squamous epithelial cells, with or without the visible presence of bacteria. The use of a Gram stain on uncentrifuged urine also increased the accuracy of the result (131). The inoculum is prepared simply by dipping a sterile cotton-tipped swab into the urine specimen, squeezing out the excess fluid against the side of the tube, and streaking a plate of plain Mueller-Hinton agar as in the standardized test. After disk placement, the plates are incubated overnight as normal. The results are interpreted using the standard criteria for those tests where the culture confirms urinary tract infection; there is adequate growth on the medium; the cultures are not mixed (even if they are all pathogens); and the quantitative culture of the original specimen is 10^4 CFU/mL. The issue whether to report results as susceptible when they are categorized as intermediate because of high urinary antibiotic concentrations remains unresolved. Doing so increases the "accuracy" of the direct test (127). Intermediate results are sometimes seen when the urine bacterial concentration is higher than the inoculum in the standardized test. Some authors have also noted that the accuracy of direct testing drops when resistance to an antibiotic class is prevalent (128) and have attributed this to the proximity of many zone diameters to breakpoint values when resistance is present. If all the just described criteria are followed, then direct results could be considered valid and should not require repeat testing by the conventional method (128).

Direct susceptibility testing of urine has also been successfully attempted using disk elution (132) and agar dilution breakpoint plates (130).

Blood Cultures

If blood cultures become positive, it is possible to use the blood culture broth to perform direct disk susceptibility testing. This method has been confirmed to perform well in a range of studies (133–141). Rates of overall agreement with standardized testing range from 90% to 95%. One study showed that these rates of agreement could be reached after 6 hours for gram-positive bacteria, although gram-negative bacteria required overnight incubation. One advantage of blood culture broth as a source for the inoculum is that the inoculum can be standardized turbidometrically, provided the blood is not lysed (a common problem with *E. coli* and *S. pneumoniae*), although at least one study showed good agreement by using the positive blood culture broth directly (137). There are several options for preparing the inoculum, including direct use of the blood culture broth (137), subculture of a fixed withdrawn volume and further broth incubation to reach Mc-Farland 0.5 (136), and mixing the blood culture broth with broth or distilled water to adjust to the McFarland standard (2). A further advantage of direct blood culture broth use is that knowledge of the Gram stain characteristics of the isolate can guide the choice of a test medium.

There are some drawbacks to direct testing from blood culture bottles: the presence of high thymidine concentrations in blood culture media will carry over and antagonize the sulfonamides and trimethoprim, and the presence of sodium polyanethol sulfonate (SPS) in older blood culture media to remove antibiotics can antagonize some penicillins, aminoglycosides, and glycopeptides (2). All results generated by direct testing should be confirmed by standardized testing the next day, as bacteremia is a serious condition requiring confident antimicrobial choices.

Other Specimens

Other specimens in fluid format are also potentially capable of direct testing when infected. Direct disk testing has also been attempted with intraocular aspirates (142) and bronchial secretions (143), with some success.

GRADIENT DIFFUSION SUSCEPTIBILITY TESTING

Gradient diffusion susceptibility testing was pioneered by a Swedish company, AB BIODISK (Solna, Sweden), under the brand name Etest and is now owned and marketed by BioMérieux, Craponne, France. Since patent expiry, a competitor product (M.I.C.E., Thermo Fisher Scientific, Basingstoke, United Kingdom) has appeared on the market.

Gradient diffusion technology exploits the properties of antibiotic diffusion in agar to generate MIC values. It achieves this by applying a gradient of antibiotic along a carrier strip placed on the inoculated surface of an agar plate in the same way that antibiotic disks are placed. The antibiotic gradient is created on the strip by applying different concentrations of antibiotics in repeated arrays of an increasing number of small dots. When applied to the agar surface, the antibiotic diffuses into the surrounding medium in high to low amounts from one end of the strip to the other. The gradient remains stable after diffusion, and the zone of inhibition created takes the form of a pointed ellipse, from which the original Etest takes its name. The MIC is read off the scale printed on the upper side of the strip at the point where the zone edge meets the strip edge (Fig. 2.5).

The first evaluations of this product proved the Etest was comparable to conventional MIC testing (144–146). The Etest has since been evaluated against a very broad range of bacteria, including mycobacteria, as well as yeasts and molds. In general, the gradient diffusion strips produce results similar to those of conventional MIC tests against almost all bacteria. Its attraction is that it is simple to set up (as simple as disk diffusion) and takes less work, time, and materials than any agar or broth dilution method. Difficulties are encountered with some organism–antibiotic combinations, because finding the end point (where the zone intersects the strip) suffers from the same problems as zone edge interpretation in disk diffusion. Indeed, the effect is sometimes exaggerated. However, as the innovator product has undergone constant reevaluation over the 14 years since its release, the company has provided an excellent range of technical guides, charts, and other visual materials to assist the user in reading and interpreting the results correctly. Problems such as microcolonies at the intersection, swarming, paradoxical effects, hemolysis, resistant subpopulations, end points for bacteriostatic drugs, and technical errors are all dealt with and examples provided.

Like all such products, gradient diffusion strips must be properly stored and handled. The details of how to store the strips are provided by the manufacturer. Although the strips can be readily handled individually by sterile (flamed) forceps, devices are available for handling single strips in particular ways. The strips are made of plastic and are flexible enough to allow misplacement if forceps are used. As in the case of routine disks, the antibiotic will commence rapid diffusion as soon as the strip is placed. Hence, it is not possible to relocate the strip once it is placed. The length of the strips is such that one fits comfortably on a 90-mm Petri dish. With careful placement, two different antibiotics can be tested on a single 90-mm plate and is necessary with combination

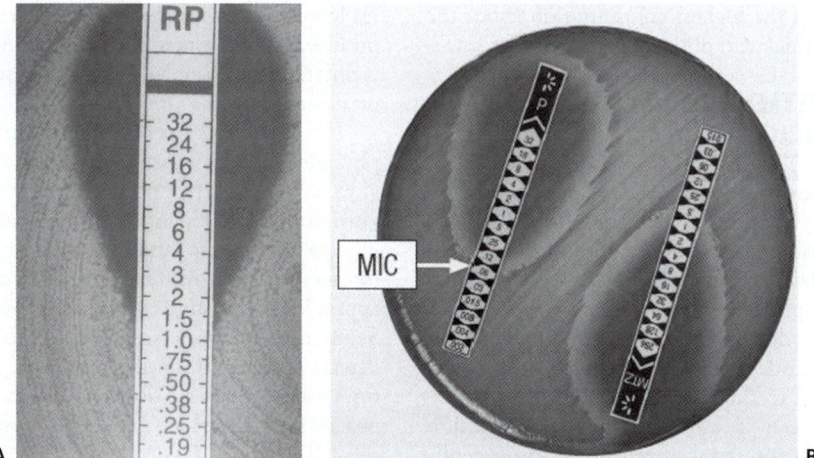

Figure 2.5 ■ **A.** Etest gradient diffusion test for *Streptococcus pneumoniae* and quinu-pristin/dalfopristin. **B.** M.I.C.E gradient diffusion test for *Helicobacter pylori* with penicillin and metronidazole. The MIC is where the growth of the strain meets the strip, ignoring the zone of hemolysis. (See Color Plate in the front of the book.)

testing. If done, the strips must be oriented in op-posite directions. Larger plates are recommended if more than one strip is to be used. A normal 150-mm Petri plate will comfortably accommo-date six strips provided that the bottoms of the strips are all facing the center of the plate.

Gradient diffusion strips have the MIC scale printed on the upper side. The scale differs between the two products. On Etest strips, the scale is modified from the conventional base 2 logarith-mic scale and includes intermediate "dilutions," such as 3 mg/L between the values of 2 and 4 mg/L. These values are not true halfway points on the $\log_2$ scale but rather rounded values, and the lines on the strip at these dilutions are placed accordingly. The scale on M.I.C.E. is arranged dif-ferently, with the intermediate values represented by a dark band rather than a line and value, requir-ing the reader to make some judgment about what that intermediate value should be.

The greatest advantage of the gradient diffu-sion strips is that they provide a laboratory with the ability to conveniently perform an MIC de-termination on a single strain without the full setup required for a conventional MIC test. If the clinical circumstances demand it, a quantita-tive susceptibility value can be easily generated. As an example, suppose a serious invasive infection such as meningitis or septicemia has been caused by *S. pneumoniae* but the categorical susceptibil-ity results (susceptible, intermediate, resistant) provide insufficient information to guide clinical

antibiotic decision making. A gradient diffusion test or tests can also be used to validate unusual resistances generated by conventional testing.

OTHER AGAR-BASED METHODS

Gradient Agar Plates
The concept of creating a single agar plate with a gradient of antibiotic concentration is an old one (147,148). Gradient plates provide a range of concentrations in a single plate and have been used principally to compare the susceptibilities of a range of strains on a single plate, especially when the MIC differences are likely to be small. More recently, gradient plates have also been used to select for resistant variants. When a gradient plate is used for this purpose, the strain being examined must be exposed to subinhibitory concentrations in one part of the plate (149).

In the most common method for preparing a gradient plate, a square Petri plate (100 mm by 100 mm usually) is tilted at a 12° angle while kept pre-cisely level along the perpendicular axis (150–151). Agar (~25 mL per 100-mm plate) containing the antibiotic of interest at a known concentration is poured into the tilted plate and allowed to set. The plate is then set flat and precisely level, and a sec-ond identical volume of agar containing no antibi-otic is poured over the top. The plate is ready to use after this second layer has set. Strains under test are usually streaked in a linear fashion starting from the lowest to the highest concentration (from the thin to the thick end of the lower layer).

POPULATION ANALYSIS PROFILING

The emergence of low-level resistance to vancomycin in a number of countries has led to the reintroduction of a research tool now called *population analysis profiling*. The technique was successfully applied to demonstrate the emergence of resistance during treatment of *P. aeruginosa* in an animal model with single agents (152). It was later applied to the characterization of methicillin resistance in *S. aureus* (153). Its application to the study of reduced vancomycin susceptibility in *S. aureus* began with Hiramatsu et al. (154), who successfully applied this technique to strains with homogeneous and heterogeneous reduced susceptibility. Refinements have been made to the technique in an attempt to minimize false positivity by comparing the area under the curve (AUC) of the population profile (log-transformed CFU/mL) with that of the original heteroresistant strain (Mu3) isolated in Japan (150). AUC ratios of 0.9 comparing the test strain with Mu3 were considered positive for heteroresistance. A ratio of 1.3 was used in a later study to define strains with homogeneous reduced resistance (155). There is ongoing uncertainty about the sensitivity and specificity for detecting hetero- and homogeneous reduced glycopeptide susceptibility in staphylococci using this test. It is very labor-intensive and consumes significant resources and thus is likely to remain a research or reference tool (156).

CLINICAL VALUE OF IN VITRO TESTING

The artificial nature of in vitro susceptibility testing frequently raises questions about the interpretation and meaning of results for patient management. Certainly, there are significant differences between the in vitro and in vivo situations on a range of factors such as (a) fixed versus varying drug concentrations, (b) no protein binding versus protein binding, (c) 16 to 24 hours of drug exposure versus days for treatment courses, (d) fixed versus variable physiologic conditions such as pH and eH, (e) absence versus presence of host immune response, (f) optimum growth conditions versus restricted growth in vivo, and

(g) low versus high inocula at the start of drug exposure. It is likely, therefore, that the MIC in vitro is different from the MIC in vivo in some, many, or all situations.

The differences between the morphologic and physiologic characteristics of bacterial growth in vitro and in vivo can be stark, suggesting that in vitro simulation of conditions might aid in getting in vitro responses to better mimic in vivo responses to therapy (157,158). Tests on solid surfaces may approximate the state of organisms in vivo closer. Standard laboratory susceptibility tests do not detect the range of antibacterial effects of an antimicrobial, such as sub-MIC effects (157,159), postantibiotic effects (160,161), postantibiotic sub-MIC effects (162), leukocyte enhancement effects (163), and supra-MIC effects.

Yet there is evidence that in vitro testing as conducted in the routine laboratory is predictive of response to therapy. Although there are very few studies that have examined test results versus patient outcomes in the routine setting (164), those that have been done, together with clinical experience and the findings of some prospective clinical studies, suggest that there is a high correlation. The question is why such correlation is possible.

The first part of the answer is that although MICs and their susceptibility testing correlates are artificial and indeed somewhat arbitrary, this does not matter. The yard and the meter are also arbitrary units of measurement, yet no one would deny their universal value for making measurements and, more importantly, comparing of measurements. Provided that there are MIC methods that are simple and reproducible and have low degrees of scatter, MICs can be used as a basis for comparing in vitro activity with the outcomes of treatment.

Second, if reproducible correlations can be shown between MICs (whatever values are generated) and bacteriologic and clinical outcomes, concerns about their poor reflection of in vivo activity can be bypassed. In essence, MICs become a convenient "yardstick" for predicting treatment outcomes. Prediction of outcomes has always been the goal of in vitro susceptibility testing. It is only then necessary to demonstrate that routine methods themselves correlate with MICs obtained using standardized methods.

Correlations between MICs and outcomes are now being generated through the emergence of the science of antimicrobial pharmacodynamics (166–169). By the use of in vitro and animal models, it has been possible to define the key pharmacodynamic parameters for a broad range of antimicrobial classes, including the β-lactams (166,170), the aminoglycosides (170,171), the macrolides (172,173), the quinolones (174,175), and the glycopeptides (166,176), and to provide guidance on the polymyxins (177), the tetracyclines (179), the lincosamides (178), and the oxazolidinones (166). Extrapolation of these findings to human infections has so far not revealed major discrepancies. Extrapolation is frequently necessary, as it is unethical to conduct clinical studies in which some patients must fail therapy in order to confirm pharmacodynamic correlates. Occasionally, failure to take into account pharmacodynamics has led to poor outcomes (180,181). Data on pharmacodynamics are now being applied as part of the development of breakpoint values.

Third, another goal of susceptibility testing is to detect the presence of resistance, defined microbiologically as the acquisition of a mutation or external genetic material or the induction of natural enzymes with an effect on the phenotype. Resistance will be reflected by an increase in MIC to above normal levels. All susceptibility testing methods include the concept of detecting abnormal phenotypes, although many have set breakpoints that will not detect all abnormal phenotypes. This reflects the tension between microbiologic and pharmacodynamic breakpoints, a tension that is not yet fully resolved. In a range of standardized methods, supplementary tests are recommended to increase the chances of detecting abnormal phenotypes, including β-lactamase detection tests and screening plates. How closely abnormal phenotypes that are below the breakpoints correlate with clinical outcomes is largely unknown, but the conservative position is to interpret them as resistant (or at least intermediate) until it is known that they are susceptible clinically.

TESTS ON AGAR FOR ANTIMICROBIAL INTERACTIONS

In clinical practice, combinations of antimicrobials are often used (a) to ensure adequate coverage of potential pathogens in empirical therapy, (b) to increase the likelihood of clinical success by achieving synergy between agents, (c) to reduce the risk of selection of resistance during treatment, and (d) to boost the efficacy of a primary agent that tests as resistant. Of these, the one of greatest interest to

the laboratory is synergy, for which a great variety of methods have been developed over the decades, most using broth systems (182) but some using agar. Important for the laboratory, there are actually only a few instances where true synergy has been shown in clinical practice (apart from old combination agents such as trimethoprim-sulfamethoxazole), the most important of these being enterococcal endocarditis (183).

Agar-Based Methods for Detection of High-Level Aminoglycoside Resistance

Cure rates of enterococcal endocarditis are higher when a cell wall–active agent (penicillin or glycopeptides) is combined with an aminoglycoside, even though *Enterococcus* species have low-level intrinsic resistance to this class. The two agents most often favored by treating clinicians are gentamicin and, when there is high-level resistance to gentamicin, streptomycin. When there is high-level aminoglycoside resistance due to the presence of an acquired resistance mechanism, the synergistic effect is abolished. Endocarditis isolates of *Enterococcus* species should therefore be tested for the presence of high-level resistance to gentamicin and streptomycin. Two agar-based methods are described by CLSI: a disk diffusion method performed on Mueller-Hinton agar using high-potency disks of gentamicin (120 μg) and streptomycin (300 μg) and an agar screening plate method performed on two different brain–heart infusion agar plates containing gentamicin 500 μg/mL and streptomycin 2,000 μg/mL (69). EUCAST describes a disk diffusion method using a different potency disk for gentamicin and with interpretive criteria (184). Other disk diffusion methods provide details of similar tests.

Disk Approximation Methods

The most time-honored agar-based method for detecting the drug interactions is that of disk approximation. This is a phenotypic test that still has application for the detection of resistance mechanisms such as inducible resistance to clindamycin, extended-spectrum β-lactamases, and some carbapenemases (27,69). When testing for the presence of synergy or antagonism, the disk approximation test will provide visual evidence of these types of interactions (Figs. 2.6 and 2.7). The test can be applied to any organism that can

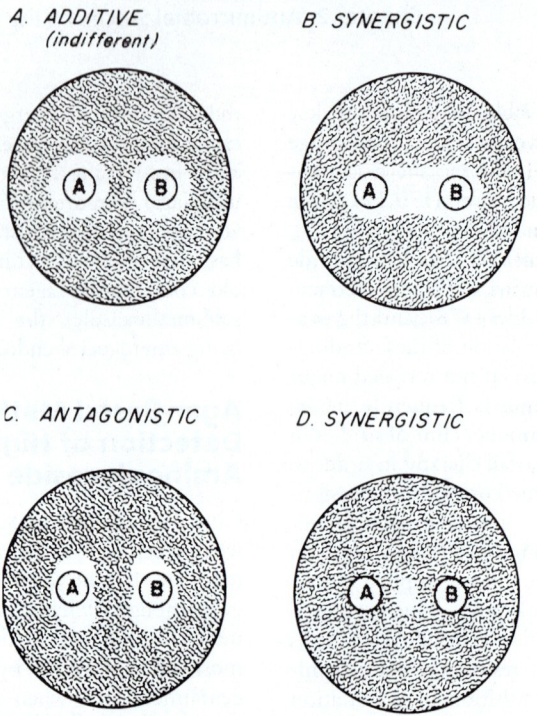

Figure 2.6 ■ **Assessment of antimicrobial combinations with the disk diffusion technique, using disks containing only one antimicrobial. A:** Additive or autonomous result. **B** and **D:** Synergism. **C:** Antagonism. *Shading,* bacterial growth; *clear areas,* zones of growth inhibition.

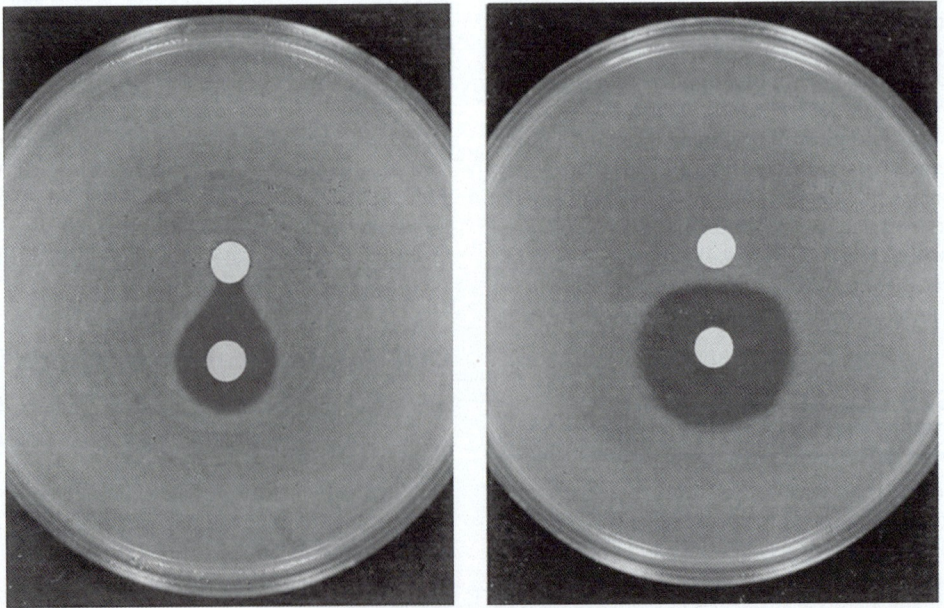

Figure 2.7 ■ **Assessment of antimicrobial combinations with the disk approximation technique.** Combinations of β-lactams were tested against one strain of *Enterobacter cloacae.* **Left:** Synergism between the two drugs. **Right:** Activity of one drug is antagonized by the second, at concentrations below those that inhibit growth of the organism.

be grown on agar plates, including those with the modifications and additives mentioned at the beginning of this chapter. Figure 2.6 shows the three different types of interaction that may be observed: indifferent, synergistic, and antagonistic. Note the two different types of synergistic interaction that may be seen. This is because interactions are critically dependent on both disk potency and separation distance. Unfortunately, there are no simple rules for determining the optimum combination of potency and separation distance of disks. This limits the value of this test to that of being indicative of a type of interaction, but it is unable to quantify the interaction further.

Disk Combination Methods

A variation on the disk approximation method is to use two disks containing the drugs individually plus a disk containing both drugs. After incubation with the test strain, the zone diameters of the three disks are compared. Interpretation is more difficult than the disk approximation method: A larger zone with the combination disk than with either single drug disk alone excludes antagonism but does not readily distinguish between indifference and synergy. A smaller zone with the combination disk than with either single drug disk alone suggests antagonism.

Gradient Diffusion Combination Methods

More recently, with the emergence of highly multiresistant organisms in clinical practice, there has been renewed interest in examining antimicrobial interactions using the application of gradient diffusion strips (184). Most interest has focused on

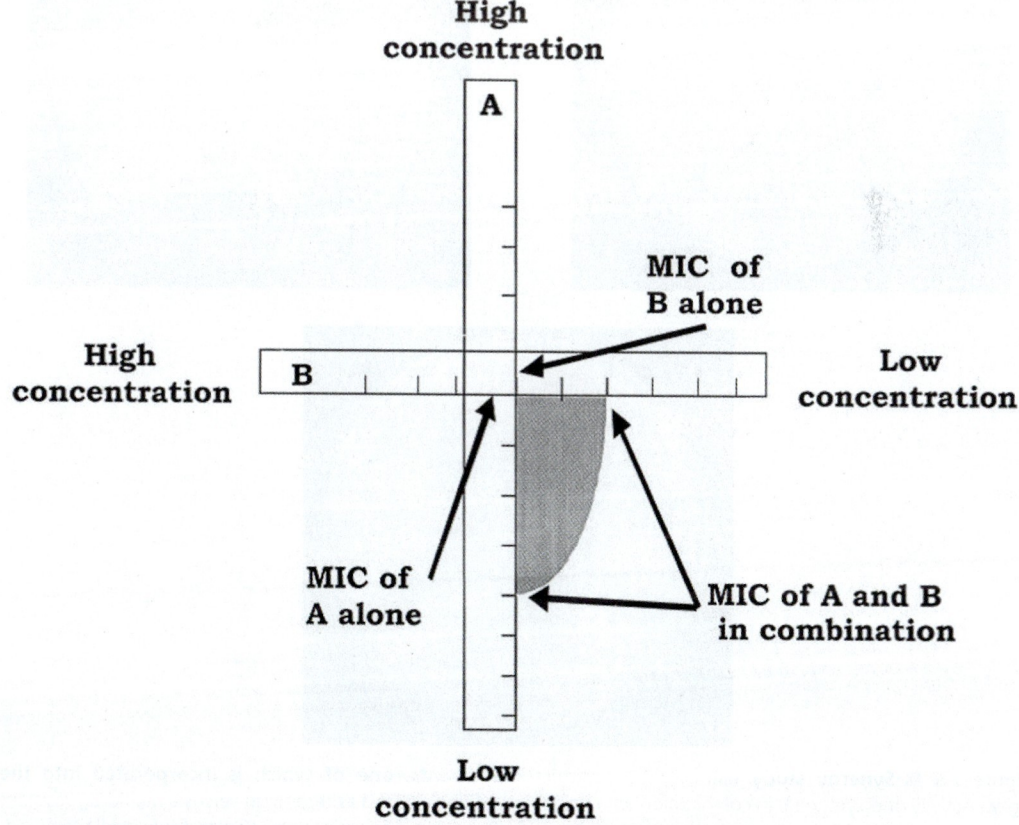

Figure 2.8 ■ Standard approach to synergy testing with gradient diffusion strips. MIC, minimum inhibitory concentration. (From White RL, Burgess DS, Manduru M, et al. Comparison of three different in vitro methods of detecting synergy: time-kill, checkerboard, and E test. *Antimicrob Agents Chemother* 1996;40[8]:1914–1918.)

multiresistant *A. baumannii* (184–195), but the method has also been used with *Enterococcus faecium* (196,197), staphylococci (198,199), *P. aeruginosa* (195,200–202), Enterobacteriaceae (195,203), and *Stenotrophomonas maltophilia* (195,204).

The features of this method are illustrated in Figure 2.8. The MICs are determined with the two gradient diffusion strips alone on the agar medium most appropriate for the test strain. The following day, two new strips are placed at right angles to other such that they intersect at the marks on their individual MICs. After a further day's incubation, when synergy is present, there will be a new zone of inhibition between the two strips, and the new lower MICs for both agents can be read off the two strips. The results are then interpreted using the same fractional inhibitory concentrations employed in checkerboard broth microdilution procedures (182).

A variation on this method has also been described. It takes advantage of the fact that an antimicrobial agent can be incorporated into the medium on which the test organism and the gradient diffusion strips are placed, making it possible to test the interaction of three antimicrobial agents at once (Fig. 2.9) (187).

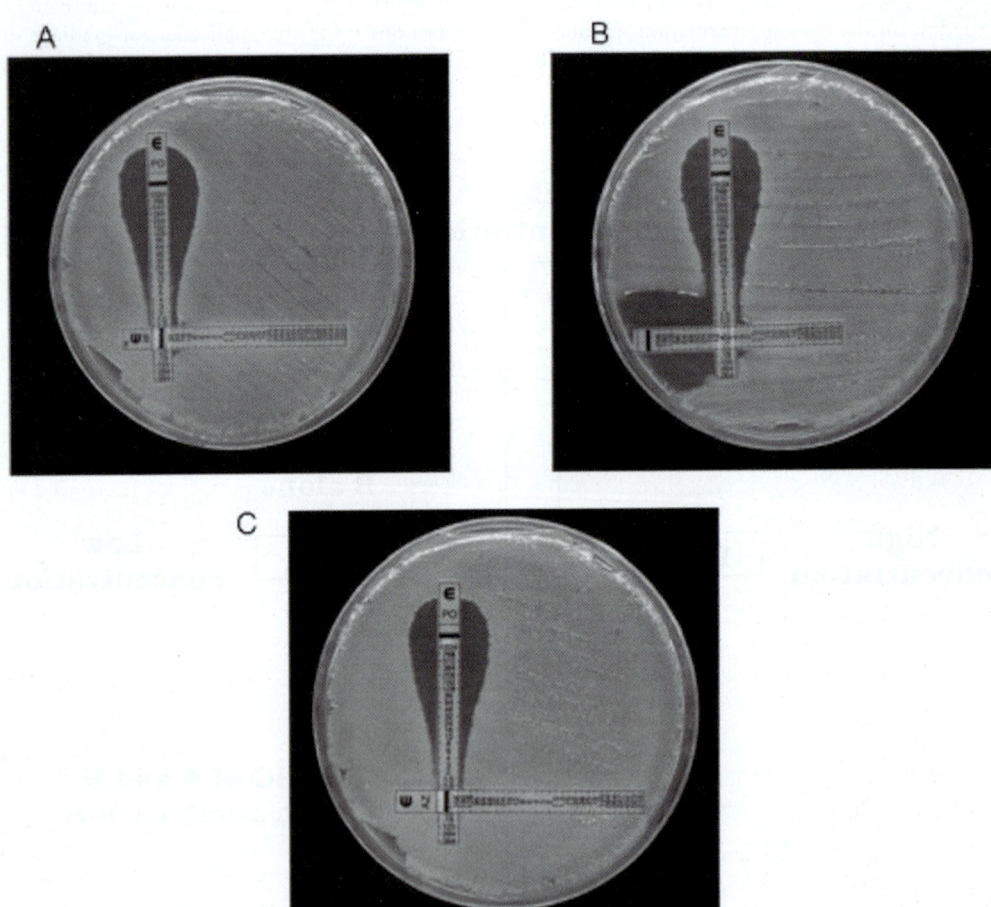

Figure 2.9 ■ Synergy study using three antimicrobial agents, one of which is incorporated into the agar. Activity of polymyxin B in combination with imipenem, rifampicin, and azithromycin versus a multidrug-resistant *A. baumannii* OXA-23 clones using the Etest method. **A:** Polymyxin and imipenem. **B:** Polymyxin and rifampicin. **C:** Polymyxin and azithromycin. (From Wareham DW, Bean DC. In-vitro activity of polymyxin B in combination with imipenem, rifampicin and azithromycin versus multidrug resistant strains of *Acinetobacter baumannii* producing Oxa-23 carbapenemase. *Ann Clin Microbiol Antimicrob* 2006;5:10.) (See Color Plate in the front of the book.)

REFERENCES

1. Acar JF, Goldstein FW. Disk susceptibility testing. In: Lorian V, ed. *Antibiotics in laboratory medicine.* 3rd ed. Baltimore: Lippincott Williams & Wilkins, 1991:17–52.
2. Acar JF, Goldstein FW. Disk susceptibility testing. In: Lorian V, ed. *Antibiotics in laboratory medicine.* 4th ed. Baltimore: Lippincott Williams & Wilkins, 1996:1–51.
3. Barry AL. Procedure for testing antibiotics in agar media: theoretical considerations. In: Lorian V, ed. *Antibiotics in laboratory medicine.* Baltimore: Lippincott Williams & Wilkins, 1980:1–23.
4. Clinical and Laboratory Standards Institute. *Susceptibility testing of mycobacteria, nocardiae and other aerobic actinomycetes—second edition.* Wayne, PA: Clinical and Laboratory Standards Institute, 2011. CLSI document M24-A2.
5. Clinical and Laboratory Standards Institute. *Methods for antimicrobial susceptibility testing for human mycoplasmas.* Wayne, PA: Clinical and Laboratory Standards Institute, 2011. CLSI document M43-A.
6. Clinical and Laboratory Standards Institute. *Method for antifungal disk diffusion susceptibility testing of yeasts—second edition.* Wayne, PA: Clinical and Laboratory Standards Institute, 2009. CLSI document M44-A2.
7. Clinical and Laboratory Standards Institute. *Method for antifungal disk diffusion susceptibility testing of nondermatophyte filamentous fungi.* Wayne, PA: Clinical and Laboratory Standards Institute, 2010. CLSI document M51-A.
8. McHugh DJ. *A guide to the seaweed industry.* In: *FAO Fisheries Technical Paper 441.* Rome, Italy: Food and Agriculture Organization of the United Nations, 2003.
9. Amisen R, Galatas F. Production, properties and uses of agar. In: HcHugh DJ, ed. *Production and utilization of products from commercial seaweeds.* Rome, Italy: Food and Agriculture Organization of the United Nations, 1987. http://www.fao.org/docrep/X5822E/X5822E00.htm. Accessed March 1, 2013.
10. European Committee on Antimicrobial Susceptibility Testing. Antimicrobial susceptibility testing—EUCAST disk diffusion method, version 2.1. http://www.eucast.org/fileadmin/src/media/PDFs/EUCAST_files/Disk_test_documents/Manual_v_2.1_EUCAST_Disk_Test.pdf. Accessed March 1, 2013.
11. Bell SM, Pham JN, Nguyen TT. Antibiotic susceptibility testing by the CDS method. http://web.med.unsw.edu.au/cdstest/GTF_CDS_site/WebPages/HomeLevel/ManualFrames.htm. Accessed March 1, 2013.
12. British Society for Antimicrobial Chemotherapy. BSAC methods for antimicrobial susceptibility testing version 11.1. May 2012. http://bsac.org.uk/wp-content/uploads/2012/02/Version-11.1-2012-Final-.pdf. Accessed March 1, 2013.
13. Bauer AW, Kirby WMM, Sherris JC, et al. Antibiotic sensitivity testing by a standardized single disk method. *Am J Clin Path* 1966;45:493–496.
14. Bridson EY, ed. *The Oxoid manual.* 9th ed. Basingstoke, United Kingdom: Oxoid Limited, 2006.
15. Members of the SFM Antibiogram Committee. Comité de l'Antibiogramme de la Société Française de Microbiologie report 2003. *Int J Antimicrob Agents* 2003;21:364–391.
16. Clinical and Laboratory Standards Institute. *Protocols for evaluating dehydrated Mueller-Hinton agar—second edition.* Wayne, PA: Clinical and Laboratory Standards Institute, 2006. CLSI document M6-A2.
17. International Organization for Standardization. *Criteria for acceptable lots of dehydrated Mueller-Hinton agar and broth for antimicrobial susceptibility testing.* Geneva: International Organization for Standardization. ISO 16782 March 8, 2013 draft.
18. European Committee for Antimicrobial Susceptibility Testing of the European Society for Clinical Microbiology and Infectious Diseases. Determination of minimum inhibitory concentrations (MICs) of antibacterial agents by agar dilution. *Clin Microbiol Infect* 2000;6:509–515.
19. Toohey M, Francis G, Stingemore N. Variation in Iso-Sensitest agar affecting β-lactam testing. *ASIGnation* 1990;1(6):5–8.
20. Swedish Reference Group on Antibiotics. Dilution methods. http://www.srga.org/RAFMETOD/Basmet2.htm. Accessed March 1, 2013.
21. Andrews JM. Determination of minimum inhibitory concentrations. *J Antimicrob Chemother* 2001;48(Suppl 1):5–16.
22. Clinical and Laboratory Standards Institute. *Methods for antimicrobial susceptibility testing of anaerobic bacteria: approved standard—fifth edition.* Wayne, PA: Clinical and Laboratory Standards Institute, 2012. CLSI document M11-A8.
23. Hecht DW, Lederer L. Effect of the choice of medium on the results of in vitro susceptibility testing of eight antimicrobials against the *Bacteroides fragilis* group. *Clin Infect Dis* 1995;20(Suppl 2):S346–S349.
24. Roe DE, Hecht DW, Finegold SM, et al. Multilaboratory comparison of anaerobe susceptibility results using three different agar media. *Clin Infect Dis* 2001;35(Suppl 1):S40–S46.
25. Roe DE, Hecht DW, Finegold SM, et al. Multilaboratory comparison of growth characteristics for anaerobes using five different media. *Clin Infect Dis* 2001;35(Suppl 1):S36–S45.
26. Waterworth PM. Sulphonamides and trimethoprim. In: Reeves DS, Phillips I, Williams JD, et al, eds. *Laboratory methods in antimicrobial chemotherapy.* Edinburgh, United Kingdom: Churchill Livingstone, 1978:82–84.
27. Clinical and Laboratory Standards Institute. *Performance standards for antimicrobial disk susceptibility tests: approved standards—eleventh edition.* Wayne, PA: Clinical and Laboratory Standards Institute, 2012. CLSI document M2-A11.
28. Kenny MA, Pollock HM, Minshew BH, et al. Cation components of Mueller-Hinton agar affecting testing of *Pseudomonas aeruginosa* susceptibility to gentamicin. *Antimicrob Agents Chemother* 1980;17:55–62.
29. Casillas E, Kenny MA, Minshew BH, et al. Effect of ionized calcium and soluble magnesium on the predictability of the performance of Mueller-Hinton agar susceptibility testing of *Pseudomonas aeruginosa* with gentamicin. *Antimicrob Agents Chemother* 1981;19:987–992.
30. Fuchs PC, Barry AL, Brown S. Daptomycin susceptibility tests: interpretive criteria, quality control, and the effect of calcium on in vitro tests. *Diagn Microbiol Infect Dis* 2000;38:51–58.
31. Fernández-Mazarrasa C, Mazarrasa O, Calvo J, et al. High concentrations of manganese in Mueller-Hinton agar increase MICs of tigecycline determined by Etest. *J Clin Microbiol* 2009;47:827–829.

32. Veenemans J, Mouton JW, Kluytmans JA, et al. Effect of manganese in test media on in vitro susceptibility of Enterobacteriaceae and *Acinetobacter baumannii* to tigecycline. *J Clin Microbiol* 2012;50:3077–3079.

33. Girardello R, Bispo PJM, Yamanaka TM, et al. Cation concentration variability of four distinct Mueller-Hinton agar brands influences polymyxin B susceptibility results. *J Clin Microbiol* 2012;50:2414–2418.

34. Waterworth PM. The aminoglycosides. In: Reeves DS, Phillips I, Williams JD, et al, eds. *Laboratory methods in antimicrobial chemotherapy*. Edinburgh: Churchill Livingstone, 1978:85–87.

35. D'Amato RF, Thornsberry C, Baker CN, et al. Effect of calcium and magnesium on the susceptibility of *Pseudomonas* species to tetracycline, gentamicin, polymyxin B, and carbenicillin. *Antimicrob Agents Chemother* 1975;7:596–600.

36. Reller LB, Schoenknecht FD, Kenny MA, et al. Antibiotic susceptibility testing of *Pseudomonas aeruginosa*: selection of a control strain and criteria for magnesium and calcium content of media. *J Infect Dis* 1974;130:454–463.

37. Washington JA, Snyder RJ, Kohner PC, et al. Effect of cation content of agar on the activity of gentamicin, tobramycin and amikacin against *Pseudomonas aeruginosa*. *J Infect Dis* 1978;137:103–111.

38. Cooper GL, Louie A, Baltch AL, et al. Influence of zinc on *Pseudomonas aeruginosa* susceptibilities to imipenem. *J Clin Microbiol* 1993;31:2366–2370.

39. Daly JS, Dodge RA, Glew RH, et al. Effect of zinc concentration in Mueller-Hinton agar on susceptibility of *Pseudomonas aeruginosa* to imipenem. *J Clin Microbiol* 1997;35:1027–1029.

40. Atmaca S. Effect of zinc concentration in Mueller-Hinton agar on susceptibility of *Pseudomonas aeruginosa* to meropenem. *J Med Microbiol* 1998;47:653.

41. Cooke P, Heritage J, Kerr K, et al. Different effects of zinc ions on the in vitro susceptibilities of *Stenotrophomonas maltophilia* to imipenem and meropenem. *Antimicrob Agents Chemother* 1996;40:2909–2910.

42. Berkman S, Henry RJ, Housewright RD. Studies on streptomycin, I: factors influencing the activity of streptomycin. *J Bacteriol* 1947;53:567.

43. Medeiros AA, O'Brien TF, Wacker WEC, et al. Effect of salt concentration on the apparent in vitro susceptibility of *Pseudomonas* and other Gram-negative bacilli to gentamicin. *J Infect Dis* 1971;124(Suppl):S59–S66.

44. Rosenblatt JE, Schoenknecht F. Effect of several components of anaerobic incubation on antibiotic susceptibility results. *Antimicrob Agents Chemother* 1972;1:433–440.

45. Bemer-Melchior P, Juvin M-E, Tassin S, et al. In vitro activity of the new ketolide telithromycin compared to those of the macrolides against *Streptococcus pyogenes*: influences of resistance mechanisms and methodological factors. *Antimicrob Agents Chemother* 2000;44:2999–3002.

46. Dibb WL, Digranes A, Bottolfson KL. Effects of carbon dioxide upon the in vitro activity of erythromycin. *Acta Pathol Microbiol Immunol Scand* 1986;94:173–176.

47. Goldstein EJC, Sutter VL, Kwok Y-Y, et al. Effect of carbon dioxide on in vitro susceptibility of anaerobic bacteria to erythromycin. *Antimicrob Agents Chemother* 1981;20:705–708.

48. Johnson MM, Hill SL, Piddock LJV. Effect of carbon dioxide on testing of susceptibilities of respiratory tract pathogens to macrolides and azalide antimicrobial agents. *Antimicrob Agents Chemother* 1999;43:1862–1865.

49. Retsema JA, Brennan LA, Girard AE. Effects of environmental factors on the in vitro potency of azithromycin. *Eur J Clin Microbiol Infect Dis* 1991;10:834–842.

50. Spangler SK, Jacobs MR, Appelbaum PC. Effect of CO_2 on susceptibilities of anaerobes to erythromycin, azithromycin, clarithromycin, and roxithromycin. *Antimicrob Agents Chemother* 1994;38:211–216.

51. Bouchillon SK, Johnson JL, Hoban DJ, et al. Impact of carbon dioxide on the susceptibility of key respiratory tract pathogens to telithromycin and azithromycin. *J Antimicrob Chemother* 2005;56:224–227.

52. Johnson J, Bourchillon S, Pontani D. The effect of carbon dioxide on susceptibility testing of azithromycin, clarithromycin and roxithromycin against isolates of *Streptococcus pneumoniae* and *Streptococcus pyogenes* by broth microdilution and Etest: Artemis Project–first-phase study. *Clin Microbiol Infect* 1999;5:327–330.

53. Spangler SK, Appelbaum PC. Oxyrase, a method which avoids CO_2 in the incubation atmosphere for anaerobic susceptibility testing of antibiotics affected by CO_2. *J Clin Microbiol* 1993;31:460–462.

54. Jansen JE, Bremmelgarrd A. Susceptibility testing of 7 antibiotics against anaerobic bacteria: comparison of 2 different media and carbon dioxide concentrations. *Acta Pathol Microbiol Scand B* 1987;95:65–73.

55. Hansen SL, Swomley P, Drusano G. Effect of carbon dioxide and pH on the susceptibility of *Bacteroides fragilis* group to erythromycin. *Antimicrob Agents Chemother* 1991;19:335–336.

56. Reynolds AV, Hamilton-Miller JM, Brumfitt W. Diminished activity of gentamicin under anaerobic or hypercapnic conditions. *Lancet* 1976;1(7957):447–449.

57. Traub WH, Leonhard B. Antibiotic susceptibility tests with fastidious and nonfastidious bacteria reference strains: effects of aerobic versus hypercapnic incubation. *Chemotherapy* 1995;41:18–33.

58. Ward PB, Palladino S, Looker JC, et al. P-nitro-phenylglycerol in susceptibility testing media alters the MICs of antimicrobials for *Pseudomonas aeruginosa*. *J Antimicrob Chemother* 1993;31:489–496.

59. Ward PB, Palladino S, Looker JC. P-nitrophenylglycerol in susceptibility testing media alters the MICs of antimicrobials for aerobic Gram-negative bacilli. *J Antimicrob Chemother* 1993;31:803–805.

60. Winstanley T, Edwards C, Limb D, et al. Evaluation of a surfactant, Dispersol LN, as an anti-swarming agent in agar dilution susceptibility testing. *J Antimicrob Chemother* 1994;33:353–356.

61. Liu M-C, Lin S-B, Chien H-F, et al. 10'(Z),13'(E)-heptadecadienylhydroquinone inhibits swarming and virulence factors and increases polymyxin B susceptibility in *Proteus mirabilis*. *PLoS One* 2012;7:e45563.

62. Clinical and Laboratory Standards Institute. *Methods for dilution antimicrobial susceptibility tests for bacteria that grow aerobically; approved standard—ninth edition*. Wayne, PA: Clinical and Laboratory Standards Institute, 2012. CLSI document M7-A9.

63. Murray CK, Walter EA, Crawford S, et al. *Abiotrophia* bacteremia in a patient with neutropenic fever and antimicrobial susceptibility testing of *Abiotrophia* isolates. *Clin Infect Dis* 2001;32:e140–e142.

64. Touhy MJ, Procop GW, Washington JA. Antimicrobial susceptibility of *Abiotrophia adiacens* and *Abiotrophia defectiva*. *Diagn Microbiol Infect Dis* 2000;38:189–191.

65. Clinical and Laboratory Standards Institute. *Methods for antimicrobial dilution and disk diffusion susceptibility tests*

for testing of infrequently isolated or fastidious bacteria—second edition. Wayne, PA: Clinical and Laboratory Standards Institute, 2010. CLSI document M45-A2.

66. Acar JF, Goldstein FW, Lagrange P. Human infections caused by thiamine- or menadione-requiring *Staphylococcus aureus. J Clin Microbiol* 1978;8:142–147.

67. Tapsall JW, Wilson E, Harper J. Thymine dependent strains of *Escherichia coli* selected by trimethoprim-suphamethoxazole during therapy. *Pathology* 1974;6:161–167.

68. Clark RB, Lewinski MA, Loeffelholz MJ, et al. Cumitech 31A, verification and validation of procedures. In: Sharp SE, ed. *Clinical microbiology laboratory.* Washington, DC: ASM Press, 2009.

69. Clinical and Laboratory Standards Institute. *Performance standards for antimicrobial susceptibility testing: fourteenth informational supplement.* Wayne, PA: Clinical and Laboratory Standards Institute, 2013. CLSI document M100-S23.

71. Ericsson HM, Sherris JC. Antibiotic sensitivity testing: report of an international collaborative study. *Acta Pathol Microbiol Scand* 1971;217(Suppl B):1–90.

72. Courvalin P, Soussy J-C, eds. Technical recommendations for in vitro susceptibility testing. 1996 Report of the Comité de l'Antibiogramme de la Société Française de Microbiologie. *Clin Microbiol Infect* 1996;2(Suppl 1):S11–S34.

73. Rousseau D, Harbec PS. Delivery volumes of the 1- and 3-mm pins of a Cathra replicator. *J Clin Microbiol* 1987;25:1311.

74. Moosdeen F, Williams JD, Secker A. Standardization of inoculum size for disc susceptibility testing: a preliminary report of a spectrophotometric method. *J Antimicrob Chemother* 1988;21:439–443.

75. Cooper KE, Gillespie WA. The influence of temperature on streptomycin inhibition zones in agar cultures. *J Gen Microbiol* 1952;7:1–7.

76. Cooper KE, Linton AH. The importance of the temperature during the early hours of incubation of agar plates in assays. *J Gen Microbiol* 1952;7:8–17.

77. Working Party on Antibiotic Sensitivity Testing of the British Society for Antimicrobial Chemotherapy. A guide to sensitivity testing. *J Antimicrob Chemother* 1991;27(Suppl D):1–50.

78. Franklin JC. Quality control in agar dilution sensitivity testing by direct assay of the antibiotic in solid medium. *J Clin Path* 1980;33:93–95.

79. McDermott SN, Hartley TF. New datum handling methods for the quality control of antibiotic solutions and plates used in the antimicrobial susceptibility test. *J Clin Microbiol* 1989;27:1814–1825.

80. Cooper KE. Theory of antibiotic inhibition zones in agar media. *Nature* 1955;176:510–511.

81. Cooper KE, Linton AH, Sehgal SN. The effect of inoculum size on inhibition zones in agar media using staphylococci and streptomycin. *J Gen Microbiol* 1958;18:670–687.

82. Cooper KE. The theory of antibiotic inhibition zones. In: Kavanaugh F, ed. *Analytical microbiology.* New York: Academic Press, 1964:1–86.

83. Humphrey JH, Lightbown J. A general theory for plate assay of antibiotics with some practical applications. *J Gen Microbiol* 1952;7:129–143.

84. Barry AL. *The antimicrobic susceptibility test: principles and practices.* Philadelphia: Lea and Febiger, 1976.

85. Lorian V. A five hour disc antibiotic susceptibility test. In: Lorian V, ed. *Significance of medical microbiology in the care of patients.* Baltimore: Lippincott Williams & Wilkins, 1977:203–212.

86. Shungu D. Chemical and physical properties of antibiotics: preparation and control of antibiotic susceptibility disks and other devices containing antibiotics. In: Lorian V, ed. *Antibiotics in laboratory medicine.* 4th ed. Baltimore: Lippincott Williams & Wilkins, 1995:766–792.

87. Casals JB, Gylling Pedersen O. Tablet sensitivity testing: a comparison of methods. *Acta Pathol Microbiol Scand* 1972;80:806–816.

88. Rosco Diagnostica A/S. Users guide: Neo-Sensitabs™ susceptibility testing, 2011. https://rosco.docontrol.com. Accessed March 1, 2013.

89. Cavenaghi LA, Biganzoli E, Danese A, et al. Diffusion of teicoplanin and vancomycin in agar. *Diag Microbiol Infect Dis* 1992;15:253–258.

89a. Barry AL, Fay GD. The amount of agar in antimicrobic disk susceptibility test plates. *J Clin Pathol* 1973;59:196–198.

89b. Davis WW, Stout TR. Disc plate method of microbiological antibiotic assay, I: Factors influencing variability and error. *Appl Microbiol* 1971;22:659–665.

90. Annear D. Full expression of methicillin resistance in *Staphylococcus aureus. J Antimicrob Chemother* 1985;15:253–254.

91. Baker CN, Huang MB, Tenover FC. Optimizing testing of methicillin-resistant Staphylococcus species. *Diagn Microbiol Infect Dis* 1994;19:167–170.

92. Comité de l'Antibiogramme de la Société Française de Microbiologie. Recommandations 2011. http://www.sfm-microbiologie.org/UserFiles/file/CASFM/casfm_2011.pdf. Accessed March 1, 2013.

93. Barry AL, Fuchs PC, Gerlach EH, et al. Multilaboratory evaluation of an agar diffusion disk susceptibility test for rapidly growing anaerobic bacteria. *Rev Infect Dis* 1990;12(Suppl 2):S210–S217.

94. Horn R, Bourgault A-M, Lamothe F. Disk diffusion susceptibility testing of the *Bacteroides fragilis* group. *Antimicrob Agents Chemother* 1987;31:1596–1599.

95. Sutter VL, Kwok YY, Finegold SM. Standardized antimicrobial disc testing of anaerobic bacteria, I: susceptibility of *Bacteroides fragilis* to tetracycline. *Appl Microbiol* 1973;3:188–193.

96. King A. Recommendations for susceptibility tests on fastidious organisms and those requiring special handling. *J Antimicrob Chemother* 2001;48(Suppl 1):77–80.

97. Hachem CY, Clarridge JE, Reddy R, et al. Antimicrobial susceptibility testing of *Helicobacter pylori. Diagn Microbiol Infect Dis* 1996;24:37–41.

98. Iovene MR, Romano M, Pilloni AP, et al. Prevalence of antimicrobial resistance in eighty clinical isolates of *Helicobacter pylori. Chemotherapy* 1999;45:8–14.

99. Midolo PD, Bell JM, Lambert JR, et al. Antimicrobial resistance testing of *Helicobacter pylori*: a comparison of Etest and disk diffusion methods. *Pathology* 1997;29:411–414.

100. McNulty C, Owen R, Tompkins D, et al. *Helicobacter pylori* susceptibility testing by disc diffusion. *J Antimicrob Chemother* 2002;49:601–609.

101. Smith C, Perkins J, Tompkins D. Conparison of Etest and disc diffusion for detection of antibiotic resistance in *Helicobacter pylori. Microbiol Digest* 1997;14:21–23.

102. Weiss K, Laverdiere M, Restieri C. Comparison of 10 antibiotics against clinical strains of *Helicobacter pylori* by three different techniques. *Can J Gastroenterol* 1998;12:181–185.

103. Shah PM. Recording zone diameters—a rare phenomenon in microbiology laboratories? [letter]. *Int J Antimicrob Agents* 2004;23:208.

104. Metzler CM, DeHaan RM. Susceptibility tests of an-aerobic bacteria: statistical and clinical considerations. *J Infect Dis* 1974;130:588–594.

105. Brunden MN, Zurenko GE, Kapik B. Modification of the error-rate bounded classification scheme for use with two MIC break points. *Diagn Microbiol Infect Dis* 1992;15:135–140.

106. Clinical and Laboratory Standards Institute. *Development of in vitro susceptibility testing criteria and quality control parameters—third edition*. Wayne, PA: Clinical and Laboratory Standards Institute, 2008. CLSI document M23-A3.

107. Craig BA. Modeling approach to diameter breakpoint determinations. *Diagn Microbiol Infect Dis* 2000;36: 193–202.

108. DePalma G, Craig BA. dBETS—diffusion Breakpoint Estimation Testing Software. http://glimmer.rstudio. com/dbets/dBETS/. Accessed March 1, 2013.

109. Barry AL, Joyce LJ, Adams AP, et al. Rapid determi-nation of antimicrobial susceptibility for urgent clinical situations. *Am J Clin Path* 1973;59:693–699.

110. Boyle VJ, Faucher ME, Ross RW. Rapid modified Kirby Bauer susceptibility test with single high concen-tration antimicrobial discs. *Antimicrob Agents Chemother* 1973;3:418–424.

111. Kluge RM. Accuracy of Kirby-Bauer susceptibility tests read at 4, 8 and 12 hours of incubation: comparison with reading at 18 to 20 hours. *Antimicrob Agents Chem-other* 1975;8:139–145.

112. Saha SK, Darmstadt GL, Baqui AH, et al. Rapid identifi-cation and antibiotic susceptibility testing of *Salmonella enterica* serovar *typhi* isolated from blood: implications for therapy. *J Clin Microbiol* 2001;39:3583–3585.

113. Shahidi M, Ellner PD. Effect of mixed cultures on antibiotic susceptibility testing. *Appl Microbiol* 1969;18:766–770.

114. Ellner PD, Johnson E. Unreliability of direct suscep-tibility testing on wound exudates. *Antimicrob Agents Chemother* 1976;9:355–356.

115. Doern GV, Vautour R, Gaudet M, et al. Clinical impact of rapid in vitro susceptibility testing and bacterial iden-tification. *J Clin Microbiol* 1994;32:1757–1762.

116. Bacteriology Committee of the Association of Clinical Pathologists. Report on antibiotic sensitivity test trial organized by the Bacteriology Committee of the Associa-tion of Clinical Pathologists. *J Clin Pathol* 1965;18:1–5.

117. Perez JR, Gillenwater JY. Clinical evaluation of testing immediate antibiotic disk sensitivities in bacteriuria. *J Urol* 1973;110:452–456.

118. Dornbusch K, Nord C-E, Olsson B, et al. Antibacte-rial susceptibility testing by the dip-slide technique: a methodological evaluation. *Chemotherapy (Basel)* 1976;22:190–202.

119. Hollick GE, Washington JA. Comparison of direct and standardized disk diffusion susceptibility testing of urine cultures. *Antimicrob Agents Chemother* 1976;9:804–809.

120. Waterworth PM, Del Piano MD. Dependability of sensitivity tests in primary culture. *J Clin Pathol* 1976;29:179–184.

121. Dornbusch K, Lindeberg B, Nord C-E, et al. Bacteriuria diagnosis and antibiotic susceptibility testing in a group practice by dip-slide techniques. *Chemotherapy (Basel)* 1979;25:227–232.

122. Källenius G, Dornbusch K, Hallander HO, et al. Comparison of direct and standardized antibiotic sus-ceptibility testing in bacteriuria. *Chemotherapy (Basel)* 1981;27:99–105.

123. Scully PG, O'Shea B, Flanagan KP, et al. Urinary tract infection in general practice: direct antibiotic sensitivity testing as a potential diagnostic method. *Irish J Med Sci* 1990;159:98–100.

124. Blue AP, Gordon DL. Is primary sensitivity testing on urine samples valid? *Pathology* 1991;23:149–152.

125. Jenschke WJ, Trevino E, Vaqnce PH, et al. Comparison of direct urine and standard Kirby-Bauer sensitivities. In: *Abstracts of the 93rd general meeting of the American Society for Microbiology*. Washington, DC: American So-ciety for Microbiology; 1993. Abstract C-190.

126. Mukerjee C, Reiss-Levy E. Evaluation of direct disc diffusion susceptibility testing for bacteriuria using di-luted urine against the standard CDS method. *Pathology* 1994;26:201–207.

127. Oakes AR, Badger R, Grove DI. Comparison of direct and standardized testing of infected urine for antimicro-bial susceptibilities by disk diffusion. *J Clin Microbiol* 1994;32:40–45.

128. Johnson JR, Tiu FS, Stamm WE. Direct antimicrobial susceptibility testing for acute urinary tract infection in women. *J Clin Microbiol* 1995;33:2316–2323.

129. Gillenwater JY, Clark MM. Tentative direct antimicrobial susceptibility testing in urine. *J Urol* 1996;156:149–153.

130. Bronnestam R. Direct antimicrobial susceptibility test-ing in bacteriuria. *APMIS* 1999;107:437–444.

131. Breteler KB, Rentenaar RJ, Verkaart G, et al. Perfor-mance and clinical significance of direct antimicrobial susceptibility testing of urine from hospitalized patients. *Scand J Infec Dis* 2011;43:771–776.

132. Heinze PA, Thrupp LD, Anselmo CR. A rapid (4–6 hour) urine-culture system for direct identification and direct antimicrobial susceptibility testing. *Am J Clin Pathol* 1979;71:177–183.

133. Johnson JE, Washington JA. Comparison of direct and standardized antimicrobial susceptibility testing of positive blood cultures. *Antimicrob Agents Chemother* 1976;10:211–214.

134. Wegner DL, Mathis CR, Neblett TR. Direct method to determine the antibiotic susceptibility of rapidly growing blood pathogens. *Antimicrob Agents Chemother* 1976;9:861–862.

135. Fay D, Oldfather JE. Standardization of direct suscep-tibility test for blood cultures. *J Clin Microbiol* 1979;9: 347–350.

136. Mirrett S, Reller LB. Comparison of direct and standard antimicrobial disk susceptibility testing for bacteria iso-lated from blood. *J Clin Microbiol* 1979;10:482–487.

137. Coyle MB, McGonagle LA, Plorde JJ, et al. Rapid an-timicrobial susceptibility testing of isolates from blood cultures by direct inoculation and early reading of disk diffusion tests. *J Clin Microbiol* 1984;20:473–477.

138. Edelmann A, Pietzcker T, Wellinghausen N. Com-parison of direct disk diffusion and standard microtitre broth dilution susceptibility testing of blood culture isolates. *J Med Microbiol* 2007;56(Pt 2):202–207.

139. Tan TY, Ng LS, Kwang LL. Evaluation of disc sus-ceptibility tests performed directly from positive blood cultures. *J Clin Pathol* 2008;61:343–346.

140. Bennett K, Sharp SE. Rapid differentiation of methi-cillin-resistant *Staphylococcus aureus* and methicillin-sus-ceptible *Staphylococcus aureus* from blood cultures by use of a direct cefoxitin disk diffusion test. *J Clin Microbiol* 2008;46:3836–3838.

141. Cuellar-Rodriguez JM, Ponce-de-León A, Quiroz-Mejia R, et al. Rapid detection of ESBL-producing

gram-negative bacteria isolated from blood: a reasonable and reliable tool for middle and low resource countries. *Rev Invest Clin* 2009;61:306–312.

142. Miño de Kaspar H, Neubauer AS, Molnar A, et al. Rapid direct antibiotic susceptibility testing in endophthalmitis. *Ophthalmology* 2002;109:687–693.

143. Kontopidou F, Galani I, Panagea T, et al. Comparison of direct antimicrobial susceptibility testing methods for rapid analysis of bronchial secretion samples in ventilator-associated pneumonia. *Int J Antimicrob Agents* 2011;38:130–134.

144. Brown DF, Brown L. Evaluation of the Etest, a novel method of quantifying antimicrobial activity. *J Antimicrob Chemother* 1991;27:185–190.

145. Jorgensen JH, Howell AW, Maher LA. Quantitative antimicrobial susceptibility testing of *Haemophilus influenzae* and *Streptococcus pneumoniae* by using the E-test. *J Clin Microbiol* 1991;29:109–114.

146. Hunt GS, Citron DM, Claros MC, et al. Comparison of Etest to broth microdilution method for testing *Streptococcus pneumoniae* susceptibility to levofloxacin and three macrolides. *Antimicrob Agents Chemother* 1996;40: 2413–2415.

147. Hunt DE, Sandham HJ. Improved agar gradient-plate technique. *Appl Microbiol* 1969;17:329–330.

148. Szybalski W. Microbial selection, I: gradient plate technique for study of bacterial resistance. *Science* 1952;116: 46–48.

149. Carsenti-Etesse H, Roger PM, Dunais B, et al. Gradient plate method to induce *Streptococcus pyogenes* resistance. *J Antimicrob Chemother* 1999;44:439–443.

150. Wootton M, Howe RA, Hillman R, et al. A modified population analysis profile (PAP) method to detect hetero-resistance to vancomycin in *Staphylococcus aureus* in a UK hospital. *J Antimicrob Chemother* 2001;47: 399–403.

151. Liu Y, Li J, Du J, et al. Accurate assessment of antibiotic susceptibility and screening resistant strains of a bacterial population by linear gradient plate. *Sci China Life Sci* 2011;54:953–960.

152. Gerber AU, Vastola AP, Brandel J, et al. Selection of aminoglycoside-resistant variants of *Pseudomonas aeruginosa* in an in vivo model. *J Infect Dis* 1982;146: 691–697.

153. Berge-Bachi B, Strassle A, Kayser FH. Characterization of an isogenic set of methicillin-resistant and susceptible mutants of *Staphylococcus aureus. Eur J Clin Microbiol* 1986;5:697–701.

154. Hiramatsu K, Arikata N, Hanaki H, et al. Dissemination in Japanese hospitals of strains of *Staphylococcus aureus* heterogeneously resistant to vancomycin. *Lancet* 1997;350:1670–1673.

155. Walsh TR, Bolmström A, Qwärnström A, et al. Evaluation of current methods for detection of staphylococci with reduced susceptibility to glycopeptides. *J Clin Microbiol* 2001;39:2439–2444.

156. Howden BP, Davies JK, Johnson PD, et al. Reduced vancomycin susceptibility in *Staphylococcus aureus*, including vancomycin-intermediate and heterogeneous vancomycin-intermediate strains: resistance mechanisms, laboratory detection, and clinical implications. *Clin Microbiol Rev* 2010;23:99–139.

157. Lorian V. Low concentrations of antibiotics. *J Antimicrob Chemother* 1985;15(Suppl A):15–26.

158. Lorian V. Differences between in vitro and in vivo studies. *Antimicrob Agents Chemother* 1988;32:1600–1601.

159. Odenholt I. Pharmacodynamic effects of subinhibitory antibiotic concentrations. *Int J Antimicrob Agents* 2001;17:1–8.

160. Craig WA. Post-antibiotic effects in experimental animal models: relationship to in-vitro phenomena and the treatment of infections in man. *J Antimicrob Chemother* 1993;31(Suppl D):149–158.

161. MacKenzie FM, Gould IM. The post-antibiotic effect. *J Antimicrob Chemother* 1993;31(Suppl D):519–537.

162. Cars O, Odenholt-Tornqvist I. The post-antibiotic sub-MIC effect in vitro and in vivo. *J Antimicrob Chemother* 1993;31(Suppl D):159–166.

163. Pruul H, McDonald PJ. Damage to bacteria by antibiotics in vitro and its relevance to antimicrobial chemotherapy. *J Antimicrob Chemother* 1988;21:695–698.

164. Lorian V, Burns L. Predictive value of susceptibility tests for the outcome of antibacterial therapy. *J Antimicrob Chemother* 1990;25:175–181.

166. Craig WA. Basic pharmacodynamics of antibacterials with clinical applications to the use of β-lactams, glycopeptides and linezolid. *Infect Dis Clin North Am* 2003;17:479–501.

167. Drusano GL. Antimicrobial pharmacodynamics: critical interactions of "bug and drug." *Nat Rev Microbiol* 2004;2: 289–300.

168. Drusano GL. Pharmacokinetics and pharmacodynamics of antimicrobials. *Clin Infect Dis* 2007;45(Suppl 1):S89–S95.

169. Ambrose PG, Bhavnani SM, Rubino CM, et al. Pharmacokinetics-pharmacodynamics of antimicrobial therapy: it's not just for mice anymore. *Clin Infect Dis* 2007; 44:79–86.

170. McNabb JJ, Bui KQ. β-lactam pharmacodynamics. In: Nightingale CH, Murakawa T, Ambrose PG, eds. *Antimicrobial pharmacodynamics in theory and clinical practice.* New York: Marcel Dekker, 2002:99–123.

171. Turnidge JD. Pharmacodynamics and dosing of aminoglycosides. *Infect Dis Clin North Am* 2003;17:503–528.

172. Nightingale CH, Mattoes HM. Macrolide, azalide and ketolide pharmacodynamics. In: Nightingale CH, Murakawa T, Ambrose PG, eds. *Antimicrobial pharmacodynamics in theory and clinical practice.* New York: Marcel Dekker, 2002:205–220.

173. Maglio D, Nicolau DP, Nightingale CH. Impact of pharmacodynamics on dosing of macrolides, azalides and ketolides. *Infect Dis Clin North Am* 2003;17:563–577.

174. Owens RC Jr, Ambrose PG. Pharmacodynamics of quinolones. In: Nightingale CH, Murakawa T, Ambrose PG, eds. *Antimicrobial pharmacodynamics in theory and clinical practice.* New York: Marcel Dekker, 2002: 155–178.

175. Ambrose PG, Bhavnani SM, Owens RC. Clinical pharmacodynamics of quinolones. *Infect Dis Clin North Am* 2003;17:529–543.

176. Ross GH, Wright DH, Rotschafer JC, et al. Glycopeptide pharmacodynamics. In: Nightingale CH, Murakawa T, Ambrose PG, eds. *Antimicrobial pharmacodynamics in theory and clinical practice.* New York: Marcel Dekker, 2002:177–204.

177. Hermsen ED, Sullivan CJ, Rotschafer JC. Polymyxins: pharmacology, pharmacokinetics, pharmacodynamics and clinical applications. *Infect Dis Clin North Am* 2003;17:545–562.

178. Lamp K, Lacy MK, Freeman C. Metronidazole, clindamycin, and streptogramin pharmacodynamics. In: Nightingale CH, Murakawa T, Ambrose PG, eds. *Antimicrobial pharmacodynamics in theory and clinical practice.* New York: Marcel Dekker, 2002:221–246.

179. Cunha BA, Mattoes HM. Tetracycline pharmacodynamics. In: Nightingale CH, Murakawa T, Ambrose PG, eds. *Antimicrobial pharmacodynamics in theory and clinical practice*. New York: Marcel Dekker, 2002:247–257.

180. Harding I, MacGowan AP, White LO, et al. Teicoplanin therapy for *Staphylococcus aureus* septicaemia: relationship between pre-dose serum concentrations and outcome. *J Antimicrob Chemother* 2000;45:835–841.

181. Snydman DR, Cucheral GJ Jr, McDermott L, et al. Correlation of various in vitro testing methods with clinical outcomes in patients with *Bacteroides fragilis* group infections treated with cefoxitin: a retrospective analysis. *Antimicrob Agents Chemother* 1992;36:540–544.

182. Pillai SK, Moellering RC Jr, Eliopoulos GM. Antimicrobial combinations. In: Lorian V, ed. *Antibiotics in laboratory medicine*. Philadelphia: Lippincott Williams & Wilkins, 2005:365–424.

183. Turnidge J. Drug-drug combinations. In: Vinks A, Derendorf H, Mouton J, eds. *Fundamentals of antimicrobial pharmacokinetics and pharmacodynamics*. New York: Springer, 2013:153–198.

184. European Committee on Antimicrobial Susceptibility Testing. Breakpoint tables for interpretation of MICs and zone diameters, version 3.1. http://www.eucast.org/fileadmin/src/media/PDFs/EUCAST_files/Disk_test_documents/Manual_v_2.1_EUCAST_Disk_Test.pdf. Accessed March 1, 2013.

185. White RL, Burgess DS, Manduru M, et al. Comparison of three different in vitro methods of detecting synergy: time-kill, checkerboard, and E test. *Antimicrob Agents Chemother* 1996;40(8):1914–1918.

186. Bonapace C, White R, Friedrich L, et al. Evaluation of antibiotic synergy against *Acinetobacter baumannii*: comparison with Etest, time kill and checkerboard methods. *Diagn Microbiol Infect Dis* 2000;38:43–50.

187. Wareham DW, Bean DC. In-vitro activity of polymyxin B in combination with imipenem, rifampicin and azithromycin versus multidrug resistant strains of *Acinetobacter baumannii* producing Oxa-23 carbapenemase. *Ann Clin Microbiol Antimicrob* 2006;5:10.

188. Tan TY, Ng LS, Tan E, et al. In vitro effect of minocycline and colistin combinations on imipenem-resistant *Acinetobacter baumannii* clinical isolates. *J Antimicrob Chemother* 2007;60:421–423.

189. Pankey GA, Ashcraft DS. The detection of synergy between meropenem and polymyxin B against meropenem-resistant *Acinetobacter baumannii* using Etest and time-kill assay. *Diagn Microbiol Infect Dis* 2009;63:228–232.

190. Gordon NC, Png K, Wareham DW. Potent synergy and sustained bactericidal activity of a vancomycin-colistin combination versus multidrug-resistant strains of *Acinetobacter baumannii*. *Antimicrob Agents Chemother* 2010;54:5613–5622.

191. Sopirala M, Mangino JE, Gebreyes WA, et al. Synergy testing by Etest, microdilution checkerboard, and time-till methods for pan-drug-resistant *Acinetobacter baumannii*. *Antimicrob Agents Chemother* 2010;54:4678–4683.

192. Tan TY, Lim TP, Lee WH, et al. In vitro synergy in extensively drug-resistant *Acinetobacter baumannii*: the effect of testing by time-kill, checkerboard, and Etest methods. *Antimicrob Agents Chemother* 2011;55:436–438.

193. Wareham DW, Gordon NC, Hornsey M. In vitro activity of teicoplanin combined with colistion versus multidrug-resistant strains of *Acinetobacter baumannii*. *J Antimicrob Chemother* 2011;66:1047–1051.

194. Miyasaki Y, Morgan MA, Chan RC, et al. In vitro activity of antibiotic combinations against multidrug-resistant strains of *Acinetobacter baumannii* and the effects of their antibiotic resistance determinants. *FEMS Microbiol Lett* 2012;328:26–31.

195. Hornsey M, Longshaw C, Phee L, et al. In vitro activity of televancin in combination with colistin versus Gram-negative bacterial pathogens, *Antimicrob Agents Chemother* 2012;56:3080–3085.

196. Pankey G, Ashcraft D, Patel N. In vitro synergy of daptomycin plus rifampicin against *Enterococcus faecium* resistant to both linezolid and vancomycin. *Antimicrob Agents Chemother* 2005;49:5166–5168.

197. Pankey GA, Ashcraft DS. In vitro synergy of telavancin and rifampin against *Enterococcus faecium* resistant to both linezolid and vancomycin. *Ochsner J* 2013;13:61–65.

198. Tsuji BT, Rybak MJ. Etest synergy testing of clinical isolates of Staphylococcus aureus demonstrating heterogeneous resistance to vancomycin. *Diagn Microbiol Infect Dis* 2006;54:73–77.

199. Hellmark B, Unemo M, Nilsdottir-Augustinsson A, et al. In vitro antimicrobial synergy testing of coagulase-negative staphylococci isolated from prosthetic joint infections using Etest and with a focus on rifampicin and linezolid. *Eur J Clin Microbiol Infect Dis* 2010;29:591–595.

200. Chachanidze V, Curbelo-Irizarry A, Ashcraft D, et al. In vitro synergy of levofloxacin plus piperacillin/tazobactam against *Pseudomonas aeruginosa*. *Interdiscip Perspect Infect Dis* 2009;2009:948934.

201. Samonis G, Maraki S, Karageogopoulos DE, et al. Synergy of fosfomycin with carbapenems, colistin, netilmicin, and tigecycline against multidrug-resistant *Klebsiella pneumoniae*, *Escherichia coli*, and *Pseudomonas aeruginosa*. *Eur J Clin Microbiol Infect Dis* 2012;31:695–701.

202. He W, Kaniga K, Lynch AS, et al. In vitro Etest synergy of doripenem with amikacin, colistin, and levofloxacin against *Pseudomonas aeruginosa* with defined carbapenem resistance mechanisms as determined by the Etest method. *Diagn Microbiol Infect Dis* 2012;74:417–419.

203. Pankey GA, Ashcraft DS. Detection of synergy using the combination of polymyxin B with either meropenem or rifampin against carbapenemase-producing *Klebsiella pneumoniae*. *Diagn Microbiol Infect Dis* 2011;70:561–564.

204. Church D, LLloyd T, Peirano G, et al. Antimicrobial susceptibility and combination testing of invasive *Stenotrophomonas maltophilia* isolates. *Scand J Infect Dis* 2013;45:265–270.

Susceptibility Testing of Antimicrobials in Liquid Media

Daniel Amsterdam

Fleming's serendipitous observation that the action of *Penicillium notatum* could repel several species of bacteria became what was to be known as the chemotherapy era. From that discovery, Fleming developed two approaches for assessing antimicrobial activity that are currently used. The initial discovery was determined by an agar diffusion methodology. Subsequent experiments that attempted to characterize this newly found antibacterial substance can be recognized as exemplifying the broth dilution method for susceptibility testing (1). One method Fleming used to obtain quantitative assessments of the degree of activity of an antimicrobial agent was to inoculate a suspension of the organism into a liquid growth medium that incorporated serial twofold dilutions of the agent. This we recognize as the broth macrodilution method. Obviously, it is not the broth that is diluted. The potentially active compound is the component that is diluted. As penicillin became available for therapeutic use, other medical microbiologists quickly adopted this procedure in order to guide therapy (2). No doubt another impetus for antimicrobial susceptibility testing became manifest as a result of financial considerations. Before World War II, the production of penicillin was limited and extremely expensive. Thus, it was evident that a procedure capable of predicting when the use of penicillin would be effective in a particular infectious disease needed to be developed. In the 1940s, several antibiotics were discovered. Although the broth susceptibility method was the first procedure developed for assessing the in vitro efficacy of antimicrobial agents (and it still serves today as a reference method), it was replaced by methods using antibiotic-impregnated filter paper strips (3) and, later, disks (4).

Toward the end of the 1950s, the status of antimicrobial susceptibility testing was in disarray as a result of the lack of acceptable standard procedures. To remedy this situation, an international group of experts was convened. They outlined general guidelines and reported on the need for standards (5). After the World Health Organization (WHO) report, an international collaborative group was formed to address the problems of standardization. The report by this group (6) was later followed by adoption of the procedures of Bauer et al. (7) in the *Federal Register* (8,9), which in large part was directed toward agar disk diffusion susceptibility testing. The International Collaborative Study (ICS) report (6) was the springboard for establishing a database and objectives of standardization for current methods (9–11).

As it evolved from Fleming's pioneering studies, the technique of using serial twofold dilutions in a liquid medium for studying the antimicrobial action of therapeutic agents is referred to as the *broth dilution method*, although the component diluted is clearly the antimicrobial agent. Initially, this technique was performed in test tubes in a final volume of 1 to 2 mL, and most laboratories followed the procedure detailed by the ICS (6). As the number of antimicrobial agents for testing increased, a more manipulative assay was automated and became popular. This procedure, referred to as the *microdilution technique* because the final volume was only 50 µL, has gained much wider acceptance than the earlier dilution methodology, known as the macrobroth or macrodilution technique.

Commercial development and application of the miniaturized technique has made it accessible to all laboratories. Thus, minimal inhibitory concentrations (MICs) can be provided by any laboratory regardless of its technical resources. Microdilution test results have been nearly equivalent to those obtained with the conventional macrodilution method, with little exception. For gram-negative microorganisms, the microdilution procedure yields MICs approximately one dilution lower than does the macrodilution method (see "Standard Broth Dilution Procedures").

The focus of this chapter is on selected elements in the design and performance of standard methods and new rapid, automated, and instrumental approaches to antimicrobial susceptibility testing in liquid media. Although reference is made to a variety of fastidious microorganisms, anaerobes and mycobacteria are not discussed (see Chapters 4 and 5).

GENERAL CONSIDERATIONS

Test Procedure

In selecting a procedure to determine the outcome of the interaction of microbe and antimicrobial compound, the laboratory must first determine whether qualitative or quantitative information is desired or required. Although, as stated, the central focus of this discussion is on the interaction of bug and drug in a liquid (broth) environment, a comparison of broth and agar diffusion methodologies is warranted (Table 3.1).

It is evident that a distinct advantage of broth methods is that they permit the determination of a minimal bactericidal concentration (MBC) end point. For those laboratories involved in special clinical pharmacologic studies, the assessment of the clinical efficacy of antimicrobial compounds (older or newly formulated); detailed assays of drug levels, distribution, and toxicity; and fully quantifiable results determined by MIC end points derived from broth dilution studies are required. The MIC can in turn be used to calculate therapeutic ratios, that is, the ratio of serum (or tissue) fluid concentration to MIC. The MIC can be determined from standard quantitative broth (or agar) dilution methods and derived from regression analysis of the diameter of zone inhibition (12,13) (Table 3.1). If the laboratory has established a database and has experience with one methodology, changing procedures for an alternative method can create new problems.

The advantages of one approach over another are summarized in Table 3.1. In certain clinical therapeutic situations (e.g., in cases of endocarditis or osteomyelitis), MICs may be indicated. When MICs are obtained, they can be used to calculate therapeutic regimens to minimize the adverse effects of potentially toxic drugs, giving added confidence in the selected therapeutic regimen. If broth is used, the simultaneous or sequential determination of MIC and MBC values can be achieved or the killing rate determined (14). Furthermore, the quantitative assay of drug combinations to detect synergy is more readily achievable in liquid systems and may be required in certain clinical situations (e.g., in cases of infection with *Enterococcus*).

Table 3.1

Comparative Feature of Disk Diffusion and Dilution Methods

Feature	Disk Diffusion	Agar Dilution	Broth Dilution[a]
Contamination readily observed	Yes	Yes	No[b]
Test for most resistant members of inoculum	No	No	Yes
Inoculum effect	No[c]	No	Yes[c]
Quantitative result	No[d]	Yes	Yes
MBC result	No	No	Yes
Direct test from clinical material	Yes	?	No
Applicable for slow-growing and fastidious organisms	No[e]	Yes	Yes
Readily amenable to automation	No	?	Yes

[a]Micro (0.1 mL) or macro (1 or 2 mL).
[b]Contaminants can be detected on subculture to appropriate medium.
[c]Slow-growing subpopulations (e.g., methicillin-resistant *S. aureus* [MRSA], methicillin-resistant *S. epidermidis* [MRSE]) require additional incubation interval and/or medium advantage.
[d]Zone diameters are inversely related to MIC and require regression analysis for development of interpretive guidelines (*S*, susceptible; *I*, intermediate or indeterminate; *R*, resistant).
[e]Current standards apply to aerobic organisms.

For clinical laboratories, combining two approaches could prove to be more useful and cost-effective. For example, antimicrobial susceptibility testing of urine samples could be done by agar disk diffusion, and broth dilution could be reserved for isolates recovered from putatively sterile compartments (blood, spinal fluid, synovial fluid, etc.). With this strategy, isolates recovered from nonsterile compartments would not require quantitative studies.

Results obtained from broth dilution susceptibility testing may be less than optimal with certain antimicrobial–microorganism combinations. The bacteria that have produced difficulties in the past decade are *Enterococcus*, methicillin-resistant *Staphylococcus aureus* (MRSA), *Pseudomonas aeruginosa*, *Haemophilus influenzae*, and *Neisseria gonorrhoeae*. Antimicrobials that delivered unreliable data included the sulfonamides, trimethoprim, nitrofurantoin, and newer combination drugs as the β-lactam–β-lactamase inhibitors. These problems were attributable to lack of appropriate standardization of inoculum and medium and have been resolved.

Several variables must be controlled to obtain accurate reproducible results. As with any assay system, deviation from standard procedure modifies the results obtained. Table 3.2 outlines some elements of the broth dilution test that have produced variable results. These are discussed in the pages that follow.

Table 3.2

Factors that Modify the Results of Broth Dilution Tests
Dilution schedule
Serial twofold versus arithmetic intervals
Medium composition
pH
Cation concentration
Osmolarity
Supplements
Volume
Inoculum size and growth phase
Temperature of incubation
Duration of incubation
Varying quality control and standardization procedures

Limitations

One must recognize that the laboratory brings together in an artificial way (in vitro) the bug and drug in a setting outside of the host environment. Whether liquid (broth) or semisolid (agar) environments more truly represent the living human milieu is a subject of ongoing discussion and controversy (15). More pointedly, is the microorganism selected for study representative of the infectious agent offending the host? Because nosocomial infections predominate in hospital settings, a key question is whether the microorganisms recovered from patient specimens are representative of infection or colonization. Usually, this question cannot be answered, but it is clear that the most likely pathogen from a specific specimen should be tested and that routine testing of mixed flora should not be done. The identity of the isolate to be tested frequently dictates or influences the methodology. For certain microorganisms, such as *Streptococcus pyogenes* and *Neisseria meningitidis*, testing may not be necessary because the outcome can be readily assured using certain antimicrobial agents or the method and interpretative standard are not yet fully established for the species. For certain rare pathogens or microorganisms with slow growth potential, clearer end points may be obtainable in broth as compared with agar.

In the final analysis, it is necessary to realize that in the laboratory setting, there is a continuous exposure of 10^5 to 10^6 colony-forming units (CFU) of microorganism per milliliter to a static (albeit minimally varying) drug concentration during the entire incubation period. These conditions do not prevail in vivo, where larger (or smaller) numbers of bacteria at the infected site are exposed to fluctuating drug concentration gradients.

ANTIMICROBIAL AGENTS

Selection of Antimicrobial Compounds for Evaluation

As the number of approved compounds continues to increase (although now at a limited rate), the challenge for the laboratory is to select rationally a limited number of antimicrobial agents for testing. To test all licensed drugs would be impractical and, in this era of constrained laboratory budgets, uneconomical. In the past, the selection of agents for testing was aided in part by the U.S. Food and Drug Administration (FDA) as it recognized class compounds or, as they apply to agar disk diffusion testing, class disks. However, as the number of chemical classes and congeners within each class increases, the unique pharmacokinetic (PK) properties frequently dictate separate disks for each newly approved compound. With the current proliferation of newer β-lactam agents and quinolones, the class idea of drug selection has become even more important for achieving economy of testing, especially given the availability of the several commercial systems.

Each laboratory and clinical setting should develop a strategy for testing compounds based on previously accrued information on resistance patterns of class agents. Patient demographics as well as patterns of antibiotic use (and abuse) will assist in this selection process. Guidelines to assist laboratories in this process have been proposed by the Clinical and Laboratory Standards Institute (CLSI), formerly named the National Committee for Clinical Laboratory Standards (NCCLS) (10,11) and are included here for convenience (Table 3.3).

It should be noted that the represented groups of organisms are those for which it is most difficult to predict, with any degree of certainty, a susceptibility result based on prior experimental data. The agents in the primary and secondary groups achieve peak levels in serum, whereas those noted in the urine group attain maximum concentrations in that compartment. Final drug selection should represent a consensus opinion at each site or medical center and should include input from the clinical microbiologist, infectious disease specialist, and clinical pharmacist. As noted, these decisions require information about the antimicrobial nature (toxicity and pharmacokinetics) and the probability of resistance for each drug–bug pair previously tested. Acquisition and use costs also need to be considered. Frequently, these data are incorporated into a quarterly or annual summary report distributed by the institution.

Although costs and test constraints may limit the number of agents tested (usually 8 to 12), hospital and/or laboratory information systems can specify the distribution of reports of susceptibility test results to the patient's chart. In a sense, the problem of selecting agents for testing prompts the following question: What information about which agent should be routinely reported? Compounds that are on restricted or limited formulary status need not be routinely reported, but the data can be stored for consultation and future consideration of routine testing and reporting. The laboratory may also wish to consider testing those

agents that are soon to be approved by the FDA, in anticipation of acquiring a database for setting new priorities.

In the performance of any susceptibility assay, the laboratory needs to define its objectives clearly. These should include the following:

1. To test organisms recovered from significant sites (e.g., blood or cerebrospinal fluid) to provide a guide for rational therapy.
2. To evaluate the susceptibility of selected nosocomial agents to determine variations in resistance patterns.
3. To determine and monitor antibiotic susceptibility (resistance) patterns as epidemiologic markers and thus as evidence of the effective use of antibiotics for coverage.
4. To study the activity of recently approved and introduced agents as well as experimental agents.

For routine clinical laboratories, an integrated approach is prudent. This approach serves to discourage the potential abuse of newer agents and thus can help minimize the selective pressure on nosocomial isolates, limiting their potential for developing resistance (Table 3.3).

Several caveats need to be mentioned in regard to Table 3.3, which represents a guide for general test selection of antimicrobial agents against selected bacterial genera.

- For bacteria recovered from cerebrospinal fluid, cefotaxime and ceftriaxone should be tested and reported. Several antimicrobial agents and types may not be effective for treatment. These include the following:
  - Agents administered orally
  - First- and second-generation cephalosporins (except cefuroxime)
  - Clindamycin
  - Macrolides
  - Tetracyclines
  - Fluoroquinolones
- Rifampin should not be used as the sole antimicrobial agent.
- The macrolides and clindamycin should not be routinely reported for microorganisms recovered from the urinary tract.

Concentration Range for Testing

When susceptibility plates are prepared in-house or ordered from a commercial supplier, specific concentrations must be selected that conform to the

(continued on page 58)

Table 3.3

Antimicrobial Agents that Should be Considered for Standard Antibiotic Susceptibility Testing and Reporting by the Clinical Microbiology Laboratory[a]

Enterobacteriaceae[b]	Pseudomonas aeruginosa Non-Enterobacteriaceae	Gram-negative Organisms		Neisseria gonorrhoeae[q]
		Haemophilus[p]		
Primary agents	*Primary agents*	*Primary agents*		*Primary agents*
Amikacin	Amikacin	Amoxicillin/clavulanic acid or ampicillin/sulbactam		Ceftriaxone
Ampicillin[d]	Aztreonam	Ampicillin		Cefixime
Amoxicillin/clavulanic acid	Cefepime	Cefotaxime or ceftazidime or ceftriaxone		Ciprofloxacin
Ampicillin/sulbactam	Ceftazidime	Chloramphenicol		Tetracycline
Cefepime	Ciprofloxacin	Meropenem		*Supplemental panel*
Cefmetazole	Doripenem	Trimethoprim-sulfamethoxazole[f]		Spectinomycin
Cefoperazone	Gentamicin	*Supplemental panel[c]*		
Cefotaxime[h] or ceftriaxone	Imipenem	Azithromycin		
Cefoxitin/cefotetan	Levofloxacin	Clarithromycin		
Cefuroxime	Meropenem	Amoxicillin/clavulanic acid		
Ciprofloxacin or levofloxacin	Mezlocillin or ticarcillin	Aztreonam		
Doripenem, ertapenem, imipenem, or meropenem	Norfloxacin[j,k]	Cefaclor		
Gentamicin	Piperacillin-tazobactam	Cefprozil		
Piperacillin	Sulfisoxazole[j,k]	Cefuroxime		
Piperacillin-tazobactam	Tetracycline[j,k]	Ciprofloxacin		
Ticarcillin/clavulanic acid	Tircarcillin	Ceftaroline		
Trimethoprim-sulfamethoxazole	Tobramycin	Levofloxacin or lomefloxacin or moxifloxacin or ofloxacin		

(Continued)

Table 3.3 (Continued)

Antimicrobial Agents that Should be Considered for Standard Antibiotic Susceptibility Testing and Reporting by the Clinical Microbiology Laboratory[a]

Gram-negative Organisms

Enterobacteriaceae[b]	Pseudomonas aeruginosa Non-Enterobacteriaceae	Haemophilus[b]	Neisseria gonorrhoeae[q]
Supplemental panel[c]	*Supplemental panel[c]*	Gemifloxacin	
Aztreonam	Lomefloxacin or ofloxacin (U)	Ertapenem or imipenem	
Ceftazidime	Norfloxacin (U)	Rifampin	
Ceftaroline		Tetracycline	
Cephalothin (U)			
Chloramphenicol			
Tetracycline			
Lomefloxacin[i] or ofloxacin (U)			
Norfloxacin (U)			
Nitrofurantoin[i] (U)			
Sulfamethoxazole (U)			
Trimethoprim (U)			

Gram-positive Cocci

Staphylococcus	Enterococcus	Stretococcus pneumoniae	Streptococcus
Primary agents	*Primary agents*	*Primary agents*	*Primary agents*
Azithromycin or clarithromycin or erythromycin	Ampicillin	Cefepime	Ampicillin
Ceftaroline	Gentamicin (high level)	Cefotaxime or ceftriaxone	Chloramphenicol
Chloramphenicol	Daptomycin	Chloramphenicol	Clindamycin
Clindamycin	Linezolid	Clindamycin	Erythromycin
Daptomycin	Penicillin	Doxycycline	Penicillin
Doxycycline or minocycline or tetracycline	Gentamicin (high level)	Erythormycin	Vancomycin
Gentamicin	Streptomycin (high level)	Gemifloxacin or levofloxacin or moxifloxacin or ofloxacin	*Supplemental panel[c]*
Linezolid	Vancomycin	Meropenem	Chloramphenicol

	Supplemental panel[c]	Penicillin (oxacillin disk)	Clindamycin
Moxifloxacin	Ciprofloxacin (U)	Tetithromycin	Erythromycin
Oxacillin[n] or methicillin	Levofloxacin (U)	Tetracycline	Linezolid
Cefoxitin	Nitrofurantoin[j]	Vancomycin	
Penicillin[m]	Norfloxacin[j] (U)	**Supplemental panel**	
Rifampin	Rifampin	Amoxicillin	
Vancomycin	Tetracycline[g] (U)	Amoxicillin/clavulanic acid	
Supplemental panel[c]		Cefuroxime	
Chloramphenicol		Ceftaroline	
Ciprofloxacin or levofloxacin or ofloxacin or gatifloxacin			
Gentamicin		Chloramphenicol	
Lomefloxacin or norfloxacin[i] (U)		Ertapenem or imipenem	
Nitrofurantoin[i] (U)		Linezolid	
Sulfisoxazole (U)		Rifampin	
Trimethoprim (U)			

[a] Final selection of appropriate antimicrobials for regular reporting must be made by each laboratory in consultation with infectious disease specialists and pharmacy staff. Susceptibility patterns of nosocomial pathogens in each hospital should be considered. "Primary" and "supplemental panels" are designed for specificity in utilization of newer expensive agents and thereby minimize costs and selection of multiresistant strains.

[b] Also applied to other gram-negative species which are not apparent on primary isolation plates (e.g., *Acinetobacter, Aeromonas,* and nonpigmented *Pseudomonas* species).

[c] Supplemental panels comprise alternative drugs to be tested (a) against strains that are resistant to multiple primary agents, especially to primary drugs in a given family (e.g., β-lactams or aminoglycosides) by initial disk diffusion or primary set of dilution tests; (b) in some institutions known to harbor multiple-resistant strains, where selected secondary agents, that is, cefoxitin or amikacin, may warrant testing with the primary set; (c) for epidemiologic purposes; or (d) as alternate treatment for patients allergic to penicillin or other primary drugs.

[d] Results generally equivalent for amoxicillin, bacampicillin, and mecillinam.

[e] Generally representative of first-generation cephalosporins such as cephapirin, cephradine, cephalexin, cefaroline, and cefazolin. *Note:* Occasional strains of Enterobacteriaceae, particularly some *E. coli,* may be more susceptible to cefazolin or to cefuroxime than to cephalothin or other first-generation cephalosporins. Thus, while cephalothin can be utilized reliably to predict susceptibility to cefazolin and cefuroxime, the reverse is not necessarily true, that is, cefazolin-susceptible enterics may occasionally be resistant to cephalothin.

[f] Usually representative also of additional second-generation cephalosporin agents such as cefamandole, cefonicid, or ceftriaxone. Generally, one agent from the group can be tested.

[g] Generally representative of the tetracycline group, although doxycycline or minocycline may be more active for selected nonfermenting gram-negative bacilli or occasional staphylococci.

[h] Usually representative also of additional third-generation cephalosporin agents such as moxalactam, ceftazidime, ceftizoxime, or cefotetan. Generally, one agent from the group can be tested.

[j] Tested only for pathogens recovered from urinary tract infections.

[k] May be useful against selected nonfermenters and *Pseudomonas* spp other than *P. aeruginosa.*

[l] Other drugs absent from this column such as cephalosporins, clindamycin, or the aminoglycosides (low-level concentrations) should not be tested against enterococci because of the prevalence of high-level resistance indicating resistance to synergy (see text and Chapter 10).

[m] Results against staphylococci are equivalent for ampicillin (see text).

[n] Representative of the semisynthetic β-lactamase–resistant penicillins. Oxacillin or nafcillin may be preferable to methicillin because of better stability characteristics.

[o] Penicillin is representative of ampicillin, ampicillin cogeners, amoxicillin, acylamino penicillins, etc. It may be used to predict susceptibility to ampicillin, amoxicillin, ampicillin–sulbactam, amoxicillin–clavulanic acid, piperacillin, and piperacillin–tazobactam for non-β-lactamase–producing enterococci.

[p] For isolates recovered from blood and cerebrospinal fluid, only results of testing with ampicillin, chloramphenicol, and a third-generation cephalosporin should be reported. Results of tests with oral agents should be reported only against isolates recovered from localized uncomplicated infection (e.g., otitis media, sinusitis).

[q] A β-lactamase test should be used to detect the most common form of penicillin resistance. It will also provide useful epidemiologic information.

microtiter configuration (conventionally, 8×12 wells) or the containers being used. The concentrations selected must satisfy several criteria.

1. The concentrations should extend over the end points of a large series of isolates, taking into consideration whether the distribution of end points is dichotomous, unimodal, or bimodal. For example, *Streptococcus pneumoniae* and other streptococci (e.g., *Streptococcus viridans*) are exquisitely susceptible to penicillin. For these organisms, limiting the lower end of the concentration range to 0.5 or 0.1 μg/mL may fail to detect minor but significant variations in the susceptibility pattern. Although such shifts may be minor, they provide a way of tracking emerging resistance. The development of emerging resistance of *S. pneumoniae* to penicillin has been documented (16,17) but has limited clinical relevance, since the large doses of penicillin that can be administered to patients will kill pneumococci with an MIC 10 times higher than the normal.

2. The concentrations tested should include and exceed (by at least one dilution step) the highest concentration found in biologic fluids. For those compounds that are concentrated in the urine in their active form, such levels can be quite high. PK data for compartmentalized antimicrobics in specific compartments must be reviewed when making these selections. Similarly, for potentially toxic agents, such as the aminoglycosides, it is pointless to test expanded upper ranges of concentrations beyond one or two dilutions above the pharmacologically toxic level. Here is one example of the failure of the twofold serial dilution schedule. Because of the narrow safety margin (therapeutic index) of aminoglycosides, rather than increasing the range above (in this case) the urinary level and taking the drug outside the therapeutic index range, it would be more prudent to prepare small arithmetic incremental dilutions for gentamicin (as well as tobramycin) in the 6 to 12 μg/mL range (18) as follows: 0.5, 1.0, 2.0, 4.0, 6.0, 8.0, 10.0, 12.0, and perhaps 16.0 μg/mL. For amikacin, a similar stepping range from 1.0 to 32 μg/mL is appropriate. Table 3.4 fails to note these figures, because the panels are not commercially available and are difficult to prepare. However, they are presented here for the reader's consideration.

3. The range of concentrations included in the panel should permit the end point detection

of quality control (QC) strains (see "Quality Control"). Although routine plates and tubes cannot be prepared in anticipation of predicting synergy-checkerboard patterns, it is worth noting that certain species, such as those in the genus *Enterococcus*, can be readily treated with a combination of penicillin G or ampicillin and an aminoglycoside, usually gentamicin, to produce synergistic bactericidal activity. Testing for synergistic and bactericidal activity is discussed elsewhere in this volume. Although dilution and synergy or killing curves in broth underscore a conventional basis for quantitative methods of testing synergy, such tests represent a special objective outside the scope of standard broth dilution procedures for routine susceptibility tests. However, the enterococci can be challenged with a single aminoglycoside concentration to determine whether the organisms demonstrate high-level resistance and would be susceptible to the synergistic action of a β-lactam and an aminoglycoside (19). Such high-level resistance can be determined with a single concentration outside of the clinically useful range included in Table 3.4. A 500- to 2,000-μg/mL concentration of aminoglycoside (usually gentamicin) could be included to screen for this type of resistance to synergy in the enterococci, as is common in some commercial systems. It is wise to consider whether this single high-level dilution should be added to the standard series or whether it should be part of a separate screening process for all gram-negative bacilli.

It is difficult to arrange a series of concentrations that satisfy all of the criteria noted earlier and that are applicable in the clinical laboratory setting. However, Table 3.4 presents a suggested outline of concentration ranges designed to approach the goals. Two series ranges are indicated in the table. The first (denoted by "X") represents a basic set of eight dilutions that cover minimum concentrations. These usually include MIC breakpoints suggested for assigning a general interpretive result to three or four categories, regardless of the terminology used to define the interpretive scheme. The use of widely spaced, selected, screening dilution steps frequently employed for certain drugs in commercial microdilution trays should be avoided. The use of widely spaced (skip-step) dilutions results in a less accurate quantitative assay than does a continuum of concentrations (see "Interpretive Guidelines

(continued on page 62)

Table 3.4

Standard Dilution Ranges of Antimicrobial Agents for Antimicrobial Testing in the Clinical Laboratory[a]

Antimicrobial Agent	Concentration (µg/mL)													
	0.015	0.03	0.06	0.12	0.25	0.5	1.0	2.0	4.0	8.0	16	32	64	128
β-Lactam penicillins														
Ampicillin[b]														
Gram-positive[c]	+	+	×	×	×	×	×	×	×	×	+		+	
Ampicillin														
Gram-negative[d]			+	+	+	×	×	×	×	×	×	×	×	+
Carbenicillin														
Gram-negative						×	×	×	×	×	×	×	×	×
Carbenicillin														
Pseudomonas[e]							×	×	×	×	×	×	×	×
Extended-spectrum penicillins[f]							(8)	(16)	(32)	(64)	(128)	(256)	(512)	
Gram-negative			+	+	×	×	×	×	×	×	×	×	+	+
Pseudomonas			+	+	+	+	×	×	×	×	×	×	×	×
Oxacillin[g] or nafcillin or		+	+	×	×	×	×	×	×	×	×	+	+	
methicillin		+	+	×	×	×	×	×	×	×	×	+	+	
Penicillin	+	+	×	×	×	×	×	×	×	×	+	+		
β-lactam–β-lactamase inhibitor combination														
Amoxicillin/clavulanic acid or ampicillin/sulbactam			+	+	×	×	×	×	×	×	×	×	+	
Piperacillin/tazobactam or ticarcillin/clavulanic acid			+	×	×	×	×	×	×	×	×	×	+	+(256)

(Continued)

Table 3.4 (Continued)

Standard Dilution Ranges of Antimicrobial Agents for Antimicrobial Testing in the Clinical Laboratory[a]

Antimicrobial Agent	Concentration (µg/mL)													
	0.015	0.03	0.06	0.12	0.25	0.5	1.0	2.0	4.0	8.0	16	32	64	128
Cephalosporins and cephems														
Cephalosporin 1[o,h,i]														
Gram-positive	+	+	×	×	×	×	×	×	×	×	+	+	+	
Gram-negative[d]			+	+	+	×	×	×	×	×	×	×	×	+
Cephalosporin 2[o,j] and 3[o,k]														
Gram-negative		+	+		×	×	×	×	×	×	×	+	+	
Cephalosporin 3[o,k]														
Pseudomonas				+	+	×	×	×	×	×	×	×	×	+
Cephalosporin 4[o]														
Cefepime				+	+	×	×	×	×	×	×	×	×	+
Carbenems/monobactams														
Aztreonam							×	×	×	×	×	×	×	×
Imipenem						×	×	×	×	×	×	×	×	
Ertapenem						×	×	×	×	×	×	×	×	
Meropenem						×	×	×	×	×	×	×	×	
Glycopeptides														
Teicoplanin	+	+	×	×	×	×	×	×	×	×	+	+		
Vancomycin	+	+	×	×	×	×	×	×	×	×	+	+		
Aminoglycosides[j]														
Amikacin[m] or kanamycin			+	+	×	×	×	×	×	×	×	×	×	+
Gentamicin or tobramycin[m]		+	+	×	×	×	×	×	×	×	×	×	×	

	(0.6)	(1.2)	(2.4)	(4.8)	(9.5)	(19)	(38)	(76)	(152)	(304)	(608)	(1216)	
Macrolides													
Azithromycin or clarithromycin, or dirithromycin			x	x	x	x	x	x	x	x	x		+
Erythromycin	+	+	x	x	x	x	x	x	x	x	+		
Telithromycin	+	+	x	x	x	x	x	x	x	x	+		
Tetracycline[n]	+	+	+	x	x	x	x	x	x	x	+	+	
Quinolones[o]	+	+	x	x	x	x	x	x	x	+			
Others													
Chloramphenicol	+	+	+	x	x	x	x	x	x	x	+	+	
Clindamycin	+	x	x	x	x	x	x	+	+				
Linezolid				x	x	x	x	x	x	x			
Nitrofurantoin[p]				x	x	x	x	x	x	x	x	x	
Quinupristin-dalfopristin			x	x	x	x	x	x					
Rifampin	+	x	x	x	x	x	x	+	+				
Trimethoprim-sulfamethoxazole	+ (0.6)	+ (1.2)	+ (2.4)	x (4.8)	x (9.5)	x (19)	x (38)	x (76)	x (152)	x (304)	x (608)	x (1216)	

[a] x = concentrations designed for a basic 8-dilution series, such as for an 8-well or tube tray (see text). + = added dilutions designed for comprehensive 12-dilution series, such as for a 12-well or tube tray (see text).

[b] Also applicable to amoxicillin and bacampicillin.

[c] Gram-positive and "sensitive" gram-negative organisms, for example, *Staphylococcus* spp, *Streptococcus* spp including *Streptococcus pneumoniae*, *Neisseria* spp, and *Haemophilus* spp (ampicillin only).

[d] Gram-negative bacilli (e.g., Enterobacteriaceae and miscellaneous nonfermentative gram-negative bacilli).

[e] If special panel is used for *Pseudomonas aeruginosa.*

[f] Applicable to ticarcillin, mezlocillin, piperacillin, and azlocillin.

[g] Interpretive results representative of penicillinase-resistant penicillin group such as nafcillin, oxacillin, cloxacillin, and dicloxacillin.

[h] Dilution ranges usually apply to all cephalosporins and monobactams. (See text and Table 3.1 for discussion of interpretive standards and of selection of representative first-, second-, and third-generation cephalosporins and analogs for testing in usual clinical microbiology procedures.)

[i] Applicable for cephalothin, cephapirin, cefazolin, cephradine, cephalexin, ceforamide, and cefadroxil.

[j] Applicable for cefamandole, cefuroxime, cefotixin, and cefonicid.

[k] Applicable for cefotaxime, moxalactam, cefoperazone, ceftazidime, ceftizoxime, and cefsulodin.

[l] Concentrations listed are for standard $\log_2$ dilutions. Some authors suggest added precision is warranted for aminoglycosides by adding "half" dilutions such as 6 (and 12) for gentamicin and tobramycin and 12 (and 24) for kanamycin and amikacin.

[m] May be reserved for secondary testing or reporting of strains resistant to gentamicin or to multiple other agents on primary tests (see text).

[n] Dilutions and interpretive results representative of the tetracycline group.

[o] Applicable to ciprofloxacin, norfloxacin (see note p), ofloxacin, gatifloxacin, gemifloxacin, levofloxacin, moxifloxacin, and sparfloxacin.

[p] To be tested only against gram-negative pathogens from urinary tract infections.

Table 3.5

		Directions for Preparing Dilutions			**Final IU or μg per mL**[a]	**Log₂ IU or μg per mL**
System for Preparing Dilutions for the Broth Dilution Method						

	Directions for Preparing Dilutions		Final IU or μg per mL[a]	Log₂ IU or μg per mL
2 mL	2,000 IU/μg per mL stock + 13.62 mL	broth = 256 μg or IU per mL	128	7
2 vols	256 IU/μg per mL (above) + 2 vols	broth = 128 μg or IU per mL	64	6
1 vol	256 IU/μg per mL (above) + 3 vols	broth = 64 μg or IU per mL	32	5
1 vol	256 IU/μg per mL (above) + 7 vols	broth = 32 μg or IU per mL	16	4
2 vols	32 IU/μg per mL (above) + 2 vols	broth = 16 μg or IU per mL	8	3
1 vol	32 IU/μg per mL (above) + 3 vols	broth = 8 μg or IU per mL	4	2
1 vol	32 IU/μg per mL (above) + 7 vols	broth = 4 μg or IU per mL	2	1
2 vols	4 IU/μg per mL (above) + 2 vols	broth = 2 μg or IU per mL	1	0
1 vol	4 IU/μg per mL (above) + 3 vols	broth = 1 μg or IU per mL	0.5	−1
1 vol	4 IU/μg per mL (above) + 7 vols	broth = 0.5 μg or IU per mL	0.25	−2
2 vols	0.5 IU/μg per mL (above) + 2 vols	broth = 0.25 μg or IU per mL	0.125	−3
1 vol	0.5 IU/μg per mL (above) + 3 vols	broth = 0.125 μg or IU per mL	0.063	−4
1 vol	0.5 IU/μg per mL (above) + 7 vols	broth = 0.063 μg or IU per mL	0.031	−5
2 vols	0.063 IU/μg per mL (above) + 2 vols	broth = 0.031 μg or IU per mL	0.016	−6
etc.	etc.	etc.		

Note: Any multiple of the volumes in the table may be used, according to the number of tests to be made, that is, 0.5 mL volumes suffice for two tests and 4 mL volumes for eight tests.
[a]The final concentration is obtained in the test tubes after 1 mL of the concentration given in the first column is diluted with 1 mL of inoculum.
Reproduced from Ericsson HM, Sherris JC. Antibiotic sensitivity testing: report of an international collaborative study. *Acta Pathol Microbiol Scand* 1971;217(Suppl B):390.

for Susceptibility or Resistance") and fails to detect upward trending of resistance. Also noted in Table 3.4 are extended concentrations (denoted by "+") for expanding the basic dilution series to provide additional relevant concentrations. These additional concentrations are added to either the upper or lower end of the range to permit better estimation of possible clinical utility against partially resistant strains in uncomplicated urinary tract infections, where high levels of drugs may be achieved in the urine (20). The addition of the end dilutions (concentrations) allows detection of modest changes in the susceptibility patterns frequently seen with highly susceptible isolates (as mentioned in the preceding section) for organisms such as *S. pneumoniae* or *N. gonorrhoeae* or occasional gram-negative bacilli that might be especially susceptible to newer agents. If the laboratory determines that the scheme outlined

in Table 3.4 is unacceptable and represents a far too customized situation, a compromise standard series of dilutions can be prepared, as outlined by the ICS (6). Table 3.5 lists dilution concentrations recommended for preparation of standard twofold dilutions in 13 × 100-mm tubes. The scheme represented in Table 3.5 can be extended to include as many end points as desired. As indicated, 14 dilution steps are included, making the scheme broad enough to address most of the problems noted earlier, but it may not be practical or necessary for the average clinical laboratory. For larger volumes of work, when more tubes are necessary, the scheme outlined in Table 3.6 is recommended (6). Here again, although the series may be customized for specific bacterial agents, employing the same standard dilution for all drugs has the advantage of simplicity and utility for routine use.

Table 3.6

Alternative Dilution System for Large Numbers of Broth Dilution Tests						
Initial Concentration Required (µg or U per mL)	Amount of Antibiotic for 50 mL	Concentration of Stock Solution (µg or U per mL)	Stock Solution (mL)	Broth or Other Diluent (mL)	Concentration after Adding Inoculum (µg or U per mL)	Log₂
256	12,800	1,280	10	40	128	64
128	6,400	1,280	5	45	64	32
64	3,200	1,280	2.5	47.5	32	16
32	1,600	1,280	1.25	48.75	16	8
16	800	80 (1:16 of 1,280)	10	40	8	4
8	400	80 (1:16 of 1,280)	5	45	4	2
4	200	80 (1:16 of 1,280)	2.5	47.5	2	1
2	100	80 (1:16 of 1,280)	1.25	48.75	1	0
1	50	5 (1:16 of 80)	10	40	0.5	−1
0.5	25	5 (1:16 of 80)	5	45	0.25	−2
etc.	etc.					

The example is for 50 tests. Diluent may be dispensed with a sterile automatic buret and volumes distributed with automatic pipettes. Reproduced from Ericsson HM, Sherris JC. Antibiotic sensitivity testing: report of an international collaborative study. *Acta Pathol Microbiol Scand* 1971;217(Suppl B):390.

Preparation and Storage of Stock Solutions

The decision to purchase commercial test systems or to prepare in-house panels depends on the laboratory type (clinical, developmental, etc.) and the objectives. Prior to the development of commercial antimicrobial susceptibility test systems, there was little choice, except for deciding whether agar or broth dilution would be used. In either case, rigorous standards have to be followed for controlling the preparation and maintenance of stock solutions of antimicrobial agents.

Reagent-quality antimicrobial powders can be obtained from the pharmaceutical manufacturer, the FDA, or the U.S. Pharmacopeia (Rockville, MD). Drug preparations stocked by pharmacies for clinical administration should not be used in the laboratory because they may contain preservatives and may not be standardized as carefully as assay-quality powders. Additionally, some clinical preparations (e.g., chloramphenicol sodium succinate) require hydrolysis in vivo to be in the active form.

Laboratories need to maintain a detailed registry of the antibiotic powders requested that indicates the date of receipt, supplier, lot number, assay potency, outdate, and storage conditions and incorporates information supplied by the manufacturer. Frequently, along with the powder, the supplier sends a material safety data sheet (MSDS) detailing the method of disposal and other pertinent information on the use of the powder and its potential danger to the user.

Once opened, sealed vials must be stored in a desiccator; some require refrigerated storage in a desiccator. Antimicrobials vary in their storage requirements. Aminoglycosides are stable at room temperature (in a desiccator), whereas β-lactams need to be kept at 20°C or lower. A general rule to heed is that the lower temperatures add to the risk of water condensation and the associated problems of ensuring adequate desiccation. When preparing to open a sealed desiccator unit, it is necessary to hold the unit and its contents at room temperature and permit both to equilibrate. Before being returned to the freezer or refrigerator, the desiccator should be resealed and the accumulated moisture desiccated. Because of their instability, some β-lactams (ampicillin, amoxicillin, and methicillin) should not be stored for longer than 6 weeks. Although there is a paucity of data on the

Table 3.7

Storage of Primary Concentrated Reconstituted Therapeutic Solutions

| Drug | Essentially Complete Stability (or Approximate Percent Original Activity) for Storage Time at Temperature | | | |
	−15°C to −20°C	4°C to 5°C	23°C to 25°C	pH of Primary Compound
Amikacin sulfate	>36 mo	>36 mo	36 mo	3.5–5.5
Ampicillin sodium (20 mg/mL in 0.9% NaCl)	92%–96%/24 h	97%/24 h	85%–92%/24 h	8–10
Carbenicillin sodium	<1 mo	6 d	80%/3 d	6–8
Cefazolin sodium	<3 mo	14 d	90%–92%/4 d	4.2–7
Cefotaxime	>3 mo	10 d	24 h	
Cefoxitin sodium	<8 mo	26 d	33–44 h	4.2–7
Cephalothin sodium	<6 wk	4 d	12 h	6–8.5
Cephapirin sodium	<2 mo	10 d	12 h	6.5–8.5
Clindamycin phosphate	>1 mo	32 d	16 d	5.5–7
Gentamicin sulfate			2 yr	3.5–5.5
Methicillin sodium	1 mo	4–24 d	24 h	6–8.5
Nafcillin sodium	3–9 mo	7 d	3 d	5–8
Oxacillin sodium	3 mo	7 d	3 d	8
Penicillin G potassium	3 mo	7 d		6–7
Tetracycline HCl	>1 mo		12–24 h	2–3
Ticarcillin disodium	>1 mo	91%/7 d	93%/24 h 63%/3 d	6–8
Tobramycin sulfate	>3 mo	4 d	24 h	6–8

Primarily reconstituted concentration solutions of therapeutic products. Most diluents sterile distilled H$_2$O. Drug concentration varied in different studies cited, but most ranged from 10 to 300 mg/mL.
From Trissel LA. *Handbook on injectable drugs*. Bethesda, MD: American Society of Hospital Pharmacists, 1983.

stability of laboratory stock standards, Table 3.7 provides some relevant information (21).

When antibiotic stock solutions are being prepared, powdered (lyophilized) material must be completely dissolved. Because all antimicrobials are not soluble in water, Table 3.8 indicates the nonaqueous solvents that are usually used. Some solvents, such as dimethylformamide (DMF), are intrinsically antibacterial. Barry and Lasner (22) found that use of DMF as a solvent for nitrofurantoin introduced errors in nitrofurantoin diluted 1:50. However, if DMF was diluted in Mueller-Hinton broth (MHB) at 1:100 to 1:200 (i.e., 0.1 to 0.2 mL of DMF), there was no detectable inhibition or antagonism associated with the residual DMF

concentration when tested against *S. aureus* or *Escherichia coli* (Fig. 3.1).

When stock solutions are prepared, they frequently need to be sterilized by filtration. At the level of concentrated stock solutions, it may not be necessary to filter-sterilize because these highly active solutions may be self-sterilizing. Aseptic precautions should be followed when further dilutions are warranted. When filtration through a matrix is needed, care should be taken to avoid the use of fiber pads owing to their absorbent nature, especially with antimicrobial agents of protein structure. The characteristics of four filter types in the retention of antimicrobial activity were studied by Murray and Niles (23) and are listed in Table 3.9.

Table 3.8

Solvents and Diluents for Preparation of Stock Solutions of Antimicrobial Agents Requiring Solvents Other Than Water[a]

Antimicrobial Agent[b]	Solvent[c]	Diluent
Amoxicillin, ticarcillin, clavulanic acid, and sulbactam	Phosphate buffer, pH 6.0, 0.1 M	Phosphate buffer, pH 6.0, 0.1 M
Ampicillin	Phosphate buffer, pH 8.0, 0.1 M	Phosphate buffer, pH 6.0, 0.1 M
Azithromycin and erythromycin	95% ethanol	Broth medium
Aztreonam	Saturated solution sodium bicarbonate	Water
Cefepime, cefadroxil, cefazolin, cefdinir, cefditoren, cefetamet, cefuroxime	Phosphate buffer, pH 6.0, 0.1 M	Phosphate buffer, pH 6.0, 0.1 M
Cefixime	Phosphate buffer, pH 7.0, 0.1 M	Phosphate buffer, pH 7.0, 0.1 M
Ceftibuten	⅒ vol DMSO	Water
Cefotetan	DMSO	Water
Cefpodoxime	0.10% aqueous sodium bicarbonate	Water
Ceftaroline	DMSO to 30% volume	0.85% saline
Ceftazidime[d]	Sodium bicarbonate[d]	Water
Ceftibuten	DMSO 1/10 volume	Water
Ceftibiprole	DMSO + glacial acetic acid	Water
Cephalexin	Phosphate buffer, pH 6.0, 0.1 mol/L	Water
Cephalothin	Phosphate buffer, pH 6.0, 0.1 M	Water
Chloramphenicol	95% ethanol	Water
Cinoxacin and nalidixic acid	½ volume of water, then add 0.1 N NaOH dropwise to dissolve	Water
Clarithromycin	Methanol or glacial acetic acid	Phosphate buffer, pH 6.5, 0.1 M
Clavulanic acid	Phosphate buffer, pH 6.0, 0.1 M	Phosphate buffer, pH 6.0, 0.1 M
Dalbavancin	DMSO	DMSO
Dirithromycin	Glacial acetic acid	Water
Doripenem	0.85% saline	Saline
Enoxacin, fleroxacin, norfloxacin, and ofloxacin	1/2 volume of water, then 0.1 N NaOH dropwise	Water
Ertapenem	Phosphate buffer, pH 7.2, 0.01 M	Phosphate buffer, pH 7.2, 0.01 M
Erythromycin	95% ethanol or glacial acetic acid	Water
Enoxacin, fleroxacin, norfloxacin, and ofloxacin	½ volume of water, then 0.1 M NaOH dropwise to dissolve	Water
Imipenem	Phosphate buffer, pH 7.2, 0.01 M	Phosphate buffer, pH 7.0, 0.1 M
Levofloxacin	½ volume of water, then 0.1 M NaOH dropwise to dissolve	Water
Metronidazole	DMSO	Water
Moxalactam[e] (diammonium salt)	0.04 N HCl (let sit for 1.5 to 2 h)[f]	Phosphate buffer, pH 7.0, 0.1 M
Nitrofurantoin[g]	Phosphate buffer, pH 8.0, 0.1 M	Phosphate buffer, pH 8.0, 0.1 M
Rifampin	Methanol	Water (with stirring)
Sulfonamides	½ volume of hot water and minimal amount of 2.5 M NaOH to dissolve	Water
Telavancin	DMSO	Water
Telithromycin	Glacial acetic acid	Water

(Continued)

Table 3.8 (Continued)

Solvents and Diluents for Preparation of Stock Solutions of Antimicrobial Agents Requiring Solvents Other Than Water[a]		
Antimicrobial Agent[b]	**Solvent[c]**	**Diluent**
Ticarcillin	Phosphate buffer 0.1 mol/L; pH 6.0	Same buffer
Trimethoprim	0.05 N lactic or hydrochloric acid, 10% of final volume	Water (may require heat)

[a] The agents known to be suitable for water solvents and diluents are amikacin, azlocillin, carbenicillin, cefaclor, cefamandole, cefmetazole, cefonicid, cefotaxime, cefoperazone, cefoxitin, cefprozil, ceftizoxime, ceftriaxone, ciprofloxacin, clinafloxacin, clindamycin, garenoxacin, gatifloxacin, gemifloxacin, gentamicin, kanamycin, linezolid, loracarbef, mecillinam, meropenem, methicillin, mezlocillin, moxifloxacin, nafcillin, netilmicin, oxacillin, penicillin G, piperacillin, quinupristin-dalfopristin, sparfloxacin, spectinomycin, streptomycin, sulbactam, tetracyclines, tobramycin, trimethoprim (lactate), and vancomycin.

[b] Some agents are included for completeness but are not listed in Table 3.4.

[c] Some of these solvents are potentially toxic; consult manufacturer's material safety data sheet (MSDS). These solvents and diluents are for making stock solutions of antimicrobial agents requiring solvents other than water. They can be further diluted as necessary with water or broth.

[d] Use anhydrous sodium carbonate at a weight exactly 10% of the ceftazidime to be used. Put the sodium carbonate in solution in most of required water. Dissolve the antibiotic in this sodium carbonate solution and add water to the desired volume. Use the solution as soon as possible, but it can be stored up to 6 hours at no more than 25°C.

[e] The diammonium salt of moxalactam is very stable but is almost pure R isomer. Moxalactam clinical is a 1:1 mixture of R and S isomers. Therefore, dissolve the salt in 0.04 N HCl and allow it to react for 1.5 to 2 hours to convert to equal parts of both isomers.

[f] Solubilize other cephalosporins and cephamycins (unless manufacturer indicates otherwise) in phosphate buffer, pH 6.0, 0.1 M, and further dilute in sterile distilled water. These include cephalothin, cefazolin, and cefuroxime.

[g] Alternatively, dissolve nitrofurantoin in dimethyl sulfoxide (DMSO).

Adapted from Baker CN, Thornsberry C, Hawkinson RW. Inoculum standardization in antimicrobial susceptibility testing: evaluation of overnight agar cultures and the Rapid Inoculum Standardization System. *J Clin Microbiol* 1983;17:450–457; Baker CN, Thornsberry C. Jones RN. In vitro antimicrobial activity of cefoperazone, cefotaxime, moxalactam (LY 127935), azlocillin, mezlocillin, and other β-lactam antibiotics against *Neisseria gonorrhoeae* and *Haemophilus influenzae*, including β-lactamase–producing strains. *Antimicrob Agents Chemother* 1980;17:757–761; National Committee for Clinical Laboratory Standards. *Methods for dilution antimicrobial susceptibility tests for bacteria that grow aerobically: approved standard*. 6th ed. Wayne, PA: National Committee for Clinical Laboratory Standards, 2003. NCCLS document M7-A6. See Shungu DL. Chemical and physical properties of antibiotics: preparation and control of antibiotic susceptibility disk and other devices containing antibiotics. In: Lorian V, ed. *Antibiotics in laboratory medicine*, 4th ed. Baltimore: Lippincott William & Wilkins, 1995:766–792.

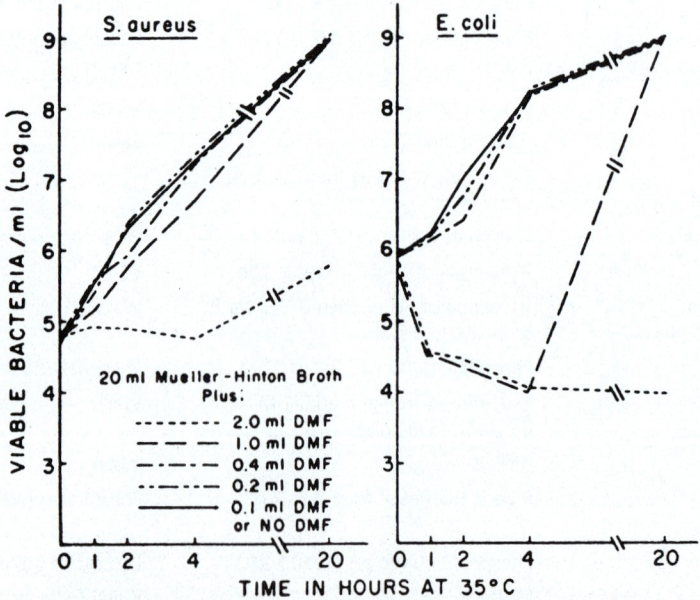

Figure 3.1 ■ Inhibition of bacterial growth by DMF. Growth curves obtained in MHB with 0.1 mL of DMF are superimposed on those obtained in control broth with no DMF. (Reproduced from Barry AL, Lasner RA. Inhibition of bacterial growth by the nitrofurantoin solvent dimethylformamide. *Antimicrob Agents Chemother* 1976;9:549–550.)

Table 3.9

Effect of Filtration on 20 Antimicrobial Agents

Antimicrobial Agent[a]	Percent Antimicrobial Activity Recovered after Filtration Through			
	Glass Fiber	Cellulose Triacetate	Mixed Esters	Polycarbonate
Amikacin	100	100	96	102
Ampicillin	99	102	97	97
Carbenicillin	99	99	97	97
Cefoxitin	96	107	96	96
Cephalothin	95	102	102	94
Clindamycin	100	101	101	102
Erythromycin	102	103	101	100
Gentamicin	97	98	100	100
Kanamycin	102	98	95	98
Methicillin	100	98	101	98
Nafcillin	98	100	99	98
Nalidixic acid	97	99	102	98
Nitrofurantoin	101	100	100	100
Oxacillin	101	102	98	98
Penicillin G	101	101	103	101
Rifampin	96	96	94	98
Sulfadiazine	104	101	101	100
Tetracycline	101	102	98	102
Tobramycin	102	102	98	100
Vancomycin	101	101	103	101

[a] Initial concentration, 100 μg/mL.
From Murray PR, Niles AC. Effect of filtration on antimicrobial solutions. *Antimicrob Agents Chemother* 1981;20:268–687.

FACTORS THAT MODIFY THE RESULTS AND REPRODUCIBILITY OF THE BROTH DILUTION TEST

Several factors influence the outcome and reproducibility of broth susceptibility results. First, the microorganism manifests its own genetic background, structure, and metabolic behavior, which strongly influence the development of resistance and disease-producing potential. Second, the antimicrobial agent possesses characteristics that affect solubility, protein binding, distribution, absorption, stability, and metabolic modification. The third factor is the milieu in which these interactions are tested and evaluated. These variables are noted in Table 3.2 and are discussed in the following pages. The problems associated with dilution schedules are discussed in "Concentration Range for Testing."

Media

Ideally, the medium in which the microorganism and antimicrobial agent interact should mimic the serum or interstitial fluid of the patient. The problem of medium influencing the results and reproducibility of susceptibility tests has long been recognized. Liquid (and agar) media suffers from variations in the lots produced by the manufacturer, in part because of the variability of raw materials and the intrinsically undefined nature of the formulations. It is clear that no single medium could ever completely satisfy the goals of providing relevant reproducible end points for all antimicrobial agents tested against all potential pathogens. The requirements for an ideal medium (liquid or solid) have been summarized by Barry (24) as follows:

1. The medium should support the growth of a variety of pathogens for which susceptibility tests are required, without the need for special supplements or enrichments.
2. Medium contents should be defined, at least to the point of specific production details for crude components such as peptone and agar.
3. Different batches of the medium prepared by different manufacturers should yield reproducible results.
4. The medium should be free of components that are known to interact with antimicrobial agents that will be tested.
5. The medium should be capable of controlling pH (especially on the acid side) during the growth of common pathogens.
6. The broth and agar versions of the medium should have the same formulation, except for the solidifying agent.
7. The medium should be approximately isotonic for bacteria, and the agar version should be able to accept the addition of blood when required for the growth of fastidious microorganisms.

Over the years, several different media representing compromises from the ideal have been used. In a coordinated effort, the ICS (6) directed a study to determine the effects of variations in medium constituents. When two media, namely Grove and Randall no. 9 medium (25) and Mueller-Hinton medium (26,27), were compared (1), it was found by the ICS that Mueller-Hinton was more suitable for supporting the rapid growth of enteric gram-negative bacilli and group A streptococci, whereas Grove and Randall no. 9 produced better growth of these gram-positive organisms: *Staphylococcus aureus*, the enterococci, and *Streptococcus viridans*, the streptococci. When two commercial sources of Mueller-Hinton were evaluated, notable differences were found only for the aminoglycosides (at that time, streptomycin and kanamycin). It is likely that varying cation content accounted for these differences (discussed later).

MHB is probably the most widely recommended liquid medium for broth dilution tests (6,28–32). However, this medium was originally intended not for susceptibility testing but for the isolation of pathogenic *Neisseria* species (33). Because MHB contained low levels of paraaminobenzoic acid (*p*-ABA), it was used in agar form to determine the susceptibility of microorganisms

to sulfonamide (34). The beef extract and casein hydrolysate in MHB are poor credentials for a reference medium. The former is difficult to standardize, and the high salt content of the latter needs to be compensated for. In spite of these deficiencies, the ICS group decided to use MHB in several studies because of the relatively good reproducibility and simplicity. An added feature was the low content of *p*-ABA, which made the medium suitable for testing sulfonamides. When MHB, brain-heart infusion (BHI), trypticase soy (TS), and Oxoid media were used in comparing tube (macrodilution) and broth microdilution results, MHB fared extremely well (35). In a replicate test series with *S. aureus*, none of the means of MICs varied by more than one dilution. For gram-negative organisms, the MICs were generally lower for MHB than for the other media tested. The greatest variation was with the Oxoid medium, which produced differences of as much as three dilutions between the macrodilution and microdilution methods. In another study in which the same four media were evaluated, Tilton et al. (36) found significant differences among the media when tested against reference strains of *E. coli* (Table 3.10), *S. aureus*, and *Pseudomonas* spp. The highest MICs were obtained in TS broth for the gram-negative strains. Differences between the media rarely exceeded 1.5 dilution steps, and the authors concluded that MHB, at cation-adjusted concentrations, was an acceptable medium. Other researchers have reached the same conclusion (37).

The issue of Mueller-Hinton being designated as a reference medium, even though its deficiencies have been recognized, has become moot. The medium has been used extensively, and there appears to be no proposals or contenders to replace it. CLSI (NCCLS) has established a reference lot for Mueller-Hinton agar (38). Cation-adjusted Mueller-Hinton broth (CAMHB), once recommended by CLSI (NCCLS) for routine testing of commonly encountered microorganisms, is now recommended when testing all species and antimicrobial agents. CAMHB is available from commercial manufacturers with Ca^{2+} (20 to 25 mg/L) and Mg^{2+} (10 to 12.5 mg/L) supplemented for convenience and uniformity. It is necessary to use CAMHB when aminoglycosides are tested against *P. aeruginosa* and when tetracycline is tested against other bacteria.

pH, Buffer, and Incubation

The mechanisms of the effect of antimicrobial pH are not precisely understood and are not consistent from drug to drug. In addition, the pH of the

Table 3.10

Effect of Growth Media on Minimum Inhibitory Concentration *(Escherichia coli)*						
	***E. coli* Control**	**Significant**	**Media**			
Antibiotic	**Organism**	**Difference**	**OST**	**BHI**	**TS**	**MH**
Ampicillin	WHO-5	$P < 0.001$	8.69	9.33	9.80	8.69
Cephalothin	WHO-5	N.S.	10.20	10.50	10.50	10.44
Chloramphenicol	WHO-5	$P < 0.001$	7.82	8.90	9.40	8.44
Kanamycin	WHO-5	$P < 0.02$	8.81	9.90	10.00	9.33
Tetracycline	WHO-16	$P < 0.001$	7.11	7.99	8.56	7.61
Gentamicin	4883	N.S.	7.94	7.99	9.10	8.19
Colistin	WHO-5	$P < 0.001$	7.62	7.34	8.56	8.61

Results expressed as $\log_2 \overrightarrow{X}$ MIC + 9.
OST, Oxoid sensitivity test; BHI, brain-heart infusion; TS, trypticase soy; MH, Mueller-Hinton.
From Tilton RC, Lieberman L, Gerlach EH. Microdilution antibiotic susceptibility test: examination of certain variables. *Appl Microbiol* 1973;26:658–665.

medium affects the activity of certain antibiotics. For some drugs, the pH variation is minor. For example, the nonionized side chain of penicillin G is slightly more active in acidic medium, but the effect is inconsequential, in that it can be demonstrated only by utilizing special experiments. The effect of the pH of the medium on the activity of six classes of antimicrobial agents is indicated in Table 3.11.

Penicillins that are nonionized or weak acids demonstrated minor variations according to the broth medium used, even when the pH was adjusted to approximately 7.0, and the MICs observed were generally within experimental error (one or two dilutions) for five different broths (39).

This situation is in contrast to that of the aminoglycosides. Streptomycin is 500 times more active in alkaline medium than in acidic medium (40). Other aminoglycosides show similar but less drastic shifts in activity with changes in pH (Table 3.12).

The buffering capacity inherent in the formulation of a medium contributes to the stability of the pH during incubation; the inclusion of glucose in the medium results in some lowering of pH during the growth of strains that can ferment the substrate. These differences were observed in medium with and without glucose when *E. coli* was used as the test organism (24). The effect of

Table 3.11

Examples of General Optimum pH for Activity of Groups of Antimicrobial Agents	
Drug Group	**Optimum pH**
Tetracycline	6.6
Penicillin and cephalosporins	6.8
Trimethoprim and sulfonamides	7.3
Erythromycin and clindamycin	7.8
Aminoglycosides	7.8
Vancomycin	7.8

Adapted from Garrod LP, Waterworth PM. Effect of medium composition on the apparent sensitivity of *Pseudomonas aeruginosa* to gentamicin. *J Clin Parthol* 1969;22:534–538.

Table 3.12

Fold Increase (+) or Decrease (−) in the Minimum Inhibitory Concentration of Different Aminoglycosides for *Staphylococcus aureus* in Broth at Different pH				
	pH			
Drug	**5.5**	**6.5**	**7.5**	**8.5**
Streptomycin	+64	+16	1	−8
Gentamicin	+16	+4	1	−2
Tobramycin	+16	+8	1	−2
Kanamycin	+16	+4	1	1
Amikacin	+32	+4	1	−2
Sisomicin	+16	+4	1	−2

From Waterworth PM. Sensitivity tests with trimethoprim-sulphonamide. *S Afr Med J* 1970;44(Suppl):10–12.

Table 3.13

Effect of pH on Antimicrobial Activity

Increased		Decreased Acidic	Variable to Little
Acidic	**Alkaline**		
Amoxicillin	Amikacin	Azithromycin	Aztreonam
Ampicillin	Azlocillin	Clarithromycin	Cefamandole
Carbenicillin	Clarithromycin	Clindamycin	Cefoperazone
Cloxacillin	Erythromycin	Metronidazole	Ceftazidime
Doxycycline	Mezlocillin	Trospectomycin	Ceftriaxone
Minocycline	Nalidixic acid		Cephalexin
Nitrofurantoin	Netilmicin		Cephalothin[a]
Piperacillin	Quinolones		Chloramphenicol
Tetracyclines	Streptomycin		Moxalactam
	Tobramycin		Nafcillin
			Penicillin[a]
			Polymixin B
			Sulfonamide[a]
			Trimethoprim

From Nicolle LE. Measurement and significance of antibody activity in the urine. In: Lorian V, ed. *Antibiotics in Laboratory Medicine,* 4th Ed, Baltimore: Williams and Wilkins, 1986;793–812.
[a]Variable effect.

adding specific buffers to stabilize a defined synthetic amino acid medium (SAAM) (41) has also been demonstrated.

Does the pH of the medium modulate the outcome of susceptibility results to the extent that the interpretation of the test and its clinical relevance would be altered? Can the pH environment of the patient be clinically manipulated significantly for therapeutic purposes? The answer to both questions is in the affirmative. Such examples probably occur more readily with the macrolide and aminoglycoside groups, which are more active in slightly basic media, and the tetracyclines, which are more active in acidic environments. Definitive changes in interpretive results have occurred with gentamicin, kanamycin, erythromycin, novobiocin, and tetracycline (15) (Table 3.13).

The marked pH effect on the aminoglycosides may be explained by the degree of ionization of these compounds. However, this explanation is not plausible for changes with the prototypic penicillin G, which is intrinsically slightly acidic but allows for minimal changes of antibacterial activity in the range pH 6 to 8. Another mechanism proposed for nonionized erythromycin may be directly responsible for antimicrobial activity (42). The antimicrobial activity of this macrolide is enhanced vividly as the pH approaches a pK_a of 8.6 (Fig. 3.2). This enhanced activity of erythromycin at alkaline pH extends the spectrum of activity of

this compound to include gram-negative organisms, particularly *E. coli* (43). These observations have been used in the clinical treatment of urinary tract infections. It has been shown that alkalinization of the urine is sufficient to activate

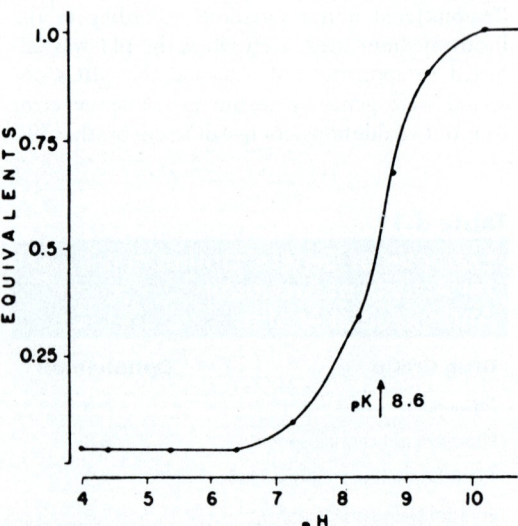

FIGURE 3.2 ■ **Ionization of erythromycin.** (Reproduced from Sabath LD, Lorian V, Gerstein D, et al. Enhancing effect on alkalinization of the medium on the activity of erythromycin against gram-negative bacteria. *Appl Microbiol* 1968;16:1288–1292.)

erythromycin and produces successful clinical treatment (42). Theoretically, laboratories should set up an environment that mimics this pH difference, but rarely is this needed or accomplished.

Another example of the effect of pH on the outcome of susceptibility test results and treatment can be found in studies with *Helicobacter* species. During the past several years, *Helicobacter* organisms have been implicated in a wide variety of conditions involving the stomach and duodenum, from gastritis to dyspepsia, as well as potentially gastric carcinoma (44). *Helicobacter pylori* was formerly referred to as *Campylobacter pylori* and is generally regarded as the agent associated with or implicated in these conditions. *H. pylori* is susceptible to a wide variety of antimicrobial agents, including penicillins, cephalosporins, macrolides, nitrofurantoins, and quinolones (44,45). The relative efficacy of these treatments is unknown, and many patients have gastric intolerance as a side effect (44). It is uncertain at which pH antimicrobial agents demonstrate maximum effectiveness in vivo. Similarly, it is questionable at what pH antimicrobial susceptibility testing should be executed. Recently, Grayson et al. (46) tested the susceptibility of 22 isolates of *H. pylori* (obtained from gastric mucosal biopsies) against eight antimicrobial agents. Antimicrobial susceptibility studies utilized the agar dilution methodology with an inoculum of 5×10^5 CFU/spot. The comparative efficacies of the agents are

shown in Table 3.14. The macrolides, quinolones, and clindamycin demonstrated diminished activity at acidic pH, compared with their activity at pH 7.4. In the alkaline pH range, MIC_{90} values were moderately but uniformly decreased (increased potency) for these same drugs. The MICs for ampicillin and metronidazole were essentially constant and within clinically achievable levels in the three pH ranges tested. The authors concluded, based on the results of their study, that if the pH of a human gastric environment was only slightly below pH 7.4, a significant loss of antimicrobial activity could result. They suggested that the modulating effect of pH on antimicrobial activity may explain the apparent discrepancy between in vitro susceptibility results and observed therapeutic failures and that clinicians need to consider the effect of pH when selecting an agent for the treatment of *H. pylori*. Added data from a study of 30 clinical isolates of *H. pylori* with trospectomycin, ampicillin, metronidazole, clarithromycin, azithromycin, and clindamycin under varying pH conditions showed that an acidic environment unfavorably affected the activity of all of the agents tested (47).

The gaseous environment is important in stabilizing the pH of media, particularly solid media; it can also affect broth. The presence of carbon dioxide (CO_2) in the incubation atmosphere, for example, may produce acidic changes, at least early in the course of incubation. Standardized susceptibility testing should not be performed

Table 3.14

Comparative Activity (MIC_{90}) of Eight Antimicrobial Agents against *Campylobacter pylori* at Three pH Ranges			
	MIC_{90} at		
Antimicrobial Agents	**pH 7.4**	**pH 5.7–6.0**	**pH 7.8–8.0**
Ampicillin	0.5	2.0	0.25
Erythromycin	0.25	>4.0	0.125
Dirythromycin	1.0	>4.0	1.0
Ciprofloxacin	0.5	4.0	0.5
Ofloxacin	1.0	2.0	0.5
Metronidazole	4.0	4.0	4.0
Doxycycline	2.0	2.0	4.0
Clindamycin	2.0	8.0	1.0

Adapted from Grayson ML, Eliopoulos GM, Ferraro MJ, et al. Effect of varying pH on the susceptibility of *Campylobacter pylori* to antimicrobial agents. *Eur J Clin Microbiol Infect Dis* 1989;8:888–889.

in a CO_2 environment. If capnophilic organisms are being tested, their growth would be scanty in an aerobic atmosphere, and so they can be incubated in CO_2, but interpretation of the results is not considered routine. When susceptibility results obtained in an aerobic environment and a 10% CO_2 incubator were compared, the MICs of aminoglycosides and erythromycins were higher (i.e., the antimicrobials were less active) and tetracyclines, methicillin, and novobiocin were more active in the CO_2 environment (6). These studies pertained to diffusion tests; however, the net effect of the 10% CO_2 environment was a lowering of pH.

Although one would expect that the target temperature for incubation of antimicrobial susceptibility tests would be between 35°C and 37°C, the temperature of incubation has been studied, particularly in regard to the detection of MRSA. Because MRSA strains are known to grow at reduced rates, it would be anticipated that these would be favored at lower incubation temperatures, compared with their more rapidly growing susceptible counterparts. In a study by Mackowiak (48), incubation at 35°C proved satisfactory for routine growth of MRSA strains as well as for all susceptibility tests. However, the heteroresistance of MRSA may be missed at 37°C. At elevated temperatures (from 35°C to 41.5°C), incubation of routine susceptibility tests (microtiter and serum bactericidal tests) indicated that more than 20% of the MIC values were lowered significantly (Fig. 3.3), and serum activity was enhanced at the higher temperatures.

The molarity (i.e., the strength) of a buffer used in the formulation of a medium can also affect the antimicrobial activity of certain compounds. In tobramycin assay systems, it was shown that the activity of the drug was generally increased with decreasing molarity, and the effect was dependent on the type of assay system used (49). For gentamicin, increasing concentrations of phosphate buffer in concert with shifts in pH produced a greater degree of error.

The extent of incubation has been studied in relationship to its effect on MIC. As incubation was prolonged, increasing MICs of cephalothin were observed beyond 12 hours (50). Such effects may be partly due to progressive antibiotic inactivation with increasing incubation interval and are more likely to be encountered with the relatively unstable penicillins and cephalosporins (51,52). Broth and agar dilution methods were compared (53) in relationship to the duration of incubation (12 and 24 hours) (Table 3.15).

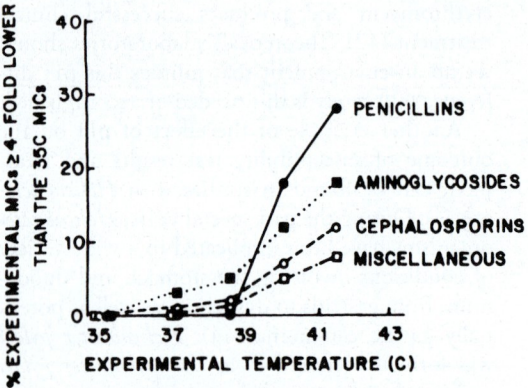

Figure 3.3 ■ **Effect of temperature on the antimicrobial susceptibility of 432 bacterial strains to classes of antimicrobial agents.** Data are the percentages of experimental MICs (determined at the indicated temperatures) that were four or more times lower than standard MICs (determined at 35°C). Comparison of the results at 40°C and 41.5°C with those at 35°C by Fisher's one-tailed exact test showed statistically significant differences for all antibiotic classes ($p < 0.05$). (Reproduced from Mackowiak RA, Marling-Cason M, Cohen RL. Effects of temperature on antimicrobial susceptibility of bacteria. *J Infect Dis* 1982;145:550–555.)

For the broth dilution techniques, the MICs increased at least twofold more than twice as often with prolonged incubation, compared with the changes that occurred between 12 and 24 with agar dilutions. This effect can be observed for ampicillin and cephalothin as well as newer broad-spectrum β-lactams. In broth dilution systems, the best reproducibility and minimal alteration in MICs from the late growth of residual persister cells can be seen if a routine is followed of reading broth dilution end points after overnight incubation (usually 18 hours). (See "Automated, Rapid, and Instrument-Associated Methods" for the adverse effects of short-term incubation.)

When microorganisms are exposed in broth to antibiotic concentrations for short durations and then the antibiotic is removed or inactivated, the resultant effect has been termed the *postantibiotic effect*, defined by Craig and Gudmundsson (54). This phenomenon may be relevant to clinical responses to therapy and can be used to establish dosage schedules (55,56). Extended incubation over a number of hours in antibiotic-deficient medium must be used to determine the residual effect of brief exposure (0.5 to 4 hours) to the antimicrobial agent, so this type of assay cannot be considered a routine or rapid test.

Table 3.15

Increase of Ampicillin and Cephalothin Minimum Inhibitory Concentration (MIC) for 18 Bacterial Strains between 12 and 24 Hours of Incubation

Antibiotic	Test Method	Fold Increase in MIC		
		0	2	4
Ampicillin	Broth[a] dilution	5[b]	9	4
	Agar[a] dilution	13	5	0
Cephalothin	Broth dilution	8	9	1
	Agar dilution	14	4	0

Strains tested were eight *Staphylococcus aureus*, four enterococci, four *Escherichia coli*, and two *Aerobacter-Klebsiella*.
[a] Mueller-Hinton broth and agar (Difco Laboratories, Detroit, MI).
[b] Number of strains.
From Sherris JC, Rashad AL, Lighthart GA. Laboratory determination of antibiotic susceptibility to ampicillin and cephalothin. *Ann NY Acad Sci* 1967;145:248–267.

Cation Concentration and Osmolality

The divalent cations calcium and magnesium have a profound modulating impact on the effects of the aminoglycosides, especially gentamicin. For example, the general results of broth dilution tests with gentamicin show MICs 1 $\log_2$ unit higher than the results for agar medium, probably reflecting variations in cation concentrations. Other aminoglycosides, as well as tetracycline, are also affected. Varying cation content has posed significant problems in agar medium (57). However, different concentrations of magnesium in broth medium have also been responsible for marked MIC variations in the activity of gentamicin against many *Pseudomonas* strains (58). Falsely low MICs are observed with media not supplemented with calcium and magnesium. A similar but less pronounced effect can be seen against other gram-negative organisms in unsupplemented media (58,59). The data in Table 3.16 indicate results obtained by varying the concentrations of magnesium, calcium, and sodium salts in nutrient broth for susceptibility studies of *Pseudomonas* with gentamicin. After extensive surveys (60), it was suggested that final concentrations of magnesium of 20 to 35 mg/L and concentrations of calcium of 50 to 100 mg/L should supplement broth. These concentrations modify the medium and bring it into the physiologic concentration range found in serum (Table 3.17). In commercial microdilution systems, the medium is cation-supplemented.

In studies with the tetracyclines, different MICs were obtained in TS broth compared with MHB (62). These differences were attributed to variations in cation concentrations. MHB produced eightfold lower MICs against *S. aureus*, *E. coli*, and *Klebsiella* species, but the antibiotic inhibitory effect of the TS broth was reversed by the apparent chelating effects of phosphate, oxalate, or citrate. The opposite effects (increased MICs) on tetracycline in MHB were produced by adding the cations magnesium, calcium, or iron (62).

Sodium chloride (NaCl) concentrations change the osmolarity of medium and have a marked effect on the activity of the aminoglycosides gentamicin (63) and tobramycin (49). A sixfold decrease in activity and increase in MIC was noted by changing (increasing) the NaCl concentration from 22 to 174 mmol/L.

β-Lactams that bind to varying penicillin-binding proteins (PBPs) may be uniquely affected by the osmolarity and, in turn, the conductivity of the test medium. This effect of osmolarity varies from strain to strain of bacterium. For some strains of *Proteus* or *Klebsiella* tested against mecillinam, a 500-fold increase in MIC as a result of increasing molarity from 185 to 402 mOsmol/L was observed. In contrast, a strain of *Enterobacter cloacae* showed no change in the MIC for mecillinam between the same osmolarity levels in the same broth (NIH medium) (64).

Supplements and Other Additives

Recently, MHB has been shown to be acceptable for a wide variety of antimicrobial susceptibility tests and to be well suited for standard, rapidly

Table 3.16

Growth of *Pseudomonas aeruginosa* 41501 in Nutrient Broth Containing Serial Dilutions of Gentamicin and Various Concentrations of Salts

Salt	Concentration of Salt (mM)	Conductivity (mΩ⁻¹) at 0°C	Gentamicin (μg/mL)											
			31.3	15.6	7.8	3.9	2.0	1.0	0.5	0.25	0.13	0.06	0.03	0.015
NaCl	174	8.1	0	0	0	0	0	0	+	+	+	+	+	+
	87		0	0	0	0	0	0	0	0	+	+	+	+
	44		0	0	0	0	0	0	0	0	0	+	+	+
	22		0	0	0	0	0	0	0	0	0	0	0	+
	11		0	0	0	0	0	0	0	0	0	0	0	+
	5.4		0	0	0	0	0	0	0	0	0	0	0	+
	2.7		0	0	0	0	0	0	0	0	0	0	0	+
MgCl₂	29.5	3.4	0	0	+	+	+	+	+	+	+	+	+	+
	14.8		0	0	0	+	+	+	+	+	+	+	+	+
	7.4	1.6	0	0	0	0	0	0	+	+	+	+	+	+
	3.7		0	0	0	0	0	0	0	+	+	+	+	+
	1.8		0	0	0	0	0	0	0	0	+	+	+	+
	0.9		0	0	0	0	0	0	0	0	0	+	+	+
	0.5		0	0	0	0	0	0	0	0	0	0	+	+
MgSO₄	29.5		0	0	+	+	+	+	+	+	+	+	+	+
	14.8		0	0	0	+	+	+	+	+	+	+	+	+
	7.4		0	0	0	0	0	0	+	+	+	+	+	+
	3.7		0	0	0	0	0	0	0	+	+	+	+	+
	1.8		0	0	0	0	0	0	0	0	+	+	+	+
	0.9		0	0	0	0	0	0	0	0	0	+	+	+
	0.5		0	0	0	0	0	0	0	0	0	0	+	+
CaCl₂	2.95		0	0	0	0	0	+	+	+	+	+	+	+
	1.5		0	0	0	0	0	0	0	+	+	+	+	+
	0.8		0	0	0	0	0	0	0	0	+	+	+	+
	0.4		0	0	0	0	0	0	0	0	0	+	+	+
	0.2		0	0	0	0	0	0	0	0	0	0	+	+
	0.1		0	0	0	0	0	0	0	0	0	0	+	+
	0.05		0	0	0	0	0	0	0	0	0	0	+	+
None	0.8		0	0	0	0	0	0	0	0	0	0	0	+

Reproduced from Medeiros AA, O'Brien T, Wacker WEC, et al. Effect of salt concentration on the apparent in vitro susceptibility of *Pseudomonas* and other Gram-negative bacilli to gentamicin. *J Infect Dis* 1971;124(Suppl):S59–S64.

growing pathogens such as enteric gram-negative bacilli, *Pseudomonas* spp, staphylococci, and *Enterococcus* spp. For organisms that grow rapidly and have been studied adequately, there are well-standardized interpretive guidelines and QC standards (10,11). For bacteria that do not grow readily on this medium, other supplements or alternative media may be required. The addition of blood or hemoglobin or of special additives such as IsoVitaleX (Baltimore Biological Laboratories,

Table 3.17

Total Concentrations of Magnesium and Calcium in Normal Serum and Commercial Batches of Mueller-Hinton Media

Medium (No. of Batches Tested)	Concentration (mg/L)[a]	
	Mg^{2+}	Ca^{2+}
MH broth		
BBL (5)	3.0 ± 0.8	10.8 ± 10.4
	(2.0–4.7)	(4.1–31.6)
Difco (5)	4.2 ± 1.0	15.0 ± 10.5
	(2.9–5.6)	(8.0–35.8)
Human serum[b] (60)	21.7 ± 1.2	98.0 ± 2.5

[a]Mean ± SD (range).
[b]Adapted from Pybus, cited by Reller et al. (60).
MH, Mueller-Hinton; BBL, Baltimore Biological Laboratories; Difco, Difco Laboratories.
Adapted from Reller LB, Schoenknecht FD, Kenny MA, et al. Antibiotic susceptibility testing of *Pseudomonas aeruginosa*: selection of a control strain and criteria for magnesium and calcium content in media. *J Infect Dis* 1974;130:454–463.

Baltimore, MD) has been proposed to enhance the growth of many fastidious organisms that may frequently require susceptibility testing (see "Fastidious and Unusual Pathogens"). Because some of the supplements produce an opacity that cannot be readily used in standard macrodilution or microdilution broth systems, they are more suitable to solid agar medium. The susceptibility testing of *H. influenzae* has long been a problem in this regard. Only recently, Jorgensen et al. (65) studied the problem and developed a special test medium, *Haemophilus* test medium (HTM), which has become commercially available and provides a solution to this problem.

The addition of various supplements of unknown chemical composition may in some instances alter antibiotic activity. However, if adequate controls are incorporated, standards are developed for appropriate interpretation, and additional control strains are utilized in the testing protocol, media supplemented with various components may be used successfully for broth dilution susceptibility tests.

Supplementation of test media with previously used (but undefined) components can result in unusual effects. Eliopoulos et al. (66) reported on the effect of 5% sheep blood added to Mueller-Hinton agar on the activity of cefotaxime and other cephalosporins against *Enterococcus faecalis*. They determined that the activities of cefotaxime and other aminothiazoyl oxime cephalosporins (e.g., cefpirome, ceftazidime, cefmenoxime, ceftriaxone, and ceftizoxime) against *E. faecalis* were enhanced by the addition of 5% sheep blood. This effect was not documented for aztreonam (a non-oxime aminothiazolyl), cefotiam, or other cephalosporins and was specific to the *syn*-configuration of the oxime moiety. Enhancement of cefotaxime activity was shown against 50% of 85 clinical isolates and could be demonstrated only with low bacterial inocula. The α-globulin fraction of serum mimicked this enhancing activity, whereas α$_1$-, β-, and γ-globulin fractions and albumin frequently antagonized or did not significantly affect the antimicrobial activity. Although these observations may not have direct clinical relevance, they present a possible explanation for the relatively infrequent occurrence of enterococcal superinfection in patients treated with cefotaxime, which demonstrates poor in vitro activity.

When 5% sheep blood or 10% fetal calf serum was added to liquid media for testing *H. pylori* susceptibility (67), sheep blood inhibited growth. When the effect of bismuth was evaluated, it was found that the compound inhibited growth in medium containing starch but that the inhibition was neutralized in medium containing serum (Fig. 3.4).

Prior to the development of HTM, broth dilution tests were satisfactorily done using MHB (68). Today, susceptibility testing of sulfonamides does not pose a serious, relevant clinical problem. Sulfonamides are rarely used in treatment, and their testing is not usually required. Media enriched with various digests or supplements may contain *p*-ABA, thus obviating sulfonamide inhibition and rendering the tests inaccurate or useless. Testing of trimethoprim or a combination of trimethoprim and sulfamethoxazole presents similar problems, in that the activity of trimethoprim or sulfamethoxazole is antagonized by the high thymidine content of enriched media. This problem exists in vitro although apparently not in vivo, because thymidine and thymine both seem to be present in sufficiently low levels in blood and urine so as not to interfere with in vivo bacteriostatic and bactericidal activity during treatment (69,70). Thus, media have to be adjusted so that the thymidine content is diminished or absent. A suitable formulation was designated SF medium base (71). Dramatic differences between a stand-

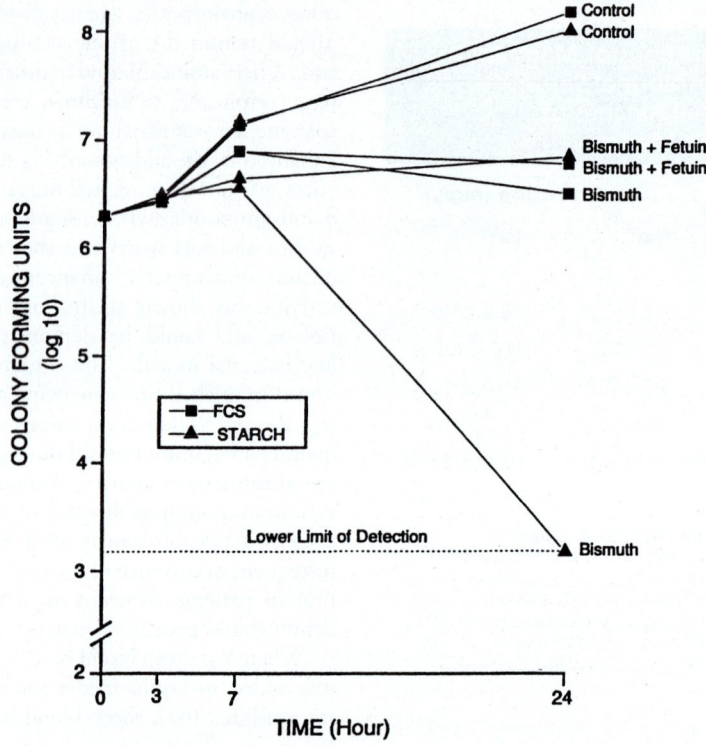

Figure 3.4 ■ **Effect of broth components, fetal calf serum (FCS) (10%), starch (0.5%), and fetuin (1.2 mg/mL) on the bactericidal activity of bismuth (32 g/mL).** (Reproduced from Coudron PE, Stratton CW. Factors affecting growth and susceptibility testing of *Helicobacter pylori* in liquid media. *J Clin Microbiol* 1995;33:1028–1030.)

ard broth medium and one enriched with 5% lysed horse blood can be seen in Figure 3.5. The supplement of 5% lysed horse blood contains sufficient thymidine phosphorylase to inactivate thymidine in various media (71,72). In the United States, most commercial lots of Mueller-Hinton medium have proven satisfactory for overnight incubation as a result of careful QC measures by the manufacturers. Other technical problems encountered with broth dilution methods when testing sulfonamides and trimethoprim result in hazy end points. These problems have been resolved by manipulation of the medium and the use of small inocula (72).

Other Media

It appears that MHB and CAMHB have established a foothold in the antimicrobial susceptibility literature. Presently, no other medium has been studied sufficiently to replace them. There have been investigations into one defined medium, namely, SAAM (41). Although this medium proved comparable in growth support and antagonism of sulfatrimethoprim, it has not gained acceptance for routine use. Similarly, another defined medium free of purines or pyrimidines (73) has been studied. However, a large proportion of *Streptococcus* and *Staphylococcus* strains failed to grow on this medium; thus, it is unsuitable for use in routine clinical laboratories. There has been little investigation into other media that would meet the ideal criteria defined by Barry (88,89). It is more likely that, with the aid of organizations like CLSI (NCCLS), reference lot media may be designed and accepted. As noted, a reference lot has been defined for Mueller-Hinton agar with regard to susceptibility testing of *H. influenzae* on agar surfaces.

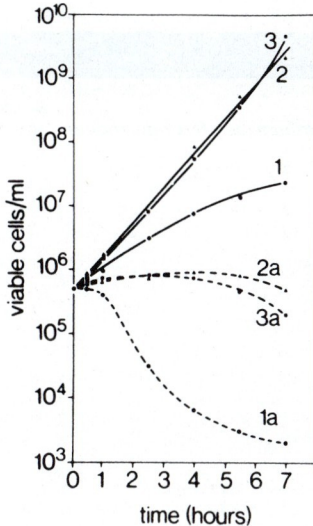

Figure 3.5 ■ Influence of 5% lysed horse blood on the effect of trimethoprim (2 g/mL) on growth of _E. coli_ B in different media. The blood-containing media were heated for 30 minutes to 56°C before inoculation. Media: _1_, sensitivity test broth (Oxoid); _1a_, medium 1 plus 5% lysed horse blood; _2_, nutrient broth no. 2 (Oxoid); _2a_, medium 2 plus 5% lysed horse blood; _3_, BHI (Difco Laboratories, Detroit, MI); _3a_, medium 3 plus 5% lysed horse blood. (Adapted from Then R. Thymidine and the assessment of co-trimoxazole. In: Williams JD, Geddes Am, eds. _Chemotherapy_. New York: Plenum Press, 1976:2.)

INOCULUM SIZE, EFFECTS, AND STANDARDIZATION

The density of inoculum in an antimicrobial susceptibility assay is critical for the generation of reliable and reproducible susceptibility test results. The adjustment of inoculum density is more important for broth dilution tests than for disk diffusion and agar dilution methods. The reason is that, with agar methods, visual (macroscopic) inspection of growth permits semiquantitative evaluation of inoculum density. In contrast, it is difficult to estimate the growth density in the growth control tubes (Table 3.1).

Susceptibility test results differ according to the species, strain, and antimicrobial agent tested (36,53,74,75). During growth of a particular bacterial strain, it can be assumed that homogeneous progeny develop. However, some degree of inoculum size effect may result from the MICs of individual bacterial cells that follow a normal

distribution. Thus, with larger inocula, there is a greater probability that there will be some cells or variants from the more resistant end of the distribution curve. In broth, the cells from this extreme of the normal distribution are more likely to survive and grow.

As mentioned, large bacterial populations are less promptly and completely inhibited than smaller ones. Also, the likelihood of the emergence of resistant mutants is greater in a large population of bacterial cells. This is exemplified by the emergence and recognition of MRSA and methicillin-resistant _Staphylococcus epidermidis_ (76). To detect and define these particular populations more accurately, it is necessary to depress the growth of the more rapidly growing, susceptible population and to extend the incubation interval beyond the usual 18 to 24 hours so as to readily detect the presence of the more slowly growing, resistant population (77). There is less chance of observing the resistant population if the critical inoculum is small. According to Sanders et al. (78–80), low-frequency mutant subpopulations of antimicrobial-resistant organisms are best detected by broth dilution systems at an inoculum concentration of more than 10^5 CFU/mL.

The inoculum effect, first reported in 1940 for the interaction of _Streptococcus haemolyticus_ and a sulfa compound (81), was later described for penicillin and _S. aureus_ (273). The effect has been found in several bacterial species and is particularly widespread among the β-lactam antimicrobial agents when their activity is directed against β-lactamase–producing bacteria. Although the inoculum effect has been most widely studied in the staphylococci, it has been shown to be associated with a variety of bacterial species and almost every class of antimicrobial agent. Table 3.18 outlines the antibiotic–organism pairs that generally exhibit an inoculum effect. This effect is generally attributed to the inactivation of the antimicrobial agent by β-lactamase (82). However, it is known to occur with antimicrobial agents lacking the β-lactam ring. Other possible causes of the inoculum effect include the selection of resistant mutants and drug breakdown by other drug-targeted inactivating enzymes. The inoculum effect can be defined as a significant increase in MIC (plus two dilutions) when the inoculum size is increased (at least by 0.5 log unit). In some studies, the effect was noted when the inoculum was varied by four orders of magnitude. Early studies investigating this phenomenon need to be considered in light of the standardized elements of testing recommended

Table 3.18

Evidence of Occurrence of an Inoculum Effect

Antimicrobial Agent	S. aureus	Enterobacteriaceae	Pseudomonas	H. influenzae	N. gonorrhoeae	Branharmella catarrhalis
Penicillins	+	+	+	+	+	+
1° Cephalosporin	+	V	V	+	+	+
2° Cephalosporin	+	V	V	+	+	+
3° Cephalosporin	−	+	+	+	+	+
Aminoglycoside	+	0	0	U	U	U
Chloramphenicol	−	0	0	+	U	U
Quinolones	V	0	0	U	U	U
Imipenem	V	U	U	+	U	U

+, effect observed; 0, effect not observed; V, variable response; U, undetermined.
Data derived from Bartlett JG. *Campylobacter pylori*: fact or fancy. *Gastroenterology* 1988;94:229–232.

by CLSI (NCCLS) (10). Additionally, studies elucidating the inoculum phenomenon have not been well standardized; they vary in incubation interval, reagent volume, and size of the test vessel.

The clinical implications of the inoculum effect are uncertain. Clearly, the inoculum standard established by CLSI (NCCLS) (5×10^5 CFU/mL final concentration for broth dilution and 10^4 CFU/spot) is not applicable to all clinical situations. At best, it represents a compromise between various clinical infections and the procedural manipulation for eliminating the potential for trailing end points. This methodologic result occurs when the inoculum exceeds a final concentration of 10^7 CFU/mL. With several of the antibiotic–organism pairs that have exhibited the inoculum effect (Table 3.18), the final MIC result, although elevated compared with the result obtained with a smaller inoculum size, would still have yielded an interpretation of susceptible based on the MIC:level ratio.

Of the several factors that can modulate the outcome of antimicrobial susceptibility tests, the inoculum size, besides being relatively easy to measure, should be among the easiest to standardize. The role of inoculum size was shown in studies of penicillin-sensitive and penicillin-resistant strains of *S. aureus* treated with cephalexin (83,84). Marked changes in MICs and MBCs were observed for 100-fold changes in inoculum density (Fig. 3.6). The effects of 10-fold dilutions of inoculum, from 10^3 to 10^7 CFU/mL, can be seen for several antibiotic groups used against *E. coli* (Table 3.19), gram-positive and gram-negative organisms (Table 3.20), and *Pseudomonas*

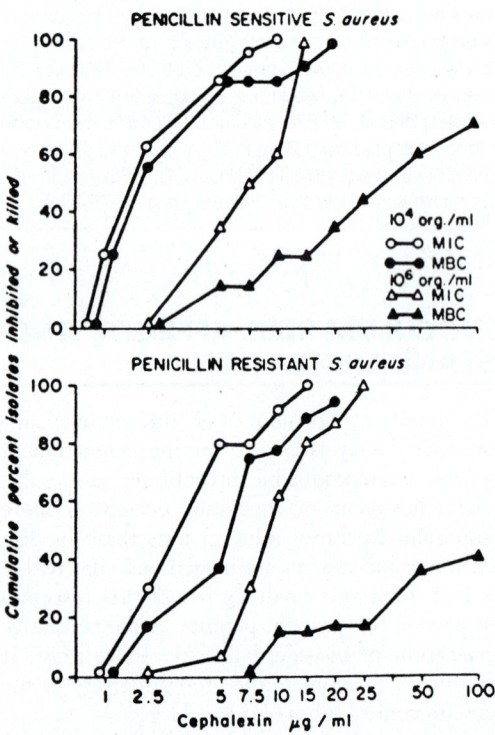

Figure 3.6 ■ Cumulative percentages of 16 isolates of penicillin-susceptible *S. aureus* and 13 isolates of penicillin-resistant *S. aureus* inhibited (MIC) or killed (MBC) by increasing concentrations of cephalexin, tested in nutrient broth medium with bacterial inocula of two different sizes. (Reproduced from Clark H, Turck M. In vitro and in vivo evaluation of cephalexin. *Antimicrob Agents Chemother* 1969;8:296–301.)

Table 3.19

Effect of the Inoculum Concentration *Escherichia coli* on Minimum Inhibitory Concentration

Antibiotic	*E. coli* Control Organism	Significant Difference	Inoculum Concentration (CFU)			
			10^4	10^5	10^6	10^7
Ampicillin	WHO-5	$P < 0.05$	8.71	8.57	8.71	10.00
Cephalothin	WHO-5	$P < 0.01$	10.28	10.28	11.00	12.00
Chloramphenicol	WHO-5	$P < 0.05$	8.76	8.58	8.91	9.54
Kanamycin	WHO-5	$P < 0.01$	8.77	9.25	10.08	10.77
Tetracycline	WHO-16	N.S.	7.40	7.50	7.29	7.86
Gentamicin	4883	$P < 0.001$	6.50	7.67	8.75	10.00
Colistin	WHO-5	$P < 0.001$	6.00	8.50	9.00	9.75

Results expressed as $\log_2 \bar{x}$ MIC + 9.
WHO, World Health Organization; CFU, colony-forming units.
Adapted from Tilton RC, Lieberman L, Gerlach EH. Microdilution antibiotic susceptibility test: examination of certain variables. *Appl Microbiol* 1973;36:658–665.

spp (Tables 3.21 and 3.22). Against *E. coli*, tetracycline was found to be the most refractory to inoculum effects, whereas significant changes were recorded with the other antimicrobial agents, especially at the high end of the inoculum range (Table 3.10). For *P. aeruginosa*, the effect of varying inoculum size on the activity of the antimicrobials tested was related to the agent tested (75). When the inoculum was increased to 5×10^5 CFU/mL, the MIC$_{90}$ values for all drugs tested were increased (Table 3.21). When the inoculum was increased further to 5×10^7 CFU/mL, the MIC$_{90}$ values could be determined only for gentamicin and thienamycin. The MBC$_{90}$ values at an inoculum of 5×10^5 CFU/mL ranged from 8 µg/mL for gentamicin and thienamycin to 128 µg/mL for cefotaxime (Table 3.21). With the largest inoculum, the MBC$_{90}$ values for gentamicin and thienamycin remained constant but the MBC$_{90}$ values for the other drugs tested were less than 128 µg/mL. The susceptibility results for *H. influenzae* are seriously influenced by the size of the inoculum (85–87). The effect is more pronounced for ampicillin-resistant isolates (β-lactamase producers?) and penicillin than for cephalosporins. Now that inoculum size and medium have been defined for *H. influenzae* susceptibility testing, variation in susceptibility test results is anticipated to diminish.

The effect of inoculum density variation on various antimicrobial agents tested against several species must be considered in any recommendation for a standard or reference method. Most investigations support the earlier work of the ICS (6), which suggested that an inoculum of 10^5 to 10^6 CFU/mL would yield acceptable results in a macrobroth dilution test. Some workers adjust the inoculum

Table 3.20

Effect of Increasing Inoculum Concentrations of Gram-positive and Gram-negative Bacteria[a] on the Minimum Inhibitory Concentrations of Cefuroxime and Four Other Cephalosporins

Cephalosporins	MIC$_{50}$ at Inoculum Concentrations (CFU/mL)		
	10^3	10^5	10^7
Cefuroxime	2	4	>32
Cefamandole	0.5	1	>32
Cefoxitin	4	4	16
Cephalothin	4	8	>32
Cefazolin	2	4	>32

[a]Includes the following species (number of strains): *Escherichia coli* (22), *Klebsiella* spp (20), *Enterobacter* spp (20), *Proteus mirabilis* (19), *Proteus* spp (20), *Pseudomonas capacia* (3), *Pseudomonas maitophilla* (5), *Aeromonas hydrophila* (4), and *Staphylococcus aureus* (26).
MIC, minimum inhibitory concentration; CFU, colony-forming units.
From Barry AL, Thornsberry C, Jones RN, et al. Cefuroxime, an in vitro comparison with six other cephalosporins. *Proc R Soc Med* 1977;70(Suppl 9):63–71.

Table 3.21

Influence of Inoculum Size on Concentrations of Gentamicin, *N*-formimidoyl Thienamycin, Moxalactam, Cefotaxime, and Piperacillin Required to Inhibit the Growth of 40 Isolates of *Pseudomonas aeruginosa* by a Broth Microtiter System

	MBC (μg/mL of Medium)								
				For % of Isolates					
	Range			50			90		
Compound	5×10^3	5×10^5	5×10^7	5×10^3	5×10^5	6×10^7	5×10^3	5×10^5	5×10^7
Gentamicin	0.06–64	0.125–64	0.5–128	0.25	0.5	1	1	2	4
N-formimidoyl thienamycin	0.06–8	0.25–16	0.5–16	0.5	1	4	2	8	8
Moxalactam	0.5–32	0.5–64	16–>128	4	8	128	16	32	>128
Cefotaxime	1–64	4–128	16–>128	4	8	>128	16	32	>128
Cefoperazone	0.5–16	1–32	16–>128	2	4	>128	4	8	>128
Piperacillin	0.5–16	2–64	32–>128	2	4	>128	8	16	>128

MIC, minimum inhibitory concentration.
From Corrado ML, Landesman SH, Cherubin CE. Influence of inoculum size on activity of cefoperazone, cefotaxime, moxalactam, piperacillin, and N-formimidoyl thienamycin (MK 0787) against *Pseudomonas aeruginosa. Antimicrob Agents Chemother* 1980;18:893–896.

Table 3.22

Influence of Inoculum Size on Concentrations of Gentamicin, *N*-formimidoyl Thienamycin, Moxalactam, Cefotaxime, Cefoperazone, and Piperacillin Required for Bactericidal Activity for 40 Isolates of *Pseudomonas aeruginosa* by a Broth Microtiter System

	MBC (μg/mL of Medium)								
				For % of Isolates					
	Range			50			90		
Compound	5×10^3	5×10^5	5×10^7	5×10^3	5×10^5	5×10^7	5×10^3	5×10^5	5×10^7
Gentamicin	0.06–128	0.25–128	0.5–128	0.5	1	2	1	8	8
N-formimidoyl thienamycin	0.25–8	0.5–16	1.0–16	1	2	4	4	8	8
Moxalactam	0.5–64	4–64	16–>128	8	16	>128	32	32	>128
Cefotaxime	1–128	8–>128	64–>128	8	16	>128	32	128	>128
Cefoperazone	0.5–32	1–>128	32–>128	2	4	>128	8	64	>128
Piperacillin	1–16	2–>128	64–>128	2	4	>128	16	32	>128

MBC, minimal bactericidal concentration.
From Corrado ML, Landesman SH, Cherubin CE. Influence of inoculum size on activity of cefoperazone, cefotaxime, moxalactam, piperacillin, and N-formimidoyl thienamycin (MK 0787) against *Pseudomonas aeruginosa. Antimicrob Agents Chemother* 1980;18:893–896.

closer to the range of 1 to 5×10^5 CFU/mL. For microdilution, the average recommended inoculum is 1×10^6 CFU (30).

Methodology for Standardizing Inocula

For the reasons mentioned earlier, it is imperative that each culture inoculum be individually standardized. The procedures frequently used for both the macrodilution and microdilution systems involve either adjustment of a logarithmic-phase broth culture to a McFarland 0.5 turbidity standard (7,10) or defined direct dilutions from 0.5-mL volumes of stationary-phase broth cultures (10). Several discrete colonies, usually three to seven, are subcultured to the inoculum growth broth, to avoid single-colony variance. The inoculum is usually cultured in the same broth medium used for the test, such as MHB or CAMHB (richer media such as TS broth and BHI can also be used satisfactorily). For rapidly growing pathogens, overnight broth cultures (4 to 8 mL) grow to approximately 10^9 CFU/mL. A 1:1,000 or 1:2,000 dilution of this growth brings the inoculum density to the range of 5×10^5 to 5×10^6 CFU/mL. Results have generally been satisfactory with such methods, because most rapidly growing pathogens achieve stationary-phase growth at density levels that fall within a reasonable range. Alternatively, one can adjust the turbidity of a 4- to 8-mL overnight culture or a 4- to 6-hour broth culture (both are considered to be in the stationary phase) to a standardized density. This can be accomplished nephelometrically with instruments frequently provided with automated units for determining susceptibility or manually by dilution to match the visual turbidity of the McFarland 0.5 $BaSO_4$ standard, which approximates 10^5 CFU/mL. The 4- to 6-hour broth culture offers a significant time advantage compared with the overnight incubation. However, for some more slowly growing, more fastidious strains, such as *Haemophilus* or *Neisseria* strains, overnight growth may be required. Satisfactory results have been obtained by emulsifying colony plate growth to match either nephelometric or McFarland turbidity standards. Then, appropriate dilutions (e.g., 1:2,000) are made for the final inoculum.

It has been shown that turbidity-adjusted direct suspensions can also yield reproducible and accurate results for commonly encountered gram-negative or gram-positive, rapidly growing microorganisms (44). When the growth phase of the inoculum was studied systematically by Barry et al. (88), they found that generally satisfactory reproducibility with control strains was dependent on whether the inoculum standard utilized required harvesting direct suspensions from overnight colonies or from logarithmic-phase (2- to 4-hour) or stationary-phase (5- to 6-hour) broth cultures.

After an inoculum has been prepared, variability has been observed in the delivery of the inoculum to the test system. In some systems, this was more dependent on a mechanical inoculum preparation and transfer system and independent of the growth phase of the organism. Inocula prepared with *Pseudomonas* strains demonstrated lower counts, perhaps due to clumping, than did those prepared with other organisms (89). Final MIC results were generally reproducible and consistent regardless of the method of inoculum preparation and despite the system-dependent inoculum variations from 2×10^4 to 1×10^6 CFU/mL (44). Table 3.19 indicates that, with some drug–organism combinations (10%), statistically significant differences in geometric mean MICs resulted from different growth or inoculum preparation methods tested in two different microdilution systems (89).

Numerous techniques have been developed for inoculum preparation, standardization, and transfer and been incorporated into the expanding range of commercial microdilution test systems (see "Standard Broth Dilution Procedures"). Several systems adjust turbidity suspensions instrumentally. However, most recommend the use of a mechanical device that involves touching five colonies directly with a wand containing grooves at its bottom crosshatch, followed by emulsification in an appropriate volume of saline. This system, referred to as *RISS* and marketed as PROMPT, eliminates prior broth incubation and turbidity adjustment (90,91). Figure 3.7 illustrates how the CFU/mL values in the inoculum are affected by increasing the number of colonies touched; a maximum colony count is achieved after selecting four colonies.

STANDARD BROTH DILUTION PROCEDURES

The focus of this chapter is on broth dilution procedures. However, it is worthwhile to note that comparisons of results of broth and agar dilution methodologies have shown them to be similar (92). In some instances, as noted by Lorian (93), the differences for quinolones have been significant. There has been a considerable range of variability in studies, depending on the method used,

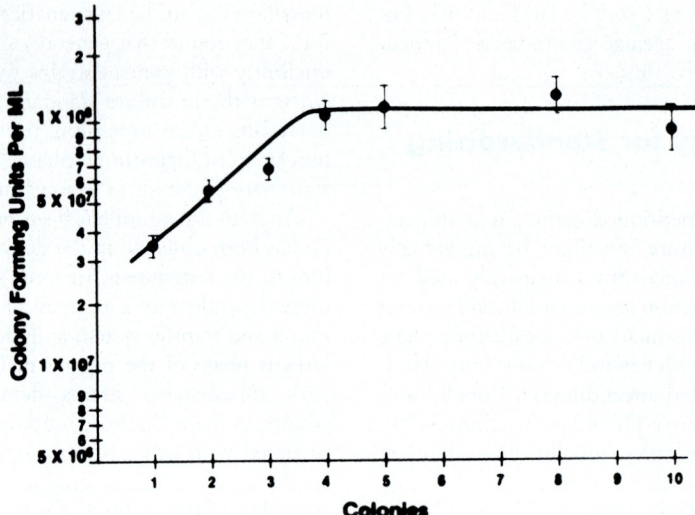

Figure 3.7 ■ Inoculum standardization with RISS. The range and mean of viable *E. coli* ATCC strain 25922 obtained with the inoculation rod versus the number of colonies picked are shown. (Reproduced from Wicks et al. [270].)

the antimicrobial agent studied, and the organisms tested. A number of investigations have also compared microdilution and macrotube dilution techniques (37,94,95). Tables 3.23 and 3.24 present some of the results. Clearly, for the majority of agents tested, there were few strains that varied by more than plus or minus one dilution.

Comparative evaluations of the microdilution and macrodilution broth procedures are noted here to provide a historical perspective. Since the 1980s, there have been no evaluations of these two broth methodologies, owing in part to the popularity of the microdilution procedure. Furthermore, commercial applications of the miniaturized technique that began in the mid-1970s have made it practical for laboratories to provide MICs for all isolates, or at least for all those they wish to report on. In general, microdilution test results are essentially equivalent to those obtained with the standardized macrobroth dilution procedure. For certain organisms, such as gram-negative bacilli, the microdilution results are approximately one dilution step lower than those obtained with the macrodilution broth technique. This seems to be a general feature of the microdilution technique and may be partially due to the way end points are read. Minimal turbidity, which is visible in a test tube, may not be readily observed in a microtiter well. Another possible explanation may involve the inoculum. Although

in their final concentrations the inocula in the two systems contain approximately 5×10^5 organisms and are comparable, the absolute number of viable cells delivered into the microtiter well is 1 log unit less than that inoculated into the test tube.

Standard Microdilution Broth Procedure

The performance of microdilution tests has been described by a number of authors using in-house panels prepared by mechanical semiautomated or automated equipment (29,94,96–101) or commercial test panels routinely prepared or customized for the user. Commercially prepared test panel systems employ either frozen antimicrobial solutions in medium or dried preparations that need to be rehydrated by adding diluent and inoculum to each well. The test panel state of some commercial preparations and their method of inoculation are noted in Table 3.25.

For preparation of standard microdilution panels in the laboratory, the following general recommendations and directions can be followed (29,102). The antimicrobial agent stock solutions are prepared and stored as noted in Tables 3.4 and 3.7 and as found in CLSI (NCCLS) standard M7-A6 (10). The recommended dilutions have been included in Table 3.4, and the flexibility

Table 3.23

Comparison of Microdilution[a] and Macrodilution[b] Results: Frequency of Agreement and Variation of Microdilution Minimum Inhibitory Concetrations when Compared with Macrodilution Minimum Inhibitory Concetrations as the Reference Standard

Antibiotic	Microdilution >Macrodilution					Microdilution and Macrodilution Identical	Microdilution <Macrodilution					Totals
	>4	4	3	2	1		1	2	3	4	>4	
Penicillin G					4	14	7					25
Methicillin					4	18	3					25
Ampicillin					5	14	5	1				25
Cephalothin				2	12	11						25
Erythromycin					2	18	5					25
Tetracycline-HCl					3	17	5					25
Kanamycin					7	14	4					25
Gentamicin					7	4	7	6	1			25
Colistin				2	10		5	6	1	1		25
Total no. (% distribution)	0	0	0	4 (2)	45 (20)	120 (54)	39 (17)	13 (6)	2 (1)	1 (0.5)	0	225 (100)

Twenty-five strains were tested by both methods with each antibiotic.
[a]Automated dilutions in Mueller-Hinton broth using microtiter trays and the Canalco Autotiter apparatus.
[b]Manual macrotube dilutions in Mueller-Hinton broth according to Ericsson and Sherris (6).
MICs, minimum inhibitory concentrations.
Adapted from Gerlach EH. Microdilution, I: A comparative study. In: Balows A, ed. *Current techniques for antibiotic susceptibility testing*. Springfield, Il: Charles C Thomas, 1973:63–76.

Table 3.24

Occurrence of Discrepant Test Results against *Pseudomonas* Strains, Based on the Susceptibility Test Method Used

Drug	Microdilution MIC > Tube MIC		Microdilution MIC = Tube MIC	Microdilution MIC < Tube MIC	
	Two Dilutions	**One Dilution**		**One Dilution**	**Two Dilutions**
Gentamicin	0	5	24	70	1
Tobramycin	0	34	51	15	0
Amikacin	1	19	61	19	0
Carbenicillin	0	13	61	26	0

MIC, minimum inhibitory concentrations.
From Jorgensen JH, Lee JC, Jones PM. Chemically defined antimicrobial susceptibility test medium for Pseudomonas aeruginosa. *Antimicrob Agents Chemother 1977;11:415–419.*

Table 3.25

Historical Overview of Automated and Instrument-Associated Antimicrobial Susceptibility Test Systems

System (Manufacturer)	Antimicrobial State	Inoculation	Instrument	Incubation Interval (Hours)
Autobac (Organon Teknika, Durham, NC)[a]	Disk	Channel distribution	Light scatter at 665 nm, 35°/log index	3–5
Avantage (Abbott, Irving, TX)[a]	Disk	Channel distribution	Absorbance at 665 nm/algorithm	3–6
AMS (Vitek Systems, Inc., McDonnell Douglas, Hazelwood, MO)[b]	Card	Channel distribution	Absorbance at 665 nm/algorithm	6–10
Sceptor (BBL)	Dry	Multitip pipet	Visual turbidity	16–18
Sensititre (Radiometer, Westlake, OH)	Dry	Sequential autoinoculation	Fluorometer/ algorithm	5–18
UniScept (API, Plainview, NY)[a]	Dry	Sequential autoinoculation	Absorbance/AC	16–24
MicroScan (Baxter, West Sacramento, CA)[c]	Frozen	Multiprong	Absorbance/AC	16–24 or 4–89[d]
Microcoder II (Beckman)[a]	Frozen	Multiprong	Visual AC	16–24
Precept (Austin Biological, TX)[a]	Dry	Multiprong	Visual growth/no growth, light pen	16–24
MIC BioPlate (Plasco/Difco)[a]	Frozen	Multiprong	Visual turbidity, light pen	16–24
Repliscan (Cathra, St. Paul, MN)	In medium	Multiprong	Visual growth/no growth, light pen	16–24

[a]These systems are no longer commercially available. See Table 3.35.
[b]Vitek bioMérieux. See Table 3.35.
[c]New corporate sponsor. See Table 3.35.
[d]Fluorogenic substrates permit rapid readings.
AC, analog conversion.
Adapted from Amsterdam D. Instrumentation for antimicrobic susceptibility testing: yesterday, today, and tomorrow. *Diagn Microbiol Infect Dis* 1988;9:167–178.

dilution schedule need not be limited to serial two-fold increments.

The recommended broth for testing is Mueller-Hinton supplemented with 50 mg/L Ca^{2+} and 25 mg/L Mg^{2+}. These concentrations are achieved by the addition of the appropriate amounts of filter-sterilized $CaCl_2$ and $MgCl_2$ stock solutions to cold sterile broth. Ideally, microdilution trays should be prepared each day they are used. However, with the availability of semiautomated dispensing devices for preparing dilutions and dispensing prediluted agent, it is possible to prepare large numbers of trays at one time and store them frozen until required. As trays are filled, they are stacked in groups of 5 to 10 and are either covered with an empty tray on top or placed and sealed in plastic bags and frozen at 20°C or 70°C. Household freezers are satisfactory, but they should not contain self-defrosting units, because fluctuations in temperature during the defrost cycle thaw and refreeze the antimicrobial agents and thus contribute to their deterioration. Trays quick-frozen at 70°C and stored at 20°C have a useful shelf life of about 6 weeks. Storage at 70°C significantly increases the shelf life to approximately 3 months. Once a group of trays is removed from the freezer, they should be allowed to warm at room temperature prior to use. Unused thawed trays should be discarded and never refrozen.

Actively growing broth cultures are diluted to a McFarland value of 0.5 (as described earlier). Multipoint plastic or metal replicators (inoculators) are used in several commercial and semiautomated systems. After inoculation, each well should contain approximately 5×10^5 CFU/mL (5×10^4 CFU/well).

After inoculation of microdilution trays, they should be covered with sealing tape to minimize evaporation. Alternatively, large numbers of trays can be stacked and covered with an empty tray. After 16 to 20 hours of incubation, trays may be examined from below with a reflective viewer and MICs determined. The trays can also be read visually from the top. The end point MIC is the lowest concentration of drug at which the microorganism tested does not demonstrate visible growth. In judging the end point, it is necessary to compare the growth (or absence of growth) in the test wells with the growth (or absence of growth) in the well without the antimicrobial agent. End points are easily read as turbid wells or clear wells. For some antimicrobials, such as the sulfonamides and trimethoprim, end points may trail. The end point

for these drugs should be read as an 80% to 90% decrease in growth compared with growth in the control well.

Standard Macrodilution Broth Procedure

The variables that affect the outcome of dilution tests were outlined earlier and were reviewed in the preceding section. The procedures for performing the macrodilution broth test have been described by several authors (6,24,25,32,103–106). Errors and statistical variability of dilution procedures have been reviewed (30). The basic methodology described in the ICS report (6) has proven satisfactory for many laboratories, and Table 3.5 presents a scheme recommended in the ICS report for the preparation of antibiotic dilutions. An alternative dilution schedule for preparing a larger number of tubes is shown in Table 3.6. Because the dilutions are pipetted directly into blocks of three dilution tubes with one pipette, the chance of error is significantly reduced. A sequential twofold dilution method is summarized from the work of Jones et al. (107) as follows. The working antimicrobial solution is prepared by diluting the drug and MHB to the highest final concentration desired. The test is performed in 13 100-mm screw-capped (or cotton-plugged, etc.) test tubes. For a limited number of tests, twofold dilutions are prepared directly in test tubes as follows: 2 mL of the working solution of the drug is added to test tube 1 of the dilution series. To each remaining tube, 1 mL of MHB is added. With a sterile pipette, 1 mL is transferred from tube 1 to tube 2. After thorough mixing, 1 mL is transferred (using a separate pipette for this and each succeeding transfer) to tube 3. This process is continued to the next to last tube, from which 1 mL is removed and discarded. The last tube receives no antimicrobial agent and serves as a growth control. The final concentrations of antimicrobial agents in this test are half those of the initial dilution series because of the addition of an equal volume of inoculum in broth. The inoculum is prepared and adjusted, as noted earlier, to contain 10^5 to 10^6 CFU/mL, by adjusting the turbidity of the broth culture to match the McFarland 0.5 standard. It is then further diluted 1:200 in broth, and 1 mL of the adjusted inoculum is added to each test tube. Tubes are incubated at 35°C for 16 to 20 hours. The lowest concentration of antimicrobial agent that results in complete inhibition of visible growth represents the MIC. A very faint haziness or a small button is usually disregarded.

Quality Control

For in vitro susceptibility test results to be meaningful for selecting appropriate antimicrobial agents and monitoring their use for the treatment of infection, they need to be accurate and reproducible. Because of the potential for variation, emphasis has been focused on strict adherence to methods and reference procedures (10,11). The development of QC parameters has played a significant role in the high level of performance obtained by most laboratories. Keys to this performance are the application of standard reference strains with known reactivity and the assessment of qualitative and quantitative end points.

The ideal reference strain for QC of dilution susceptibility methods should have MIC end points near the middle of the range of concentrations being tested for a given drug, or at least no closer than two dilutions from the extremes of the test range included (102). Thus, in QC for dilution testing, it has been necessary to deviate from established QC strains that have been used for disk diffusion testing. For example, *S. aureus* American Type Culture Collection (ATCC) strain 29213, a weak β-lactamase producer, is recommended instead of ATCC strain 25923. Additionally, *S. faecalis* ATCC strain 29212 and *E. coli* ATCC strain 35218 have been recommended as controls for β-lactamase inhibitors such as clavulanic acid and sulbactam. A sixth control strain, *H. influenzae* ATCC strain 49247, has recently been proposed (by CLSI [NCCLS]) for testing drugs against *H. influenzae* (10).

Studies of the precision and accuracy of macrodilution and microdilution MIC end points with the older established QC strains have shown that reproducibility should be within plus or minus 1 $\log_2$ dilution interval for 95% of the replicates (32,103) and that most tests should fall at the modes. The ranges of MICs expected for several contemporary antimicrobial agents against the reference strains are indicated in Table 3.26.

Control reference strains should remain genetically and phenotypically stable over many replications and long-term storage. Control strains must be stored using procedures designed to minimize chances of mutation or variant selection (32). It is suggested that, for long-term storage, QC strains

be lyophilized or frozen in a stabilizing medium such as whole sheep blood or 15% glycerol in an enriched broth such as BHI or 50% serum in broth. Freezing at 60°C (or below) is preferable to storing in conventional freezers (20°C). Strains can be maintained for short-term storage at 4°C for approximately 2 weeks on agar (soybean digest casein).

When new batches or lots of microdilution trays are received from a commercial source or prepared, they should be tested with reference strains to determine their acceptability. The MICs resulting from QC testing should be no more than one dilution interval above or below the anticipated MIC. If the difference is greater, either the batch is rejected or the results with the affected antimicrobial agent are not recorded or reported. Additionally, representative uninoculated trays should be tested for sterility of the medium. QC should be done on a periodic basis after reproducibility and accuracy have been documented by daily QC practice (10,108). These QC procedures provide a review of variables such as antimicrobial potency and stability, instrument function, and technical proficiency. The MICs obtained with each reference strain should be maintained in a record book for ongoing review.

Some additional QC procedures are necessary for broth dilution tests but are less critical for agar or disk diffusion tests. A purity control plate for each isolate tested is subcultured, for isolation on an appropriate agar medium, directly from the final inoculum suspension to detect potential contamination or mixed cultures. A growth control tube (or well) free of antimicrobial agents is included within each panel set to ensure adequate growth. This also serves as a turbidity control (a comparative aid) when reading end points. The inoculum should be measured periodically by a direct dilution plate count of the time 0 inoculum from the growth tube or well. Finally, the proficiency of the observers determining end points should be monitored periodically by comparing their results with those from a standard reader to ensure uniformity between different observers reading the same plate.

There are several types of susceptibility test results that, when obtained, require further confirmation or investigation. Forty-five nonsusceptible phenotypes are listed in Table 3.27, and these may be associated with pre- or postanalytical (test) errors. In any event, these phenotypes warrant follow-up study.

(continued on page 90)

Table 3.26

Acceptable Quality Control Ranges NCCLS[a] of Minimum Inhibitory Concentrations (μg/mL)[b] for Reference Strains

Antimicrobial Agent	Staphylococcus aureus ATCC 29213	Enterococcus faecalis ATCC 29212	Escherichia coli ATCC 25922	Pseudomonas aeruginosa ATCC 27853	Escherichia coli ATCC 35218
Amikacin	1–4	64–256	0.5–4	1–4	
Amoxicillin-clavulanic acid	0.12/0.06–0.5/0.25	0.25/0.12–1.0/0.5	2/1–8/4		4/2–16/8
Ampicillin	0.5–2	0.5–2	2–8		
Ampicillin-sulbactam	—	2/1–8/4	8/4–32/16		
Azlocillin	2–8	1–4	8–32	2–8	
Azithromycin	0.5–2				
Aztreonam			0.06–0.25	2–8	
Carbenicillin	2–8	16–64	4–16	16–64	
Cefaclor	1–4		1–4		
Cefamandole	0.25–1		0.25–1		
Cefazolin	0.25–1		1–4		
Cefdinir	0.12–0.5		0.12–0.5		
Cefditoren	0.25–2		0.12–1		
Cefepime	1–4		0.016–0.12	1–8	
Cefetamet			0.25–1		
Cefixime	8–32		0.25–1		
Cefmetazole	0.5–2		0.25–1	>32	
Cefonicid	1–4		0.25–1		
Cefoperazone	1–4		0.12–0.5	2–8	
Cefotaxime	1–4		0.03–0.12	8–32	
Cefotetan	4–16		0.06–0.25		
Cefoxitin	1–4		2–8		
Cefpodoxime	1–8		0.25–1		
Cefprozil	0.25–1		1–4		
Ceftazidime	4–16		0.06–0.5	1–4	
Ceftibuten			0.12–0.5		
Ceftizoxime	2–8		0.03–0.12	16–64	
Ceftriaxone	1–8		0.03–0.12	8–64	
Cefuroxime	0.5–2		2–8		
Cephalothin	0.12–0.5		4–16		
Chloramphenicol	2–8	4–16	2–8		
Cinoxacin			2–8		

(Continued)

Table 3.26 (Continued)

Acceptable Quality Control Ranges NCCLS[a] of Minimum Inhibitory Concentrations (μg/mL)[b] for Reference Strains

Antimicrobial Agent	Staphylococcus aureus ATCC 29213	Enterococcus faecalis ATCC 29212	Escherichia coli ATCC 25922	Pseudomonas aeruginosa ATCC 27853	Escherichia coli ATCC 35218
Ciprofloxacin	0.12–0.5	0.25–2	0.004–0.016	0.25–1	
Clarithromycin	0.12–0.5				
Clinafloxacin	0.008–0.06	0.03–0.25	0.002–0.016	0.06–0.5	
Clindamycin	0.06–0.25	4–16			
Daptomycin	0.25–1	1–8			
Dirithromycin	1–4				
Doxycycline			0.5–2		
Doripenem	0.015–0.00	1–4	0.015–0.06	0.12–0.5	
Enoxacin	0.5–2	2–16	0.06–0.25	2–8	
Ertapenem	0.06–0.25	4–16	0.004–0.016	2–8	
Erythromycin	0.25–1	1–4			
Fleroxacin	0.25–1	2–8	0.03–0.12	1–4	
Fostomycin	0.5–4	32–128	0.5–2	2–8	
Garenoxacin	0.004–0.03	0.03–0.25	0.004–0.03	0.5–2	
Gatifloxacin	0.03–0.12	0.12–1.0	0.008–0.03	0.5–2	
Gemifloxacin	0.008–0.03	0.016–0.12	0.004–0.016	0.25–1	
Gentamicin	0.12–1	4–16	0.25–1	0.5–2	
Grepafloxacin	0.03–0.12	0.12–0.5	0.004–0.03	0.25–2.0	
Imipenem	0.016–0.06	0.5–2	0.06–0.25	1–4	
Kanamycin	1–4	16–64	1–4		
Levofloxacin	0.06–0.5	0.25–2	0.008–0.06	0.5–4	
Linezolid	1–4	1–4			
Lomefloxacin	0.25–2	2–8	0.03–0.12	1–4	
Loracarbef	0.5–2		0.5–2	>8	
Mecillinam			0.03–0.25		
Meropenem	0.03–0.12	2–8	0.008–0.06	0.25–1	
Methicillin	0.5–2	>16			
Meziocillin	1–4	1–4	2–8	8–32	
Minocycline	0.06–0.5	1–4	0.25–1		
Moxalactam	4–16		0.12–0.5	8–32	
Moxifloxacin	0.016–0.12	0.06–0.5	0.008–0.06	1–8	
Nafcillin	0.12–0.5	2–8			
Nalidixic acid			1–4		
Netilmicin	≤0.25	4–16	≤0.5–1	0.5–8	

(Continued)

Table 3.26 *(Continued)*

Acceptable Quality Control Ranges NCCLS[a] of Minimum Inhibitory Concentrations (μg/mL)[b] for Reference Strains

Antimicrobial Agent	*Staphylococcus aureus* ATCC 29213	*Enterococcus faecalis* ATCC 29212	*Escherichia coli* ATCC 25922	*Pseudomonas aeruginosa* ATCC 27853	*Escherichia coli* ATCC 35218
Nitrofurantoin	8–32	4–16	4–16		
Norfloxacin	0.5–2	2–8	0.03–0.12	1–4	
Ofloxacin	0.12–1	1–4	0.015–0.12	1–8	
Oritavancin	0.5–2	0.12–1			
Oxacillin	0.12–0.5	8–32			
Penicillin	0.25–2	1–4			
Piperacillin	1–4	1–4	1–4	1–8	
Piperacillin-tazobac-tam	0.25/4–2/4	1/4–4/4	1/4–4/4	1/4–8/4	0.5/4–2/4
Quinupristin-dalfo-pristin	0.25–1	2–8			
Rifampin	0.004–0.016	0.5–4	4–16	16–64	
Sparfloxacin	0.03–0.12	0.12–0.5	0.004–0.016	0.5–2	
Sulfisoxazole	32–128	32–128	8–32		
Teicoplanin	0.25–1	0.06–0.25			
Telavancin	0.12–1	0.12–0.5			
Telithromycin	0.06–0.25	0.016–0.12			
Tetracycline	0.12–1	8–32	0.5–2	8–32	
Ticarcillin	2–8	16–64	4–16	8–32	
Ticarcillin-clavulanic acid	0.5/2–2/2	16/2–64/2	4/2–16/2	8/2–32/2	8/2–32/2
Tigecycline	0.03–0.25	0.03–0.12	0.03–0.25		
Tobramycin	0.12–1	8–32	0.25–1	0.25–1	
Trimethoprim	1–4	≤1	0.5–2	>64	
Trimethoprim-sulfamethoxazole	≤0.5/9.5	≤0.5/9.5	≤0.5/9.5	8/152–32/608	
Trospectomycin	2–16	2–8	8–32		
Trovafloxacin	0.008–0.03	0.06–0.25	0.004–0.016	0.25–2	
Vancomycin	0.5–2	1–4			

[a]Adapted from National Committee for Clinical Laboratory Standards. *Methods for dilution antimicrobial susceptibility tests for bacteria that grow aerobically: approved standard.* 6th ed. Wayne, PA: National Committee for Clinical Laboratory Standards. 2003. NCCLS document M7-A6.
[b]MICs were obtained from several reference laboratories by broth microdilution with CAMHB.
NCCLS, National Committee for Clinical Laboratory Standards; MICs, minimum inhibitory concentrations; ATCC, American Type Culture Collection.

Table 3.27

Antimicrobial Test Results that Require Confirmation and/or Investigation[a]

Microorganism[b]	Nonsusceptible Phenotypes[c]
Gram-negative	
Enterobacteriaceae	Amikacin, carbapenems,[d] fluoroquinolones
Pseudomonas aeruginosa	Aminoglycosides (multiple)
Stenotrophomonas maltophilia	Trimethoprim-sulfamethoxazole
Haemophilus influenzae	Ampicillin, amoxicillin-clavulanic acid,[e] aztreonam, carbapenem, third-generation cephalosporins, fluoroquinolones
Neisseria gonorrhoeae	Third-generation cephalosporins, fluoroquinolones
Neisseria meningitidis	Penicillin, ciprofloxacin
Gram-positive	
Enterococcus faecalis	Ampicillin or penicillin, linezolid, high-level aminoglycosides, quinupristin-dalfopristin
Enterococcus faecium	High-level aminoglycoside, linezolid, quinupristin-dalfopristin
Staphylococcus aureus	Linezolid, oxacillin, quinupristin-dalfopristin, vancomycin
Staphylococcus, coagulase-negative	Linezolid, vancomycin
Streptococcus pneumoniae	Fluoroquinolones, linezolid, meropenem, third-generation cephalosporins, penicillin, vancomycin
Streptococcus, beta	Ampicillin or penicillin, third-generation cephalosporins, linezolid, vancomycin
Streptococcus viridans	Penicillin, linezolid, vancomycin

[a]See Livermore DM, Winstanley TG, Shannon KP. Interpretative reading: recognizing the unusual and inferring resistance mechanisms from resistant phenotypes. *J Antimicrobial Chemother* 2001;48(Suppl 1):87–102; National Committee for Clinical Laboratory Standards. *Performance standards for antimicrobial disk susceptibility tests: approved standard*. 8th ed. Wayne, PA: National Committee for Clinical Laboratory Standards, 2003. NCCLS document M2-A8.
[b]Any microorganism that is resistant to all agents tested warrants review and investigation.
[c]Microorganisms that fail to meet the interpretive criteria for S (susceptible); they may be I or R.
[d]*Proteus* spp are an exception for imipenem.
[e]β-Lactamase negative.

FASTIDIOUS AND UNUSUAL PATHOGENS

The standard broth procedures described thus far are applicable to routine antimicrobial susceptibility testing. The term routine reflects the fact that the testing is of rapidly growing, nonfastidious pathogens frequently encountered in the clinical setting. Routine susceptibility procedures, however, may not be applicable to predictably slow-growing microorganisms with prolonged lag times and/or slow generation times (109). Some clinically significant bacteria have characteristics that preclude their being tested by standard methods. They may grow too slowly, may require special nutrients or atmospheres, or simply may not have been tested with enough frequency to demonstrate that they can

be tested accurately and reproducibly by the standard methods. These microorganisms have been termed *fastidious* and/or *unusual*. Specifically, fastidious organisms do not readily grow on Mueller-Hinton medium without supplementation. Unusual organisms may grow well on Mueller-Hinton medium, but studies have not been completed to demonstrate that they can be tested reliably by standard methods. Testing the susceptibility of unusual organisms to antimicrobial agents may also present special problems.

In the past, many of these organisms did not require susceptibility tests because they were known to be universally susceptible to an appropriate antimicrobial agent that was not toxic and could reach sufficient levels to effect a clinical cure. "Resistant" strains have emerged, however. Resistance to β-lactams is most often due to production of β-lactamase, which may be constitutive or inducible and may be mediated by either chromosomal or plasmid genes (80,110). In some species, such as *H. influenzae* and *N. gonorrhoeae*, penicillin and ampicillin resistance has been typically caused by the acquisition of plasmids that mediate constitutive β-lactamase production by the organisms (111,112). In other species, such as *S. pneumoniae*, penicillin resistance is not due to β-lactamase production caused by plasmids but is chromosomally mediated and is due to the alteration of PBPs (113).

These developments have produced challenges for clinicians because previously employed empirical therapies associated with these fastidious or unusual organisms may not be adequate. Additional laboratory testing is sometimes required to support a prediction of therapeutic success.

For some organisms, such as group A streptococci, susceptibility tests are not necessary because these organisms have maintained (with some exceptions) universal susceptibility to penicillin, the drug of choice. However, for *S. pneumoniae*, especially if it was isolated from a putatively sterile site, a test to determine susceptibility to penicillin is indicated, because some of the strains may be relatively or completely resistant to penicillin. If it becomes necessary to perform susceptibility tests on clinical isolates for which no standard method has been described, it is usually best to determine the MIC using the general broth dilution method described earlier and in CLSI (NCCLS) standard M7-A6. For testing of infrequently isolated or fastidious, see CLSI document M45-A2. Table 3.28 details the antimicrobial susceptibility methods that can be used for these fastidious or unusual organisms. It is obvious that certain microorganisms have been omitted, notably anaerobes, *Mycobacterium tuberculosis*, *Chlamydia* spp, *Mycoplasma* spp, and spirochetes. For these groups, readers can refer to appropriate chapters in this volume.

For the antimicrobial susceptibility testing of fastidious and/or infrequently encountered bacteria, the CLSI has published guidelines for testing with interpretive breakpoints (114). These guidelines encompass the following bacterial groups.

Aeromonas spp
Bacillus spp (other than *Bacillus anthracis*)
Campylobacter coli and *Campylobacter jejuni*

Corynebacterium spp
Erysipelothrix rhusiopathiae
HACEK group (*Aggregatibacter actinomycetemcomitans* and *Aggregatibacter aphrophilus*, *Cardiobacterium hominis*, *Eikenella corrodens*, and *Kingella kingae*)
Lactobacillus spp
Leuconostoc spp
Listeria monocytogenes
Moraxella catarrhalis
Pasteurella spp
Pediococcus spp
Plesiomonas shigelloides
Streptococci, nutritional dependent spp (now *Abiotrophia* and *Granulicatellas* spp)

In addition to the microorganisms listed earlier, the CLSI has proposed guidelines for the standardized testing of the generally recognized agents of bioterrorism, namely *Bacillus anthracis*, *Francisella tularensis*, *Brucella* spp, *Yersinia pestis*, and *Burkholderia pseudomallei*. (See Table 2 of CLSI M45-A2 [114].) As of this writing, standardized testing for other fastidious bacteria, for example, *Legionella* and *Bordetella*, are unavailable because these less frequently encountered bacterial infections generally respond to clinically recommended antimicrobial agents.

Haemophilus influenzae

H. influenzae and other *Haemophilus* species are examples of common clinical pathogens with special growth requirements. The widespread emergence of β-lactamase–producing strains has made rapid detection of β-lactamase production and, in turn, detection of ampicillin resistance in *Haemophilis* important objectives (102,115–117).

Antimicrobial resistance among clinical isolates of *H. influenzae* has been monitored in the United States, Canada, and Europe. In a comprehensive study (118) involving isolates in the United States, 20% of all *H. influenzae* isolates were ampicillin-resistant by virtue of β-lactamase production. Enzyme-mediated resistance to ampicillin is approximately twice as common in serotype B strains (31.7%) as in non–B strains (15.6%). As a result of the production of the inactivating enzyme chloramphenicol acetyltransferase (119), occasional resistance has been noted with chloramphenicol, as well as resistance to tetracycline, trimethoprim-sulfamethoxazole, rifampin, and first-generation cephalosporins.

Because of the worldwide prevalence of β-lactamase–producing strains of *H. influenzae*, it

(continued on page 98)

Table 3.28

Susceptibility Testing of Fastidious and Unusual Pathogens[a]

Organism	Method	Medium	Incubation/ Environment	Comments
Campylobacter spp	Broth microdilution (258) Agar dilution	CAMHB + 5% LHB[b] MHA + 5% blood	35°C, 18–24 h in 85% N₂ 10% CO₂ 5% O₂	Some strains may require 48 h for adequate growth. Does not require routine testing, as many cases of gastrointestinal disease are self-limiting. Empirical treatment with a macrolide is usually successful.
Corynebacterium spp	Broth microdilution (258) Agar dilution	CAMHB MHA	35°C, 18–24 h	Some strains may require a more nutritive medium (e.g., blood or serum additives). Test JK against vancomycin and rifampin.
Haemophilus spp	Broth microdilution (65,102,117,258) QC: *H. influenzae* ATCC 49247 and 49766	HTM[c] (inoculum from choc)	35°C, 20–24 h	See the most recent NCCLS dilution standard for recommendations on drugs and breakpoints.
	β-lactamase (102)		Room temperature up to 1 h	Do not need induction. Any β-lactamase method can be used. Some strains may be ampicillin-resistant but β-lactamase–negative.
Helicobacter pylori	Agar dilution NCCLS QC: *H. pylori* ATCC 43504	MHA	35°C, 3 d in special *Campylobacter* gas systems	Interpretive criteria only for clarithromycin.
Legionella spp	Do not test routinely (259)			Therapy can be empirical (macrolide and/ or rifampin). Susceptibility testing should be done only in reference laboratories.
Listeria monocytogenes	Broth microdilution (258) Agar dilution QC: *Streptococcus pneumoniae* ATCC 49619	CAMHB + 5% LHB MHA + 5% sheep blood	35°C, 16–20 h	*L. monocytogenes* may be susceptible to cephalosporins in vitro but they are not effective clinically. Drugs of choice are ampicillin and TMP-SMX. Ampicillin MICs are usually 0.5–1.0 µg/mL. Ampicillin is usually the drug of choice in meningitis.

Organism	Method	Medium	Conditions	Comments
Moraxella catarrhalis	Broth microdilution (258) Agar dilution β-lactamase (102,259)	CAMHB MHA	35°C, 18–24 h Room temperature up to 1 h	Some strains may require a more nutritive medium. Use only the nitrocefin method. Other methods must be proven to be equivalent. Eighty percent or more of strains are β-lactamase–positive. The β-lactamase is not the TEM type but is inhibited by clavulanic acid and sulbactam.
Mycobacterium fortuitum and *Mycobacterium chelonae*	Broth microdilution; inoculum is prepared from overnight growth in MHB + 0.02% Tween 80 (259)	CAMHB	35°C, 72 h	Avoid creating aerosols. Test aminoglycosides, doxycycline, cefoxitin, crythromycin, and sulfonamides. Ciprofloxacin also has activity against *M. fortuitum*. Other *Mycobacterium* spp are not tested by this method.
Neisseria meningitidis	Broth microdilution (258)	CAMHB+ 2%–5% LHB	35°C, 24 h in CO_2	Test penicillin, rifampin, and sulfonamide. Organisms in broth may lyse after 24 h. Rifampin and sulfa data are for decisions on prophylaxis and not therapy (260).
	Agar dilution (258)	MHA	35°C, 18–24 h in CO_2	
Neisseria gonorrhoeae	Agar dilution or disk diffusion (See text and Jones et al. [124])	GC agar base with "XV" supplement	35°C, 24 h in CO_2	Ideally, test for penicillin, tetracycline, spectinomycin, and ceftriaxone.
	β-lactamase (102)	From isolation media	Room temperature up to 1 h	Occasional strains may be resistant to penicillin but β-lactamase–negative. Induction not required: any β-lactamase method can be used.
Nocardia spp	Broth microdilution (258)	CAMHB	35°C, 48 h	*Nocardia asteroides* has four or five different susceptibility patterns; *Nocardia brasiliensis* has one. Sulfas are generally drugs of choice, but intolerance or allergy is fairly common. Test a variety of antimicrobials including third-generation cephalosporins and β-lactam–β-lactamase inhibitor combinations (personal communication from Dr. Richard Wallace, University of Texas Health Science Center, Tyler, TX).

(Continued)

Table 3.28 (Continued)

Susceptibility Testing of Fastidious and Unusual Pathogens[a]

Organism	Method	Medium	Incubation/Environment	Comments
Nonfermentative bacteria (other than *Acinetobacter* spp)	Broth microdilution (258)	CAMHB or CSMHB + supplements if needed	35°C, 18–24 h or longer; use CO_2 if necessary	Some of these isolates may require a more enriched medium.
	Agar dilution (258)	MHA + supplements if needed		
"Organisms causing endocarditis": nonenterococcal streptococci	See *Streptococcus* spp section for MIC methods			If penicillin MIC >0.1 µg/mL, β-lactam plus aminoglycoside (streptomycin or gentamicin) therapy should be considered.
Enterococcus spp	See *Streptococcus* spp section for MIC methods			Use β-lactam and aminoglycoside (streptomycin or gentamicin) for therapy. Some strains will not respond synergistically to the combination (see below).
	High-level aminoglycosides test for synergy *E. faecalis* ATCC 29212 (S) ATCC 51299 (R)	BHI broth	35°C, 24 h; additional 24 h if necessary	Test streptomycin at 1,000 µg/mL and gentamicin at 500 µg/mL. If there is no growth, synergy between the β-lactam and the aminoglycoside is likely to occur; if there is growth, synergy is unlikely. Blood may influence susceptibility tests with aminoglycosides and cephalosporins and some enterococci (183).
				It is assumed that most oxacillin-resistant staphylococci can be detected by agar dilution, although there are no data or recommendations for adding NaCl (33).
S. pneumonia	Broth microdilution (258,259) QC: *S. pneumoniae* ATCC 49619	CAMHB + 5% LHB	35°C, 18–24 h	MIC breakpoints for penicillin are susceptible, ≤0.06; intermediate, 0.12–1.0; and oxacillin disk diffusion zone diameter of ≥20 MICs indicate susceptibility.

Streptococcus spp	Broth microdilution (258) QC: *S. pneumoniae* ATCC 49619	CAMHB + 5% LHB	35°C, 18–24 h in CO$_2$ if necessary	Nonenterococcal streptococci that grow well in this medium (and may require CO$_2$) may also be tested by the standard NCCLS disk diffusion methods (261). The oxacillin screen test as used for pneumococci (i.e., to indicate penicillin resistance) does not work for these organisms. Penicillin resistance occurs most often in *S. mitis* but does occur in other species. For group A streptococci, erythromycin resistance occurs; zones of ≥18 mm correlate well with MICs of ≤0.12 µg/mL, and zones of <18 mm with MICs of ≥2 µg/mL (33).
Streptococci, pyridoxal-dependent	Broth microdilution (126,258)	CAMHB + 5% LHB + 0.001% pyridoxal HCl	35°C, 18–24 h in CO$_2$ if necessary	Grow organisms on agar containing 0.001% pyridoxal HCl. Alternatively, 1% pyridoxal HCl can be swabbed onto the surface of a blood agar plate prior to inoculation. Prepare inoculum suspension from growth on plate.
Fastidious or unusual organisms not mentioned previously	Broth dilution (258) Agar dilution (258)	Use CAMHB/A plus supplements as necessary. Trial and error may be necessary to determine needs	35°C, 18–24 h or longer. Use required atmosphere. Trial and error may be necessary to determine needs	If unusual supplements or atmosphere is necessary, report MIC as not done with a standardized test.

(Continued)

Table 3.28 (Continued)

Susceptibility Testing of Fastidious and Unusual Pathogens[a]

Organism	Method	Medium	Incubation/Environment	Comments
Staphylococcus aureus, oxacillin-resistant (methicillin-resistant)[d,e]	Agar screen (77,123) S. aureus 29213 (OS) S. aureus ATCC 433000 (OR)	MHA + 4% NaCl and 6 μg/mL oxacillin or 10 μg/mL methicillin	35°C, full 24 h but no longer	Use as a screening test for methicillin, oxacillin, nafcillin, or cloxacillin resistance. Oxacillin is the preferred test agent in most institutions. Inoculate plate by "pie-plating" or by "spot" inoculation with swab. Growth indicates chromosomal intrinsic resistance. Use as a second test in addition to the broth microdilution or disk diffusion test. *Note:* This method is not reliable for detecting oxacillin-resistant coagulase-negative staphylococci.
	Broth microdilution—for methicillin and oxacillin and methicillin and oxacillin only (cephalothin or other β-lactams, excluding cefamandole, if desired) (77,123,258)	CAMHB + 2% NaCl	35°C, full 24 h but no longer	For S. aureus, S ≤ 2 and R ≥ 4. For coagulase-negative staphylococci, S ≤ 0.25 and R ≥ 0.5. The above breakpoints are to be used only with this MIC method. Oxacillin is the preferred test agent. To prepare inoculum, suspend colonies from an overnight agar plate into broth or saline to equal the turbidity of a 0.5 McFarland standard (88,90). Final inoculum should be 3–5 × 10^5 CFU/mL. Some strains are hyperproducers of β-lactamase and yield resistant or borderline MICs to oxacillin and methicillin but will not be intrinsically resistant. These strains are not usually multiresistant to drugs other than β-lactams. These strains are usually susceptible to amoxicillin-clavulanic acid (intrinsically oxacillin-resistant strains are not).

Clues (flags) indicating resistance to methicillin, oxacillin, or nafcillin:

1. Multiple resistance to any or all of the following:
   - erythromycin
   - aminoglycosides
   - chloramphenicol
   - tetracycline
   - clindamycin
2. Intermediate MIC to methicillin or oxacillin.
3. Failure to show cross-resistance between methicillin, nafcillin, and oxacillin.

[a] In general, the inoculum for most of these tests is preferably prepared directly from growth off of agar plates (262). It is best to use a fresh plate, but some organisms may require 48 hours for adequate growth. Suspend the growth into a clear broth and standardize the suspension to match a 0.5 McFarland standard. Then make appropriate dilutions depending on type of system or method being used (see directions for specific organisms). Inoculum for broth microdilution should be 10^5 to 5×10^5 CFU/mL and for agar, 10^4 to 5×10^4 CFU/spot.

[b] The lysed blood used in these tests is lysed by freezing, thawing at least six times, and then adding an equal volume of sterile distilled water. The solution is clarified by centrifugation (10,000 × g) for 20 minutes and subsequent decantation of the supernate (not necessary if it is to be added to agar). Sheep blood is not recommended for tests with *Haemophilus* spp or with sulfonamides.

[c] To make *Haemophilus* test medium (HTM), first prepare a fresh hematin stock solution by dissolving 50 mg of powder in 100 mL of 0.01 N NaPH with heat and stirring until the powder is thoroughly dissolved. Add 30 mL of the hematin stock. After autoclaving and cooling, cations are added aseptically, if needed as in CAMHB, and 3 mL of NAD stock solution (50 mg of NAD dissolved in 10 mL of filter-distilled water), also aseptically added. If sulfonamides or trimethoprim are to be tested, 0.2 IU/mL thymidine phosphorylase should also be aseptically added to the medium.

[d] *S. aureus* exhibiting resistance to one of the penicillinase-resistant penicillins (MRSA) must be reported as resistant to cephalosporin-like antimicrobial agents, regardless of *in vitro* dilution test results, because in most cases of documented MRSA infections, patients have responded poorly to cephalosporin chemotherapy. Methicillin-resistant, coagulase-negative *Staphylococcus* spp also appear not to respond well to cephalosporin treatment, but the data are less clear than with *S. aureus*.

[e] Also applies to other *Staphylococcus* spp.

CAMHB, cation-adjusted Mueller-Hinton broth (26); MHA, Mueller-Hinton agar; QC, quality control; ATCC, American Type Culture Collection; NCCLS, National Committee for Clinical Laboratory Standards; TMP-SMX, trimethoprim-sulfamethaxazole; CSMHB, cation-supplemented Mueller-Hinton broth; BHI, brain-heart infusion; CFU, colony-forming unit; NAD, nicotinamide adenine dinucleotide.

is imperative that clinical laboratories routinely perform β-lactamase studies on all clinically significant isolates. Several media formulations have been employed for dilution or diffusion susceptibility testing with *H. influenzae* (65,120). Although individual methods may have been useful in individual laboratories, a common problem with these media formulations has been the complexity of their preparation and their opaque nature. Recently, a new simplified medium, HTM, has been developed; it avoids many of these problems (65). HTM is optically clear, stable, and reproducible from lot to lot and is currently available commercially from several manufacturers. The use of HTM has been advocated by CLSI (NCCLS) for both dilution and diffusion tests with *H. influenzae* (10). Guidelines for the interpretation of MIC and QC results with an *H. influenzae* reference strain are included in this chapter and are contained in Table 3.28.

In addition to *H. influenzae*, other problem organisms have been tested, as indicated in Table 3.28. Following is a discussion of current approaches to the testing of MRSA, *N. gonorrhoeae*, *S. pneumoniae*, *S. viridans*, *L. monocytogenes*, *E. corrodens*, and *Chlamydia* spp, along with appropriate references.

In general, the use of a full incubation interval of 24 hours and the addition of 2% NaCl to cation-supplemented MHB have facilitated the testing of MRSA and have greatly enhanced the reliability of standard microdilution tests in detecting such organisms (121–123). Variable results have been obtained with different dilution methods for testing MRSA strains with cephalosporins, and many strains appear fully susceptible to cephalosporins, which is inconsistent with treatment results. This has led to the standard recommendation that cephalosporin tests not be reported for MRSA and methicillin-resistant *S. epidermidis* (11).

Neisseria gonorrhoeae

The changing antimicrobial susceptibility of *N. gonorrhoeae* is an example of how clinical laboratories have had to modify their approaches and strategies in susceptibility testing. *N. gonorrhoeae* has developed resistance to all of the agents that have been recommended for gonorrhea therapy. When penicillin was the recommended therapy for *N. gonorrhoeae* infection, most isolates were initially susceptible. From the mid-1940s to the 1970s, there was a 24-fold increase in the dosage of pro-

Table 3.29

Broth Phenotypic Resistance Screening Tests in *Staphylococcus aureus*				
	mecA-Mediated Oxacillin Resistance	**Vancomycin MIC ≥8 µg/mL**	**Inducible Clindamycin Resistance**	**High-level Mupirocin Resistance**
Antimicrobial	4 µg/mL cefoxitin	No "standard" screening methodology documented	4 µg/mL erythromycin + 0.5 µg/mL clindamycin (in same well)	256 µg/mL mupirocin
Medium	Cation-adjusted Mueller-Hinton broth		Cation-adjusted Mueller-Hinton broth	Cation-adjusted Mueller-Hinton Broth
Inoculum	Standard broth microdilution		Standard broth microdilution	Standard broth microdilution
Incubation conditions	33°C–35°C ambient air 16–20 h		35°C ± 2°C ambient air	35°C ± 2°C ambient air 24 h
Results	>4 µg/mL = *mecA* positive		Growth = inducible clindamycin resistance	Growth = high-level mupirocin resistance
	≤4 µg/mL = *mecA* negative		No growth = no inducible clindamycin resistance	No growth = absence of high-level mupirocin resistance
Result reporting	Report as oxacillin resistant (not cefoxitin, which is used as surrogate)		Isolate presumed clindamycin resistant based on detection of inducible clindamycin resistance	High-level mupirocin detected (or *not* detected)
QC recommendation	*S. aureus* ATCC 43300 (MIC >4 µg/mL)		*S. aureus* ATCC 20213	*S. aureus* ATCC 29213 or *E. faecalis* ATCC 29212

QC, quality control; ATCC, American Type Culture Collection; MIC, minimum inhibitory concentration.

caine penicillin (2×10^5 units to 4.8×10^6 units). Penicillin is no longer the recommended therapy.

The resistance of *N. gonorrhoeae* to antibacterials is due either to multiple chromosomal mutations or to R factor plasmids. In 1987, the increasing prevalence of strains with β-lactamase plasmids prompted discontinuation of the use of penicillin as a single-dose therapy. Determining resistance, which is primarily a laboratory responsibility, affects epidemiologic surveillance and patient care.

A standardized laboratory method for monitoring the susceptibilities of gonococcal isolates was formulated and has been recommended by CLSI (NCCLS) based on a multicenter laboratory study whose purpose was to standardize disk diffusion and agar susceptibility tests (124). The recommended test medium is GC agar base with a defined XV-like supplement. Three QC organisms are required: *N. gonorrhoeae* ATCC strain 49226 (CDC F-18), *N. gonorrhoeae* WHO strain V, and *S. aureus* ATCC strain 25923.

The publication of the multicenter guidelines does not alter the need or methodology for detecting penicillinase-producing *N. gonorrhoeae*. Penicillinase-producing *N. gonorrhoeae* strains may be identified by detection of β-lactamase with a nitrocefin substrate (Table 3.28). Strains of *N. gonorrhoeae* that have chromosomally mediated resistance to antimicrobial agents or plasmid-mediated resistance to penicillin and/or tetracycline may be detected by measuring their susceptibilities by disk diffusion (124) and are not discussed here. Agar dilution methodology is preferred to broth dilution, as *N. gonorrhoeae* is known to autolyze in liquid media.

Streptococcus pneumoniae

Throughout the world, there have been increasing reports of the relative resistance of *S. pneumoniae* to penicillin as well as to other drugs such as tetracycline, erythromycin, clindamycin, and chloramphenicol (16,17). Nonsusceptible strains have been isolated in the United States with increasing frequency; thus, routine testing of isolates of *S. pneumoniae* is probably warranted. Satisfactory broth dilution tests can be performed with *S. pneumoniae*, provided that the broth medium is appropriately supplemented by adding 5% defibrinated sheep blood to freshly thawed MHB in microdilution trays that have been stored for no more than 2 months at 20°C. Commercially prepared test systems are available but have limitations and need to be verified and validated (125). Tests for other streptococci are indicated in Table 3.28.

Special studies related to susceptibility testing of several other species have been performed and are noted here. MICs, MBCs, and killing curves have been studied for *L. monocytogenes* using TS broth (126,127). *Pasteurella multocida* was tested in microtiter panels using MHB supplemented with 10% horse serum (128). Vanhoof et al. (129) evaluated inhibition and killing of *Campylobacter jejuni* in MHB. *E. corrodens* susceptibility testing has been accomplished using MHB supplemented with 0.5% lysed sheep blood (130). *Mycoplasma* spp have also been studied (131) in macrotube systems and by microdilution susceptibility testing (132,133). Unlike conventional bacteria, which can grow in artificial media, *Chlamydia trachomatis* has been tested against a variety of antimicrobial agents by incorporating antibiotic dilutions in cycloheximide-treated McCoy cell cultures (134,135). Utilizing this approach, MICs and MBCs can be determined (see Chapter 7).

Nocardia spp and Actinomycetes

In large part, problems associated with the susceptibility testing of this group of microorganisms relates to the new directions in the methods used for their identification. In the last 15 years, newer approaches such as molecular testing using 16S ribosomal RNA sequencing and Matrix-Assisted Laser Desorption Ionization-Time of Flight (MALDI-TOF) methodologies have been adopted (136,137). Although broth microdilution is the recommended methodology, false resistance using this approach has been documented, specifically for *Nocardia* spp (138). The generally recommended antimicrobial agents for primary testing are amikacin, amoxicillin-clavulanate, ceftriaxone, ciprofloxacin, clarithromycin, imipenem, linezolid, minocycline, moxifloxacin, trimethoprim-sulfamethoxazole and tobramycin. Secondary testing compromises cefepime, cefotaxime, doxycycline, rifampin, and vancomycin. Susceptibility testing for the aerobic actinomycetes requires 2 to 5 days, contrasted to 24 to 48 hours for species of *Rhodococcus*.

METHODS FOR DETECTION OF ANTIMICROBIAL RESISTANCE

Although there has been limited development of new antimicrobial agents and classes over the past 10 years, microorganisms have developed novel and, in some cases, multiresistant mechanisms to limit the clinical use of the available compounds. Several phenotypic and genotypic methods are available as screening tests, which do not result in an MIC but possess the necessary accuracy that confirmatory testing is not required and results can be used to guide antimicrobial therapy. Molecular, that is, genotypic, methods are reviewed by Hegstad et al. in Chapter 9 of this volume "Molecular Methods for Detection of Antibacterial Resistance Genes: Rationale and Applications"; phenotypic approach will be discussed here.

β-Lactamase Detection

Three iterations of this assay are available: acidometric, iodometric, and chromogenic; the latter being the most common. Results are typically available within 60 minutes. Although β-lactamase production inactivates ampicillin, amoxicillin, and penicillin for *N. gonorrhoeae*, it detects only one form of resistance and for chromosomally mediated resistance with PBPs, resistance can only be detected by disk diffusion or agar dilution methods. Because some β-lactamase–producing organisms (e.g., *Staphylococcus*) may produce detectable levels of the enzyme after induction, it is generally recommended that for serious infections requiring penicillin therapy an MIC be performed following the rapid phenotypic β-lactamase assay.

Detection of Methicillin Resistance: Methicillin-Resistant *Staphylococcus aureus* and Related Resistance Phenotypes

Rapid and early diagnosis of MRSA is necessary for prompt initiation of appropriate antimicrobial therapy. The most common method is culture modified more recently with the application of chromogenic agars (139). Other than molecular approaches there are no equivalent rapid "broth" phenotypic approaches. However, broth phenotypic resistance screening tests for *S. aureus* are extant and address *mecA*-mediated oxacillin resistance, inducible clindamycin resistance, and high-level murpirocin resistance (Table 3.29).

Rapid approaches for detection of methicillin resistance in *S. aureus* has become a major concern in hospital and community settings as the potential for this organism to become a multidrug-resistant pathogen capable of causing mild to severe infections poses a high risk of mortality (140). Although β-lactam antimicrobials are the drugs of choice for *S. aureus* whenever possible, glycopeptides—specifically, vancomycin—has become frontline therapy. The increased use of vancomycin associated with higher incidences of MRSA has resulted in reduced susceptibility to vancomycin.

In 1977, the initial strain of *S. aureus* with reduced susceptibility to vancomycin was reported in Japan (141). Strains considered to have reduced susceptibility are the following: vancomycin-resistant *Staphylococcus aureus* (VRSA) are characterized by MICs greater than or equal to 16 μg/mL; vancomycin-intermediate *Staphylococcus aureus* (VISA), characterized by MICs 4 to 8 μg/mL; and heterogeneously vancomycin-intermediate *Staphylococcus aureus* (h-VISA), defined as the presence of isolated populations of VISA with concentrations of organism at $1/10^5$ to 10^6 susceptible to vancomycin. h-VISA appears to be the stage before the development of VISA. The presence of h-VISA significantly compromises the treatment of patients with bacteremia and frequently escapes detection in the clinical laboratory. Population analysis profile/area under curve (PAP-AUC) ratio is considered to be the gold standard for detection; however, due to its complexity, it is not feasible to routinely perform in clinical settings. An expedient alternative is the E-test macromethod (MET) (140).

Clindamycin Resistance in Streptococci and Staphylococci

In streptococci, clindamycin and/or erythromycin resistance may be associated with the *erm* genes, which enable production of macrolide ribosomal methylases or to the expression of the *mef* gene, which turn on an efflux pump targeting only macrolides. Alternatively, *erm* enzymes cause decreased binding of macrolides and lincosamides (e.g., clindamycin and streptogramin antibiotics—the macrolide-lincosamide-streptogramin [MLS] phenotype). The MLS resistance phenotype can be either induced or constitutively expressed. Inducible clindamycin resistance cannot be determined by routine susceptibility testing. A suggested approach is the use of a single-well microdilution test containing 4 μg/mL erythromycin and 0.5 μg/mL clindamycin. Any growth in the well is an indication of inducible clindamycin resistance; no growth indicates the absence of inducible clindamycin resistance (see Table 3.29).

Aminoglycoside (High-Level Resistance) in Enterococcus

Typically, enterococci are innately resistant to low levels of aminoglycosides owing to their facultative anaerobic metabolism, which limits the uptake of drug. Cases of serious enterococcal infections and endocarditis mandate the use of an aminoglycoside plus a cell wall–directed agent such as ampicillin, penicillin, or vancomycin, or specifically in the latter case, an aminoglycoside and streptomycin.

The antibiotic combination allows for the increased uptake of drugs and leads to the directed bactericidal activity against the organism in the absence of high-level aminoglycoside resistance (HLAR). To determine the potential for HLAR, CLSI recommends HLAR screening of enterococci with gentamicin and streptomycin using a broth microdilution method by determining the growth capability of the recovered enterococcal isolate in the presence of 1,000 µg/mL of streptomycin or 500 µg/mL of gentamicin in BHI broth; other approaches are also described (142). (See Tables 3.29 and 3.30.)

Vancomycin-Resistant Enterococci

Vancomycin-resistant enterococci, common colonizers of the gastrointestinal tract represent opportunistic pathogens in health care facilities.

Two common patterns of enterococcal resistant are extant; both demonstrate elevated vancomycin MICs. The most clinically important type is vancomycin resistance associated with the acquisition of genomic elements in the form of a plasmid or other transmissible genetic element. Representation of this acquired trait is more frequently encountered in strains of *Enterococcus faecium* and *E. faecalis* harboring *van A* or *van B* genes that erode high levels of vancomycin resistance expressed as MICs greater than 128 µg/mL for the *van A* gene and lower MICs of 16 to 64 µg/mL for the *van B* gene. Another pattern of vancomycin resistance is intrinsic in nature and associated with *van C* and potentially other *van* genes; for example, *van E*, *van G*, and *van L* observed in species of *Enterococcus gallinarum* and *Enterococcus casseliflavus*. This expression of resistance results in low to intermediate levels typically in the range of 2 to 16 µg/mL. Guidelines for the susceptibility testing of enterococci to vancomycin are in the 2012 CLSI document (143).

Table 3.30

Broth Phenotypic Resistance Screening Tests for High-level Aminoglycoside Resistance and Inducible Clindamycin Resistance in *Streptococcus*

	High-level Aminoglycoside Resistance		Inducible Clindamycin Resistance	
	Gentamicin HLAR	**Streptomycin HLAR**	**β-Hemolytic Streptococci**	**S. pneumoniae**
Antimicrobials	Gentamicin 500 µg/mL	Streptomycin 1,000 µg/mL	1 µg/mL erythromycin and 0.5 µg/mL clindamycin in same well	1 µg/mL erythromycin and 0.5 µg/mL clindamycin in same well
Medium	BHI broth	BHI broth	Cation-adjusted Mueller-Hinton broth + LHB (2.5%–5%)	Cation-adjusted Mueller-Hinton broth + LHB (2.5%–5.0%)
Inoculum	Standard broth microdilution	Standard broth microdilution	Standard broth microdilution	Standard broth microdilution
Incubation conditions	35°C ± 2°C ambient air 24 h	35°C ± 2°C ambient air 24–48 h (if susceptible at 24 h, reincubate)	35°C ± 2°C ambient air 20–24 h	35°C ± 2°C ambient air 20–24 h
Results	Any growth = resistant	Any growth = resistant	*Any growth* = inducible clindamycin resistance *No growth* = no inducible clindamycin resistance	
Result/ Reporting	*Resistant* = not synergistic with cell wall active agents (e.g., ampicillin, penicillin, and vancomycin) *Susceptible* = synergistic with cell wall active agents (e.g., ampicillin, penicillin, and vancomycin)		Report inducible clindamycin resistant as "clindamycin resistant."	
QC recommendation	*E. faecalis* ATCC 29212 = susceptible	*E. faecalis* ATCC 29212 = susceptible	*S. pneumonia* ATCC 49619 or *S. aureus* ATCC BAA-976 = no growth	

HLAR, high-level aminoglycoside resistance; BHI, brain-heart infusion; ATCC, American Type Culture Collection.

Detection of Extended-Spectrum β-Lactamases in Enterobacteriaceae

Several genera among the Enterobacteriaceae and *P. aeruginosa* are capable of producing β-lactamases referred to as *extended-spectrum β-lactamases* (ESBLs), which have the capacity of hydrolyzing penicillins, aztreonam, and the cephalosporin groups encompassing the extended spectrum moieties as cefotaxime, ceftriaxone, ceftizoxime, and ceftazimine. Guidelines are available that specify screening and confirmatory approaches for detecting ESBL production in *E. coli, Klebsiella pneumoniae*, and *Proteus mirabilis* (144). (See Table 3.31.) ESBL screening should not be performed for *Enterobacter* spp and *Serratia* spp, which produce Amp C–type hydrolyzing enzymes; ESBL screening is not advised because false-negative results can occur. The need to screen and confirm the presence of ESBLs was necessitated because standard MIC (and disk diffusion) susceptibility testing were not uniformly capable of identifying isolates capable of producing ESBLs. As ESBLs are typically inhibited by clavulanic acid, this property was used to detect ESBLs and interpret that presence as potential for conferring resistance to all penicillins, cephalosporins, and the monobactam aztreonam. The establishment of new lower interpretive criteria for the three aforementioned drug groups based mainly on PK and pharmacodynamic (PD) data permitted clinical laboratories to abandon screening tests and that testing results for the three drug groups be reported as tested. The European Committee on Antimicrobial Susceptibility Testing (EUCAST) has adopted similar breakpoints for the cephalosporins (see Tables 3.32 and 3.33) and recommends that laboratories continue to screen and confirm ESBL production due to limited clinical data and that cephalosporin reporting results be diminished by one category of interpretation (i.e., "susceptible" to "intermediate") if ESBLs are detected (145).

Detection of Carbapenemase Activity in Enterobacteriaceae

Enzymes that hydrolyze the carbapenem class of antimicrobials, doripenem, ertapanem, meropenem, and imipenem—referred to as *carbapenemases*—usually hydrolyze other currently used β-lactams with the exception of aztreonam. Carbapenemases have been identified in a wide range of gram-negative genera and are subdivided into three classes composed of serine class A (including KPC, SME,

IMI, GES, and NMC); class B enzymes, the metallo-β-lactamases (VIM, IMP, and NDM); and class D OXA enzymes (146). KPC is recognized as the most frequently identified class A carbapenemase in the United States and can be found in the Enterobacteriaceae and in *P. aeruginosa* (147). Metallo-β-lactamases are typically detected in *Acinetobacter* spp and *P. aeruginosa*; however, the NDM group is widespread among Enterobacteriaceae, particularly *K. pneumoniae*. The OXA group is associated with *Acinetobacter* spp but has also been reported in the Enterobacteriaceae.

Other than in 2009, the modified Hodge test was the recommended methodology for the detection of carbapenemase activity in Enterobacteriaceae (148). The assay is an agar diffusion methodology, which uses the reduced activity of a carbapenem, ertapenem, or meropenem observed by an indentation of the zone of inhibition against known stock strain of carbapenemase-producing *K. pneumoniae*. This test was originally recommended when carbapenem MICs were elevated or resistant. In 2010, the CLSI lowered the breakpoints for carbapenems to identify carbapenemase-producing strains, which would test as intermediate or resistant to this antimicrobial group. Use of the revised breakpoints eliminates the need to routinely perform the modified Hodge test, although such testing may be of value for epidemiologic or infection control.

An overview of the guidance for detection of ESBLs and carbapenemases as suggested by Livermore et al. (149) appears in Table 3.34.

Detection of Plasmid-Mediated AMPC-Type β-Lactamases

This group of β-lactamases, in some cases chromosomally mediated, are produced by a wide range of gram-negative species. Although detection of this group of enzymes is deemed important for epidemiologic and infection control initiatives, no sufficiently standardized testing regimens has been developed to use a screening approach.

AUTOMATED, RAPID, AND INSTRUMENT-ASSOCIATED METHODS

Direct Microscopy and Observation of Bacterial Morphology

Early in the use of penicillin, it was noted that cultures of either spinal fluid or blood taken from individuals who had been treated with penicillin

(continued on page 112)

Table 3.31

Broth Phenotypic Resistance Screening/Confirmatory Tests

	ESBLs		Carbapenemase[a]	
	Screen	**Confirmatory**	**Screen**	**Confirmatory**
Antimicrobials	*K. pneumoniae, K. oxytoca,* and *E. coli* Cefpodoxime 4 µg/mL or Ceftazidime 1 µg/mL or Aztreonam 1 µg/mL or Cefotaxime 1 µg/mL or Ceftriaxone 1 µg/mL *P. mirabilis* Cefpodoxime 1 µg/mL Ceftazidime 1 µg/mL Cefotaxime 1 µg/mL	Ceftazidime 0.25–128 µg/mL Ceftazidime-clavulanic acid 0.25/4–128/4 µg/mL and Cefotaxime 0.25–64 µg/mL Cefotaxime-clavulanic acid 0.25/4–64/4 µg/mL Use of both cefotaxime and ceftazidime alone and in combination with clavulanic acid	Ertapenem 1 µg/mL or Imipenem 1 µg/mL or Meropenem 1 µg/mL	A confirmatory test in broth is not available. Use Mueller-Hinton agar and the modified Hodge test (144).
Medium	Cation-adjusted Mueller-Hinton broth	Cation-adjusted Mueller-Hinton broth	Cation-adjusted Mueller-Hinton broth	
Inoculum	Standard broth microdilution	Standard broth microdilution	Standard broth microdilution	
Incubation conditions	35°C ± 2°C 16–20 h	35°C ± 2°C ambient air 16–20 h	35°C ± 2°C ambient air 16–20 h	
Results	Growth at or above test concentrations may indicate ESBL production.	A ≥3 twofold decrease in MIC for either antimicrobial tested in combination with clavulanic acid versus the MIC when tested alone	Growth at or above test concentration may indicate carbapenemase production.	
Result/Reporting	Screen-positive for ESBLs or reflex to confirmatory test.	For confirmed ESBL-producing strains report as resistant to penicillins, cephalosporins, and aztreonam		
QC recommendation	*K. pneumoniae,* ATCC 700603 *E. coli* ATCC 25922	A <3 twofold concentration decrease in MIC for combo testing with clavulanic acid.	*E. coli* ATCC 25922	

[a]Use with "old" interpretive criteria for carbapenems and CLSI M100-S20, January 2010 (114).
ESBLs, extended-spectrum β-lactamases; MIC, minimum inhibitory concentration; ATCC, American Type Culture Collection.

TABLE 3.32

2013 Clinical and Laboratory Standards Institute Minimum Inhibitory Concentration Interpretive Standards for Enterobacteriaceae, *Pseudomonas aeruginosa*, *Acinetobacter* spp, and *Stenotrophomonas maltophilia*

Drug Class	Antimicrobial Agents	Enterobacteriaceae		P. aeruginosa		Acinetobacter spp		S. maltophilia		Other Nonfermenters	
		CLSI	EUCAST	CLSI	EUCAST	CLSI	EUCAST	CLSI	EUCAST	CLSI	EUCAST
		R	R	R	R	R	R	R	R	R	R
Penicillins	Ampicillin	≥32	≥8	NA	NA	NA	NA	NA	NA	NA	NA
	Piperacillin	≥128	≥16	≥128	≥16	≥128	NA	NA	NA	≥128	NA
	Ticarcillin	≥128	≥16	≥128	≥16	≥128	NA	NA	NA	≥128	NA
	Mezlocillin	≥32	≥8	NA	NA	≥128	NA	NA	NA	≥128	NA
β-Lactamase inhibitors	Amoxicillin/clavulanic acid	≥32/16	≥8/2	NA	NA	NA	NA	NA	NA	NA	NA
	Ampicillin/sulbactam	≥32/16	≥8/4	NA	NA	≥32/16	NA	NA	NA	NA	NA
	Piperacillin/tazobactam	≥128/4	≥16/4	≥128/4	≥16/4	≥128/4	NA	NA	NA	≥128/4	NA
	Ticarcillin/clavulanic acid	≥128/2	≥16/2	≥128/2	≥16/2	≥128/2	NA	≥128/2	NA	≥128/2	NA
Cephems (parenteral)	Cefazolin	≥8	NA	NA	NA	NA	NA	NA	NA	NA	NA
	Cephalothin	≥32	NA	NA	NA	NA	NA	NA	NA	NA	NA
	Cefepime	≥32	≥4	≥32	≥8	≥32	NA	NA	NA	≥32	NA
	Ceftriaxone	≥4	≥2	NA	NA	≥64	NA	NA	NA	≥64	NA
	Cefotaxime	≥4	≥2	NA	NA	≥64	NA	NA	NA	≥64	NA
	Cefotetan	≥64	NA	NA	NA	NA	NA	NA	NA	NA	NA
	Cefoxitin	≥32	NA	NA	NA	NA	NA	NA	NA	NA	NA
	Cefuroxime	≥32	≥8	NA	NA	NA	NA	NA	NA	NA	NA
	Ceftaroline	≥2	≥0.5	NA	NA	NA	NA	NA	NA	NA	NA
	Ceftazidime	≥16	≥4	≥32	≥8	≥32	NA	≥32	NA	≥32	NA
	Cefamandole	≥32	NA	NA	NA	NA	NA	NA	NA	NA	NA
	Cefmetazole	≥32	NA	NA	NA	NA	NA	NA	NA	NA	NA
	Cefonicid	≥32	NA	NA	NA	NA	NA	NA	NA	NA	NA
	Cefoperazone	≥64	NA	NA	NA	NA	NA	NA	NA	≥64	NA

Class	Drug	1	2	3	4	5	6	7	8	9
	Ceftizoxime	≥4	NA	NA	NA	NA	NA	NA	≥64	NA
	Moxalactam	≥64	NA	NA	NA	NA	NA	NA	≥64	NA
Cephems (oral)	Cefuroxime	≥32	≥8	NA	NA	NA	NA	NA	NA	NA
	Loracarbef	≥32	NA	NA	NA	NA	NA	NA	NA	NA
	Cefaclor	≥32	NA	NA	NA	NA	NA	NA	NA	NA
	Cefdinir	≥4	NA	NA	NA	NA	NA	NA	NA	NA
	Cefixime	≥4	≥1	NA	NA	NA	NA	NA	NA	NA
	Cefpodoxime	≥8	≥1	NA	NA	NA	NA	NA	NA	NA
	Cefprozil	≥32	NA	NA	NA	NA	NA	NA	NA	NA
	Cefetamet	≥16	NA	NA	NA	NA	NA	NA	NA	NA
	Ceftibuten	≥32	≥1	NA	NA	NA	NA	NA	NA	NA
Monolactam	Aztreonam	≥16	≥4	≥32	≥16	NA	NA	NA	≥32	NA
Carbapenems	Doripenem	≥4	≥4	≥8	≥4	≥4	NA	NA	NA	NA
	Ertapenem	≥2	≥1	NA	NA	NA	NA	NA	NA	NA
	Imipenem	≥4	≥8	≥8	≥8	≥8	NA	NA	≥16	NA
	Meropenem	≥4	≥8	≥8	≥8	≥8	NA	NA	≥16	NA
Tetracyclines	Tetracycline	≥16	NA	NA	≥16	≥16	NA	NA	≥16	NA
	Doxycycline	≥16	NA	NA	≥16	≥16	NA	NA	≥16	NA
	Minocycline	≥16	NA	NA	≥16	≥16	≥16	NA	≥16	NA
Aminoglycosides	Gentamicin	≥16	≥4	≥16	≥4	≥16	≥16	NA	≥16	NA
	Tobramycin	≥16	≥4	≥16	≥4	≥16	≥16	NA	≥16	NA
	Amikacin	≥64	≥16	≥64	≥16	≥64	≥64	NA	≥64	NA
	Kanamycin	≥64	NA	NA	NA	NA	NA	NA	NA	NA
	Netilmicin	≥32	≥4	≥32	≥4	≥32	≥32	NA	≥32	NA

(Continued)

TABLE 3.32 (Continued)

2013 Clinical and Laboratory Standards Institute Minimum Inhibitory Concentration Interpretive Standards for Enterobacteriaceae, *Pseudomonas aeruginosa*, *Acinetobacter* spp, and *Stenotrophomonas maltophilia*

Drug Class	Antimicrobial Agents	Enterobacteriaceae CLSI	Enterobacteriaceae EUCAST	P. aeruginosa CLSI	P. aeruginosa EUCAST	Acinetobacter spp CLSI	Acinetobacter spp EUCAST	S. maltophilia CLSI	S. maltophilia EUCAST	Other Nonfermenters CLSI	Other Nonfermenters EUCAST
		R	R	R	R	R	R	R	R	R	R
Fluoroquinolones	Ciprofloxacin	≥4	≥1	≥4	≥1	≥4	≥1	NA	NA	≥4	NA
	Levofloxacin	≥8	≥2	≥8	≥2	≥8	≥2	≥8	NA	≥8	NA
	Lomefloxacin	≥8	NA	≥8	NA	NA	NA	NA	NA	≥8	NA
	Ofloxacin	≥8	≥1	≥8	NA	NA	NA	NA	NA	≥8	NA
	Norfloxacin	≥16	≥1	≥16	NA	NA	NA	NA	NA	≥16	NA
	Enoxacin	≥8	NA	NA	NA	NA	NA	NA	NA	NA	NA
	Gatifloxacin	≥8	NA	≥8	NA	≥8	NA	NA	NA	≥8	NA
	Gemifloxacin	≥1	NA	NA	NA	NA	NA	NA	NA	NA	NA
	Grepafloxacin	≥4	NA	NA	NA	NA	NA	NA	NA	NA	NA
	Fleroxacin	≥8	NA	NA	NA	NA	NA	NA	NA	NA	NA
Quinolones	Cinoxacin	≥64	NA	NA	NA	NA	NA	NA	NA	NA	NA
	Naladixic acid	≥32	NA	NA	NA	NA	NA	NA	NA	NA	NA
Folate pathway inhibitors	TMP-SXT	≥4/76	≥4	NA	NA	≥4/76	≥4	≥4/76	≥4	≥4/76	NA
	Sulfonamides	≥512	NA	NA	NA	NA	NA	NA	NA	≥512	NA
	Trimethoprim	≥16	≥4	NA	NA	NA	NA	NA	NA	NA	NA
Phenicols	Cholramphenicol	≥32	≥8	NA	NA	NA	NA	≥32	NA	≥32	NA
Fosfomycin	Fosfomycin	≥256	≥32	NA	NA	NA	NA	NA	NA	NA	NA
Nitrofurans	Nitrofurantoin	≥128	≥64	NA	NA	NA	NA	NA	NA	NA	NA
Lipopeptides	Colistin	NA	≥2	≥8	≥4	≥4	≥2	NA	NA	≥8	NA
	Polymyxin B	NA	NA	≥8	≥4	≥4	NA	NA	NA	≥8	NA

From Clinical and Laboratory Standards Institute. Performance standards for antimicrobial susceptibility testing. Twenty-third informational supplement. Wayne, PA: Clinical and Laboratory Standards Institute, 2013. CLSI publication M100-S23; European Committee on Antimicrobial Susceptibility Testing. Expert Rules. Version 2.0. 29 October 2011. www.eucast.org/expertrules. Accessed July 2013.

Table 3.33

2013 Clinical and Laboratory Standards Institute Minimum Inhibitory Concentration Interpretive Standards for *Staphylococcus*, *Enterococcus*, *Streptococcus pneumoniae*, and *Streptococcus* spp other than SPNE

Drug Class	Antimicrobial Agents	Staphylococcus CLSI R	Staphylococcus EUCAST R	Enterococcus CLSI R	Enterococcus EUCAST R	S. pneumoniae CLSI R	S. pneumoniae EUCAST R	α-Hemolytic Streptococci CLSI R	α-Hemolytic Streptococci EUCAST R	β-Hemolytic Streptococci CLSI R	β-Hemolytic Streptococci EUCAST R
Penicillins	Penicillin	≥0.25	≥0.12	≥16	NA	≥8	≥2	≥4	≥2	≥0.12	≥0.25
	Oxacillin	≥4	≥2	NA	NA	NA	NA	NA	NA	NA	NA
	Ampicillin	NA	NA	≥16	≥8	≥8	≥2	≥8	≥2	≥0.25	NA
	Methicillin	NA	NA	NA	NA	NA	NA	NA	NA	NA	NA
	Nafcillin	NA	NA	NA	NA	NA	NA	NA	NA	NA	NA
β-Lactamase inhibitors	Amoxicillin/clavulanic acid	≥8/4	NA	NA	≥8/2	≥8/4	NA	NA	NA	NA	NA
	Ampicillin/sulbactam	≥32/16	NA	NA	≥8/4	NA	NA	NA	NA	NA	NA
	Piperacillin/tazobactam	≥16/4	NA	NA	NA	NA	NA	NA	NA	NA	NA
	Ticar/clav	≥16/2	NA	NA	NA	NA	NA	NA	NA	NA	NA
Cephems (parenteral)	Cefamandole	NA	NA	NA	NA	NA	NA	NA	NA	NA	NA
	Cefazolin	NA	NA	NA	NA	NA	NA	NA	≥0.5	NA	NA
	Cefepime	NA	NA	NA	NA	≥4	≥2	≥4	≥0.5	NA	NA
	Cefmetazole	NA	NA	NA	NA	NA	NA	NA	NA	NA	NA
	Cefonicid	NA	NA	NA	NA	NA	NA	NA	NA	NA	NA
	Cefoperazone	NA	NA	NA	NA	NA	NA	NA	NA	NA	NA
	Cefotaxime	NA	NA	NA	NA	≥4	≥2	≥4	≥0.5	NA	NA
	Cefotetan	NA	NA	NA	NA	NA	NA	NA	NA	NA	NA
	Ceftaroline	NA	≥1	NA	NA	NA	≥0.25	NA	NA	NA	NA
	Ceftazidime	NA	NA	NA	NA	NA	NA	NA	NA	NA	NA
	Ceftizoxime	NA	NA	NA	NA	NA	NA	NA	NA	NA	NA
	Ceftriaxone	NA	NA	NA	NA	≥4	≥2	≥4	≥0.5	NA	NA
	Cefuroxime	NA	NA	NA	NA	≥2	≥1	≥4	≥0.5	NA	NA

(Continued)

Table 3.33 (Continued)

2013 Clinical and Laboratory Standards Institute Minimum Inhibitory Concentration Interpretive Standards for *Staphylococcus, Enterococcus, Streptococcus pneumoniae,* and *Streptococcus* spp other than SPNE

Drug Class	Antimicrobial Agents	*Staphylococcus*		*Enterococcus*		*S. pneumoniae*		α-Hemolytic Streptococci		β-Hemolytic Streptococci	
		CLSI	EUCAST	CLSI	EUCAST	CLSI	EUCAST	CLSI	EUCAST	CLSI	EUCAST
		R	R	R	R	R	R	R	R	R	R
Cephems (oral)	Cephalothin	NA	NA	NA	NA	NA	NA	NA	NA	NA	NA
	Moxalactam	NA	NA	NA	NA	NA	NA	NA	NA	NA	NA
	Cefoxitin	≥8	≥4	NA	NA	NA	NA	NA	NA	NA	NA
	Cefaclor	NA	NA	NA	NA	≥4	≥0.5	NA	NA	NA	NA
	Cefdinir	NA	NA	NA	NA	≥2	NA	NA	NA	NA	NA
	Cefpodoxime	NA	NA	NA	NA	≥2	≥0.5	NA	NA	NA	NA
	Cefprozil	NA	NA	NA	NA	≥8	NA	NA	NA	NA	NA
	Cefuroxime	NA	NA	NA	NA	≥4	NA	NA	NA	NA	NA
	Loracarbef	NA	NA	NA	NA	≥8	NA	NA	NA	NA	NA
Carbapenems	Doripenem	NA	NA	NA	NA	NA	≥1	NA	≥1	NA	NA
	Ertapenem	NA	NA	NA	NA	≥4	≥0.5	NA	≥0.5	NA	NA
	Imipenem	NA	NA	NA	≥8	≥1	≥2	NA	≥2	NA	NA
	Meropenem	NA	NA	NA	NA	≥1	≥2	NA	≥2	NA	NA
Tetracyclines	Tetracycline	≥16	≥2	≥16	NA	≥4	≥2	≥8	NA	≥8	≥2
	Doxycycline	≥16	≥2	≥16	NA	≥1	≥2	NA	NA	NA	≥2
	Minocycline	≥16	≥1	≥16	NA	NA	≥1	NA	NA	NA	≥1
Aminoglycosides	Gentamicin	≥16	≥1	NA	NA	NA	NA	NA	NA	NA	NA
	Amikacin	≥64	≥16	NA	NA	NA	NA	NA	NA	NA	NA
	Kanamycin	≥64	NA	NA	NA	NA	NA	NA	NA	NA	NA
	Netilimicin	≥32	≥1	NA	NA	NA	NA	NA	NA	NA	NA
	Tobramycin	≥16	≥1	NA	NA	NA	NA	NA	NA	NA	NA

Macrolides	Azithromycin	≥8	≥2	NA	NA	≥2	≥0.5	≥2	NA	≥2	≥0.5
	Clarithromycin	≥8	≥2	NA	NA	≥1	≥0.5	≥1	NA	≥1	≥0.5
	Erythromycin	≥8	≥2	≥8	NA	≥1	≥0.5	≥1	NA	≥1	≥0.5
	Telithromycin	≥4	NA	NA	NA	≥4	≥0.5	≥4	NA	NA	≥0.5
	Dirithromycin	≥8	NA	NA	NA	≥2	NA	≥2	NA	≥2	NA
Fluoroquinolones	Ciprofloxacin	≥4	≥1	≥4	NA	NA	≥2	NA	NA	NA	NA
	Levofloxacin	≥4	≥2	≥8	NA	≥8	≥2	≥8	NA	≥8	≥2
	Ofloxacin	≥4	≥1	NA	NA	≥8	≥4	≥8	NA	≥8	NA
	Moxifloxacin	≥2	≥1	NA	NA	≥4	≥0.5	NA	NA	NA	≥1
	Lomefloxacin	≥8	NA	≥8	NA	NA	NA	NA	NA	NA	NA
	Norfloxacin	≥16	NA	≥16	NA	NA	NA	NA	NA	NA	NA
	Enoxacin	≥8	NA	NA	NA	NA	NA	NA	NA	NA	NA
	Gemifloxacin	NA	NA	NA	NA	≥0.5	NA	NA	NA	NA	NA
	Gatifloxacin	≥2	NA	≥8	NA	≥4	NA	≥4	NA	≥4	NA
	Grepafloxacin	≥4	NA	NA	NA	≥2	NA	≥2	NA	≥2	NA
	Sparfloxacin	≥2	NA	NA	NA	≥2	NA	≥2	NA	NA	NA
	Fleroxacin	≥8	NA	NA	NA	≥4	NA	≥4	NA	NA	NA
	Trovafloxacin	NA	NA	NA	NA	≥4	NA	≥4	NA	≥4	NA
Glycopeptides	Vancomycin	Saur ≥16 CNS ≥32	Saur ≥2 CNS ≥4	≥32	≥4	NA	≥2	NA	≥2	NA	≥2
	Teicoplanin	≥32	Saur ≥2 CNS ≥4	≥32	≥2	NA	≥2	NA	≥2	NA	≥2
Lincosamides	Clindamycin	≥4	≥0.5	NA	NA	≥1	≥0.5	≥1	≥0.5	≥1	≥0.5
Folate pathway inhibitors	TMP-SXT	≥4/76	≥4	NA	≥1	≥4/76	≥2	NA	NA	NA	≥2
	Sulfonamides	≥512	NA	NA	≥1	NA	NA	NA	NA	NA	NA
	Trimethoprim	≥16	≥4	NA	≥1	NA	NA	NA	NA	NA	≥2

(Continued)

Table 3.33 (Continued)

2013 Clinical and Laboratory Standards Institute Minimum Inhibitory Concentration Interpretive Standards for *Staphylococcus, Enterococcus, Streptococcus pneumoniae,* and *Streptococcus* spp other than SPNE

Drug Class	Antimicrobial Agents	Staphylococcus		Enterococcus		S. pneumoniae		α-Hemolytic Streptococci		β-Hemolytic Streptococci	
		CLSI	EUCAST	CLSI	EUCAST	CLSI	EUCAST	CLSI	EUCAST	CLSI	EUCAST
		R	R	R	R	R	R	R	R	R	R
Phenicols	Cholramphenicol	≥32	≥8	≥32	NA	≥8	≥8	≥16	NA	≥16	≥8
Fosfomycin	Fosfomycin	NA	≥32	≥256	NA	NA	NA	NA	NA	NA	NA
Nitrofurans	Nitrofurantoin	≥128	≥64	≥128	≥64	NA	NA	NA	NA	NA	≥64
Lipopeptides	Daptomycin	NA	≥1	NA	NA	NA	NA	NA	NA	NA	≥1
Ansamycins	Rifampin	≥4	NA	≥4	NA	≥4	NA	NA	NA	NA	NA
Streptogramins	Quinupristin-dalfopristin	≥4	≥2	≥4	≥4	≥4	NA	≥4	NA	≥4	NA
Oxazolidinones	Linezolid	≥8	≥4	≥8	≥4	NA	≥4	NA	NA	NA	≥4

From Clinical and Laboratory Standards Institute. Performance standards for antimicrobial susceptibility testing. Twenty-third informational supplement. Wayne, PA: Clinical and Laboratory Standards Institute, 2013. CLSI publication M100-S23; European Committee on Antimicrobial Susceptibility Testing. Expert Rules. www.eucast.org/expertrules. Version 2.0. 29 October 2011. Accessed July 2013.

Chapter 3: Susceptibility Testing of Antimicrobials in Liquid Media**111**

Table 3.34

Guidance and Interpretive Breakpoints for Testing and Detecting Extended-Spectrum β-Lactamases and Carbapenemase for Enterobacteriaceae

Organization	Guidance Pre-2011	Guidance Post-2011	Breakpoints (µg/mL) Pre-2011 CTX/CRO	FEP	CAZ	IPM/MEM	ETP	Post-2011 CTX	FEP	CAZ	IPM/MEM	ETP
CLSI	Test for ESBL by clavulanate synergy or carbapenemases by Hodge test; report ESBL producers as cephalosporin resistant	No test for ESBL or carbapenemase; report as tested.	S≤8	S≤8	S≤8	S≤4	S≤2	S≤1	S≤8	S≤4	S≤1	S≤0.25
			R≥64	R≥32	R≥32	R≥16	R≥8	R≥4	R≥32	R≥16	R≥4	R≥1
EUCAST	ESBL producers, edit correct: cephalosporin	Report as tested.	S≤1	S≤1	S≤1	S≤2	S≤0.5	S≤1	S≤1	S≤1	S≤1	S≤0.5
	S to I and I to R		R>2	R>8	R>8	R>8	R>1	R>2	R>4	R>4	R>4	R>1

CLSI, Clinical and Laboratory Standards Institute; EBSL, extended-spectrum β-lactamase; CTX, cefotaxime; CRO, ceftriaxone; FEP, cefepime; CAZ, ceftazidime; IPM, imipenem; MEM, meropenem; ETP, ertapenem; S, susceptible; I, intermediate; R, resistant; EUCAST, European Committee on Antibiotic Susceptibility Testing.

demonstrated aberrant forms in these clinical specimens. Observations of morphologic alterations in bacteria produced during early exposure to various antimicrobial agents were recorded by several investigators (150,151). Growth can be observed by a variety of means, including light, phase-contrast, and electron microscopy, with different changes being produced by an antibiotic, depending on the bacterial species and the mode of action and concentration of the agent. Antibiotics, especially those of the β-lactam class, which interfere with cell wall synthesis and bind to the lytic PBPs (see "Minimal Bactericidal Concentration"), can produce various filamentous forms or protoplasmic enlargements (152). Similar morphologic alterations can be seen in inocula exposed to concentrations that are below the MIC but that nonetheless modify the characteristics of the affected bacterial population (153).

The minimum amount of antimicrobial agent necessary to induce such alterations has been termed the *minimal antibacterial concentration* (MAC) (153,154). When visualized by light microscopy, this approach represents a rapid method because the changes may occur rapidly, occasionally within minutes. However, these observations are qualitative, the methods are not standardized, and the observations are labor-intensive.

Clinical data demonstrating the relevance of a given alternative antibiotic susceptibility test method in the care and management of infectious disease are based primarily on the MIC of the agent against the infecting organism. Additional investigation is needed to establish the interpretive significance of a standard derived from the new approach. Thus, in the MAC approach, one would have to study the MAC/MIC ratios (153,155) to determine the MAC's clinical utility.

Early Reading of Conventional Tests

Like in the early reading of disk diffusion tests, where the kinetics of growth and zone formation are fairly well stabilized for many drug–bug interactions within 8 hours of incubation and frequently within 5 hours (156) or 6 hours (88), results of rapid or early reading can be estimated in liquid media. It is suggested, however, that early estimated results be confirmed by a later reading or by retesting with conventional incubation intervals. Lampe et al. (157) determined the accuracy of early reading compared with standard ICS macrotube dilution (i.e., 3 hours in comparison with the conventional

18-hour incubation time). Values from the conventional incubation were at least four times higher than those from the early 3-hour reading for 43% of the strains tested. Agreement was improved with the 8-hour incubation period. When procedural modifications were initiated for the purpose of producing rapid results that would conform to conventional end points, comparisons of different media, shaking versus static cultures, and reading by particle count versus visually did not eliminate the discrepancies (157). However, increasing the inoculum size to possibly 10^7 CFU/mL produced better agreement, with 14% of the test isolates demonstrating fourfold dilution errors (Table 3.35). Because this approach is not applicable to all species, especially in view of variable mechanisms of resistance, additional clinical investigations of these interpretations are warranted. Until such investigations for establishing clinical guidance in earlier time frames are completed, the focus will be on the reference overnight method.

There have been attempts over the years to develop methods that could enhance the apparent growth of bacteria and thereby reduce the conventional overnight incubation required to determine an MIC. Investigators have used colorimetric indicators and leuco dyes to amplify the macroscopic observation of turbidity. In macrodilution assays, phenol red was added to assay tubes containing glucose and yeast extract to enhance growth. If the test organism grew utilizing the glucose, tubes would turn yellow as a result of the pH change. If the antimicrobial agent inhibited the organism, the indicator would remain red. Nonfermenter organisms could be detected by an orange-red color if they grew in the antibiotic-free tubes.

Redox indicators such as resazurin, triphenyltetrazolium chloride, and methylene blue have been used as indicators of growth (158). Because these dyes may be antibacterial, the strategy was to add them to the control tube after a brief (3- to 5-hour) incubation period. If sufficient growth was then detectable, the indicator would be added to all assay tubes. Bartlett and Mazens (159) enhanced the sensitivity of triphenyltetrazolium chloride by the addition of phenazine methosulfate, which accelerated formation of the red formazan precipitate resulting from growth of the bacteria. The indophenol reagent dichlorophenolindophenol is another redox dye that has been tested (93). A proprietary tetrazolium-type reagent (Alamar blue) incorporated into commercially prepared antibiotic-containing testing panels has received some attention (160).

Table 3.35

Comparison of Overnight Minimum Inhibitory Concentration Readings with Inocula of 10^5/mL[a] to 3-Hour Readings with Inocula of 10^7/mL

					Ratio of 18- to 3-Hour Readings				
Determinants	**0.03**	**0.125**	**0.25**	**0.5**	**1**	**2**	**4**	**8**	**Total Strains**
Three- and 18-hour MICs within range tested		2	5	20	32	9	2	1	71[c]
One of the two MICs above the range tested[b]	1	1	2	6	—[c]		1		11[c]
One of the two MICs below the range tested[b]				4					4[c]
Subtotals	1	3	7	30	32[c]	9	3	1	
Total		11			71[c]		4		86[c]

[a]ICS broth tube dilution method (6).
[b]Ratios calculated by considering MIC readings of, for example, >128 as 256 and <0.25 as 0.125.
[c]In 22 cases, both MICs were above the range tested and were excluded.
MIC, minimum inhibitory concentration.
Adapted from Lampe MR, Aitken CL, Dennis PG, et al. Relationship of early readings of minimal inhibitory concentrations to the results of overnight tests. *Antimicrob Agents Chemother* 1975;8:429–433.

In a unique approach, bacterial respiration was detected utilizing the respiration of hemoglobin as an indicator. A 3% suspension of red blood cells (outdated human or animal) served as the indicator (161).

The rapid approaches described in these early reports have not been accepted by and are not applied in clinical or reference laboratories. Had they received some commercial impetus and if ample reference and QC measures had been developed to ensure reliability, they might have achieved acceptance.

Alternative Rapid Instrumental Methods

Detection of Bacteria and Bacterial Products

In the search for rapid methods for determining the interaction of antimicrobial agents and organisms, microbiologists have examined the products of bacterial metabolism (intermediate and end products) as well as the interaction of the organism with various energy sources. In addition to the more complex products of bacterial metabolism detectable by gas chromatographic methods (162), there are the more immediate end products of glucose degradation (i.e., CO_2, water, energy, adenosine triphosphate [ATP], and heat). Thus, if glucose is tagged with radioactive carbon or some other substrate is similarly tagged, then the CO_2 released via bacterial metabolism is radioactive and can be detected by radiometry (163–166). Alternatively, the CO_2 produced can be monitored by infrared spectroscopy to detect growth (266). Also, the ATP produced by metabolism can be measured by the luciferin-luciferase reaction, and the energy quanta derived from this interaction can be measured with an ATP luminometer (167). Similarly, heat in the form of nonutilizable energy derived from the enzymatic degradation of glucose can be detected (Fig. 3.8) and measured by microcalorimetry (27). As bacteria replicate in the growth medium, they decrease the measured electrical resistance (impedance in alternating-current circuits) in the medium (Fig. 3.9). Impedance has been measured in bacterial cultures by passing a high-voltage, alternating-current signal through the medium and monitoring its effect (168–170). All of these approaches are bacteriologically sound, in that any method used to detect bacterial growth can be applied to the measurement of the interaction of antimicrobial and bacterium and thus to the testing of susceptibility (27,171).

Of the several methods noted here, two persist in commercial instrumentation suitable for clinical laboratories: radiometry and ATP luminometry. Only the former is currently applied to antimicrobial susceptibility testing, specifically with mycobacteria (172,173,269).

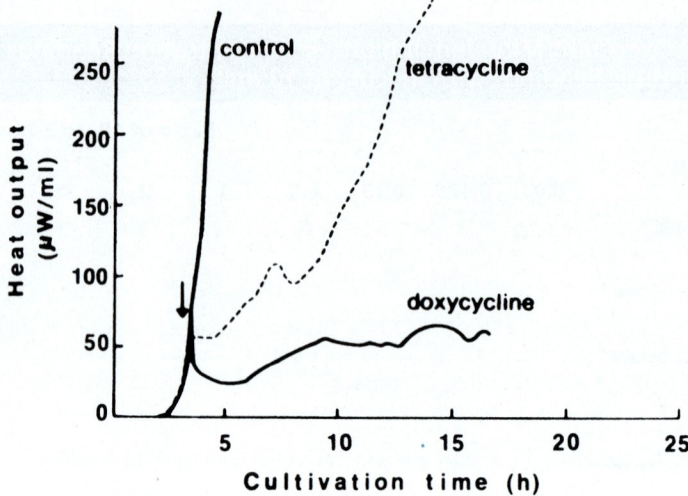

Figure 3.8 ■ **Microcalorimetric response of logarithmic-phase cells of** **_E. coli_ toward two antibiotics.** _Arrow_, time of addition of drugs. (Reproduced from Mardh PA, Anderson KE, Wadso I. Kinetics of the actions of tetracyclines on _Escherichia coli_ as studied by microcalorimetry. _Antimicrob Agents Chemother_ 1976;10:604–609.)

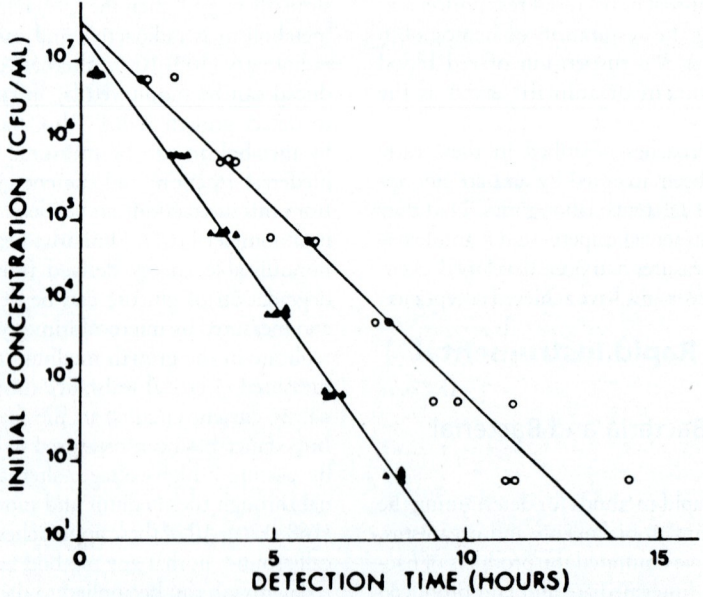

Figure 3.9 ■ **Detection times by electrical impedance monitoring graphed** **against initial concentrations of microorganisms for _E. coli_ (▲) and _S. aure-_** **_us_ (○), both growing in TS broth at 35°C.** The _solid lines_ represent least-squares linear fits to the data points for each organism. The slopes of the lines reflect the organisms' generation times (26 minutes for _E. coli_ and 38 minutes for _S. aureus_). The correlation between log initial concentration and detection time was 0.95 for _E. coli_ and 0.94 for _S. aureus_. (Reproduced from Cady PS, Dufour W, Draeger SJ. Electrical impedance measurements: rapid method for detecting and monitoring microorganisms. _J Clin Microbiol_ 1978;7:265–272.)

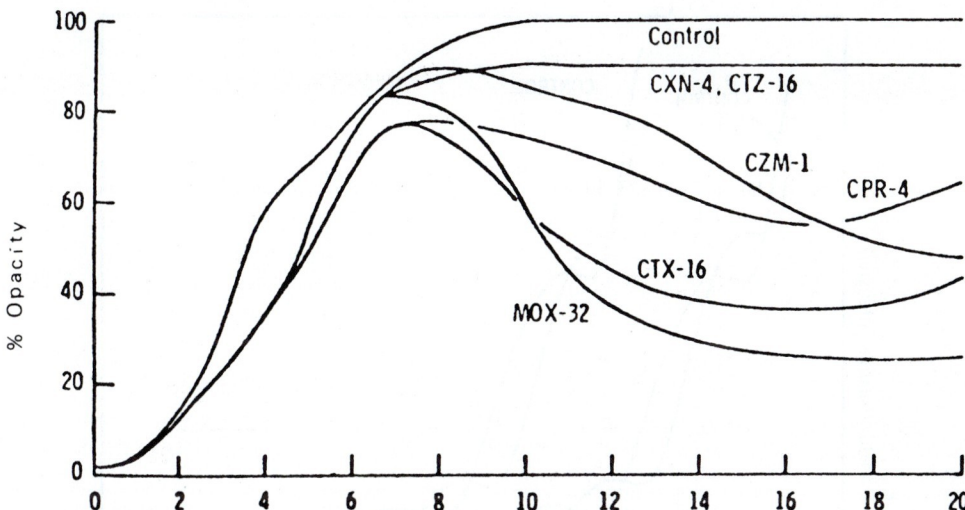

Figure 3.10 ■ Growth response, as measured by turbidity (opacity) of *P. aeruginosa* toward several β-lactam antibiotics. The drop in turbidity due to lysis varied depending on the antibiotic. Regrowth was observed with cefoperazone at 4 μg/mL and cefotaxime at 16 μg/mL. The initial population at time 0 was about 10^6 cells/mL, at which time drugs were added. MOX, moxalactam; CTX, cefotaxime; CPR, cefoperazone; CZM, ceftazidime; CXN, ceftriaxone; CTZ, ceftizoxime. Numerals refer to concentrations in μg/mL, which were equivalent to twice the MIC for each of the drugs. (Reproduced from Greenwood D, Eley A. A turbidimetric study of the responses of selected strains of *Pseudomonas aeruginosa* to eight antipseudomonal β-lactam antibiotics. *J Infect Dis* 1982;145:110–117.)

Another approach to the detection of bacteria and, in turn, the determination of susceptibility involves measuring bacteria interacting with some component of the electromagnetic spectrum. Theoretically, one can measure single particles (individual bacteria) or, for better accuracy, a population of particles (bacteria). The origin of using densitometry (turbidity and visual turbidity) (Fig. 3.10) can be traced to the hallmark works of McFarland (174) and Longsworth (175). Specialized light-scattering methods (Fig. 3.11) using coherent light emanating from a laser have also been applied (176,177). Infrared light (126) and ultraviolet light have been used as energy sources to detect bacteria. Radiation of the latter type interacts with nucleic acids at 260 nm. The uptake of thymidine, a DNA precursor, by microorganisms in the presence and absence of antimicrobial agents has been assessed by Amaral et al. (178). In this assay, labeled thymidine (with either tritium or carbon as the label) is used to determine susceptibility profiles directly from a patient's specimen, thereby obviating the need for a primary culture and the time delay associated with the initial culture. The assay determines the amount of radioactive thymidine incorporated into DNA compared with control and antibiotic-containing cultures. Clear drawbacks of this approach include the potential contamination of the workplace and technical staff and the costs associated with the necessity to routinely monitor the environment and personnel and dispose of materials.

Flow Cytometry

A recent significant development in antimicrobial susceptibility testing is the application of flow cytometry (179). The technology of flow cytometry encompasses aspects of immunology, biochemistry, molecular biology, and histology. Any cellular analyte or metabolic event that can be tagged with a fluorescent dye is a potential candidate for analysis by flow cytometry. Flow cytometers are complex instruments linked to powerful computers still largely dependent on manual procedures. The essence of current multiparameter flow cytometry resides in the capability of the instrument to analyze individual cells (and cell types) of a subpopulation within a larger heterogeneous population without the need for separating or isolating the subpopulation. During flow cytometric analyses, cells in suspension are pushed (flow) single file through a flow cell (Figs. 3.12 and 3.13), where the cells are exposed to monochromatic light emanating

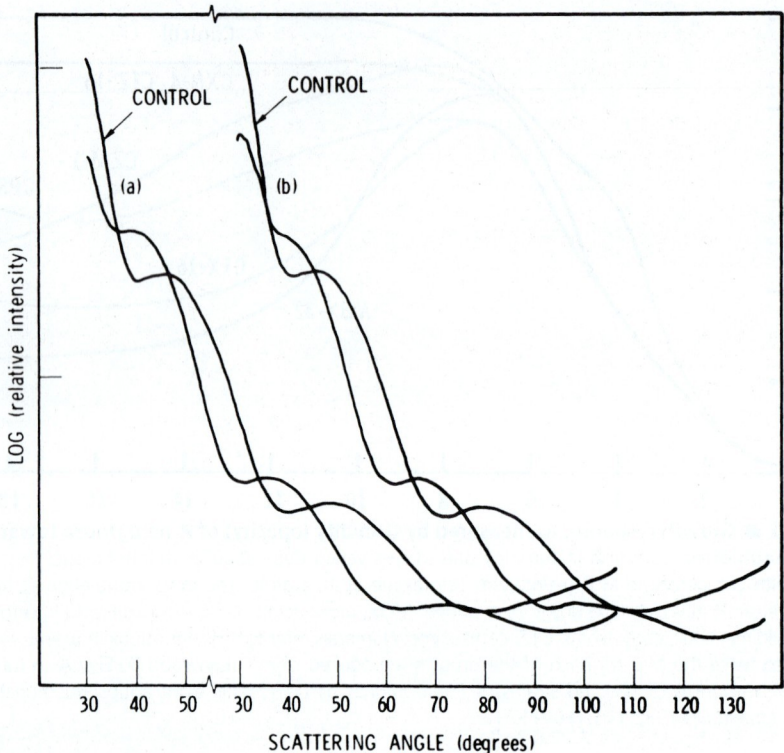

Figure 3.11 ■ Effects of *(a)* ampicillin (0.20 µg/mL) and *(b)* penicillin (0.14 µg/mL) on the light-scattering patterns from a suspension of susceptible *S. aureus*. (Reprinted from Wyatt [177].)

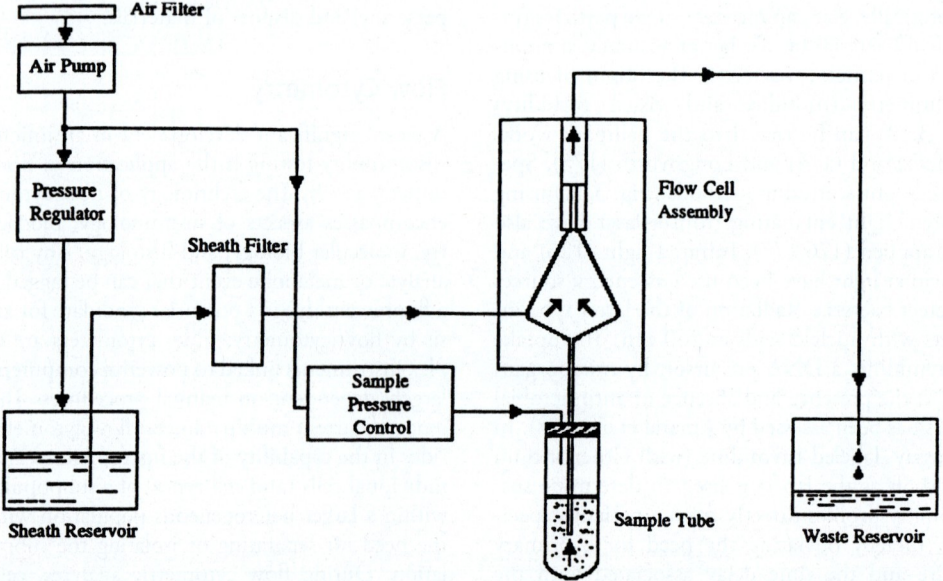

Figure 3.12 ■ **Simplified fluidics system of a flow cytometer concerned with moving the cells.** The sample moves in a uniform stream across the laser intersection. (Reproduced from National Center for Infectious Diseases. *Flow cytometric immunophenotyping procedure manual*. Atlanta: U.S. Department of Health and Human Services, 1993.)

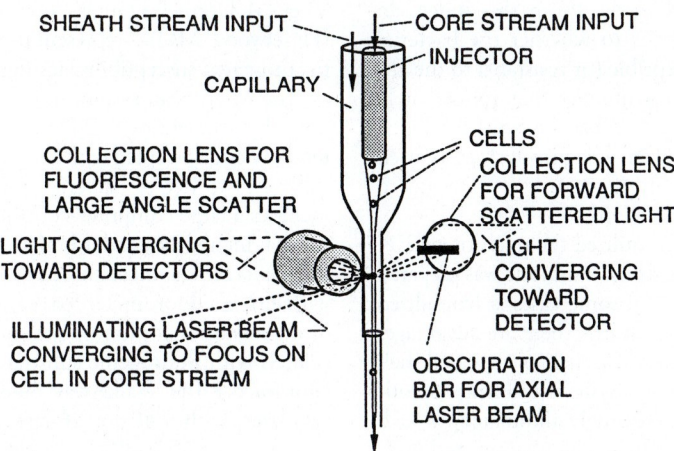

Figure 3.13 ■ **Schematic diagram of a typical flow cytometer.** (Reproduced from Shapiro HM. *Practical flow cytometry*, 2nd ed. New York: Alan R. Liss, 1988.)

from a laser beam, usually of the argon-ion type (180,181). Two cellular parameters derived from the scatter of the laser light are measured: size (forward light scatter) and internal complexity or surface irregularity (right-angle scatter). Detectors in the flow cytometers are sensitive to the colors emitted by fluorochrome-tagged antibodies or fluorescent tracers after excitation by the laser beam.

The technique, as applied to antimicrobial susceptibility testing of microbes, exposes the organism to an antimicrobial agent for 2 to 6 hours at an appropriate incubation temperature. After exposure, organisms are stained with a fluorescent stain like ethidium bromide, which results in increased fluorescence due to breakdown of the cells. The increased fluorescence is then interpreted as death and could be used to determine the MIC. This approach has been applied to *M. tuberculosis* (182). There is no commercial instrument exclusively for this specific application. The current drawbacks of using flow cytometry for bacterial susceptibility testing are the cost of the system and the limited data accumulated for bacteria.

Automated Antimicrobial Susceptibility Test Systems

During the 1980s, clinical microbiology laboratories increased their use of commercial instrument-associated antimicrobial susceptibility testing methods. The growing acceptance of these commercial

instruments by laboratories parallels progress in electronics, robotics, and microcomputers—progress that permitted manufacturers to develop instrumentation able to identify routine gram-negative and gram-positive bacteria of medical importance, determine the associated antimicrobial susceptibility, and combine the results into a single report. The broth microdilution susceptibility tests and associated identification component have become the most popular of the systems currently available to clinical microbiology laboratories in the United States (183).

Background, Development, and Description of Automated Susceptibility Test Systems

The earliest automated and probably rapid susceptibility test system was the TAAS (Technicon Automated Antimicrobial Susceptibility) system. It was developed in the early 1970s by Technicon Instrument Corporation (Tarrytown, NY). It was never marketed. In this system, an antimicrobial agent was delivered by dropping antibiotic-impregnated disks into broth. Through the process of elution, the antimicrobial agent was free to act in a short period of time. After bacterial inoculation and growth for 3 hours in the presence of the single antimicrobial concentration, growth was compared with a control broth without antibiotic. A growth index was calculated based on the ratio of the growth in the presence and absence of the antimicrobial agent. From this index, an evaluation was made as to whether the bacterial population was susceptible (or resistant) to the antimicrobial agent. Instruments that immediately followed, such as the Autobac system (developed and marketed by Pfizer Diagnostics), also used antibiotic elution from paper disks as a means to initiate antimicrobial activity.

Subsequent systems utilized the microtiter 12 × 8 (96-well) format, in which antibiotic was prepared and frozen until used. In some cases, a lyophilized dry powder was used. Clearly, there are advantages associated with dry powders, such as increased shelf life and storage flexibility. Systems utilizing microtiter formats became increasingly automated, to such an extent that the inoculation, incubation, and readout could be handled without human intervention. Once microcomputers with expanded memory became available, along with the capability of printing susceptibility results with bacterial identification and associated patient demographics, data management systems that could be used for the generation of cumulative susceptibility profiles were developed.

An abbreviated list of automated susceptibility systems available during the past two decades is presented in Table 3.25. As noted, most systems are no longer manufactured, and the commercial sponsors of the viable systems have changed.

Of the several antimicrobial susceptibility testing systems listed in Table 3.25, all but one use visible light as a measuring parameter (184). The Sensititre system uses fluorometric monitoring for determining the interaction of antimicrobial agent and bacterium (185). The systems that detect early growth with limited incubation (less than 6 hours) are the Autobac, the Avantage, and the AMS Vitek and Sensititre systems. If one considers the operational definition of rapid as 4 to 6 hours, then only the Autobac and Avantage systems fall into this category. All of the other systems require 6-hour or overnight incubation. However, the effects of limited incubation intervals, especially with β-lactam drugs, warrant serious evaluation (186). The accuracy of these systems (plus or minus one dilution) ranges from 87.6% to 98.3% (124).

It is not productive to describe in detail the varied commercial systems that were available, because frequent changes and corporate direction have modified the design and features of these instruments. Table 3.36 outlines contemporary instruments currently available and widely used. The descriptions of the two systems that follow—the MicroScan system, originally developed by Baxter, and the system from Vitek/McDonnell Douglas, now Vitek bioMérieux (Hazelwood, MO)—represent different approaches to automated susceptibility testing.

The MicroScan system developed in the 1980s uses the conventional 96-well format or an extended design coupled with fluorogenic or standard substrates to detect bacterial growth. The system includes a large computer-controlled microprocessor that incubates standard microdilution trays and interprets biochemical and/or susceptibility results with either a fluorometer for fluorogenic substrates or a conventional photometer for standard plates. (Panels with fluorogenic substrates have been discontinued.) The WalkAway model is available in two sizes, with a 40- or 96-test panel capacity. It consists of a large, self-contained incubator/reader with humidifier, a carousel that rotates towers containing the panels, a bar code scanner, photometers (spectrophotometer/fluorometer), and associated robotic mechanisms to move panels and perform designated computer-controlled robotic steps to access and position trays, add reagents, and position trays for reading. The instrument is associated with a microcomputer, a video display terminal, and a printer. The database management system is capable of producing a patient report and storing that information to subsequently reproduce cumulative reports, epidemiologic reports, and antibiograms. Although the instrument discussed is automated, preparation of the inoculum is done individually and manually using a seed trough, which is transferred to the test panel with a rehydrator/inoculator (RENOK). This approach is more conventional, using the microtiter format with multiple antibiotic concentrations directed by microcomputer-controlled robotics (except for inoculum preparation) to achieve a final MIC result.

In contrast to the microtiter panel approach platform is the specialized design and concept of the Vitek system. The essence of this system is the reagent card, a small thin plastic unit that contains 30 wells or microcuvettes in the Legacy version and 45 wells in the Vitek II version. The wells are connected by capillaries in which bacterial test suspension passes for rehydration and inoculation. The cards are available with a variety of predetermined configurations of antimicrobial agents and reagents to identify gram-positive or gram-negative organisms. The MIC end point is determined by an algorithm from results of testing one to five antimicrobial concentrations. Cards are stored at 4°C, with a shelf life of approximately 12 months. The system includes integrated hardware consisting of a filler/sealer that serves as the inoculator

Table 3.36

Contemporary Automated Susceptibility Test Systems					
System (Manufacturer)	**Test Panel**	**Inoculation**	**Readout**	**System Components**	**Expert System**
MicroScan WalkAway (Dade Behring Inc, Deerfield, IL)	Conventional 8 × 12 microdilution trays; 40/96 panel capacity	Multiprong manual device	Turbidometric direct MIC or breakpoint	Incubator/reader, PC with video monitor and printer; data management system	Yes
Phoenix (Becton, Dickinson and Company, Franklin Lakes, NJ)	Proprietary test panel with 136 wells; 100 panel capacity	Manual by self-filling transfer device into opening of test panel	Turbidometric with redox indicator system for direct MIC	Incubator/reader with integrated PC/monitor	EpiCenter software package available separately
Sensititre ARIS (Trek Diagnostics Inc, Cleveland, OH)	Conventional 8 × 12 microdilution trays; 64 panel capacity	Autoinoculator	Fluorometric direct MIC or breakpoint	Incubator/reader PC with video monitor and printer; autoin-oculator	
Vitek Legacy (bioMérieux)	Proprietary plastic reagent cards with microchannels to 30/45 wells; 120 card capacity	Manual inoculum prep, filler-seal module, density verification	Turbidometric kinetic measurements of growth perform linear regression plots and derive MICs algorithmically	Incubator/reader; PC with video monitor and printer	Yes
Vitek 2 (bioMérieux)	Proprietary plastic reagent cards with microchannels to 64 wells; 60/120 card capacity	Automated inoculum dilution, density verification, card filling and sealing	As for legacy, some agents are direct MICs	Incubator/reader; filler-sealer; PC with video monitor and printer; data management system	Yes

and sealer for up to 10 cards; a reader/incubator that contains the robotic system to move the cards on a timely basis from a carousel to a position in the instrument where optical density or biochemical reactions are determined by a photometer; and a computer module that contains software, a video display terminal, and a printer. Systems are available in different capacities and can hold from 30 to 240 cards. Growth is determined turbidometrically at hourly intervals for up to 15 hours and is compared to the baseline and expressed as a ratio. Normalized linear regression of the growth is used to calculate a best fit to determine the MIC. The user can opt to print susceptibility results as discrete MICs or qualitative breakpoint results (susceptible to resistant).

Each of the systems described here can be linked to the main laboratory information system through a standard RS232 interface. The data

management system is designed for storing and retrieving data for laboratory pharmacy and infection control purposes as well as printing chartable patient reports.

In addition to the instruments listed in Table 3.36, there are available several semiautomated devices that only turbidometrically or fluorometrically read/scan test panels inoculated manually and incubated overnight (18 to 24 hours). These include the AutoScaptor (Becton, Dickinson and Company, Franklin Lakes, NJ), MicroScan autoSCAN-4 (Dade Behring Inc, Deerfield, IL), mini API (bioMérieux, France), and Sensititre AutoReader (Trek Diagnostics Inc, Cleveland, OH). Also not included in Table 3.36 are the several computer-assisted semiautomated devices that measure disk diffusion zone diameters by image analysis (see Chapter 2). This latter group of instruments interprets zone diameter readings according to a user-selected database for reporting S, I, and R categories. One system, BIOMIC (Giles Scientific, Santa Barbara, CA), determines MICs by regression analysis of measured zone diameters. Clear advantages of this instrument group are that they generally provide results that are more reproducible than those achieved by manual observation, measurement, and recording and that they can be interfaced to laboratory information systems, thereby reducing the potential for transcription errors in patient reports.

Advantages of Automated Systems

A perceived advantage of the automated approach to antimicrobial susceptibility testing is the apparently more efficient use of robotics, rather than humans, in executing these tests. However, the gain in labor savings is not extensive. Perhaps a more meaningful advantage is the reproducibility of results obtained by using this type of instrumentation. Because procedures for inoculum preparation, the specified duration of incubation, and the assessment of growth are standardized in these systems, subjective components are removed and intralaboratory and interlaboratory standardization is readily achieved. For high-volume laboratories that demand high throughput, the time required for reading and interpreting routine susceptibility tests is diminished. The associated capability of performing identifications is an additional advantage. Considerable labor savings are also derived from the potential to establish a link between the computer and the laboratory information system. This capability precludes technologist error in transcribing, sorting, and entering results in individual reports.

Limitations and Problems of Automated Systems

Systems that mimic and merely robotize a multi-well approach to performing conventional MICs seem to have only minor disadvantages. However, when the systems associated with these instruments offer limited testing panel capacity are not applicable to all groups of bacteria and fail to incorporate QC end points that are on scale (i.e., within the MIC range of the test panel), their flexibility and precision are questionable. Furthermore, the capital outlay required for purchase and the high cost per test for reagent rental acquisition need to be assessed and compared with the expense of manual test methods. If the clinical impact significantly improves the quality of patient care and reduces hospital costs overall, then the financial costs of the testing itself become irrelevant.

The design of automated instruments that utilize extremely small volumes, modify the inoculum, and reduce the incubation interval has created several problems in the detection of resistance. The detection of type 1 inducible β-lactamase resistance associated with *Citrobacter*, *Enterobacter*, *Serratia*, *Providencia*, *Pseudomonas*, and indole-positive *Proteus* strains is hampered by short detection (incubation) intervals. Owing to their inherent nature, inducible-type resistors are missed because a longer incubation is required for induction and expression and subsequent detection of spontaneous mutants.

Because of the failure to detect emerging vancomycin resistance in enterococci, the FDA had imposed prohibitions for automated testing of enterococci with vancomycin. Similarly, these restrictions have been applied to *S. pneumoniae* susceptibility testing. As noted earlier, the limitations associated with short incubation times contribute to these problems.

Other specific problems related to automated susceptibility systems have been encountered. These include false resistance to aztreonam, especially for *Proteus* and *Morganella* spp, and false resistance to imipenem associated with *Pseudomonas* spp.

A serious limitation of contemporary instrumentation concerns the newly recognized need to verify methicillin resistance. This is especially pertinent when testing coagulase-negative staphylococci. Verification can be accomplished by molecular detecting of *mecA* or its surrogate encoded protein product, PBP-2A, by latex agglutination. *MecA* detection is the gold standard. Alternatively, CLSI (NCCLS) has previously recommended a cefoxitin agar diffusion methodology (11).

During the development and evaluation of each commercial automated systems, reports have cited problems. As problems are identified, the manufacturer has attempted to address then by modifying the system by adjusting the growth support and cation content of the growth medium, modifying the reagents, and revising the software and/or algorithms associated with the optical reading device. Due to ongoing modifications, it is difficult to compare and evaluate the accuracy of the systems. As clinical microbiology laboratories come to understand the limitations of these systems, they may rethink the apparent benefit of automation and return to classical approaches, which are more flexible, less fraught with resistance problems, and less costly.

Verification of Antimicrobial Susceptibility Test Systems

When the laboratory considers endorsing a newly acquired automated test system or transitions from an extant system or conventional microdilution method to a new system, it is critical that the test performance of the new system is verified. Verification is accomplished by using the new or revised test method in parallel with a reference method with a known and satisfactory level of performance. The evaluation of susceptibility test methods should be done using a distribution of organisms typically encountered at the institution, ideally including susceptible and resistant strains for each antimicrobial agent. Guidelines are available, but generally the evaluation should be designed to include at least 100 strains and detect three types of errors categorized as *very major* (reference method R; new system S), *major* (reference method S, new system R), and *minor* (reference method R or S, new system I). Very major errors should be less than or equal to 3% and major and minor errors should less than or equal to 7% (187).

Clinical Impact of Automated or Rapid Testing

Early evaluations of automated systems now more than 20 years old have failed to show that rapid susceptibility tests produce a sustained significant positive impact on patient care. In studies of patients with bacteremia, Doern et al. (188) found that, among 173 patients who were receiving antibiotics, rapid susceptibility testing indicated a change in therapy for 48 of these patients. For 32 of the 48 patients, the change in therapy was made 24 hours earlier as the result of 1-day earlier testing. Trenholme et al. (189) found that, for 226 bacteremic patients, rapid automated susceptibility results were associated with a greater likelihood of administration of appropriate antimicrobial therapy, a change to more effective therapy, and/or use of less costly therapy. These studies failed to find a change in patient outcome.

In a follow-up study, Doern et al. (190) evaluated two controlled patient groups in a tertiary care institution. One group was tested with conventional overnight microbiologic procedures for identification and susceptibility testing. The other group had the benefit of rapid, same-day procedures. The investigators found that, with regard to mortality rates, the patients receiving the advantage of rapid, same-day testing experienced a lower mortality rate (8.8% vs. 15.3% in the conventional testing group).

Other advantages associated with rapid testing were fewer laboratory studies, fewer days of incubation, fewer days in critical care units, and shortened times prior to modifications in antimicrobial therapy. In a more recent study, Barenfanger et al. (191) documented clinical and financial benefit (reduced length of stay) of rapid identification and antimicrobial susceptibility testing.

Schifman et al. (192) determined that a significant issue impacting patient outcome was the slow reporting of and response to results in the postanalytical phase of testing. These authors found that the value of susceptibility test results in initiating or modifying therapy was reduced by inefficient reporting practices. In many institutions, getting clinicians to respond promptly to actionable health care information is an ongoing quality improvement concern.

Rapid methods to determine susceptibility (actually resistance) have been used and no doubt will continue to be used as an adjunct to conventional susceptibility testing. Mention has been made of the use of β-lactamase testing using nitrocefin disks and the detection of chloramphenicol resistance by chloramphenicol acetyltransferase assay (119,193). Tests modeled on this strategy have been designed using the breakthroughs in recombinant nucleic acid technology to promptly assess resistant mechanisms (194) (see Chapter 9). For example, by testing for the presence of a plasmid product (an enzyme) or the nucleotide sequence that directs the synthesis of the product, a laboratory can report results within hours. Several nucleic acid probes for detecting and identifying specific infectious agents are already FDA-approved, and they are useful in the clinical laboratory. At recent count, 106 plasmids have been identified, and the gene products probed can be used to detect resistance for 16 classes of antimicrobial agents (195,196). Recently, York et al. (197) evaluated the molecular detection of *mecA* by polymerase chain reaction and the standard method for determining methicillin resistance in coagulase-negative staphylococci. Since *mecA* encodes for a low-affinity PBP, PBP-2a, one could alternatively detect this protein product using a commercially available latex agglutination kit. It can be anticipated that commercial probes for resistance markers may be available in the near future. This approach to susceptibility testing (actually determining resistance) can be extremely useful, especially in therapeutic situations in which meningitis is present. A note of caution: the presence of a particular nucleotide sequence that indicates the potential for producing the plasmid-mediated resistance product does not always mean that the product is expressed by the bacterium.

Indirect guides to determine the susceptibility of *S. viridans* group streptococci associated with endocarditis have been proposed (198). Studies have shown that the quantity of glycocalyx produced by these organisms is correlated with the size of infected cardiac vegetations and resistance to antimicrobial therapy (276). Other approaches to screening resistance of selected pathogens using antimicrobial agents incorporated into agar have been used successfully.

INTERPRETIVE GUIDELINES FOR SUSCEPTIBILITY OR RESISTANCE

It is clear that in contemporary medical practice, antimicrobial susceptibility testing is necessary component for the delivery of effective, cost-efficient medical care. The MIC is of major import in the comparative evaluation of antimicrobial agents and in the ability to predict their clinical effectiveness by gauging bacteriologic outcome. Ever since Fleming's discovery of the activity of penicillin and the subsequent development of antimicrobial agents, methods have been evaluated to measure and define the true value and meaning of this interaction—the MIC. The testing of the interaction between microorganism and antimicrobial agent is clinically applicable when it defines a breakpoint that parts the susceptible from the resistant. Test conditions and parameters can indeed modulate the outcome of test results, as discussed. In basic microbiology research laboratories, the end point of a standardized test, with the resultant MIC, yields an operational definition that identifies the organism tested as susceptible to the lowest concentration in the series. This does not require further clarification. However, in clinical microbiology laboratories, the medical relevance of that susceptibility test result is paramount. The variables and considerations that form the basis of the recommendations for the development of susceptibility testing interpretive guidelines were discussed in a landmark report by Ericsson and Sherris (6) and formed the basis for the interpretive categories recommended by Bauer et al. (7) and the CLSI (NCCLS) documents on dilution susceptibility testing (10). A commonly held misconception is that the MIC and its interpretation are based solely on the ratio of the MIC and the peak achievable serum level. This is incorrect. In fact, the interpretive guidelines, as evaluated by

CLSI and EUCAST, although somewhat different are based on a tripartite set of databases, as originally recommended by Ericsson and Sherris (6), Bauer et al. (7), and CLSI (NCCLS). The database for evaluating interpretive standards is dependent on the susceptibility of isolates in a large population distribution, the clinical pharmacology of the drug, and the drug's clinical efficacy. When examining the MIC of new drugs for isolates or reviewing the efficacy of older drugs, the results are compared with the mode (or modes), range, and character (i.e., unimodal, bimodal, or skewed) of the distribution of MICs for populations of strains of the same species being tested. These ranges are then compared with the distribution of MICs of other species within the same group for the same drug and other agents of the same class.

In evaluating the clinical pharmacology of the drug, one includes the range, peak, mean, and trough serum levels expected from the variety of dosage schedules and also considers other PK parameters such as protein binding, volume of distribution, tissue level, and level of the active drug in urine. The range of mean serum levels rather than peak values more appropriately reflects overall tissue levels and avoids inappropriately amplified therapeutic ratios that result from comparing transient, maximally achievable peak serum levels with the MIC of the organism. Lastly, data are collected and evaluated from prospective clinical investigations that reflect the in vivo response to treatment of patients with specific infections caused by various strains of species with known MICs. Guidelines for performing these types of experiments have been included in a CLSI (NCCLS) document (199).

The problems of developing the interpretive breakpoints are usually more difficult for disk diffusion assays, where one has to establish the appropriate disk mass to produce zones of inhibition of a range usable in clinical microbiology laboratories. This is often done initially with customized or handmade disks and then confirmed later with commercially prepared formulations. The usual practice is to construct regression lines of a zone of inhibition versus MIC for about 500 separate isolates covering the spectrum of the new antimicrobial agent. These studies often include one or more comparative agents of the same class as the test agent. The bacterial strains used are obtained from geographic areas within the United States and represent the major routine isolates that would be expected to be treated with the agent under development. Breakpoints are selected based on the pharmacokinetics of the agent in humans, the ability to separate resistant and susceptible bacterial species, and the minimization of major errors of interpretation (false-susceptible or false-resistant). Additionally, for disk development, the paper containing the antimicrobial reagent has to be evaluated for content and stability over time and under storage conditions.

Differences in breakpoint determinations are extant between CLSI and EUCAST. These differences can readily be seen in Tables 3.32 and 3.33. Table 3.32 documents comparisons for 14 drug classes against five gram-negative microbial groups. Generally, EUCAST data demonstrate lower MICs than CLSI with the exception of the carbapenems. Of note is the threefold lower MIC listed for cefepime ($\geq$4.0 µg/mL vs. $\geq$32.0 µg/mL) than CLSI. These variations are highlighted as a result of the 2011/2012 changes by CLSI as related to the detection of ESBLs.

For gram-positive bacteria (Table 3.33), notably *Staphylococcus*, there is dichotomy among the standard organizations for vancomycin, EUCAST indicating a threefold lower breakpoint for *S. aureus* and a fourfold lower concentration for the coagulase-negative staphylococci.

Over time, the criteria that have been used to establish breakpoints have changed, and various countries and organizations have adapted differing criteria (see Chapter 1). Early in antimicrobial susceptibility studies, it was observed that all strains of a bacterial species do not demonstrate the same degree of susceptibility and that the susceptibilities (i.e., MICs) for a population of strains are distributed according to a bimodal or normal distribution. Eventually, national committees and organizations such as CLSI came to conclude that in the derivation of a breakpoint, the PK properties (e.g., drug distribution in the host) and PD properties (e.g., activity against the infecting agent) of the antimicrobial compound indicated that the MIC (interpreted as susceptible) would suggest the possibility—perhaps the probability (not quantitatively defined)—of antimicrobial therapy success and resistant would connote failure. It is of interest to note the differing approaches used in various countries by the empowered organized committees that oversee or regulate antimicrobial susceptibility testing. The Dutch committee for regulating antimicrobial susceptibility testing, the CRG, states, "Micro-organisms are categorized susceptible (S), as opposed to resistant (R) to an antimicrobial agent; if concentrations of the non-protein bound fraction in vivo, based on the dosing regimen proposed, are above the MIC of a microorganism

for a sufficient time-period in order to eradicate the microorganism, and thereby cure of the patient can be reasonably expected." In contrast, the British Society for Antimicrobial Chemotherapy uses this formula: breakpoint concentration = $C_{max} \cdot csf$ (e.t), where C_{max} is the maximum serum concentration following a stated dose at steady state, e is the factor by which the C_{max} should exceed the MIC, f is a protein-binding factor, s is a reproducibility factor, and t represents the serum half-life. Clearly, organized groups have used varied data and criteria in establishing breakpoints, although the trend is toward the inclusion of PK and PD information.

In the United States, the FDA and the CLSI Subcommittee on Antimicrobial Susceptibility Testing have the responsibility for the development of standards that promote accurate and reproducible antimicrobial susceptibility testing and appropriate reporting. Data reviewed for establishing susceptibility breakpoints include in vitro drug characteristics, necessary distributions of microorganisms, PK/PD parameters, and the correlation of test results with outcome statistics.

As suggested, organizing committees in several countries are now using PK/PD relationships in their breakpoint estimations. For many drugs, data were accumulated documenting the relationship between drug concentration and effect. Three major characteristics of the concentration time curve (AUC) of a drug have been delineated: concentration (C_{max}), area under the AUC, and the time the concentration remains above the MIC (T>MIC) (Fig. 3.14). From these are derived

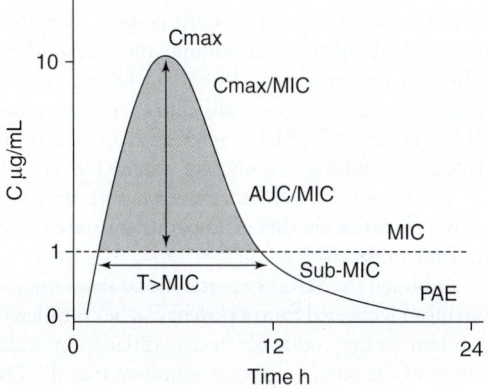

Figure 3.14 ■ **Relationship of PK and PD properties of antimicrobial agents.** C_{max}, peak concentration; MIC, minimum inhibitory concentration; AUC, area under the curve; T>MIC, time over the MIC; PAE, postantibiotic effect.

Table 3.37

PK/PD Parameters of Seven Fluoroquinolones with Derived Breakpoints						
					S-Breakpoint[a] µg/mL	
Fluoroquinolone[b]	**Dosing Regimen**	**C_{max} µg/mL**	**AUC µg h/mL**	**Protein Binding %**	**Pd[a]**	**NCCLS**
Ciprofloxacin	500 mg/12 h	2.6	22.2	22	0.25	1.0
Sparfloxacin[c]	200 mg/24 h	0.6	16.4	45	0.125	0.5
Levofloxacin	500 mg/24 h	5.2	61.1	30	0.5	2.0
Ofloxacin	200 mg/12 h	2.2	29.2	30	0.25	2.0
Grepafloxacin[c]	400 mg/24 h	0.9	11.4	50	0.125	0.5
Trovofloxacin[c]	200 mg/24 h	2.2	30.4	70	0.125	1.0
Moxifloxacin	400 mg/24 h	4.5	48.0	40	0.5	1.0

[a]Based on AUC/MIC of 100–125 h and a C_{max}/MIC of 8–12.
[b]Does not include recently FDA-approved gemifloxacin.
[c]Discontinued in the United States.
AUC, area under the curve; NCCLS, National Committee for Clinical Laboratory Standards.
Adapted from Lampe MR, Aitken CL, Dennis PG, et al. Relationship of early readings of minimal inhibitory concentrations to the results of overnight tests. *Antimicrob Agents Chemother* 1975;8:429–433; Forrest A, Nix DE, Ballow CH, et al. Pharmacodynamics of intravenous ciprofloxacin in seriously ill patients. *Antimicrob Agents Chemother* 1993;37:1073–1081.

PK/PD indices by relating the drug parameter to the MIC: AUC/MIC, C_{max}/MIC, and T>MIC. Studies of animal models of infection show an evident relationship between the PK/PD indices and efficacy. The setting of these breakpoints is derived from highest generally achieved indices: 100 to 125 for the AUC/MIC and 8 to 12 for the C_{max}/MIC (19). Examples of PK/PD relationships and breakpoints are shown in Table 3.37.

Although it was generally considered instructive and meaningful to classify antimicrobial agents as bacteriostatic or bactericidal (all antibiotics are bacteriostatic but not necessarily bactericidal), contemporary interpretation identifies two patterns of bacterial killing: time-dependent killing or concentration-dependent killing. Time-dependent killing agents are characterized by the PD parameter T>MIC, whereas concentration-dependent killing agents are characterized by C_{max}/MIC or AUC/MIC. Several antimicrobial classes classified by these PD parameters are listed in Table 3.38.

Although the MIC of a particular strain of microorganism recovered from a patient can be considered constant and reproducible (it may differ from other strains of the same species), it is known that the PK parameters of absorption rate, volume of distribution, and clearance can differ among individuals. Drusano and colleagues (202) acknowledged these variations and presented an integrated approach to population pharmacokinetics and microbiologic

Table 3.38

Pharmacodynamic Indices as Surrogate Markers of Time-Dependent and Concentration-Dependent Antimicrobial Agents	
Antibiotic Class	**PD Index**
Time-dependent	
β-Lactams Penicillins Cephalosporins Monobactams Carbapenem	T>MIC
Glycopeptides	T>MIC C_{max}-free/MIC
Concentration-dependent	
Aminoglycosides	C_{max}/MIC AUC/MIC
Fluoroquinolones	C_{max}/MIC AUC/MIC
Macrolides Azithromycin Clarithromycin Crythromycin	C_{max}/MIC AUC/MIC
Ketolides	C_{max}/MIC
Telithromycin	AUC/MIC

PD, pharmacodynamic; T>MIC, time over the minimum inhibitory concentration; C_{max}, concentration; AUC, area under the curve; MIC, minimum inhibitory concentration.

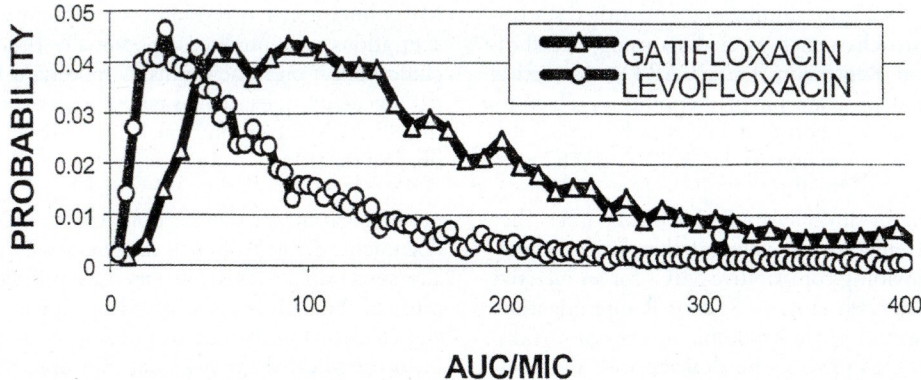

Figure 3.15 ■ Probability distribution curves for two quinolones, gatifloxacin, and levofloxacin, depicting AUC. Solidus MIC ratios against *S. pneumoniae*. Distributions integrate AUC and MIC. If an AUC/MIC of 120 (or less) is associated with a positive clinical outcome, then gatifloxacin has a greater probability of achieving that ratio (275).

susceptibility information. Statistical simulation Monte Carlo (using a computer-generated program that integrates variously attainable PK/PD indices and MICs) can provide insight into the proportion of the population who can achieve an effective AUC/MIC and for whom clinical success can be quantitative by predicted (200–202). Monte Carlo simulation incorporates a probability function to generate random AUC and MIC values from a sampling distribution. Thousands of single-point estimates are made and their probabilities plotted (Fig. 3.15). Whereas single-point AUC/MIC estimates provide information on what is possible, Monte Carlo simulations can determine probability. Thus, one could predict the probability of achieving a targeted AUC/MIC ratio at different MIC breakpoints (Fig. 3.16).

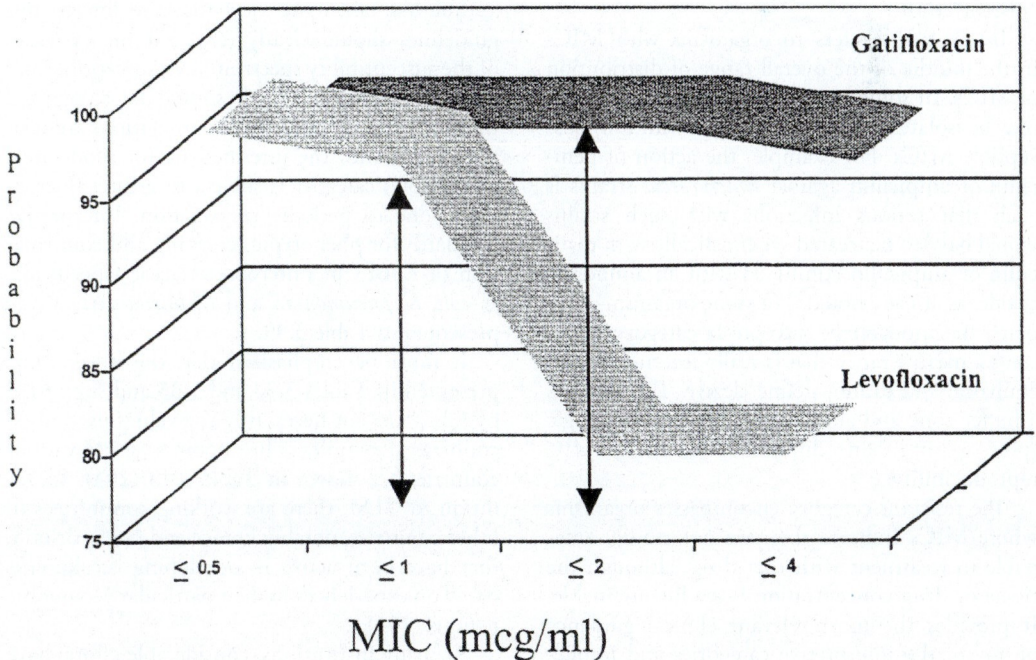

Figure 3.16 ■ Probability of achieving an AUC/MIC ratio of 30 at differing MICs for two quinolones, gatifloxacin and levofloxacin. Note gatifloxacin maintains a near 90% probability from 0.5 to 3.0 µg/mL, whereas levofloxacin declines abruptly at 0.75 µg/mL (275).

Monte Carlo simulations and other statistical approaches, such as analysis using Classification and Regression Tree (CART), a statistical computer program for predicting the probability of a clinical response to infection by a microorganism as a function of the peak-C_{max}/MIC ratio (203), are and will be useful in developing more meaningful clinically applicable breakpoints. They do not enhance the value of the clinical laboratory providing comparative MICs for an infective organism with only an S, I, or R interpretation. What would prove applicable in light of this discussion is to provide the clinician with the number of $\log_2$ concentrations below the S breakpoint concentration that was achieved; indirectly, this would be relative to AUC/MIC and C_{max}/MIC.

These considerations have led, at least in the United States, to the separation of data into three (or possibly four) interpretive categories: susceptible, intermediate (or "moderately susceptible"), and resistant. Susceptible organisms attain MICs that fall into the susceptible range of MICs and would generally be below serum or tissue levels of the drug achievable with usual dosage regimens; the implication is that infections attributable to such organisms may be appropriately treated with that drug. Strains classified as resistant would not be inhibited by typically achievable systemic concentrations.

Intermediate refers to organisms with MICs in the middle of the overall range of distribution of MICs. In some population distributions, there may be isolates that have no strains with fully susceptible MICs. For example, the action of penicillin or ampicillin against *Enterococcus* strains is such that serious infections with such strains would have to be treated synergistically with penicillin or ampicillin combined with an aminoglycoside, as already noted. For some organism–drug pairs, the moderately susceptible category represents a narrow range that is really intermediate or equivocal and cannot define clearly. This range is a buffer zone and allows for technical or biologic (plus or minus one dilution) variation in MIC reproducibility.

The resistant category encompasses organisms whose MICs indicate they are not readily amenable to treatment with that drug, although the tissue or drug concentration is readily attainable. It provides the most relevant clinical guidance of any of the interpretive categories and implies with reasonable assurance that normally a serious infection would not respond to treatment. However, it should be noted that, for the typical

MICs interpreted as resistant, subinhibitory concentrations may produce a potentially beneficial clinical effect on some strains by modifying some pathogenicity traits such as rate of growth, ability to adhere, toxin production, or susceptibility to phagocytic action.

In the past, for selected multiresistant strains producing urinary tract infections, CLSI (NCCLS) documents defined a fourth category, "conditionally susceptible." This category was utilized because of the high levels achieved by certain drugs and the occasional value of utilizing these drugs in uncomplicated urinary tract infections associated with multiresistant enteric bacteria with high MICs. This interpretive category is absent from current documents, and the intermediate category now encompasses this group.

A new term has emerged, "nonsusceptible," which has two different interpretations. CLSI (NCCLS) uses this term for characterizing some organism–antimicrobial combinations where there are or very few resistant strains to define a resistant category. "Clinically nonsusceptible" refers to that population of microorganisms that qualify as either intermediate or resistant.

Because the interpretation of these guidelines cannot be arithmetically quantified and cannot be agreed upon with a great deal of reliability, this author has taken the view that the interpretive guidelines should clearly represent the extremes of the susceptibility spectrum (i.e., susceptible and resistant). Additionally, it should be recognized that the extreme categoric interpretations are relatively constant. The intermediate (or moderately susceptible) category is subject to greater fluctuations, due to periodic reevaluation. Interpretive standards for phenotypic screening and confirmation of ESBLs in Enterobacteriaceae (specifically *E. coli*, *K. pneumoniae*, and *Klebsiella oxytoca*) are presented in Table 3.39.

It must be emphasized that the breakpoints presented in Tables 3.32 and 3.33 and supported by CLSI are not necessarily the values used in all countries. Examples of breakpoints used in various countries are shown in Table 3.40 (204). In addition to CLSI, there are working committees in other countries, notably France and Great Britain, that have been active in developing breakpoints based on experiences in their particular geographic regions (204).

At many institutions, considerable efforts have been made to educate physicians not trained as infectious disease specialists in the utilization of MICs. However, one frequently sees that in daily

Table 3.39

Screening and Confirmatory Tests[a] for Extended-Spectrum β-Lactamases[b]

Initial/Screen		Confirmatory	
Antimicrobial Agent[c]	**MIC**	**Antimicrobial Agent[d]**	**MIC**
Aztreonam	≥2	Cefotaxime	>8 or
Cefotaxime	≥2	Cefotaxime-clavulanic acid (4 μg/mL)	≥3 twofold decrease
Cefpodoxime	≥8	AND	
Ceftazidime	≥2	Ceftazidime	>8 or
Ceftriaxone	≥2	Ceftazidime-clavulanic acid (4 μg/mL)	≥3 twofold decrease

[a]Standard broth dilution with CAMB. For QC: *E. coli* ATCC 25922 for screening and *K. pneumoniae* ATCC 700603 for confirmatory testing.
[b]Although several species of Enterobacteriaceae produce extended-spectrum β-lactamases, these interpretations are for *K. pneumoniae*, *K. oxytoca*, and *E. coli*.
[c]The use of multiple antimicrobial agents will improve detection.
[d]Confirmatory testing requires the use of cefotaxime and ceftazidime alone *and* in combination with clavulanic acid.
MIC, minimum inhibitory concentration.

practice, MICs are poorly understood and interpreted. One type of error involves the choice of the wrong class of drug. For instance, an aminoglycoside might unnecessarily be used to treat a relatively benign infection with *E. coli* that is susceptible to multiple drugs merely because an MIC of 1 for amikacin appears to indicate greater susceptibility than the MIC of 2 for tetracycline or the MIC of 4 for ampicillin. Another type of error leads to a false categorical interpretation of the wrong drug within a class when the absolute values of the MICs are seemingly different. For these

Table 3.40

Examples of Breakpoints Used in Various Countries Compared with Breakpoints Determined by the Proposed Method for the Species *Yersinia enterocolitica*[a]

	CAR[b]		MEZ		CXT	
	≤	≥[c]	≤	≥	≤	≥
United States[b]	32.16		16.64		8.8	
France	128		8	21	8	
FRG	32		4	22	1	
Great Britain	32		16			
Sweden	16	24			4	25
Netherlands	16	22	8	23	4	25
Proposed method	8	24	4	30[c]	4	29

[a]The breakpoints shown separate the sensitive strains from the others. These data were published in the papers cited in references (Swedish Reference Group on Antibiotics [1981], US National Committee for Clinical Laboratory Standards 1983 and 1984, European Committee on Antimicrobial Susceptibility Testing [1985], British Society for Antimicrobial Chemotherapy [1985], and Comité de l'Antibiogramme de la Société Française de Microbiologie [1985]).
[b]In the United States, the interpretive standards proposed for dilution tests (first number) should not be confused with the values of approximate MIC correlates obtained from diffusion tests (second number).
[c]This value is proposed in the meantime, until new cluster(s) eventually appear.
CAR, carbenicillin: MEZ, mezlocillin; CXT, cefoxitin; MIC, minimum inhibitory concentration; FRG, Federal Republic of Germany; ≤, a strain is sensitive when its MIC expressed in μg/mL is inferior or equal to the breakpoint concentration; ≥, a strain is sensitive when its diameter expressed in mm is superior or equal to the breakpoint diameter. This is indicated only when the same breakpoint concentration and the same ICS diffusion technique (164) are used.

reasons, it is recommended that the appropriate interpretive category always be reported along with the numerical value of the MIC. In some clinical settings, there has been a tendency to report the ratio of the MIC to theoretical peak serum (or urine) levels for various dosages. The reports are sometimes computerized and are semiquantitated by a single plus sign or several plus signs, indicating the degree of susceptibility (or resistance). Such reports really are somewhat arbitrary and falsely quantitative. Although theoretically, such calculations are possible, they omit other PK parameters such as the possibility of protein binding (Should it be subtracted?), the use of peak or mean levels, and the use of trough levels in the numerator. What about renal or liver function tests, and in whom have the levels been determined? The patient under consideration has a specific disease and may not be compartmentalizing the drug in the typical way that the manufacturer's product insert indicates for that antibiotic. Such specific pseudoquantitative reporting systems are based on oversimplified pharmacologic assumptions and may be misleading.

The general concept of therapeutic ratios is useful in teaching antimicrobial management. Thus, it may be appropriate and informative for laboratories to include, in their quarterly or annual reports, tables summarizing the standard interpretive breakpoints (as noted in Tables 3.32 and 3.33) and the ranges of mean serum levels. Additionally, this information can be placed at the back of a patient's report. Lastly, since the bottom line is always cost, it is often necessary in many clinical settings for the laboratory, through the pharmacy and therapeutics committee, to supply clinicians with the average daily cost of an antibiotic, as determined at that institution, for treatment of severe to moderate infections. The clinicians can then use the laboratory susceptibility data along with the cost data to determine the most clinically efficacious and least expensive therapy.

Minimum Inhibitory Concentrations: Predictive Value of Clinical Outcome

Earlier, reference was made to the inoculum concentration, rate of replication, and phase as modifying factors in obtaining accurate, reproducible MIC results. Recently, it has been learned that microbial interactions in biofilms can confound the interpretation and predictive value of in vitro systems using homogenous bacterial populations.

The model of the way bacteria reproduce and grow as free-swimming planktonic cells is not truly realized in nature. Planktonic cells attach to inanimate surfaces (e.g., plastic catheters or sand) or to the epithelial cells of an airway system. Their ability to detach or remain attached is dependent on several characteristics of the host system. Typically, the ability of clusters of bacteria to remain attached and form biofilms relates to availability of a foreign object (catheter) or dead tissue and to protection from host defenses and antibodies. Microbial biofilms are slow to develop, cause collateral damage to tissues, and are persistent. They are regarded as communities of bacteria that grow on surfaces, as opposed to microorganisms that are dispersed or free floating, and they complicate several medical problems, namely, periodontitis, osteomyelitis, infected catheters (pacemaker leads and urinary catheters), and cystic fibrosis.

It is expected that within communities the bacteria communicate. In the 1960s, marine microbiologists discovered that for *Vibrio fischeri*, the ability to produce light (bioluminescence) is dependent on a critical population size. The signal that turned on the light was genetically controlled by an autoinducer. Infectious disease specialists and microbiologists who study pathogenic mechanisms and virulence have learned that the changes in gene expression patterns in response to the host environment are a prerequisite for bacterial infection, and autoinducers and associated genes have been found in gram-positive and gram-negative bacteria. In studies of *P. aeruginosa* in cystic fibrosis patients, it was found that the prophylactic administration of macrolides that do not kill *P. aeruginosa* (e.g., azithromycin) can bring about clinical relief. This might be attributable to the activity of the drug on the normal oropharyngeal flora, thus minimizing the release of autoinducer-2 (AI-2) of *P. aeruginosa*. AI-2 is responsible for the induction of virulence genes for exotoxin and elastase (205). For glycopeptide intermediate-level resistant *Staphylococcus aureus* (GISA), the majority of infections originate on biomedical devices. The loss of accessory gene regulator (*agr*), a gene cluster comprising five different genes, involved in quorum sensing (the mechanism bacteria use to communicate with each other) has been suggested as contributing to their ability to produce biofilms. All VISA/GISA strains tested belong to *agr* group II and have defective *agr* function (206). In *E. faecalis*, the gene locus *fsr* has been identified as present in 70% of clinical isolates. It appears responsible for regulation of two virulence genes, for gelatinase and a serine protease (207). Homology between *fsr* and the *agr* gene of *Staphylococcus* has been noted (208).

The role of these virulence genes in diverse bacterial groups interacting with normal or commensal microflora and/or growing as biofilms poses challenging questions for medical microbiologists. What is the value of isolating a single offending species and determining the MICs of a variety of antimicrobial agents when, in situ, its role may be regulated by other bacterial populations within the community it resides in?

Given this background, what is the reliability of an MIC and its S/R interpretation in predicting the clinical outcome of antimicrobial therapy? Apart from pharmaceutical-sponsored studies of directed single-agent activity against a particular bacterial target or group, there is a paucity of reports on the relevance of in vitro bacterial susceptibility to the outcome of antimicrobial therapy.

In a retrospective study (209) of 510 patients who received antimicrobial therapy, 382 (75%) had susceptibility tests performed on at least one culture prior to the administration of antimicrobial therapy. Eighteen bacterial species (~75% due to gram-negative rods) were recovered from 298 patients, and of these patients, 271 (91%) received antimicrobial therapy to which the organisms were susceptible and 219 (81%) improved. Of the 271 patients who received therapy to which the bacteria were resistant, 3% demonstrated improvement and 82% did not improve. This study clearly shows the value of selecting therapy according to in vitro susceptibility test results. Similarly, a prospective observational study of 2,634 septic patients showed that "adequate antibiotic treatment" defined on the basis of in vitro susceptibility of an isolated microorganism (at least five species were identified) and/or initiation of antibiotic treatment between 24 hours before and 72 hours after study enrollment resulted in a 10% decrease (33% vs. 43%) in mortality (210). In contrast, an international prospective observational study (211) of 844 hospitalized patients with blood cultures positive for *S. pneumoniae* reported that "discordant therapy" (inactive in vitro susceptibility with penicillins, cefotaxime, and ceftriaxone but not cefuroxime), as compared with "concordant antibiotic therapy" (i.e., receipt of a single antibiotic with in vitro activity against *S. pneumoniae*), did not result in a higher mortality rate. Similarly, the time required for defervescence and the frequency of suppurative complication did not result in a higher mortality rate. The conclusion from these data is that β-lactam antibiotics could prove useful for pneumococcal bacteremia regardless of in vitro susceptibility as defined by CLSI (NCCLS) breakpoints.

Research on acute exacerbation of chronic bronchitis (AECB) includes several studies that compared the activity of quinolones and macrolides against *H. influenzae*. There are differences in the impact of compounds of these two types. Apart from the direct antibacterial PD properties of these agents, the macrolides appear to possess an immunomodulatory effect that prevents recurrence of infection. A conclusion of Martinez in cases of AECB is that in vitro antimicrobial resistance is of unclear significance (212,213).

Against nosocomial pneumonia, antimicrobial agents are the mainstay of pharmacologic measures. It is worth noting that in these studies gram-negative bacteria were the most frequently isolated microorganisms. Several studies examined the mortality rate in association with inadequate antimicrobial therapy. When antibiotic therapy was "appropriate" (i.e., the infective organisms were susceptible), there was a 60% decrease in mortality from 90% (inappropriate) therapy to 30% (appropriate) (214–216).

Prior to the publication of the Yu et al.'s (211) study cited earlier, Rex and Pfaller (217) reviewed multiple reports examining the correlation of therapeutic outcome with in vitro susceptibility. They proposed the "90–60 rule," which states that infections that are due to susceptible isolates respond to appropriate therapy about 90% of the time, whereas infections that are due to resistant isolates or are treated inappropriately respond about 60% of the time.

ASSAY OF BACTERICIDAL ACTIVITY

MIC values estimate the bacteriostatic or inhibitory activity of antimicrobial agents. An MIC, when determined according to the standards and references detailed, is a reproducible parameter for a given antimicrobial agent against a variety of rapidly growing pathogens. In clinical practice, the MIC usually suffices for guiding chemotherapy. The success of in vivo antimicrobial action depends to a large extent on the host's defense mechanisms, which ultimately sequester and kill the microorganisms that have been reduced by the bacteriostatic action of the chemotherapeutic agent. The main body of medical microbiology, clinical pharmacology, and infectious disease literature utilizes MIC data in studying the effects of antimicrobials and in establishing criteria for application in therapy.

For antimicrobial agents that possess bactericidal action (mainly aminoglycosides and β-lactams), it is sometimes necessary to perform additional quantitative assessments of the killing effect on a given offending microorganism. The parameter known as the MBC can be determined in several ways:

1. By estimating the MBC as a result of the MIC for an infecting organism.
2. By estimating the titer of serum of a patient receiving antimicrobial therapy that kills the infecting organism after fences (i.e., the serum bactericidal titer or test [SBT]).
3. By determining the number of surviving bacteria in a fixed concentration of the drug using the average obtainable blood level at defined time intervals (i.e., the killing curve).

The assessment of bactericidal activity, although methodologically feasible, is fraught with microbiologic phenomena and technical problems requiring consummate understanding on the part of those who consider their application and those who execute the assays.

Microbiologic Factors

Since the interactions of bacteria and antimicrobial agents began to be gauged, investigators have observed unusual and complex phenomena that remain incompletely understood in the modern molecular era. One such phenomenon is known as the paradoxical effect (or the Eagle phenomenon) (55). Discovered in the early days of penicillin therapy, the paradoxical effect manifests as the puzzling appearance of increasing numbers of bacterial survivors at concentrations higher than the MBC. Since its discovery, it has been observed for several species of bacteria and for antimicrobial agents other than the β-lactam group and is believed to be the result of interference with protein synthesis of the organism by higher concentrations of the β-lactam. The paradox occurs when the proportion of surviving cells increases significantly even as the concentration of antimicrobial agent increases beyond the MBC. It has been theorized that the high concentration of antimicrobial agent inhibits protein synthesis to a degree that prevents the growth necessary for expression of the lethal effect of the drug. No therapeutic implications appear associated with this effect.

A second complexity involving incomplete killing has been referred to as the *persistence phenomenon* and relates to the small proportion (usually less than 0.1%) of the inoculum cells that persist (survive) despite the lethal activity of antimicrobial agents. Again, this is especially common with β-lactam agents. If the persisters are subcultured and retested, they appear as susceptible to the effects of the antimicrobial agent as the original isolate, and no greater proportion of cells persist. Persisters have been considered to be metabolically inactive forms that were not actively growing at the time of the interaction of the drug with the inoculum and consequently were not killed by the β-lactam compound.

Of the several mechanisms by which bacteria seemingly evade the killing effect of antimicrobial agents, perhaps the least understood is that of tolerance. The term was coined in 1970 by Tomasz et al. (218) to describe the atypical in vitro response of pneumococcal strains to penicillin. This response was later recognized as genotypic tolerance. The more common and perhaps more clinically relevant type of tolerance, phenotypic tolerance, was described earlier, in 1942, by Hobby et al. (219).

Reports related to the phenomenon of tolerance have accumulated rapidly over the past few years, and several reviews deal with it (220–223). Operationally, tolerance can be defined as the ability of bacteria to grow in the presence of high concentrations of antimicrobials, so that the killing action of the drug is avoided but the MIC remains the same. In Tomasz's (218,226) original observation, typical pneumococcal isolates were quickly lysed and lost viability at penicillin concentrations greater than the MIC. However, the selected tolerant strain was not lysed and lost viability at a significantly reduced rate. Recently, it has been suggested that four different mechanisms may contribute to the ability of organisms to survive (or survive at a higher rate) during treatment with penicillin or other cell wall–directed compounds. Tuomanen et al. (223) proposed the term *survivor mutation* and attributed the mechanism of survival to ancillary bactericidal and lytic processes. Moreover, they cautioned against using the term *tolerant* to describe all of these isolates. The relationship between the killing rates in different bacterial populations and the MBC is depicted in Figure 3.17.

Tolerance in the main has been associated with -lactam agents and has been reported for a number of genera, including *Streptococcus*, *Staphylococcus*, *Listeria*, *Lactobacillus*, and *Clostridium*. A growing

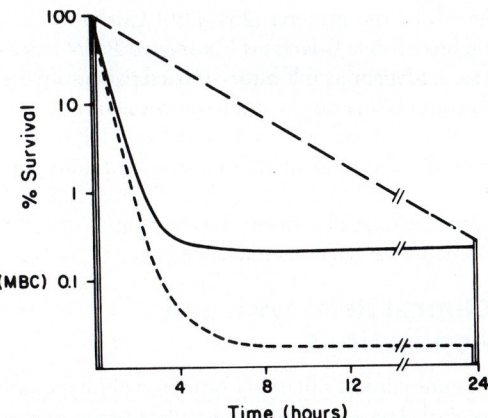

Figure 3.17 ■ Relationship between killing rates and MBC values. Curves show three possible types of kinetics for the loss of viability during treatment with penicillin at a concentration of one time the MIC value. The *vertical bar* at 0 minutes indicates the inoculum; the *bars* at 24 hours represent percent survival, as determined by the MBC value. The *lower bar* represents less than 0.1% survival reached along the rapidly declining killing curve of the nontolerant bacterium (– – –). The *higher bars* indicate survival of more than 0.1% of the cells, which indicates tolerance by the MBC test. However, rates (and mechanisms) of killing in the two tolerant cultures are different. The truly tolerant mutant undergoes slow loss of viability (– – –), whereas the other culture (——) has an initially rapid rate of killing typical of nontolerant cells but a higher survival rate, which may be due to a physiologically heterogeneous inoculum (e.g., higher percentage of dormant cells that are phenotypically tolerant). Alternatively, these cells may represent increased persisters or a subpopulation of resistant cells. (Reprinted from Handwerger S, Tomasz A. Antibiotic tolerance among clinical isolates of bacteria. *Rev Infect Dis* 1985;7:368–386.)

debate revolves around the criteria used to define tolerance. The generally acceptable definition has been a ratio of the MBC to the MIC of more than 32, as originally defined by Sabath et al. (224). However, differences among investigators have led to an assortment of values ranging from 8 to 32 to 100 (221). A more precise approach for detecting tolerant strains is to use quantitative killing curve methods. More than 20 bacterial species recovered from clinical material have been implicated as tolerant strains. However, because of a lack of consensus, the true incidence of tolerance among clinical isolates remains to be determined. The problem is muddied by the variable application of adequate bacteriologic techniques, the variable definition of tolerance, and the lack of suitable reference strains.

To study the effects of antimicrobials on bacteria with decreased or arrested division rates, two new parameters have been suggested for assessing the efficacy of killing. One of them, the MnBC, is analogous to the MBC but applicable to conditions (phenotypic) of slower growth; it is defined as the concentration of drug that achieves a 1-log killing in 24 hours of cells starved for 10 minutes before the addition of antibiotic (223).

Whatever the terms and categories used to describe these events, it is necessary to recognize that the organisms involved may be present in various clinical situations. Although it is generally accepted that rapidly growing and dividing organisms are more susceptible to the inhibiting effects of cell wall–directed antimicrobial agents, it is recognized that rapidly growing bacteria flourish under broth-related clinical conditions like bacteremia. In other clinical conditions, specifically osteomyelitis, it has been demonstrated that microorganisms divide at a much reduced rate and thus would be less susceptible to the effects of antimicrobial agents. A perceived problem in dealing with this clinical dilemma is how to select antimicrobial agents that would be well targeted in arrested growth situations (222). It is of utmost interest and importance to determine whether these isolates are the result of technical manipulation in the laboratory or are indicative of a real clinical phenomenon (Fig. 3.18).

The concept of tolerance is derived from the bactericidal mode of action of β-lactam antibiotics. β-Lactam compounds are bactericidal because they inhibit bacterial cell wall synthesis. Basically, their mode of action is to interfere with the transpeptidation process that links the individual peptidoglycan components of the bacterial cell wall to each other (35,68,225–227). β-Lactams bind to and inactivate specific targets on the inner surface of the bacterial cell membranes. These targets are referred to as the *PBPs* (160,226–229). The PBPs are enzymes—transpeptidases, carboxypeptidases, and endopeptidases—involved in the terminal stages of assembling the bacterial cell wall and maintaining the structure of the cell wall during growth and division (230,277). β-Lactam compounds have different attachment sites and binding capacities for the various PBPs and, depending on the specific PBP bound, have different effects on bacteria (231–233). The inactivation of some PBPs (PBPs 1A, 1BS, 2, and 3) contributes to bacterial death. In contrast, other PBPs (PBPs 4, 5, and 6) are not essential for bacterial viability, and their inactivation by β-lactam molecules is not

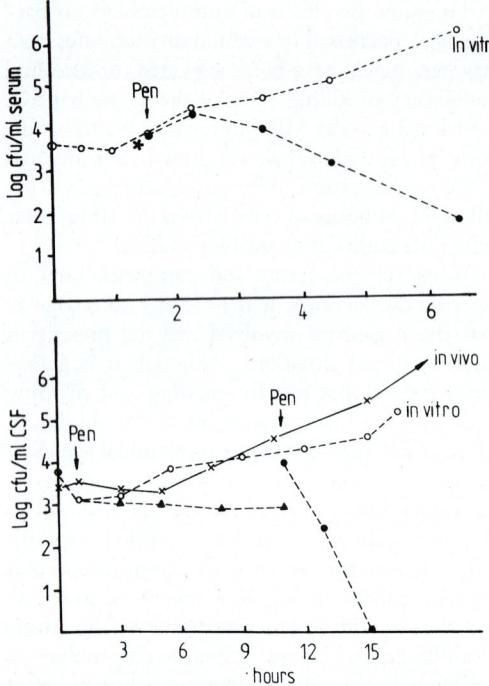

Figure 3.18 ■ Phenotypic tolerance of nongrowing *S. pneumoniae* upon their transfer from serum to cerebrospinal fluid (CSF). (Top) *S. pneumoniae* strain S₁₁₁ was grown in a chemically defined medium (167), filtered, and resuspended in heat-treated rabbit serum. During growth (*), the culture was divided into six aliquots. One aliquot was maintained as a control (o), and one was exposed to penicillin at 20 times the MIC (●). Viability was determined over 6 hours. The remaining aliquots were filtered, resuspended in saline, and used in the experiment, whose results are shown in the bottom panel. **(Bottom)** Pneumococci were either injected into the subarachnoid space of rabbits, as described (2) (×), or suspended in normal CSF in vitro (o). Viability was determined over 17 hours. Benzylpenicillin *(Pen)*, at 20 times the MIC, was added at two time points *(arrows)* to the ex vivo culture aliquots: at 1 hour of the initial 5-hour lag phase (▲) or at 10 hours during the growth phase in CSF (●). In vivo and in vitro growth rates in the CSF were comparable. Transfer of growing pneumococci from the serum to the CSF resulted in a temporary halt in bacterial growth. Benzylpenicillin was not able to kill the nongrowing, phenotypically tolerant pneumococci. Bacteria actively growing in serum or CSF were killed rapidly. (Reproduced from Tuomanen E. Phenotypic tolerance: the search for β-lactam antibiotics that kill nongrowing bacteria. *Rev Infect Dis* 1986;8[Suppl]:S279–S291.)

lethal for the bacteria (234,279). Currently, it is theorized that β-lactams binding to PBPs inactivate endogenous inhibitors of bacterial autolysins. The autolysins can then disrupt covalent bonds in the bacterial cell wall and cause bacteriolysis. The growth of certain organisms that lack autolysins can be inhibited by β-lactam antibiotics, but such organisms are not killed, thus leading to the phenomenon of bacterial tolerance (44).

Clinical Relevance and Applications

In some clinical situations, both microbiologic and clinical data have been accumulated that suggest that MBC determinations or other bactericidal assays may be interpretable and relevant. These have been referred to earlier and include directed activity against *Enterococcus* strains associated with endocarditis (235) and occasional cases of bacterial endocarditis (236) caused by other organisms that may not be fully susceptible, particularly *Pseudomonas* species, MRSA, various species of coagulase-negative *Staphylococcus*, and *S. aureus*. The MBC may also be of value in the management of osteomyelitis (237) and bacteremic infections in granulocytopenic patients (238).

Technical Factors

The application of the MBC (which is founded on the MIC and its derivative, the MBC/MIC ratio) to determine the microbicidal activity of antimicrobial agents has been questioned because the end points are based on arbitrary definitions and are often poorly reproducible. Even within a particular methodology, such as macrodilution versus microdilution procedures (239), there is great biologic variability and different end points may be obtained (Table 3.41).

Dilution methods suffer from several technical problems such as antibiotic carryover, bacteria adhering to the surface of the test vessel, and variations in the medium and growth phase of the inoculum, all of which affect the CFU recovered from subculture plates (240,241) (see "Minimal Bactericidal Concentration Procedure"). One step in performing the assay is critical because of an unusual condition that occurs at the surface (meniscus) of the assay container. At the medium interface, viable organisms flourish, perhaps to escape the potential lethal action of the antimicrobial agent. This potential for error is diminished by mixing and reincubating (see "Minimal Bactericidal Concentration" steps 13 and 14).

Table 3.41

Technical Factors Influencing Minimal Bactericidal Concentration Tests	
Variable Factor	**Effect**
Phase of growth	Increases survivors in stationary phase; paradoxical (Eagle) effect exaggerated in late logarithmic phase
Type of tube or glassware	Adhesion to inside of test vessel varies with material and may elevate counts of survivors, leading to false results
Mode of inoculation	Eliminates adhesion above meniscus by using a small-volume inoculum below the meniscus and avoid shaking
Mixing at 20 h	Vortexing is needed to resuspend all cells
Reincubation for 4 h and vortex again	Allows all cells resuspended at 20 h from above meniscus to be killed before sampling
Antibiotic carryover	Gives falsely low counts of survivors at higher antibiotic concentrations
Reincubation of recovery media	Total of 48 h for staphylococci (72 h for fastidious organisms) may be necessary for final results

Adapted from Schoenknecht FD, Sabath LD, Thornsberry C. Susceptibility tests: special tests. In: Lennette EH, Balows A, Hausler WH Jr, et al, eds. *Manual of clinical microbiology*, 3rd ed. Washington, DC: American Society for Microbiology, 1985:1000–1008.

As for MIC assays, the recommended broth is MHB supplemented with Ca^{2+} and Mg^{2+} for testing *P. aeruginosa*. NaCl (2% final concentration) should be added for testing *S. aureus*. MHB can be used with human serum (HS) in a 1:1 ratio. The use of HS depends on the antimicrobial agent to be tested (and its potential for protein binding), the organism, and the bactericidal test executed. The selection of medium may be altered for research needs in order to grow fastidious microorganisms. For the serum bacterial titer, a 1:1 combination of MHB and HS is the recommended medium (242).

Adherence to the details outlined in the preceding sections with respect to inoculum size, strain storage, growth phase, assay medium, cation content, and incubation duration and temperature must be strict.

Whereas it is anticipated that for bactericidal drugs the MIC and MBC would be similar, it is accepted that for bacteriostatic drugs the MBC could be several dilutions greater. A procedural problem related to the MBC is the definition of the end point as it relates to the number of survivors that remain in the population, because 100% elimination is an impossible goal to achieve (241,243). Several investigators have utilized the definition of a reduction of the number of bacteria present in the inoculum to 99.99% of the original population. This represents a 10^{-3} ($-\log 10^3$) reduction and is somewhat arbitrary, since there is no convincing evidence that a 99.0% or 98.0% reduction actually portrays the outcome and is more clinically relevant. In the United States, CLSI (NCCLS) (180) has written a proposed standard for these tests in which a 1,000-fold reduction of the original inoculum is used as a conventional standard. When the ratio of MBC to MIC is 32 or greater for a given bacterium–antimicrobial combination, the organism is said to be tolerant to the action of the antimicrobial and it is questionable whether a favorable clinical response or outcome can be achieved. The popular definition of tolerance (MBC/MIC greater than 32) has little scientific basis and results in organisms whose response to penicillin is close to the 99.9% definition of kill being artificially divided into susceptible and tolerant categories (240) (Fig. 3.19). In view of the lack of reproducibility of conventional MBC methods, the definition should be treated with caution.

Minimum Bactericidal Concentration

The important studies by Taylor et al. (244) on the MBC determination for staphylococci have shown that much of the variability in the assay results is due to procedural details. In the United States, most of the contention regarding the assay revolves around the issue of whether to use the

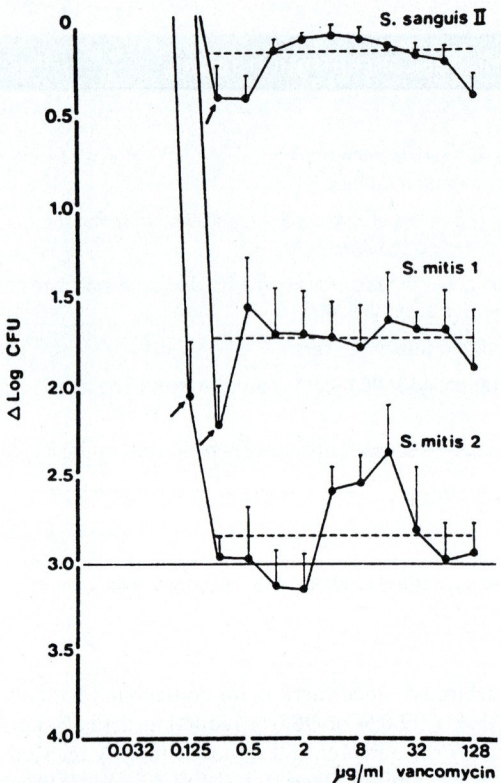

Figure 3.19 ■ Actual reduction of the viable counts for three representative strains after standard broth dilution testing with vancomycin. *Arrows*, MIC. The *solid line* at 3 log$_{10}$ represents the cutoff value of 99.9% killing defining the MBC. The *dashed lines* for each strain represent the mean Δlog CFU. The mean Δlog CFU values for *Streptococcus sanguis* II, *Streptococcus mitis* 1, and *S. mitis* 2 were 0.1 (MBC, more than 128 μg/mL), 1.72 (MBC, more than 128 μg/mL), and 2.84, respectively. The MBC for *S. mitis* 2 was difficult to define because of more than 99.9% killing with 1 and 2 μg/mL vancomycin but not above 4 μg/mL vancomycin. (Reproduced from Meylan PR, Francioli P, Glauser MP. Discrepancies between MBC and actual killing of viridans group streptococci by cell-wall-active antibiotics. *Antimicrob Agents Chemother* 1986;29:418–423.)

macrodilution or microdilution method. In an extensive investigation, James (245) compared four methods for determining the MIC and MBC of penicillin against *S. viridans*. In his studies, the macrodilution and microdilution methods were compared, along with the membrane and gradient plate methods. The author studied 28 strains of *S. viridans* streptococci by these methods and determined the MICs and MBCs. From these data, he calculated the mean error span shown in

Table 3.42. Note that conventional MIC methods are expected to yield reproducibility between tests within one doubling dilution, which equates to a mean error span of less than 0.5 tube errors. If this criterion is applied, then the macrodilution, membrane, and gradient methods gave acceptable reproducibility, whereas the microdilution method did not and therefore should not be used for the determination of the MIC, at least with *S. viridans* streptococci. When one applies the same criterion to MBC determinations, only the gradient method gave acceptable reproducibility, and it was the most reliable method for predicting penicillin tolerance. James (245) concluded from his studies that the mean error spans for all methods were acceptable, except for the microdilution technique. However, correct and reproducible results were obtained for all control organisms by the gradient method and, to a lesser extent, the membrane method. His study clearly indicated that the microdilution results were unacceptable.

In deciding on a method to adopt for determining the MBC, it is thus best, as shown by the work of James (245), to avoid the microdilution method. Because many reference and clinical laboratories may not have accumulated experience with the gradient or membrane methods, the macrodilution method is the logical choice. It is described here in detail, as adapted from Schoenknecht et al. (241).

Minimum Bactericidal Concentration Procedure

Minimum Inhibitory Concentration

1. Subculture organisms onto appropriate medium (usually a blood agar plate) and incubate overnight at 35°C.
2. Inoculate a tube containing 3 mL of saline or MHB with five or more colonies from the overnight plate to achieve a turbidity equivalent to a no. 1 McFarland standard (approximately 10^8 organisms/mL).
3. Transfer 0.1 mL of turbid inoculum (patient's pathogen) into 10 mL of MHB or other appropriate broth. Incubate in a shaking waterbath or equivalent at 35°C until turbid. This corresponds to an end point between a no. 1 McFarland standard and an overnight suspension and requires 5 or 6 hours for rapid growers.
4. Inoculate the standard control organism (*E. coli*, *S. aureus*, etc.) into 3 mL of broth and incubate (without shaking) at 35°C until turbid.

Table 3.42

Test Variation for 28 Strains of Viridans Streptococci Tested for Minimal Inhibitory Concentration and Minimal Bactericidal Concentration by Four Methods[a]

Method	No. of Strains Tolerant[b,c]	MIC Tube Error (Range)	MBC Tube Error (Range)
Microdilution	13	±1.56	±4.24
		± (0–9)	± (0–18)
Macrodilution	11	±0.48	±3.47
		± (0–6)	± (0–23)
Membrane	12	±0.50	±2.50
		± (0–4)	± (0–20)
Gradient	12	±0.23	±0.22
		± (0–1)	± (0–3)

[a]Mean error span for each method (±2 SD) expressed as the number of twofold dilutions.
[b]On the basis of mean MBC/MIC >32, 6 strains were tolerant by all methods.
[c]No single organism was responsible for major discrepancies in all methods.
MIC, minimum inhibitory concentration; MBC, minimum bactericidal concentration.
Adapted from James PA. Comparison of four methods for the determination of MIC and MBC of penicillin for viridans streptococci and the implications for penicillin tolerance. *J Antimicrob Chemother* 1990;25:209–216.

5. Prepare twofold serial dilutions of the antibiotic in 2 mL of MHB (total volume per acid-washed borosilicate glass tube); 16 × 100-mm glass tubes with loose-fitting metal caps are preferred.
6. Standardize the inocula (patient's organism and control organism) to equal a 0.5 McFarland turbidity standard (approximately 5×10^7 organisms/mL) in 3 mL of saline or broth.
7. Dilute adjusted inocula 1:10 (0.2 mL in 1.8 mL of MHB or appropriate substitute). This equals about 5×10^6 organisms/mL.
8. Dispense, using an Eppendorf or equivalent pipette, 100 µL of diluted inoculum into tubes containing serial dilutions of the antibiotic. To inoculate, insert the pipette tip well under the surface of the antibiotic-containing broth. Avoid any contact between the tip and the walls of the tube. Rinse the tip five times in solution. The same tip may be used throughout the test if inoculating from lowest to highest concentration of antibiotic. The final inoculum size is approximately 2.5×10^5 organisms/mL.
9. Incubate for 20 hours at 35°C.
10. From the 1:10 dilution of the 0.5 McFarland-adjusted inoculum, which should be about 5×10^6 organisms/mL (step 7), dilute serially 1:10 in MHB four times to achieve a final inoculum of 5×10^2 organisms/mL as follows: 0.2 mL (5×10^6 CFU/mL) + 1.8 mL MHB; 0.2 mL (5×10^6 CFU/mL) + 1.8 mL MHB

5×10^5 CFU/mL; 0.2 mL (5×10^6 CFU/mL) + 1.8 mL MHB 5×10^4 CFU/mL; 0.2 mL (5×10^4 CFU/mL) + 1.8 mL MHB 5×10^3 CFU/mL; 0.2 mL (5×10^3 CFU/mL) + 1.8 mL MHB 5×10^2 CFU/mL.
11. Aliquot 0.1 mL of this suspension, dispense either into a tube of melted agar for the preparation of pour plates or onto an appropriate agar plate (e.g., blood agar) and distribute evenly using sterile bent glass rods. This procedure should be done in duplicate. Incubate overnight at 35°C.
12. Observe and record MIC of control organisms.
13. For patient's sample only, vigorously vortex-mix tubes without visible growth for 15 seconds and reincubate for an additional 4 hours.
14. Vortex-mix again and sample tubes for MBC determination; spread 100-µL samples across the surface of dried TS agar plates with sterile bent glass rods.
15. Record patient's MIC.

Minimum Bactericidal Concentration

16. Incubate plates overnight at 35°C for the MBC test.
17. After 1 day (or 2 days), count the number of colonies per plate from the original inoculum plates or pour plates and average. Determine a colony count that represents 0.1% of the original inoculum (i.e., 99.9% reduction).

18. Count colonies from MBC plates. Any number equal to or less than the determined colony count from step 17 is considered as a 99.9% kill or bactericidal result.

When counting the number of colonies to determine the plate average, the mean is referred to as N. Apply the formula $N/2 + 2(\sqrt{N/2})$ to determine the upper limit of a colony count that represents 0.1% of the original inoculum (approximately 95% confidence limits). Therefore, any colony counts from MBC plates equal to or less than the determined inoculum colony count upper limit are considered 99.9% kill or bactericidal results.

Alternatively, rejection values can be determined from a chart that takes into account the final inoculum size, dual sampling, pipetting error, and the Poisson distribution of sample responses (Table 3.43).

Hacek et al. (246), recognizing the potential variability and complexity imposed by this assay, proposed a modified scheme. Their modified bactericidal testing protocol includes omitting serum supplementation, incubation without agitation, running tests in duplicate with a reduced number of dilutions (six instead of nine), extending the incubation interval for 24 hours to resolve discrepancies, using single 0.1-mL aliquots, and adopting an alternate end point calculation. The authors found a 91% agreement between the standard and their modified protocol and suggest the alternative procedure is practical for the clinical laboratory.

Serum Bactericidal Titer/Test

Clinical Relevance and Applications

The seminal work on and application of this test were done by Schlichter and MacLean (247). In its original form, the test determined bacteriostatic activity; it was later modified to include bactericidal activity. However, in the nearly 50 years that the test has been available and used, there has been no clear, universally accepted criteria for its application. Critical reviews of the SBT have not found the test clinically useful and have stressed the need for standardization of the methodology (237,248). CLSI (NCCLS) has developed a proposed guideline (249), and in a thoughtful review, Stratton (91) addressed the specific application and clinical relevance of the test.

Assessing the antimicrobial activity in a patient's serum during treatment by using the offending organisms isolated from the patient as the test strain would appear to be the most logical approach to evaluating and monitoring chemotherapy. The SBT measures the combined effects of absorption and elimination of the antimicrobial agent; its potential binding to serum proteins; the effect of metabolic congeners of the parent compound against the microorganisms; and, if dual antimicrobial therapy is administered, the effects

Table 3.43

Rejection Value (Number of Colonies) and Calculated Sensitivity and Specificity for Each Initial Inoculum Concentration on the Basis of Duplicate 0.01-mL Samples[a]

Final Inoculum (CFU/mL)	Rejection Value[b]	Sensitivity (%)[c]	Specificity (%)[c]
1×10^5	4	77	97
2×10^5	8	89	99
3×10^5	15	99	99
4×10^5	20	99	99
5×10^5	25	99	99
6×10^5	29	99	99
7×10^5	33	99	99
8×10^5	38	99	99
9×10^5	42	99	99
1×10^6	47	99	99
2×10^6	91	99	99
3×10^6	136	99	99
4×10^6	182	99	99
5×10^6	227	99	99
6×10^6	273	99	99
7×10^6	318	99	99
8×10^6	364	99	99
9×10^6	409	99	99
1×10^7	455	99	99

[a]A 5% error (pipette plus full sampling) is considered for determination of final inoculum based on *duplicate* sampling of final inoculum size.
[b]Number of colonies. When the sum of colonies from duplicate samples is equal to or less than the rejection value, the antibiotic is determined to be lethal (a 0.999 or greater reduction in the final inoculum).
[c]Sensitivity and specificity calculated for each specific final inoculum concentration and rejection value.
Adapted from National Committee for Clinical Laboratory Standards. *Methods for determining bactericidal activity of antimicrobial agents.* Wayne, PA: National Committee for Clinical Laboratory Standards, 1999. NCCLS document M26-A.

of drug interactions, including synergistic, additive, and antagonistic effects.

As with the determination as MBC, the SBT can be helpful in monitoring the treatment of bacterial endocarditis (235,236), bacteremia in patients with cancer (150), osteomyelitis or septic arthritis (237,250), and bacterial meningitis (251).

As an experimental tool, the SBT has been used in evaluating new drugs and drug combinations and detecting antimicrobial potency in infected body fluids other than blood. When the SBT has been used for drug evaluation (in humans or animals), analysis of the results can be aided by using the titer to measure the area under the bactericidal curve (AUBC) (252).

Although the SBT approach seems to be a logical integration of physiologic (pharmacokinetic) and in vitro susceptibility, this test, as well as other bacterium-antimicrobial assays, fails to evaluate the cellular and humoral defenses of the host, the site and severity of the infection, the quantity of bacteria present and their virulence, and the continually changing concentration of the antimicrobial agent in the host.

Serum Bactericidal Titer/Test Methodology

As with the MBC procedures, many variations of this test exist. The same care and attention to details and materials used in executing the MBC procedures should be used here. The method that follows is adapted from several sources (241,243,249).

Collection of Patient Serum

Inherent in this procedure is the use of the patient's serum to represent the physiologic concentration of the antimicrobial agent. For this purpose, a peak level and a trough level are generally obtained. The peak level is considered the level obtained 30 to 45 minutes after an intravenous infusion, 60 minutes after an intramuscular infusion, or 90 minutes after an oral dose. The peak level is obtained 30 to 60 minutes after the drug is absorbed and distributed. The trough level is the level that is considered to occur 30 minutes prior to the following dose.

After the specimen has been collected, it should be transported to the laboratory properly and promptly, to separate the blood and serum. Serum collected from the specimen should be frozen if a delay of more than 2 hours in performing the SBT is anticipated. Ideally, trough and peak serum specimens should be pair-matched rather than collected on different days of therapy.

Patient Organism

The SBT must be anticipated so that the patient's clinical isolate can be saved. Because it is the practice of many clinical laboratories to save bacteremic isolates as well as isolates from spinal and other body fluids, these can be retrieved early. On the other hand, if it is anticipated that the isolate will be needed, this should be kept frozen at 70°C in a TS broth or in a cryoprotectant medium (e.g., glycerol).

Serum Bactericidal Titer/Test Procedure

1. Serially dilute the patient's serum twofold at least 1:64, using MHB as diluent. The final volume per tube should be 1 mL.
2. Add the patient's organism to a 0.1-mL volume of a carefully prepared inoculum (see steps 10 and 11 of the MBC procedure).
3. Prepare pour plates for establishing original inoculum CFU counts (see steps 7 through 11 of the MBC procedure).
4. Include a growth control tube containing MHB and inoculum but no serum.
5. Incubate for 18 to 24 hours.
6. Subculture for the 99.9% bactericidal end point, as described for the MBC procedure.

Interpretation

The interpretation of end points is controversial. The CLSI (NCCLS) guidelines (249) offer the following: peak titer of 1:2 and trough titer of 1:2, interpretation of inadequate; peak titer of 1:4 to 1:16 and trough titer of 1:4, interpretation of intermediate; and peak titer of 1:32 and trough titer of 1:8, interpretation of adequate. According to Stratton (237), in orthopedic infections, a titer of 1:8 is prognostic of cure, although higher titers do not necessarily preclude positive outcomes.

Killing Curve

The killing curve or killing rate is represented by a plot of the number of survivors in the host after administration of a typical therapeutic regimen. It has been used to evaluate and compare new drugs and to study differences and changes in the antimicrobial susceptibility of clinically important bacterial isolates. These determinations are rarely used for guiding chemotherapy; they are mainly applied in experimental situations to animal models and are generally used to assess classes of drugs. One concentration of antibiotic is tested, usually that which is representative of an average level

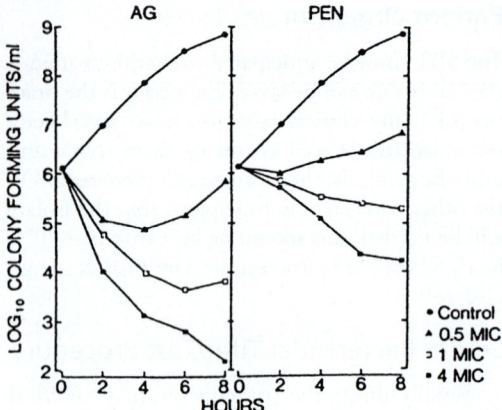

Figure 3.20 ■ **Killing curves.** At periodic intervals, usually at 0, 4, 12, and 24 hours of incubation, colony counts are performed and charted on semilogarithmic paper, with the survivor colony count on the ordinate (logarithmic scale) and time on the abscissa (arithmetic scale). *AG*, aminoglycoside; *PEN*, penicillin.

obtainable during therapy. At periodic intervals, usually at 0, 4, 12, and 24 hours of incubation, colony counts are performed and charted on semilogarithmic paper, with the survivor colony count on the ordinate (logarithmic scale) and time on the abscissa (arithmetic scale) (Fig. 3.20). For example, when one compares the β-lactam antimicrobial agents with the aminoglycosides, the former are characterized by slower, dose-dependent initial bactericidal activity. The extent of the bactericidal action is related to the time during which the serum level exceeds the MIC. If this level falls below the MIC, there is immediate regrowth of the microorganisms. In contrast, aminoglycosides demonstrate rapid, dose-dependent initial bactericidal activity, followed by a bacteriostatic phase that can last several hours after the serum concentration falls below the MIC.

The kinetics of antimicrobial activity, as described, provides a theoretical basis for dosing frequency and depends on the pathogen and the antibiotic used. Only one antibiotic concentration, representing the average obtainable blood level, or a limited number of concentrations, representing multiples or fractions of the blood level, are used. In the plot in Figure 3.20, the aminoglycoside is shown to be a drug with concentration-dependent bactericidal activity. At increasing drug concentrations, there is an increase in the magnitude and rate of killing. β-lactam compounds (penicillin in Fig. 3.20) demonstrate little concentration-dependent bactericidal activity. At

least for two antimicrobial agents, ampicillin and ciprofloxacin, their activities (expressed as killing rates) were similar in MHB and human urine, as judged by an in vitro PD model (40).

Although the protocol outlined in the following text relates to evaluating the lethal activity of individual antimicrobial agents, agents combined for their potential synergistism can also be tested (see Chapter 10).

More recently, modified killing curve investigations have been used to elucidate anticipated multiple resistance mechanisms expressed by *S. pneumoniae* and *Mycobacteria* species against fluoroquinolone compounds (253,254). In this variation of the killing curve procedure, large numbers of microorganisms (10^8 to 10^{10}) are plated on increasing concentrations of antibiotic—in this case, fluoroquinolones—and the fraction of cells that can be recovered are then treated as CFU. The fraction that survive or grow are plotted against the concentration (i.e., the MIC). As can be seen in Figure 3.21, the first dip in the plot occurs at the MIC; a second inflection point in mutant

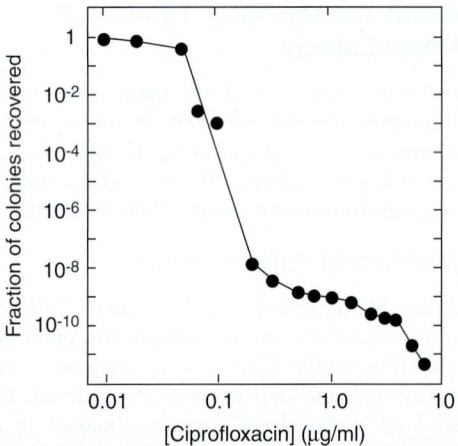

Figure 3.21 ■ **Effect of increasing concentrations of a quinolone (e.g., ciprofloxacin) on selection of resistant mutants.** As drug concentration increases, note two inflections in the number of colonies recovered. The first drop equals the MIC. The second drop in mutant recovery occurs at the concentration required to block the growth of first-step mutants—the MPC (From Blondeau JM, Zhao X, Hansen G, et al. Mutant prevention concentrations of fluoroquinolones for clinical isolates of *Streptococcus pneumoniae*. *Antimicrob Agents Chemother* 2001;45:433–438; Dong Y, Zhao X, Domagala J, et al. Effect of fluoroquinolone concentration on selection of resistant mutants of *Mycobacterium bovis* BCG and *Staphylococcus aureus*. *Antimicrob Agents Chemother* 1999;43[7]:1756–1758.).

recovery occurs at a concentration the authors refer to as the mutant prevention concentration (MPC), the concentration required to block first-step mutants. This approach has proved valuable in studying the design of the fluoroquinolones in order to anticipate the possible development of stepwise mutants.

Killing Curve Procedure

1. Prepare inoculum of approximately 5×10^7 CFU/mL, as in steps 1 through 3 and 5 and 6 of the MBC procedure.
2. Inoculate according to step 8 of the MBC procedure. The final concentration should be 5×10^5 CFU/mL for each tube.
3. Immediately vortex-mix for 15 seconds the zero growth tube and dispense 0.1 mL into a tube of melted agar for the preparation of agar pour plates. Incubate at 35°C for 18 to 24 hours.
4. Similarly, for each subsequent time interval, prepare pour plates.
5. For testing at 24 hours, vortex-mix the last tube at 20 hours and reincubate for an additional 4 hours.
6. At 24 hours, vortex-mix again and prepare pour plates.

Serum Bactericidal Rate

The time-kill curve evaluates the rate at which single or multiple drugs kill bacteria. The serum bactericidal rate represents the rate of serum killing; the method used integrates in vitro activity and the in vivo pharmacokinetics of antimicrobial drugs and therefore reflects very accurately what happens in the host.

In a novel approach to the application of the serum bactericidal rate, Barriere et al. (252) measured the AUBC to determine the total synergistic bactericidal activity. When the calculated value of the AUBC for a combination was greater than the sum of the values for the individual drugs, the combination was judged to be synergistic.

A therapeutic role for the use of killing curves was shown by Small and Chambers (255). They studied the clinical failure of vancomycin when treating intravenous drug users with *S. aureus* endocarditis. In vitro studies with 10 strains of *S. aureus* recovered from this patient group demonstrated that, at four times the MIC, vancomycin was less rapidly bactericidal than nafcillin (Fig. 3.22). At 4 hours after incubation, the mean decreases in bacterial counts for vancomycin and the β-lactam were similar. However, after 24 hours,

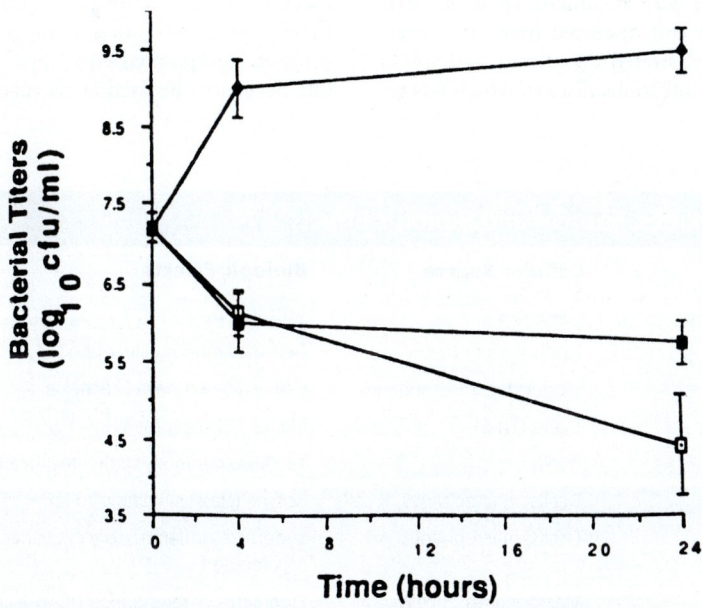

Figure 3.22 ■ Time-kill curves for nafcillin (▪) and vancomycin (●) at a concentration of four times the MIC for 10 clinical isolates of *S. aureus*. ♦, Control. (Reproduced from Small PM, Chambers HF. Vancomycin for *Staphylococcus aureus* endocarditis in intravenous drug users. *Antimicrob Agents Chemother* 1990;34:1227–1231.)

the mean count for vancomycin had not significantly changed from the 4-hour titration, although there was a significant reduction (2.8 log$_{10}$ CFU/mL) for nafcillin. It was on this basis that the authors explained relapses and persistent bacteremia in the vancomycin-treated group and concluded that vancomycin was less effective than nafcillin for treating this infection.

CYTOKINES AND CYTOKINE ACTIVITY

Cytokines represent a broad group of soluble mediators of cell-to-cell communication; the group includes interleukins, interferons, and colony-stimulating factors (172,272). Cytokine molecules are mediators of specific and nonspecific host defense responses. As such, they play a critical role in effector mechanisms that eliminate foreign antigens such as microorganisms. Advances in our understanding of cytokines have focused on two primary biologic activities: the regulation of inflammation with effective immune responses to pathogen invasions and a wide array of hemopoietic activities that serve to modulate the growth of immune cells. Table 3.44 lists some cytokines and their biologic effects. It is with the understanding that cytokines may play a supportive or synergistic role in conjuction with antimicrobial agents that they are included and discussed here. The interferons have demonstrated significant activity in different types of infectious disease, which has re-

sulted in several FDA-approved indications (256). Interferon- has shown antiviral activity, and some interleukins are known to demonstrate protection against intracellular pathogens. Interleukin-1 receptor antagonist serves as an active mediator during severe bacterial infection or septic shock. As recombinant forms of these compounds become available, no doubt clinical trials will be attempted to determine effectiveness.

The cytokines can be readily assayed in human biologic fluids by an enzyme-linked immunosorbent assay–type sandwich immunoassay that recognizes both natural human and *E. coli*–derived human cytokines. A typical standard curve from a commercial kit assay is shown in Figure 3.23.

FUTURE CONSIDERATIONS

Laboratory assessments of antimicrobial activity will no doubt attempt to more broadly incorporate microbiologic and pharmacologic attributes of antibiotics. Advances in PK/PD modeling have made significant contributions to establishing breakpoint determinations that are more clinically relevant. However, the application to direct patient care in real time has not been fully realized. As currently conceived, some of the approaches that use computer-simulated models are too tedious to execute as part of actionable health care. Aspects of these interactive models as suggested have not as yet been incorporated into "apps" available on mobile devices to be used at the patient's bedside to

TABLE 3.44

Selected Cytokines: Sources and Biologic Effects[a]		
Cytokine	**Cellular Source**	**Biologic Effects**
Interferon (IFN)-α, -β	Phagocytes	Antiviral, pyrogenic
IFN-γ	T cells	Activates mononuclear phagocytes
Interleukin (IL)-1[b]	Monocytes, macrophages	Cell activation, fever, cachexia
IL-1 ra	T cells (Th-1)	Blocks IL-1 receptor
IL-2[c]	T cells	T-cell proliferation, stimulates B-cell proliferation
IL-4	T cells, macrophages, B cells	Isotype (class) switching to IgE
IL-10	T cells, macrophages	Suppresses inflammatory cytokines, enhances B-cell proliferation
IL-12	Macrophages, B cells	Stimulates differentiation of Th 1 cells
Tumor necrosis factor (TNF)-α	Numerous cell types	Wide range of inflammatory and immune responses

[a]Compiled from various sources (e.g., Howard, Miyajima, and Coffman [172]).
[b]Lymphocyte activating factor.
[c]T-cell growth factor.

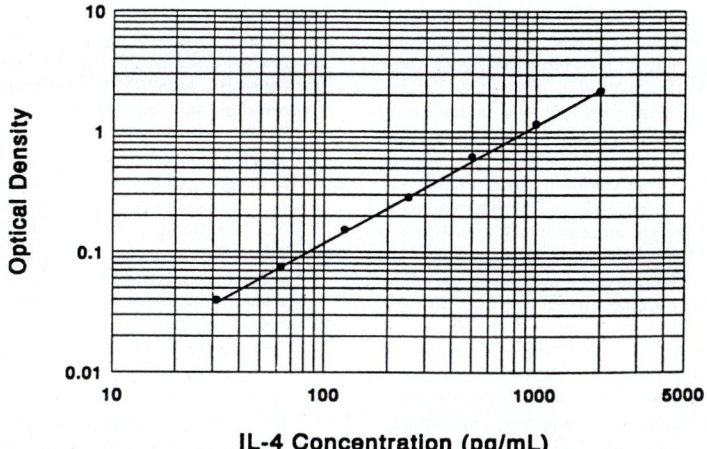

Figure 3.23 ■ Typical sandwich enzyme-linked immunosorbent assay standard curve obtainable with a commercial kit that recognizes natural human and *E. coli*–derived recombinant interleukin-4 (IL-4).

help in the delivery of rational, safe, and effective therapy (257). As new pathogens emerge, many associated with resistance mechanisms that threaten to limit the effective therapeutic use of antimicrobial agents, clinical laboratories will be called upon to move rapidly and accurately to screen for the presence of resistant members. Toward this end, methods for detecting genetic markers of resistance such as those discussed in this volume will be used. Additionally, the use of multiple probes directed

toward more than one gene target (multiplexing) need to be designed as panels to detect the several antimicrobial-resistant phenotypes. Lastly, as the pipeline for the development of new antimicrobial compounds maintains its constricted development, pharmaceutical companies may consider developing additional innovative, antiinflammatory, antisepsis medicines. At that time, clinical laboratories will have the capability to titrate inflammatory cytokines and their immunotherapeutic targets.

REFERENCES

1. Fleming A. On the antibacterial action of cultures of a penicillium with special reference to their use in the isolation of *B. influenzae*. *Br J Exp Pathol* 1929;10:226–236.
2. Rammelkamp CH, Maxon T. Resistance of *Staphylococcus aureus* to the action of penicillin. *Proc Soc Exp Biol Med* 1942;51:386–389.
3. Foster JW, Woodruff HB. Microbiological aspects of penicillin. *J Bacteriol* 1943;46:187–202.
4. Vincent JG, Vincent HW. Filter paper modification of the Oxford cup penicillin determination. *Proc Soc Exp Biol Med* 1944;55:162–164.
5. World Health Organization. *Standardization of methods for conducting microbic sensitivity tests: second report of the Expert Committee on Antibiotics.* World Health Organization technical reports series, no. 210. New York: World Health Organization, 1961.
6. Ericsson HM, Sherris JC. Antibiotic sensitivity testing: report of an international collaborative study. *Acta Pathol Microbiol Scand* 1971;217(Suppl B):390.
7. Bauer AW, Kirby WMM, Sherris JC, et al. Antibi-

otic susceptibility testing by a standardized single disk method. *Am J Clin Pathol* 1966;45:493–496.
8. Federal Register. Rules and regulations: antibiotic susceptibility disks: correction. *Federal Register* 1973;38:2576.
9. Federal Register. Rules and regulations: antibiotic susceptibility discs. *Federal Register* 1972;37:20525–20529.
10. National Committee for Clinical Laboratory Standards. *Methods for dilution antimicrobial susceptibility tests for bacteria that grow aerobically: approved standard.* 6th ed. Wayne, PA: National Committee for Clinical Laboratory Standards. 2003. NCCLS document M7-A6.
11. National Committee for Clinical Laboratory Standards. *Performance standards for antimicrobial disk susceptibility tests: approved standard.* 8th ed. Wayne, PA: National Committee for Clinical Laboratory Standards, 2003. NCCLS document M2-A8.
12. D'Amato RF, Hochstein L, Vernaleg JR, et al. Evaluation of the BIOGRAM antimicrobial susceptibility test system. *J Clin Microbiol* 1985;22:793–798.

13. Matsen J, Koepcke M, Quie P. Evaluation of the Bauer-Kirby-Sherris-Turck and single-disk diffusion methods of antibiotic susceptibility testing. *Antimicrob Agents Chemother* 1970;9:445–453.

14. Amsterdam D. Principles of antibiotic testing in the laboratory. In: Balows A, Hausler WJ Jr, Lennette EH, eds. *Laboratory diagnosis of infectious disease: principles and practice*. Vol 1. New York: Springer-Verlag, 1988:22–38.

15. Lorian V. In vitro simulation of in vivo conditions: physical state of the culture medium. *J Clin Microbiol* 1989;27:2403–2406.

16. Appelbaum PC. Worldwide development of antibiotic resistance in pneumococci. *Eur J Clin Microbiol* 1987;6:367–377.

17. LaForce FM. Pneumonia3—41987: new developments. *Eur J Clin Microbiol* 1987;6:613–617.

18. Woolfrey BF, Fox JMK, Lally RT, et al. Broth microdilution testing of Pseudomonas aeruginosa and aminoglycosides: need for employing dilutions differing by small arithmetic increments. *J Clin Microbiol* 1982;16:663–667.

19. Moellering RC, Wennersten C, Medrek T, et al. Prevalence of high level resistance to aminoglycosides in clinical isolates of enterococci. *Antimicrob Agents Chemother* 1970;10:335–340.

20. Brumfitt W, Percival A. Laboratory control of antibiotic therapy in urinary tract infection. *Ann NY Acad Sci* 1967;145:329–343.

21. Trissel LA. *Handbook on injectable drugs*. Bethesda, MD: American Society of Hospital Pharmacists, 1983.

22. Barry AL, Lasner RA. Inhibition of bacterial growth by the nitrofurantoin solvent dimethylformamide. *Antimicrob Agents Chemother* 1976;9:549–550.

23. Murray PR, Niles AC. Effect of filtration on antimicrobial solutions. *Antimicrob Agents Chemother* 1981;20:686–687.

24. Barry AL. *The antimicrobic susceptibility test: principles and practices*. Philadelphia: Lea & Febiger, 1976.

25. Grove DC, Randall WA. *Assay methods of antibiotics: methods for the determination of bacterial susceptibility to antibiotics*. New York: Medical Encyclopedia, 1955.

26. Bauer AW, Sherris JC. The determination of sulfonamide susceptibility of bacteria. *Chemotherapia* 1964;9:1–19.

27. Binford JS Jr, Binford LF, Adler P. A semiautomated microcalorimetric method of antibiotic sensitivity testing. *Am J Clin Pathol* 1973;59:86–94.

28. Barry AL, Jones RN, Gavan TL. Evaluation of the micromedia system for quantitative antimicrobial drug susceptibility testing: a collaborative study. *Antimicrob Agents Chemother* 1978;13:61–69.

29. Gavan TL, Barry AL. Microdilution test procedures. In: Lennette EH, Spaulding EH, Truant JP, eds. *Manual of clinical microbiology*. 3rd ed. Washington, DC: American Society for Microbiology, 1980:359–362.

30. Gavan TL, Jones RN, Barry AL. Evaluation of the Sensititre system for quantitative antimicrobial drug susceptibility testing: a collaborative study. *Antimicrob Agents Chemother* 1980;17:464–469.

31. MacLowry JD, Jaqua MJ, Selepak ST. Detailed methodology and implementation of a semi-automated serial dilution microtechnique for antimicrobial susceptibility testing. *Appl Microbiol* 1970;20:46–53.

32. Washington JA II, Sutter VL. Dilution susceptibility test: agar and macro-broth dilution procedures. In: Lennette EH, Spaulding EH, Truant JI, eds. *Manual of clinical microbiology*. Washington, DC: American Society for Microbiology, 1980:453–458.

33. Mueller JH, Hinton J. A protein-free medium for the primary isolation of the gonococcus and meningococcus. *Proc Soc Exp Biol Med* 1941;48:330–333.

34. Chow BF, McKee CM. Interaction between crystalline penicillin and human plasma proteins. *Science* 1945;101:67–68.

35. Tilton RC, Newberg L. Standardization of the microdilution susceptibility test. In: Balows A, ed. *Current techniques for antibiotic susceptibility testing*. Springfield, IL: Charles C Thomas Publisher, 1973:77–87.

36. Tilton RC, Lieberman L, Gerlach EH. Microdilution antibiotic susceptibility test: examination of certain variables. *Appl Microbiol* 1973;26:658–665.

37. Neussel H. Problems of standardization of media. In: Williams JD, Geddes AM, eds. *Chemotherapy*. New York: Plenum Press, 1976:2.

38. National Committee for Clinical Laboratory Standards. *Protocols for evaluating dehydrated Mueller-Hinton agar*. Villanova, PA: National Committee for Clinical Laboratory Standards, 1996. NCCLS document M6-A.

39. Pursiano TA, Misiek M, Leitner F, et al. Effect of assay medium on the antibacterial activity of certain penicillins and cephalosporins. *Antimicrob Agents Chemother* 1973;3:33–39.

40. Drobot GR, Karlowsky JA, Hoban DJ, et al. Antibiotic activity in microbiological media versus that in human urine: comparison of ampicillin, ciprofloxacin, and trimethoprim-sulfamethoxazole. *Antimicrob Agents Chemother* 1996;40:237–240.

41. Hoeprich PD, Barry AL, Fay GD. Synthetic medium for susceptibility testing. *Antimicrob Agents Chemother* 1970;1969:494–497.

42. Sabath LD, Lorian V, Gerstein D, et al. Enhancing effect on alkalinization of the medium on the activity of erythromycin against Gram-negative bacteria. *Appl Microbiol* 1968;16:1288–1292.

43. Lorian V, Sabath LD. Effect of pH on the activity of erythromycin against 500 isolates of Gram-negative bacilli. *Appl Microbiol* 1970;20:754–756.

44. Bartlett JG. *Campylobacter pylori*: fact or fancy. *Gastroenterology* 1988;94:229–232.

45. McNulty CAM, Dent J, Wise R. Susceptibility of clinical isolates of *Campylobacter pyloridis* to 11 antimicrobial agents. *Antimicrob Agents Chemother* 1985;28:837–838.

46. Grayson ML, Eliopoulos GM, Ferraro MJ, et al. Effect of varying pH on the susceptibility of *Campylobacter pylori* to antimicrobial agents. *Eur J Clin Microbiol Infect Dis* 1989;8:888–889.

47. Debets-Ossenkopp YJ, Namarar F, MacLaren DM. Effect of an acidic environment on the susceptibility of *Helicobacter pylori* to trospectomycin and other antimicrobial agents. *Eur J Clin Microbiol Infect Dis* 1995;14:353–355.

48. Mackowiak RA, Marling-Cason M, Cohen RL. Effects of temperature on antimicrobial susceptibility of bacteria. *J Infect Dis* 1982;145:550–555.

49. Lamb JW, Mann JM, Simmons RJ. Factors influencing the microbiological assay of tobramycin. *Antimicrob Agents Chemother* 1972;1:323–328.

50. Wick WE. Delineation of the differences of various bacterial susceptibility tests with cephalexin. *Antimicrob Agents Chemother* 1969;1968:435–441.

51. Selwyn S, Lam C. Combined effect on protein-binding and β-lactamases on the activity of penicillins and cephalosporins. In: Williams JD, Gedes AM, eds. *Chemotherapy*. Vol 2. New York: Plenum Press, 1976:325–330.

52. Wick WE. Influence of antibiotic stability on the results of in vitro testing procedures. *J Bacteriol* 1964;87:1162–1170.

53. Sherris JC, Rashad AL, Lighthart GA. Laboratory determination of antibiotic susceptibility to ampicillin and cephalothin. *Ann NY Acad Sci* 1967;145:248–267.

54. Craig WA, Gudmundsson S. The postantibiotic effect. In: Lorian V, ed. *Antibiotics in laboratory medicine.* 2nd ed. Baltimore: Williams and Wilkins, 1985:515–536.

55. Eagle H, Musselman A. The rate of bactericidal action of penicillin in vitro as a function of its concentration, and its paradoxically reduced activity at high concentrations against certain organisms. *J Exp Med* 1948;88:99–131.

56. McDonald PJ, Craig WA, Kunin CM. Brief antibiotic exposure and effect on bacterial growth. In: Williams JD, Geddes AM, eds. *Chemotherapy.* Vol 2. New York: Plenum Press, 1976:95–102.

57. Kenny MA, Pollock HM, Minshew BH, et al. Cation components of Mueller-Hinton agar affecting testing of *Pseudomonas aeruginosa* susceptibility to gentamicin. *Antimicrob Agents Chemother* 1980;17:55–62.

58. Garrod LP, Waterworth PM. Effect of medium composition on the apparent sensitivity of *Pseudomonas aeruginosa* to gentamicin. *J Clin Pathol* 1969;22:534–538.

59. Fass RJ, Barnishan J. Effect of divalent cation concentrations on the antibiotic susceptibilities of nonfermenters other than *Pseudomonas aeruginosa. Antimicrob Agents Chemother* 1979;16:434–438.

60. Reller LB, Schoenknecht FD, Kenny MA, et al. Antibiotic susceptibility testing of *Pseudomonas aeruginosa*: selection of a control strain and criteria for magnesium and calcium content in media. *J Infect Dis* 1974;130:454–463.

62. Weinberg ED. The mutual effects of antimicrobial compounds and metallic cations. *Bacteriol Rev* 1957;21:46–68.

63. Medeiros AA, O'Brien T, Wacker WEC, et al. Effect of salt concentration on the apparent in vitro susceptibility of *Pseudomonas* and other Gram-negative bacilli to gentamicin. *J Infect Dis* 1971;124(Suppl):S59–S64.

64. Neu H. Mecillinam, a novel penicillanic acid derivative with unusual activity against Gram-negative bacteria. *Antimicrob Agents Chemother* 1976;9:973–999.

65. Jorgensen JH, Redding JS, Maher LA, et al. Improved medium for antimicrobial susceptibility testing of *Haemophilus influenzae. J Clin Microbiol* 1987;25:2105–2113.

66. Eliopoulos GM, Reiszner E, Willey S, et al. Effect of blood product medium supplements on the activity of cefotaxime and other cephalosporins against *Enterococcus faecalis. Diagn Microbiol Infect Dis* 1989;12:149–156.

67. Coudron PE, Stratton CW. Factors affecting growth and susceptibility testing of *Helicobacter pylori* in liquid media. *J Clin Microbiol* 1995;33:1028–1030.

68. Neu HC. Penicillins: new insights into their mechanisms of activity and clinical use. *Bull NY Acad Med* 1982;58:681–695.

69. Van Klingeren B, Rutgers A. Usefulness of commercially available media to MIC determinations of trimethoprim. In: Williams JD, Geddes AM, eds. *Chemotherapy.* Vol 2. New York: Plenum Press, 1976:2.

70. Waterworth PM. Sensitivity tests with trimethoprim-sulphonamide. *S Afr Med J* 1970;44(Suppl):10–12.

71. Then R. Thymidine and the assessment of co-trimoxazole. In: Williams JD, Geddes AM, eds. *Chemotherapy.* New York: Plenum Press, 1976:2.

72. Ferone RS, Bushby RM, Burchall JJ, et al. Identification of Harper-Cawston factor as thymidine phosphorylase and removal from media of substances interfering with susceptibility testing to sulfonamides and diaminopyrimidines. *Antimicrob Agents Chemother* 1975;7:91–98.

73. Dougherty PF, Yotter DW, Matthews TR. Chemically defined medium for susceptibility testing of antimicrobial agents. *Antimicrob Agents Chemother* 1976;10:923–925.

74. Brook I. Inoculum effect. *Rev Infect Dis* 1989;11:361–368.

75. Corrado ML, Landesman SH, Cherubin CE. Influence of inoculum size on activity of cefoperazone, cefotaxime, moxalactam, piperacillin, and N-formimidoyl thienamycin (MK 0787) against *Pseudomonas aeruginosa. Antimicrob Agents Chemother* 1980;18:893–896.

76. Seligman SJ, Hewitt WL. Resistance to penicillins and cephalosporins. *Antimicrob Agents Chemother* 1965;5:387–391.

77. Thornsberry C. Methicillin-resistant (heteroresistant) staphylococci. *Antimicrob Newslett* 1984;1:43–47.

78. Minami S, Yotsuji A, Inoue M, et al. Induction of β-lactamase by various β-lactam antibiotics in *Enterobacter cloacae. Antimicrob Agents Chemother* 1980;18:382–385.

79. Sanders CC, Sanders WE. Emergence of resistance to cefamandole: possible role of cefoxitin-inducible S. aureus lactamases. *Antimicrob Agents Chemother* 1979;7:1521.

80. Sanders CC, Sanders WE. Emergence of resistance during therapy with newer (-lactam antibiotics: role of inducible lactamases and implications for the future. *Rev Infect Dis* 1983;5:639–648.

81. Woods DD. The relation of p-aminobenzoic acid to the mechanism of action of sulphanilamide. *Br J Exp Pathol* 1940;21:74–90.

82. Chapman SW, Steigbigel RT. Staphylococcal (β-lactamase and efficacy of (β-lactam antibiotics: in vitro and in vivo evaluation. *J Infect Dis* 1983;143:1078–1089.

83. Clark H, Turck M. In vitro and in vivo evaluation of cephalexin. *Antimicrob Agents Chemother* 1969;8:296–301.

84. Kind AC, Kestle DG, Standiford HC, et al. Laboratory and clinical experience with cephalexin. *Antimicrob Agents Chemother* 1969;8:361–365.

85. Eickhoff TC, Ehret JM. In vitro comparison of cefoxitin, cefamandole, cephalexin, and cephalothin. *Antimicrob Agents Chemother* 1976;9:994–999.

86. Emerson BB, Smith AL, Harding AL, et al. *Haemophilus influenzae* type B susceptibility of seventeen antibiotics. *Pediatrics* 1975;86:617–620.

87. Syriopoulou V, Scheifele DW, Sack CM, et al. Effect of inoculum size on the susceptibility of *Haemophilus influenzae* b to β-lactam antibiotics. *Antimicrob Agents Chemother* 1979;16:510–513.

88. Barry AL, Joyce LJ, Adams AP. Rapid determination of antimicrobial susceptibility for urgent clinical situations. *Am J Clin Pathol* 1973;59:693–699.

89. Barry AL, Badal RE, Hawkinson RW. Influence of inoculum growth phase on microdilution susceptibility tests. *J Clin Microbiol* 1983;18:645–651.

90. Aldridge KE, Janney A, Sanders CV, et al. Interlaboratory variation of antibiograms of methicillin-resistant and methicillin-susceptible *Staphylococcus aureus* strains with conventional and commercial testing systems. *J Clin Microbiol* 1983;18:142–147.

91. Stratton CW. Serum bactericidal test. *Clin Microbiol Rev* 1988;1:1926.

92. MacLowry JD, Young MJ, Selepak ST, et al. A semiautomated microtechnique for serial dilution antimicrobial sensitivity testing in the clinical laboratory. *Int J Clin Pharmacol* 1970;3:70–72.

93. Lorian V. *Antibiotics and chemotherapeutic agents in clinical and laboratory practice.* Springfield, IL: Charles C Thomas, 1966.

94. Gerlach EH. Microdilution, I: a comparative study. In: Balows A, ed. *Current techniques for antibiotic susceptibility testing.* Springfield, IL: Charles C Thomas, 1973:63–76.

95. Gerlach EH. Dilution test procedures for susceptibility testing. In: Bondi A, Bartola JT, Prier JD, eds. *The clinical laboratory as an aid in chemotherapy of infectious disease.* Baltimore: University Park Press, 1977:45–50.

96. Gavan TL, Butler D. An automated microdilution method for antimicrobial susceptibility testing. In: Balows A, ed. *Current techniques for antibiotic susceptibility testing.* Springfield, IL: Charles C Thomas, 1973:88–93.

97. Jones RN, Gavan TL, Barry AL. Evaluation of the Sensititre microdilution antibiotic susceptibility system against recent clinical isolates: three-laboratory collaborative study. *J Clin Microbiol* 1980;11:426–429.

98. Jones RN, Thornsberry C, Barry AL, et al. Evaluation of the Sceptor microdilution investigation. *J Clin Microbiol* 1981;13:184–194.

99. McMaster PRB, Robertson E, Witebsky F, et al. Evaluation of a dispensing instrument (Dynatech MIC-2000) for preparing microtiter antibiotic plates and testing potency during storage. *Antimicrob Agents Chemother* 1978; 13:842–844.

100. Waterworth PM. In: Reeves DS, Phillips I, Williams JD, et al, eds. *Laboratory methods in chemotherapy.* Edinburgh: Churchill Livingstone, 1978:4.

101. Woolfrey BF, Ramadel WA, QUail CO. Evaluation of a semiautomated micro-broth dilution system for determining minimum inhibitory concentrations of antimicrobics. *Am J Clin Pathol* 1980;73:374–379.

102. Thornsberry C, Gavan TL, Gerlach EH. *New developments in antimicrobial agent susceptibility testing.* Cumitech 6. Washington, DC: American Society for Microbiology, 1977.

103. Gavan TL. Broth dilution methods. In: Gavan TL, Cheatle EL, McFadden HW, eds. *Antimicrobial susceptibility testing.* Chicago: American Society of Clinical Pathology, 1971:105–124.

104. Jackson GG, Finland M. Comparison of methods for determining sensitivity of bacteria to antibiotics in vitro. *Arch Intern Med* 1951;88:446–460.

105. Waisbren BA, Carr C, Dunnette J. The tube dilution method of determining bacterial sensitivity to antibiotics. *Am J Clin Pathol* 1951;21:884–891.

106. Washington JA II. *Laboratory procedures in clinical microbiology.* Boston: Little, Brown and Co, 1974.

107. Jones RN, Barry AL, Gavan TL, et al. Susceptibility tests: microdilution and macrodilution broth procedures. In: Lennette EH, Balows A, Hausler WJ Jr, et al, eds. *Manual of clinical microbiology.* 4th ed. Washington, DC: American Society for Microbiology, 1985.

108. Miller JM, Andersen BV, Caudill SP. New quality control frequency guidelines for antimicrobic susceptibility testing. *Antimicrob Newslett* 1986;3:77–79.

109. Lebek G, Zund P. R-factors affecting host generation time: their influence on sensitivity testing. *Infection* 1981;9:76.

110. Richmond MH, Sykes RB. The β-lactamases of Gram-negative bacteria and their possible physiological role. In: Rose AH, Tempesti DW, eds. *Advances in microbiology and physiology.* Vol 9. New York: Academic Press, 1973:31–88.

111. Elwell LP, DeGraff J, Seibert D, et al. Plasmid-linked ampicillin resistance in *Haemophilus influenzae* type b. *Infect Immun* 1975;12:404–410.

112. Elwell LP, Roberts M, Mayer L, et al. Plasmid-mediated (β-lactamase production in *Neisseria gonorrhoeae. Antimicrob Agents Chemother* 1977;11:533–538.

113. Zigheiboin S, Tomasz A. Penicillin binding proteins of multiply antibiotic-resistant South African strains of Streptococcus pneumoniae. *Antimicrob Agents Chemother* 1980;17:434–441.

114. Clinical and Laboratory Standards Institute. Performance standards for antimicrobial susceptibility testing. Nineteenth informational supplement. Wayne, PA: Clinical and Laboratory Standards Institute, 2009. CLSI publication M100-S19.

115. Baker CN, Thornsberry C, Jones RN. In vitro antimicrobial activity of cefoperazone, cefotaxime, moxalactam (LY 127935), azlocillin, mezlocillin, and other (β-lactam antibiotics against *Neisseria gonorrhoeae* and *Haemophilus influenzae,* including (β-lactamase–producing strains. *Antimicrob Agents Chemother* 1980;17: 757–761.

116. Needham CA. *Haemophilus influenzae*: antibiotic susceptibility. *Clin Microbiol Rev* 1988;1:218–227.

117. Thornsberry C, Baker CN, Kirven LA, et al. Susceptibility of ampicillin-resistant *Haemophilus influenzae* to seven ampicillins. *Antimicrob Agents Chemother* 1976;9: 70–73.

118. Doern GV, Jorgensen JH, Thornsberry C, et al. National collaborative study of the prevalence of antimicrobial resistance among clinical isolates of *Haemophilus influenzae. Antimicrob Agents Chemother* 1988;32:180–185.

119. Azemun P, Stall T, Roberts M, et al. Rapid detection of chloramphenicol resistance in *Haemophilus influenzae. Antimicrob Agents Chemother* 1981;20:168–170.

120. Jorgensen JH, Doern GV, Thornsberry C, et al. Susceptibility of mutliple-resistant *Haemophilus influenzae* to newer antimicrobial agents. *Diagn Microbiol Infect Dis* 1988;9:27–32.

121. Dillon LK, Howe SE. Early detection of oxacillin-resistant staphylococcal strains with hypertonic broth diluent for microdilution panels. *J Clin Microbiol* 1984;19: 473–476.

122. McDougal LK, Thornsberry C. The role of (β-lactamase in staphylococcal resistance to penicillinase-resistant penicillins and cephalosporins. *J Clin Microbiol* 1986; 23:832–839.

123. Thornsberry C, McDougal LK. Successful use of broth microdilution in susceptibility tests for methicillin-resistant (heteroresistant) staphylococci. *J Clin Microbiol* 1983;18:1084–1091.

124. Jones RN, Gavan TL, Thornsberry C, et al. Standardization of disk diffusion and agar dilution susceptibility tests for *Neisseria gonorrhoeae*: interpretive criteria and quality control guidelines for ceftriaxone, penicillin, spectinomycin, and tetracycline. *J Clin Microbiol* 1989;27:2758–2766.

125. Tenover FC, Baker CN, Swenson JM. Evaluation of commerical methods for determining antimicrobial susceptibility of *Streptococcus pneumoniae. J Clin Microbiol* 1996;34:10–14.

126. Cooksey RC, Swenson JM. In vitro antimicrobial inhibition patterns of nutritionally variant streptococci. *Antimicrob Agents Chemother* 1979;16:514–518.

127. Winslow DL, Damme J, Dieckman E. Delayed bactericidal activity of β-lactam antibiotics against Listeria monocytogenes: antagonism of chloramphenicol and rifampin. *Antimicrob Agents Chemother* 1983;23:555–558.

128. Stevens DL, Higbee JW, Oberhofer TR, et al. Antibiotic susceptibilities of human isolates of *Pasteurella multocida. Antimicrob Agents Chemother* 1979;16:322–324.

129. Vanhoof R, Gordts B, Diedickx R, et al. Bacteriostatic and bactericidal activities of 24 antimicrobial agents against *Campylobacter fetus* subsp jejuni. *Antimicrob Agents Chemother* 1980;18:118–121.

130. Goldstein EJC, Cherubin CE, Shulman M. Comparison of microtiter broth dilution and agar dilution methods for susceptibility testing of *Eikenella corrodens*. *Antimicrob Agents Chemother* 1983;23:42–45.

131. Jao RL, Finland M. Susceptibility of *Mycoplasma pneumoniae* to 21 antibiotics in vitro. *Am J Med Sci* 1967; 253:639–650.

132. Smith TF. *In vitro* susceptibility of *Ureaplasma urealyticum* to rosaramicin. *Antimicrob Agents Chemother* 1979; 16:106–108.

133. Spaepern MS, Kundsin RB. Simple direct broth-disk method for antibiotic susceptibility testing of *Ureaplasma urealyticum*. *Antimicrob Agents Chemother* 1977; 11:267–270.

134. Bowie WR. Lack of in vitro activity of cefoxitin, cefamandole, cefuroxime, and piperacillin against *Chlamydia trachomatis*. *Antimicrob Agents Chemother* 1982;21:339–340.

135. Hammerschlag M, Gleyzer A. In vitro activity of a group of broad-spectrum cephalosporins and other (β-lactam antibiotics against *Chlamydia trachomatis*. *Antimicrob Agents Chemother* 1983;23:493–494.

136. Brown-Elliott BA, Brown JM, Conville PS, et al. Clinical and laboratory features of the *Nocardia* spp. Based on current molecular taxonomy. *Clin Microbiol Rev* 2006; 19:259–282.

137. Verroken A, Janssens M, Berhin C, et al. Evaluation of matrix-assisted laser description ionization-time of flight mass spectrometry for identification of *Nocardia* species. *J Clin Microbiol* 2010;48:4015–4021.

138. Clinical and Laboratory Standards Institute. Susceptibility testing of mycobacteria, nocardiae, and other aerobic actinomycetes; approved standard—2nd ed. Wayne, PA: Clinical and Laboratory Standards Institute. CLSI publication M24-A2.

139. Malhotra-Kumar S, Haccuria K, Michiels M, et al. Current trends in rapid diagnostics for methicillin-resistant *Staphylococcus aureus* and glycopeptide-resistant *Enterococcus* species. *J Clin Microbiol* 2008;46:1577–1587.

140. Rong SL, Leonard SN. Heterogenous vancomycin resistance in *Staphylococcus aureus*: a review of epidemiology, diagnosis and clinical significance. *Ann Pharmacol* 2010;44:844–850.

141. Hiramatsu K, Hanaki H, Ino T, et al. Methicillin-resistant *Staphylococcus aureus* clinical strain with reduced vancomycin susceptibility. *J Antimicrob Chemother.* 1997; 40:135–136.

142. Swenson JM, Ferraro MJ, Sahm DF, et al. National Committee for Clinical and Laboratory Standards Study Group on Enterococci. Multi-laboratory evaluation of screening methods for detection of high-level aminoglycoside resistance in enterococci. *J Clin Microbiol* 1995;33:3008–3018.

143. Clinical and Laboratory Standards Institute. Performance standards for antimicrobial susceptibility testing. 21st informational supplement. Wayne, PA: Clinical and Laboratory Standards Institute, 2012. CLSI publication M100-S22.

144. Clinical and Laboratory Standards Institute. Performance standards for antimicrobial susceptibility testing. Twenty-third informational supplement. Wayne, PA: Clinical and Laboratory Standards Institute, 2013. CLSI publication M100-S23.

145. European Committee on Antimicrobial Susceptibility Testing. Expert rules. Version 2.0. www.eucast.org/expertrules. Accessed July 15, 2013.

146. Queenan AM, Bush K. Carbapenemases: the versatile β-lactamases. *Clin Microbiol Rev* 2007;20:440–458.

147. Villegas MV, Lolans K, Correa A, et al. First identification of *Pseudomonas aeruginosa* isolates producing a KPC-type carbapenem-hydrolyzing β-lactamase. *Antimicrob Agents Chemother* 2007;51:1553–1555.

148. Clinical and Laboratory Standards Institute. Performance standards for antimicrobial susceptibility testing. Nineteenth informational supplement. Wayne, PA: Clinical and Laboratory Standards Institute, 2009. CLSI publication M100-S19.

149. Livermore DM, Andrews JM, Hawkey PM, et al. Are susceptibility tests enough, or should laboratories still seek ESBLs and carbapenemeases directly? *J Antimicrob Chemother* 2012;67:1569–1577.

150. Duguid JP. The sensitivity of bacteria to the action of penicillin. *Edinb Med J* 1946;53:401–412.

151. Gardner AD. Morphological effects of penicillin on bacteria. *Nature* 1940;146:837–838.

152. Greenwood D, Eley A. A turbidimetric study of the responses of selected strains of *Pseudomonas aeruginosa* to eight antipseudomonal β-lactam antibiotics. *J Infect Dis* 1982;145:110–117.

153. Lorian V. Some effects on subinhibitory concentrations of antibiotics on bacteria. *Bull NY Acad Med* 1975;51: 1046–1055.

154. Lorian V. Effect of low antibiotic concentrations on bacteria. In: Lorian V, ed. *Antibiotics in laboratory medicine.* 2nd ed. Baltimore: Williams and Wilkins, 1986:596–668.

155. Zanon U. Sub-inhibitory levels of antibiotics. *J Antimicrob Chemother* 1977;3:106–107.

156. Lorian V, Waluschka A, Carruth C, et al. A five-hour disc susceptibility test. In: Lorian V, ed. *The significance of medical microbiology in the care of patients.* Baltimore: Williams & Wilkins, 1982.

157. Lampe MR, Aitken CL, Dennis PG, et al. Relationship of early readings of minimal inhibitory concentrations to the results of overnight tests. *Antimicrob Agents Chemother* 1975;8:429–433.

158. Sorensen RH. Rapid antibiotic sensitivity test using a redox indicator. *Med Technol Bull* 1959;10: 144–148.

159. Bartlett RC, Mazens MF. Rapid antimicrobial susceptibility test using tetrazolium reduction. *Antimicrob Agents Chemother* 1979;15:769–774.

160. Baker CN, Banerjee SH, Tenover FC. Evaluation of Alamar colorimetric MIC method for antimicrobial susceptibility testing Gram-negative bacteria. *J Clin Microbiol* 1994;32:1261–1267.

161. Sellers W. Antibiotic sensitivity testing. In: Graber CD, ed. *Rapid diagnostic methods in medical microbiology.* Baltimore: Williams and Wilkins, 1970:163–178.

162. Mitruka BM. *Gas chromatographic applications in microbiology and medicine.* New York: John Wiley and Sons, 1975.

163. DeLand FH, Wagner HN Jr. Early detection of bacterial growth with carbon 14-labeled glucose. *Radiology* 1969;92:154–155.

164. DeLand F, Wagner HN Jr. Automated radiometric detection of bacterial growth in blood culture. *J Lab Clin Med* 1970;75:529–534.

165. Levin GV. Rapid microbiological determinations with radioisotopes. *Adv Appl Microbiol* 1963;5:95–133.

166. Levin GV, Hein AH, Clendenning JR, et al. Gulliver: a quest for life on Mars. *Science* 1962;138:114–121.

167. Chappelle EW, Levin GV. Use of firefly bioluminescent reaction for rapid detection and counting of bacteria. *Biochem Med* 1968;2:41–52.

168. Cady P. Progress in impedance measurements in microbiology. In: Sharpe AN, Clarke DS, eds. *Mechanizing microbiology*. Springfield, IL: Charles C Thomas, 1978:199–239.

169. Cady PS, Dufour W, Draeger SJ. Electrical impedance measurements: rapid method for detecting and monitoring microorganisms. *J Clin Microbiol* 1978;7:265–272.

170. Ur A, Brown D. Monitoring of bacterial activity by impedance measurements. In: Heden C, Illeni T, eds. *New approaches to the identification of microorganisms*. New York: John Wiley and Sons, 1975:61–71.

171. Colvin HJ, Sherris JC. Electrical impedance measurements in the reading and monitoring of broth dilution susceptibility tests. *Antimicrob Agents Chemother* 1977;2:61–66.

172. Howard MC, Miyajima A, Coffman R. T-cell derived cytokines and their receptors. In: Paul WE, ed. *Fundamental immunology*. 3rd ed. New York: Raven Press, 1993:763–800.

173. Johnston Laboratories. Drug susceptibility of *M. tuberculosis* cultures by the Bactec system: Bactec data JL1—664. In: Bactec news. Cockeysville, MD: Johnston Laboratories, 1979.

174. McFarland J. The nephelometer: an instrument for estimating the numbers of bacteria in suspensions used for calculating the opsonic index and for vaccines. *JAMA* 1907;49:1176–1178.

175. Longsworth LG. The estimation of bacterial populations with the aid of a photoelectric densitometer. *J Bacteriol* 1936;32:307–328.

176. Wyatt PJ. Identification of bacteria by differential light scattering. *Nature* 1969;221:1257–1258.

177. Wyatt PJ. Automation of differential light scattering for antibiotic susceptibility testing. In: Heden CG, Illeni T, eds. Automation in microbiology and immunology. New York: John Wiley and Sons, 1975:267–291.

178. Amaral L, Trigenis B, Atkinson BA. The radioactive thymidine incorporation method for the determination of antibiotic susceptibility of Gram-negative bacilli. *Eur J Clin Microbiol* 1982;1:149–154.

179. Pore RS. Antibiotic susceptibility testing by flow cytometry. *J Antimicrob Chemother* 1994;34:613–627.

180. National Center for Infectious Diseases. *Flow cytometric immunophenotyping procedure manual.* Atlanta: US Department of Health and Human Services, 1993.

181. Shapiro HM. *Practical flow cytometry.* 2nd ed. New York: Alan R. Liss, 1988.

182. Nicolle Norden MA, Kurzyski TA, Bounds SE, et al. Rapid susceptibility testing of *Mycobacterium tuberculosis* (H37Ra) by flow cytometry. *J Clin Microbiol* 1995;33:1231–1237.

183. College of American Pathologists. *Proficiency survey program: College of American Pathologists surveys final critique for set D-A 199.* Northfield, IL: College of American Pathologists, 1991.

184. Amsterdam D. Instrumentation for antimicrobic susceptibility testing: yesterday, today, and tomorrow. *Diagn Microbiol Infect Dis* 1988;9:167–178.

185. Staneck JL, Allen SD, Harris EE, et al. Automated reading of MIC microdilution trays containing fluorogenic enzyme substrates with the Sensititre autoreader. *J Clin Microbiol* 1985;22:187–191.

186. Eng RHK, Cherubin CM, Smith SM, et al. Inoculum effect of β-lactam antibiotics on Enterobacteriaceae. *Antimicrob Agents Chemother* 1985;28:601–606.

187. Elder LB, Hansen SA, Kellogg JA, et al. *Verification and validation of procedures in the clinical microbiology laboratory Cumitech 31.* Washington, DC: ASM Press, 1997.

188. Doern GV, Scott DR, Rashad AL. Clinical impact of rapid antimicrobial susceptibility testing of blood culture isolates. *Antimicrob Agents Chemother* 1982;21:1023–1024.

189. Trenholme GM, Kaplan RL, Karakusis PH, et al. Clinical impact of rapid identification and susceptibility testing of bacterial blood culture isolates. *J Clin Microbiol* 1989;27:1342–1345.

190. Doern GV, Vaator R, Gaudet M, et al. Clinical impact of rapid in vitro susceptibility testing and bacterial identification. *J Clin Microbiol* 1994;32:1757–1762.

191. Barenfanger J, Drake C, Kacich G. Clinical and financial benefits of rapid identification and antimicrobial susceptibility testing. *J Clin Microbiol* 1999;37:1415–1418.

192. Schifman RB, Pindur A, Bryan JA. Laboratory practices for reporting bacterial susceptibility tests that affect antibiotic therapy. *Arch Pathol Lab Med* 1997;121:1168–1170.

193. de la Maza K, Miller ST, Ferraro MJ. Use of commercially available rapid chloramphenicol acetyltransferase test to detect resistance in *Salmonella* species. *J Clin Microbiol* 1990;28:1867–1869.

194. Tenover FC. Studies of antimicrobial resistance genes using DNA probes. *Antimicrob Agents Chemother* 1986;29:721–725.

195. Rasheed JK, Tenover FC. Detection and characterization of antimicrobial resistance genes in bacteria. In: Murray PR, Baron EJ, Pfaller MA, et al, eds. *Manual of clinical microbiology.* 8th ed. Washington, DC: ASM Press, 2003:1196–1212.

196. Tenover FC, Popovic T, Olsvik O. Genetic methods for detecting antibacterial resistance genes. In: *Manual of clinical microbiology.* 6th ed. Washington, DC: ASM Press, 1995;1368–1378.

197. York MK, Gibbs L, Chehab F, et al. Comparison of PCR detection of mecA with standard susceptibility testing methods to detennine methicillin resistance in coagulasenegative staphylococci. *J Clin Microbiol* 1996;34:249–253.

198. Dall LR, Herndon BL. Association of cell-adherent glycocalyx and endocarditis production by viridans group streptococci. *J Clin Microbiol* 1990;28:1698–1700.

199. National Committee for Clinical Laboratory Standards. *Proposed guidelines for pharmaceutical and susceptibility test reagent manufacturers.* Villanova, PA: National Committee for Clinical Laboratory Standards, 1986. NCCLS document M23-P.

200. Ambrose PG, Grasela DM. The use of Monte Carlo simulation to examine pharmacodynamic variance of drugs: fluoroquinolone pharmacodynamics against *Streptococcus pneumoniae*. *Diagn Microbiol Infect Dis* 2000;38:151–157.

201. Drusano GL, Johnson DE, Rosen M, et al. Pharmacodynamics of a fluoroquinolone antimicrobial agent in a neutropenic rat model of Pseudomonas sepsis. *Antimicrob Agents Chemother* 1993;37:483–490.

202. Drusano GL, Preston SL, Hardalo C, et al. Use of preclinical data for selection of a phase II/III dose for evernimicin and identification of a preclinical MIC breakpoint. *Antimicrob Agents Chemother* 2001;45:13–22.

203. Mouton JW. Breakpoints: current practice and future perspectives. *Int J Antimicrobial Agents* 2002;19:323–331.

204. Scavizzi MR, Bronner FD. A statistical model for the interpretation of antibiotic susceptibility tests. *Int J Exp Clin Chemother* 1988;1:23–42.

205. Duan K, Dammel C, Stein J, et al. Modulation of *Pseudomonas aeruginosa* gene expression by host microflora through interspecies communication. *Molec Microbiol* 2003;50:1477–1491.

206. Sakoulas G, Eliopoulos GM, Moellering RC Jr, et al. *Staphylococcus aureus* accessory gene regulator (agr) group II: is there a relationship to the development of intermediate-level glycopeptide resistance? *J Clin Infect Dis* 2003;187:929–938.

207. Pillai SK, Sakoulas G, Gold HS, et al. Prevalence of the fsr locus in *Enterococcus faecalis* infections. *J Clin Microbiol* 2002;40:2651–2652.

208. Qin X, Singh KV, Weinstock GM, et al. Effects of *Enterococcus faecalis fsr* genes on production of gelatinase and a serine protease and virulence. *Infect Immun* 200;68:2579–2586.

209. Lorian V, Burns L. Predictive value of susceptibility tests for the outcome of antibacterial therapy. *J Antimicrob Chemother* 1990;25:175–181.

210. MacArthur RD, Miller M, Albertson T, et al. Adequacy of early antimicrobic antibiotic treatment and survival in severe sepsis: experience from the MONARCS trial. 2004;38:284–288.

211. Yu VL, Chiou CC, Feldman C, et al. An international prospective study of pneumococcal bacteremia: correlation with in vitro resistance, antibiotics administered and clinical outcome. *Clin Infect Dis* 2003;37:230–237.

212. Flaherty KR, Saint S, Fendrick AM, et al. The spectrum of acute bronchitis. *Postgrad Med* 2001;109:39–47.

213. Lynch JP III, Fernandez JM. Clinical relevance of macrolide-resistant Streptococcus pneumoniae for community-acquired pneumonia. *Clin Infect Dis* 2002; 34(Suppl 1):S27–S46.

214. Alvarez-Lerma F. Modification of empiric antibiotic treatment in patients with pneumonia acquired in the intensive care unit. ICU-Acquired Pneumonia Study Group. *Intensive Care Med* 1996;22:387–394.

215. Kollef MH, Sherman G, Ward S, et al. Inadequate antimicrobial treatment of infections: a risk factor for hospital mortality among critically ill patients. *Chest* 1999;115:462–474.

216. Luna CM, Vujacich P, Niederman MS, et al. Impact of BAL data on the therapy and outcome of ventilator-associated pneumonia. *Chest* 1997;111:676–685.

217. Rex JH, Pfaller MA. Has antifungal susceptibility come of age? *Clin Infect Dis* 2002;35:982–989.

218. Tomasz A, Albino A, Zanati E. Multiple antibiotic resistance in a bacterium with suppressed autolytic system. *Nature* 1970;227:138–140.

219. Hobby GL, Meyer K, Chaffee E. Observations on the mechanism of action of penicillin. *Proc Soc Exp Biol Med* 1942;50:281–285.

220. Handwerger S, Tomasz A. Antibiotic tolerance among clinical isolates of bacteria. *Rev Infect Dis* 1985;7:368–386.

221. Sherris JC. Problems in in vitro determination of antibiotic tolerance in clinical isolates. *Antimicrob Agents Chemother* 1986;30:633–637.

222. Tuomanen E. Phenotypic tolerance: the search for β-lactam antibiotics that kill nongrowing bacteria. *Rev Infect Dis* 1986;8(Suppl):S279–S291.

223. Tuomanen E, Durack DT, Tomasz A. Antibiotic tolerance among clinical isolates of bacteria. *Antimicrob Agents Chemother* 1986;30:521–527.

224. Sabath LD, Wheeler N, Laverdiere M, et al. A new type of penicillin resistance of *Staphylococcus aureus*. *Lancet* 1977;1:443–447.

225. Tipper DJ. Mode of action of beta-lactam antibiotics. In: Queener SF, Webber JA, Queener SW, eds. *Beta-lactam antibiotics for clinical use*. New York: Marcel Dekker Inc, 1986:17–47.

226. Tomasz A. The mechanism of the irreversible antimicrobial effects of penicillins: how the β-lactam antibiotics kill and lyse bacteria. *Annu Rev Microbiol* 1979;33: 113–137.

227. Yocum RR, Rasmussin JR, Strominger SL. The mechanism of action of penicillin: penicillin activates the active site of Bacillus stearothermophilus D-alanine carboxypeptidase. *J Biol Chem* 1980;255:3977–3986.

228. Blumberg PM, Strominger JL. Interaction of penicillin with the bacterial cell: penicillin-binding proteins and penicillin-sensitive enzymes. *Bacteriol Rev* 1974;38: 291–335.

229. Spratt BG. Biochemical and genetical approaches to the mechanism of action of penicillin. *Philos Trans R Soc Lond [Biol]* 1980;289:273–283.

230. Tipper DJ, Wright A. The structure and biosynthesis of bacterial cell walls. In: Sokatch JR, Ornston LN, eds. *Mechanisms of adaptations*. New York: Academic Press,

231. Georgopapadakou NH, Liu FY. Binding of β-lactam antibiotics to penicillin-binding proteins of *Staphylococcus aureus* and *Streptococcus faecalis*: relation to antibacterial activity. *Antimicrob Agents Chemother* 1980;18:834–836.

232. Neu HC. Penicillin-binding proteins and role of amdinocillin in causing bacterial cell death. *Am J Med* 1983;75(Suppl 2A):9–20.

233. Spratt BG. Properties of the penicillin-binding proteins of Escherichia coli K 12. *Eur J Biochem* 1977;72:341–352.

234. Tomasz A. Penicillin-binding proteins and the antibacterial effectiveness of β-lactam antibiotics. *Rev Infect Dis* 1986;8(Suppl 3):S260–S278.

235. Wilson WR, Geraci JE. Antibiotic treatment of infective endocarditis. Annu Rev Med 1983;34:413–427.

236. Dormer AE. The treatment of bacterial endocarditis. *Br Med Bull* 1960;16:61–66.

237. Stratton CW. The usefulness of the serum bactericidal test in orthopedic infections. *Orthopedics* 1984;7:1579–1580.

238. Sculier JP, Klastersky J. Significance of serum bactericidal activity in gram-negative bacillary bacteremia in patients with and without granulocytopenia. *Am J Med* 1984;76:429–435.

239. Reimer LG, Stratton C, Reller LB. Minimum inhibitory and bactericidal concentrations of 44 antimicrobial agents against three standard control strains in broth with and without human serum. *Antimicrob Agents Chemother* 1981;19:1050–1055.

240. Meylan PR, Francioli P, Glauser MP. Discrepancies between MBC and actual killing of viridans group streptococci by cell-wall-active antibiotics. *Antimicrob Agents Chemother* 1986;29:418–423.

241. Schoenknecht FD, Sabath LD, Thornsberry C. Susceptibility tests: special tests. In: Lennette EH, Balows A, Hausler WH Jr, et al, eds. *Manual of clinical microbiology*. 3rd ed. Washington, DC: American Society for Microbiology, 1985:1000–1008.

242. National Committee for Clinical Laboratory Standards. *Methods for determining bactericidal activity of antimicrobial agents*. Wayne, PA: National Committee for Clinical Laboratory Standards, 1999. NCCLS document M26-A.

243. Anhalt JP, Washington JW II. Bactericidal tests. In: Washington JA, ed. *Laboratory procedures in clinical microbiology.* 2nd ed. New York: Springer-Verlag, 1985: 431–745.

244. Taylor PC, Schoenknecht FD, Sherris JC, et al. Determination of minimum bactericidal concentration of oxacillin for Staphylococcus aureus: influence and significance of technical factors. *Antimicrob Agents Chemother* 1983;23:142–150.

245. James PA. Comparison of four methods for the determination of MIC and MBC of penicillin for viridans streptococci and the implications for penicillin tolerance. *J Antimicrob Chemother* 1990;25:209–216.

246. Hacek DM, Dressel DC, Peterson LR. Highly reproducible bactericidal activity test results by using a modified rational committee for clinical laboratory standards broth microdilution technique. *J Clin Microbiol* 1999;37: 1881–1884.

247. Schlichter JG, MacLean H. A method of determining the effective therapeutic level in the treatment of subacute bacterial endocariditis with penicillin. *Am Heart J* 1947;34:209–211.

248. Stratton CW, Weinstein MP, Reller LB. Correlation of serum bactericidal activity with antimicrobial agent level and minimal bactericidal concentration. *J Infect Dis* 1982;145:160–168.

249. National Committee for Clinical Laboratory Standards. *Methodology for the serum bactericidal test.* Wayne, PA: National Committee for Clinical Laboratory Standards, 1999. NCCLS document M21-A.

250. Prober CG, Yeager AS. Use of the serum bactericidal titer to assess the adequacy of oral antibiotic therapy in the treatment of acute hematogenous osteomyelitis. *J Pediatr* 1979;95:131–135.

251. Sande MA. Antibiotic therapy of bacterial meningitis: lessons we've learned. *Am J Med* 1981;7:507–510.

252. Barriere SL, Ely E, Kapusnik JE, et al. Analysis of a new method for assessing activity of combinations of antimicrobials: area under the bactericidal curve. *J Antimicrob Chemother* 1985;16:49–59.

253. Blondeau JM, Zhao X, Hansen G, et al. Mutant prevention concentrations of fluoroquinolones for clinical isolates of *Streptococcus pneumoniae. Antimicrob Agents Chemother* 2001;45:433–438.

254. Dong Y, Zhao X, Domagala J, et al. Effect of fluoroquinolone concentration on selection of resistant mutants of *Mycobacterium bovis* BCG and *Staphylococcus aureus. Antimicrob Agents Chemother* 2000;

255. Small PM, Chambers HF. Vancomycin for *Staphylococcus aureus* endocarditis in intravenous drug users. *Antimicrob Agents Chemother* 1990;34:1227–1231.

256. Baron S, Tyring SK, Fleischman R, et al. The interferons: mechanisms of action and clinical applications. *JAMA* 1991;266:1375–1383.

257. Mohr JF, Wanger A, Rex JH. Pharmacokinetic/pharmacodynamic modeling can help guide targeted antimicrobial therapy for nosocomial Gram-negative infections in critically ill patients. *Diag Microbiol Infect Dis* 2004;48:125–130.

258. National Committee for Clinical Laboratory Standards. *Evaluation of lots of Mueller-Hinton broth for antimicrobial susceptibility testing: proposed guideline.* Wayne, PA: National Committee for Clinical Laboratory Standards, 2001. NCCLS document M32-P.

259. Thornsberry C, Swensen JM, Baker CN, et al. Susceptibility testing of fastidious and unusual pathogens. *Antimicrob Newslett* 1987;4:47–55.

260. Stull VR. Clinical laboratory use of differential light scattering, I: antibiotic susceptibility testing. *Clin Chem* 1973;19:883–890.

261. Jorgensen JH, Lee JC, Jones PM. Chemically defined antimicrobial susceptibility test medium for Pseudomonas aeruginosa. *Antimicrob Agents Chemother* 1977;11:415–419.

262. Baker CN, Hollis G, Thornsberry C. Antimicrobial susceptibility testing of Francisella tularensis with a modified Mueller-Hinton broth. *J Clin Microbiol* 1988; 22:212–215.

263. Baker CN, Thornsberry C, Hawkinson RW. Inoculum standardization in antimicrobial susceptibility testing: evaluation of overnight agar cultures and the Rapid Inoculum Standardization System. *J Clin Microbiol* 1983;17:450–457.

266. Dugan DL, Wright DN. Quantitative infrared photoanalysis of selected bacteria. *Appl Microbiol* 1974;28: 205–211.

267. Forrest A, Nix DE, Ballow CH, et al. Pharmacodynamics of intravenous ciprofloxacin in seriously ill patients. *Antimicrob Agents Chemother* 1993;37:1073–1081.

269. Inderlied CB, Young LS. Radiometric in vitro susceptibility testing of Mycobacterium tuberculosis. *Antimicrob Newslett* 1986;3:55–60.

270. Wicks JH, Nelson RL, Krejcarek GE. Rapid inoculum standardization system: a novel device for standardization of inocula in antimicrobial susceptibility testing. *J Clin Microbiol* 1983;17:1114–1119.

272. Kushner I. Regulation of the acute phase response by cytokines. In: Oppenheim JJ, Rossio JL, Geaniny AH, eds. *Clinical application of cytokines.* New York: Oxford University Press, 1993:27–34.

273. Luria SE. A test for penicillin sensitivity and resistance in Staphylococcus. *Proc Soc Exp Biol Med* 1946; 61:46–51.

274. Mardh PA, Anderson KE, Wadso I. Kinetics of the actions of tetracyclines on Escherichia coli as studied by microcalorimetry. *Antimicrob Agents Chemother* 1976;10:604–609.

275. Preston SL, Drusano GL, Berman AL, et al. Pharmacodynamics of levofloxacin: a new paradigm for early clinical trials. *JAMA* 1998;279:125–129.

276. Pulliam L, Dall L, Inokuchi S, et al. Effects of exopolysaccharide production by viridans streptococci on penicillin therapy of experimental endocarditis. *J Infect Dis* 1985;151:153–156.

277. Spratt BG. Distinct penicillin binding proteins involved in the division, elongation, and shape of Escherichia coli, K 12. *Proc Natl Acad Sci USA* 1975;72:2999–3003.

279. Waxman DJ, Strominger JL. Penicillin-binding proteins and the mechanisms of action of β-lactam antibiotics. *Annu Rev Biochem* 1983;52:825–869.

Chapter 4

Antimicrobial Susceptibility Testing of Anaerobic Bacteria

Anilrudh A. Venugopal and David W. Hecht

Anaerobic bacteria have been well established in the literature as causing significant infection in humans (1). In certain situations, a single anaerobic organism can be the cause of a specific infection or sequelae, such as tetanus (*Clostridium tetani*), botulism (*Clostridium botulinum*), or food poisoning (*Clostridium perfringens*). However, the majority of infections due to anaerobes occur most often as mixed infections involving intraabdominal, skin and soft tissue, pulmonary, or central nervous system sites (1). Anaerobes have been recognized as either a causative agent or contributor to infection, and appropriate treatment is required for a good clinical outcome (2,3).

Recently, much attention has been given to antibiotic resistance among numerous aerobic and facultative anaerobic bacteria, with clear evidence of clinical failure when an ineffective antibiotic is used (4–7). Much less attention has been given to the role of antibiotic resistance among anaerobes and adverse clinical outcome. In fact, clinical trials that assess the efficacy of new antibiotics with good in vitro activity against anaerobic bacterial pathogens generally show favorable outcomes when compared with less active agents (8). However, until recently, there have been few studies demonstrating a correlation of antibiotic-resistant anaerobes with poor clinical outcome. Factors that have limited the ability to draw such conclusions from any study include the nature of the infection (mixed aerobes and anaerobes), lack of identification of anaerobic bacteria from specimens, absence of clinical data, effects of surgical drainage or debridement (a major factor that obscures the importance of a resistant organism), and previous inaccurate or modified susceptibility testing methods (9,10).

Several retrospective clinical studies were published in the 1980s and early 1990s that supported the association of antibiotic resistance among *Bacteroides* sp and clinical failure (11–13). However, a sentinel prospective, observational, *Bacteroides fragilis* group bacteremia study published in 2000 confirmed these previous suppositions and conclusions (14). In that study, mortality rate for patients receiving ineffective therapy (for resistant *B. fragilis*) was significantly higher than those receiving therapy that was active in vitro against the organism. Similarly, clinical failure and microbiologic persistence were greater for patients receiving ineffective therapy. These findings, along with numerous reports of increased antibiotic resistance (15), have prompted the Clinical and Laboratory Standards Institute (CLSI) (formerly the National Committee for Clinical Laboratory Standards [NCCLS]) to make recommendations for susceptibility testing of anaerobic bacteria in certain situations in their most recent standards publication (10). These recommendations have also been echoed in other publications (3,16).

To accomplish the most recent consensus document, the CLSI working group on antimicrobial susceptibility testing of anaerobic bacteria had previously conducted several multicenter collaborative studies to establish a highly reproducible agar dilution reference standard and comparable broth microdilution method (17,18). Coupled with the commercially available Etest (AB Biodisk, Solna, Sweden), there are now three reproducible and reliable methods for susceptibility testing of anaerobic bacteria (19). These different but comparable methods each have their pros and cons, depending on the testing needs.

INDICATIONS FOR SUSCEPTIBILITY TESTING

Susceptibility testing has been rarely employed at most hospitals and medical centers. Despite the increasing prevalence of resistance among anaerobes, the frequency of testing was reported to be declining in the last survey conducted in the early 1990s partly because of budgetary reductions, a concomitant loss of expertise at these institutions, a lack of automated testing for anaerobes, and a failure to consider resistance as important to clinicians (20,21).

The recent and varied trends in antibiotic resistance, spread of resistance genes, and poor clinical outcomes resulting from ineffective antibiotic therapy argue strongly for more susceptibility testing of anaerobes. The most recent CLSI recommendations suggest that clinical laboratories should strongly consider susceptibility testing to assist in the management of individual cases of serious or life-threatening infections, to test for surveillance purposes for local and regional resistance rates, and to determine the rates of susceptibility of anaerobes when newer antimicrobial agents are introduced (10). The current major indications for testing individual isolates should be based on persistent infection despite an adequate treatment regimen, or difficulty in making empiric decisions based on precedent and known resistance of an organism or species (10). Organisms recognized as highly pathogenic and for which antimicrobial resistance cannot be predicted include members of the *B. fragilis* group, *Prevotella* sp, *Fusobacterium* sp, *Clostridium* sp, *Bilophila wadsworthia*, and *Sutterella wadsworthensis* (10).

Surveillance Testing

Annual surveillance testing is now recommended for clinical laboratories that routinely identify anaerobic bacteria to establish local patterns of resistance for commonly encountered anaerobes (3,10,16). Proper identification of anaerobes is, of course, an important first step in this process. Laboratories should be aware of recent taxonomic changes that have occurred within gram-negative anaerobic bacteria (based on 16S recombinant DNA techniques) that have resulted in regrouping of some organisms and the identification of new species. The reader is referred to excellent descriptions of these changes, as well as a strategy for identification of anaerobic species (22–25).

Strains to be tested for surveillance purposes should be collected over several months and stored until at least 50 to 100 are available for batch testing, allowing for the most efficient use of time, training, and materials. In general, anaerobic isolates to be tested should reflect the distribution of bacteria isolated in the laboratory. Because of the high frequency of resistance among the *B. fragilis* group, it is recommended that at least 20 isolates be selected from the various species, along with the testing of 10 isolates from other frequently isolated anaerobic genera. When choosing antibiotics to test, laboratories should consider at least one agent from each antibiotic class, and that should also reflect their respective hospital's formulary (10,16).

Routine Testing

Individual isolate testing may also be appropriate in certain clinical situations. Isolates obtained from severe infections including brain abscess, bacteremia, endovascular infections, and bone and joint infections should be strongly considered for testing (10). Consultation with the physician about the clinical situation will be important in deciding on the need for susceptibility testing of these isolates (10).

Strategy for Testing

The anaerobe working group suggests a strategy for testing gram-positive and gram-negative groups of anaerobes. This includes a listing of primary and supplemental choices for testing *B. fragilis* group and other gram-negative anaerobes and gram-positive anaerobes (10). Examples of primary choices include one each of the β-lactam–β-lactamase (BLA) inhibitor combinations, carbapenems, clindamycin, and metronidazole for *B. fragilis* group and gram-negative rods. For the gram-positive anaerobes, penicillin (or ampicillin), β-lactam/BLA inhibitors, clindamycin, carbapenems, and metronidazole are recommended for routine primary testing.

MECHANISMS OF ACTION OF ANTIANAEROBIC ANTIMICROBIAL AGENTS

The mechanism of action for most antianaerobic antimicrobial agents is either proven or presumed the same as that demonstrated for other nonanaerobic organisms. Although many of the pathogenic anaerobic bacteria are gram-negative, the either high or low degree of activity of some agents does not always closely match that of aerobic or facultative anaerobic bacteria. Cases where differences in activity are known are included in the discussion. The mechanism of action of clindamycin (and lincomycin), metronidazole, quinolones, aminoglycosides, and tetracyclines are discussed here. The mechanism of action of β-lactam antibiotics is not presented in this section, as this is thoroughly discussed in Chapter 11.

Clindamycin and lincomycin both work by binding to the 50S ribosomal subunit of bacteria, resulting in a disruption of protein synthesis by interfering with the transpeptidation reaction, preventing peptide chain elongation (26). Of note, chloramphenicol and macrolides compete for binding at the same site and are thought to be potentially antagonistic when used together. In aerobic bacteria, clindamycin may potentiate opsonization and phagocytosis of bacteria, presumably by the resulting changes in the cell wall surface decreasing adherence of bacteria to host cells and increasing intracellular killing (27,28). This phenomenon has not been demonstrated for anaerobes but could also occur. Clindamycin is considered bactericidal against *B. fragilis*, although its activity can be inconsistent. Resistance to this agent is discussed in the next section.

Metronidazole activity against anaerobes is mediated through a four-step process. In the first step, metronidazole must enter the cell, which it does efficiently as a low molecular weight compound that diffuses easily across cell membranes (29). The second step includes reductive activation by intracellular transport proteins. Metronidazole is reduced by the pyruvate:ferredoxin oxidoreductase system in the mitochondria of obligate anaerobes altering its chemical structure. Metronidazole is reduced when its nitro group acts as an electron sink, capturing electrons and reducing the compound, which also results in a concentration gradient driving its own uptake as well as forming intermediate compounds and free radicals toxic to the cell (30,31). In the third step, reduced intermediate particles interact with host cell DNA, resulting in fatal DNA strand breakage (32,33). Lastly, breakdown of cytotoxic intermediates occurs, resulting in inactive end products (34). Metronidazole is rapidly bactericidal in a concentration-dependent manner, killing *B. fragilis* and *C. perfringens* more rapidly than does clindamycin (35,36).

Fluoroquinolones directly inhibit bacterial DNA synthesis by binding to the complex of both DNA gyrase and topoisomerase IV, which are required for bacterial replication (37). The key event in quinolone action is reversible trapping of gyrase-DNA and topoisomerase IV–DNA complexes. Complex formation with gyrase is followed by a rapid, reversible inhibition of DNA synthesis

and growth, resulting in damage to bacterial DNA and cell death. Thus, quinolones are also bactericidal agents.

Aminoglycosides bind 30S ribosomal subunits of aerobic bacteria but have no activity against anaerobes. Uptake of aminoglycosides by bacteria requires an energy-dependent phase normally provided by an oxygen- or nitrogen-dependent electron transport system that is absent in strictly anaerobic bacteria (38). Thus, anaerobes do no import aminoglycosides. However, aminoglycosides do bind to the ribosomes of *B. fragilis* and *C. perfringens* from cell-free extracts, indicating likely activity if they could gain entry into cells (39). Tetracyclines, on the other hand, are able to enter bacteria passively, including anaerobes, and also bind the 30S ribosomal subunit, preventing protein synthesis (40). However, resistance to this agent is widespread among anaerobes and, therefore, not frequently used. Specific resistance mechanisms are discussed in the next section.

ANTIMICROBIAL RESISTANCE AMONG ANAEROBES

As noted previously, antibiotic resistance among some anaerobes has increased significantly over the last few decades and parallels that of nonanaerobic bacteria (41). Organisms for which the most significant change has occurred are members of the *B. fragilis* group. Three major surveillance studies have reported significant changes in resistance among these bacteria since the 1980s (42–46). All three surveys confirm that resistance is increasing with hospital-to-hospital variation, even within the same geographic area. The most recent anaerobe survey conducted at eight medical centers throughout the United States reporting data from 2006 to 2009 confirms the presence of increasing resistance among anaerobes in geographically diverse areas (47).

Clindamycin Resistance

Clindamycin resistance among *Bacteroides* sp has increased the most significantly in the last two decades. Starting at only 3% in 1987, resistance to clindamycin in 2000 ranged from 16% to 44% resistance among the members of the *B. fragilis* group (42,46,48). In the 2006 to 2009 survey, the rates of clindamycin resistance remained stable at 19% to 50%, suggesting that this is not a good empiric initial choice without specific susceptibilities for this group of organisms (47). For many non-*Bacteroides* anaerobes, resistance has also increased, albeit not as significantly as in the *B. fragilis* group (48). Other reports have found up to 10% clindamycin resistance for *Prevotella* sp, *Fusobacterium* sp, *Porphyromonas* sp, and *Peptostreptococcus* sp, with higher rates for some *Clostridium* sp (especially *Clostridium difficile*) (44,49).

β-Lactam Antibiotic Resistance

Resistance to β-lactam agents among anaerobes is fairly widespread for the penicillins, cephamycins, and third-generation cephalosporins. Around 97% of the *B. fragilis* group is resistant to penicillin G by virtue of BLA production. In contrast, cefoxitin retains activity against most *B. fragilis* group members, although resistance has ranged between 8% and 22% over the period of 1987 to 2000 and similarly it ranged between 6% and 20% from 2006 to 2009 (47). Cefotetan activity is very similar to that of cefoxitin against *B. fragilis* but is much less potent against other members of the *B. fragilis* group (30% to 87% resistant) (43). Resistance to piperacillin, the most active ureidopenicillin against anaerobes, is also now widespread among members of the *B. fragilis* group (average 25% resistant). Resistance is also found among non-*Bacteroides* anaerobes (42,46,48).

Fortunately, activity of other more potent β-lactams, the β-lactam–BLA inhibitor combinations and carbapenems, remains excellent. The three combination agents of ampicillin/sulbactam, ticarcillin/clavulanate, and piperacillin/tazobactam are highly active against members of the *B. fragilis* group, with less than 4% resistance reported in the most recent survey (47). The carbapenem class of antibiotics including doripenem, imipenem/cilastatin, meropenem, and ertapenem remain potent agents against members of the *B. fragilis* group, with rates of resistance being less than 3% in recently tested isolates (47).

Resistance to β-lactam agents among non-*Bacteroides* anaerobes is generally much lower than that of *Bacteroides*. However, similar to that of *Bacteroides* organisms, *Prevotella* spp are also potent BLA producers, with more than 50% resistant to penicillin and ampicillin (50). Aldridge et al. (44) have reported penicillin resistance for *Fusobacterium* sp, *Porphyromonas* sp, and *Peptostreptococcus* sp. at 9%, 21%, and 6%, respectively. In the same survey, resistance to cefoxitin, cefotetan, β-lactam–BLA inhibitor combinations, and carbapenems was 0%, except for resistance to ampicillin/sulbactam in *Peptostreptococcus* sp and *Porphyromonas* sp, which were 4% and 5%, respectively (44).

5-Nitro-Imidazole Resistance

Although metronidazole resistance among gram-negative anaerobes had been reported in a single case in the United States, from a patient returning from Europe, and occasionally but rarely in European countries (51–53), however, more recent reports from United States and Europe have shown resistance rates of less than 1% for metronidazole among tested *B. fragilis* group isolates (47,54). Metronidazole resistance among gram-positive anaerobes is far more common, especially for most isolates of *Propionibacterium acnes* and *Actinomyces* sp (21).

Tetracycline and Glycylcycline Resistance

Among other antibiotic classes, tetracycline resistance is now nearly universal among *Bacteroides* sp and many other anaerobes, limiting its use in therapy. Tigecycline is the first agent in a newer glycylcycline class that was created by adding on a side chain to minocycline (55). It was designed to overcome the tetracycline-specific efflux pump and increase its activity over both aerobic and anaerobic bacteria (55). Although tigecycline has anaerobic activity against *C. difficile*, *Fusobacterium* sp, *Prevotella* sp, *Porphyromonas* sp, and the *B. fragilis* group, resistance in the latter has been reported at 0% to 8% (47,55).

Resistance to Other Antibiotics

Fluoroquinolone resistance among anaerobes has increased the most significantly and rapidly. Moxifloxacin is approved by the U.S. Food and Drug Administration (FDA) for treatment of complicated intraabdominal infections. Currently, use of this agent is very limited due to increasing resistance among the *B. fragilis* group. In the most recent anaerobe survey, the rates of resistance in the *B. fragilis* group ranged from 30% to 80% (47).

Resistance to aminoglycosides is universal among anaerobes, with this antibiotic restricted to combination therapy for mixed infections. Chloramphenicol resistance is very rare, but this agent is also rarely used in the clinical setting (56).

MECHANISMS OF ANTIMICROBIAL RESISTANCE AMONG ANAEROBES

Table 4.1 summarizes the current known mechanisms of resistance and resistance genes for anaerobic bacteria. Not surprisingly, antibiotic resistance mechanisms are quite different for each class of

Table 4.1

Anaerobic Bacterial Gene Transfer Factors Contributing to Antibiotic Resistance

Bacterial Group	Antibiotic	Gene Designation	Transferable	Transfer Factor
B. fragilis group	Clindamycin	*ermF,*	+	Plasmid
		ermS		
	Tetracycline	*tetQ, tetX[a]*	+	Plasmid
	Cephalosporin	*cepA, cblA*	ND[b]	
	Cefoxitin	*cfxA*	+	Transposon
	Carbapenems	*ccrA, cfiA*	+	Plasmid[c]
	Metronidazole	*nimA,*	+	Plasmid
		nimB,	(*nimA, C, D*)	
		nimC,		
		nimD,		
		nimE, nimF		
		gyrA,		
		gyrB,		
		parC,		
		parE		
	Quinolones		??	
	Streptomycin	*aadS[a]*	+	Transposon
C. perfringens	Chloramphenicol	*catQ,[d]*	+	Plasmid
		catP		
	Clindamycin	*ermQ,*	ND	
		ermP		
	Tetracycline	*tetA(P)*	+	Plasmid
		tetB(P)		
C. difficile	Tetracycline	*tcr*	+	Transposon?[e]
	Chloramphenicol	*catD*	+	Transposon
	Clindamycin	*ermZ, ermBZ*	+	Transposon
Clostridium butyricum	Chloramphenicol	*catA, catB*	ND	
Prevotella spp.	Tetracycline	*tetQ, tetO, tetM*	+	Transposon (*tetQ*)
Fusobacterium spp.	Tetracycline	*tetM*	+	Transposon

[a]cryptic
[b]Not determined.
[c]A plasmid-borne imipenem/cilastatin resistance determinant has been isolated, but the gene has not been characterized.
[d]*catQ* was characterized from a nonconjugative strain.
[e]The exact nature of the transfer factor is unknown.

antibiotics. Clindamycin resistance is mediated by a macrolide-lincosamide-streptogramin (MLS) type 23S methylase similar to that of staphylococci (48) and is typically encoded by one of several erythromycin ribosome methylation (*erm*) genes that are typically regulated and expressed at high levels. However, some isolates that contain *erm* genes demonstrate only moderately elevated minimum inhibitory concentrations (MICs) that would not otherwise be designated as resistant. Some of these latter strains can be detected by testing for erythromycin resistance. It is possible that these isolates could be induced to higher levels of resistance under selective pressure. At the current time, however, there is no specific recommendation to screen for resistance using erythromycin. Transfer of *erm* genes by conjugation in *B. fragilis* group organisms is easily demonstrated in the laboratory and likely explains the rapid emergence of this resistance phenotype (57–59). Of note, clindamycin is no longer recommended as empiric therapy for intraabdominal infections in the latest published guidelines, presumably because of the high rate of resistance (3).

Resistance to β-lactam antibiotics can occur by one of three major mechanisms: inactivating enzymes (BLAs), low-affinity penicillin-binding proteins (PBPs), or decreased permeability. BLA is by far the most common mechanism associated with resistance to β-lactam antibiotics. The most common BLAs found among *Bacteroides* sp and *Prevotella* sp are cephalosporinases of the type 2e class. These BLAs are inhibited by sulbactam, clavulanic acid, or tazobactam, thus the increased potency of the β-lactam–BLA inhibitor combinations. Cefoxitin- and cefotaxime-inactivating enzymes and other BLAs have also been reported in many *B. fragilis* group species (60). The most potent BLAs are the zinc metalloenzymes encoded by either *ccrA* or *cfiA* genes of the *B. fragilis* group (61). These enzymes are responsible for the rare resistance to carbapenems, are active against all β-lactam antibiotics with known activity against anaerobes, and are not inactivated by current BLA inhibitors. Although resistance to carbapenems is currently quite rare in the United States, up to 3% of *Bacteroides* strains have been found to carry one of the genes expressed at a very low level. These strains can be induced to a higher level of resistance in the laboratory under selective pressure caused by a promoter (contained in an insertion sequence) that has inserted upstream of the *ccrA* or *cfiA* genes (29,62).

Production of BLAs by other anaerobic bacteria has been generally less well studied, but strains of *Clostridium*, *Porphyromonas*, and *Fusobacterium* organisms express resistance by one or more of these enzymes. Penicillin-resistant *Fusobacterium* and *Clostridium* organisms express penicillinases that are typically inhibited by clavulanic acid, although exceptions among some *Clostridium* sp have been reported (56,63).

Other mechanisms of resistance to β-lactam antibiotics are far less frequent in occurrence and less well studied. Decreased binding to PBP2 or PBP1 complex has been reported in rare clinical

isolates in cefoxitin resistance among *B. fragilis* strains (64). Alterations in pore-forming proteins of gram-negative anaerobes are a third type of resistance, with the absence of one or more outer membrane proteins associated with high MICs to ampicillin/sulbactam in some strains of *B. fragilis* (65,66).

Metronidazole resistance occurs by the lack of reduction to its active form in anaerobic bacteria. Metronidazole-resistant *B. fragilis* group organisms, although rare, carry one of six known *nim* genes that appear to encode a nitroimidazole reductase that converts 4- or 5-nitroimidazole to 4- or 5-aminoimidazole, preventing the formation of the toxic drug form necessary for the agents' activity (67,68). These genes have been identified on both the chromosome and on transferable plasmids. High-level expression of the *nim* genes requires an insertion sequence with a promoter, similar to that of carbapenem resistance (69). Differential gene expression affecting cell metabolism in *Bacteroides* has also been reported as an alternative mechanism for resistance (70). In contrast to *Bacteroides*, the mechanism of resistance to metronidazole for non-*Bacteroides* anaerobes is currently not known. Interestingly, metronidazole resistance in the microaerophilic organism *Helicobacter pylori* has been partially solved for some strains that contain mutations in the *rdxA* gene, an oxygen-insensitive nitroreductase that converts metronidazole to its active form in this organism (71). Other candidate genes for resistance include the flavin oxidoreductase (*frxA*), ferredoxin-like proteins (*fdxA*, *fdxB*), and pyruvate oxidoreductase (*porA*, *porB*) (72). Metronidazole also has activity against *Mycobacterium tuberculosis*, although apparently only in dormant cells, when reduction of the drug can occur. Resistance among actively growing *Mycobacterium* organisms is presumed secondary to a lack of sufficient reducing potential (73).

Fluoroquinolone resistance among *Bacteroides* sp has been attributed to either a mutation in the quinolone resistance–determining region of the gyrase A gene (*gyrA*) from single or multiple mutations, or an alteration in efflux of the antibiotic (74–77). High-level resistance may be secondary to both mechanisms in the same cell, although only a few strains have been tested to date. Both of these mechanisms appear to be responsible for the cross-class resistance to newer quinolones.

The lack of activity of aminoglycosides against anaerobes is related to the lack of uptake by the bacteria under anaerobic conditions and a failure to reach their ribosome targets (39). Tetracycline resistance is widespread, especially among *B. fragilis* group and *Prevotella* sp (15). Several genes encoding resistance have been identified among various anaerobes, which encode protective proteins, resulting in protection of the ribosomes. More importantly, however, is the association of tetracycline resistance and the inducible transfer of this resistance determinant upon exposure to low levels of the antibiotic. Chloramphenicol resistance is extremely rare but, when found, is associated with inactivation of the drug by nitroreduction or acetyltransferase (78).

METHODS FOR ANTIMICROBIAL SUSCEPTIBILITY TESTING OF ANAEROBIC BACTERIA

Several different methods, spanning five decades, have been utilized in antimicrobial susceptibility testing (AST) of anaerobic bacteria. During that time, more than 16 methods, 16 different media, and a host of other variables have been described to test susceptibility of anaerobes. NCCLS took the lead in developing a consensus for AST of anaerobes starting with the first approved standard in 1985, along with alternative methods published in a second document the same year. Subsequently, several revisions have been published that modified, added, or eliminated some methods (10). Following extensive multilaboratory collaborative studies sanctioned by the NCCLS in the late 1990s, a consensus was reached culminating in a single agar dilution standard and one broth microdilution method, both using the same medium (10,17,18). In addition to NCCLS methods, a very useful and highly correlated user-friendly method, Etest (AB Biodisk), has been FDA approved and available for

several years (19,79). As a proprietary product, the Etest is not included in the CLSI documents. Of note, all methods can be performed in ambient air but require incubation in an anaerobic jar or glove box.

Choosing a method from among these three recognized and approved methods may depend on a number of factors (Table 4.2). The agar dilution standard has a very high degree of reproducibility but is fairly labor-intensive. A laboratory can test up to 30 isolates plus two controls, making it useful for batch testing. However, individual sets of dilution plates must be pored for each antibiotic, increasing material and labor costs. As the reference standard, agar dilution is most often used for evaluation of new antimicrobial agents. The broth microdilution method is more user-friendly than agar dilution and has the flexibility to test multiple antibiotics using the same microtiter plate, albeit only one isolate at a time. Based on available comparative studies of broth microdilution to the standard, results are considered equivalent when testing members of the *B. fragilis* group. However, results are not as comparable for non-*Bacteroides* anaerobes because of poor growth, and broth microdilution is not used for this group at this time. It should be noted that previously published studies testing non-*Bacteroides* anaerobes using a different broth (anaerobe MIC broth) were able to grow non-*Bacteroides* anaerobes with MIC results within twofold of those for agar dilution. Thus, broth microdilution testing for non-*Bacteroides* anaerobes can be considered but only if correlated with the current agar dilution standard. The third method, Etest, is relatively easy to perform and is well suited for testing individual isolates of any anaerobe. For surveillance testing, costs could be prohibitive.

Table 4.2

Methods for Antimicrobial Susceptibility Testing of Anaerobic Bacteria

Method	Medium	Inoculum	Advantages	Disadvantages
Agar dilution	*Brucella* blood agar	10^5 CFU/spot	Reference method, suitable for surveillance	Labor-intensive
Broth microdilution	*Brucella* broth supplemented with blood	10^6 CFU/mL	Multiple antibiotics/isolate, commercially available	Limited to *B. fragilis* group, panel shelf life
Etest	*Brucella* blood agar	1 McFarland swab plate	Precise MIC values, convenient	Expensive for surveillance

CFU, colony-forming unit; MIC, minimum inhibitory concentration.

CLINICAL AND LABORATORY STANDARDS INSTITUTE REFERENCE AGAR DILUTION METHOD

For the agar dilution reference standard, each test concentration of an antibiotic is mixed into molten agar and poured into separate Petri dishes to which an inoculum of an organism is applied, incubated anaerobically, and examined to determine the MIC for the antimicrobial agent tested. Methods described here are adapted from those of CLSI standards (10). For laboratories inexperienced with this method and anaerobe AST, a useful time table for setup and testing is provided as an appendix in the CLSI standards document.

Testing Medium

Brucella blood agar supplemented with 5 μg hemin, 1% vitamin K_1, and 5% laked sheep blood is the recommended testing medium (10). Brucella agar blanks (17 mL) can be prepared in advance containing hemin and vitamin K_1, and flash-autoclaved or microwaved and placed in an approximately 50°C water bath on the day of use (10). One milliliter of laked sheep blood is then added to each melted blank while still in the water bath. Two milliliters of each twofold diluted test antibiotic is then added to the agar, mixed by inverting the tubes, and poured into sterile Petri dishes (10). Following hardening of the plates, and drying briefly in an inverted position in a 37°C incubator, the plates are ready for use. Preferably, plates should be made on the day of testing but can be sealed in plastic bags and stored at 2°C to 8°C for periods of up to 72 hours if necessary (10). Exceptions to storage include plates containing clavulanic acid or imipenem/cilastatin, which must be made on the day of use.

Inoculum Preparation

The inoculum can be prepared by either a direct colony suspension or growth method. Direct colony suspension requires 24- to 48-hour growth on a *Brucella* blood agar plate (10). Several colonies are touched lightly with an inoculating needle or cotton swab and suspended in reduced *Brucella* broth to achieve a turbidity equivalent to a McFarland standard of 0.5 (10). The alternative growth method involves the inoculation of enriched thioglycollate medium (without indicator) with portions of five or more colonies from a *Brucella* blood agar plate, incubating for 6 to 24 hours at 37°C, and adjusting the turbidity to a McFarland standard of 0.5 by addition of reduced *Brucella* broth (10).

Inoculation and Incubation of Plates

Once the inoculum is prepared, it is most often applied using an inoculum-replicating apparatus, such as a Steers-Foltz replicator, to deliver 1 to 2 μL on the agar surface, corresponding to 1 × 10^5 colony-forming units (CFUs) per spot. Depending on the device, either 32 or 36 wells can be filled with different test organisms and controls using a Pasteur or other pipette (10). Application of inoculum to plates includes repeated stamping of plates, starting with lowest to highest dilution of each antibiotic set. One plate of supplemented *Brucella* blood agar without antibiotic should be stamped prior to and after each set of antibiotics for growth control. Contamination by aerobic bacteria during the inoculation procedure can be detected by inoculating a drug-free plate and incubated aerobically. Once plates are inoculated, they should sit until liquid is absorbed into the medium and then incubated in an anaerobic environment at 35°C to 37°C for 42 to 48 hours (10).

Interpretation of Results

End points are determined by reading each plate against a dark, nonreflecting background and comparing it with the control growth plate. Any growth on the aerobic control should eliminate further interpretation of that test organism. The end point for a given test organism is where a marked reduction occurs in the appearance of growth compared with control. A marked change includes a haze, multiple tiny colonies, or one to several normal-sized colonies. These descriptions have been problematic for those inexperienced with using this method. To that end, CLSI recommends the use of two figures containing 28 full-dilution color photographic examples of end point readings to illustrate the written descriptions (10).

Interpretative categories approved by CLSI for MICs derived for anaerobic bacteria are shown in Table 4.3. This table includes agents that are the most frequently used in the clinical setting and were updated through 2012. Interpretative categories for any organism have been determined based on the population distribution of the bacteria, the pharmacokinetics, and pharmacodynamic properties of the antibiotic with verification of efficacy by clinical studies (see an in-depth description in Chapter 1). This works particularly well for single-organism infections. However, this is rarely the case for anaerobic bacteria, which are typically isolated from mixed infections. Many of the published anaerobic breakpoints were

Table 4.3

Interpretive Categories for Minimum Inhibitory Concentrations for Anaerobic Bacteria[a]			
	MIC (µg/mL)		
Antimicrobial Agent	**Susceptible**	**Intermediate**	**Resistant**
Penicillin/ampicillin	<0.5	1	≥2
Ampicillin/sulbactam	<8/4	16/8	≥32/16
Piperacillin/tazobactam	<32/4	64/4	≥128/4
Cefoxitin	<16	32	≥64
Ertapenem	<4	8	≥16
Imipenem/cilastatin	<4	8	≥16
Meropenem	<4	8	≥16
Metronidazole	<8	16	≥32
Clindamycin	<2	4	≥8
Moxifloxacin	<2	4	≥8

[a]Breakpoints as listed in the CLSI M11-A08 Standards document (10).

determined on the basis of animal models or the result of clinical trials involving patients with polymicrobial infections as well as pharmacokinetic data. Despite these potential limitations, the use of maximum dosages of antibiotics along with appropriate ancillary therapy (debridement or drainage) should be effective for organisms with susceptible breakpoints, although those with intermediate susceptibilities should be monitored closely (10).

CLINICAL AND LABORATORY STANDARDS INSTITUTE–RECOMMENDED BROTH MICRODILUTION METHOD

The broth microdilution method has been validated by CLSI for susceptibility testing of the *B. fragilis* group.

Media

Brucella broth supplemented with hemin (5 µg/mL), vitamin K₁, and lysed horse blood is the recommended medium, which is essentially equivalent to that of agar dilution (10). Trays can be prepared fresh and then frozen or purchased commercially. Trays should be kept at −70°C. Antibiotics are diluted according to an algorithm recommended by CLSI in volumes of 15 to 100 mL (10) and delivered using a device that can simultaneously dispense aliquots of 0.1 mL per well

(or 0.05 mL per well if a pipette will be used to deliver an equal volume of inoculum) (10). When a pipette is used for inoculation, antibiotic concentrations should be prepared at 2× the final desired concentration. Volumes of less than 0.1 mL are not recommended (10).

Inoculum Preparation, Inoculation Procedure, and Incubation

Inoculum preparation is the same as for agar dilution to achieve a turbidity of a McFarland standard of 0.5 (10). Commercially available inoculating devices can be used that deliver 10 µL of a 1:15 dilution of a 0.5 McFarland inoculum (10). For commercially prepared trays, follow the manufacturer's recommendations. The final concentration of inoculum should be 1×10^7 CFU/mL.

Before inoculation, frozen trays should be brought to room temperature and inoculated within 15 minutes of inoculum preparation. It is advisable to perform a colony count and purity check of the inoculum by removing 10 µL from the growth control well and diluting it into 10 mL of saline, streaking 0.1 mL onto the surface of an anaerobic blood agar plate, and incubating anaerobically (10). One hundred colonies on the plate correspond to 1×10^6 CFU/mL. Trays are then incubated for 46 to 48 hours at 35°C in an anaerobic atmosphere (see previous discussion), ensuring sufficient humidity to prevent drying (10).

Interpretation of Results

The MIC values are read by viewing the plates from the bottom using a stand and a mirror. A sufficient growth control is required to interpret results. The MIC end point is read as the concentration where no growth, or the most significant reduction of growth, is observed. A trailing effect may be observed for some drug–organism combinations. Again, two figures containing 28 examples of broth microdilution end points are provided by CLSI (10). Breakpoints for broth microdilution interpretation are the same as those for agar dilution (see Table 4.3).

QUALITY CONTROL

A quality control program to monitor accuracy of testing, reagents, equipment, and persons conducting tests is essential. The quality control strains chosen for anaerobic bacteria are limited to two *Bacteroides* sp, a nontoxigenic *C. difficile* strain, and an *Eggerthella* strain. *B. fragilis* ATCC 25285 and *Bacteroides thetaiotaomicron* ATCC 29741 are appropriate for testing using any of the methods listed. *C. difficile* ATCC 700057 is preferred over *Eggerthella lenta* ATCC 43055 when testing gram-positive anaerobes (10). Two of the four quality control strains should be used for each assessment when agar dilution is used. When an individual strain is being tested by broth microdilution or Etest, one strain should be included. Expected values for end points for both agar and broth microdilution methods are published by CLSI.

ETEST

The Etest is an excellent and convenient choice for testing individual anaerobic organisms. Several studies have validated this method, demonstrating good correlation with the agar dilution method (19,79). However, Rosenblatt and Gustafson (79) have noted that some *Prevotella* and *Bacteroides* strains show false susceptibility when testing penicillin and ceftriaxone that is minimized if BLA-producing strains are eliminated. A more significant warning is potential false resistance to metronidazole as a result of test conditions and medium quality (80). This aberrant result can be avoided by prereducing test plates in an anaerobic chamber the night before testing.

Procedure

The Etest is a familiar technique to most clinical laboratories and does not differ significantly in its application to anaerobic bacteria. The Etest strips are coated with a gradient of antimicrobial on one side with an MIC interpretative scale on the other. The organism to be tested is prepared to a McFarland standard of 1 and applied to a 150-mm diameter Petri dish of supplemented *Brucella* blood agar, with the strips applied in a radial fashion. Smaller plates can be used with fewer strips. Incubation is recommended for 48 hours at 35°C and read where an elliptical zone of inhibition intersects the strip on the scale of MIC values.

β-LACTAMASE TESTING

The BLA testing deserves mention, although it is not a true AST test. Testing for BLA activity can be performed on anaerobic organisms, although it is not recommended for the *B. fragilis* group because of the high prevalence of positivity. This test can be used as a first step to drive additional testing choices. Any BLA-producing anaerobe should be considered resistant to penicillin and ampicillin. However, as noted in the section on antimicrobial resistance, alternative mechanisms of resistance to β-lactams are known, and a negative test does not assure susceptibility to penicillin.

The recommended method for testing is chromogenic and cephalosporin-based, either by a nitrocefin disk assay (Cefinase; BBL Microbiology Systems, Cockeysville, MD) or the S1 chromogenic disk (International BioClinical, Inc., Portland, OR). Tests are performed according to manufacturers' directions. A positive reaction is denoted by a change in color from yellow to red that typically occurs within 5 to 10 minutes. However, some *Bacteroides* strains may react more slowly (up to 30 minutes) (10).

REFERENCES

1. Finegold SM, George WL. *Anaerobic infections in humans*. San Diego, CA: Academic Press, 1989.
2. Proceedings of the 1st North American Congress on Anaerobic Bacteria and Anaerobic Infections. Marina del Rey, California, 24–26, 1992. *Clin Infect Dis* 1993; 16(Suppl 4):S159–S457.
3. Solomkin JS, Mazuski JE, Bradley JS, et al. Diagnosis and management of complicated intra-abdominal infection in adults and children: guidelines by the Surgical Infection Society and the Infectious Diseases Society of America. *Clin Infect Dis* 2010;50: 133–164.
4. Martinez E, Miro JM, Almirante B, et al. Effect of penicillin resistance of *Streptococcus pneumoniae* on the presentation, prognosis, and treatment of pneumococcal endocarditis in adults. *Clin Infect Dis* 2002;35:130–139.

5. Paterson DL, Ko WC, Von Gottberg A, et al. International prospective study of *Klebsiella pneumoniae* bacteremia: implications of extended-spectrum beta-lactamase production in nosocomial infections. *Ann Intern Med* 2004;140:26–32.

6. Peres-Bota D, Rodriguez H, Dimopoulos G, et al. Are infections due to resistant pathogens associated with a worse outcome in critically ill patients? *J Infect* 2003;47:307–316.

7. Yu Y, Zhou W, Chen Y, et al. Epidemiological and antibiotic resistant study on extended-spectrum beta-lactamase-producing *Escherichia coli* and *Klebsiella pneumoniae* in Zhejiang Province. *Chin Med J (Engl)* 2002;115:1479–1482.

8. Rosenblatt JE, Brook I. Clinical relevance of susceptibility testing of anaerobic bacteria. *Clin Infect Dis* 1993;16(Suppl 4):S446–S448.

9. National Committee for Clinical Laboratory Standards. *Methods for antimicrobial susceptibility testing of anaerobic bacteria*. 4th ed. M11-A4. Villanova, PA: National Committee for Clinical Laboratory Standards, 1997.

10. Clinical and Laboratory Standards Institute. *Methods for antimicrobial susceptibility testing of anaerobic bacteria*. 8th ed. M11-A8. Wayne, PA: Clinical and Laboratory Standards Institute, 2012.

11. Bieluch VM, Cuchural GJ, Snydman DR, et al. Clinical importance of cefoxitin-resistant Bacteroides fragilis isolates. *Diagn Microbiol Infect Dis* 1987;7:119–126.

12. Dalmau D, Cayouette M, Lamothe F, et al. Clindamycin resistance in the *Bacteroides fragilis* group: association with hospital-acquired infections. *Clin Infect Dis* 1997;24:874–877.

13. Snydman DR, Cuchural GJ Jr, McDermott L, et al. Correlation of various in vitro testing methods with clinical outcomes in patients with *Bacteroides fragilis* group infections treated with cefoxitin: a retrospective analysis. *Antimicrob Agents Chemother* 1992;36:540–544.

14. Nguyen MH, Yu VL, Morris AJ, et al. Antimicrobial resistance and clinical outcome of *Bacteroides* bacteremia: findings of a multicenter prospective observational trial. *Clin Infect Dis* 2000;30:870–876.

15. Nikolich MP, Shoemaker NB, Salyers AA. A *Bacteroides* tetracycline resistance gene represents a new class of ribosome protection tetracycline resistance. *Antimicrob Agents Chemother* 1992;36:1005–1012.

16. Citron DM, Hecht DW. Susceptibility test methods: anaerobic bacteria. In: Murray PR, Baron EJ, Jorgensen JH, et al, eds. *Manual of clinical microbiology*. 8th ed. Washington, DC: ASM Press, 2003:1141–1148.

17. Roe DE, Finegold SM, Citron DM, et al. Multilaboratory comparison of anaerobe susceptibility results using 3 different agar media. *Clin Infect Dis* 2002;35:S40–S46.

18. Roe DE, Finegold SM, Citron DM, et al. Multilaboratory comparison of growth characteristics for anaerobes, using 5 different agar media. *Clin Infect Dis* 2002;35:S36–S39.

19. Citron DM, Ostovari MI, Karlsson A, et al. Evaluation of the E test for susceptibility testing of anaerobic bacteria. *J Clin Microbiol* 1991;29:2197–2203.

20. Goldstein EJ, Citron DM, Goldman RJ. National hospital survey of anaerobic culture and susceptibility testing methods: results and recommendations for improvement. *J Clin Microbiol* 1992;30:1529–1534.

21. Goldstein EJC. United States national hospital survey of anaerobic culture and susceptibility methods. *Anaerobe* 1995;1:309–314.

22. Citron DM, Hecht DW. Susceptibility test methods: anaerobic bacteria. In: Murray PR, Baron EJ, Jorgensen JH, et al, eds. *Manual of Clinical Microbiology*. 8th ed. Washington, DC: ASM Press, 2003:343.

23. Jousimies-Somer H, Summanen P. Recent taxonomic changes and terminology update of clinically significant anaerobic gram-negative bacteria (excluding spirochetes). *Clin Infect Dis* 2002;35:S17–S21.

24. Song Y, Liu C, McTeague M, et al. Rapid identification of Gram-positive anaerobic coccal species originally classified in the genus Peptostreptococcus by multiplex PCR assays using genus- and species-specific primers. *Microbiology* 2003;149:1719–1727.

25. Song Y, Liu C, McTeague M, et al. 16S ribosomal DNA sequence-based analysis of clinically significant gram-positive anaerobic cocci. *J Clin Microbiol* 2003;41:1363–1369.

26. Chang FN, Weisblum B. The specificity of lincomycin binding to ribosomes. *Biochemistry* 1967;6:836–843.

27. Veringa EM, Ferguson DA Jr, Lambe DW Jr, et al. The role of glycocalyx in surface phagocytosis of *Bacteroides* spp. in the presence and absence of clindamycin. *J Antimicrob Chemother* 1989;23:711–720.

28. Veringa EM, Verhoef J. Influence of subinhibitory concentrations of clindamycin on opsonophagocytosis of *Staphylococcus aureus*, a protein-A-dependent process. *Antimicrob Agents Chemother* 1986;30:796–797.

29. Edwards R, Read PN. Expression of the carbapenemase gene (cfiA) in *Bacteroides fragilis*. *J Antimicrob Chemother* 2000;46:1009–1012.

30. Edwards DI. Reduction of nitroimidazoles in vitro and DNA damage. *Biochem Pharmacol* 1986;35:53–58.

31. Muller M. Reductive activation of nitroimidazoles in anaerobic microorganisms. *Biochem Pharmacol* 1986;35:37–41.

32. Tocher JH, Edwards DI. The interaction of reduced metronidazole with DNA bases and nucleosides. *Int J Radiat Oncol Biol Phys* 1992;22:661–663.

33. Tocher JH, Edwards DI. Evidence for the direct interaction of reduced metronidazole derivatives with DNA bases. *Biochem Pharmacol* 1994;48:1089–1094.

34. Goldman P, Koch RL, Yeung TC, et al. Comparing the reduction of nitroimidazoles in bacteria and mammalian tissues and relating it to biological activity. *Biochem Pharmacol* 1986;35:43–51.

35. Ralph ED, Kirby WM. Unique bactericidal action of metronidazole against *Bacteroides fragilis* and *Clostridium perfringens*. *Antimicrob Agents Chemother* 1975;8:409–414.

36. Stratton CW, Weeks LS, Aldridge KE. Comparison of the bactericidal activity of clindamycin and metronidazole against cefoxitin-susceptible and cefoxitin-resistant isolates of the Bacteroides fragilis group. *Diagn Microbiol Infect Dis* 1991;14:377–382.

37. Drlica K, Zhao X. DNA gyrase, topoisomerase IV, and the 4-quinolones. *Microbiol Mol Biol Rev* 1997;61:377–392.

38. Bryan LE, Van Den Elzen HM. Streptomycin accumulation in susceptible and resistant strains of *Escherichia coli* and *Pseudomonas aeruginosa*. *Antimicrob Agents Chemother* 1976;9:928–938.

39. Bryan LE, Kowand SK, Van Den Elzen HM. Mechanism of aminoglycoside antibiotic resistance in anaerobic bacteria: *Clostridium perfringens* and *Bacteroides fragilis*. *Antimicrob Agents Chemother* 1979;15:7–13.

40. Craven GR, Gavin R, Fanning T. The transfer RNA binding site of the 30 S ribosome and the site of tetracycline inhibition. *Cold Spring Harb Symp Quant Biol* 1969;34:129–137.

41. Hecht DW. Prevalence of antibiotic resistance in anaerobic bacteria: worrisome developments. *Clin Infect Dis* 2004;39(1):92–97.

42. Snydman DR, Jacobus NV, McDermott LA, et al. National survey on the susceptibility of *Bacteroides fragilis* group: report and analysis of trends for 1997–2000. *Clin Infect Dis* 2002;35:S126–S134.

43. Snydman DR, Jacobus NV, McDermott LA, et al. Multicenter study of in vitro susceptibility of the *Bacteroides*

fragilis group, 1995 to 1996, with comparison of resistance trends from 1990 to 1996. *Antimicrob Agents Chemother* 1999;43:2417–2422.

44. Aldridge KE, Ashcraft D, Cambre K, et al. Multicenter survey of the changing in vitro antimicrobial susceptibilities of clinical isolates of *Bacteroides fragilis* group, *Prevotella*, *Fusobacterium*, *Porphyromonas*, and *Peptostreptococcus* species. *Antimicrob Agents Chemother* 2001;45:1238–1243.

45. Hecht DW, Osmolski JR, O'Keefe JP. Variation in the susceptibility of *Bacteroides fragilis* group isolates from six Chicago hospitals. *Clin Infect Dis* 1993;16(Suppl 4):S357–S360.

46. Hecht DW, Vedantam G. Anaerobe resistance among anaerobes: what now? *Anaerobe* 1999;5:421–429.

47. Snydman DR, Jacobus NV, McDermott LA, et al. Update on resistance of *Bacteroides fragilis* group and related species with special attention to carbapenems 2006–2009. *Anaerobe* 2011;17:147–151.

48. Jimenez-Diaz A, Reig M, Baquero F, et al. Antibiotic sensitivity of ribosomes from wild-type and clindamycin resistant *Bacteroides vulgatus* strains. *J Antimicrob Chemother* 1992;30:295–301.

49. Ackermann G, Degner A, Cohen SH, et al. Prevalence and association of macrolide-lincosamide-streptogramin B (MLS(B)) resistance with resistance to moxifloxacin in *Clostridium difficile*. *J Antimicrob Chemother* 2003;51:599–603.

50. Hecht DW. Anaerobes: antibiotic resistance, clinical significance, and the role of susceptibility testing. *Anaerobe* 2006;12:115–121.

51. Breuil J, Dublanchet A, Truffaut N, et al. Transferable 5-nitroimidazole resistance in the *Bacteroides fragilis* group. *Plasmid* 1989;21:151–154.

52. Urban E, Soki J, Brazier JS, et al. Prevalence and characterization of nim genes of *Bacteroides* sp. isolated in Hungary. *Anaerobe* 2002;8:175–179.

53. Ricci V, Peterson ML, Rotschafer JC, et al. Role of topoisomerase mutations and efflux in fluoroquinolone resistance of *Bacteroides fragilis* clinical isolates and laboratory mutants. *Antimicrob Agents Chemother* 2004;48(4):1344–1346.

54. Nagy E, Urban E, Nord CE, et al. Antimicrobial susceptibility of *Bacteroides fragilis* group isolates in Europe: 20 years of experience. *Clin Microbiol Infect* 2011;17(3):371–379.

55. Stein GE, Craig WA. Tigecycline: a critical analysis. *Clin Infect Dis* 2006;43:518–524.

56. Rasmussen BA, Bush K, Tally FP. Antimicrobial resistance in anaerobes. *Clin Infect Dis* 1997;24(Suppl 1):S110–S120.

57. Bachoual R, Dubreuil L, Soussy CJ, et al. Roles of gyrA mutations in resistance of clinical isolates and in vitro mutants of *Bacteroides fragilis* to the new fluoroquinolone trovafloxacin. *Antimicrob Agents Chemother* 2000;44:1842–1845.

58. Privitera G, Dublanchet A, Sebald M. Transfer of multiple antibiotic resistance between subspecies of *Bacteroides fragilis*. *J Infect Dis* 1979;139:97–101.

59. Welch RA, Jones KR, Macrina FL. Transferable lincosa-mide-macrolide resistance in *Bacteroides*. *Plasmid* 1979;2:261–268.

60. Rogers MB, Parker AC, Smith CJ. Cloning and characterization of the endogenous cephalosporinase gene, cepA, from *Bacteroides fragilis* reveals a new subgroup of Ambler class A beta-lactamases. *Antimicrob Agents Chemother* 1993;37:2391–2400.

61. Yang Y, Rasmussen BA, Bush K. Biochemical characterization of the metallo-beta-lactamase CcrA from *Bacteroides fragilis* TAL3636. *Antimicrob Agents Chemother* 1992;36:1155–1157.

62. Podglajen I, Breuil J, Collatz E. Insertion of a novel DNA sequence, 1S1186, upstream of the silent carbapenemase gene cfiA, promotes expression of carbapenem resistance in clinical isolates of *Bacteroides fragilis*. *Mol Microbiol* 1994;12:105–114.

63. Appelbaum PC, Spangler SK, Pankuch GA, et al. Characterization of a beta-lactamase from *Clostridium clostridioforme*. *J Antimicrob Chemother* 1994;33:33–40.

64. Fang H, Edlund C, Nord CE, et al. Selection of cefoxitin-resistant *Bacteroides thetaiotaomicron* mutants and mechanisms involved in beta-lactam resistance. *Clin Infect Dis* 2002;35:S47–S53.

65. Wexler HM. Outer-membrane pore-forming proteins in gram-negative anaerobic bacteria. *Clin Infect Dis* 2002;35:S65–S71.

66. Wexler HM, Halebian S. Alterations to the penicillin-binding proteins in the *Bacteroides fragilis* group: a mechanism for non-beta-lactamase mediated cefoxitin resistance. *J Antimicrob Chemother* 1990;26:7–20.

67. Carlier JP, Sellier N, Rager MN, et al. Metabolism of a 5-nitroimidazole in susceptible and resistant isogenic strains of *Bacteroides fragilis*. *Antimicrob Agents Chemother* 1997;41:1495–1499.

68. Haggoud A, Reysset G, Azeddoug H, et al. Nucleotide sequence analysis of two 5-nitroimidazole resistance determinants from *Bacteroides* strains and of a new insertion sequence upstream of the two genes. *Antimicrob Agents Chemother* 1994;38:1047–1051.

69. Trinh S, Haggoud A, Reysset G, et al. Plasmids pIP419 and pIP421 from *Bacteroides*: 5-nitroimidazole resistance genes and their upstream insertion sequence elements. *Microbiology* 1995;141(Pt 4):927–935.

70. Diniz CG, Farias LM, Carvalho MA, et al. Differential gene expression in a *Bacteroides fragilis* metronidazole-resistant mutant. *J Antimicrob Chemother* 2004;54(1):100–108.

71. van der Wouden EJ, Thijs JC, Kusters JG, et al. Mechanism and clinical significance of metronidazole resistance in *Helicobacter pylori*. *Scand J Gastroenterol Suppl* 2001;10–14.

72. Chisholm SA, Owen RJ. Mutations in *Helicobacter pylori* rdxA gene sequences may not contribute to metronidazole resistance. *J Antimicrob Chemother* 2003;51:995–999.

73. Wayne LG, Sramek HA. Metronidazole is bactericidal to dormant cells of *Mycobacterium tuberculosis*. *Antimicrob Agents Chemother* 1994;38:2054–2058.

74. Oh H, Hedberg M, Edlund C. Efflux-mediated fluoroquinolone resistance in the *Bacteroides fragilis* group. *Anaerobe* 2002;8:277–282.

75. Onodera Y, Sato K. Molecular cloning of the gyrA and gyrB genes of *Bacteroides fragilis* encoding DNA gyrase. *Antimicrob Agents Chemother* 1999;43:2423–2429.

76. Ricci V, Piddock L. Accumulation of garenoxacin by *Bacteroides fragilis* compared with that of five fluoroquinolones. *J Antimicrob Chemother* 2003;52:605–609.

77. Schapiro JM, Gupta R, Stefansson E, et al. Isolation of metronidazole-resistant *Bacteroides fragilis* carrying the nimA nitroreductase gene from a patient in Washington State. *J Clin Microbiol* 2004;42(9):4127–4129.

78. Britz ML, Wilkinson RG. Chloramphenicol acetyltransferase of *Bacteroides fragilis*. *Antimicrob Agents Chemother* 1978;14:105–111.

79. Rosenblatt JE, Gustafson DR. Evaluation of the Etest for susceptibility testing of anaerobic bacteria. *Diagn Microbiol Infect Dis* 1995;22:279–284.

80. Cormican MG, Erwin ME, Jones RN. False resistance to metronidazole by E-test among anaerobic bacteria investigations of contributing test conditions and medium quality. *Diagn Microbiol Infect Dis* 1996;24:117–119.

Chapter 5

Antimycobacterial Agents: In Vitro Susceptibility Testing and Mechanisms of Action and Resistance

Clark B. Inderlied and Edward Desmond

Worldwide, tuberculosis (TB) remains a leading cause of morbidity and mortality, with an estimated 9 million new cases of symptomatic disease leading to 2 or 3 million deaths each year. Dwarfing these numbers is the estimated 2 billion people infected by *Mycobacterium tuberculosis*, the primary causative agent of TB. However, TB is infrequent in the general population in many developed countries (<20 per 100,000), including North America. This relatively low incidence is offset by the staggering epidemics occurring in many poorer countries. For instance, in the African countries of Botswana and South Africa, the incidence of TB is approximately 500 and 1,000 per 100,000 people, respectively as reported by the World Health Organization (WHO) in 2011 (1).

Despite these figures, over the last few years, there have been several major advances in the global fight against TB. Between 1995 and 2010, 55 million TB patients have been treated in countries with directly observed therapy, short course(DOTS) programs and, of these, 46 million (84%) have been treated successfully (1) and since 2006, the numbers of new cases worldwide appears to be declining. However, at the same time, the WHO reported there was a significant increase in cases of multidrug-resistant tuberculosis (MDRTB), defined minimally as the simultaneous resistance to isoniazid (INH) and rifampin (2) (Fig. 5.1). To counter this ominous trend, the WHO recommended an expansion of the number of laboratories which perform culture and drug susceptibility testing so that there is at least one such laboratory per 5 million population (1).

As with TB control, there have been numerous other advances in our understanding of *M. tuberculosis*. Perhaps the most notable advances emanated from the complete genome sequencing of multiple serovars of *M. tuberculosis*. Genome sequencing and other molecular genetic approaches led to a rapid increase in our knowledge of the genetic basis of drug resistance in *M. tuberculosis* including both identification of the target genes and the nature of the mutations that confer resistance (3). This led to a new generation of molecular techniques for rapid, direct detection of drug-resistant tubercle bacilli in clinical samples using nucleic acid amplification techniques (4). Two such methods, the Hain line probe assay (5) and the Cepheid GeneXpert (6) were emphatically endorsed by the WHO.

The *Mycobacterium avium* complex (MAC) was once a major cause of morbidity and mortality in patients with AIDS. However, with the implementation of highly active antiretroviral therapy and effective anti-MAC prophylaxis, disseminated MAC disease in HIV-positive patients has all but disappeared. In contrast, MAC continues to be a cause of difficult to treat pulmonary disease and appears to be more prevalent (7–9). Rapidly growing mycobacteria continue to be important causes of respiratory disease and disseminated cutaneous infections, although the antimicrobial armamentarium that is available for treating these infections

Percentage of previously treated tuberculosis cases with MDR-TB*

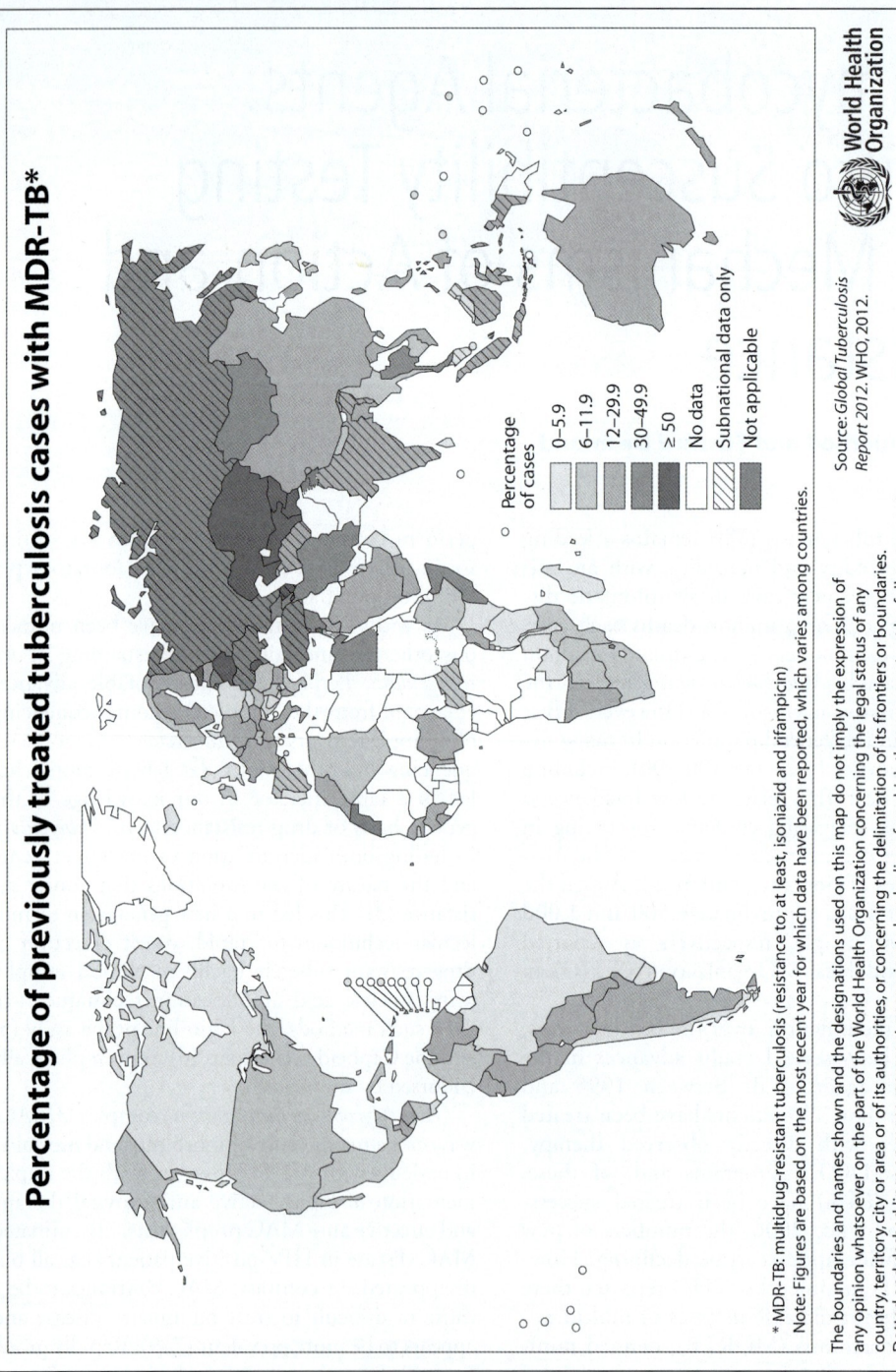

Percentage
of cases

- 0–5.9
- 6–11.9
- 12–29.9
- 30–49.9
- ≥ 50
- No data
- Subnational data only
- Not applicable

Source: Global Tuberculosis Report 2012. WHO, 2012.

World Health
Organization

* MDR-TB: multidrug-resistant tuberculosis (resistance to, at least, isoniazid and rifampicin)
Note: Figures are based on the most recent year for which data have been reported, which varies among countries.

The boundaries and names shown and the designations used on this map do not imply the expression of
any opinion whatsoever on the part of the World Health Organization concerning the legal status of any
country, territory, city or area or of its authorities, or concerning the delimitation of its frontiers or boundaries.
Dotted and dashed lines on maps represent approximate border lines for which there may not yet be full agreement.

Figure 5.1 ■ Multiple Drug Resistant Tuberculosis, minimally defined as resistance to isoniazid and rifampin, has emerged as the most difficult complicating factor in the worldwide effort to control and eventually eliminate tuberculosis. The small circles on the map indicate results for areas of the world
where the land mass is too small to be shown on a map of this scale. (From Global Tuberculosis Report 2012, WHO 2012. Reprinted with permission.)

has greatly improved (10). Phylogenetically, the rapidly growing mycobacteria are distinct and separate from the other mycobacteria. But, even within the slowly growing mycobacteria, there are considerable phylogenetic distinctions. These distinctions are reflected in the diverse relationships between mycobacterial species and a wide range in susceptibility and resistance to antimicrobial agents.

The authors of this chapter have strived to integrate conventional wisdom with new knowledge in an effort to provide reliable practical information about antimicrobial agents and mycobacteria for the use of both mycobacteriology specialists and clinicians.

IN VITRO SUSCEPTIBILITY TESTING METHODS

Mycobacterium tuberculosis Complex

M. tuberculosis is the most clinically important member of the *M. tuberculosis* complex, which includes *M. tuberculosis*, *Mycobacterium bovis*, *M. bovis* bacillus Calmette-Guérin (BCG), *Mycobacterium africanum*, *Mycobacterium microti*, and *Mycobacterium caprae* (11). The members of the complex are closely related based on DNA homology (12,13). Indeed, the degree of DNA homology indicates that the complex is more properly considered a collection of serovars or pathovars of the same species. Disease caused by *M. bovis* and *M. africanum* is clinically indistinguishable from disease caused by *M. tuberculosis*, and treatment is the same for all three "species" with the exception that *M. bovis* is inherently resistant to treatment with pyrazinamide (PZA). However, with pasteurization of milk, the isolation of *M. bovis* is uncommon and *M. africanum* is only rarely isolated from clinical specimens in the United States. *M. microti* causes a TB-like disease in voles and *M. caprae* is typically isolated from goats, but neither of these latter serovars is considered pathogenic for humans. Clearly, *M. tuberculosis* is the most common cause of both pulmonary and extrapulmonary TB in humans.

Treatment

The Centers for Disease Control and Prevention (CDC), the American Thoracic Society (ATS), and the Infectious Diseases Society of America (IDSA) in the United States now recommend the use of four drugs for the initial phase of treatment of *M. tuberculosis* pulmonary disease caused by drug-susceptible organisms that includes isoniazid, rifampin, ethambutol and PZA for two months of treatment (14). The initial phase should be followed by a "continuation phase" of 4 or 7 months of additional treatment with INH and rifampin or INH and rifapentine (15). Modifications of these regimens is dependent on a variety of factors, including HIV status, confirmation of drug susceptibility, and complicating factors such as young age, pregnancy, liver disease, and HIV infection (14). Recommendations are provided for appropriate modifications of the initial phase as well as the continuation phase of treatment, including when continuation treatment is appropriate (16).

Clearly, however, the treatment of pulmonary TB has become significantly more difficult because of the emergence of multiple drug resistance (MDR) and extensively drug resistance (XDR) as well as the large and growing numbers of TB patients coinfected with HIV.

The use of four drugs is the preferred regimen for compliant patients with a fully susceptible *M. tuberculosis* isolate. Ethambutol for adults or perhaps streptomycin for children who cannot be monitored for visual acuity should be included in the regimen until susceptibility results are known. At least two additional active agents should be added to failing treatment regimens in any patients with TB (1,17).

The early detection of drug resistance is essential for the successful management of MDRTB. In this regard, rifampin resistance is the most useful indicator of an MDR phenotype. A commercially available, highly automated real-time polymerase chain reaction (PCR) assay (Cepheid Xpert MTB/RIF) has been developed and has shown good performance in detection of rifampin resistance (18). Because the Xpert MTB/RIF assay is highly automated, it can be used in many settings, including laboratories where the level of training and expertise may not be sufficient to offer TB culture and drug susceptibility testing. This has led the WHO to strongly recommend that the "Xpert MTB/RIF be used *as the initial diagnostic test* in individuals suspected of MDRTB or HIV-associated TB" (6). Indeed, the XPERT MTB/RIF is likely to have broad application not only because of its ability to predict resistance to rifampin but also because it can simultaneously detect the presence of TB complex bacilli, including in HIV-infected patients and in children with a sensitivity that exceeds that of acid-fast microscopy for direct specimen testing (19–21). However, caution must be exercised in the interpretation of XPERT MTB/RIF results because this system also detects mutations in the *rpoB* gene that are not associated with rifampin resistance. These unassociated mutations can have a significant effect on predictive values in settings where the prevalence of rifampin resistance is not high (22).

Also, commercial PCR-based line probe assays have been developed which simultaneously detect the presence of *M. tuberculosis* complex and the presence or absence of mutations associated with first- or second-line drug resistance (23–25). These assays require greater technical expertise than the XPERT MTB/RIF assay but yield more information, including the ability to predict susceptibility or resistance to INH and some second-line drugs. For this reason, line probe assays also have been endorsed by WHO for use when drug-resistant TB is suspected, according to country-specific algorithms (5).

Real-time PCR assays such as XPERT MTB/RIF use molecular beacon probes to detect the presence or absence of wild-type nucleotide sequences as markers of rifampin susceptibility or resistance. One weakness of this approach is that not all polymorphisms within the target result in phenotypic rifampin resistance or may only cause small changes in quantitative drug susceptibility but the change may be sufficient to prevent hybridization to the reporter and the system will report such isolates as rifampin-resistant. Hain line probe assays incorporate DNA probes, which are directed against some of the most commonly occurring mutations associated with rifampin resistance. These mutant-specific probes improve the ability of the assay to specifically detect mutations associated with phenotypic resistance. However, inevitably, some mutations may be detected by probe-based systems, which are not associated with drug resistance. DNA sequencing systems, therefore, provides the most definitive detection of resistance compared with probe-based systems. Databases are already available and increasing in size, which associate particular gene sequences with drug susceptibility, resistance, and, in some cases, quantitative associations between nucleotide sequences and likely minimal inhibitory concentrations (MIC) (3).

Finally, the cost of DNA sequencing is rapidly decreasing, and applications have been developed for determining the nucleotide sequences of previously identified targets directly from clinical specimens (26–28).

Molecular versus Phenotypic Testing

Differences in genotypic (nucleotide sequence) and phenotypic (growth or inhibition of growth) test results are expected and observed. Where resources permit, it is sometimes best to use both genotypic and phenotypic testing to obtain the best prediction of drug efficacy. Among the differences that are known to result in such discrepancies are the following:

1. Not all mutations associated with drug resistance are known. For example, mutations in the *katG* gene and *inhA* promoter region account for most INH resistance, typically 80% to 90%, but not all (3,29,30).
2. Culture-based susceptibility testing will often use a class drug to predict susceptibility or resistance to several drugs within a class. For example, testing rifampin may serve to predict susceptibility to other rifamycins, and testing one fluoroquinolone drug may be used to predict susceptibility or resistance to all fluoroquinolones. However, specific mutations have been identified that genotypically distinguish rifampin-resistant versus rifabutin-susceptible isolates and ofloxacin-resistant versus moxifloxacin-susceptible isolates (31,32).
3. Mixed populations of drug-susceptible and drug-resistant bacilli may be simultaneously present as drug resistance develops. A molecular test may detect the predominant wild-type population at a point in time, whereas a growth-based test may reveal the emerging drug-resistant subpopulation of tubercle bacilli. Because resistant bacilli in a proportion of greater than 1% is associated with treatment failure, failure to detect minority populations of resistant bacilli can be considered a weakness of current molecular methods (33). However, in practical terms, given the selective presence of anti-TB drugs, the persistence of a mixed population of drug-susceptible and drug-resistant bacilli in a patient's tissue is relatively brief, and correlations between phenotypic and genotypic results are high.
4. Molecular methods may reveal nucleotide polymorphisms of unknown significance within sequences previously associated with drug resistance. Some of these polymorphisms could

lead to drug resistance even though the affected strain tests as susceptible in a growth-based test. For example, mutations in the *rpoB* gene have been described which lead to small MIC increases (34,35).

5. Finally, because susceptibility test results may not be reported for days to weeks depending on the availability of resources and location, patients with suspected MDRTB should be empirically treated with an injectable drug (e.g., amikacin or kanamycin), a fluoroquinolone, ethambutol, PZA, and perhaps a fifth drug (e.g., ethionamide, p-aminosalicylic acid [PAS], linezolid, clarithromycin, amoxicillin-clavulanate, rifabutin, or cycloserine) (36).

Despite the aforementioned limitations, there is increasing evidence that the sensitivity and specificity of molecular tests are in excess of 85% for several drugs. A compilation of sequence-based results in comparison with proportion susceptibility testing is shown in Table 5.1. For the first-line drugs, the sensitivities and specificities varied significantly depending on gene target, method, and perhaps operator.

Drug Resistance and Critical Concentrations

An in vitro susceptibility test of *M. tuberculosis* is fundamentally a test to detect drug resistance, and the most reliable in vitro susceptibility test result

Table 5.1

Detection of Drug Resistance in *Mycobacterium tuberculosis* by Molecular Methods							
Drug	**Gene Targets**	**Sequencing by ABI 3130xl**		**MTBDR*sl***		**Pyrosequencing or Sequencing by ABI 3730**	
		Sensitivity	**Specificity**	**Sensitivity**	**Specificity**	**Sensitivity**	**Specificity**
Rifampin	*rpoB*	97.1	93.6			97.1	97.9
Isoniazid	*inhA katG*	85.4	100			76.9	100
	katG and/or inhA	90.6	100				
Fluoroquinolones	*gyrA*	81.6	97.7	85.1	100	85.1	100
Kanamycin	*rrs*	57.7	99.0				
	eis	28.8	97.0	43.2	100	70.3	100
	rrs or *eis*	86.5	96.1				
Amikacin	*rrs*	90.0	98.8	84.2	100	84.2	100
Capreomycin	*rrs*	55.1	88.6	71.4	97.3		
	tlyA	10.1	98.8	71.4	97.3		
	rrs and/or *tlyA*	60.9	87.3				
Pyrazinamide	*pncA*	84.6	85.8				
Ethambutol	*embB*	78.6	93.1	56.2	100	90.7	95.8
MDR (rif + INH)	*rpoB + katG and/or inhA*	90.8	94.7				

Data are a compilation of three different studies that compared drug susceptibility testing using a growth-based method with a molecular method, using the genotype MTBDRs*l* and ABI 3730 DNA sequencing, Huang et al. (427): ABI 3130xl DNA sequencing, Campbell et al. (3); and DNA pyrosequencing (rifampin and isoniazid results only), Garcia-Sierra et al. (27). The results demonstrate that the sensitivity (ability of the test to be positive for a resistant genotype) varies significantly between genotypes, methods, and investigators. The specificity (ability of the test to be negative in the absence of the resistant genotype) of the methods is generally high. In addition, the data suggest that all mechanisms of drug resistance may not be attributable to the gene sequences targeted by these molecular tests.

that mycobacterial laboratories can report is that an isolate of *M. tuberculosis* is resistant to a drug (i.e., an isolate that tests susceptible to a drug may not be effectively treated for a variety of reasons, such as impaired drug uptake) because treatment with a drug to which *M. tuberculosis* is resistant invariably leads to therapeutic failure. Drug resistance is defined for *M. tuberculosis* in terms of the critical concentrations of drugs, and this concept is the basis for the most common *M. tuberculosis* drug susceptibility tests. David (37) showed in the early 1970s that the mutation frequencies for single-drug resistance to INH, rifampin, ethambutol, or streptomycin ranged from 1×10^{-7} to 2×10^{-10}. The clinical significance of these numbers is clear when one considers that a single caseous lesion commonly found in pulmonary TB can contain 10^8 to 10^{10} tubercle bacilli. Thus, it is apparent why treatment of TB with a single agent invariably results in relapse due to a resistant isolate. Conversely, two or more agents prevent resistance because the frequency of multiple drug resistance is the product of the single-drug frequencies of mutation, that is, 10^{-14} to 10^{-17}. If the frequency of resistant bacilli within a population is greater than 1% (usually much greater than 1%) in a previously untreated patient, this constitutes *primary resistance*. In most areas of the United States, for example, primary resistance to INH or streptomycin occurs in less than 7% of patients; however, in other areas of the world, primary resistance may occur in more than 50% of patients. If resistant bacilli are isolated from a patient in whom the initial isolates were susceptible, this constitutes *secondary resistance*; the transmission of these resistant organisms represents the most likely source of primary resistance in previously untreated patients.

The MDR phenotype develops as a result of the sequential accumulation of chromosomal mutations (38,39) and neither transposable elements nor plasmids have been associated with an MDR phenotype. In addition, the genetic basis for resistance is the same in MDR *M. tuberculosis* isolates from both HIV-positive and HIV-negative patients (38). No MDR genotypes have been described as being associated with a single genetic event or a single novel resistance determinant such as drug efflux.

Thus, the definition of critical concentrations is derived from two important observations. First, 95% or more of wild-type strains of *M. tuberculosis* are fully susceptible to first-line antimycobacterial agents, including INH, rifampin, ethambutol,

PZA, and streptomycin, where a wild type refers to a strain of *M. tuberculosis* that has never been exposed to antimycobacterial agents. Second, the percentage of a population of tubercle bacilli that would make an isolate different from wild-type strains was defined by the WHO as ranging from 1% (INH and rifampin) to 10% (ethambutol and streptomycin) based, in part, on a correlation with therapeutic efficacy. For reasons of uniformity, 1% was adopted by the CDC as the threshold for all drugs tested in the United States. The critical concentration of a drug is then defined as the concentration of drug required to prevent growth above the 1% threshold of the test population of tubercle bacilli. The critical concentration for an antituberculous agent closely approximates the MIC for wild-type *M. tuberculosis* because the convention has been to define MICs in terms of an end point of 99% inhibition of growth (Table 5.1). Finally, it is important to understand that drugs are used in combination primarily to prevent the emergence of resistance. However, there is some evidence to indicate that first-line agents may act in a synergistic manner. This synergism may reflect combined effects on tubercle bacilli but most likely also reflects the fact that different drugs may act on tubercle bacilli in different physiologic states.

Special (Local) Populations Hypothesis

In considering the susceptibility of *M. tuberculosis* to antimicrobial agents, it is important to appreciate that the organism is likely to exist in the tissue under different physiologic conditions: (a) rapidly growing cells in the aerobic and neutral-pH environment of the pulmonary cavity; (b) slowly growing cells in the oxygen-depleted and low-pH environment of the caseous lesions, where the burden of tubercle bacilli is highest; (c) cells within macrophages; and (d) dormant tubercle bacilli, which are the most intractable to treatment and the likely source of reactivation. Mitchison (40) conceptualized this phenomenon as a *special populations hypothesis*, which posits that INH, rifampin, and streptomycin are most active against the relatively rapidly dividing bacilli; rifampin is likely to also be active against bacilli that grow in spurts, and PZA is active against bacilli in the acidic milieu of caseous lesions and in acidified vacuoles of macrophages. At present, there are no agents that are known to be active against dormant bacilli. Wayne and Sramek (41) provided laboratory evidence that metronidazole (a nitro-imidazole) is active against dormant bacilli, but without therapeutic activity (42,43), but newer nitroimidazoles have promising activity (see the following texts).

Detection and Identification

The rapid and accurate detection and identification of *M. tuberculosis* not only is important for the diagnosis of disease but also for monitoring the response to therapy and for effective control of disease by public health authorities. In addition, the identification of *M. tuberculosis* is essential for accurate and reliable susceptibility testing; for example, the misidentification of *M. avium* as *M. tuberculosis* could result in a false report of MDR *M. tuberculosis* because *M. avium* is inherently resistant to INH and only variably susceptible to rifampin and ethambutol. Specimens submitted for culture include respiratory, urine, stool, sterile tissue (e.g., bone marrow), and blood samples. There are several commercial methods available for the detection of *M. tuberculosis* and other mycobacteria in clinical specimens including Septi-Chek (Becton Dickinson, Cockeysville, MD), Bactec MGIT 960 (Becton Dickinson, Sparks, MD), MB Redox (Heipha Diagnostica Biotest, Heidelberg, Germany), VersaTREK II (Trek Diagnostic Systems, Cleveland, OH), ALERT 3D (bioMerieux, Durham, NC), and Bactec 460 (Becton Dickinson, Heidelberg, Germany) (44).

The identification of several clinically significant mycobacteria can be achieved within a few hours using commercially available DNA probes (such as AccuProbe, Hologic/ Gen-Probe, Inc, San Diego, CA) that hybridize to species-specific ribosomal RNA (rRNA) sequences (45,46). AccuProbes have proven to be a reliable, fast, and cost-effective method for identifying certain specific mycobacteria isolated from clinical specimens. However, other rapid and reliable methods are available that potentially can identify a broader range of mycobacteria. These methods include transcription-mediated amplification, strand displacement amplification, 16S rDNA sequencing, multiplex PCRs, PCR restriction analysis, line probe assays high performance, liquid chromatography of mycolic acid derivatives, and matrix-assisted laser desorption/ionization time-of-flight mass spectroscopy (MALDI-TOF).

By combining a semiautomated method of detection and one of the newer methods of identification, a definitive laboratory diagnosis of mycobacterial infection should not take longer than 4 weeks. Indeed, it is not unreasonable for a clinician to expect reliable detection and (at least) presumptive identification of mycobacterial infection within 7 to 14 days. If it is not feasible to use a molecular or other rapid method for identification of mycobacteria, standard methods of identification can be improved by using a strategy that limits the number of biochemical tests (47).

SUSCEPTIBILITY TESTING

Methods and Standardization

There are four traditional methods for measuring the susceptibility of *M. tuberculosis* to the antimicrobial agents used for the treatment of TB: (a) agar proportion, (b) broth proportion, (c) absolute concentration, and (d) resistance ratio. Although there are advantages and disadvantages to each of these methods, there is some consensus that the proportion method is presently the most reliable test because the proportion procedure best controls for the inoculum size (48). Because the absolute concentration and resistance ratio methods are no longer widely used and not generally recommended, those methods are not discussed in detail.

The agar proportion method can be applied as either a direct or indirect test. In the direct test, a specimen that is smear-positive for acid-fast bacilli (AFB) is used as the source of inoculum for the susceptibility test and the specimen is inoculated directly onto the test media with and without drugs. In the indirect test, a pure culture, usually a subculture, of *M. tuberculosis* is used as the source of inoculum for the susceptibility test. On average, the results of the direct test are available 3 to 4 weeks before the results of an indirect test, using agar media.

Criteria for Performing Susceptibility Tests

The current recommendation is that all initial isolates of *M. tuberculosis* from a patient, regardless of the source of the specimen, should be tested and the results promptly reported to the health care provider and the health department/TB control (16). Beyond this, susceptibility tests should be performed on subsequent isolates if the patient's cultures fail to convert to negative within 3 months or if there is clinical evidence of a failure to respond to therapy. Other indications for susceptibility testing include the following: (a) A patient produces specimens that contain an increased number of AFB after an initial decrease; (b) a patient is suspected to have primary resistance, that is, lives in an area with a high incidence of resistant TB or was exposed to resistant TB; or (c) the isolate is from a patient with meningitis or disseminated TB (49). The susceptibility testing of initial isolates is recommended for all patients, regardless of the (local) incidence of resistance. The testing of all initial isolates provides for the continuous surveillance of drug susceptibility patterns, which is important because these patterns provide the basis for initial empiric therapy. The issue of laboratory experience in susceptibility testing is controversial. Although the original recommendation that susceptibility tests be performed only in laboratories that are capable of species identification and that perform at least 10 susceptibility tests per week (50) was reasonable several years ago, most public health and many private laboratories test primary agents because of the reliability of commercial systems and the compelling need for a rapid turnaround time. Nevertheless, a laboratory that performs susceptibility tests should be able to identify the isolate as to species as a measure of competence. However, testing should be limited to first-line drugs, but the testing of second-line drugs should be referred to a qualified reference laboratory. Indeed, it is prudent to confirm resistance to first-line drugs, especially for initial isolates, by referring the isolate to another laboratory with more experience in susceptibility testing of mycobacteria.

Choice of Antimycobacterial Agents

Primary and secondary antimycobacterial agents are listed in Table 5.2, along with important pharmacokinetic information and the average MIC for susceptible strains of *M. tuberculosis*. Although the recommendation is to test PZA as a first-line agent, PZA testing remains somewhat problematic. If PZA is not routinely tested along with first-line agents, testing must be done as soon as there is evidence for resistance to the other first-line agents. While PZA monoresistant strains of *M. tuberculosis* are uncommon, the prevalence may be increasing (51). Second-line agents are usually tested only if an isolate is resistant to the primary agents or if the patient has failed therapy with first-line agents. An isolate of *M. tuberculosis* complex may be considered resistant to primary agents if it is resistant to rifampin or to any two first-line agents (49). Three different fluoroquinolones are commonly included as second-line agents (49). However, many laboratories do not test second-line agents and appropriately refer such requests to an experienced reference laboratory.

Sources of Antimycobacterial Agents

Antimicrobial reference powders can be obtained from commercial sources or from the manufacturer. In addition, most antimicrobial reference powders are available from the United States Pharmacopeial Convention (http://www.usp.org) or in Europe from the Zentrallaboratorium Deutscher Apotheker (http://www.zentrallabor.com). Antimicrobial agents formulated for therapeutic use in humans or animals should not be used for susceptibility testing. The potency (usually micrograms per milligram of powder) and expiration date must be known for each lot of drug, and the drugs should be stored as recommended by the manufacturer or, in the absence of recommendations, at −20°C in a desiccator under vacuum. The desiccator should be brought to room temperature before opening in order to avoid condensation and inadvertent hydration of the powders, which may affect the weight and activity of the drugs. The potency of a compound should take into account purity, water content, and active fraction (e.g., free base or acid vs. salt) (49).

Stock Solutions of Antimycobacterial Agents

Stock concentrations of drugs should be prepared on the basis of the potency and purity of the drug, which may vary from lot to lot. The required weight (using a fixed volume) or volume (using a fixed weight) for preparing a stock solution can be calculated using one of the following equations:

$$\text{weight (mg)} = [\text{volume (mL)} \times \text{concentration} \\ (\mu g/mL)]/\text{potency} (\mu g/mg)$$

$$\text{volume (mL)} = [\text{weight (mg)} \times \text{potency} \\ (\mu g/mg)]/\text{concentration} (\mu g/mL)$$

Stock solutions should be prepared at a concentration of at least 1,000 μg/mL, preferably 10,000 μg/mL or 10-fold higher than the highest concentration to be tested, whichever is greater. The drug should be dissolved in water or the smallest amount of solvent necessary to produce a clear solution. The solvent and diluent should be water, dimethyl sulfoxide, or buffer. In general,

Table 5.2

Antimycobacterial Agents Commonly Tested against *Mycobacterium tuberculosis*

Generic Name	Trade or Other Names	Average MIC (µg/ml) Wild-Type (Susceptible) MTB	Serum and CSF Concentration for Selected Doses			Dosage Recommendations					Half-Life (h) Normal Adult
						Adults Dose/Interval			Children Dose/Interval		
			Dose	Peak Serum Level (µg/mL) @ Time (h) or % of Serum	Peak CSF	Oral	Parenteral	Maximum Daily Dose	Oral	Parenteral	
Primary agents											
Isoniazid (INH)[a]	Niadox, INH, Hyzyd, Niconyl	0.05–0.2	7 mg/kg PO	4.5–1[b] @ 1–2 h	100%	0.3 g q24h or 5 mg/kg or 15 mg/kg 1–3×/wk	0.3 g q24h IM	0.3 g/d or 0.9 g/dose	10–20 mg/kg/d q12–24h	10–20 mg/kg/d q12–24h IM	0.5–4[b,c]
Ethambutol (EMB)	Myambutol, Servambutol	1–5	25 mg/kg PO	2–5 @ 2–4 h	25%–50%	15 mg/kg/d[d]		15 mg/kg	15 mg/kg/d (not recommended)		3–4
Rifampin (RMP)	Rifampicin (UK), Rifadin, Rimactane	0.5	0.6 g PO 0.6 IV[e]	7 17.5	10%–20%	0.6 g/24 h	0.6 g/24 h	0.6 g	10–20 mg/kg/d q12–24h		2–5
Pyrazinamide (PZA)	Zinamide	20	0.5 g PO	9–12 @ 1–4 h	100%	15–30 mg/kg/d		3 g	30 mg/kg/d q12–24h (not approved)		10–16
Secondary agents											
Amikacin (AN)	Amikin, Biclin, Biklin, Likacin	0.25–1	0.5 g IM 7.5 mg/kg IV	38 @ 1 h	15%–24%		15 mg/kg/d q8–12h	1.5 g		15 mg/kg/d q8–12h	2–3
Streptomycin (SM)		2	1 g IM	25–50 @ 1–2 h	20%		1 IM q24h	2 g		20–40 mg/kg q24h	2–3

(Continued)

Table 5.2 (Continued)

Antimycobacterial Agents Commonly Tested against *Mycobacterium tuberculosis*

Generic Name	Trade or Other Names	Average MIC (µg/ml) Wild-Type (Susceptible) MTB	Serum and CSF Concentration for Selected Doses			Dosage Recommendations					Half-Life (h) Normal Adult
						Adults			Children		
				Peak Serum	Peak CSF	Dose/Interval		Maximum Daily Dose	Dose/Interval		
			Dose	Level (µg/mL) @ Time (h) or % of Serum		Oral	Parenteral		Oral	Parenteral	
Kanamycin (KM)[d]	Kantrex	0.5–4	7.5 mg/kg IM 7.5 mg/kg IV	22 @ 1 h	43%		15 mg/kg q8–12h	1.5 g		15 mg/kg q8–12h	2–4
Capreomycin (CM)[f]	Capastat	1–4	1 g IM	20–47 @ 1–2 h	NA		1 g IM q24h 15–20 mg/kg/d IM[g]	20 mg/kg/d		10–20 mg/kg/d IM (not approved)	4–6
Viomycin[h]	Viocin, Vinactane, Tuberactinomycin B	0.5–2	1 g IM	25–50 @ 2 h			1 g q12h twice weekly	2g			
Ciprofloxacin	Cipro, Ciflox	0.25–3	0.5 g PO 0.75 g PO 0.2 g IV	2.9 4 3.8		0.25–0.75 g q12h	0.2–0.3 g q12h				3.5
Ofloxacin	Floxin, Eoxin, Ocuflox, Tarivid	0.5–2.5	0.2 g PO 0.4 g PO 0.6 g PO	2.6 8.6 11		0.2–0.4 g q12h					5.8
Moxifloxacin	Avelox, Vigamox	0.03–0.125	400 mg PO/IV q24h	4.2–4.6	>2.1–2.3						
Rifapentine	Priftin	0.125–0.25	600 mg PO	15.05	NA	600 mg q72h					13–19

Drug	Trade names								
Rifabutin	Mycobutin, Ansamycin	0.06 g[i]	0.3 g PO	0.2–0.5		0.3 g/d	0.3 g	4–18.5 mg/kg q24h	2–5
Paraamino-salicylic acid (PAS)	PAS, Parasal, Para, Pamisyl, Pascorbic, Respias	1	4 g PO (free acid)	76–104 @ 1–2 h	10%–50%	150 mg/kg/d q6–12h	12 g	150–360 mg/kg/d q6–8h	1
Cycloserine (CS)	Oxamycin, Seromycin	5–20	0.25 g PO	10 @ 3–4 h	80%–100%	0.25–0.5 g q12h	1 g	10–20 mg/kg q12h (not approved)	3.3
Ethionamide (ETA)	Trecator-SC	0.6–2.5	1 g PO	20 @ 2–3 h	100%	0.25–0.5 g q12h	1 g	15–20 mg/kg/d q12h (not approved)	3
Linezolid[k]	Zyvox, Zyvoxam	0.5–2	600 mg/IV q12h	15–20	9%–14%	600 mg IV q12h	600 mg/IV q12h	10 mg/kg q12h	5
Amithiozone (Not available in USA)	Thiacetazone, Panthrone	1	150 mg PO	1.6–3.2 @ 4–5 h		150 mg/d			

[a]To minimize the risk of polyneuritis from isoniazid-induced pyridoxine deficiency, pyridoxine (15 to 50 mg) is often given concurrently.
[b]Should be taken with food, which decreases the rate and absorption of drug.
[c]Elimination kinetics of isoniazid depend on the "acetylator phenotype" of the patient. The half-life for "rapid acetylators" is 0.5 to 1.5 hours and for "slow acetylators," 2 to 4 hours.
[d]Amikacin is the preferred to kanamycin because serum levels are much higher, serum levels are readily available, and amikacin is more widely distributed. Both drugs can have significant adverse effects.
[e]Infused over 30 minutes.
[f]Pharmacokinetics similar to streptomycin.
[g]The dosage is 1 g IM daily for 2 to 4 months and is reduced to 1 g two to three times weekly thereafter.
[h]Capreomycin is the preferred to streptomycin. Both drugs can have significant adverse effects.
[i]Rifampin-susceptible M. tuberculosis.
[j]Rifampin-resistant M. tuberculosis.
[k]Although there is evidence that linezolid is effective in the treatment of XDR pulmonary tuberculosis, patients must be monitored closely for adverse reactions.

Adapted from Amsden GM. Tables of antimicrobial agent pharmacology. In: Mandell GL, Bennett JE, Dolin R, eds. Principles and practice of infectious diseases. Vol 1. 7th ed. Philadelphia: Churchill Livingstone Elsevier, 2010; Wallace RJ Jr, Griffith DE. Antimycobacterial agents. In: Mandell GL, Bennett JE, Dolin R, eds. Principles and practice of infectious diseases. Vol 1. 7th ed. Philadelphia: Churchill Livingstone Elsevier, 2010; Mitnick CD, McGee B, Peloquin CA. Tuberculosis pharmacotherapy: strategies to optimize patient care. Expert Opin Pharmacother 2009;10(3):381–401; http://www.medicalletter.org, The Handbook of Antimicrobial Therapy, Tuberculosis, p. 99, 2014. Please refer to the original references for additional information regarding displayed values, recommendations and footnotes. Dosage schedules may change, review the manufacturer's packages information for definitive directions and information.

it is more accurate to carefully weigh a quantity of drug that is slightly in excess of the desired amount (50 to 100 mg) and adjust the volume of the solvent to achieve the desired final concentration. If necessary, the stock solution should be sterilized by aseptic filtration through a 0.22-μm pore membrane. Some drug solutions, such as rifampin, autosterilize. The stock solutions should be dispensed into screw-capped polypropylene tubes and stored at −70°C. Thawed tubes of stock drug solution should not be refrozen. Stock solutions prepared and stored in this manner have an expiration date of 1 year (or less) from the time of preparation or a length of time that is in accordance with the manufacturer's recommendations (52). To add drug to media, a tube of the frozen stock solution is thawed and diluted with water or buffer to yield a solution of 100 to 10,000 μg/mL. The appropriate volume of diluted stock solution is added to 200 mL of sterile 7H10 medium to achieve the desired final concentration (Table 5.3).

Preparation of Media

Three solid media have been commonly used for *M. tuberculosis* susceptibility testing: Middlebrook and Cohn 7H10 and 7H11 agar supplemented with oleic acid/albumin/dextrose/catalase (OADC), and Löwenstein-Jensen egg-based medium. All of these media are usually commercially available. The Middlebrook 7H10 agar is preferable because of the simple composition and ease of preparation of this medium. Some resistant isolates of *M. tuberculosis* may grow more luxuriantly on Middlebrook 7H11 agar, but the concentrations of certain drugs must be adjusted and routine use of Middlebrook 7H11 medium is not encouraged. Egg-based media, including Löwenstein-Jensen, Wallenstein, and Ogawa media, are not recommended for susceptibility testing. However, it is important to note that this recommendation (i.e., to not use Löwenstein-Jensen) is not universally accepted and may not always be practical. Löwenstein-Jensen medium (International Union Tuberculosis Medium [IUTM] modification) with or without INH (0.2 mg/L), rifampicin (40 mg/L), dihydrostreptomycin (4 mg/L), and ethambutol (2 mg/L) incorporated into 28 mL universal containers or screw-capped tubes is recommended by the International Union Against Tuberculosis and Lung Disease for proportion testing of *M. tuberculosis* (48). Indeed, this medium may be more readily available where the incidence of TB is highest and the International Union procedures have proven to be effective in treating and controlling TB in those parts of the world.

The 7H10 agar medium is prepared according to the manufacturer's directions. The antimicrobial agents are incorporated into 200-mL aliquots of 7H10 agar held at 50°C to 56°C, following the schedule in Table 5.4. The medium is supplemented with OADC and dispensed (in 5-mL aliquots) into sterile plastic quadrant plates. One quadrant is filled with 7H10 medium without drug, which is for the growth control. The medium should be dispensed quickly, the agar allowed to solidify, and either used immediately or stored at 4°C in sealed plastic bags for not more than 28 days (52). The plates should be protected from light during storage and thoroughly equilibrated to room temperature. The agar surface must be dry before inoculation.

Disk Elution Alternative

The disk elution alternative method for preparing media for the proportion method of susceptibility testing is both convenient and practical. The disk elution method was originally developed by Wayne and Krasnow (53) and was critically evaluated in comparison with an agar dilution method (52,54). Commercially available disks (e.g., BD Diagnostic Systems, BBL Sensi-Disk Antimycobacterial, Cockeysville, MD) impregnated with standardized amounts of first-line antimycobacterial drugs are placed in separate quadrants of sterile plastic plates. The amounts of drug contained in the disks, the distribution of disks into the quadrants of the plate, and the final concentrations of drug are shown in Table 5.5. The disks are aseptically placed in the center of the quadrant and 5 mL of 7H10 agar (without drug) at about 52°C is dispensed into each quadrant. The disks should remain submerged and centered in the quadrant until the medium solidifies. The plates should be incubated overnight at room temperature to allow for complete diffusion of the drug through the medium. Plates containing antimicrobial agents should be used immediately or stored in plastic bags, in the dark, at 4°C for not more than 4 weeks. At 37°C, more than 50% of the initial concentration of INH, ethambutol, rifampin, ethionamide, and cycloserine in agar plates is lost to deterioration in 2 days (ethambutol) to 1 to 2 weeks (52); these values emphasize the need for proper storage of plates.

Table 5.3

Antimycobacterial Agents: Chemical Properties and Preparation of Stocks for Agar Proportion Method

Antimicrobial Agent	Potency[a] (μg/mg)	Solvent	Molecular Weight	Molecular Structure	Volume (mL) to Add to 200 mL 7H10 Agar[b]	Final Conc. (μg/mL)
Amikacin sulfate	Varies	SDW[c]	781.76		0.8	4
Capreomycin sulfate[d]	Varies	SDW	IA 864.9 IB 848.9 IIA 735.7 IIB 719.7		2	10
Ethambutol HCl	1,000	SDW	277.23		1, 2	5, 10
Ethionamide	1,000	DMSO[e]	166.24		1	5

(Continued)

Table 5.3 *(Continued)*

Antimycobacterial Agents: Chemical Properties and Preparation of Stocks for Agar Proportion Method

Antimicrobial Agent	Potency[a] (μg/mg)	Solvent	Molecular Weight	Molecular Structure	Volume (mL) to Add to 200 mL 7H10 Agar[b]	Final Conc. (μg/mL)
Isoniazid	1,000	SDW	127.14		0.2, 1	0.2, 1
Kanamycin sulfate	Varies	SDW	582.58		1	5
Levofloxacin	Varies	Dilute[f] base	370.38	See Ofloxacin	1	1
Moxifloxacin HCl	Varies	Dilute[f] base	437.89		0.5	0.5
Ofloxacin	1,000	Dilute[f] base	361.38		0.4	2
p-Aminosalicylic acid	1,000	SDW	153.14		0.4	2
Rifabutin	Varies	MeOH[g]	847.00	See rifampin	1	0.5

Rifampin	1,000	DMSO	822.94		0.2	1
Streptomycin sulfate	Varies	SDW	1457.41		0.4, 2	2, 10

[a]Calculate weight based on potency (μg/mg) if less than 100%. The potency of a reference standard varies with the lot number and typically varies between 85% and 98%. The actual potency is noted on the manufacturer's label.

[b]Stock solutions are prepared at 10,000 μg/mL for storage (e.g., 100 mg in 10 mL SDW). Sterilize stock solutions by filtration through 0.22 μm pore membranes, dispense into vials, and store at −70°C for up to 12 months. "Working stock solutions" are prepared at 1,000 μg/mL or as follows: isoniazid, 200 μg/mL; levofloxacin at 200 μg/mL; moxifloxacin at 200 μg/mL; and rifabutin at 100 μg/mL. The solvent for rifabutin is methanol. "Volume to Add" is the milliliter of "Working Stock Solutions" added to 200 mL of 7H10 agar to achieve the "Final Conc." Discard remainder and do not refreeze.

[c]SDW, sterile distilled water. Unless otherwise noted, the drug is freely soluble in SDW.

[d]Capreomycin sulfate is the disulfate salt of capreomycin, a polypeptide mixture produced by the growth of *Streptomyces capreolus*. Structure shows capreomycin IA where the R₁ group is a hydroxyl and the R₂ group is a β-lysyl. Capreomycin IB where the R₁ group is a hydrogen and the R₂ group is a β-lysyl. Capreomycin is greater than or equal to 90% IA and IB.

[e]DMSO, dimethylsulfoxide.

[f]Dilute base. Suspend the drug in one-half the total volume to be prepared, then, using a dropper, add 0.1M NaOH until the drug dissolves and the solution is clear or only slightly cloudy.

[g]MeOH, methanol.

Table 5.4

Concentrations of First- and Second-line Drugs Utilizing Agar and Broth Proportion Methods

	Growth Medium/Test System and Drug Concentration[a] (µg/mL)				
	Agar Proportion Method		Broth Proportion Methods[b]		
Drug	**7H10**	**7H11**	**MGIT 960**	**VersaTREK (ESP)**	**Bactec 460**
Isoniazid	0.2	0.2	0.1	0.1	0.1
Isoniazid (high)	1	1	0.4	0.4	0.4
Rifampin	1	1	1	1	2
Ethambutol	5	7.5	5	5	2.5
Ethambutol (high)	10.0	NR	NR	8	7.5
Pyrazinamide	NR	NR	100	300	100.0
Amikacin	4.0		1	NA	1
Capreomycin	10.0	10.0	2.5	NA	1.25
Ethionamide	5.0	10.0	5	NA	2.5
Kanamycin	5.0	6.0	2.5	NA	5
Levofloxacin	1.0	NR	2	NA	2
Linezolid	NR	NR	1	NA	NA
Moxifloxacin	0.5	0.5	0.25/2	NA	NA
Ofloxacin	2.0	2.0	2	NA	2
Rifabutin	0.5	0.5	0.5	NA	0.5
Streptomycin	2.0	2.0	1	NA	2
Streptomycin (high)	10.0	10.0	4	NA	6

[a]The lowest concentrations shown correspond to "critical concentrations"; high concentrations are usually tested only if an isolate is "resistant" to the critical concentration.
[b]Bactec MGIT 960 SIRE Kit (BD Diagnostic Systems, Franklin Lakes, NJ); VersaTREK Mycobacteria Detection and Susceptibility Testing (Thermo Fisher Scientific, Waltham, MA); Bactec 460TB, radiometric microbial growth detection system that is no longer manufactured (Becton Dickinson, Sparks, MD). Drug concentrations for the Bactec 460 systems are provided for historical comparison.
NR, not recommended; NA, not available.
Adapted from Woods GL, Lin SY, Desmond EP. Susceptibility test methods: mycobacteria, Nocardia, and other actinomycetes. In: *Manual of clinical microbiology.* Vol 1. 10th ed. Washington, DC: ASM Press, 2011:1215–1238; Clinical and Laboratory Standards Institute. *Susceptibility testing of mycobacteria, nocardiae, and other aerobic actinomycetes; approved standard—second edition.* CLSI document M24-A2. Wayne, PA: Clinical and Laboratory Standards Institute, 2011.

Table 5.5

Distribution of Drug-Containing Disks for Disk Elution Susceptibility Test

Plate	Quadrant	Drug	Amount (µg)/Disk	Final Concentration (µg/mL)
1	I	Control	—	—
	II	Isoniazid	1	0.2
	III	Isoniazid	5	1.0
	IV	Ethambutol	25	5.0
2	I	Control	—	—
	II	Rifampin	5	1.0
	III	Streptomycin	10	0.2
	IV	Streptomycin	50	10.0

Quality Control Strains

No strains of *M. tuberculosis* have been as rigorously standardized for controlling the quality of susceptibility tests as are available for testing rapidly growing gram-negative bacilli and gram-positive cocci. However, there are several strains of *M. tuberculosis* with different resistance phenotypes that can be used for quality control (QC) testing. At least one fully susceptible strain should be considered for QC testing (e.g., *M. tuberculosis* H37Rv [ATCC strain 27294], which is susceptible to the primary agents). The choice of a resistant strain is more problematic. Many of the resistant strains of *M. tuberculosis* that are available from ATCC have very high levels of resistance, which is not particularly useful when confirming the ability of a method to distinguish resistant from susceptible. A strain with a stable low-level resistance phenotype to a single drug is preferred for QC strain (e.g., ATCC BAA-812). The BAA-812 strain has a stable mutation in the *inhA* promoter and consistently yields an MIC for INH between 0.2 and 0.8 μg/mL. Multiple resistant isolates (i.e., MDR *M. tuberculosis*) should *not* be used because of the risk of laboratory-acquired infection. The QC strains are grown in liquid medium, diluted to a standard turbidity, dispensed into 1-mL aliquots, and frozen at −70°C. Once each week, or whenever a new lot of medium is prepared, one or more aliquots of the control strains should be thawed and two dilutions prepared according to the standard dilution protocol. One dilution should yield 200 to 300 colonies and the other dilution should yield 20 to 30 colonies on the control plates. In this manner, both the quality of the medium and the dilution technique are tested.

Media Components

Guthertz et al. (55) examined the effects of different lots of Middlebrook 7H10 agar, OADC, and 0.5% glycerol on standard susceptibility test results using a modified proportion method. Three assays were used to measure the comparative quality of the components: (a) a comparative resistance assay to monitor drug stability in solution and in agar, (b) a disk potency assay to monitor the potency of disks impregnated with antimycobacterial agents, and (c) a standard concentration assay to monitor changes in antibiograms caused by changes in the test medium. Rejection criteria included both changes in the size of colonies and changes in the number of colonies; a 20% change in either colony size or number was considered significant. The test strains included *M. tuberculosis* H37Rv (ATCC strain 27294) and several strains of *M. tuberculosis*, *M. avium*, and other slowly growing mycobacteria. By this method, the authors concluded that 30% of lots of OADC and 15% of lots of Middlebrook 7H10 agar were unacceptable, leading to interpretations of both false susceptibility and false resistance. The primary reasons for rejection were reduced colony size and drug binding. This study emphasizes the importance of recording the lot numbers of all components and testing new lots of medium components, especially OADC and 7H10 powder, with standard strains of *M. tuberculosis* and other slowly growing mycobacteria, to ensure the reliability of results from batch to batch. A convenient protocol for monitoring OADC was described by Butler et al. (56). They established a correlation between the ability of OADC to support the growth of *Bacillus subtilis* (measured as a change in optical density over 24 hours) in a heart infusion broth supplemented with a test lot of OADC and the ability of OADC to support mycobacterial growth. Acceptable lots of OADC support the growth of *B. subtilis* (biomass turbidity increase of 0.2 OD_{650} in 24 hours) and good growth of mycobacteria, whereas failure to support growth of *B. subtilis* correlates with poor growth of mycobacteria.

Sterility Tests

A representative sample (10%) of each lot of plates (agar dilution or disk elution) should be incubated for 48 hours at 35°C and checked for sterility.

Agar Proportion Method: Direct Test

The principle of the "direct test" is to inoculate drug-containing media directly with a smear-positive, processed (digested, decontaminated, and concentrated) specimen. The advantages of the direct test are decreased time to reporting of susceptibility test results, a potentially more accurate measure of the percentage of resistant tuberculous bacilli in the specimen, and decreased cost. The direct test should be performed only with specimens that are smear-positive for AFB and only using the agar proportion method or a commercial method that has been specifically approved for use as a direct test. The inoculum should be carefully controlled because overinoculation may lead to false resistance and underinoculation may lead to false susceptibility. The direct method may be most appropriate when there is a high prevalence of drug resistance with a patient population, but logically, this would require that second-line drugs be tested as soon as possible or feasible (49).

An agar proportion direct method includes the following steps:

1. Digest, decontaminate, and concentrate the specimen, as appropriate, according to an accepted procedure.
2. Prepare, stain, and examine a smear using either a fluorochrome or carbol-fuchsin method. Record the number of bacilli in each of 20 fields and calculate the average number per field. Because the test is based on measuring a reduction in colony-forming units (CFU), count any clump as a single organism; however, it is important to emphasize that the suspension should be completely homogenized. Dilute the specimen in water (e.g., 0.5 mL of specimen in 4.5 mL of water) based on the stain, using the dilution scheme shown in Table 5.6 as a guide. Choose two concentrations so there is a 100-fold difference between the concentrations of the two inocula.
3. Use a sterile safety pipette to inoculate 0.1 mL of each dilution onto each quadrant of duplicate plates and use separate sets of plates for each dilution of the inoculum. Let the plates stand for 1 hour to absorb the inoculum. If the patient has received anti-TB medications, include an undiluted inoculum regardless of the smear results because AFB observed in the smears of specimens from treated patients may be nonviable.
4. Place the plates into CO_2-permeable polyethylene bags (6 × 8 inches) with the medium on the bottom, that is, do not invert the plates. Heat-seal the bags and incubate the plates at 35°C to 37°C in 5% to 10% CO_2.
5. Read the plates weekly for 3 weeks; however, do not report a result as "susceptible" before 3 weeks. Colonies of "resistant" isolates often develop more slowly than the colonies of susceptible isolates. If growth is not apparent, examine each quadrant with a dissecting microscope (30× to 60× magnification) for the presence of slowly growing microcolonies; however, take care not to overinterpret the results because the deterioration of drugs may lead to the appearance of microcolonies. Grade the results, at both dilutions, according to the following criteria: (a) confluent (too numerous to count), record 3+ or 4+; (b) in the range of 100 to 200 colonies, record 2+; (c) in the range of 50 to 100 colonies, record 1+; (d) less than 50 colonies, record the actual number (note the presence of microcolonies). The control plate, at one dilution or the other, should contain 50 to 100 colonies, and the percentage of resistant colonies is based on this number. If the control plate contains insufficient growth or confluent growth, the test must be repeated unless the isolate is fully susceptible to all drugs tested. The susceptibility test should be terminated at 3 weeks because even susceptible isolates may eventually grow in the presence of bacteriostatic drugs.
6. Retain the control plate (quadrant) as an additional source of the isolate because this plate was directly inoculated with the specimen.

Mycobacteria Growth Indicator Tube

Beginning in 1993, drug susceptibility testing in liquid medium became the standard of practice (57). Because some patients with drug-resistant TB, particularly those with AIDS, were dying before results of solid medium proportion testing became available, an emphasis was placed on the relatively rapid testing methods, including Bactec 12B medium, TREK Diagnostics ESP medium, and others. Bactec 12B medium permitted rapid and accurate drug susceptibility testing of *M. tuberculosis* complex, but it had several drawbacks including use of radioactive carbon-14 and the requirement to use needles for inoculation, growth detection, and removal of samples for acid-fast smear or other purposes.

Table 5.6

Dilution of Sputum Concentrate for Inoculation of Susceptibility Test Medium-Direct Proportion Method

Dilution	Fluorochrome Stain[a]
Undiluted	<25[b]
Undiluted, 1:10	25–50
Undiluted, 1:100	50–250
1:100, 1:1,000	>250

[a]Number of fluorochrome-positive bacilli observed at 200 to 400× microscopic field.
[b]Increase inoculum to 0.2 mL if less than five bacilli per 200 to 400× microscopic field.
Adapted from Clinical Laboratory Standards Institute (CLSI), 2011, Susceptibility Testing of Mycobacteria, Nocardiae, and Other Aerobic Actinomycetes; Approved Standard-Second Edition. M24-A2, Wayne, PA.

For these reasons, Becton Dickinson discontinued the production of Bactec 12B medium and now produces a nonradioactive broth culture system, the Mycobacteria Growth Indicator Tube (MGIT), along with reader/incubator instruments with a capacity for 960 or 320 tubes (cultures). At the bottom of each MGIT broth tube is silicon rubber impregnated with ruthenium pentahydrate, which serves as a fluorescence quenching–based oxygen sensor. When oxygen is depleted due to growth of mycobacteria, this is detected as fluorescence by the automated 960 reader. Fluorescence is measured every 60 minutes by the 960 TB instrument and expressed as fluorescence units unique to this instrument. When primary, pure culture of *M. tuberculosis* bacilli consumes a sufficient amount of oxygen to generate a defined threshold of fluorescence, the culture is reported as "positive" by the 960 TB instrument. The positive threshold for the 960 TB instrument is equivalent to 10^5 or 10^6 CFU/mL of medium.

In 2002, the 960 TB system was approved by the U.S. Food and Drug Administration (FDA) for susceptibility testing of *M. tuberculosis* complex against the primary drugs: INH, rifampin, ethambutol, streptomycin, and PZA (58). The concentrations of primary drugs were chosen to give results equivalent to previous reference methods, and the 960 TB test performance characteristics were found to be accurate and reproducible (59–61). However, a recent meta-analysis and review of the 960 TB system by Horne et al. (62) found that ethambutol testing may not be equivalent to other methods. In this study, the sensitivity for detecting ethambutol resistance was only moderate, and the investigators suggested that a review and possible revision of the ethambutol test concentration in MGIT 960 TB test may be warranted. This suggestion is supported by data from a review of proficiency testing results, which showed that when isolates were expected to be resistant to ethambutol, based on previous tests, the MGIT 960 TB test reported the isolates as resistant only 79% of the time, a performance markedly poorer than that seen with other drugs (63).

For the MGIT 960 TB test, lyophilized drug preparations are provided, which are reconstituted with water to prepare stock solutions for streptomycin, INH, rifampin, ethambutol (SIRE), and PZA drugs. Although streptomycin is provided in the MGIT SIRE kit, the Clinical and Laboratory Standards Institute (CLSI) M24A2 standard recommends making streptomycin a second-line drug to be tested only on request. MGIT drug susceptibility testing kits from Becton Dickinson include a growth supplement, which is composed of OADC (oleic acid/bovine albumin/dextrose/catalase) in the case of SIRE kits, and OADC supplemented with polyoxyethylene stearate (POES) in the case of PZA test kits. The supplements should not be interchanged between SIRE and PZA test kits.

The source of inocula can be either a pure culture of fresh growth on solid medium or a positive MGIT 960 vial containing actively growing bacilli. Separate protocols are provided for inocula from MGIT broth and solid medium. Careful adherence to the manufacturer's protocol in preparation of inocula is essential. From MGIT 960 broth, if testing is performed at 1 or 2 days following detection of growth by the 960 instrument, the broth may be mixed and used directly as inoculum for MGIT 960 drug susceptibility testing. However, if testing is delayed 3 to 5 days from the time of initial growth detection, it is likely the concentration of TB bacilli will be too high and the culture must be diluted 1:5 before being used as an inoculum. From solid medium, a suspension is made from fresh growth not more than 14 days after the first appearance of colonies on the medium. The suspension is adjusted to a turbidity equivalent to a McFarland 0.5 standard and then diluted 1:5 using 7H9 broth or MGIT 960 medium.

When primary MGIT broths inoculated with patient specimens are detected by the MGIT 960 instrument as positive, laboratory protocols may vary in terms of the amount of growth removed for acid-fast microscopy, verification of growth purity, and identification (e.g., Gen-Probe AccuProbe, San Diego, CA). Thus, the amount of growth remaining for drug susceptibility testing can vary. For this reason, a proposal was made to use the turbidity-based inoculum technique as described for solid media, with liquid media as well as with solid media (64).

Control vials are inoculated with a 1:100 dilution (for SIRE drugs) or 1:10 dilution (for PZA) of the inoculum in sterile saline. Control and drug-containing test vials are then registered into the reader/incubator system in sets. The growth in each MGIT tube is then monitored by the instrument by periodic measurements of fluorescence. When the control vial fluorescence reaches a level of 400 growth units (GU) within 4 to 13 days, the MGIT system flags the completion of a drug test and interprets the susceptibility or resistance to each drug using a threshold of greater than

100 GU for resistance or less than or equal to 100 GU in the drug-containing tubes to indicate susceptibility.

When growth is detected in a drug-containing MGIT tube, it is important to confirm that it is *M. tuberculosis* complex and not a non-TB *Mycobacterium* or other contaminant. Visual inspection of the tube should show clumps settled at the bottom of the tube (Fig. 5.2). Acid-fast microscopy should generally show AFB cording or in tight clumps. When visual or acid-fast observations are not what is expected, a subculture or "purity plate" can be inoculated to confirm whether a contaminant is present. If a culture contains nonmycobacterial contaminants or is suspected to contain non-TB mycobacteria, it may be possible to prepare a pure inoculum of *M. tuberculosis* complex from the purity plate.

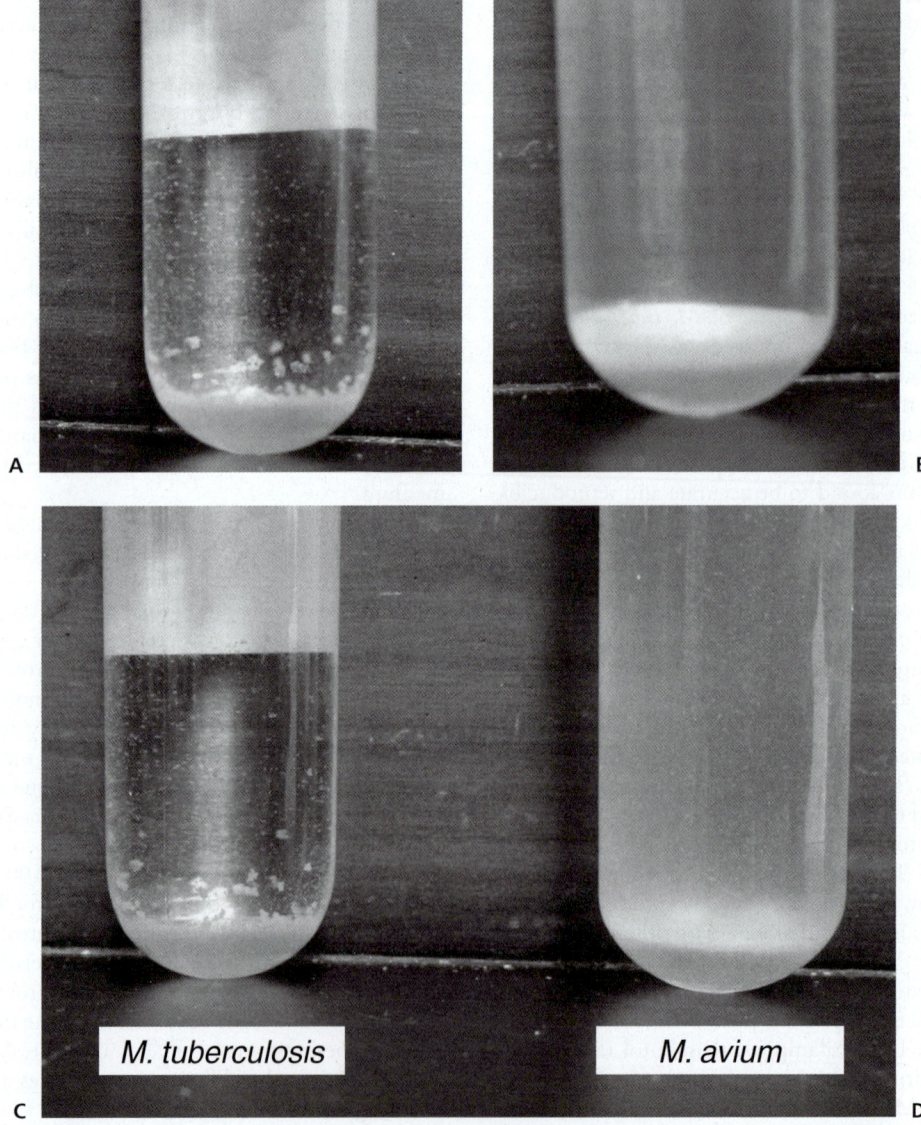

Figure 5.2 ■ Growth in MGIT 960 medium comparing *M. tuberculosis* with *M. avium* before **(A,B)** and after **(C,D)** slight swirling. *M. tuberculosis* **(A, C)**. *M. avium* **(B, D)**. (Photographs courtesy of Jane Wenger, California Department of Public Health.) (See Color Plate in the front of the book.)

Each laboratory must develop a protocol for how and when to confirm unusual or unexpected drug susceptibility testing results. For example, resistance to rifampin in an isolate which is INH susceptible or monoresistance to ethambutol or PZA may be questionable and indicate the need for retesting, preferably by a different method. Alternative methods could include testing in agar medium by the proportion method or molecular methods such as DNA sequencing or use of DNA probes to detect common resistance-conferring mutations. If an alternative method is not available, repeat testing by the same method may sometimes be expected to determine whether an error has been made. Although confirmatory testing is underway, the health care provider caring for the patient should be made aware of preliminary results and the timing of expected confirmatory testing.

Protocols have been developed for testing TB complex isolates for susceptibility to second-line drugs as well (64–66). These and other studies were considered in the preparation of a consensus document by the WHO, which makes recommendations for test concentrations for first- and second-line drugs in various media including Middlebrook agars, Löwenstein-Jensen medium, and MGIT (67). For MGIT, critical test concentrations (μg/mL) recommended are 1.0 for amikacin, 2.5 for capreomycin, 2.0 for levofloxacin, 0.25 for moxifloxacin, 5.0 for ethionamide, and 1.0 for linezolid. Testing levofloxacin or moxifloxacin is recommended in order to encourage the use of these fluoroquinolones, which are more active than ofloxacin against *M. tuberculosis*. Testing of moxifloxacin at the WHO-recommended concentration of 0.25 μg/mL has been shown to correlate with the presence of mutations in the quinolone resistance-determining region (QRDR) of the *gyrA* gene and to predict resistance to ofloxacin (32). However, moxifloxacin may retain clinical activity despite the presence of some mutations associated with MICs less than 2 μg/mL. Clinical evidence for use of moxifloxacin for treatment of cases in which the isolate is resistant at a concentration of 0.25 μg/mL but susceptible at 2 μg/mL is slight (68), but treatment using high-dosage moxifloxacin may be considered for the most difficult to treat cases.

PZA testing is a particular challenge by culture-based methods (69,70). PZA is active in acidic environments, so its activity is evaluated in an acidified version of MGIT broth at a pH at or near 6 where growth of *M. tuberculosis* is suboptimal. Precise adherence to inoculum protocol is critical for PZA since the inoculum can influence pH of the medium. Piersimoni et al. (71) have recommended a reduced inoculum volume of 0.25 mL rather than 0.5 mL and presented data indicating that a reduced inoculum leads to more accurate results (71). Another factor is the age of the culture because PZA has been shown to be more active against older cultures than it is in inhibiting log phase cultures (70). A further confounding factor may be inhibition of some strains by the POES incorporated into the MGIT test system (72). These variables render culture-based testing of PZA in MGIT or other media less reliable than the testing of INH or rifampin. A test of susceptibility to nicotinamide at a neutral pH has been proposed as an alternative, but sequencing of the *pncA* gene is more promising because of quick and reliable results (69,72). Assay for pyrazinamidase activity has also been shown to predict PZA resistance with a sensitivity of approximately 89% and a specificity of 97% or greater (73,74).

Other Culture-Based Commercially Available Systems for Drug Susceptibility Testing of *M. tuberculosis* in Liquid Medium

ESP/VersaTREK

The VersaTREK system, formerly known as ESP, is available for testing susceptibility of isolates of *M. tuberculosis* complex for susceptibility to INH, rifampin, ethambutol, streptomycin, and PZA. It gives results similar to MGIT 960 (75–77). The VersaTREK system is an automated broth culture system with detection of growth by means of detecting changes in gas pressure in the head space over the culture broth. The PZA concentration (300 μg/mL) is higher than that used in MGIT, and in the study by Espasa et al. (77), VersaTREK gave slightly fewer resistant results than MGIT.

Sensititre MYCOTB Minimal Inhibitory Concentration Panel

This system is also manufactured by TREK Diagnostics. It tests susceptibility of *M. tuberculosis* complex isolates using a 96-well microtiter plate format to three first-line (INH, rifampin, ethambutol) and nine second-line (amikacin, cycloserine, ethionamide, kanamycin, moxifloxacin, ofloxacin, PAS, rifabutin, and streptomycin) drugs. This selection of drugs offers the advantage that two drugs are tested in the fluoroquinolone class, two aminoglycosides, and two rifamycin drugs. It is therefore not necessary to rely on a "class drug" to predict susceptibility or resistance to another drug in the same class. This has several possible advantages. For example, moxifloxacin may retain activity in spite of the presence of a *gyrA* mutation which causes resistance to ofloxacin, amikacin may still have activity and be useful in the treatment of infections by strains which are resistant to kanamycin due to G-10A mutations in the *eis* promoter region (78), and rifabutin may be active against some strains of *M. tuberculosis* which have *rpoB* mutations which make them resistant to rifampin.

There is controversy regarding the reporting of MIC results for susceptibility testing of *M. tuberculosis* complex. Some clinicians may be unprepared to interpret MIC results and apply them to decision making regarding design of treatment regimens for TB. There is a danger that clinicians may be unaware of the significance of intracellular infections by TB bacilli or of the presence of special populations of TB bacilli in walled-off lesions and in varying metabolic states. Comparisons of MIC values with serum or tissue achievable levels, as is done for many types of extracellular infections, may be poorly predictive for treatment of TB (79). On the other hand, MIC values may assist a well-informed clinician in making decisions about whether to use rifabutin versus rifampin in some patients whose TB bacilli have an *rpoB* mutation or whether to use moxifloxacin, perhaps at a higher dose, in the presence of some *gyrA* gene mutations.

Two studies evaluating the Sensititre system have recently been published, which were supported by the manufacturer (80,81). These studies compared Sensititre results with those obtained using the agar proportion method. When Sensititre drug concentrations which match closely the drug concentrations in agar are chosen for interpretation, high levels of correlation are seen with the agar proportion method, ranging from 94% to 100% for different drugs. More studies are needed to establish the accuracy, reproducibility, and utility of this method. Reading of end points is performed using a mirror or video camera linked to a computer screen.

Microscopic Observation Drug Susceptibility Method

Hardy Diagnostics manufactures a microscopic observation drug susceptibility (MODS) test kit, which uses a 24-well plate with Middlebrook 7H9 broth and OADC supplement. Detection of *M. tuberculosis* complex is performed starting with decontaminated, concentrated sputum sediments. To make the broth medium more selective for *M. tuberculosis* complex, a selective "NAPTA" (nalidixic acid, azlocillin, polymyxin B, trimethoprim, amphotericin B) antibiotic solution is mixed with the specimens at the time of inoculation. Drug-free wells serve as growth controls, and specimens are also inoculated into wells containing final concentrations of 0.4 µg/mL INH and 1 µg/mL rifampin. The culture plates are sealed with a "safety lid" and incubated at 37°C. A CO_2 atmosphere is not required.

As indicated by the name of this procedure, growth is detected by microscopic observation using an inverted microscope. Growth of *M. tuberculosis* is observed as cords after approximately 5 to 10 days incubation. *Mycobacterium chelonae* may also exhibit cording in broth growth but will typically grow in less than 5 days.

MODS can also be performed using reagents, drugs, media, and supplies from various sources in order to reduce cost. MODS requires substantially less time (5 to 10 days) than culture in solid medium followed by drug susceptibility testing in solid medium, which often requires approximately 2 months to complete. MODS, therefore, permits much earlier changes in patient therapy when drug resistance is detected (82–84). Detailed assistance with the protocol may be obtained online at http://www.jove.com/video/845/the-mods-method-for-diagnosis-tuberculosis-multidrug-resistant.

A recent study has tentatively established test concentrations for second-line drugs in the MODS assay (85). The drugs included capreomycin, ciprofloxacin, cycloserine, ethambutol, ethionamide, kanamycin, PAS, and streptomycin. Further testing is required before the test concentrations proposed by this study can be confirmed.

Colorimetric Redox Indicator Methods

Colorimetric redox (reduction/oxidation) methods have been developed to assist the detection of *M. tuberculosis* growth in drug susceptibility testing, allow resistance to be reported earlier, and standardize reporting. Redox indicators have been proposed for use in low-resource countries, where more expensive systems such as MGIT may not be considered affordable. Broth or agar media are used, with standardized inoculum and drug concentrations (86,87), and a redox indicator such as alamar blue, MTT [3(4,5-dimethylthiazole-2-yl)-2,5-diphenyltetrazolium-bromide], or resazurin. Commonly, a microtiter plate broth culture format is used, with drug-free control wells and drug-containing wells. After incubation for a few days, the redox indicator is added, and growth is detected as a color change. The additional step of adding the redox indicator and the potential biohazard involved with opening a culture following incubation may make these methods less attractive for laboratories which can afford MGIT or other system which permits detection of growth in a sealed tube or plate. However, the fact that media and reagents are nonproprietary may lead to lower prices for redox methods. Martin et al. (86) evaluated a microtiter plate assay with resazurin indicator for detection of extensively drug-resistant TB in a multicenter study. Critical concentrations were 0.5 μg/mL for rifampin, 0.25 μg/mL for INH, 2 μg/mL for ofloxacin, and 2.5 μg/mL for kanamycin and capreomycin. Overall accuracy figures for the five drugs, compared with the Löwenstein Jensen proportion method, were 98.4%, 96.6%, 96.7%, 98.3%, and 90%, respectively.

NONTUBERCULOUS MYCOBACTERIA

The nontuberculous mycobacteria have been divided historically into two groups: (a) slowly growing mycobacteria with generation times of approximately 24 hours and that take more than 7 days to form visible colonies on solid media and (b) rapidly growing mycobacteria (RGM) with generation times less than 24 hours and that form visible colonies in 7 days or less. However, these historical distinctions are not absolute. Slowly growing mycobacteria can fluctuate in growth rate from a latent nonreplicating state to a comparatively fast rate of replication in patients with active disease. Even RGM may take much longer than 7 days for growth to be detected during primary isolation (the definition of rapidly growing refers more specifically to the growth on solid medium inoculated from a dilute suspension from a primary culture). Nevertheless, the terms *rapidly* and *slowly growing mycobacteria* continue to be used and continue to have relevance to the diagnosis and treatment of mycobacterial infections. Indeed, taxonomic studies based on sequence analysis (e.g., 16S rRNA, *hsp*65, *rpoB*, and *sod* genes) have validated the phenotypic classification of slowly and rapidly growing mycobacteria (11).

Based on molecular taxonomic methods, there are more than 120 species of nontuberculous mycobacteria, but the majority (90%) of infections in humans are caused by two species of slowly growing mycobacteria (MAC and *Mycobacterium kansasii*) and three species of RGM (*Mycobacterium fortuitum*, *M. chelonae*, and *Mycobacterium abscessus*) (8,88,89). The two slowly growing mycobacteria are important causes of pulmonary disease; MAC is the predominant cause. The RGM species are important causes of skin and soft tissue, pulmonary, and nosocomial infections, especially following catheter insertions, augmentation mammaplasty, and cardiac bypass surgery (90). Disseminated MAC disease was an important coinfection in HIV-infected patients prior to the advent of effective antiretroviral therapy. Disseminated disease caused by RGM is rare and is usually associated with immunodeficiency, including that associated with corticosteroid therapy, but not HIV infection (91).

The ATS in conjunction with the IDSA established diagnostic criteria for nontuberculous mycobacterial lung disease: (a) chest radiograph or high-resolution computed tomography scan, (b) three or more sputa positive for acid-fast bacteria, and (c) exclusion of TB or other disorders. However, even these criteria are most applicable to disease caused by MAC, *M. kansasii*, and *M. abscessus* and application of the criteria to other nontuberculous mycobacteria may not be appropriate (10).

There are a variety of antimicrobial agents recommended for the treatment of infections caused by nontuberculous mycobacteria (Table 5.7) (88,89,92). However, the activity of these antimicrobial agents varies considerably from species to species, which reflects differences in inherent and acquired resistance. The different mechanisms of resistance include (a) lack of cell wall penetration; (b) biotransformation by ribosylation, acetylation, nitrosation, and hydrolysis; (c) induction of inactivating enzymes; (d) presence of efflux pumps; and (e) mutation of the gene that encodes the structural or enzymatic target. Therefore, drug susceptibility testing is often an important component of a successful treatment strategy. The mechanisms of resistance to antimicrobial agents in nontuberculous mycobacteria are both the same and different compared with the *M. tuberculosis* complex. Most

Table 5.7

Antimycobacterial Agents and Antibiogram Data for Various Nontuberculous Mycobacterial Diseases

	Isoniazid	Rifampin[a]	Ethambutol	Pyrazinamide	Azithromycin[b]	Clarithromycin[b]	Amikacin[c]	Streptomycin	Imipenem	Cefoxitin	Clofazimine	Cycloserine	Rifabutin	Ciprofloxacin[d]	Moxifloxacin[d]	Levofloxacin or ofloxacin	Trimeth/Sulfa	Doxycycline	Minocycline	Linezolid	Tigecycline	Typical Regimen[e]
M. abscessus cutaneous					20%	20%				70%				+								CLM only for 6 mo, but inducible *erm* may be present.
M. abscessus pulmonary or disseminated					20%	20%	+		~50%	70%				+	~15%	<5%				50%	+	AMK + IMP or CFX + CLM for 4–6 mo, but inducible *erm* may be present.
M. bovis[f]	+	+	+																			Use *M. tuberculosis* doses, 9–12 mo.
BCG[f]	+	+	+																			INH only or INH + RIF + EMB for 3 or 6 mo.
M. avium complex immunocompromised			+		+	+	+															Prophylaxis (AZM or CLM), treatment (CLM + EMB ± RBT), post Tx suppression (CLM or AZM + EMB).
M. avium complex immunocompetent			+		+	+	+	+														AZM or CLM + EMB + RIF; AZM or CLM + EMB ± SM or AMK.
M. celatum					+	+							+	+	+							CLM + EMB + CIP ± RBT.
M. chelonae					+	+			+	+					+	+				+	+	CLM only or add AMK or CFX or add Mox or Lev.

Species	Regimen / Comments
M. fortuitum	AMK + CFX + probenecid then T/S or Dox for 6–12 mo. Inducible *erm* may mitigate use of macrolides. Min or Dox or Cip for nail salon infections.
M. haemophilum	CLM + RBT or CLM + CIP + RBT. No standard regimen identified.
M. genavense	CLM + EMB + RBT.
M. gordonae	RIF + EMB + Kan or CIP. No standard regimen identified.
M. kansasii	INH + RIF + EMB.
M. marinum	CLM or MIN or Dox or T/S or RIF + EMB.
M. scrofulaceum	CLM + CLF ± EMB or INH or RIF or SM + CS.
M. simiae	Treat like MAC. No standard regimen identified.
M. ulcerans	RIF + AMK or EMB + T/S or RIF + SM. Surgery usually needed.
M. xenopi	CLM + RIF or RBT + EMB ± SM or INH + RIF + EMB. No standard regimen identified.
M. leprae	RIF + dapsone or RIF + OFX + MIN. USA and WHO doses differ.

[a] Rifampin is likely to be active against the *Mycobacterium* spp as indicated, especially if not previously treated with a rifamycin.

[b] Clarithromycin or azithromycin are likely to be active, if not previously treated with a macrolide, but macrolides should not be used as monotherapy.

[c] Amikacin, in general, is the most active aminoglycoside against nontuberculous mycobacteria, but activity is quite variable between species.

[d] Moxifloxacin is more active than ciprofloxacin against nontuberculous mycobacteria, but clinical efficacy has not been firmly established.

[e] Typical regimens may or may not be endorsed by a professional organization as noted.

[f] *M. bovis* and BCG are members of the *M. tuberculosis* complex.

Data taken or adapted from http://www.sanfordguide.com, The Sanford Guide Web Edition, Anti-infective Drugs, Antimycobacterial; Wallace RJ Jr, Griffith DE. Antimycobacterial agents. In: Mandell GL, Bennett JE, Dolin R, eds. *Principles and practice of infectious diseases*. Vol 1. 7th ed. Philadelphia: Churchill Livingstone Elsevier, 2010:533–548; Brown-Elliott BA, Nash KA, Wallace RJ Jr. Antimicrobial susceptibility testing, drug resistance mechanisms, and therapy of infections with nontuberculous mycobacteria. *Clin Microbiol Rev* 2012;25(3):545–582.

Table 5.8

Antimicrobial Agent Resistance: Nontuberculous Mycobacteria

Agent	Cell Wall/ Penetration	Biotransformation	Induction	Efflux Pump Gene	Target/Gene
Amikacin Tobramycin Tigecycline		Nucleotidyltransferases Phosphotransferases Acetyltransferases		*tetV* *tap* P55	16S RNA *rrs*
Clarithromycin/ macrolides/ketolides	+		*erm(38)* *erm(39)* *erm(40)* *erm(41)*		*rrl* 23S rRNA
Imipenem Meropenem	+				
Penicillins	+		β-lactamase (*blaS*, *blaE*)	*lfrA*	
Cefoxitin	+				
Ciprofloxacin Moxifloxacin	+	Acetylation Nitrosation		*lfraA* *efpA* *pstB*	Gyrase A or B subunit *gyrA* *gyrB*
Linezolid					23S rRNA
Doxycycline/ tetracyclines				*tetV* *tap* P55	
Rifampin/rifamycins	+	ADP ribosyltransferase		*efpA*	*rpoB*
Ethambutol	+				*embA* *embB* *embR*

Adapted from van Ingen J, Boeree MJ, van Soolingen D, et al. Resistance mechanisms and drug susceptibility testing of nontuberculous mycobacteria. *Drug Resist Updat* 2012;15(3):149–161.

of these mechanisms of resistance are discussed in greater detail elsewhere in this chapter, but a summary of the mechanisms of resistance that are specific to nontuberculous mycobacteria are shown in Table 5.8. The role of the mycobacterial cell wall and the presence of porins, efflux pumps, and cell wall maintenance mechanisms appear to be important sources of "inherent" antimicrobial resistance among the nontuberculous mycobacteria, perhaps to a greater extent than in the *M. tuberculosis* complex (93).

The newer macrolides (clarithromycin, azithromycin, roxithromycin) and perhaps the ketolides are important drugs for the treatment of many nontuberculous mycobacterial infections, for example, *M. chelonae* and *M. abscessus* and perhaps 80% of *M. fortuitum* (89). However, the apparent susceptibility of the RGM to macrolides may be misleading as several harbor an inducible *erm* gene (e.g., *erm* [39]), that can confer a high-level clarithromycin resistance (94,95). In addition, most isolates of *M. chelonae* have clarithromycin MICs of 0.25 µg/mL or less, but resistance develops quickly with monotherapy (96); in these cases, resistance is conferred by mutation in the 23S rRNA gene (97).

RAPIDLY GROWING MYCOBACTERIA SUSCEPTIBILITY TESTING

It is important to quickly distinguish the RGM from other mycobacteria because all first- and most second-line antituberculous drugs are ineffective against the RGM (88,89,92), which may not always be appreciated by the clinician with limited experience in treating these infections. As previously noted, a more difficult consideration is assessing the clinical significance of RGM isolated from clinical specimens. The nontuberculous mycobacteria that commonly cause most clinical disease are *M. abscessus*, *M. fortuitum* group, *M. kansasii*, *M. chelonae*, *Mycobacterium haemophilum*, *Mycobacterium ulcerans*, *Mycobacterium terrae* complex, and *Mycobacterium marinum* (8–10,98). The following species are rarely a cause of clinical disease: *Mycobacterium gordonae*, *Mycobacterium mucogenicum*, *Mycobacterium botniense*, *Mycobacterium cookie*, *Mycobacterium chlorophenolicum*, *Mycobacterium frederiksbergense*, *Mycobacterium hodleri*, and *Mycobacterium murale* (98).

In order to optimize the susceptibility testing and facilitate interpretation of the RGM susceptibility results, the CLSI recommends (99) that isolates be identified to at least differentiate the *M. fortuitum* group from the *M. abscessus-chelonae* group. Preferably, identification should be to the species level. Several methods have been described

for measuring the in vitro susceptibility of RGM, including (a) agar dilution, (b) agar disk elution, (c) Etest, (d) disk diffusion, and (e) broth microdilution (98,99). However, the standard recommended by the CLSI is a broth microdilution assay using cation-supplemented Mueller-Hinton broth (CSMHB) plus 5% OADC supplement as the preferred medium (98,99) and only this method is discussed further. Dry, microdilution plates are commercially available, on a research use only basis, for testing rapidly growing and slowly growing nontuberculous mycobacteria, that is, RAPMYCO and SLOMYCO, TREK Diagnostic Systems (Fig. 5.3).

Antimicrobial Agents

Antimicrobial standard reference powders can be obtained commercially from the manufacturer, from United States Pharmacopeia or the Zentrallaboratorium Deutscher Apotheke. Drug stock solutions, based on the potency of the drug, should be prepared as specified by the CLSI procedure (99) or as specified by the manufacturer.

Plate Code:	SLOMYCO								
	1	2	3	4	5	6	7	8	9
A	CLA 0.06	CLA 0.12	CLA 0.25	CLA 0.5	CLA 1	CLA 2	CLA 4	CLA 8	CIP 16
B	CLA 16	CLA 32	CLA 64	MXF 8	RIF 8	SXT 8/152	AMI 64	LZD 64	CIP 8
C	RFB 8	EMB 16	INH 8	MXF 4	RIF 4	SXT 4/76	AMI 32	LZD 32	CIP 4
D	RFB 4	EMB 8	INH 4	MXF 2	RIF 2	SXT 2/38	AMI 16	LZD 16	CIP 2
E	RFB 2	EMB 4	INH 2	MXF 1	RIF 1	SXT 1/19	AMI 8	LZD 8	CIP 1
F	RFB	EMB	INH 1	MXF 0.5	RIF 0.5	SXT	AMI	LZD	CIP

Drug	Code	Dilution Range
Amikacin	AMI	1-64
Ciprofloxacin	CIP	0.12-16
Clarithromycin	CLA	0.06-64
Doxycycline	DOX	0.12-16
Ethambutol	EMB	0.5-16
Ethionamide	ETH	0.3-20
Isoniazid	INH	0.25-8
Linezolid	LZD	1-64
Moxifloxacin	MXF	0.12-8
Rifabutin	RFB	0.25-8
Rifampin	RIF	0.12-8
Streptomycin	STR	0.5-64
Trimethoprim/ Sulfamethoxazole	SXT	0.12/2.3 8-8/152

Figure 5.3 ■ Sensititre SLOMYCO plate. Microtiter plate format designed to be used with CSMHB with 5% OADC for susceptibility testing of slowly growing nontuberculous mycobacteria against 13 drugs that may be used in treating infections caused by nontuberculous mycobacteria. Note that drug susceptibility testing is not recommended for many nontuberculous mycobacteria because of a lack of correlation with clinical efficacy, poor test performance by any test method, and limited experience treating certain types of infections. Designated as for research use only in the United States. Other plate conformations are available for *M. tuberculosis* (MYCOTB) and rapidly growing mycobacteria (RAPMYCO) from TREK Diagnostic Systems. (Adapted from TREK Diagnostic Systems. Sensititre custom plate format. http://www.trekds.com/products/sensititre/files/SLOMYCO.pdf. Accessed October 2012.)

The agents that should be tested are shown in Table 5.9. Clarithromycin is considered a class representative for newer macrolides (e.g., azithromycin and roxithromycin). Test both ciprofloxacin and moxifloxacin because the spectrums of activity are not identical. Testing of carbapenems can be problematic and should be performed to experienced laboratory, but even then the results are often difficult to reproduce. Imipenem, meropenem, and ertapenem should be tested separately; imipenem is the most active carbapenem against RGM.

The drug-containing 96-well plates can be prepared fresh for each susceptibility assay or batch prepared ahead of time and stored until needed. Two approaches are recommended for the batch production and storage of drug-containing plates.

1. Drug dilution series can be prepared in broth and 0.1-mL aliquots added to the wells of a 96-well microplate; the plates should then be sealed in plastic bags and stored at −70°C for up to 6 months. The plates should not be stored in a frost-free freezer (such freezers have

Table 5.9

Susceptibility Testing of Rapidly Growing Mycobacteria: Recommended Test Ranges, Interpretive Criteria, and Suggested Quality Control Reference Ranges

Antimicrobial Agent	Recommended Test Ranges (µg/mL)	MIC (µg/mL) Breakpoints			Reference Range End Points (µg/mL) for Quality Control Strains	
		Susceptible	Intermediate	Resistant	*M. peregrinum* ATCC 700686	*S. aureus* ATCC 29213
Amikacin[a]	8–128	≤16	32	≥64	≤1–4	1–4
Cefoxitin	8–256	≤16	32–4	≥128	16–32	1–4
Ciprofloxacin[b]	0.5–8	≤1	2	≥4	≤0.125–0.5	0.125–0.5
Clarithromycin[c]	1–16	≤2	4	≥8	≤0.06–0.5	0.125–0.5
Doxycycline[d]	0.5–32	≤1	2–8	≥16	0.125–0.5	0.125–0.5
Imipenem[e]	2–32	≤4	8	≥16	2–16	—
Linezolid	4–64	≤8	16	≥32	≤2–4	1–4
Meropenem	2–64	≤4	8–16	≥32	2–16	0.03–0.12
Moxifloxacin	0.5–8	≤1	2	≥4	≤0.06–0.25	4–16
Tobramycin[f]	2–32	≤4	8	≥16	2–8	0.125–1
Trimethoprim/ sulfamethoxazole[g]	1/19–8/152	≤2/38	—	≥4/76	≤0.25/4.8–2/38	≤0.5/9.5

Breakpoint interpretations taken from Table 7 of CLSI document M24-A2, Vol 35, No. 5. Footnotes are similar but not identical in all instances. See the CLSI document for additional information and MIC ranges for alternate quality control strains (i.e., *P. aeruginosa* ATCC 27853 and *E. faecalis* ATCC 29212). Recommended test ranges are one dilution lower and one dilution higher than breakpoints in order to better define the observed MIC and monitor for drift in MICs upon retesting.
[a] Amikacin is active against only ~80% of *M. chelonae* and ~70% of *M. abscessus* isolates and MICs 64 µg/mL or more against *M. abscessus* are very uncommon and should be reported with appropriate caution and be confirmed by repeat testing and referral to an experienced reference lab.
[b] Ciprofloxacin is considered a class drug for methoxyfluoroquinolones, but ciprofloxacin and levofloxacin are less active than newer methoxyfluoroquinolones such as moxifloxacin against susceptible strains of mycobacteria.
[c] Clarithromycin is the class drug for azithromycin and roxithromycin. Pulmonary infections caused by rapidly growing mycobacteria should not be treated with clarithromycin alone. Macrolide resistance among nonpigmented rapidly growing mycobacteria may be inducible and in vitro susceptibility tests should be held for 14 days to ensure detection of such resistance.
[d] Minocycline can be substituted for doxycycline.
[e] Breakpoints are tentative and testing should be performed at an experienced reference laboratory. Imipenem results are NOT predictive of results for meropenem and ertapenem. Imipenem is the most active carbapenem against rapidly growing mycobacteria.
[f] Tobramycin is the aminoglycoside of choice for *M. chelonae* only and should not be used to treat *M. abscessus* or *M. fortuitum* group. In vitro testing should be referred to an experienced reference laboratory.
[g] Trailing is common and growth inhibition has been defined as an 80% reduction in growth compared with the no-drug control.

defrost cycles), and thawed plates should not be refrozen.

2. Drug dilution series can be prepared in sterile distilled water (or other suitable diluent—should not significantly affect the constituents of the broth medium when reconstituted), aliquoted, and the material lyophilized in situ. With this approach, the amount a drug added per well should give the required concentration in a final volume of 0.1 mL.

The commercially available RAPMYCO, dry, extended shelf life microtiter plates include the following drugs: amikacin, amoxicillin/clavulanic acid, cefepime, cefoxitin, ceftriaxone, ciprofloxacin, clarithromycin, doxycycline, imipenem, linezolid, minocycline, moxifloxacin, tigecycline, tobramycin, and trimethoprim-sulfamethoxazole.

The CLSI guidelines are based on the use of flat-bottomed 96-well microplates, which allows the quantitation of microcolonies or bacterial clumps in wells with low-level growth. This ability may aid in determining the end point for some antimicrobial agents. Alternatively, "U"- or "V"-bottomed plates can be used. The benefit of these styles of plate is that all the sedimented bacteria collect in a small area, which helps distinguish wells with low-level growth from wells with no growth. The disadvantage of "U"- or "V"-bottomed wells is that quantitation of microcolonies or bacterial clumps is not feasible.

Inoculation

Susceptibility tests should be performed only on pure cultures. The organisms can be stored on Löwenstein-Jensen slants before testing and then subcultured to a nonselective medium such as trypticase soy or blood agar plates and incubated in air for 2 to 4 days at 30°C to 35°C to obtain discrete colonies. A sterile swab should be used to transfer a sweep of organisms to tubes containing 4.5 mL of sterile water to give a turbidity equivalent to a McFarland no. 0.5 standard. To aid the dispersion of bacteria clumps, 3-mm glass beads (7 to 10 should be sufficient) should be added to the tube and the suspensions vortexed aggressively for 15 to 20 seconds. Any remaining large bacterial clumps should be allowed to settle. RGM that are adjusted to a McFarland no. 0.5 standard contain 1×10^7 to 2×10^8 CFU/mL (100).

The final inoculum preparation depends on the nature of the drug-containing plates. (a) If plates containing lyophilized agents are used, then the bacterial suspension described· earlier must be diluted 200-fold to give a final density of approximately 5×10^5 CFU/mL, for example, 50 μL of suspension (turbidity equivalent to a McFarland no. 0.5 standard) mixed with 10 mL of CAMHB broth for RGM or 10 mL CAMHB plus 5% OADC for slowly growing nontuberculous mycobacteria. Aliquots of 0.1 mL per well (approximately 5×10^4 CFU) are then dispensed into each well of the assay plates. (b) If the plates contain drugs already reconstituted in growth medium (0.1 mL per well), the inoculum should be diluted to a density of approximately 5×10^5 CFU/mL. Aliquots of 0.1 mL per well (approximately 5×10^4 CFU) are then dispensed into the assay plate. Appropriate adjustments should be made if multipronged inoculators are used to deliver an inoculum of 0.01 mL per well. The plates are sealed in plastic bags or placed in another sealed storage container and incubated at a temperature appropriate for the test microorganism. Inoculate a nutrient agar plate to check for purity of the inoculum.

Reading of Results

The plates should be examined after 3 days (72 hours) and then daily up to day 5 (120 hours). Usually, the MICs can be read at day 3 with most *M. fortuitum* group isolates. In contrast, some strains of *M. chelonae* may require an incubation time of 4 days (96 hours). Minimally, the no-drug controls should be visibly turbid with clumps of bacteria at the bottom of the wells. The most reliable results are likely to be obtained with the shortest incubation period that gives acceptable growth in control wells. This is especially important for drugs that are unstable in broth media, for example, imipenem. It is advisable to repeat the testing of isolates that have MIC interpreted as being indicative of resistance, either in-house or sent out to a reference laboratory. Testing carbapenems, tetracyclines, and tigecycline may be problematic because of drug instability. Isolates that test susceptible to clarithromycin should be incubated for a total of 14 days to assure detection of inducible macrolide resistance (94,95).

The MIC is the lowest concentration of antimicrobial agent that completely inhibits the growth of the organism as detected by the unaided eye. End points are easy to read for most drugs; however, a faint haze of growth is common with sulfonamides. Consequently, the sulfamethoxazole MIC is usually determined from the well showing approximately 80% inhibition of growth compared to the no-drug control well.

Quality Control

QC procedures should reflect regulatory requirements and acceptable standards of practice. Well-characterized reference strains should be used for QC, for example, *Mycobacterium peregrinum* ATCC 700686, *Staphylococcus aureus* ATCC 29213, *Pseudomonas aeruginosa* ATCC 27853, and *Enterococcus faecalis* ATCC 29212. The importance of inoculum preparation cannot be overemphasized because overinoculation may result in false resistance and underinoculation in false susceptibility. QC strains should be set up at least weekly for laboratories that perform more than one test per week. In laboratories performing fewer tests, the QC strain should be always included. With stored drug-containing microplates, each batch should be validated with the QC strain and tested for sterility before use.

As with all clinical tests, reliability and reproducibility are critical. Thus, laboratory personnel who score susceptibility assays should be monitored by comparing end points with that determined by an experienced reader. All personnel should agree ±1 dilution with the experienced reader.

MYCOBACTERIUM AVIUM COMPLEX

The MAC is traditionally defined as a serologic complex divided into 30 or more serovars (101) based on the composition of the cell surface oligosaccharide linked to a peptidoglycolipid core that is produced by all members of the complex (102). In the postgenomic era, the taxonomy and clinical significance of MAC is more complex but better understood. It is now clear that the MAC includes both strictly environmental mycobacteria and host-associated pathogenic mycobacteria with specific genetic distinctions. In taxonomic terms, *M. avium* and *Mycobacterium intracellulare* are distinct species and the MAC consists of a single species, *M. avium*, with multiple subspecies, notable *M. avium* subsp *avium*, *M. avium* subsp *paratuberculosis*, and *M. avium* subsp *silvaticum* (103,104). *M. avium* subsp. *avium* is a cause of avian TB, cervical lymphadenitis in children (scrofula), chronic pulmonary disease in cystic fibrosis patients and elderly women, and the cause of disseminated disease in AIDS patients with

extremely depleted T cells (105,106). *M. avium* subsp *paratuberculosis* is an important animal pathogen and the cause of Johne's disease in ruminants and *M. avium* subsp *silvaticum* cause disease in wood pigeons. *M. intracellulare* causes pulmonary disease in immunocompetent humans and has been isolated from animals and from the environment. Drug susceptibility testing has focused on *M. avium* subsp *avium* and to a much lesser degree on *M. intracellulare*.

Mycobacterium avium Complex Resistance

MAC isolates are predictably resistant to INH and only variably susceptible to rifampin and ethambutol, and the susceptibility patterns are considerably more variable than those of *M. tuberculosis* (107,108), emphasizing the potential importance of susceptibility testing. The inherent antimicrobial resistance is most likely due to the impermeability of the MAC cell wall and membrane (109), and in vitro cell-free studies confirmed that drug targets (e.g., ribosomes, ribosomal subunits, and RNA polymerase) in MAC cells bind the drugs and the corresponding target functions are inhibited. MAC isolates, like most mycobacteria, produce low levels of β-lactamase (110), but there is no evidence that MAC isolates actively degrade or inactivate β-lactams or possess inactivating enzymes for other antimicrobials. Most MAC isolates have plasmids of varying size and, while plasmids have been associated with antimicrobial resistance in some MAC isolates, specific resistance transfer factors have not been identified (111,112).

Colony Variants

Susceptibility testing of the MAC is complicated by the observation that MAC isolates display two colony variants on agar-based media (113). One colony variant is flat, spreading, and translucent in appearance, while the second colony variant is raised, condensed, and opaque (Fig. 5.4). The translucent variant is more resistant to antimicrobial agents (113) and is more virulent in animal models of infection (114). Stormer and Falkinham (115) showed that nonpigmented variants of *M. avium*, isolated from both the environment and patients with disseminated *M. avium* disease, are significantly more resistant to a variety of antimicrobial agents than are pigmented segregants of the same strains. Because

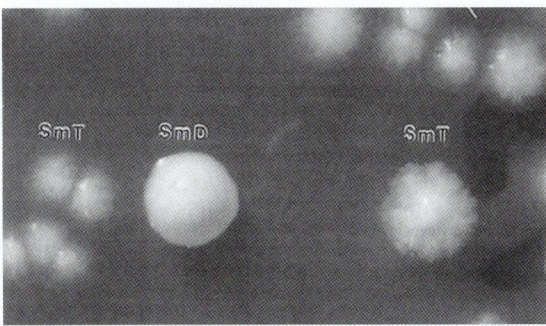

Figure 5.4 ■ **Smooth-domed (*SmD*) and smooth-transparent (*SmT*) colony variants of *M. avium*.** (From Inderlied C, Nash KA. Microbiology and in vitro susceptibility testing. In: Benson C, Korvick J, eds. *Mycobacterium avium complex infection: progress in research and treatment.* New York: Marcel Dekker, 1995:109–140.)

the pigmented and more susceptible variants appear more quickly and are more prominent on culture plates, nonpigmented variants could be overlooked in the selection of *M. avium* colonies for susceptibility testing.

When to Test

In most situations, it is unnecessary to perform in vitro susceptibility tests on initial MAC isolates. However, establishing baseline MIC values may assist in interpreting susceptibility test results weeks or months after the start of therapy. Testing is appropriate for patients on prior macrolide therapy or patients who develop bacteremia while on macrolide prophylaxis for MAC. Also, susceptibility testing may be useful if a patient relapses or if the infection is intractable and the clinical situation desperate. Testing for macrolide resistance may help in deciding whether to add drugs to a treatment regimen. However, it is not clear whether the macrolide should be withdrawn in the face of resistance. Little is known about the effects of multiple drug regimens on such resistant strains, and the chance of polyclonal MAC infections leads to the possibility of mixed susceptible and resistant strains (3). Susceptibility testing should be repeated 3 months after the start of treatment for disseminated disease or after 6 months for patients with pulmonary disease (116).

Antimicrobial Agents

While MAC infections are usually treated with a combination of antimicrobial agents, in vitro susceptibility testing is often restricted to clarithromycin

and perhaps moxifloxacin and linezolid. There is animal (117,118) and limited human data (119) on the use of mefloquine to treat MAC infections in humans (120), but no clinical trials have been performed to validate in vitro susceptibility testing methods or interpretive criteria for these agents. CLSI recommends that *M. avium* isolates be tested if isolated from patients previously treated with a macrolide; if isolated from blood during prophylaxis; from patients with culture-positive relapse; and clinically significant isolates at baseline or to hold such isolates for future testing.

Methods

MAC is most commonly tested using a broth microdilution method and Mueller-Hinton broth supplemented with cations and 5% OADC and adjusted to pH 7.3 or 7.4 as recommended by the CLSI (99). The 2011 CLSI document also recommends use of Bactec 12B medium and the Bactec 460 instrument, but the Bactec 12B medium is no longer available (98). Clarithromycin is the only drug that should be routinely tested. MAC also has been tested using SLOMYCO Sensititre Panels and JustOne Strips (TREK Diagnostic Systems, Cleveland, OH), but these latter methods are designated as "for research use only" and neither method has been evaluated in multisite studies (Fig. 5.3) (121). The SLOMYCO microtiter plates are designed to test a variety of slowly growing mycobacteria and includes several drugs, including clarithromycin (0.06 to 64 μg/mL). As the name implies, the JustOne Strips only test clarithromycin (0.12 to 128 μg/mL).

Inoculum

Collect colonies (especially transparent colony variants, if present) from the surface of a Middlebrook 7H11 plate and suspend in 5 mL of sterile deionized water to match a McFarland no. 0.5 turbidity standard. Transfer 25 μL of the suspension to 5 mL of Middlebrook 7H9 broth with casein or Mueller-Hinton broth with 5% OADC to yield ~5 × 10^5 CFU/mL in each well of a microtiter plate.

Broth Microdilution Method

Microtiter trays should be inoculated (100 μL/well) within 30 minutes of preparing the inoculum. The trays are sealed with adhesive and incubated at 35°C in ambient air. The plates are first read at 7 days but read with interpretation only when there is sufficient growth in the growth control well. If necessary, the plates are incubated for an additional 7 days. The MIC is defined as the lowest concentration of drug necessary to inhibit visible growth. Interpretive criteria for clarithromycin are shown in Table 5.10 along with tentative interpretive criteria for moxifloxacin and linezolid.

Quality Control

M. avium (ATCC 700898) is clarithromycin-susceptible and recommended for QC. QC strains should be stored at −70°C or for 3 months at −20°C or at ambient temperature for 30 days and subcultured each week or at the time of testing. *M. avium* ATCC 700898 can be used for quality control and should yield a clarithromycin MIC of 1 to 4 μg/mL; *M. avium* ATCC 8-700897 is clarithromycin-resistant.

MYCOBACTERIUM KANSASII

M. kansasii is closely related to *Mycobacterium gastri*; however, the isolation of the former is nearly always clinically significant, while isolation of the latter is rarely of clinical importance (103). In general, the incidence of *M. kansasii* disease is low and usually responds well to therapy (122,123). *M. kansasii* isolates from patients who have not been previously treated with rifampin are likely to be susceptible to rifampin at 1 μg/mL (124), and infections have been successfully treated with a combination of rifampin, INH, and a third agent (e.g., ethambutol) (125,126). Rifabutin should be substituted for rifampin in HIV-infected patients treated with a protease inhibitor (127). Clarithromycin can be used in place of INH. *M. kansasii* isolates can be tested using the proportion method or a broth microdilution method, but the latter is recommended by the CLSI. Initial drug testing should be limited to rifampin and clarithromycin, since treatment failure is mostly associated with rifampin resistance and most *M. kansasii* isolates will test resistant to INH at 0.2 μg/mL and many test resistant to 1.0 μg/mL (116). INH MICs for *M. kansasii* are 0.5 to 5 μg/mL, which makes testing somewhat problematic but helps explain the good efficacy of treatment regimen that include INH. Treatment failure is associated with rifampin and/or clarithromycin resistance; thus, testing of initial isolates is recommended. Alternative drugs are listed in Table 5.11.

Table 5.10

Mycobacterium avium Complex Susceptibility Testing and Interpretive Criteria

Antimicrobial Agent	MIC Test Range[a] μg/mL	Susceptible μg/mL	Intermediate μg/mL	Resistant μg/mL	Quality Control[b] μg/mL
Clarithromycin[c]	1–64	≤8	16	≥32	0.5–2
Moxifloxacin[d]	0.5–8	≤1	2	≥4	
Linezolid[d]	4–64	≤8	16	≥32	

[a]Broth microdilution using cation-supplemented Mueller-Hinton broth (pH 7.3 or 7.4). Macrolides and azalides are more active at pH 7.3 or 7.4, but MAC grows more poorly at this pH range; carefully check no drug and quality control results.
[b]Expected MIC ranges for *M. avium* (ATCC 700898).
[c]Clarithromycin is the class drug for expanded spectrum macrolides and azalides such as azithromycin and roxithromycin. Although an "intermediate" result may indicate the emergence of resistance in an *M. avium* complex isolate, it remains unclear if the macrolide should be withdrawn from the treatment regimen because the infecting population may remain heterogeneous.
[d]Proposed interpretive criteria but not yet verified.
Adapted from Clinical Laboratory Standards Institute (CLSI), 2011, Susceptibility Testing of Mycobacteria, Nocardiae, and Other Aerobic Actinomycetes; Approved Standard-Second Edition. M24-A2, Wayne, PA.

Table 5.11

Antimicrobial Agents for Potential Testing against *Mycobacterium kansasii* and *Mycobacterium marinum*

Antimicrobial Agent	Resistant[a] at (µg/mL)		Quality Control[b] (µg/mL)	
	M. kansasii	*M. marinum*	*M. peregrinum* ATCC 700686	*E. faecalis* ATCC 29212
Amikacin	>32	>32	≤1–4	64–256
Ciprofloxacin	>2	>2		0.25–2
Clarithromycin[c]	>16	>16	≤0.06–0.5	—
Doxycycline/minocycline		>4	0.12–0.5	2–8/1–4
Ethambutol	>4	>4		—
Isoniazid	Note[d]			—
Linezolid	>16		1–8	1–4
Moxifloxacin	>2	>2	0.06–0.25	0.06–0.5
Rifabutin	>2	>2		—
Rifampin	>1	>1		0.5–4
Streptomycin	Note[d]			—
Trimethoprim/sulfamethoxazole	>2/38	>2/38	≤0.25/4.8–2/38	≤0.5/9.5

[a]Suggested resistant breakpoints for *M. kansasii* and *M. marinum*. Routine susceptibility testing of *M. marinum* is usually unnecessary and not advised.
[b]Expected results for *M. peregrinum* using the broth microdilution method for RGM. *Enterococcus faecalis* can be used to quality control drug solutions using the CLSI method for aerobic rapidly growing bacteria. *M. kansasii* ARCC 12478 and *M. marinum* ATCC 927 may be used to quality control rifampin with expected MICs of 1 µg/mL or less and 0.25 to 4 µg/mL or less, respectively.
[c]Clarithromycin is the class drug for extended spectrum macrolides and azalides such as azithromycin and roxithromycin.
[d]Isoniazid and streptomycin have proven efficacy in treating *M. kansasii* infections, but breakpoints (susceptible or resistant) have not been established for RGM. The alternative short-course or intermittent regime is clarithromycin, rifampin, and ethambutol.
Adapted from Clinical Laboratory Standards Institute (CLSI), 2011, Susceptibility Testing of Mycobacteria, Nocardiae, and Other Aerobic Actinomycetes; Approved Standard-Second Edition. M24-A2, Wayne, PA.

MYCOBACTERIUM XENOPI

Pulmonary infections caused by *Mycobacterium xenopi* have been described, and the disease occurs more frequently in immunocompromised patients (103,123). Extrapulmonary infections are rare. Pseudo-outbreaks of *M. xenopi* infections have been reported and the significance of the isolation of this species, especially from a nonsterile body site, should be carefully examined (128,129) because *M. xenopi* can be mistakenly identified as *M. avium* if only biochemical tests are used for identification. In vitro susceptibility test results appear to be important in the management of this disease (130); however, the correlation between in vitro susceptibility test results and therapeutic response has been reported to be inconsistent (124). Some indicate that *M. xenopi* is susceptible to INH, rifampin, streptomycin, and cycloserine, while others dispute these results (131). A treatment regimen of clarithromycin, rifampin, and ethambutol is recommended by the ATS/IDSA

(10). The CLSI recommends that in vitro susceptibility test of *M. xenopi* follow the guidelines for *M. kansasii* (see earlier discussion) (99), although *M. xenopi* is reported to not grow well in CSMHB with OADC. *M. xenopi* also is considered a thermophile and grows better at 42°C to 45°C.

MYCOBACTERIUM SZULGAI

Mycobacterium szulgai is a scotochromogen at 37°C and a photochromogen at 25°C and was first reported to cause pulmonary disease in the early 1970s. Along with the other uncommon species of slowly growing, nontuberculous mycobacteria, *M. szulgai* appears to cause disease primarily in persons with a history of chronic lung disease (99,123). *M. szulgai* is not considered an environmental *Mycobacterium* and isolation from clinical specimen is probably always significant (99). These infections are reported to respond to INH, rifampin, and ethambutol (131); Woods and Washington (124) characterized *M. szulgai* as only slightly more resistant than *M. tuberculosis* to anti-TB agents, and they suggested that streptomycin, capreomycin, and viomycin are potential alternatives to the three previously mentioned first-line agents.

MYCOBACTERIUM MALMOENSE

Mycobacterium malmoense is a nonpigmented environmental *Mycobacterium* that is closely related to *Mycobacterium shimoidei*, but in clinical laboratories, it may be more important to distinguish *M. malmoense* from *M. gastri* and *M. terrae* because of the difference in clinical significance (103). *M. malmoense* has been reported as a frequent cause of pulmonary infection mostly in elderly patients with underlying lung disease, including TB and malignancy, but disseminated disease was reported in an HIV-infected patient (123,132). *M. malmoense* is second to *M. avium* as the most common cause of cervical lymph node infections in children (10). Although *M. malmoense* is reported to be variably susceptible to antimycobacterial agents, it is generally considered to be more susceptible than *M. avium*. Although there are some recommendations for treatment (133) and there are conflicting reports regarding the susceptibility of *M. malmoense* to INH (134) and rifampin (131), Hoffner et al. (135) showed that combinations of ethambutol with aminoglycosides, quinolones, or rifamycins were synergistic against *M. malmoense*. This observation is in agreement with reports on the clinical effectiveness of ethambutol, rifampin, and INH in combination in the treatment of pulmonary disease (136). Banks and Jenkins (133) showed that, although *M. malmoense* was resistant to rifampin and ethambutol, all strains were susceptible to the combination of these drugs at the lowest concentration.

MYCOBACTERIUM SIMIAE

Mycobacterium simiae is an environmental mycobacterium and an uncommon cause of disease. It is regarded as highly resistant to antimycobacterial agents, perhaps with the exception of ethionamide and cycloserine (124); however, there are exceedingly few cases of disease caused by *M. simiae* on which to base any firm conclusions about susceptibility to antimycobacterial agents. In an animal test system, clarithromycin in combination with ethambutol and perhaps a quinolone such as ofloxacin was potentially effective (137). As with *M. szulgai*, disease in humans appears to occur mostly

in persons with a history of chronic lung disease, and persons with pulmonary lesions are probably predisposed to colonization with potentially pathogenic environmental mycobacteria (103).

MYCOBACTERIUM MARINUM

This photochromogen is a cause of skin, joint, and deeper infections, primarily of the hand or limbs; infection is usually associated with exposure to water (138,139). The optimum growth temperature for *M. marinum* is 30°C to 35 °C. The successful management of *M. marinum* infections requires rapid diagnosis and the avoidance of steroid treatments (138,139). *M. marinum* is largely considered predictably susceptible to rifampin, rifabutin, and ethambutol, although most infections spontaneously resolve or respond to localized treatment without chemotherapy. Disseminated cutaneous infections respond to rifampin and ethambutol; alternative agents are tetracycline, doxycycline, minocycline, trimethoprim-sulfamethoxazole, ciprofloxacin, and clarithromycin (140,141). *M. marinum* is resistant to INH and PZA. Routine susceptibility testing using methods and interpretive criteria described for *M. tuberculosis* is inappropriate, and the methods and interpretive criteria for testing RGM are more likely to provide clinically useful results. Drug susceptibility testing should be restricted to treatment failures.

MYCOBACTERIUM ULCERANS

Detection of *M. ulcerans* by culture is difficult and may take several weeks at 25°C to 33°C. Chemotherapy plays a role secondary to surgical treatment of indolent, necrotic skin lesions that extend into the derma in infections caused by *M. ulcerans* (124). However, rifampin may be useful prior to ulceration. Clarithromycin plus rifampin can be a useful adjunct to excision (142) to prevent relapse or other complications (10). In vitro susceptibility testing is inappropriate, but it appears that rifampin resistance is likely to develop with monotherapy (143).

MYCOBACTERIUM HAEMOPHILUM

M. haemophilum is a slowly growing, nonpigmented mycobacterium that requires hemin or ferric ammonium citrate for growth, optimally at 28°C to 30°C. Early reports on the in vitro susceptibility of *M. haemophilum* were inconsistent, and the role of chemotherapy in the treatment of *M. haemophilum* infections was unclear. Woods and Washington (124) concluded that this species is resistant to INH, streptomycin, and ethambutol but susceptible to rifampin and/or PAS. *M. haemophilum* emerged as an important cause of disseminated skin infections in immunocompromised patients, including renal transplant, lymphoma, and AIDS patients (144). The organism also causes disease in immunocompetent hosts, where it causes mild, self-limited, skin infections (145). Correlations have been established between susceptibility test results and clinical efficacy, although virtually all treatment regimens examined included combinations of agents (146). Wild-type isolates of *M. haemophilum* appear to be susceptible to amikacin, quinolones, rifamycins, clarithromycin, and azithromycin and resistant to PZA and ethambutol and are likely to be resistant to INH and streptomycin (144,146). Surgical excision is usually sufficient for immunocompetent patients (10).

MYCOBACTERIUM GORDONAE

M. gordonae is commonly found in the environment and is readily isolated from water supplies and ice machines. Wayne and Sramek (103) pointed out that, because *M. gordonae* is so common (30% of nearly 20,000 nontuberculous mycobacteria studied) and disease is rare and cases of *M. gordonae* infection with clear and compelling clinical correlations are difficult, if not impossible, to find, the pathogenic potential of this species must be extremely low, even in patients with AIDS (147). Nevertheless, it is not uncommon for clinical mycobacteriology laboratories to receive requests for susceptibility testing of *M. gordonae* isolates. In response to such requests, one could pose the questions offered by Wayne and Sramek (103): (a) Is the isolate truly *M. gordonae*? (b) Is there convincing evidence that the isolate is playing a role in the disease? In the vast majority of cases, susceptibility testing is inappropriate and may only further mislead the clinician as to the true cause of the disease. The rare occurrence of true *M. gordonae* infection in patients with AIDS makes this decision more difficult. *Mycobacterium interjectum* emerged as a potential pathogen and it has been confused with both *M. gordonae* and *Mycobacterium scrofulaceum* (148,149). Drug susceptibility testing is not recommended. The ATS/IDSA suggest that ethambutol, rifabutin, clarithromycin, linezolid, and fluoroquinolones be considered in formulating a combination regimen for infections with clear and compelling evidence of cause by *M. gordonae* (10).

ANTIMYCOBACTERIAL AGENTS: MODES OF ACTION AND MECHANISMS OF RESISTANCE

Isoniazid

The inhibitory activity of INH (isonicotinic acid hydrazide) against *M. tuberculosis* is remarkably specific and potent. Indeed, no other single antimycobacterial agent has proved to be as active against the *M. tuberculosis* complex, with such comparatively low toxicity, as INH. However, the activity of INH is less for other species of mycobacteria, and the drug has little or no role in the treatment of certain types of infections, notably, disease caused by RGM and disseminated *M. avium* infection. INH has no activity against non–acid-fast bacteria and eukaryotic cells. The activity against *M. tuberculosis* is bactericidal for dividing bacilli but does not kill bacilli in stationary phase or bacilli growing under anaerobic conditions (150–152). However, it is important to note that based on extensive clinical trials, INH is an effective therapeutic and prophylactic agent for clinical latent TB (153). The effect of INH is irreversible within only a few hours of exposure of tubercle bacilli to the drug. INH can bind irreversibly to protein, which is an important interfering factor in the measurement of INH concentrations in biologic fluids.

Isoniazid Activation

INH is a prodrug that the target organism must gratuitously activate in order for it to exert an antibacterial effect. Indeed, the relative inability of most bacteria to activate INH is the primary underlying reason for the selective action of this agent against the *M. tuberculosis* complex.

The mechanism of INH activation is now reasonably well understood. INH is converted in the presence of nicotinamide adenine dinucleotide (NAD) to an INH-NAD adduct by a catalase-peroxidase encoded by the *katG* gene (Fig. 5.5A). This process is enhanced by presence of manganese ions, probably involving a shift in redox state from Mn^{2+} to Mn^{3+} and back (154). In fact, activation of INH can occur in an enzyme-free system in the presence of Mn^{3+} ions and nicotinamide coenzymes (155). The derivative generated by this oxidation is either an isonicotinic acyl radical or anion; evidence supporting the production of the free acyl radical (as

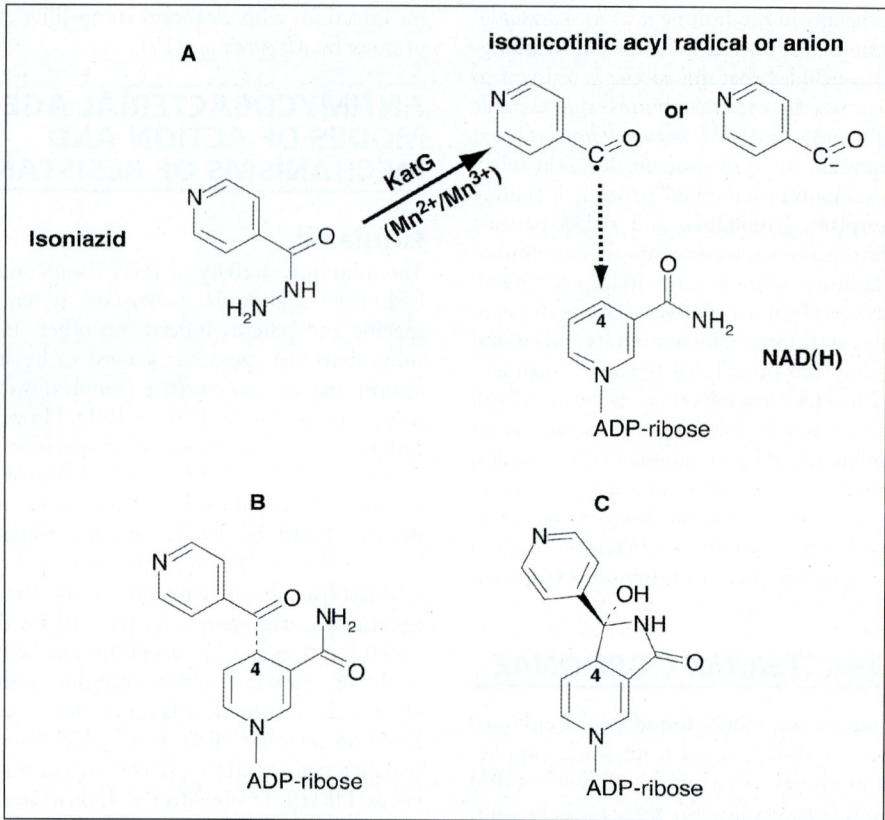

Figure 5.5 ■ Activation of isoniazid. A: The catalase/peroxidase enzyme, KatG, oxidizes isoniazid, probably forming either a free radical or anion. This catalysis is enhanced by the presence of manganese (Mn) ions. The oxidized isoniazid reacts with the nicotinamide moiety of NAD(H). The consequence of this is the formation of a covalent bond between the reactive carbon of the oxidized isoniazid and carbon at position 4 of the nicotinamide ring; the resulting molecule is referred to as an isoniazid-NAD(H) adduct. **B:** The isoniazid-NAD(H) adduct predicted from the crystal structure of the isoniazid target enzyme, InhA. **C:** An alternative isoniazid-NAD(H) adduct produced by the reaction of oxidized isoniazid and NAD(H); this adduct is inhibitory to InhA. (Structures adapted from Rozwarski DA, Grant GA, Barton DH, et al. Modification of the NADH of the isoniazid target [InhA] from Mycobacterium tuberculosis. *Science* 1998;279[5347]:98–102; Nguyen M, Quemard A, Broussy S, et al. Mn[III] pyrophosphate as an efficient tool for studying the mode of action of isoniazid on the InhA protein of Mycobacterium tuberculosis. *Antimicrob Agents Chemother* 2002;46[7]:2137–2144.)

well as the hydrazyl, peroxo, and pyridyl radical) was reported by Wengenack and Rusnak (156). The oxidized INH forms a covalent link to the carbon at position 4 of the nicotinamide moiety of nicotinamide adenine dinucleotide (hydrogen) (NAD[H]). The kinetics of INH activation and InhA inhibition suggests that the INH-NAD(H) adducts form outside of InhA and then compete with NAD(H) for the InhA binding site (157).

A possible structure of the active form of INH (Fig. 5.5A) was proposed from the X-ray crystal structure of the primary drug target, InhA, an enoyl-acyl carrier protein (ACP) reductase (158).

However, it is possible that there is more than one active form of INH. Nguyen et al. (155) isolated another INH-NAD(H) adduct with significant inhibitory activity for InhA (Fig. 5.5B).

Isoniazid Mechanism of Action

The first insights into the mechanism of action of INH were made by studying the sequence of events that occur following exposure of mycobacteria to this drug. Within 15 minutes of exposure to INH, radioactively labeled drug is taken into the cells and there is a decrease in the ratio of NAD to protein and inhibition of mycolic acid synthesis (159). Within 30 minutes, there is noticeable production of yellow pigment (peroxidase product), and by 60 to 90 minutes, there is a decline in cell viability (159). The bactericidal activity of INH is decreased in growth media depleted of trace metals, and the lethal action of INH appears to be suppressed under anaerobic conditions (159).

Over two decades ago, the demonstration that INH exposure leads to the inhibition of mycolic acid synthesis led to the hypothesis that this is the major cause of mycobacterial cell death. Winder (160) summarized the effects of INH as follows: (a) cells become more fragile and cellular material, including polysaccharides normally acylated to mycolic acids, leaks into the growth medium; (b) intracellular viscosity increases, perhaps due to an increase in cell volume or accumulation of cell wall precursors; (c) cell hydrophobicity decreases; and (d) cells lose the property of acid-fastness. Takayama et al. (161) demonstrated that INH did indeed inhibit mycolic acid synthesis in *M. tuberculosis*, leading to the accumulation of saturated C_{26} fatty acids. Central to the process of mycolic acids synthesis are the fatty acid synthesis (FAS) I and II enzyme systems.

The FAS I enzyme system synthesizes saturated fatty acid chains of 16 and 24 carbon atoms.

Interestingly, the FAS I system involves a single, multisubunit protein. The FAS II system modifies the $C_{16:0}$ and $C_{24:0}$ FAS I products, leading to the formation of mycolic acid chains of up to C_{56}. Unlike FAS I, the FAS II system involves a series of independent enzymes. The range of structures of the α-mycolic acids produced vary between species; consequently, mycolic acid profiling (by high-performance liquid chromatography [HPLC]) can be used for speciating mycobacteria.

One of the FAS II enzymes, the enoyl-ACP reductase or InhA, is the primary target for activated INH (162). The enoyl-ACP reductase catalyzes the saturation of terminal C=C double bond of the growing lipid chain prior to chain elongation by the β-ketoacyl-ACP synthases, KasA and KasB, and subsequent recycling by the β-ketoacyl-ACP reductase (MabA) and β-hydroxyacyl-ACP dehydrase (Fig. 5.6).

In summary, although there has been controversy regarding the primary target for the INH-NAD adduct, the existing biochemical and genetic evidence indicates that InhA is the primary and most physiologically relevant target for activated INH.

Isoniazid Resistance

The activity of INH is entirely dependent on activation of the prodrug, binding of the INH-NAD

Figure 5.6 ■ Isoniazid mechanisms of action. The INH-NAD adduct produced by the KatG enzyme inhibits the enoyl-ACP reductase, encoded by the inhA gene, of the fatty acid synthase II system. The inhibition of the enoyl-ACP reductase blocks the synthesis of mycolic acids, which are necessary for synthesis of the *M. tuberculosis* cell wall. The inhibition of cell wall synthesis is ultimately bactericidal for growing tubercle bacilli. (Adapted from Vilchèze C, Jacobs WR Jr. The mechanism of isoniazid killing: clarity through the scope of genetics. *Ann Rev Microbiol* 2007;61:35–50.)

adduct to the target, and exerting an inhibitory effect on that target. Thus, changes at any of these steps may lead to a change in susceptibility to INH.

Loss of Isoniazid Activation. An early observation of INH-resistant clinical isolates of *M. tuberculosis* was the changes in the catalase-peroxidase system of a significant proportion of these organisms (163), and these changes were mapped subsequently to the *kat*G gene (hydroperoxidase I) (164). Such changes in the *kat*G gene (2223 bp) prevent or reduce activation of INH. Indeed, high level INH resistance (MIC >5 μg/mL) correlates with the complete loss of catalase-peroxidase activity while low-level INH resistance (MIC <1 μg/ mL) isolates often retain catalase-peroxidase activity. The changes in the *kat*G gene range from point mutations to small deletions, through to the loss of most or all of the gene (165), although the latter case is rare. The frequency of INH resistance is high (1 in 10^5 or 10^6 tubercle bacilli) compared with the other first-line antimycobacterial agents. Point mutations are the most common genetic cause for INH resistance and more than 130 different mutations in *kat*G have been reported that result in amino acid changes and changes in the MIC for INH ranging from 0.2 to 256 μg/mL. The most common mutation in *kat*G is at codon 315 (S315T) accounting for 50% to 95% of INH resistance in clinical isolates (166).

The presence of a nonfunctional *kat*G gene increases susceptibility of *M. tuberculosis* to oxidative damage. Consequently, in such organisms, compensatory mutations in the regulatory region of the *ahp*C gene may be present (167,168). However, increased expression of *ahp*C plays little or no direct role in INH resistance (167).

Altered or Overexpressed inhA Protein. Although mutations in *kat*G account for the majority of INH resistance in *M. tuberculosis*, mutations in other genes must be involved in approximately 30% of INH-resistant isolates. Several studies have shown that resistance to INH also can be associated with mutations within the *inhA* gene (S94A) (38,162,169–172). Such mutations appear to alter the hydrogen bonding within the NAD(H) binding site, explaining the reduced affinity of NADH for the inhA protein. Such mutations confer resistance to both INH and ethionamide (173). However, mutations within the *inhA* gene of the *M. tuberculosis* complex appear to cause comparatively low-level INH resistance (174,175). Furthermore, the most common *inhA*-associated mutations in clinical isolates of *M. tuberculosis* were found to be in the promoter region of the *inh*A operon (165). In *M. tuberculosis*, the *inh*A gene is expressed as an operon with its upstream partner, *mab*; the Mab protein is a 3-ketoacyl reductase involved in mycolic acid synthesis but not in INH resistance (176). Overall, *inh*A mutations are rarely the cause of INH resistance and usually occur concurrently with a *kat*G and/or mutation. Indeed, the second most common mutation that causes INH resistance is a mutation in the inhA promoter region (C-15T). The result is an overexpression of *inh*A messenger RNA (mRNA) and InhA protein (172,177,178).

Other Mechanisms of Isoniazid Resistance. Mutations in *kas*A, *ndh*, and *glf* have been linked with increased resistance to INH (179–182). Furthermore, overexpression of the arylamine *N*-acetyltransferase (NAT) encoded by the *nho*A gene may inactivate INH and cause low-level INH resistance (183,184). However, multiple nucleotide polymorphisms appear to be common in all the genes that have been associated with INH resistance (185), including *kat*G, *inh*A, *kas*A and *ndh*. There is evidence that mycobacteria may have an efflux pump (*efpA*) that can transport INH out of the cell (186,187) and INH appears to induce increased expression and synthesis of this efflux protein (188).

In summary, although it appears there are several mechanisms of INH resistance and a genetic basis has been established for many of these mechanisms, the predominant cause of INH resistance is associated with mutations in the *kat*G gene, which results in the loss or decreased expression of catalase-peroxidase that is necessary to activate INH.

Rifamycins

The rifamycins (e.g., rifampin, rifapentine, rifabutin, rifaximin, and rifalazil) are potent inhibitors of prokaryotic DNA-dependent RNA polymerases (189), with little activity against the equivalent mammalian enzymes. However, only rifampin (Rifadin, Rimactane, Rifampicin, etc.) and rifapentine (Priftin) are approved (United States) for the treatment of TB. Rifabutin (Mycobutin) is only approved for the treatment/prophylaxis of disseminated MAC disease. Rifalazil (Kaneka Corporation, Osaka, Japan), a benzoxazinorifamycin, is significantly more active against *M. tuberculosis* compared with other rifamycins, but development of rifalazil for treating TB was discontinued because of an adverse drug effect (viz., flu-like symptom). Rifamixin is only approved for the treatment of enteropathogenic *Escherichia coli*. The rifamycins are composed of aromatic rings linked by an aliphatic bridge, more specifically an ansa polyhydroxylated bridge connecting two naphthoquinones or naphthhydroquinones (190). Most likely, the lipophilic properties of these molecules aid in the penetration of the drug across the mycobacterial cell wall and are important for binding of the drugs to the target RNA polymerase.

The susceptibility of mycobacteria to rifampin is well documented, and the drug is a first-line component of anti-TB therapy, including DOTS and DOTS-plus (191–193). However, there is significant variation in susceptibility to rifampin between MAC isolates, with the majority being intrinsically resistant. Despite this, the DNA-dependent RNA polymerases isolated from *M. intracellulare* and *M. avium* are to be sensitive to rifampin (194,195). Furthermore, substances believed to increase the permeability of the mycobacterial cell wall, such as Tween 80, also cause a significant increase in susceptibility to rifampin. Thus, it appears that the impermeability of the cell wall results in the intrinsic resistance to rifamycins among the mycobacteria where it occurs.

Rifapentine was approved in the United States in 1998 for use against *M. tuberculosis* (196). In vitro, rifapentine is more active than rifampin, and its metabolite, 25-*O*-desacetylrifapentine, has equivalent activity to rifampin (197,198). Rifapentine has a significantly longer half-life than rifampin—13.2 to 14.1 hours versus 1.5 to 5 hours, respectively (199–202). Consequently, rifapentine-containing anti-TB regimens are focused on a reduced dosing regimen compared with rifampin, for instance, twice-weekly dosing during the induction phase of therapy (i.e., the first 2 months) and once-weekly dosing during the continuation phase (203). Randomized controlled trials showed that a combination of INH and rifapentine administered weekly for 12 weeks as directly observed therapy (DOT) is as effective for preventing TB as other regimens and is more likely to be completed than a regimen of 9 months of INH daily without DOT (204). An open-label, multicenter, phase III clinical trial was designed to compare the effectiveness and tolerability of a 3-month (12-dose) regimen of weekly rifapentine and INH to the effectiveness of a 9-month regimen of daily INH to prevent TB among high-risk tuberculin skin test reactors, including children and HIV-infected persons, who require treatment of latent TB infection (205). Rifapentine is a weaker inducer of the cytochrome P450 CYP3A system than rifampin (200) and, thus, rifapentine interferes less with drugs metabolized by this system (e.g., protease inhibitors).

Rifabutin has potent activity in vitro against MAC (206) and has equivalent activity as rifapentine against *M. tuberculosis* (198). However, rifabutin failed to demonstrate efficacy in the treatment of MAC disease in some uncontrolled trials but yielded moderate benefit in other trials (207,208). Rifabutin has been shown to reduce the incidence of MAC disease in HIV-infected patients when used as a prophylactic agent, and the drug has been approved for this use (209,210). Although the basis of the prophylactic activity of rifabutin is not known, this drug has been shown to inhibit the binding of MAC to HT-29 human intestinal carcinoma cells in vitro (211). Thus, rifabutin may prevent colonization of the gastrointestinal tract, which is believed to be a major portal of entry for disseminated MAC disease. Compared with rifampin, rifabutin also has a longer half-life in vivo and is concentrated in tissues, especially the lungs, where levels can be 10 times higher than in serum.

The target site of rifamycins in all bacteria that have been studied is the β-subunit of the prokaryotic RNA polymerase. The β-subunit is one of the five subunits that comprise the polymerase and includes the catalytic center of the enzyme. Rifampin (and presumably the other rifamycins) does not bind in the catalytic center of the β-subunit but at a site upstream from the catalytic center. Thus, rifampin acts as a "plug" rather than a direct catalytic inhibitor and physically blocks (by steric occlusion) de novo RNA from elongating out of the RNA polymerase complex (Fig. 5.7). In this respect, rifamycins have similarity to macrolides (see the following discussion).

Resistance to rifamycins in *M. tuberculosis* (and many other microorganisms) is the result of mutations within the *rpoB* gene, although inactivation of rifampin via adenosine diphosphate ribosylation occurs in some mycobacteria (212). The *rpoB* gene mutations cluster in a hot spot or rifampin resistance-determining region (RRDR) and usually result in a single amino acid change in the protein sequence, and reduce the binding affinity of rifamycins to the RNA polymerase (Fig. 5.8). Since the original study by Telenti et al. (213), there have been numerous reports describing the *rpoβ* gene mutations in rifampin-resistant *M. tuberculosis* isolated in different regions of the world. Mutations in or near the RRDR of the *rpoβ* gene account for about 94% of rifampin-resistant

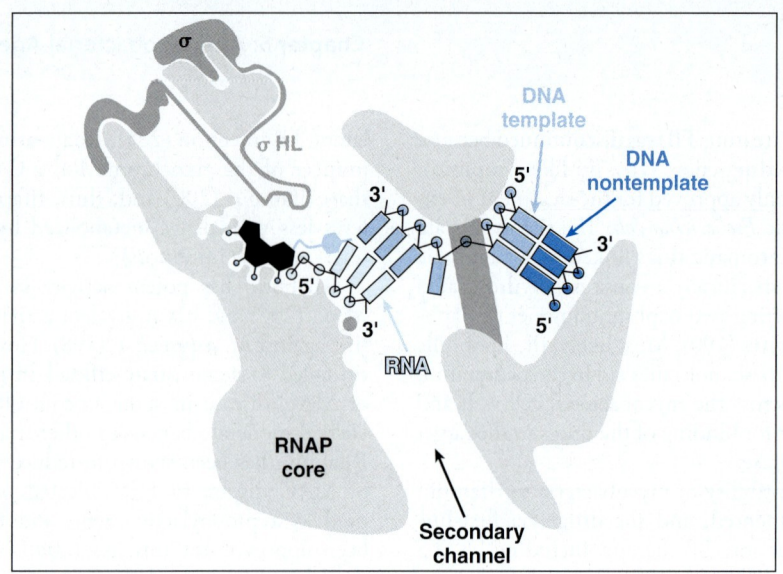

Figure 5.7 ■ Rifampin mechanism of action. The steric block model for the mechanism of action of rifamycins. The drawing illustrates the binding of rifampin sterically blocking the growing RNA chain in the transcription initiation complex of RNAP. (Adapted from Aristoff PA, Garcia GA, Kirchhoff PD, et al. Rifamycins—obstacles and opportunities. *Tuberculosis [Edinb]* 2010;90[2]:94–118; Artsimovitch I, Vassylyev DG. Is it easy to stop RNA polymerase? *Cell Cycle* 2006;5[4]:399–404.) (See Color Plate in the front of the book.)

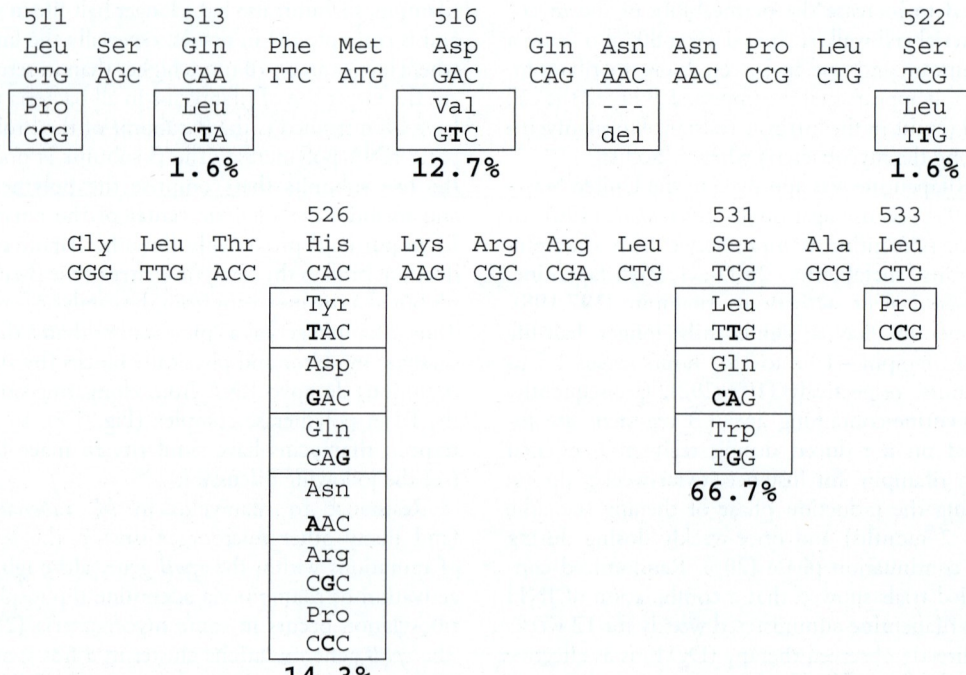

Figure 5.8 ■ Clustering of mutations in the β-subunit (*rpoβ* gene) of the RNA polymerase found in greater than 90% of rifampin-resistant *M. tuberculosis*. Shown is the *rpoβ* gene of *M. tuberculosis* from codon 511 to codon 533. The *boxes* below the sequence show the positions of 15 common gene mutations (specific bases changes are shown in bold) and the resulting amino acid changes that result in the production of a rifampin-resistant RNA polymerase. The percentage distribution for 96.9% of mutations identified in a collection of 63 clinical isolates of *M. tuberculosis* are shown below the respective boxes. (Adapted from Heep M, Brandstätter B, Rieger U, et al. Frequency of *rpoB* mutations inside and outside the cluster I region in rifampin-resistant clinical Mycobacterium tuberculosis isolates. J Clin Microbiol 2001;39(1):107–110; Telenti A, Imboden P, Marchesi F, et al. Detection of rifampicin-resistance mutation in *Mycobacterium tuberculosis*. Lancet 1993;341(8846):647–650.

M. tuberculosis. Infrequent mutations outside of the RRDR account for the remainder of rifamycin-resistant *M. tuberculosis*, notable mutations V146F and I572F (214). Such rare mutations may occur more frequently in cases of relapsed or previously treated TB (215). Although previously undescribed mutations are often reported, the most frequently identified mutations associated with rifampin-resistant clinical isolates have a mutation in codons 516, 526, or 531 (Fig. 5.8) of the β-subunit (216,217), especially mutations causing a serine to leucine change at codon 531 (S531L). Intriguingly, the predominant rifampin-resistant *M. tuberculosis* mutants selected in vitro also tend to have S531L substitutions (218). This suggests that pressures other than rifampin inhibition of RNA synthesis are involved in the appearance of stable resistant mutants. In support of this is the finding that an S531L substitution has a smaller impact on the activity of the RNA polymerase than other less common mutations (219). In addition, mutations in codons 511, 516, 518, and 522 confer a lower level of rifampin and rifapentine resistance and an unchanged susceptibility to rifabutin and rifalazil (220,221). Strains with some of these mutations may test as "susceptible" in the MGIT system, but have been associated with treatment failures in Africa and the Far East (221a).

Interestingly, the mutations associated with resistance to different rifamycins do not always match, an observation that appears to explain why rifamycins such as rifapentine, rifabutin, and rifalazil are active in vitro against some *M. tuberculosis* strains that are resistant to rifampin (220,222–224). However, the most common *rpoβ* mutations in rifampin-resistant *M. tuberculosis* (i.e., codons 526 and 531) also confer high-level resistance to the other rifamycins. Unlike most other antimycobacterial agents, evidence suggests that active rifamycin efflux in mycobacteria is minimal at best (225). Thus, increased efflux is unlikely to be a significant mechanism of clinical rifamycin resistance.

Macrolides and Ketolides

The development of new-generation macrolides has had a significant impact on the treatment of mycobacterial diseases, especially those caused by MAC, *Mycobacterium leprae*, and RGM; however, macrolides appear to be of little benefit in the treatment of TB (226–228). Azithromycin (an azalide macrolide), clarithromycin, and roxithromycin are structurally related to erythromycin, with modifications that improve acid stability, tissue accumulation, and bioavailability and lengthen elimination half-life without increasing toxicity. Although adverse drug effects are less frequent, compared to erythromycin, gastrointestinal intolerance (abdominal pain, nausea, and diarrhea) does occur with the new macrolides. Roxithromycin is not available in the United States.

Of the macrolides, clarithromycin is the most active against MAC isolates in vitro (on a weight basis), with 90% of MAC isolates having MICs of 0.5 to 4 μg/mL under mildly acidic conditions (pH 6.8). Under similar conditions, the MIC values for azithromycin and roxithromycin are both 8 to 32 μg/mL. The activity of macrolides in vitro, however, is strongly affected by pH, with MICs being one or two dilutions lower at pH 7.4 compared with at pH 6.8 (99,229). This phenomenon led to controversy in establishing interpretive standards for assessing susceptibility to macrolides in vitro. Testing of macrolides under sightly alkaline conditions, however, may be misleading because MAC strains grow more slowly under such conditions and, thus, MIC values may reflect synergy between pH and drug (206). The conditions within the phagolysosomes of MAC-infected macrophages (i.e., pH 6.0 to 6.5) suggest that susceptibility testing of macrolides under mildly acidic conditions would be more clinically relevant. Nevertheless, for reasons of uniformity and consistency, the CLSI recommends to perform testing only at pH 7.3 or 7.4 (99).

Although clarithromycin is, in general, more active than the other macrolides in vitro, the comparative pharmacokinetics suggests a different picture in vivo. Following a 500-mg dose of clarithromycin, the maximum serum level achieved is 2 or 3 μg/mL, with an elimination half-life of 7 hours. Tissue concentrations are usually four or five times those in serum, with the levels in macrophages being 20 to 30 times higher. After a similar dose of azithromycin, the maximum serum level is 0.4 to 0.6 μg/mL; however, accumulation within leukocytes approaches 200 to 800 times serum concentrations (230). This high tissue accumulation reflects the extraordinarily long elimination half-life (68 hours) of azithromycin. Roxithromycin achieves the highest serum levels of the three macrolides (11 μg/mL), with a half-life of 19 hours. Little is known about tissue accumulation of roxithromycin, although evidence suggests that roxithromycin achieves poor tissue to serum concentration ratios (231–233).

The ketolides are semisynthetic erythromycin derivatives, with replacement of the neutral L-cladinose with a keto group at position 3 of the macrolatone ring (234,235). In addition, many ketolides have other changes to the basic erythromycin framework. These changes were introduced to improve on the antimicrobial activity and pharmacokinetics compared with macrolides. Furthermore, ketolides may be active against some macrolide-resistant bacteria (236) and may continue to inhibit methylated ribosomes that are refractory to macrolides (236,237). This activity may result from the higher binding affinity of ketolides for ribosomes compared with macrolides (234,235,237). Although ketolides do not upregulate expression of inducible *erm* genes in some other bacteria (238), ketolides are good *erm* inducers in several species of mycobacteria (98). Telithromycin, a ketolide, is approved for clinical use in the United States and Europe but carries an important "black box" warning for patients with myasthenia gravis.

Ketolides have been tested against mycobacteria with some success, although the MICs for telithromycin against mycobacteria tend to be higher than for clarithromycin (239–241), and mycobacteria with mutation-acquired macrolide resistance are also resistant to ketolides (242). Nevertheless, studies with ketolides using mouse models of mycobacterioses suggest that ketolides with higher MICS are therapeutically efficacious (242–244). This discrepancy between in vitro susceptibility and activity in vivo is reminiscent of azithromycin and is based, at least in part, on the accumulation of these agents in tissues and their long half-lives.

Macrolides and ketolides are bacteriostatic agents that bind to the 50S subunit of the prokaryotic ribosome and block protein synthesis. Within the 50S subunit, the critical macrolide binding site is at the peptidyltransferase region (245), and the agents appear to interact with the adenine residues at positions 2058 and 2059 (A2058 and A2059, *E. coli* numbering) of the 23S rRNA. Macrolides bind to the ribosome in the cleft where the growing peptide chain exits the peptidyltransferase region. Thus, inhibition is the result of a physical obstruction rather than a direct inhibition of peptidyltransferase activity; such an indirect mode of action is similar to that of rifamycins (see previous discussion). That said, there is some evidence that 16-membered macrolides (e.g., spiramycin) may inhibit peptidyltransferase reactions and that 14-membered macrolides (e.g., clarithromycin) may prevent the translocation of transfer RNA

(tRNA) and increase tRNA dissociation from the ribosome (246). However, it is not clear if these are direct or indirect effects of macrolide binding. Macrolides reversibly bind to the ribosome, which is probably a major reason why these agents are primarily bacteriostatic.

Resistance to macrolides has been studied with a range of microorganisms, and three basic mechanisms have been identified (247,248): (a) ribosome modification, (b) drug efflux, and (c) drug inactivation. The predominant mechanism of clinically significant resistance is ribosome modification by methylation of the A2058 residue within the 23S rRNA. This methylation occurs prior to assembly of the 50S ribosomal subunit, which means that organisms must replace their susceptible ribosomes with nascently methylated ribosomes in order to express resistance. The methylase activity is rRNA sequence-specific and encoded by *erm* genes. Methylation of A2058 reduces the binding affinity of macrolides to the ribosome, thus explaining the resistance. Other agents, such as lincosamides and streptogramin B, associate with the A2058 residue, and thus, methylation of this site usually confers cross-resistance to these agents (i.e., MLS resistance). Efflux-based macrolide resistance is conferred by expression of the *mef*A gene of streptococci or the *msr*A gene of staphylococci (248).

There are several other potential mechanisms of macrolide resistance, including inactivating enzymes and ribosomal protein gene mutations (247,248); however, their association with clinically significant resistance is not clear.

Unlike most other bacterial pathogens, clinically acquired macrolide resistance in mycobacteria can be conferred by point mutations at residue A2058 or A2059 within the 23S rRNA gene (97,249,250), and like rRNA methylation, such mutations reduce the binding of macrolides to the ribosome (251). In mycobacteria, macrolide resistance–associated mutations also confer resistance to ketolides, lincosamides, and streptogramin B (98,242). The 23S rRNA gene mutations confer macrolide resistant because slowly growing mycobacteria only have one copy, and most RGM only have two copies of the rRNA gene operon per genome. Other bacterial pathogens have multiple copies of the *rrn* operon. A notable exception is *Helicobacter pylori* which only has two copies, and clinically acquired macrolide resistance *H. pylori* is also conferred by the 23S rRNA gene mutation (252–254).

Although macrolides are the foundation for treatment regimens for many mycobacterial infections, innate resistance to macrolides is expressed by some pathogenic mycobacteria, most notably *M. tuberculosis* (227,228). This resistance is not due to sequence divergence in the peptidyltransferase region of the 23S rRNA but to the intrinsic macrolide resistance conferred by novel *erm* genes: *erm*(41), *erm*(39), *erm*(38), and *erm*(37) genes as seen in *M. abscessus* (255), *M. fortuitum* (95), *Mycobacterium smegmatis* (94), and *M. tuberculosis* (111,112). These rRNA methylase genes are chromosomal and inducible with macrolide and lincosamide agents but not streptogramin B. The inducible nature of these *erm* methylases complicates in vitro susceptibility testing (see the following texts). Molecular detection of *erm* genes, as a drug susceptibility test, is also likely to be problematic because in some mycobacteria, the *erm* genes are inactive or have been deleted (98). Finally, although there is evidence for active macrolide efflux in mycobacteria (256), the clinical significance is not clear.

Aminoglycosides and Peptide Antibiotics

The aminoglycosides that are used in the treatment of mycobacterial infections include streptomycin, kanamycin, and amikacin. Streptomycin is active against growing *M. tuberculosis* with MICs of 2 to 4 µg/mL. Streptomycin inhibits protein synthesis in several types of bacteria, including *M. tuberculosis*, by binding to the 30S ribosome subunit at the S12 ribosomal protein and 16S rRNA site (166). Amikacin and kanamycin have very similar structures and both of these injectable aminoglycosides are second-line drugs. Capreomycin and viomycin are polypeptide antibiotics that are active against *M. tuberculosis* and are often discussed along with the aminoglycosides because of similarities in mechanisms of action and resistance. Capreomycin is preferred to viomycin because it has a better therapeutic index than viomycin. Amikacin, kanamycin, and capreomycin are second-line agents that are reserved for the treatment of MDR *M. tuberculosis* and for the prevention of extreme or total resistance (14,257). Amikacin also can be useful for the treatment of infections caused by RGM.

The mechanism of action of aminoglycosides and peptide antibiotics is well accommodated by the allosteric three-site model for the ribosomal elongation cycle (258). According to the model, the ribosome contains three binding sites: the A-site or aminoacyl-tRNA site, the P-site or peptidyl-tRNA site, and the E-site or exit site for deacylated tRNA (Fig. 5.9). The A- and E-sites are allosterically linked, such that occupation of one site decreases the affinity for the other site. The result is that the A- and P-sites have high affinity for tRNA before translocation, while the P- and E-sites have high affinity after translation. Deacylated tRNA is released upon occupation of the A-site, not during translocation. Thus, during initiation reactions, the E-site is not occupied and the A-site is said to undergo an initiation-type occupation equivalent to formation of the 70S initiation complex; however, once translocation occurs and the E-site is occupied, the A-site undergoes an elongation-type occupation. During the initiation reaction, only the P-site carries a tRNA, while during the elongation cycle, the ribosome complex carries two tRNAs, that is, a peptidyl-tRNA and deacylated tRNA. The mechanism of action of aminoglycosides and peptide antibiotics can be understood in terms of the allosteric interactions involving these binding sites (see the following discussion). There is also compelling evidence to support the conclusion that protein synthesis and the effects of protein synthesis inhibitors occur in an identical manner in mycobacteria and rapidly growing bacteria such as *E. coli* (259–261).

Viomycin resistance is reported to cross to capreomycin resistance in mycobacteria (262), and viomycin blocks the binding of capreomycin to ribosomes. Viomycin and capreomycin are bacteriostatic agents with potent activity against mycobacteria but have little activity against gram-negative bacteria. Nevertheless, viomycin is an active inhibitor of cell-free protein synthesis using extracts of gram-negative bacteria. Viomycin blocks translocation and, surprisingly, impedes elongation-type A-site binding; therefore, in the presence of viomycin, the ribosome cannot be transferred back to the pretranslocational state via A-site binding of the elongation-type (258). Thus, viomycin and capreomycin are inhibitors of translocation that block both allosteric transitions of the ribosome elongation cycle. Earlier evidence indicated that the mechanism of resistance to basic peptides was associated with ribosome mutation (263) and more recent evidence associated capreomycin, kanamycin, amikacin, and viomycin resistance with 3 to 6 *rrs* mutations and may or may not be associated with *tlyA* mutations (*tlyA* encodes a putative rRNA methyltransferase) (264,265).

In 1943, streptomycin became the first antimicrobial agent used to effectively treat TB; however, trials with PAS were also completed that same year, and there is some controversy as

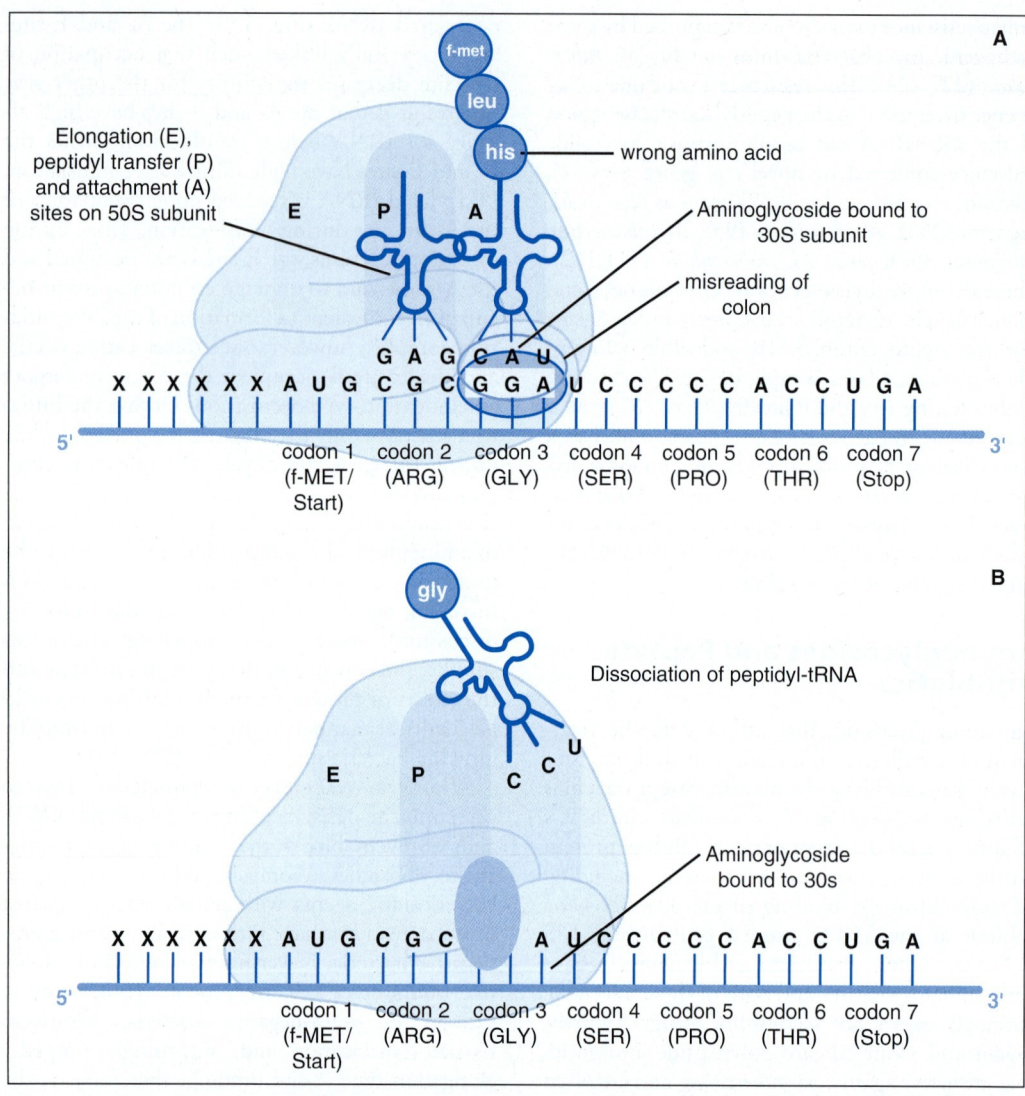

Figure 5.9 ■ Aminoglycosides prevent protein synthesis by (A) causing translation errors (proofreading errors) and the misreading of codons and insertion of incorrect amino acids) or (B) translocation errors or the dissociation of peptidyl-tRNA. Aminoglycoside resistance in *M. tuberculosis* is most commonly caused by three mutations in the *rrs* gene (16S rRNA): A1401G, C1402T, and G1484T. (Graphics adapted from http://pharmaxchange.info/press/2011/05/mechanism-of-action-of-aminoglycosides/ by Akul Mehta with animation by G. Kaiser.) (See Color Plate in the front of the book.)

to which drug was actually used first for a clinical purpose (266). Other aminoglycosides, such as kanamycin and gentamicin, have been used to treat mycobacterioses, although their therapeutic indices are less favorable than streptomycin and amikacin. The aminoglycosides are generally less bactericidal for mycobacteria than for other types of bacteria (267).

Streptomycin and dihydrostreptomycin are derivatives of streptamine, and kanamycin is a glycoside of 2-deoxystreptamine. Amikacin is a semisynthetic kanamycin derivative with a butyric acid moiety at the R3-position of kanamycin. All of the aminoglycosides reduce A-site binding of aminoacyl-tRNA of the elongation-type, while A-site binding of the initiation-type is minimally affected, as is the puromycin reaction (chain termination). Thus, the primary mechanism of action of the aminoglycosides is to inhibit the posttranslocational to pretranslocational transition, with only variable effects on the pretranslocational to posttranslocational transition. Aminoglycosides, particularly streptomycin, affect the proofreading function of the A-site, leading to the mistranslation of proteins. The pleiotropic effects of the aminoglycosides that are more difficult to explain include irreversible uptake, membrane damage, and ribosomal blockage. However, Hausner et al. (268) hypothesized that the primary molecular mechanism of aminoglycoside bactericidal activity is ribosomal blockage, with the pleiotropic effects occurring as a consequence of the disruption of protein synthesis.

Since aminoglycosides, capreomycin, and viomycin target the ribosome, it is not surprising that modification of this organelle confers high-level acquired resistance (269–278). For instance, the mechanism of resistance to streptomycin in *M. tuberculosis* is associated with mutations within the 16S rRNA *rrs* gene and the *rpsL* gene, which encodes the S12 ribosomal protein (263,274–277,279–283). Mutations in codon 43 of the *rpsL* gene and in *rrs* gene account for streptomycin resistance in approximately 50% and 20% of *M. tuberculosis* isolates, respectively (166,280,281). These mutations tend to confer high-level resistance (streptomycin MIC >500 μg/mL). The other common site for *rpsL* mutations is in codon 88. The 16S rRNA gene mutations tend to cluster in or near the loop 18 region (position 530) and the loop 27 region (position 915) for the 16S rRNA structure as shown by Brimacombe et al. (284). Other mutations have been described mostly in-between these two loop regions. The localizing of resistance-associated mutations in the loop 18 and 27 regions and the *rpsL* gene (i.e., the S12 ribosomal protein) suggests that streptomycin binds in or near the A-site. Although base substitution at position 491 of the 16S rRNA gene was found in streptomycin-resistant *M. tuberculosis* (277), this appears to be a polymorphism that does not actually confer resistance (285). A mutation in *gid*B, which encodes methyltransferase specific for 16S rRNA, is associated with low-level resistance in 33% of *M. tuberculosis*–resistant isolates (166). The 16S rRNA mutations tend to confer a lower level of streptomycin resistance than *rpsL* mutations. Low-level streptomycin resistance also is associated with mutations that cause increased efflux (286).

The known *rpsL* and 16S rRNA gene mutations account for 60% to 90% of streptomycin resistance. *M. tuberculosis* isolates with low-level streptomycin resistance (MIC ~10 μg/mL) tend to have wild-type *rpsL* and 16S rRNA genes (at least in the loop 18 and 27 regions) (280,287). This suggests that there is a third mechanism of streptomycin resistance, which may be based on changes in cell wall permeability (287).

Despite the similarity between aminoglycosides, the mechanisms of resistance may not completely overlap. For instance, clinically acquired resistance to 2-deoxystreptamine aminoglycosides (e.g., amikacin and kanamycin) in *M. abscessus* is associated with 16S rRNA gene mutation at position 1408 (278); this position is equivalent to the 16S rRNA methylation site that confers resistance to the aminoglycoside-producing bacteria (288). However, this mutation does not confer resistance to streptomycin.

Resistance to aminoglycosides in bacteria can be due to the presence of aminoglycoside-modifying enzymes (289). From studies two decades ago, RGM are known to produce aminoglycoside-acetylating enzymes (290), and a substrate profile analysis revealed two patterns of 3-NAT, with broad and narrow specificities (291). The broad-specificity enzyme was found only in *M. fortuitum*, while the narrow-specificity enzyme was found in *M. smegmatis*, *Mycobacterium vaccae*, and *Mycobacterium phlei*. However, the ubiquitous presence and activity of these enzymes in RGM does not correlate with acquired aminoglycoside resistance (292).

DNA homology studies identified putative aminoglycosides acetyltransferases in the chromosomes of both rapidly growing and slowly growing mycobacteria, including *M. tuberculosis* (293). Cloning and overexpression of the aminoglycosides acetyltransferase gene, aac(2′)-Id, of *M. smegmatis* conferred a 4- to 16-fold increase in MIC for a range of aminoglycosides, and disrupting the gene resulted in an equivalent drop in the magnitude of the MIC (293). However, expression of the *M. tuberculosis* putative aminoglycosides acetyltransferase in *M. smegmatis* did not increase resistance to this class of agent. Thus, the role of these enzymes in either intrinsic or acquired resistance to aminoglycosides is not entirely clear.

Ethambutol

Ethambutol is active against *M. tuberculosis*, with MICs in the range of 0.5 to 5 μg/mL, although its antimicrobial activity requires active growth of susceptible cells. The drug has much more variable activity against the other species of slowly growing mycobacteria and is significantly less active against

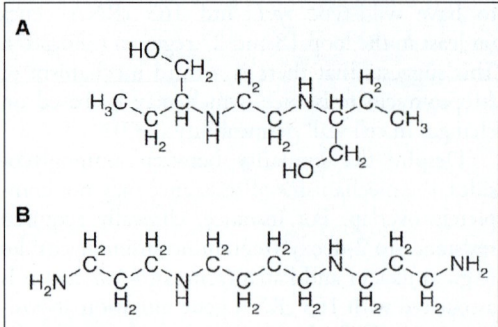

Figure 5.10 ■ Structures of ethambutol **(A)** and spermine **(B).**

RGM. On the whole, ethambutol is inactive against other microorganisms. Studies of the mechanism of action of ethambutol have focused on two targets: polyamine function and metabolism and cell wall synthesis. The influence of ethambutol on polyamine metabolism was inferred, in part, from the similarity of the chemical structures of ethambutol (d-2,2-[ethylenediimino]di[1-butanol]) and spermine (N,N'-bis[3-aminopropyl]1,4-butanediamine) (Fig. 5.10). In addition, early studies showed that the growth inhibition caused by ethambutol could be reversed by the addition of spermidine or Mg^{2+} and that cells could be protected from the effect of ethambutol by the addition of high concentrations of Mg^{2+} or by increases in the ionic strength of the growth medium. Additional studies suggested that the effect of ethambutol was on the synthesis and stability of RNA. However, a later study showed that ethambutol caused a disaggregation of cells, which most likely reflected a reduction in the lipid content of the cell wall (294). Indeed, Takayama et al. (295) showed that ethambutol inhibited the transfer of mycolic acid into the cell wall and stimulated trehalose dimycolate synthesis.

The problem with many of these studies was that the time between the addition of the drug and the observed effect was often long (hours), thus preventing distinction between primary and secondary effects. Subsequently, several studies demonstrated that the spermidine synthase enzyme from mycobacteria was inhibited by ethambutol (296,297), specifically the *dextro*-isomer and not the *levo*-isomer (only the *dextro*-isomer inhibits the growth of mycobacteria). The synthases from a *Pseudomonas* sp and an *E. coli* isolate (both are intrinsically ethambutol-resistant) were not inhibited by either form of ethambutol. In addition, the spermidine synthase from a strain of *M. fortuitum*,

with an ethambutol MIC of 8 µg/mL, required 80 µmol/L *d*-ethambutol to inhibit 50% of enzyme activity, compared with 30 µmol/L for the enzymes from strains of *M. bovis* and *Mycobacterium flavescens* with ethambutol MICs of 1 µg/mL. However, using an *M. bovis* strain, the effect of ethambutol on polyamine metabolism in vivo required an ethambutol concentration eightfold above the MIC in order to achieve a 46% reduction in spermidine synthesis after 48-hour exposure to the drug. This casts doubt on the relevance of inhibition of polyamine metabolism as the primary antimycobacterial activity of ethambutol, although it may lead to secondary effects.

In contrast, the effect of ethambutol on cell wall synthesis and, more specifically, trehalose dimycolate synthesis was later shown to occur within 15 minutes of exposure to the drug (298). In that study, precursors such as monomycolate, dimycolate, and mycolic acid began to accumulate within 1 to 12 minutes. These observations led Takayama and Kilburn (299) to identify a more specific metabolic target for ethambutol. They showed a decrease in the incorporation of $[^{14}C]$glucose into a 55% to 85% ethanol-insoluble fraction of whole cells of an ethambutol-sensitive strain of *M. smegmatis* within 15 minutes of the addition of 3 µg/mL ethambutol. The ethanol-insoluble fraction was shown to contain cell wall arabinomannan and arabinogalactan. The effect of ethambutol on the incorporation of $[^{14}C]$glucose into the arabinose residue of these complex sugars was virtually instantaneous. HPLC analysis of $[^{14}C]$-alditol acetates derived from the polysaccharide fraction of treated and control cells showed 90% and 53% inhibition of the transfer of $[^{14}C]$glucose label into arabinose and mannose, respectively. Maximal inhibition of glucose incorporation was observed with 5 µg/mL ethambutol, which was in contrast to the 60 µg/mL required to achieve an equivalent level of inhibition in an isogenic ethambutol-resistant strain of *M. smegmatis*. The in vivo studies were complemented by preliminary cell-free assays for the effect of ethambutol on arabinose metabolism. Thus, the primary mechanism of action of ethambutol appears to be the inhibition of arabinogalactan synthesis and, to a lesser degree, the inhibition of arabinomannan synthesis (300). The metabolic intermediates that accumulate in the presence of inhibitory concentrations of ethambutol include decaprenyl-P-arabinose (301), which suggests that ethambutol inhibits transfer of arabinose from its' donor molecule to the relevant polysaccharide of the cell wall (302). The proposed disruptive effects of ethambutol on cell wall synthesis are consistent with evidence for a synergistic effect of ethambutol on the activity of other antimycobacterial agents (303,304).

The target(s) of ethambutol in mycobacteria is believed to be one or more of the putative arabinosyl transferases encoded within the *emb* operon. Inhibition of these enzymes would be consistent with the accumulation of arabinosyl-donor molecules in ethambutol-treated cells. The *emb* operon comprises either two genes in *M. avium* (*emb*A and *emb*B) or three genes in *M. tuberculosis*, *M. leprae*, and *M. smegmatis* (*emb*C, *emb*A, and *emb*B [in this order]) (305,306), and the product of the *emb*R gene probably regulates expression of this operon (Fig. 5.11) (305).

Mutations in the *emb*B gene confer high-level (MICs ≥20 μg/mL) resistance to ethambutol (307), suggesting that this encodes the primary target for this drug. Although mutations in other regions associated with the *emb* operon have been described (308), perhaps, as many as 65% of *M. tuberculosis* isolates with acquired ethambutol resistance have mutations in the *emb*B gene (307), particularly at codon 306. Ethambutol-resistant strains of *M. tuberculosis* have MICs greater than 7.5 μg/mL and mutations that result in resistance occur with a frequency of 10^{-5} (166).

Polymorphisms in the *emb*B gene appear to be linked with intrinsic resistance to ethambutol in mycobacteria (309). However, even mutations in the codon 306 region have been reported in MDRTB that are still susceptible to ethambutol (310). The significance of this is unclear but may suggest that ethambutol has a target other than the *emb*B gene product.

Early studies of the frequency of resistance to ethambutol in *M. tuberculosis* cultures showed that low-level resistance occurs relatively frequently (approximately 1 in 10^{5} organisms) but that high-level resistance was extremely rare (311). This suggested that high-level resistance is most likely the result of a multistep process. Further evidence of a stepwise acquisition of high-level ethambutol resistance was reported by Telenti et al. (306). The first step appears to be an increase in expression of the *emb* operon, followed by a mutation in *emb*B. Alternatively, the second step may involve a further increase in *emb* expression (306).

Pyrazinamide

PZA in combination with INH is considered to be rapidly bactericidal for *M. tuberculosis*, and consequently, this agent is a critical component to short-course (i.e., 6 months) treatments including DOTS. However, PZA has no activity against other mycobacteria, including other members of the *M. tuberculosis* complex and the MAC (312).

The study of the anti-TB activity of PZA in vitro is problematic in that it is active only at an acidic pH (pH 5.6), which itself suppresses growth of mycobacteria. In an absolute sense, PZA MICs are high compared with other drugs, that is, 6.25 to 50 μg/mL; but PZA activity increases under anaerobic or semianaerobic conditions and also

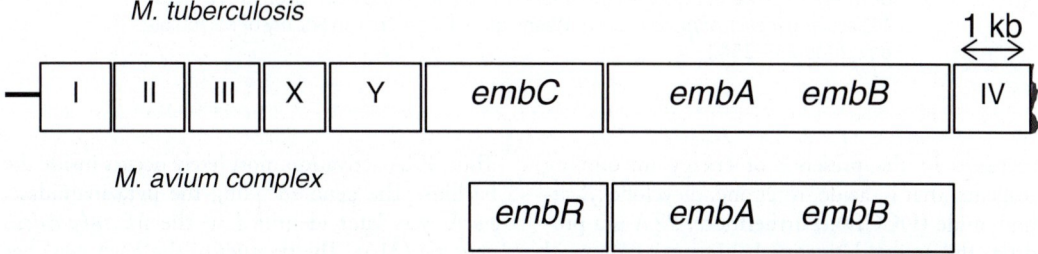

Figure 5.11 ■ Organization of the 14-kb *M. tuberculosis* emb resistance-determining region (ERDR). Three homologous *emb* genes preceded by a predicted coding region (*Y*) and by *orfX*, encoding a putative protein (*X*). *I* through *IV* represent sequences for hypothetical proteins. The *embCAB* genes encode for integral membrane proteins, most likely arabinosyl transferases. The majority of mutations that result in ethambutol resistance (MICs ≥20 g/mL) are found in within the *embB* gene. Ethambutol resistance not associated with the ERDR generally have MICs ≤10 g/mL. The intrinsic resistance to ethambutol frequently observed in non-tuberculous mycobacteria are commonly associated with amino acid changes encoded in the ERDR. Organization of the *M. avium* complex region includes only *embAB* and a putative regulator sequence (*embR*). (Adapted from Telenti A, Philipp WJ, Sreevatsan S, et al. The emb operon, a gene cluster of Mycobacterium tuberculosis involved in resistance to ethambutol. *Nature Med* 1997;3[5]:567–570; Alcaide F, Pfyffer GE, Telenti A. Role of embB in natural and acquired resistance to ethambutol in mycobacteria. *Antimicrob Agents Chemother* 1997;41[10]:2270–2273.)

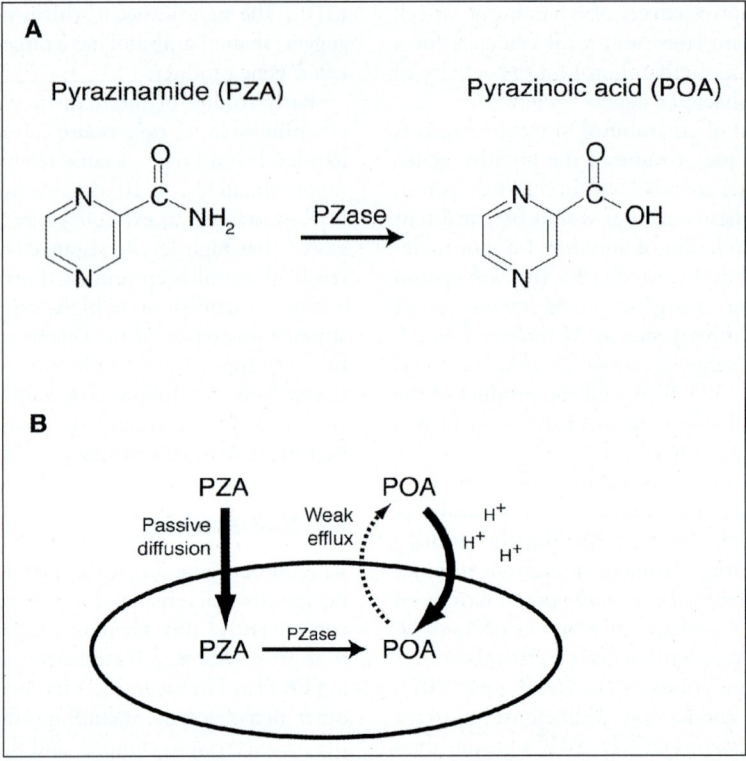

Figure 5.12 ■ **Activation and mobilization of pyrazinamide. A:** Pyrazinamide (PZA) is converted to pyrazinoic acid (POA) by the cytosolic enzyme, pyrazinamidase/nicotinamidase or PZase (encoded by the *pncA* gene). **B:** PZA enters the bacterium by passive diffusion and is converted to POA, which leaves the bacterium by diffusion aided by a weak efflux pump. Under acidic extracellular conditions, approximately 50% of the exported POA may exist in its protonated (i.e., undissociated) form, that is, at a concentration several orders of magnitude higher than intracellular concentration of this form. Thus, protonated POA will readily reenter the cell down this concentration gradient. (Based on a model proposed by Zhang Y, Telenti A. Genetics of drug resistance in *Mycobacterium tuberculosis*. In: Hatfull GF, Jacobs Jr WR, eds. *Molecular genetics of mycobacteria*. Washington, DC: American Society of Microbiology, 2000:235–254.)

increases in the presence of energy uncoupling reagents, that is, azide, rotenone, dicyclohexylcarbodiimide (DCCD). Furthermore, PZA is a prodrug, the active derivative being pyrazinoic acid (or pyrazinecarboxylic acid) (Fig. 5.12A).

The conversion of PZA to pyrazinoic acid was shown to be catalyzed by human enzymes, and thus, it was suggested that PZA activation occurs within the acidic environment of the caseous lesion and phagolysosome (313). However, it was subsequently shown that pyrazinamidase activity in mycobacteria was associated with susceptibility to PZA (314,315); most strains of *M. tuberculosis* that are resistant to PZA lack pyrazinamidase activity.

Thus, PZA activation most likely occurs inside the bacillus. The gene encoding the pyrazinamidase, *pncA*, was later identified in the *M. tuberculosis* genome (316). The product of the *pncA* gene has both pyrazinamidase and nicotinamidase activity, which explains previously reported association between these two enzyme activities (317). Furthermore, Speirs et al. (318) showed that *M. tuberculosis* isolates resistant to PZA were usually still susceptible to the PZA derivatives, pyrazinoic acid and *n*-propyl pyrazinoate, thus supporting the hypothesis that the primary mechanism of inherent resistance in the other mycobacteria involves the lack of an appropriate PZA-modifying enzyme.

The activity of PZA is not only dependent on the presence of a pyrazinamidase but also the organism needs to be in an acidic environment (external pH ≤5) because intracellular accumulation of pyrazinoic acid, but not PZA, is inversely related to the external pH (319). In addition, the relative resistance of *M. smegmatis* to pyrazinoic acid is at least partly the result of active efflux of this compound. Intriguingly, *M. tuberculosis* also has an efflux system for pyrazinoic acid, but this appears to be weak compared to *M. smegmatis* (319).

These findings lead Zhang and Telenti (216) to propose a model of PZA/pyrazinoic acid dynamics in *M. tuberculosis* (Fig. 5.12B). Briefly, PZA enters the bacterium by passive diffusion and is converted to pyrazinoic acid by the *pnc*A pyrazinamidase (PZase). Independent of external pH, the internal pH of *M. tuberculosis* is maintained at approximately pH 7 (319), and thus, pyrazinoic acid will be predominantly (>99.9%) in its dissociated form, $C_4H_3N_2\text{-}COO^-$ (i.e., minus its H^+ ion or proton). Once formed, the pyrazinoic acid diffuses out of the cell (aided by a weak efflux system). If the extracellular and intracellular conditions are comparable (i.e., pH neutral), then the total pyrazinoic acid concentration (ionic and protonated) inside and outside the bacterium will be equivalent. However, if the extracellular environment is acidic, the protonated form of pyrazinoic acid ($C_4H_3N_2\text{-}COOH$) may represent 50% of the total extracellular pyrazinoic acid. Thus, there will be a large concentration gradient of protonated pyrazinoic acid between the outside and the inside of the bacterium (perhaps >1,000-fold), leading to a net intracellular diffusion of this form of pyrazinoic acid. The weak pyrazinoic acid efflux pump of *M. tuberculosis* would have little impact on this influx, and thus, the internal concentration of total pyrazinoic acid will be considerably higher than outside. This model provides a rational explanation for why the activity of PZA and pyrazinoic acid is dependent on an acidic environment.

The inhibitory mechanism of pyrazinoic acid is not known, and attempts to isolate pyrazinoic acid–resistant mutants of *M. tuberculosis* have largely failed. It is likely that this compound affects multiple systems. Zhang et al. (320) demonstrated that pyrazinoic acid disrupts the membrane potential or proton motif force (PMF) of *M. tuberculosis*. This will have a profound effect on processes that depend on the PMF, such as some types of active transmembrane transport (320).

As stated previously, acquired resistance to PZA in *M. tuberculosis* is primarily the result of loss of PZase activity, conferred by mutation in the *pnc*A gene or its promoter. The known resistance-conferring *pnc*A mutations are strewn throughout the gene, and unlike INH resistance–associated *kat*G mutations, there does not seem to be a restricted number of principal genotypes. Interestingly, *M. bovis*, which is intrinsically resistant to PZA and is PZase-negative, has a characteristic polymorphism in the *pnc*A gene (C to G at position 169) leading to a histidine to aspartic acid change at codon 57 (321).

Although there have been reports of PZA-resistant *M. tuberculosis* without *pnc*A mutations, PZA susceptibility testing is problematic and can lead to an inaccurate indication of resistance. Thus, it is unclear whether mutations in other genes are associated with the acquisition of PZA resistance. However, the relatively strong efflux of pyrazinoic acid in intrinsically resistant *M. smegmatis* (319) suggests that mutations that enhance efflux in *M. tuberculosis* may lead to increased resistance to PZA.

Quinolones

Fluoroquinolones (e.g., ciprofloxacin, ofloxacin, levofloxacin, and moxifloxacin) are now considered essential second-line agents for the treatment of *M. tuberculosis* and especially important for the treatment of MDRTB (322). Quinolones are bactericidal for most bacteria and have moderate to excellent bactericidal activity against most, but not all rapidly growing and slowly growing mycobacteria (Table 5.1). The MICs for the aforementioned quinolones against *M. tuberculosis* isolates range from 0.03 to 4 μg/mL, with moxifloxacin being the most active on a per weight basis (323). The MICs of these quinolones are at or below their maximum serum concentrations and all show good tissue penetration, reaching concentrations in lung tissue, especially alveolar macrophages, several times those in serum (324). The elimination half-life is approximately 5 hours for ciprofloxacin, ofloxacin, and levofloxacin and about 14 hours for moxifloxacin. The use of quinolones in the treatment of nontuberculous mycobacteria is best guided by drug susceptibility testing or reliable antibiogram data (Table 5.7). For example, most isolates of *M. fortuitum* are susceptible to ciprofloxacin, whereas there is a high degree of inherent resistance among isolates of *M. chelonae*. Only 30% of MAC isolates are susceptible to ciprofloxacin at 2 μg/mL, and the MIC 90% for MAC is 16 μg/mL (206).

The main target of quinolones is bacterial DNA topoisomerase II (gyrase) and topoisomerase IV, which are enzymes that relax, uncoil, unlink, and recoil DNA during transcription, replication, and recombination. Bacterial DNA gyrase is a bifunctional tetrameric enzyme that consists of two subunits encoded by *gyrA* and *gyrB*. Common mycobacterial pathogens (*M. tuberculosis*, MAC, and *M. abscessus*) appear to only have topoisomerase II but lack a homolog topoisomerase IV (e.g., *grlA* and *grlB*) (166). Other species of mycobacteria appear to have both topoisomerases as do most other bacteria. The binding of quinolones to the gyrase results in the inhibition of mycobacterial DNA synthesis and rapid cell death. Mutations within a conserved region of the *gyrA* (320 bp) and *gyrB* (375 bp) genes, the QRDRs, cause amino acid substitutions within the translated polypeptides and result in resistance to most, if not all, methoxyfluoroquinolones (325–329). However, there is some evidence that natural polymorphisms exist in this region (e.g., codon 95), and these may be associated with low-level natural resistance in some mycobacteria (217,330).

High levels of quinolone resistance in *M. tuberculosis* are most commonly associated with two mutations in the QRDR of *gyrA* or a combination of a mutation in each of the two QRDRs (166). Resistance-associated mutations only in the QRDR of *gyrB* are rare and have unknown clinical significance. Indeed, rather than a role in acquired resistance, the mutations in the QRDR of *gyrB* may be associated with intrinsic, low-level quinolone resistance in mycobacteria. Finally, the frequency of mutations in the QRDRs appears to depend on fluoroquinolone concentration, and mutations within the *gyrA* QRDR may primarily occur at high quinolone concentrations. A possibly related observation is the variable correlation between *gyrA* mutations and phenotypic resistance; that is, quinolone resistance has been attributed to *gyrA* mutations in less than 50% of resistant isolates in some studies but to nearly 100% of isolates in other studies (331–333).

Although the DNA gyrase appears to be the main target of quinolones, there is other evidence for an alternative site of action (334). There also may be alternative mechanisms of quinolone resistance including cell wall permeability, drug efflux, drug inactivation, or subcellular sequestration (335–338).

Oxazolidinones

The oxazolidinones are relatively new antimicrobials that target the ribosome causing an inhibition of protein synthesis. Based on in vitro susceptibilities, several oxazolidinones have activity against slowly growing and rapidly growing mycobacteria (339–344). Linezolid, perhaps the first approved drug in this class, may act synergistically with rifampin, INH, PZA, and moxifloxacin against *M. tuberculosis* (345,346). Several oxazolidinones, including linezolid, were shown to significantly reduce bacterial loading in a murine model of TB (347). Linezolid has been also used "off label" in the treatment of intractable MDRTB (348,349) as well as in the treatment of other human mycobacterioses (119,350).

Oxazolidinones bind to the 50S ribosomal subunit at the P-site and overlap into the A-site blocking formation of the 70S ribosome initiation complex (351–356). This complex is composed of the 50S and 30S subunits, fMet-tRNA, initiating factors (IF1, IF2, and IF2), and the mRNA. Since the initiation complex is a transitory structure, the oxazolidinones are primarily bacteriostatic, not bactericidal. This mode of action is distinct from that of other protein synthesis inhibitors, such as macrolides and aminoglycosides, and thus, oxazolidinone resistance was expected to be distinct. Indeed, in mycobacteria, the mutations associated with linezolid resistance were at residues that do not confer resistance to macrolides and ketolides. Oxazolidinone resistance also has been linked to mutations in *rplC* and *rplD*, which encode for ribosomal proteins, in other bacteria but not as yet in mycobacteria. There are very few studies of oxazolidinone/linezolid resistance in clinical isolates of mycobacteria, partly because of limited use of the drug. In those few studies, resistance was not associated with any of the previously described mechanisms of resistance. Therefore, alternative mechanisms of resistance (e.g., methylation of 23S rRNA) in mycobacteria are suspected but as yet not reported.

p-Aminosalicylic Acid

PAS is active against *M. tuberculosis*; however, nontuberculous mycobacteria and most other microorganisms are considered resistant to this agent. The mechanism of action of PAS in mycobacteria is not entirely clear; however, two targets have been considered: inhibition of folic acid synthesis and inhibition of salicylic acid metabolism (160). PAS inhibits the synthesis of folic acid, and p-aminobenzoic acid reverses the effect of PAS in *M. tuberculosis*. Thus, the mechanism of action of this agent appears to be analogous to that of the sulfonamides and other antifolates (357). Winder

(160) argued, however, that these and other observations indicating that PAS was an antifolate agent could be attributed to effects other than those on folic acid metabolism.

Ratledge and Brown (358) suggested that the mechanism of action of PAS may be to inhibit mycobactin synthesis. Mycobactins are lipid-soluble iron chelators (359) that contain a salicylate or a 6-methylsalicylate moiety; therefore, PAS may act as a salicylate analog and block mycobactin biosynthesis. However, salicylic acid itself may be involved in iron transport, and with mycobactin-dependent strains of *M. smegmatis*, mycobactin does not overcome the effect of PAS (360,361). Brown and Ratledge (361) proposed that PAS interfered with salicylic acid metabolism, perhaps by inhibiting the transfer of iron from mycobactin to the sites of heme synthesis. Winder (160) concluded that the evidence that PAS acts as an antifolate in mycobacteria is inconclusive and, at the same time, there is good evidence that PAS interferes with salicylic acid metabolism but probably not by inhibiting mycobactin synthesis.

The mechanism of PAS resistance is unclear; however, there is evidence that PAS is acetylated by mycobacteria to yield acetyl-PAS, a compound that is not biologically active (362).

Cycloserine

D-Cycloserine (4-amino-3-isooxazolidinone) is a rigid cyclic analog of D-alanine and is active against all mycobacteria as well as a number of other microorganisms. D-Cycloserine irreversibly inhibits pyridoxal phosphate-dependent enzymes and competitively inhibits the enzymes D-alanylalanine synthetase, D-alanine racemase, and D-alanine permease (363). These latter enzymes catalyze the conversion of L-alanine to D-alanine and of D-alanine to D-alanyl-D-alanine. The dipeptide is essential for the biosynthesis of mycobacterial cell walls (peptidoglycan formation), and inhibition of its synthesis leads to lysis and cell death. The effect of D-cycloserine is antagonized by exogenous D-alanine (364,365).

Resistance to D-cycloserine is conferred by overexpression of the D-alanine racemase (encoded by the *alr*A gene) (366), whereas organisms with a defective gene are hypersusceptible to this agent (367). Low-level resistance to D-cycloserine may be conferred by mutations in the D-alanine permease, which is involved in the transport of both D-alanine and D-cycloserine. However, the D-alanine racemase is most likely the primary target for D-cycloserine.

Cross-resistance between D-cycloserine and vancomycin appears to be conferred by alterations in the mycobacterial homolog of the penicillin-binding protein 4 (PBP4) (368), although it is not known if these agents directly inhibit this protein. Other effects of D-cycloserine on mycobacterial cell wall synthesis include the inhibition of D-peptidoglycolipid synthesis in *M. tuberculosis* (37).

Mammalian enzymes such as serine hydroxymethyltransferase are inhibited by D-cycloserine, and these are most likely the targets for the antineoplastic activity of this compound. D-Cycloserine has a high toxic-to-therapeutic ratio for the treatment of mycobacterial disease; therefore, the drug is considered a choice of last resort (369,370). Terizidone consists of two molecules of cycloserine bridged by a terephthalaldehyde. Terizidone has broad-spectrum activity and retains activity against *M. tuberculosis*. Reported adverse events are less than with cycloserine, tolerance is improved, the severity of adverse symptoms is decreased, and the drug has better in vitro activity.

Ethionamide

Isonicotinyl thioamide and a variety of derivatives, including ethionamide (2-ethylpyridine-4-carbonic acid thioamide), collectively referred to as *thioamides* are potent inhibitors of *M. tuberculosis* and certain other mycobacteria. Ethionamide inhibits the synthesis of mycolic acids and stimulates oxidation-reduction reactions. Treated cells lose acid-fastness, and overall, the mechanism of action of ethionamide appears to be identical to that of INH (371). Mutations within the *inhA* gene that confer low-level resistance to INH also confer resistance to ethionamide (162). Furthermore, overexpression of the wild-type *inhA* protein in *M. tuberculosis* increased the MIC of ethionamide. Thus, like INH, the primary target for ethionamide is the *inhA* enzyme (enoyl-ACP reductase). However, unlike for INH, mutations within the *katG* gene do not confer resistance to ethionamide, which explains why most *M. tuberculosis* isolates with clinically acquired INH resistance are still susceptible to ethionamide.

Like INH, ethionamide is a prodrug that is activated by the EtaA/EthA monooxygenase (372,373). The activation pathway of ethionamide is inducible, with Rv3854c gene expression being regulated by an adjacent gene, Rv3855. The proposed activation pathway (Fig. 5.13) may generate a radical similar to the isonicotinic acyl radical derivative of INH. However, it is unclear whether ethionamide-NAD(H)

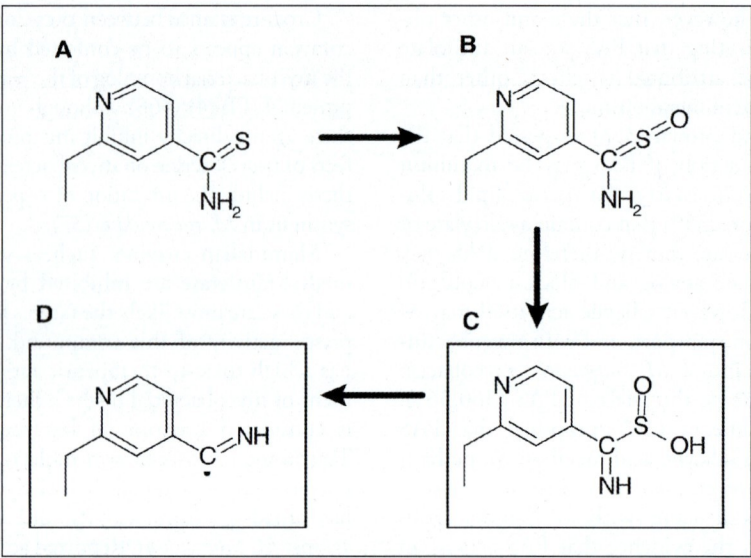

Figure 5.13 ■ **Proposed activation pathway of ethionamide. Ethionamide (A) is converted to ethionamide-S-oxide (B) by the flavin adenine dinucleotide (FAD)–dependent EtaA enzyme (encoded by gene Rv3854bc).** This enzyme then converts the oxide further, possibly to sulfinic acid **(C)** and radical **(D)** species. These later forms are unstable and probably represent the active derivative of ethionamide. (Pathway adapted from DeBarber AE, Mdluli K, Bosman M, et al. Ethionamide activation and sensitivity in multidrug-resistant *Mycobacterium tuberculosis. Proc Nat Acad Sci USA* 2000;97[17]:9677–9682; Metushi IG, Cai P, Zhu X, et al. A fresh look at the mechanism of isoniazid-induced hepatotoxicity. *Clin Pharmacol Ther* 2011;89[6]:911–914.)

adducts are formed. Prothionamide is virtually identical to ethionamide in structure and activity. EtaA also activates thiacetazone, thiocarlide, and thiobenzamide (166). Therefore, mutations in the genes encoding the EtaA/EthA activating enzyme result in resistance to not only ethionamide but also all the thioamides. Mutations that cause a change in the active site of the InhA enzyme confer both ethionamide and INH resistance.

Other Mechanisms of Drug Resistance

In *M. tuberculosis* and most other species of mycobacteria, drug resistance is a consequence of mutations or the accumulation of mutations in target genes or regulatory domains. There is no evidence that drug resistance occurs as a consequence of any mechanism of horizontal transfer of genetic material. Although specific genetic mutations have been identified that result in resistance to first-line and some second-line drugs, the frequencies of these mutations varies over a wide range (Table 5.1). Therefore, it is reasonable to assume there are

alternative mechanisms of resistance or additional unidentified mutations. Zaunbrecher et al. (374) identified mutations in the promoter region of the enhanced intracellular survival (*eis*) protein which cause low-level kanamycin resistance but not amikacin resistance. The *eis* mutation is distinct and different from the *rrs* mutations that cause high-level kanamycin and amikacin resistance, but the *eis*-encoded protein appears to be able to multiacetylate several different aminoglycosides (375). Maus et al. (257) identified a mutation in the *tlyA* gene that confers resistance to capreomycin and viomycin. The *tlyA* gene encodes a putative rRNA methyltransferase that alters the ribosome structure such that capreomycin does not bind (376). It appears that other patterns of *tlyA* and *rrs* mutations can account for various other capreomycin-, viomycin-, kanamycin-, and amikacin-resistant and -susceptible phenotypes that were previously difficult to understand (264,265). The clinical significance of these various mutations awaits further studies.

One mechanism that is well recognized is the inability of many drugs to penetrate the mycobacterial cell wall and membrane. This innate resistance varies with the type of drug and the composition of the cell wall and membrane of the mycobacterium, but it is unlikely that penetrability alone accounts for drug resistance that cannot be ascribed to a mutation. Drug exclusion in mycobacteria is also controlled by the presence of drug efflux pumps that are known to transport INH, fluoroquinolones, aminoglycosides, and tetracyclines (336,377,378). The efflux pumps along with lack of permeability are likely to be the primary mechanisms of low-level resistance. In addition, it appears that efflux pumps contribute to the survival of mycobacteria in the presence of drugs for periods of time sufficient to allow for the accumulation of mutations that confer high-level drug resistance (379,380). As a result, efflux transporters are now recognized as potential targets for new drug development (380).

MULTIPLE AND EXTENSIVELY DRUG-RESISTANT *MYCOBACTERIUM TUBERCULOSIS*

Drug resistance was recognized shortly after the introduction of INH and streptomycin for the treatment of TB in the late 1940s and early 1950s. It was quickly realized that a combination of drugs was the most effective way to prevent the development of resistance. As discussed elsewhere in this chapter, the proportion method of susceptibility testing of *M. tuberculosis* was based on preventing resistance as well as clinical efficacy. Critical concentrations of INH, rifampin, ethambutol, and PZA were defined by a threshold of 10% or 1% of resistance in a population of bacilli isolated from a patient with TB. If, depending on the particular drug, the percentage of resistance was less than 10% or 1% in a population of wild-type tubercle bacilli, it was likely that a patient would respond to a multidrug treatment regimen. Conversely, if the percentage was greater than 10% or 1%, the drug was unlikely to contribute to clinical efficacy.

It is not entirely clear when MDRTB, defined as simultaneous resistance to INH and rifampin, first emerged in the United States or worldwide. Frieden et al. (381) reported that MDRTB in previously untreated patients increased from 3% to 9% during the period from 1982 to 1991. Currently, the worldwide proportion of MDRTB ranges from 0% to less than 3% to 12% or more (382). Extensively drug-resistant tuberculosis (XDRTB) was first defined by the CDC in 2005, but subsequently modified in 2006 (383), to mean resistance to INH and rifampin plus resistance to any fluoroquinolone and at least one of three injectable drugs (amikacin, capreomycin, or kanamycin) (3). It is important to follow this recommended definition in order to ensure uniform surveillance, assist in predicting clinical outcomes, and to facilitate the reproducibility of susceptibility testing. Although there are reports of "pan-resistant" or "totally" resistant *M. tuberculosis*, which refer to isolates that are resistant to all first- and second-line drugs, others recommend against the use of these terms because of the lack of standardized drug susceptibility testing for existing, new, and investigational anti-TB drugs as well as a lack of clinical correlations (384,385).

The genetic basis for the MDRTB and XDRTB phenotypes is the same, that is, the selection of resistance during chemotherapy. Jassal and Bishai (382) described the mechanisms of epidemic drug resistance: (a) acquired resistance by a wild-type susceptible strain during treatment, (b) amplified resistance in already resistant strains because of inappropriate therapy, and (c) transmitted resistance in which the primary infection is with an already resistant strain. Sensitive, specific, reliable, robust, and inexpensive drug susceptibility testing protocols are needed for new and newly identified anti-TB drugs. Although in many cases the mechanisms of resistance for new drugs have been identified, the studies have been with laboratory-derived mutants and the primary objective may have been to help elucidate the drug's mechanism of action. Thus, for most new drugs, it is not clear if resistance that develops during the selective pressure of treatment is or is not the same as the resistance that develops under laboratory conditions.

In response to the emergence and spread of MDRTB and XDRTB, a worldwide effort was begun to identify new or newly identified drugs for the treatment of TB. Although fluoroquinolones were added as second-line drugs in 1982 (ofloxacin), 1992 (gatifloxacin), and 1996 (moxifloxacin), no drugs were added or elevated to the first-line drugs for treating TB. However, it seems likely in the very near future this situation will change. Table 5.12 lists many, but not all, of the new and newly identified drugs with activity against *M. tuberculosis*. Several of the drugs are in various stages of clinical trials. Although there is considerable optimism that some or many of these drugs will be approved and made available for treating drug-resistant *M. tuberculosis*, the timeline is unclear. In the meantime, the WHO and others recommend that drug-resistant TB be treated with combinations of drugs chosen from the groups shown in Table 5.13 (17,386).

Table 5.12

New and Newly Identified Agents with Activity against Wild-Type (Susceptible) and Multidrug-Resistant *Mycobacterium tuberculosis*

Drug Name/Number Mol Wt (MW)	Drug Class	Manufacturer/Sponsor	Mechanism of Action/ Resistance	In Vitro Activity MIC (μg/mL) 90% or Range or as Noted	Reference(s)
PA-824 MW 359.26	Nitroimidazo-oxazine	TB Alliance	Protein and cell wall lipid synthesis inhibitor; stimulates NO production	Mtb^S 0.015–0.25 Mtb^{MDR} 0.03–0.25 Mtb^S 0.0312–0.25	Stover et al. (431) Feuerriegel et al. (432)
Delamanid (OPC-67683) MW 534.48	Nitro-dihydro-imidazo-oxazole	Otsuka Pharmaceutical	Methoxy- and keto-mycolic acid synthesis inhibitor	Mtb^S 0.006–0.024 Mtb^{MDR} 0.006–0.024	Matsumoto et al. (433)
TBA-354 MW 436.34	Nitroimidazole	TB Alliance, Johns Hopkins University	Cell wall synthesis inhibitor; stimulates NO production	Mtb^S 0.034–0.279 Mtb^{MDR} ≤0.017– 0.037	Ma, Z. from Workshop on Clinical Pharmacology of TB Drugs, Preceding 2012 ICAAC Meeting, San Francisco
CPZEN-45 Caprazene MW ~1118	Nucleoside Lipouridyl antibiotic	Microbial Chemistry Research Foundation, Tokyo; Lilly TB Drug Discovery Initiative, etc.	Bacterial translocase inhibitor	Mtb^S 6.25–12.5 Mtb^{MDR} 6.25–12.5	Igarashi et al. (434) Hirano et al. (435)
DC-159a MW 419.42	8-Methoxy-fluoroquinolone	Japan Anti-Tuberculosis Association, Daiichi-Sankyo Pharmaceutical	Gyrase A/gyrA QRDR double mutation	Mtb^S 0.06 Mtb^{MDR} 0.5	Disratthakit and Doi (436) Sekiguchi et al. (437)
SQ609 MW 332.52	Dipiperidine Diamine derivative	Sequella	Cell wall synthesis inhibitor	Mtb^S 6.25–15.6 H37Rv only Mtb^S 4.0	Bogatcheva et al. (438) Bogatcheva (439) Villemagne (440)

Drug / MW	Class	Company	Mechanism	MIC	References
SQ109 MW 330.55	Ethylenediamine	Sequella, NIH	Cell wall inhibitor: membrane transporter of trehalose monomycolate (MmpL3)	Mtb^S and Mtb^{MDR} 0.2–0.52 or 0.63–1.56 μM	Protopopova et al. (441) Tahlan et al. (442)
SQ641 MW 787.2	Capuramycin derivative Nucleoside antibiotic	Sequella, Sankyo	Translocase I inhibitor: peptidoglycan biosynthesis	Mtb^S 4.0	Reddy et al. (443) Bogatcheva et al. (444) Murakami et al. (445)
BTZ043 MW 431.39	Benzothiazinone	New Medicines for Tuberculosis	Cell wall synthesis inhibitor: a 2′-epimerase	Mtb^S and Mtb^{MDR} 0.001–0.004	Villemagne (440)
Sutezolid (PNU-100480) MW 353.41	Oxazolidinone	Pfizer/Upjohn	Protein synthesis inhibitor: 50S unit, initiation	Mtb^S and Mtb^{MDR} 0.0625–0.50	Alffenaar et al. (446)
AZD5847 MW465.4	Oxazolidinone	Astrazeneca	Protein synthesis inhibitor: 50S unit, initiation	NA	Villemagne (440)
Bedaquiline (TMC207) MW 555.50	Diarylquinoline	TB Alliance, Janssen	ATP synthase inhibitor	Mtb^S 0.032–0.1 Mtb^{MDR} 0.032–0.1	Andries et al. (447) Huitric et al. (448)
Gatifloxacin MW 375.39	Fluoroquinolone	Bristol-Meyers Squibb (Gatifloxacin withdrawn from United States and Canada in 2006)	DNA gyrase inhibitor	Mtb^S 0.007–0.12	Villemagne et al. (440)
LL3850, BM212 MW ~350	1,5-diarylpyrrole derivative	Lupin Pharmaceuticals	MmpL3 mycobacterial protein	Mtb^S 0.7–1.5 Based on very limited data	La Rosa et al. (449) Deidda et al. (450) Biava et al. (451)
Imipenem/cilastatin[a]	Carbapenem and stabilizing agent	Merck & Co.	Cell wall synthesis inhibitor	Mtb^S 2–4[b] Mtb^{MDR} 4 (?)	Chambers et al. (452) Watt et al. (453)

[a]There is limited information on the the in vitro activity and clinical efficacy of imipenem against *M. tuberculosis*. The WHO classifies imipenem as a group 5 medication with an "unclear role" in the treatment of drug-resistant *M. tuberculosis*.
[b]MIC determined using continuous dosing to overcome inherent instability of the drug.

Table 5.13

Groups of Drugs to Treat Multiple Drug–Resistant Tuberculosis

Group	Drug	Daily Dose	Notes/Caveats
Group 1 First-line oral drugs	Isoniazid[a] Rifampin[a] Rifabutin Ethambutol (EMB) Pyrazinamide (PZA)	5 mg/kg 10 mg/kg 5 mg/kg 15–25 mg/kg 30 mg/kg	Use all possible but question if DST result is "susceptible" and drug was used in a previous failed regimen. Rifampin resistance often crosses to all rifamycins, i.e., rifabutin.
Group 2 Injectable drugs	Amikacin (AMK) Kanamycin (KAN) Capreomycin (CAP) Streptomycin (SM)	15 mg/kg 15 mg/kg 15 mg/kg 15 mg/kg	Use if DST result is or is likely to be "susceptible." Order of use: AMK > KAN = CAP > SM.
Group 3 Fluoroquinolones	Levofloxacin[b] Moxifloxacin[b] Ofloxacin[b]	15 mg/kg 7.5–10 mg/kg 15 mg/kg	All patients should receive levo- or moxifloxacin if DST result is or is likely to be "susceptible."
Group 4 Oral bacteriostatic second-line drugs	p-Aminosalicylic acid Cycloserine[c] Terizidone[c] Ethionamide Protionamide	150 mg/kg 15 mg/kg 15 mg/kg 15 mg/kg 15 mg/kg	Adverse reactions and interactions can be problematic. Cycloserine and terizidone are equivalent. Ethionamide, protionamide, and other thioamides: resistance caused by loss of EtaA/EthA activating enzyme, not katG.
Group 5	Clofazimine Linezolid Amoxicillin/clavulanate Thioacetazone Imipenem/cilastatin Isoniazid (high dose) Clarithromycin	100 mg 600 mg 875/125 mg/12 h 150 mg 500–1,000 mg/6 h 10–15 mg/kg 500 mg/12 h	Drugs in this group have an unclear role in the treatment of MDRTB. May be considered "salvage therapy" for XDRTB.

[a]Although it is assumed that MDRTB is resistant to isoniazid and rifampin, repeat drug susceptibility testing should be considered if the treatment history is unknown or unclear and/or previous drug susceptibility test results are not available and an isolate is available for testing. Also, rifampin resistance alone may be used as a surrogate for MDR (e.g., Xpert MTB/RIF test) and an isolate may remain susceptible to isoniazid.
[b]Approximately 50% of ofloxacin-resistant isolates may be susceptible to moxifloxacin or high-dose levofloxacin. Moxifloxacin is reported to have better sterilizing activity than standard-dose levofloxacin.
[c]Terizidone consists of two molecules of cycloserine and one molecule of terephthalaldehyde. The mechanisms of action are identical and the MICs are similar. The maximum serum concentration is higher and the half-life is longer for terizidone than for cycloserine. Adverse effects of terizidone are less but similar in nature to cycloserine.
DST, drug susceptibility testing; MDRTB, multidrug-resistant tuberculosis; XDRTB, extensively drug-resistant tuberculosis.
Table adapted from World Health Organization. *Treatment of tuberculosis: guidelines.* Geneva: World Health Organization, 2010; Caminero JA, Sotgiu G, Zumla A, et al. Best drug treatment for multidrug-resistant and extensively drug-resistant tuberculosis. *Lancet Infect Dis* 2010;10(9):621–629.

ASSAYS FOR ACTIVITY IN BIOLOGIC FLUIDS

The first-line TB drugs (i.e., INH, rifampin, PZA, and ethambutol) have predictable pharmacokinetic features when patients comply with standard doses and frequencies, for example, DOT. Certain second-line drugs (i.e., ethionamide, cycloserine, capreomycin, PAS) have a narrow therapeutic window compared with the first-line drugs and there may be a greater need for monitoring those agents (14). In addition, there are a variety of

other reasons to measure the concentrations of antimycobacterial drugs in biologic fluids, especially serum, including (a) in compliant patients who have not adequately responded to treatment; (b) to prevent toxicity reactions that occur with drugs such as aminoglycosides and cycloserine; (c) to monitor patient compliance; (d) to monitor the metabolism of certain drugs, such as in the assessment of INH acetylator phenotype; and (e) for research purposes. Patients with malabsorption syndromes, renal impairment (the excretion of INH, rifampin, and PAS is relatively unaffected by renal impairment), or liver function abnormalities; patients who are not responsive to therapy for disease caused by susceptible isolates; or patients with particularly serious disease may require monitoring to assess the toxicity or efficacy of a treatment regimen. MDRTB and patients with impaired intestinal absorption (e.g., AIDS patients) fit these aforementioned criteria (387,388). Therapeutic drug monitoring is routinely performed in all cases of MDRTB at the National Jewish Center for Immunology and Respiratory Medicine, in order to ensure that maximal concentration levels exceed the MICs of the infecting *M. tuberculosis* (389) (Table 5.14). At the same time, there are reasons to restrict the testing of first-line drugs, including the time required to obtain a proper specimen, specimen transport, test and report, results, and cost.

Again, in the vast majority of cases of TB and nontuberculous infections, there is no need or only an infrequent need to measure the levels of antimycobacterial agents in serum, that is, for therapeutic drug monitoring. Because the need is infrequent, procedures such as those described here are best performed in specialized and experienced reference laboratories. Also, it is important to point out that these procedures are based on published information and that other proprietary procedures used in reference laboratories are likely to differ from these procedures or are modified for use with other body fluids or sera that contain other drugs.

In the past, the accurate measurement of antimycobacterial drugs in biologic fluids and tissues was confounded by (a) the use of time-consuming methods with inadequate lower limits of detection; (b) reliance on bioassays that failed to distinguish metabolites or required the withholding of components of a multiple drug treatment regimen; (c) metabolism of the drug; and (d) interaction of the drug, especially protein binding. Many of these problems have been overcome with the development of new chromatographic and nonchromatographic methods for the identification and quantitation of virtually all of the primary and secondary antimycobacterial agents. Holdiness (390) has reviewed the analytical methodology, and Holdiness (391) and Peloquin (389) have reviewed the pharmacology of antimycobacterial agents.

There are three analytical methods for measuring the concentrations of antituberculous agents in biologic material: (a) HPLC and other chromatographic methods, (b) spectrophotometric and fluorometric methods, and (c) bioassays. Serum should be collected at the time of peak concentration.

However, there are a variety of factors that may influence the absorption and bioavailability of these drugs, including surgical procedures, food, and pharmacologic formulations. In addition to the problems created by the simultaneous administration of several drugs, the metabolism of antimycobacterial agents can vary considerably from patient to patient. Most of the metabolites of antimycobacterial drugs lack antimicrobial activity; however, there are important exceptions; that is, desacetylrifampin, the acetylated and glycylated forms of PAS, and the sulfoxide metabolites of ethionamide are active against *M. tuberculosis*.

Sample Timing and Preparation

Peloquin (392) has provided a general guide for the timing of samples for therapeutic drug monitoring of the first-line agents. Peak levels have the most meaning, and trough levels are usually impossible because the levels are below the limit of detection of the available assays. Peloquin (392) recommends to obtain two samples, the first at 2 hours (3 hours for ethambutol and rifabutin) and the second at 6 hours following a dose. Typically, the level at 2 hours is substantially higher than at 6 hours and malabsorption should be suspected if the levels are low or undetectable at both time points. Delayed absorption might be indicated if the level at 6 hours is higher than at 2 hours. Finally, there is insufficient information about the pharmacokinetics and pharmacodynamics of first-line agents in humans to identify precise targets such as the ratio of C_{max} to MIC or time above the MIC (392). Improper specimen preparation can result in the loss of drug activity as a consequence of protein binding or conversion of drugs to inactive or labile derivatives. Deproteination of serum samples is necessary to ensure the stability of INH even at $-20°C$ because in the presence of protein, INH activity is rapidly lost as a consequence of irreversible protein binding. Furthermore, protein frequently interferes with fluorometric methods for the detection and quantitation of INH. Depending on the analytical method, protein can be removed by treatment with 5% to 10% trichloroacetic acid or ammonium sulfate. The protein should be extracted on the day the sample is obtained, and the sample can then be stored at 4°C for up to 2 weeks or frozen at $-20°C$ (or lower) for indefinite periods. Samples collected for rifampin analysis should be treated with ascorbic acid and then stored at $-20°C$ for up to 3 months. Ethambutol, PZA,

(continued on page 228)

Table 5.14

Activity of Antimycobacterial Agents			
Agent	**MIC 50% (µg/mL)**	**MIC 90% (µg/mL)**	**Reference**
M. abscessus			
Erythromycin	8	>8	454
Amoxicillin-clavulanate	64	64	455
Azithromycin	2	8	454
Cefmetazole	32	64	455
Cefoxitin	32	64	455
Clarithromycin	0.125	0.25	454
Imipenem	8	16	455
Linezolid	32	64	344
Roxithromycin	0.5	2	454
M. asiaticum			
Cycloserine	30	—	456
Ethambutol	5–10	—	456
Isoniazid	5	—	456
Kanamycin	5	—	456
Streptomycin	10	—	456
M. avium complex			
Amifloxacin	10	≥16	457,458
Amikacin	4	16	108,267
Ampicillin	8	16	459
Azithromycin	16	32–16	108,460
Capreomycin	4–8	12	267,461
Ciprofloxacin	4–8	≥16	108
Clarithromycin	2	4	458,460
Clofazimine	—	1	462
Cycloserine	—	50	456
Erythromycin	32	64	463
Ethambutol	4	8	108,456
Ethionamide	4	—	456
Gatifloxacin	8	16	464
Gentamicin	4–8	—	465
Imipenem	8–16	≥32	459
Isoniazid	R	R	456
Kanamycin	4	12	456
Linezolid	32	64	342
Moxifloxacin	2	4	464
Minocycline	>25	>25	463
Norfloxacin	16	>16	466

Table 5.14 *(Continued)*

Activity of Antimycobacterial Agents

Agent	MIC 50% (µg/mL)	MIC 90% (µg/mL)	Reference
Ofloxacin	8	>16	462
p-Aminosalicylic acid	R	R	461
Pyrazinamide	R	R	456
Rifabutin	0.25	2	462
Rifampin	4	≥8	456
Streptomycin	4–8	8	456
Sulfisoxazole	10	20	465
Vancomycin	25	>25	457
M. bovis			
Capreomycin	—	10	456
Cycloserine	—	30	456
Ethambutol	—	5–10	456
Ethionamide	—	5–10	456
Isoniazid	0.2	0.2–1	456
Kanamycin	—	5–10	(456)
p-Aminosalicylic acid	—	2–10	456
Pyrazinamide	R	R	456
Rifampin	—	1	456
Streptomycin	—	2	456
M. bovis-BCG			
Capreomycin	—	10	456
Cycloserine	—	≥30	456
Ethambutol	—	5	456
Ethionamide	5	—	456
Isoniazid	0.2	0.2–1	456
Kanamycin	—	5	456
p-Aminosalicylic acid	—	2	456
Pyrazinamide	R	R	456
Rifampin	—	1	456
Streptomycin	—	2	456
M. celatum			
Gatifloxacin	1	1	464
Moxifloxacin	1	1	464
M. chelonae			
Amoxicillin/clavulanate	64	64	455
Amikacin	1	1	467
Azithromycin	1	2	454
Cefoxitin	≥256	≥256	100,455

(Continued)

Table 5.14 *(Continued)*

Activity of Antimycobacterial Agents

Agent	MIC 50% (µg/mL)	MIC 90% (µg/mL)	Reference
Cefmetazole	≥256	≥256	455
Ciprofloxacin	12	12	457
Clarithromycin	0.125	0.125	454
Clofazimine	1	1	468
Cycloserine	R	R	456
Erythromycin	2	8	454
Ethambutol	R	R	456
Ethionamide	R	R	456
Gatifloxacin	4	8	464
Gentamicin	8	32	100
Imipenem	16	32	455
Isoniazid	R	R	456
Linezolid	8	16	344
Moxifloxacin	8	16	464
Minocycline	>25	>25	457
Norfloxacin	8	>16	466
Ofloxacin	12	50	469
p-Aminosalicylic acid	R	R	456
Pyrazinamide	R	R	456
Rifabutin	2	4	467
Rifampin	8	>8	456
Roxithromycin	1	2	454
Tobramycin	8	16	100
Trimethoprim	>16	>16	100
Vancomycin	25	>25	457
M. flavescens			
Capreomycin	—	10	456
Cycloserine	30	—	456
Ethambutol	5	—	456
Ethionamide	R	R	456
Gatifloxacin	0.06	0.06	464
Isoniazid	1	5	456
Kanamycin	—	5	456
Moxifloxacin	0.06	0.06	464
p-Aminosalicylic acid	R	R	456
Pyrazinamide	R	R	456
Rifampin	1	—	456
Streptomycin	2	>10	456

Table 5.14 (Continued)

Activity of Antimycobacterial Agents

Agent	MIC 50% (μg/mL)	MIC 90% (μg/mL)	Reference
M. fortuitum			
Amikacin	1	8	100
Azithromycin	8	>8	454
Capreomycin	16	16	100
Cefoxitin	32	64	455
Ciprofloxacin	1	2	457
Clarithromycin	2	4	454
Clofazimine	0.5	0.5	468
Cycloserine	R	R	456
Doxycycline	8	32	100
Erythromycin	6	>25	457
Ethambutol	16	≥64	100
Ethionamide	R	R	456
Gatifloxacin	0.25	0.25	464
Gentamicin	8	16	100
Imipenem	2	4	455
Isoniazid	R	R	456
Kanamycin	5–10	—	456
Minocycline	4	16	100
Moxifloxacin	0.25	0.5	464
Linezolid	4	16	344
Norfloxacin	1	4	466
p-Aminosalicylic acid	R	R	456
Pyrazinamide	R	R	456
Rifabutin	1	2	467
Rifampin	R	R	456
Roxithromycin	4	>8	454
Streptomycin	R	R	456
Sulfamethoxazole	5	152	100
Tetracycline	8	16	100
Tobramycin	16	32	100
Vancomycin	32–64	≥64	457
M. gastri			
Capreomycin	10	—	456
Cycloserine	30	—	456
Ethambutol	5	—	456
Ethionamide	5	—	456
Isoniazid	—	5	456

(Continued)

Table 5.14 *(Continued)*

Activity of Antimycobacterial Agents

Agent	MIC 50% (µg/mL)	MIC 90% (µg/mL)	Reference
Kanamycin	5	—	456
p-Aminosalicylic acid	R	R	456
Pyrazinamide	R	R	456
Rifampin	1	—	456
Streptomycin	2	—	456
M. gordonae			
Capreomycin	10	—	456
Cycloserine	30	—	456
Ethambutol	5	—	456
Ethionamide	R	—	456
Gatifloxacin	0.5	1	464
Isoniazid	5	—	456
Kanamycin	—	5	456
Linezolid	≤2	4	342
Moxifloxacin	0.25	0.5	464
p-Aminosalicylic acid	R	R	456
Pyrazinamide	R	R	456
Rifabutin	0.5	0.5	456
Rifampin	1	1	456
Streptomycin	10	—	456
M. immunogenum			
Linezolid	32	50	344
M. haemophilum			
Rifabutin	≤0.03	≤0.03	470
Rifampin	0.5	1	470
Clarithromycin	≤0.25	≤0.25	470
Erythromycin	2	4	470
Azithromycin	4	8	470
Clofazimine	2	2	470
Amikacin	4	4	470
Ciprofloxacin	2	8	470
Ofloxacin	4	8	470
Sparfloxacin	2	4	470
Isoniazid	8	>32	470
M. intracellulare			
Ciprofloxacin	1	2	471
Gatifloxacin	4	4	464
Moxifloxacin	1	2	464
Isoniazid	50	>100	472

Table 5.14 (Continued)

Activity of Antimycobacterial Agents

Agent	MIC 50% (μg/mL)	MIC 90% (μg/mL)	Reference
Ofloxacin	4	12	471,472
Rifabutin	0.25	1	473
Rifampin	≥2	>2	472
Rifapentine	0.5	2	473
Streptomycin	25	>100	472
M. kansasii			
Amifloxacin	2	4	457
Amikacin	2	4	467
Capreomycin	10		456
Ciprofloxacin	4	8	457,474
Cycloserine	—	20–30	456
Erythromycin	3	6	457
Ethambutol	5	10	456
Ethionamide		5 (68)	456
Gatifloxacin	1	4	464
Isoniazid	1	5	456
Kanamycin	R	R	456
Minocycline	6	12	456
Linezolid	≤2	≤2	456
Moxifloxacin	0.125	2	464
Norfloxacin	8	16	466
Ofloxacin	2	3	472
p-Aminosalicylic acid	—	5–10	456
Pyrazinamide	R	R	456
Rifabutin	0.5	1	467
Rifampin	—	0.5–1	456
Streptomycin	12	50	456
Vancomycin	12	50	457
M. kansasii (rifampin-resistant)			
Rifabutin	2	>16	475
Isoniazid	1	16	475
Streptomycin	2	4	475
Amikacin	4	8	475
Ciprofloxacin	1	2	475
Clarithromycin	≤0.125	≤0.25	475
Sulfamethoxazole	≤1	4	475
M. malmoense			
Amikacin	—	4	135
Capreomycin	10	—	456

(Continued)

Table 5.14 *(Continued)*

Activity of Antimycobacterial Agents

Agent	MIC 50% (µg/mL)	MIC 90% (µg/mL)	Reference
Ciprofloxacin	—	2–4	135
Cycloserine	30	—	456
Ethambutol	5–10	—	456
Ethionamide	5	—	456
Gatifloxacin	0.25	0.25	464
Moxifloxacin	0.25	0.25	464
Isoniazid	R	R	456
Kanamycin	5	—	456
p-Aminosalicylic acid	R	R	456
Pyrazinamide	R	R	456
Rifampin	1	—	456
Streptomycin	2	—	456
M. marinum			
Amifloxacin	12.5	25	457
Amikacin	1	2	467
Capreomycin	—	10	456
Ciprofloxacin	1	2	457
Cycloserine	—	30	393
Doxycycline	4	4	476
Erythromycin	—	>25	457
Ethambutol	—	5	393
Ethionamide	—	5	393
Gatifloxacin	4	8	340
Gentamicin	20	40	141
Isoniazid	R	R	393
Kanamycin	2	5	456
Linezolid	≤2	2	340,342
Moxifloxacin	4	8	340
Minocycline	2	8	476
Pyrazinamide	R	R	456
Rifabutin	0.25	0.5	467
Rifampin	1	1	456
Streptomycin	—	10	456
Tetracycline	4	16	476
Tobramycin	32	64	476
Vancomycin	>25	>25	457
M. mucogenicum			
Linezolid	4	100	344

Table 5.14 *(Continued)*

Activity of Antimycobacterial Agents

Agent	MIC 50% (µg/mL)	MIC 90% (µg/mL)	Reference
M. scrofulaceum			
Amikacin	1	8	467
Capreomycin	10	—	456
Ciprofloxacin	4	8	467
Cycloserine	30	—	456
Ethambutol	10	—	456
Ethionamide	10	—	393
Gatifloxacin	1	1	464
Isoniazid	R	R	393
Kanamycin	5	—	393
Moxifloxacin	1	1	464
Pyrazinamide	R	R	456
Rifabutin	<0.12	<0.12	467
Rifampin	1	≥2	467
Streptomycin	10	—	393
M. simiae			
Cycloserine	30	—	456
Ethambutol	R	R	456
Ethionamide	R	R	456
Isoniazid	R	R	456
Kanamycin	R	R	456
Linezolid	32	>32	342
Pyrazinamide	R	R	456
Rifabutin	R	R	477
Rifampin	R	R	456
Streptomycin	R	R	456
M. szulgai			
Capreomycin	10	—	456
Cycloserine	30	—	456
Ethambutol	5	—	456
Isoniazid	5	—	456
Linezolid	≤2	4	342
Pyrazinamide	R	R	456
Rifampin	1	—	456
Streptomycin	4	10	456
M. terrae complex			
Capreomycin	10	—	456
Cycloserine	30	—	456

(Continued)

Table 5.14 *(Continued)*

Activity of Antimycobacterial Agents

Agent	MIC 50% (µg/mL)	MIC 90% (µg/mL)	Reference
Ethambutol	5–10	—	456
Gatifloxacin	0.25	32	464
Isoniazid	R	—	456
Moxifloxacin	0.25	16	464
Linezolid	16	32	342
Pyrazinamide	R	R	456
Rifabutin	0.5	R	456
Rifampin	1	1	456
Streptomycin	10	—	456
M. triplex			
Linezolid	≤4	8	342
M. triviale			
Capreomycin	10	—	456
Cycloserine	30	—	456
Ethionamide	5	—	456
Isoniazid	R	R	456
Kanamycin	—	5	456
Pyrazinamide	R	R	456
Rifampin	—	1	456
Streptomycin	—	2	456
M. tuberculosis (susceptible wild type)			
Amifloxacin	4	8	471
Amikacin	0.5	1	467
Azithromycin	>8	>8	478
Capreomycin	2	2	456,479
Ceftizoxime	64	>64	480
Ciprofloxacin	2	4	471
Clarithromycin	>10	>10	478,481
Clinafloxacin	0.125	0.25	478
Cycloserine	—	30	393
Difloxacin	4	8	480
Erythromycin	>25	>25	457
Ethambutol	2.5	5	393
Ethionamide	—	5	393
Gatifloxacin	0.25	0.25	343,482
Isoniazid	0.2	1	472
Kanamycin	2	4	393,479
Linezolid	0.5	1	343

Table 5.14 *(Continued)*

Activity of Antimycobacterial Agents

Agent	MIC 50% (μg/mL)	MIC 90% (μg/mL)	Reference
Levofloxacin	0.25	2	478,483
Minocycline	>25	>25	457
Moxifloxacin	≤0.25	1	478
Norfloxacin	4	8	466
Ofloxacin	0.5	1	471,478
p-Aminosalicylic acid	—	2	393
Pyrazinamide	—	25	456
Rifabutin	0.5	1	477,478
Rifampin	1	2	472
Sparfloxacin	0.25	0.5	474
Streptomycin	0.5	2	472,479
Vancomycin	25	>25	457
Viomycin	0.5	1	479
M. tuberculosis (resistant)			
Azithromycin	>8	>8	478
Ciprofloxacin	0.25	0.5	478
Clarithromycin	>8	>8	478
Clinafloxacin	0.125	0.5	478
Levofloxacin	0.25	0.25	478
Linezolid	0.5	1	339
Ofloxacin	0.5	1	478
Sparfloxacin	0.06	0.125	478
M. tuberculosis (multidrug-resistant)			
Azithromycin	>8	>8	478
Ciprofloxacin	2	4	478
Clarithromycin	>8	>8	478
Clinafloxacin	1	2	478
Levofloxacin	2	4	478
Ofloxacin	4	8	478
Sparfloxacin	0.5	1	478
M. ulcerans			
Amikacin	<0.12	0.25	467
Ciprofloxacin	0.25	0.5	467
Rifabutin	<0.12	<0.12	467
Rifampin	<0.12	<0.12	467
M. xenopi			
Amifloxacin	25	>25	457
Capreomycin	—	10	456

(Continued)

Table 5.14 *(Continued)*

Activity of Antimycobacterial Agents

Agent	MIC 50% (μg/mL)	MIC 90% (μg/mL)	Reference
Ciprofloxacin	1	4	457
Cycloserine	30	—	456
Ethambutol	5	—	456
Ethionamide	—	5	456
Gatifloxacin	0.06	0.06	464
Isoniazid	0.2	1	456
Kanamycin	—	5	456
Minocycline	25	>25	457
Moxifloxacin	0.06	0.06	464
Norfloxacin	2	8	466
p-Aminosalicylic acid	2	—	456
Pyrazinamide	R	R	456
Rifabutin	—	1	477
Rifampin	—	1	456
Streptomycin	—	2	456
Vancomycin	25	>25	457

R, resistant at all concentrations tested.

pyrazinoic acid, ethionamide, and prothionamide are unlikely to be affected by either protein binding or oxidation, and samples can be stored frozen for indefinite periods. Samples collected for PAS determination should first be chromatographed on a weak cation-exchange column to remove the breakdown product *m*-aminophenol, which can interfere with certain assays. Thiacetazone is acid labile but is stable at −20°C if extracted with ethyl acetate. Alternatively, thiacetazone can be completely hydrolyzed with 2 mol/L HCl to the stable hydrolysis product p-aminobenzaldehyde. There is little information about the stability of the other primary and secondary antituberculous drugs.

Assays

Bioassays and certain nonchromatographic assays for measuring the concentrations of INH, ethionamide, ethambutol, and rifampin in biologic fluids and tissues have been described (393). By and large, bioassays are both sensitive and inexpensive but require experience, frequently take several days to complete, and are relatively imprecise. Furthermore, bioassays cannot distinguish between the various species of active and inactive metabolites. The remainder of this section contains descriptions of relatively new methods

for detecting and quantifying antimycobacterial drugs and the clinically important metabolites of these drugs. The emphasis is on HPLC methods, which is the most common method for measuring therapeutic serum or plasma concentrations of probably most antiinfective agents. It is beyond the scope of this chapter to provide detailed information about these methods. Indeed, the accurate and precise measurement of antimycobacterial agents is a subspecialty within the field of clinical mycobacteriology and an area of expertise for a relatively small number of investigators. Simple and convenient qualitative methods for detecting INH, PAS, PZA, cycloserine, ethionamide, and ethambutol in urine are described at the end of this section. These latter methods are primarily designed for monitoring patient adherence to treatment.

Isoniazid

INH or isonicotinic acid hydrazide is metabolized to a variety of products, as shown in Figure 5.14. Acetylation of INH is the primary and clinically most significant pathway of metabolism. The major products of INH metabolism are *N*-acetylisoniazid, pyruvic hydrazone, α-ketoglutaric hydrazone, isonicotinic acid, isonicotinoyl glycine, monoacetylhydrazine, and 1,2-diacetylhydrazine. The enzyme NAT

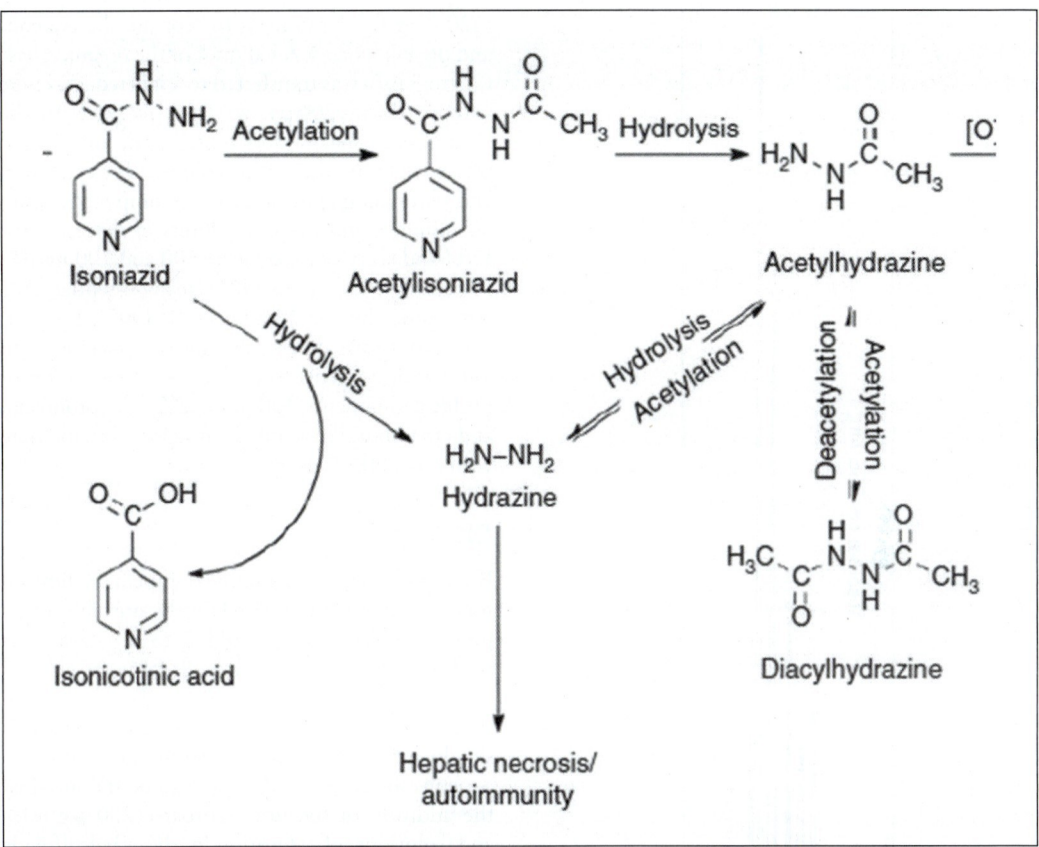

Figure 5.14 ■ Proposed isoniazid metabolic pathways. The acetylation of isoniazid is a reflection of differences in pharmacogenomics, that is, "fast" and "slow" acetylators. Acetylhydrazine and hydrazine are considered the primary cause of isoniazid-associated hepatotoxicity. (Adapted from Metushi IG, Cai P, Zhu X, et al. A fresh look at the mechanism of isoniazid-induced hepatotoxicity. *Clin Pharmacol Ther* 2011;89[6]:911–914.)

(EC 2.3.1.5) catalyzes the acetylation reaction and is located primarily in the liver and intestine. The activity of NAT can vary significantly from person to person, with a bimodal distribution within populations, and genetic analysis showed that the distribution of enzyme activity type is autosomal and dominant (394).

None of these metabolites of INH possesses antimicrobial activity; however, monoacetylhydrazine is considered hepatotoxic when hydroxylated by the cytochrome P450 mixed-function oxidase. Nevertheless, individuals with a rapid INH acetylator phenotype do not appear to be at greater risk for hepatotoxicity (395,396). The level of NAT in a patient (acetylator status) does influence the concentration of monoacetylhydrazine and diacetylhydrazine in the urine, and this is the basis for assays to determine the acetylator status (phenotype) of patients (397–399).

Several HPLC assays for measuring the concentrations of INH and acetylisoniazid in fluids and tissues have been described (397,400–404). The specific assay that is used to measure INH and/or acetylisoniazid may depend on the purpose of the assay. The method of El-Sayed and Islam (397) was used to specifically measure the concentrations of INH and acetylisoniazid in urine for acetylator phenotyping (Fig. 5.15), and the assays described by Moulin et al. (405) used small volumes of serum and may be particularly useful for testing pediatric patients. In a typical assay, Saxena et al. (406) measured INH and acetylisoniazid in serum and urine using a Bondapak C_{18} column and a mobile phase of methanol/water (3:2), with dioctyl sodium sulfosuccinate as the ion-pairing reagent. The lower limit of detection for this assay was 200 ng for INH and 50 ng for acetylisoniazid, using 1-benzoyl-2-isonicotinoylhydrazine as the internal standard. Moulin et al. (405) used a μBondapak C_{18} column and nicotinic amide as the internal standard (Fig. 5.13). The mobile phase was 5% methanol/95% 0.1 mol/L

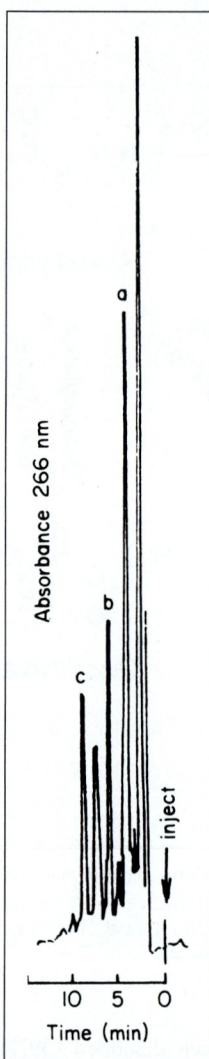

Absorbance 266 nm

a

b

c

inject

10   5   0
Time (min)

Figure 5.15 ■ **Liquid chromatogram of a patient's urine sample (slow acetylator) in which the isoniazid concentration is 36.5 µg/mL and the N-acetylisoniazid concentration is 63.5 µg/mL (inactivation index of 1.7).** *Peak a, N-acetylisoniazid; peak b, internal standard; peak c, isoniazid.* (Adapted from El-Sayed YM, Islam SI. Acetylation phenotyping of isoniazid using a simple and accurate high-performance liquid chromatography. *J Clin Phar Ther* 1989;14:197–205.)

KH$_2$PO$_4$, pH 6.9, degassed and run in an isocratic mode at 2 mL/minute. The serum sample was prepared by adding 2.5 µg of internal standard to 500 µL of serum in a 10-mL, screw-capped, glass tube. The mixture was treated in gradual increments with 150 µL of 0.1 mol/L NaOH and 0.5 g of (NH$_2$)$_2$SO$_4$, with gentle shaking. The mixture was shaken with 3 mL of chloroform and centrifuged

(520 × g for 5 minutes) to separate the aqueous and organic phases. An aliquot of the organic phase (2.5 to 3 mL) was transferred to a tapered glass tube and mixed with 200 µL of 0.05 mol/L H$_2$SO$_4$. The mixture was shaken and centrifuged, and 30 µL was loaded onto the HPLC column. The extraction and chromatography steps were completed within 30 minutes, and the lower limits of detection for INH and acetylisoniazid were 300 and 100 ng/µL, respectively. Holdiness (401), using essentially the same procedure as Moulin et al. (405), found it necessary to use dioctyl sodium sulfosuccinate (an ion-pairing reagent) to achieve good separation of profile components. Rifampin, PZA, streptomycin, and ethambutol have not been reported to interfere with these HPLC assays.

Rifampin

Rifampin or 3-(4-methyl-1-piperazinyliminomethyl) rifamycin is a relatively unstable compound in water, and at pH 2 to 3, rifampin is readily hydrolyzed to 3-formylrifamycin SV and 1-amino-4-methylpiperazine. At alkaline pH, in the presence of atmospheric oxygen, rifampin is slowly oxidized to rifampin-quinone. However, aqueous solutions of rifampin can be stabilized by the addition of sodium ascorbate (200 µg/mL), and solutions of rifampin in dimethylsulfoxide (10 mg/mL) are stable for several weeks. Rifampin is metabolized in the liver to yield 25-O-desacetylrifampin, which is readily excreted by the biliary system. In urine, rifampin is hydrolyzed to yield 3-formylrifampin (407). The pathways of rifampin metabolism are shown in Figure 5.16. Desacetylrifampin is the major metabolite of rifampin; the other metabolites are infrequently detected in fluids or tissues. Cocchiara et al. (408) showed that the major urinary metabolite of rifabutin, a spiropiperidylrifamycin with broad-spectrum antimycobacterial activity (including activity against rifampin-resistant *M. tuberculosis*), was 25-O-desacetylrifabutin; the minor metabolites of rifabutin were oxidized and oxidized/deacetylated forms of 25-O-desacetylrifabutin.

Ratti et al. (409) described a reverse-phase HPLC method for the quantitation of rifampin and 25-O-desacetylrifampin in serum. In this method, 0.5 mL of heparinized serum was added to a tube with butyl-*p*-hydroxybenzoate in acetonitrile/2-propanol (1:1) as an internal standard. The mixture was diluted 1:10 with 1 mol/L KH$_2$PO$_4$ containing 1 mg/mL sodium ascorbate and adjusted to pH 4 with 1 N HCl. The sample was extracted into 15 mL of ethyl acetate and the phases were

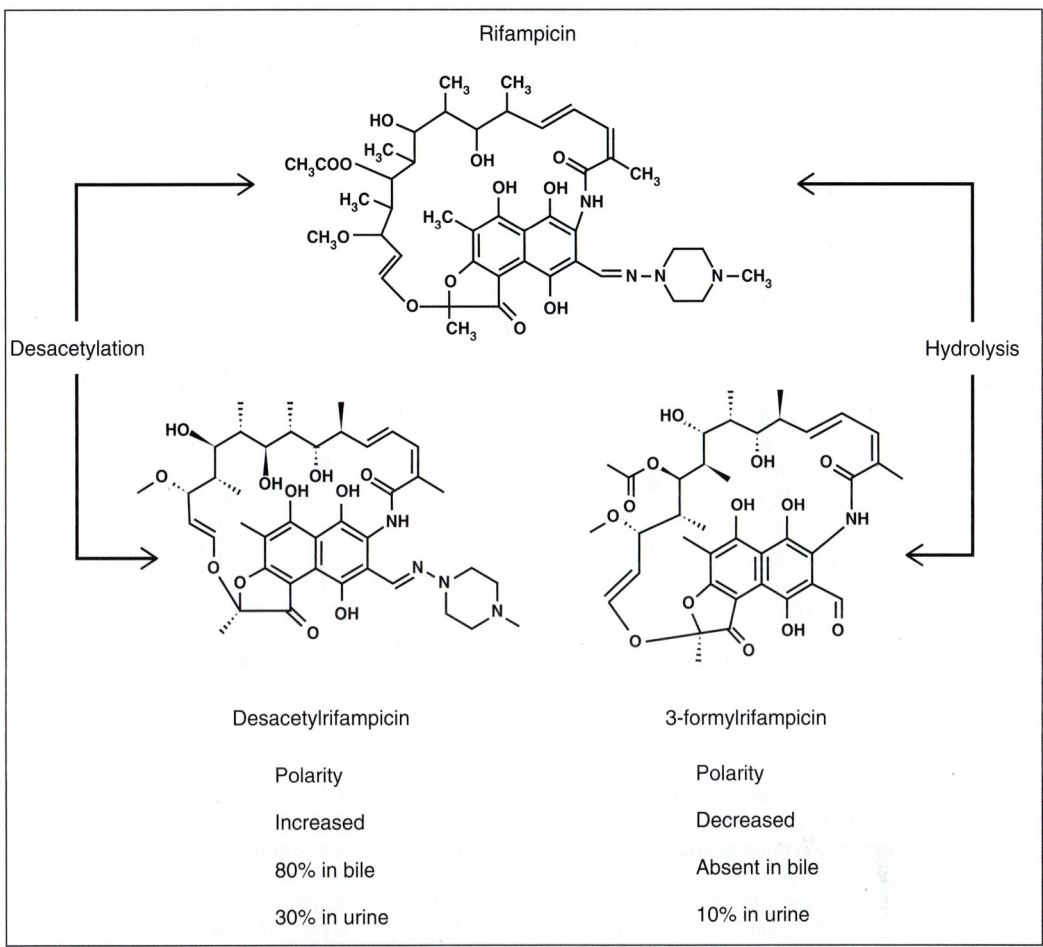

Figure 5.16 ■ Principal metabolic derivatives of rifampin in humans, polarity, and percentage recovery in bile and urine. (Adapted from Holdiness MR. Clinical pharmacokinetics of the antituberculosis drugs. *Clin Pharmacokinet* 1984;9:511–544.)

separated by centrifugation. The organic phase was concentrated by evaporation under a stream of nitrogen, resuspended in 3.5 mL of 90% aqueous acetonitrile, and then extracted with 3 mL of *n*-heptane. The *n*-heptane phase was discarded, the acetonitrile phase was concentrated by evaporation under a stream of nitrogen, and the residue was resuspended in 25 to 100 μL of acetonitrile/2-propanol (1:1) and loaded onto the HPLC column. The column was a 10-m RP-8 column (Brownlee Laboratories, Santa Clara, CA) using an isocratic mobile phase of 0.1 mol/L KH_2PO_4, pH 3.5, with 0.2 mol/L H_3PO_4 and acetonitrile. The conditions varied slightly depending on the type of instrument, and compounds were detected by ultraviolet (UV) absorbance at 254 nm. The method allowed for the separation of rifampin, 25-*O*-desacetylrifampin, 3-formylrifamycin SV, 3-formyl-25-*O*-

desacetylrifamycin, and *N*-desmethylrifampicin with a sensitivity of 0.2 μg/mL.

Ishii and Ogata (410) described an improved HPLC method that used a single extraction step and detection at 340 nm (Fig. 5.17). In this method, 3 mL of heparinized blood was drawn directly into a tube containing 10 mg of ascorbic acid. The plasma was separated and stored at −20°C in the dark. To an aliquot of 0.5 mL of plasma was added 2 mL of 0.5 mol/L phosphate buffer, pH 7.2, containing 100 L of papaverine HCl (20 μg/mL) as an internal standard. This mixture was extracted with chloroform, the phases were separated by centrifugation, and the lower organic phase was drawn off and concentrated under a stream of nitrogen at 50°C. The residue was dissolved in 300 μL of acetonitrile/2-propanol (1:1) and loaded onto the column. The HPLC column was a

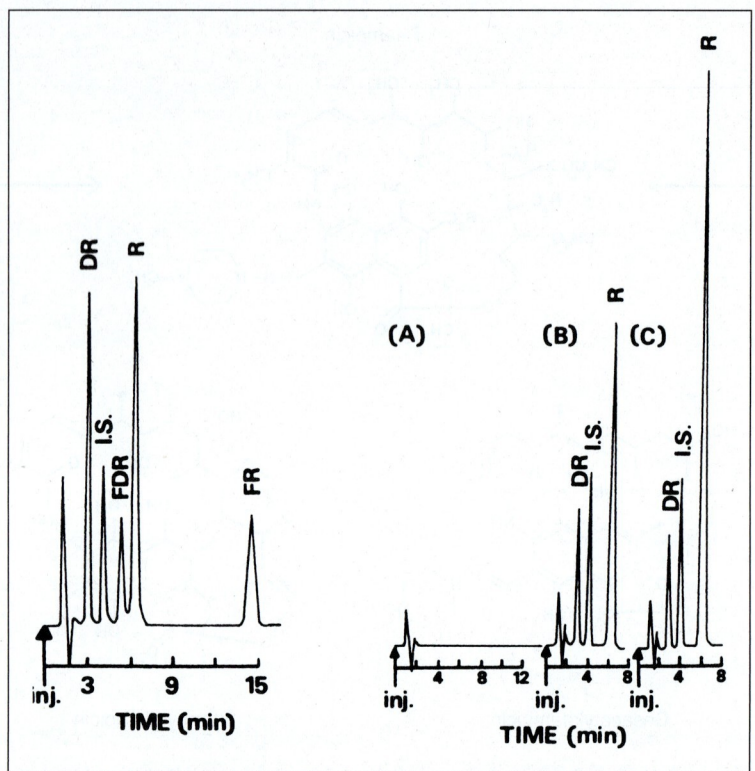

Figure 5.17 ■ Left chromatogram: rifampicin (*R*), 25-desacetyl rifampicin (*DR*), 3-formyl-25-desacetylrifamycin SV (*FDR*), 3-formylrifamycin SV (*FR*), and papaverine as the internal standard (*I.S.*). **Right chromatogram:** *(A)* blank plasma extract; *(B)* rifampicin (*R*), 25-desacetylrifampicin (*DR*), and papaverine as the internal standard (*I.S.*), spiked to a blank plasma sample. The spiked concentrations of rifampicin and 25-desacetylrifampicin were 3 and 1 µg/mL in plasma, respectively. Chromatogram of plasma extracted from a tuberculosis patient treated with 450 mg of rifampicin, 300 mg of isoniazid, and 1.0 g of ethambutol *(C)*. The concentrations of rifampicin and 25-desacetyrifampicin were estimated at 5.46 and 0.85 µg/mL, respectively. (Adapted from Ishii M, Ogata H. Determination of rifampicin and its main metabolites in human plasma by high-performance liquid chromatography. *J Chromatogr* 1988;426:412–416.)

7-µm Nucleosil C_{18} column and the mobile phase was acetonitrile/0.1 mol/L potassium phosphate buffer, pH 4.0 (38:62). This method readily separated rifampin, 25-*O*-desacetylrifampin, 3-formyl-25-descetylrifamycin SV, 3-formylrifamycin, and the internal standard over a period of less than 10 minutes. There was excellent baseline separation of all peaks, and detection at 340 nm obviated the influence of many plasma-derived interfering substances. The sensitivity of the assay was 0.1 µg/mL for rifampin and 0.06 µg/mL for 25-*O*-desacetylrifampin, with good accuracy and precision. INH and ethambutol did not interfere with the detection of rifampin or the rifampin metabolites using this method (410).

Ethambutol

Ethambutol or dextro-2,2′-(ethylenediimino)-di(1-butanol) is presumably metabolized in the liver to a dicarboxylic acid and a dialdehyde (411); however, the drug is generally considered not to be extensively metabolized in humans. Neither of the known metabolites is active against *M. tuberculosis* nor are the metabolites noted to be toxic to humans. Spectrophotometric assays have been described for the quantitation of ethambutol in cerebrospinal fluid (CSF) (412) and urine (413). Samples were extracted with chloroform and reacted with bromthymol blue, with a lower limit of detection of 500 ng/mL. A variety of gas chromatographic and gas chromatographic-mass spectrometric methods have been described for measuring the concentration of ethambutol in biologic fluids (414–417).

Pyrazinamide

PZA, which is the amide of pyrazinoic acid, is rapidly absorbed from the gastrointestinal tract and metabolized to 5-hydroxypyrazinamide, which most probably undergoes microsomal deamination to 5-hydroxypyrazinoic acid and pyrazinoic acid, which can be hydroxylated to 5-hydroxypyrazinoic acid. PZA alone has no activity against *M.*

tuberculosis; however, PZA-susceptible strains of *M. tuberculosis* readily deaminate PZA to the active metabolite pyrazinoic acid. It can be of value to monitor the concentrations of both PZA and pyrazinoic acid to prevent side effects, especially hyperuricemia. Yamamoto et al. (418,419) described an HPLC method for the rapid determination of PZA and the various metabolic products, to levels as low as 3 ng (5-hydroxypyrazinoic acid and 5-hydroxypyrazinamide) or 30 ng (pyrazinoic acid and PZA), in plasma and urine (Fig. 5.18). The method employed a 10-μm μBondapak C_{18} column (Waters Associates, Milford, MA) using a mobile phase of

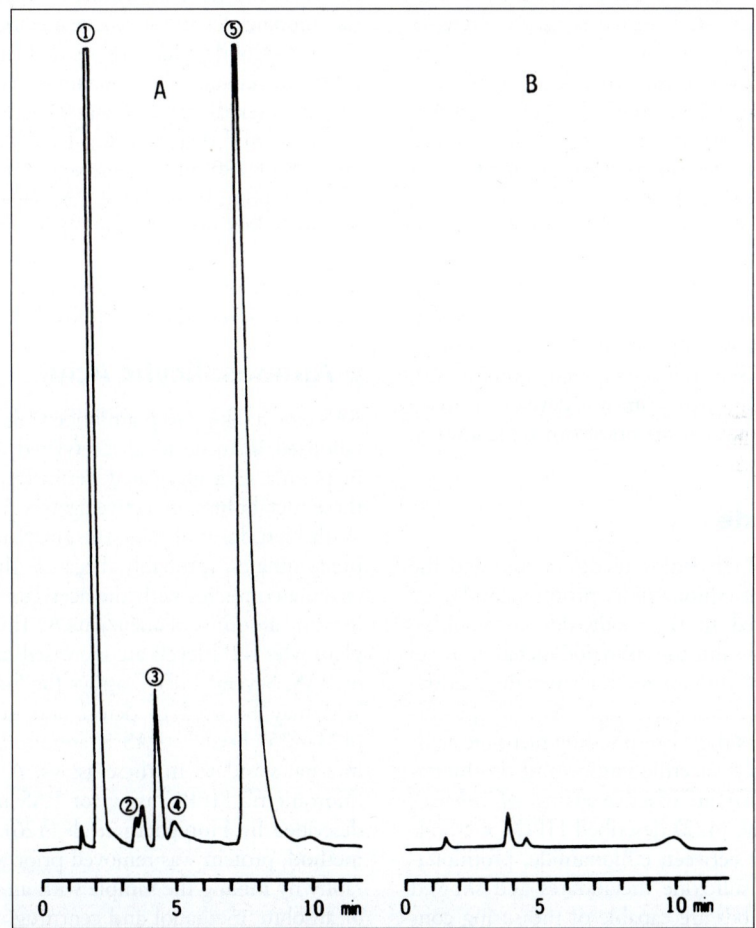

Figure 5.18 ■ A: Chromatogram of plasma extract containing pyrazinamide and its metabolites 4 hours after administration. B: Chromatogram of blank plasma. *Peak 1,* 2,3-pyrazinedicarboxamide; *peak 2,* 5-hydroxypyrazinoic acid (0.36 μg/mL); *peak 3,* 5-hydroxypyrazinamide (5.74 μg/mL); *peak 4,* pyrazinoic (6.14 μg/mL); *peak 5,* pyrazinamide (73.91 μg/mL). (Adapted from Yamamoto T, Moriwaki Y, Takahashi S, et al. Rapid and simultaneous determination of pyrazinamide and its major metabolites in human plasma by high-performance liquid chromatography. *J Chromatogr* 1987;413:342–346.)

0.02 mol/L KH_2PO_4, pH 2.56, and a fluorescence detector at 410/265 nm. Serum samples (0.5 mL) were treated with 2 mol/L perchloric acid and centrifuged, and an aliquot of the supernatant was neutralized with NaOH and loaded onto the column. Urine was stored at −20°C, thawed, and centrifuged, and a 1:10 dilution of the supernatant was loaded onto the column without further treatment. The internal standard was 2,3-pyrazinedicarboxamide and the chromatogram was developed over 10 minutes. Woo et al. (420) described another HPLC method for the simultaneous detection of PZA and rifampin in the serum of patients with tuberculous meningitis. Samples were treated with ascorbic acid and extracted into dichloromethane/diethyl ether (2:3). The treated samples were concentrated and loaded onto a reverse-phase, 5-μm, C_8 analytical column, using a mobile phase of 6% to 48% acetonitrile in 10 mmol/L KH_2PO_4, pH 3.5, and compounds were detected at 215 nm. Donald and Seifart (421) described an HPLC method for the determination of PZA in CSF from patients receiving three additional antimycobacterial drugs (INH, rifampin, and ethionamide) and phenobarbitone. This method used a Whatman Partisil 5-C_8 column, with a gradient of phosphate buffer, acetonitrile, and isopropanol and UV detection at 280/254 nm. CSF was loaded directly onto the column, and the chromatogram was developed over a period of 20 minutes, using prazepam as the internal standard.

Ethionamide

Ethionamide (2-ethylthiosonicotinamide) and the propyl analog of ethionamide, prothionamide, are readily converted to their sulfoxide metabolites. Both the analogs and the sulfoxide metabolites are active against *M. tuberculosis*; however, the 2-ethyl- and 2-propyl-nicotinamide derivatives of the sulfoxides, as well as the corresponding nicotinic acids (the end products of ethionamide and prothionamide metabolism), are inactive against *M. tuberculosis*. Jenner et al. (422) described HPLC methods that distinguish between ethionamide, prothionamide, and the sulfoxide metabolites and showed that these methods are capable of measuring concentrations as low as 10 to 50 ng/mL. Aliquots of plasma or urine (3 mL) were added to tubes containing 0.1 mL of either 150 ng or 600 ng of the appropriate internal standard. Prothionamide was used as the internal standard for the ethionamide assay and vice versa. The samples were extracted with 6 mL of diethyl ether and centrifuged to separate the organic and aqueous phases. The organic phase was extracted with 1 mL of 0.1 mol/L HCl, transferred to another tube, treated with 0.1 mL of ammonium phosphate, and then adjusted to pH 7 to 8 with 10% aqueous ammonia. The thionamides were extracted with 2 mL of ethyl acetate and concentrated by evaporation under a stream of nitrogen at 50°C. The residue was dissolved in 1 mL of dichloromethane and dried under nitrogen. Prior to chromatography, the residue was dissolved in 100 μL of the mobile phase. The chromatographic methods employed a Hypersil column of 5-m spherical silica (Shandon Southern, Runcorn, United Kingdom), with a mobile phase of chloroform/2-propanol/water (916:8:4) to separate the thionamides and sulfoxide metabolites (method 1) or a mobile phase of diethyl ether/methanol (96:4) to separate the thionamides alone (method 2). The internal standard was 2-methylthioisonicotinamide, and detection was by UV absorption at 340 nm or 280 nm, respectively. Separation of the four compounds in plasma can be achieved in approximately 8 minutes using method 1. Method 2 is suitable for distinguishing ethionamide and prothionamide in urine; interfering substances prevent determination of the two sulfoxides in urine.

p-Aminosalicylic Acid

PAS, an analog of p-aminobenzoic acid, is metabolized in urine to an acetylated derivative and in plasma to a glycylated derivative, and both of these metabolites are active against *M. tuberculosis*. With high doses of PAS, the glycylated metabolite predominates, probably because the glycylating enzyme competes with the acetylating enzyme for limiting amounts of coenzyme A. This may also explain why INH levels are increased in the presence of PAS. Several HPLC assays for 5-aminosalicylic acid may be used to detect and quantitate PAS (423–425) because PAS is commonly used as an internal standard in these assays. A nonextractive fluorometric HPLC assay for PAS in plasma was described by Honigberg et al. (426). In the latter method, protein was removed prior to chromatography by mixing the sample with an equal volume of absolute methanol and centrifuging the flocculent precipitate. An aliquot (50 μL) of the supernatant was mixed with 100 μL of the mobile phase containing internal standard, and this mixture was directly loaded onto the column. The column was a LiChrosorb C_{18} column, with a mobile phase of absolute methanol/distilled water (20:80) containing 0.005 mol/L tetrabutylammonium hydroxide and

0.01 mol/L disodium acid phosphate, pH 5.5. Tetrabutylammonium was added as an ion-pairing reagent to increase the capacity factor for PAS and to improve resolution. The internal standard was anthranilic acid, and detection was by fluorometry using an excitation wavelength of 270 nm and an emission wavelength of 385 nm, based on the native fluorescence of PAS. Plasma volumes as small as 100 μL could be tested, and the lower limit of detection was 500 pg of PAS.

Conclusions

Holdiness (390) concluded that stability studies should always be performed when evaluating an assay for antimycobacterial agents in order to ensure the stability of the agent during storage and under the conditions of the assay. Furthermore, the extraction of samples appears to generally improve the sensitivity and precision of most assays by either eliminating interfering substances contained in the biologic matrix, increasing the concentration of the agent, or separating the agent from other drugs or metabolites. Finally, the reliability of the assays, in particular the HPLC assays, is dependent on the expertise of the laboratory staff and on the type and quality of instruments. Thus, the same admonition applies to the analysis of antimycobacterial agents in biologic tissues and fluids as to the susceptibility testing of mycobacteria: Experience is the most compelling factor in ensuring that assays are performed in an accurate and precise manner.

REFERENCES

1. World Health Organization. *WHO report 2011, global tuberculosis control.* Geneva: World Health Organization, 2011.
2. Dalton T, Cegielski P, Akksilp S, et al. Prevalence of and risk factors for resistance to second-line drugs in people with multidrug-resistant tuberculosis in eight countries: a prospective cohort study. *Lancet* 2012;380(9851):1406–1417.
3. Campbell PJ, Morlock GP, Sikes RD, et al. Molecular detection of mutations associated with first- and second-line drug resistance compared with conventional drug susceptibility testing of Mycobacterium tuberculosis. *Antimicrob Agents Chemother* 2011;55(5):2032–2041.
4. Palomino JC. Molecular detection, identification and drug resistance detection in Mycobacterium tuberculosis. *FEMS Immunol Med Microbiol* 2009;56(2):103–111.
5. World Health Organization. *Molecular line robe assays for rapid screening of patients at risk of multidrug-resistant tuberculosis (MDR-TB).* Geneva: World Health Organization, 2008.
6. World Health Organization. *Automated real-time nucleic acid amplification technology for rapid and simultaneous detection of tuberculosis and rifampicin resistance: Xpert MTB/RIF system.* Geneva: World Health Organization, 2011.
7. Winthrop KL. Pulmonary disease due to nontuberculous mycobacteria: an epidemiologist's view. *Future Microbiol* 2010;5(3):343–345.
8. Winthrop KL, McNelley E, Kendall B, et al. Pulmonary nontuberculous mycobacterial disease prevalence and clinical features: an emerging public health disease. *Am J Respir Crit Care Med* 2010;182(7):977–982.
9. Griffith DE. Nontuberculous mycobacterial lung disease. *Curr Opin Infect Dis* 2010;23(2):185–190.
10. Griffith DE, Aksamit T, Brown-Elliott BA, et al. An official ATS/IDSA statement: diagnosis, treatment, and prevention of nontuberculous mycobacterial diseases. *Am J Respir Crit Care Med* 2007;175(4):367–416.
11. Devulder G, Perouse de Montclos M, Flandrois JP. A multigene approach to phylogenetic analysis using the genus Mycobacterium as a model. *Int J Syst Evol Microbiol* 2005;55(Pt 1):293–302.
12. Imaeda T. Deoxyribonucleic acid relatedness among selected strains of *Mycobacterium tuberculosis, Mycobacterium bovis BCG, Mycobacterium microti,* and *Mycobacterium africanum. Int J Syst Bacteriol* 1985;35:147–150.
13. van Soolingen D, Hoogenboezem T, de Haas PE, et al. A novel pathogenic taxon of the *Mycobacterium tuberculosis* complex, Canetti: characterization of an exceptional isolate from Africa. *Int J Syst Bacteriol* 1997;47(4):1236–1245.
14. Blumberg HM, Burman WJ, Chaisson RE, et al. American Thoracic Society/Centers for Disease Control and Prevention/Infectious Diseases Society of America: treatment of tuberculosis. *Am J Respir Crit Care Med* 2003;167(4):603–662.
15. Treatment Guidelines from The Medical Letter. Drugs for tuberculosis. 2012. http://secure.medicalletter.org/TG-article-116a. Accessed October 2012.
16. Centers for Disease Control and Prevention. Tuberculosis (TB). 2011. http://www.cdc.gov/tb/topic/treatment/. Accessed October 2012.
17. World Health Organization. *Treatment of tuberculosis: guidelines.* Geneva: World Health Organization, 2010.
18. Boehme CC, Nabeta P, Hillemann D, et al. Rapid molecular detection of tuberculosis and rifampin resistance. *N Engl J Med* 2010;363(11):1005–1015.
19. Van Rie A, Page-Shipp L, Scott L, et al. Xpert(®) MTB/RIF for point-of-care diagnosis of TB in high-HIV burden, resource-limited countries: hype or hope? *Expert Rev Mol Diagn* 2010;10(7):937–946.
20. Scott LE, McCarthy K, Gous N, et al. Comparison of Xpert MTB/RIF with other nucleic acid technologies for diagnosing pulmonary tuberculosis in a high HIV prevalence setting: a prospective study. *PLoS Med* 2011;8(7):e1001061.

21. Nicol MP, Workman L, Isaacs W, et al. Accuracy of the Xpert MTB/RIF test for the diagnosis of pulmonary tuberculosis in children admitted to hospital in Cape Town, South Africa: a descriptive study. *Lancet Infect Dis* 2011;11(11):819–824.
22. Drobniewski F, Nikolayevskyy V, Balabanova Y, et al. Diagnosis of tuberculosis and drug resistance: what can new tools bring us? *Int J Tuberc Lung Dis* 2012;16(7):860–870.
23. Ling DI, Flores LL, Riley LW, et al. Commercial nucleic-acid amplification tests for diagnosis of pulmonary tuberculosis in respiratory specimens: meta-analysis and meta-regression. *PLoS One* 2008;3(2):e1536.
24. Ling DI, Zwerling AA, Pai M. GenoType MTBDR assays for the diagnosis of multidrug-resistant tuberculosis: a meta-analysis. *Eur Respir J* 2008;32(5):1165–1174.
25. Ignatyeva O, Kontsevaya I, Kovalyov A, et al. Detection of resistance to second-line antituberculosis drugs by use of the genotype MTBDRsl assay: a multicenter evaluation and feasibility study. *J Clin Microbiol* 2012;50(5):1593–1597.
26. Halse TA, Edwards J, Cunningham PL, et al. Combined real-time PCR and rpoB gene pyrosequencing for rapid identification of Mycobacterium tuberculosis and determination of rifampin resistance directly in clinical specimens. *J Clin Microbiol* 2010;48(4):1182–1188.
27. Garcia-Sierra N, Lacoma A, Prat C, et al. Pyrosequencing for rapid molecular detection of rifampin and isoniazid resistance in Mycobacterium tuberculosis strains and clinical specimens. *J Clin Microbiol* 2011;49(10):3683–3686.
28. Engstrom A, Morcillo N, Imperiale B, et al. Detection of first- and second-line drug resistance in Mycobacterium tuberculosis clinical isolates by pyrosequencing. *J Clin Microbiol* 2012;50(6):2026–2033.
29. Zhang J, Mi L, Wang Y, et al. Genotypes and drug susceptibility of Mycobacterium tuberculosis isolates in Shihezi, Xinjiang Province, China. *BMC Res Notes* 2012;5:309.
30. Yuan X, Zhang T, Kawakami K, et al. Molecular characterization of multidrug- and extensively drug-resistant Mycobacterium tuberculosis strains in Jiangxi, China. *J Clin Microbiol* 2012;50(7):2404–2413.
31. Chen HY, Yu MC, Huang WL, et al. Molecular detection of rifabutin-susceptible Mycobacterium tuberculosis. *J Clin Microbiol* 2012;50(6):2085–2088.
32. Sirgel FA, Warren RM, Streicher EM, et al. gyrA mutations and phenotypic susceptibility levels to ofloxacin and moxifloxacin in clinical isolates of Mycobacterium tuberculosis. *J Antimicrob Chemother* 2012;67(5):1088–1093.
33. Canetti G, Froman S, Grosset J, et al. Mycobacteria: laboratory methods for testing drug sensitivity and resistance. *Bull WHO* 1963;29:565–578.
34. Van Deun A, Barrera L, Bastian I, et al. Mycobacterium tuberculosis strains with highly discordant rifampin susceptibility test results. *J Clin Microbiol* 2009;47(11):3501–3506.
35. Williamson DA, Roberts SA, Bower JE, et al. Clinical failures associated with rpoB mutations in phenotypically occult multidrug-resistant Mycobacterium tuberculosis. *Int J Tuberc Lung Dis* 2012;16(2):216–220.
36. Centers for Disease Control and Prevention ATS, Infectious Diseases Society of America. Treatment of tuberculosis. *MMWR Morb Mortal Wkly Rep* 2003;52(RR-11):1–77.
37. David HL. Probability distribution of drug-resistant mutants in unselected populations of Mycobacterium tuberculosis. *Appl Microbiol* 1970;20:810–814.
38. Cole ST. Mycobacterium tuberculosis: drug-resistance mechanisms. *Trends Microbiol* 1994;2(10):411–415.
39. Heym B, Honore N, Truffot-Pernot C, et al. The implications of multidrug resistance for the future of short course chemotherapy of tuberculosis: a molecular study. *Lancet* 1994;344:293–298.
40. Mitchison DA. The Garrod lecture. Understanding the chemotherapy of tuberculosis—current problems. *J Antimicrob Chemother* 1992;29:477–493.
41. Wayne LG, Sramek HA. Metronidazole is bactericidal to dormant cells of Mycobacterium tuberculosis. *Antimicrob Agents Chemother* 1994;38(9):2054–2058.
42. Brooks JV, Furney SK, Orme IM. Metronidazole therapy in mice infected with tuberculosis. *Antimicrob Agents Chemother* 1999;43(5):1285–1288.
43. Dhillon J, Allen BW, Hu YM, et al. Metronidazole has no antibacterial effect in Cornell model murine tuberculosis. *Int J Tuberc Lung Dis* 1998;2(9):736–742.
44. Pfyffer GE, Palicova F. Mycobacterium: general characteristic, laboratory detection, and staining procedures. In: Versalovic J, ed. *Manual of clinical microbiology*. Vol 1. 10th ed. Washington, DC: ASM Press, 2012.
45. Picken RN, Plotch SJ, Wang Z, et al. DNA probes for Mycobacteria. I. Isolation of DNA probes for the identification of *Mycobacterium tuberculosis* complex and for mycobacteria other than tuberculosis (MOTT). *Mol Cell Probes* 1988;2:111–124.
46. Sherman I, Harrington N, Rothrock A, et al. Use of a cutoff range in identifying mycobacteria by the Gen-Probe Rapid Diagnostic System. *J Clin Microbiol* 1989;27(2):241–244.
47. Wayne LG. The "atypical" mycobacteria: recognition and disease association. *CRC Crit Rev Microbiol* 1985;12(3):185–222.
48. Rieder HL, Van Deun A, Kam KM, et al. *Priorities for tuberculosis bacteriology services in low-income countries*. 2nd ed. Paris: International Union Against Tuberculosis and Lung Disease, 2007.
49. Clinical and Laboratory Standards Institute. *Susceptibility testing of mycobacteria, nocardiae, and other aerobic actinomycetes; approved standard—second edition*. CLSI document M24-A2. Wayne, PA: Clinical and Laboratory Standards Institute, 2011.
50. Kent PA, Kubica GP. *Public health mycobacteriology—a guide for the level III laboratory*. Atlanta: U.S. Department of Health and Human Services, Public Health Service, Centers for Disease Control, 1985.
51. Hannan MM, Desmond EP, Morlock GP, et al. Pyrazinamide-monoresistant Mycobacterium tuberculosis in the United States. *J Clin Microbiol* 2001;39(2):647–650.
52. Griffith ME, Bodily HL. Stability of antimycobacterial drugs in susceptibility testing. *Antimicrob Agents Chemother* 1992;36:2398–2402.
53. Wayne LG, Krasnow I. Preparation of tuberculosis susceptibility testing mediums by means of impregnated disks. *Am J Clin Pathol* 1966;45:769–771.
54. Griffith M, Barrett HL, Bodily HL, et al. Drug susceptibility tests for tuberculosis using drug impregnated discs. *Am J Clin Pathol* 1967;47:812–817.
55. Guthertz LS, Griffith ME, Ford EG, et al. Quality control or individual components used in Middlebrook 7H10 medium for mycobacterial susceptibility testing. *J Clin Microbiol* 1988;26(11):2338–2342.
56. Butler WR, Warren NG, Kubica GP, et al. Modified method for testing the quality of albumin-containing enrichments used in growth media for mycobacteria. *J Clin Microbiol* 1990;28:1068–1070.

57. Tenover FC, Crawford JT, Huebner RE, et al. The resurgence of tuberculosis: is your laboratory ready? *J Clin Microbiol* 1993;31:767–770.

58. Woods GL, Lin SY, Desmond EP. Susceptibility test methods: mycobacteria, Nocardia, and other actinomycetes. In: *Manual of clinical microbiology.* 10th ed. Washington, DC: ASM Press, 2011:1215–1238.

59. Bemer P, Palicova F, Rusch-Gerdes S, et al. Multicenter evaluation of fully automated BACTEC Mycobacteria Growth Indicator Tube 960 system for susceptibility testing of Mycobacterium tuberculosis. *J Clin Microbiol* 2002;40(1):150–154.

60. Johansen IS, Thomsen VO, Marjamaki M, et al. Rapid, automated, nonradiometric susceptibility testing of Mycobacterium tuberculosis complex to four first-line antituberculous drugs used in standard short-course chemotherapy. *Diagn Microbiol Infect Dis* 2004;50(2):103–107.

61. Scarparo C, Ricordi P, Ruggiero G, et al. Evaluation of the fully automated BACTEC MGIT 960 system for testing susceptibility of Mycobacterium tuberculosis to pyrazinamide, streptomycin, isoniazid, rifampin, and ethambutol and comparison with the radiometric BACTEC 460TB method. *J Clin Microbiol* 2004;42(3):1109–1114.

62. Horne DJ, Pinto LM, Arentz M, et al. Diagnostic accuracy and reproducibility of WHO-endorsed phenotypic drug susceptibility testing methods for first-line and second-line anti-tuberculosis drugs: a systematic review and meta-analysis. *J Clin Microbiol* 2013;51(2):393–401.

63. Angra PK, Taylor TH, Iademarco MF, et al. Performance of tuberculosis drug susceptibility testing in U.S. laboratories from 1994 to 2008. *J Clin Microbiol* 2012;50(4):1233–1239.

64. Lin SY, Desmond E, Bonato D, et al. Multicenter evaluation of Bactec MGIT 960 system for second-line drug susceptibility testing of Mycobacterium tuberculosis complex. *J Clin Microbiol* 2009;47(11):3630–3634.

65. Kruuner A, Yates MD, Drobniewski FA. Evaluation of MGIT 960-based antimicrobial testing and determination of critical concentrations of first- and second-line antimicrobial drugs with drug-resistant clinical strains of Mycobacterium tuberculosis. *J Clin Microbiol* 2006;44(3):811–818.

66. Rüsch-Gerdes S, Pfyffer GE, Casal M, et al. Multicenter laboratory validation of the BACTEC MGIT 960 technique for testing susceptibilities of Mycobacterium tuberculosis to classical second-line drugs and newer antimicrobials. *J Clin Microbiol* 2006;44(3):688–692.

67. World Health Organization. *Guidance on drug-susceptibility testing (DST) of second-line antituberculosis drugs.* Geneva: World Health Organization, 2008.

68. Feasey NA, Pond M, Coleman D, et al. Moxifloxacin and pyrazinamide susceptibility testing in a complex case of multidrug-resistant tuberculosis. *Int J Tuberc Lung Dis* 2011;15(3):417–420.

69. Zhang Y, Chang K, Leung C-C, et al. "ZS-MDR-TB" versus "ZR-MDR-TB": improving treatment outcome of MDR-TB by identifying pyrazinamide susceptibility. Emerging Microbes and Infections Web site. http://www.nature.com/emi. Accessed October 2012.

70. Zhang Y, Mitchison D. The curious characteristics of pyrazinamide: a review. *Int J Tuberc Lung Dis* 2003;7(1):6–21.

71. Piersimoni C, Mustazzolu A, Giannoni F, et al. Prevention of false resistance results obtained testing susceptibility of Mycobacterium tuberculosis to pyrazinamide with the Bactec MGIT 960 system using a reduced inoculum. *J Clin Microbiol* 2013;51(1):291–294.

72. Miller MA, Thibert L, Desjardins F, et al. Growth inhibition of Mycobacterium tuberculosis by polyoxyethylene stearate present in the BACTEC pyrazinamide susceptibility test. *J Clin Microbiol* 1996;34(1):84–86.

73. Singh P, Wesley C, Jadaun GP, et al. Comparative evaluation of Löwenstein-Jensen proportion method, BacT/ALERT 3D system, and enzymatic pyrazinamidase assay for pyrazinamide susceptibility testing of Mycobacterium tuberculosis. *J Clin Microbiol* 2007;45(1):76–80.

74. Chang KC, Yew WW, Zhang Y. Pyrazinamide susceptibility testing in Mycobacterium tuberculosis: a systematic review with meta-analyses. *Antimicrob Agents Chemother* 2011;55(10):4499–4505.

75. Ruiz P, Zerolo FJ, Casal MJ. Comparison of susceptibility testing of Mycobacterium tuberculosis using the ESP culture system II with that using the BACTEC method. *J Clin Microbiol* 2000;38(12):4663–4664.

76. LaBombardi VJ. Comparison of the ESP and BACTEC systems for testing susceptibilities of Mycobacterium tuberculosis complex isolates to pyrazinamide. *J Clin Microbiol* 2002;40(6):2238–2239.

77. Espasa M, Salvado M, Vicente E, et al. Evaluation of the VersaTREK system compared to the Bactec MGIT 960 system for first-line drug susceptibility testing of Mycobacterium tuberculosis. *J Clin Microbiol* 2012;50(2):488–491.

78. Georghiou SB, Magana M, Garfein RS, et al. Evaluation of genetic mutations associated with Mycobacterium tuberculosis resistance to amikacin, kanamycin and capreomycin: a systematic review. *PLoS One* 2012;7(3):e33275.

79. Burman WJ. The value of in vitro drug activity and pharmacokinetics in predicting the effectiveness of antimycobacterial therapy: a critical review. *Am J Med Sci* 1997;313(6):355–363.

80. Abuali MM, Katariwala R, LaBombardi VJ. A comparison of the Sensititre(R) MYCOTB panel and the agar proportion method for the susceptibility testing of Mycobacterium tuberculosis. *Eur J Clin Microbiol Infect Dis* 2012;31(5):835–839.

81. Hall L, Jude KP, Clark SL, et al. Evaluation of the Sensititre MycoTB plate for susceptibility testing of the *Mycobacterium tuberculosis* complex against first- and second-line agents. *J Clin Microbiol* 2012;50(11):3732–3734.

82. Minion J, Leung E, Menzies D, et al. Microscopic-observation drug susceptibility and thin layer agar assays for the detection of drug resistant tuberculosis: a systematic review and meta-analysis. *Lancet Infect Dis* 2010;10(10):688–698.

83. Moore DA, Shah NS. Alternative methods of diagnosing drug resistance—what can they do for me? *J Infect Dis* 2011; 204(Suppl 4):S1110–S1119.

84. Shah NS, Moodley P, Babaria P, et al. Rapid diagnosis of tuberculosis and multidrug resistance by the microscopic-observation drug-susceptibility assay. *Am J Respir Crit Care Med* 2011;183(10):1427–1433.

85. Fitzwater SP, Sechler GA, Jave O, et al. Second-line anti-TB drug concentrations for susceptibility testing in the MODS assay. *Eur Respir J* 2013;41(5):1163–1171.

86. Martin A, Paasch F, Docx S, et al. Multicentre laboratory validation of the colorimetric redox indicator (CRI) assay for the rapid detection of extensively drug-resistant (XDR) Mycobacterium tuberculosis. *J Antimicrob Chemother* 2011;66(4):827–833.

87. Martin A, Portaels F, Palomino JC. Colorimetric redox-indicator methods for the rapid detection of multidrug resistance in Mycobacterium tuberculosis: a systematic review and meta-analysis. *J Antimicrob Chemother* 2007;59(2):175–183.

88. Brown-Elliott BA, Griffith DE, Wallace RJ Jr. Newly described or emerging human species of nontuberculous mycobacteria. *Infect Dis Clin North Am* 2002;16(1):187–220.

89. Brown-Elliott BA, Wallace RJ Jr. Clinical and taxonomic status of pathogenic nonpigmented or late-pigmenting rapidly growing mycobacteria. *Clin Microbiol Rev* 2002; 15(4):716–746.

90. Piersimoni C, Scarparo C. Extrapulmonary infections associated with nontuberculous mycobacteria in immunocompetent persons. *Emerg Infect Dis* 2009;15(9): 1351–1358; quiz 1544.

91. McFarland EJ, Kuritzkes DR. Clinical features and treatment of infection due to mycobacterium fortuitum/chelonae complex. *Curr Clin Top Infect Dis* 1993;13:188–202.

92. Inderlied CB. Mycobacteria. In: Cohen J, Powderly WP, et al, eds. *Infectious diseases*. Vol II. London: Mosby; 2004:2285-2308.

93. van Ingen J, Boeree MJ, van Soolingen D, et al. Resistance mechanisms and drug susceptibility testing of nontuberculous mycobacteria. *Drug Resist Updat* 2012;15(3):149–161.

94. Nash KA. Intrinsic macrolide resistance in *Mycobacterium smegmatis* is conferred by a novel *erm* gene, *erm*(38). *Antimicrob Agents Chemother* 2003;47(10):3053–3060.

95. Nash KA, Zhang Y, Brown-Elliott BA, et al. Cloning of erm(39), a gene conferring intrinsic macrolide resistance to Mycobacterium fortuitum. *J Antimicrob Chemother* 2004.

96. Tebas P, Sultan F, Wallace RJ Jr, et al. Rapid development of resistance to clarithromycin following monotherapy for disseminated *M. chelonae* infection in a heart transplant patient. *Clin Infect Dis* 1995;20:443–444.

97. Wallace RJ Jr, Meier A, Brown BA, et al. Genetic basis for clarithromycin resistance among isolates of *Mycobacterium chelonae* and *Mycobacterium abscessus*. *Antimicrob Agents Chemother* 1996;40(7):1676–1681.

98. Brown-Elliott BA, Nash KA, Wallace RJ Jr. Antimicrobial susceptibility testing, drug resistance mechanisms, and therapy of infections with nontuberculous mycobacteria. *Clin Microbiol Rev* 2012;25(3):545–582.

99. Clinical and Laboratory Standards Institute. *Susceptibility testing of mycobacteria, nocardiae, and other aerobic actinomycetes; approved standard—second edition.* CLSI document M24-A2. Wayne, PA: Clinical and Laboratory Standards Institute, 2011.

100. Swenson JM, Thornsberry C, Silcox VA. Rapidly growing mycobacteria: testing of susceptibility to 34 antimicrobial agents by broth microdilution. *Antimicrob Agents Chemother* 1982;22(2):186–192.

101. Tsang AY, Drupa I, Goldberg M, et al. Use of serology and thin layer chromatography for the assembly of an authenticated collection of serovars within the Mycobacterium avium-Mycobacterium intracellulare-Mycobacterium scrofulaceum complex. *Int J Sys Bact* 1983;33:285–292.

102. Brennan PJ. Structure of mycobacteria: recent developments in defining cell wall carbohydrates and proteins. *Rev Infect Dis* 1989;11:S420–S430.

103. Wayne LG, Sramek HA. Agents of newly recognized or infrequently encountered mycobacterial diseases. *Clin Microbiol Rev* 1992;5:1-25.

104. Turenne CY, Wallace R Jr, Behr MA. Mycobacterium avium in the postgenomic era. *Clin Microbiol Rev* 2007;20(2):205–229.

105. Drake TA, Herron RM, Hindler JA, et al. DNA probe reactivity of Mycobacterium avium complex isolates from patients without AIDS. *Diagn Microbiol Infect Dis* 1988;11:125–128.

106. Kiehn TE, Edwards FF. Rapid identification using a specific DNA probe of *Mycobacterium avium complex* from patients with acquired immunodeficiency syndrome. *J Clin Microbiol* 1987;25:1551–1552.

107. Heifets L. MIC as a quantitative measurement of the susceptibility of *Mycobacterium avium* strains to seven antituberculosis drugs. *Antimicrob Agents Chemother* 1988;32(8):1131–1136.

108. Inderlied CB, Young LS, Yamada JK. Determination of in vitro susceptibility of *Mycobacterium avium* complex isolates to antimicrobial agents by various methods. *Antimicrob Agents Chemother* 1987;31:1697–1702.

109. Rastogi N, Frehel C, Ryter A, et al. Multiple drug resistance in *Mycobacterium avium*: is the wall architecture responsible for the exclusion of antimicrobial agents? *Antimicrob Agents Chemother* 1981;20(5):666–677.

110. Mizuguchi Y, Ogawa M, Udou T. Morphological changes induced by beta-lactam antibiotics in Mycobacterium avium-intracellular complex. *Antimicrob Agents Chemother* 1985;27(4):541–547.

111. Crawford JT, Falkinham JO III. Plasmids of the *Mycobacterium avium* complex. In: McFadden J, ed. *Molecular biology of the mycobacteria*. London: Surrey University Press, 1990:97–119.

112. Falkinham JO 3rd. Epidemiology of infection by nontuberculous mycobacteria. *Clin Microbiol Rev* 1996;9 (2):177–215.

113. Saito H, Tomioka H. Susceptibilities of transparent, opaque, and rough colonial variants of Mycobacterium avium complex to various fatty acids. *Antimicrob Agents Chemother* 1988;32(3):400–402.

114. Schaefer WB, Davis CL, Cohn ML. Pathogenicity of transparent, opaque and rough variants of Mycobacterium avium in chickens and mice. *Am Rev Respir Dis* 1970; 102:499–506.

115. Stormer RS, Falkinham JOI. Differences in antimicrobial susceptibility of pigmented and unpigmented colonial variants of Mycobacterium avium. *J Clin Microbiol* 1989;27:2459–2465.

116. National Committee for Clinical Laboratory Standards. *Susceptibility testing of mycobacteria, nocardiae, and other aerobic actinomycetes; approved standard.* NCCLS document M24-A. Wayne, PA: National Committee on Clinical Laboratory Standards, 2003.

117. Bermudez LE, Kolonoski P, Petrofsky M, et al. Mefloquine, moxifloxacin, and ethambutol are a triple-drug alternative to macrolide-containing regimens for treatment of Mycobacterium avium disease. *J Infect Dis* 2003; 187(12):1977–1980.

118. Bermudez LE, Kolonoski P, Wu M, et al. Mefloquine is active in vitro and in vivo against Mycobacterium avium complex. *Antimicrob Agents Chemother* 1999;43(8): 1870–1874.

119. Nannini EC, Keating M, Binstock P, et al. Successful treatment of refractory disseminated *Mycobacterium avium* complex infection with the addition of linezolid and mefloquine. *J Infect* 2002;44(3):201–203.

120. Bermudez LE, Inderlied CB, Kolonoski P, et al. Identification of (+)-erythro-mefloquine as an active enantiomer with greater efficacy than mefloquine against Mycobacterium avium infection in mice. *Antimicrob Agents Chemother* 2012;56(8):4202–4206.

121. Babady NE, Hall L, Abbenyi AT, et al. Evaluation of Mycobacterium avium complex clarithromycin susceptibility testing using SLOMYCO Sensititre panels and JustOne strips. *J Clin Microbiol* 2010;48(5):1749–1752.

122. British Thoracic Society. Mycobacterium kansasii pulmonary infection: a prospective study of the results of nine months of treatment with rifampicin and ethambutol. Research Committee, British Thoracic Society. *Thorax* 1994;49(5):442–445.

123. Hoffner SE. Pulmonary infections caused by less frequently encountered slow-growing environmental mycobacteria. *Eur J Clin Microbiol Infect Dis* 1994;13(11): 937–941.

124. Woods GL, Washington JAI. Mycobacteria other than Mycobacterium tuberculosis: review of microbiologic and clinical aspects. *Rev Infect Dis* 1987;9:275–294.

125. Johanson WGJ, Nicholson DP. Pulmonary disease due to Mycobacterium kansasii. An analysis of some factors effecting prognosis. *Am Rev Respir Dis* 1969;99:73–85.

126. Pezzia W, Raleigh JW, Bailey MC, et al. Treatment of pulmonary disease due to Mycobacterium kansasii: recent experience with rifampin. *Rev Infect Dis* 1981;3: 1035–1039.

127. American Thoracic Society. Diagnosis and treatment of disease caused by nontuberculous mycobacteria. *Am J Respir Crit Care Med* 1997;156(2 Pt 2):S1–S25.

128. Bennett SN, Peterson DE, Johnson DR, et al. Bronchoscopy-associated *Mycobacterium xenopi* pseudoinfections. *Am J Respir Crit Care Med* 1994;150(1):245–250.

129. Sniadack DH, Ostroff SM, Karlix MA, et al. A nosocomial pseudo-outbreak of *Mycobacterium xenopi* due to a contaminated potable water supply: lessons in prevention. *Infect Control Hosp Epidemiol* 1993;14(11): 636–641.

130. Terashima T, Sakamaki F, Hasegawa N, et al. Pulmonary infection due to Mycobacterium xenopi. *Intern Med* 1994;33(9):536–539.

131. Davidson PT. The diagnosis and management of disease caused by *M. avium* complex, *M. kansasii*, and other mycobacteria. In: Snider DE Jr, ed. *Clinics in chest medicine*. Vol 10. Philadelphia: W.B. Saunders, 1989: 431–443.

132. Zaugg M, Salfinger M, Opravil M, et al. Extrapulmonary and disseminated infections due to *Mycobacterium malmoense*: case report and review. *Clin Infect Dis* 1993;16(4):540–549.

133. Banks J, Jenkins PA. Combined versus single antituberculosis drugs on the in vitro sensitivity patterns of nontuberculous mycobacteria. *Thorax* 1987;42(11):838–842.

134. Hoffner SE, Hjelm U. Increased growth of Mycobacterium malmoense in vitro in the presence of isoniazid. *Eur J Clin Microbiol Infect Dis* 1991;10(9):787–788.

135. Hoffner SE, Hjelm U, Kallenius G. Susceptibility of *Mycobacterium malmoense* to antibacterial drugs and drug combinations. *Antimicrob Agents Chemother* 1993;37(6):1285–1288.

136. Banks J, Jenkins PA, Smith AP. Pulmonary infection with *Mycobacterium malmoense*—a review of treatment and response. *Tubercle* 1985;66(3):197–203.

137. Valero G, Moreno F, Graybill JR. Activities of clarithromycin, ofloxacin, and clarithromycin plus ethambutol against Mycobacterium simiae in murine model of disseminated infection. *Antimicrob Agents Chemother* 1994;38(11):2676–2677.

138. Edelstein H. *Mycobacterium marinum* skin infections. Report of 31 cases and review of the literature. *Arch Intern Med* 1994;154(12):1359–1364.

139. Kozin SH, Bishop AT. Atypical Mycobacterium infections of the upper extremity. *J Hand Surg* 1994;19(3): 480–487.

140. Forsgren A. Antibiotic susceptibility of *Mycobacterium marinum*. *Scand J Infect Dis* 1993;25(6):779–782.

141. Sanders WJ, Wolinsky E. In vitro susceptibility of *Mycobacterium marinum* to eight antimicrobial agents. *Antimicrob Agents Chemother* 1980;18:529–531.

142. Marsollier L, Prevot G, Honore N, et al. Susceptibility of Mycobacterium ulcerans to a combination of amikacin/rifampicin. *Int J Antimicrob Agents* 2003;22(6): 562–566.

143. Marsollier L, Honore N, Legras P, et al. Isolation of three Mycobacterium ulcerans strains resistant to rifampin after experimental chemotherapy of mice. *Antimicrob Agents Chemother* 2003;47(4):1228–1232.

144. Straus WL, Ostroff SM, Jernigan DB, et al. Clinical and epidemiologic characteristics of Mycobacterium haemophilum, an emerging pathogen in immunocompromised patients. *Ann Intern Med* 1994;120(2):118–125.

145. Kiehn TE, White M. Mycobacterium haemophilum: an emerging pathogen. *Eur J Clin Microbiol Infect Dis* 1994;13(11):925–931.

146. Bernard EM, Edwards FF, Kiehn TE, et al. Activities of antimicrobial agents against clinical isolates of Mycobacterium haemophilum. *Antimicrob Agents Chemother* 1993;37(11):2323–2326.

147. Lessnau KD, Milanese S, Talavera W. Mycobacterium gordonae: a treatable disease in HIV-positive patients. *Chest* 1993;104(6):1779–1785.

148. Emler S, Rochat T, Rohner P, et al. Chronic destructive lung disease associated with a novel mycobacterium. *Am J Respir Crit Care Med* 1994;150(1):261–265.

149. Springer B, Kirschner P, Rost-Meyer G, et al. Mycobacterium interjectum, a new species isolated from a patient with chronic lymphadenitis. *J Clin Microbiol* 1993;31(12):3083–3089.

150. Betts JC, Lukey PT, Robb LC, et al. Evaluation of a nutrient starvation model of Mycobacterium tuberculosis persistence by gene and protein expression profiling. *Mol Microbiol* 2002;43(3):717–731.

151. Herbert D, Paramasivan CN, Venkatesan P, et al. Bactericidal action of ofloxacin, sulbactam-ampicillin, rifampin, and isoniazid on logarithmic- and stationary-phase cultures of Mycobacterium tuberculosis. *Antimicrob Agents Chemother* 1996;40(10):2296–2299.

152. Yamori S, Ichiyama S, Shimokata K, et al. Bacteriostatic and bactericidal activity of antituberculosis drugs against Mycobacterium tuberculosis, Mycobacterium avium-Mycobacterium intracellulare complex and Mycobacterium kansasii in different growth phases. *Microbiol Immunol* 1992;36(4):361–368.

153. American Thoracic Society and Centers for Disease Control and Prevention. Targeted tuberculin testing and treatment of latent tuberculosis infection. *Am J Respir Crit Care Med* 2000;161:S221–S247.

154. Magliozzo RS, Marcinkeviciene JA. The role of Mn(II)-peroxidase activity of mycobacterial catalase-peroxidase in activation of the antibiotic isoniazid. *J Biol Chem* 1997;272(14):8867–8870.

155. Nguyen M, Quemard A, Broussy S, et al. Mn(III) pyrophosphate as an efficient tool for studying the mode of action of isoniazid on the InhA protein of Mycobacterium tuberculosis. *Antimicrob Agents Chemother* 2002;46(7):2137–2144.

156. Wengenack NL, Rusnak F. Evidence for isoniazid-dependent free radical generation catalyzed by Mycobacterium tuberculosis KatG and the isoniazid-resistant mutant KatG(S315T). *Biochemistry* 2001;40(30):8990–8996.

157. Rawat R, Whitty A, Tonge PJ. The isoniazid-NAD adduct is a slow, tight-binding inhibitor of InhA, the Mycobacterium tuberculosis enoyl reductase: adduct affinity and drug resistance. Proc Natl Acad Sci USA 2003;100(24):13881–13886.

158. Rozwarski DA, Grant GA, Barton DH, et al. Modification of the NADH of the isoniazid target (InhA) from Mycobacterium tuberculosis. Science 1998;279(5347):98–102.

159. Takayama K, Davidson LA. Isonicotinic acid hydrazide. In: Hahn FE, ed. Mechanism of action of antibacterial agents. Vol V. Berlin: Springer-Verlag, 1979:98–119.

160. Winder FG. Mode of action of the antimycobacterial agents and associated aspects of the molecular biology of the mycobacteria. In: Ratledge C, Stanford J, eds. The biology of the mycobacteria. Vol 1 (Physiology, Identification and Classification). New York: Academic Press, 1982:353–438.

161. Takayama K, Schnoes HK, Armstrong EL, et al. Site of inhibitory action of isoniazid in the synthesis of mycolic acids in Mycobacterium tuberculosis. J Lipid Res 1975;16:308–317.

162. Banerjee A, Dubnau E, Quemard A, et al. inhA, a gene encoding a target for isoniazid and ethionamide in Mycobacterium tuberculosis. Science 1994;263(5144):227–230.

163. Middlebrook G. Isoniazid-resistance and catalase activity of tubercle bacilli. A preliminary report. Am Rev Tuberc 1954;69:471–472.

164. Zhang Y, Heym B, Allen B, et al. The catalase-peroxidase gene and isoniazid resistance of Mycobacterium tuberculosis. Nature 1992;358(6387):591–593.

165. Musser JM, Kapur V, Williams DL, et al. Characterization of the catalase-peroxidase gene (katG) and inhA locus in isoniazid-resistant and -susceptible strains of Mycobacterium tuberculosis by automated DNA sequencing: restricted array of mutations associated with drug resistance. J Infect Dis 1996;173(1):196–202.

166. Zhang Y, Yew WW. Mechanisms of drug resistance in Mycobacterium tuberculosis. Int J Tuberc Lung Dis 2009;13(11):1320–1330.

167. Sreevatsan S, Pan X, Zhang Y, et al. Analysis of the oxyR-ahpC region in isoniazid-resistant and -susceptible Mycobacterium tuberculosis complex organisms recovered from diseased humans and animals in diverse localities. Antimicrob Agents Chemother 1997;41(3):600–606.

168. Wilson TM, Collins DM. ahpC, a gene involved in isoniazid resistance of the Mycobacterium tuberculosis complex. Mol Microbiol 1996;19(5):1025–1034.

169. Morris S, Bai GH, Suffys P, et al. Molecular mechanisms of multiple drug resistance in clinical isolates of Mycobacterium tuberculosis. J Infect Dis 1995;171(4):954–960.

170. Zhang Y, Young D. Molecular genetics of drug resistance in Mycobacterium tuberculosis. J Antimicrob Chemother 1994;34(3):313–319.

171. Basso LA, Zheng R, Musser JM, et al. Mechanisms of isoniazid resistance in Mycobacterium tuberculosis: enzymatic characterization of enoyl reductase mutants identified in isoniazid-resistant clinical isolates. J Infect Dis 1998;178(3):769–775.

172. Vilchèze C, Jacobs WR Jr. The mechanism of isoniazid killing: clarity through the scope of genetics. Annu Rev Microbiol 2007;61:35–50.

173. Vilcheze C, Wang F, Arai M, et al. Transfer of a point mutation in Mycobacterium tuberculosis inhA resolves the target of isoniazid. Nature Med 2006;12(9):1027–1029.

174. Heym B, Alzari PM, Honore N, et al. Missense mutations in the catalase-peroxidase gene, katG are associated with isoniazid resistance in Mycobacterium tuberculosis. Mol Microbiol 1995;15(2):235–245.

175. Wilson TM, Lisle d, Collins DM. Effect of inhA and katG on isoniazid resistance and virulence of Mycobacterium bovis. Mol Microbiol 1995;15(6):1009–1015.

176. Banerjee A, Sugantino M, Sacchettini JC, et al. The mabA gene from the inhA operon of Mycobacterium tuberculosis encodes a 3-ketoacyl reductase that fails to confer isoniazid resistance. Microbiology 1998;144(Pt 10):2697–2704.

177. Slayden RA, Lee RE, Barry CE 3rd. Isoniazid affects multiple components of the type II fatty acid synthase system of Mycobacterium tuberculosis. Mol Microbiol 2000;38(3):514–525.

178. Larsen MH, Vilcheze C, Kremer L, et al. Overexpression of inhA, but not kasA, confers resistance to isoniazid and ethionamide in Mycobacterium smegmatis, M. bovis BCG and M. tuberculosis. Mol Microbiol 2002;46(2):453–466.

179. Miesel L, Weisbrod TR, Marcinkeviciene JA, et al. NADH dehydrogenase defects confer isoniazid resistance and conditional lethality in Mycobacterium smegmatis. J Bacteriol 1998;180(9):2459–2467.

180. Lee AS, Teo AS, Wong SY. Novel mutations in ndh in isoniazid-resistant Mycobacterium tuberculosis isolates. Antimicrob Agents Chemother 2001;45(7):2157–2159.

181. Mdluli K, Slayden RA, Zhu Y, et al. Inhibition of a Mycobacterium tuberculosis beta-ketoacyl ACP synthase by isoniazid. Science 1998;280(5369):1607–1610.

182. Chen P, Bishai WR. Novel selection for isoniazid (INH) resistance genes supports a role for NAD+-binding proteins in mycobacterial INH resistance. Infect Immun 1998;66(11):5099–5106.

183. Payton M, Auty R, Delgoda R, et al. Cloning and characterization of arylamine N-acetyltransferase genes from Mycobacterium smegmatis and Mycobacterium tuberculosis: increased expression results in isoniazid resistance. J Bacteriol 1999;181:1343–1347.

184. Upton AM, Mushtaq A, Victor TC, et al. Arylamine N-acetyltransferase of Mycobacterium tuberculosis is a polymorphic enzyme and a site of isoniazid metabolism. Mol Microbiol 2001;42:309–317.

185. Ramaswamy SV, Reich R, Dou SJ, et al. Single nucleotide polymorphisms in genes associated with isoniazid resistance in Mycobacterium tuberculosis. Antimicrob Agents Chemother 2003;47(4):1241–1250.

186. Viveiros M, Portugal I, Bettencourt R, et al. Isoniazid-induced transient high-level resistance in Mycobacterium tuberculosis. Antimicrob Agents Chemother 2002;46(9):2804–2810.

187. Choudhuri BS, Sen S, Chakrabarti P. Isoniazid accumulation in Mycobacterium smegmatis is modulated by proton motive force-driven and ATP-dependent extrusion systems. Biochem Biophys Res Commun 1999;56(3):682–684.

188. Wilson M, DeRisi J, Kristensen HH, et al. Exploring drug-induced alterations in gene expression in Mycobacterium tuberculosis by microarray hybridization. Proc Natl Acad Sci USA 1999;96(22):12833–12838.

189. Levin ME, Hatfull GF. Mycobacterium smegmatis RNA polymerase: DNA supercoiling, action of rifampicin and mechanism of rifampicin resistance. Mol Microbiol 1993;8(2):277–285.

190. Aristoff PA, Garcia GA, Kirchhoff PD, et al. Rifamycins—obstacles and opportunities. Tuberculosis (Edinb) 2010;90(2):94–118.

191. Bastian I, Stapledon R, Colebunders R. Current thinking on the management of tuberculosis. *Curr Opin Pulm Med* 2003;9(3):186–192.

192. Farmer P. DOTS and DOTS-plus: not the only answer. *Ann NY Acad Sci* 2001;953:165–184.

193. Frieden TR, Sterling TR, Munsiff SS, et al. Tuberculosis. *Lancet* 2003;362(9387):887–899.

194. Hui J, Gordon N, Kajioka R. Permeability barrier to rifampin in mycobacteria. *Antimicrob Agents Chemother* 1977;11:773–779.

195. Fuji K, Saito H, Tomioka H, et al. Mechanism of action of antimycobacterial activity of the new benzoxazinorifamycin KRM-1648. *Antimicrob Agents Chemother* 1995;39(7):1489–1492.

196. Roehr B. FDA approves rifapentine for the treatment of pulmonary tuberculosis.. . . Food and Drug Administration. *J Int Assoc Physicians AIDS Care* 1998;4(8):19–25.

197. Bemer-Melchior P, Bryskier A, Drugeon HB. Comparison of the in vitro activities of rifapentine and rifampicin against Mycobacterium tuberculosis complex. *J Antimicrob Chemother* 2000;46(4):571–576.

198. Rastogi N, Goh KS, Berchel M, et al. Activity of rifapentine and its metabolite 25-O-desacetylrifapentine compared with rifampicin and rifabutin against Mycobacterium tuberculosis, Mycobacterium africanum, Mycobacterium bovis and M. bovis BCG. *J Antimicrob Chemother* 2000;46(4):565–570.

199. Conte JE Jr, Golden JA, McQuitty M, et al. Single-dose intrapulmonary pharmacokinetics of rifapentine in normal subjects. *Antimicrob Agents Chemother* 2000; 44(4):985–990.

200. Burman WJ, Gallicano K, Peloquin C. Comparative pharmacokinetics and pharmacodynamics of the rifamycin antibacterials. *Clin Pharmacokinet* 2001;40(5): 327–341.

201. Keung A, Eller MG, McKenzie KA, et al. Single and multiple dose pharmacokinetics of rifapentine in man: part II. *Int J Tuberc Lung Dis* 1999;3(5):437–444.

202. Keung AC, Owens RC Jr, Eller MG, et al. Pharmacokinetics of rifapentine in subjects seropositive for the human immunodeficiency virus: a phase I study. *Antimicrob Agents Chemother* 1999;43(5):1230–1233.

203. Temple ME, Nahata MC. Rifapentine: its role in the treatment of tuberculosis. *Ann Pharmacother* 1999;33 (11):1203–1210.

204. Centers for Disease Control and Prevention. Recommendations for use of an isoniazid-rifapentine regimen with direct observation to treat latent Mycobacterium tuberculosis infection. *MMWR Morb Mortal Wkly Rep* 2011;60(48):1650–1653.

205. Sterling TR, Villarino ME, Borisov AS, et al. Three months of rifapentine and isoniazid for latent tuberculosis infection. *N Engl J Med* 2011;365(23):2155–2166.

206. Inderlied CB. Antimycobacterial susceptibility testing: present practices and future trends. *Eur J Clin Microbiol Infect Dis* 1994;13(11):980–993.

207. Inderlied CB, Kemper CA, Bermudez LEM. The Mycobacterium avium complex. *Clin Microbiol Rev* 1993;6: 266–310.

208. Benson CA, Williams PL, Currier JS, et al. A prospective, randomized trial examining the efficacy and safety of clarithromycin in combination with ethambutol, rifabutin, or both for the treatment of disseminated Mycobacterium avium complex disease in persons with acquired immunodeficiency syndrome. *Clin Infect Dis* 2003;37(9):1234–1243.

209. Masur H. Recommendations on prophylaxis and therapy for disseminated *Mycobacterium avium* complex disease in patients infected with the human-immunodeficiency-virus. *N Eng J Med* 1993;329:898–904.

210. Nightingale SD, Cameron WD, Gordin FM, et al. Two controlled trials of rifabutin prophylaxis against *Mycobacterium avium* complex infection in AIDS. *N Eng J Med* 1993;329:828–833.

211. Bermudez LE, Young LS, Inderlied CB. Rifabutin and sparfloxacin but not azithromycin inhibit binding of Mycobacterium avium complex to HT-29 intestinal mucosal cells. *Antimicrob Agents Chemother* 1994;38(5):1200–1202.

212. Quan S, Imai T, Mikami Y, et al. ADP-ribosylation as an intermediate step in inactivation of rifampin by a mycobacterial gene. *Antimicrob Agents Chemother* 1999;43(1):181–184.

213. Telenti A, Imboden P, Marchesi F, et al. Detection of rifampicin-resistance mutations in *Mycobacterium tuberculosis*. *Lancet* 1993;341(8846):647–650.

214. Siu GK, Zhang Y, Lau TC, et al. Mutations outside the rifampicin resistance-determining region associated with rifampicin resistance in Mycobacterium tuberculosis. *J Antimicrob Chemother* 2011;66(4):730–733.

215. Van Deun A, Martin A, Palomino JC. Diagnosis of drug-resistant tuberculosis: reliability and rapidity of detection. *Int J Tuberc Lung Dis* 2010;14(2):131–140.

216. Zhang Y, Telenti A. Genetics of drug resistance in *Mycobacterium tuberculosis*. In: Hatfull GF, Jacobs Jr WR, eds. *Molecular genetics of mycobacteria*. Washington, DC: American Society of Microbiology, 2000:235–254.

217. Ramaswamy S, Musser JM. Molecular genetic basis of antimicrobial agent resistance in Mycobacterium tuberculosis: 1998 update. *Tuberc Lung Dis* 1998;79(1):3–29.

218. Morlock GP, Plikaytis BB, Crawford JT. Characterization of spontaneous, In vitro-selected, rifampin-resistant mutants of Mycobacterium tuberculosis strain H37Rv. *Antimicrob Agents Chemother* 2000;44(12):3298–3301.

219. Billington OJ, McHugh TD, Gillespie SH. Physiological cost of rifampin resistance induced in vitro in Mycobacterium tuberculosis. *Antimicrob Agents Chemother* 1999;43(8):1866–1869.

220. Williams DL, Spring L, Collins L, et al. Contribution of rpoB mutations to development of rifamycin cross-resistance in Mycobacterium tuberculosis. *Antimicrob Agents Chemother* 1998;42(7):1853–1857.

221. Bodmer T, Zurcher G, Imboden P, et al. Mutation position and type of substitution in the beta-subunit of the RNA polymerase influence in-vitro activity of rifamycins in rifampicin-resistant Mycobacterium tuberculosis. *J Antimicrob Chemother* 1995;35(2):345–348.

221a. Van Deun A, Aung KJ, Bola V, et al. Rifampin drug resistance tests for tuberculosis: Challenging the gold standard. *J Clin Microbiol* 2013;51(8):2633–2640.

222. Moghazeh SL, Pan X, Arain T, et al. Comparative antimycobacterial activities of rifampin, rifapentine, and KRM-1648 against a collection of rifampin-resistant Mycobacterium tuberculosis isolates with known rpoB mutations. *Antimicrob Agents Chemother* 1996;40(11):2655–2657.

223. Yang B, Koga H, Ohno H, et al. Relationship between antimycobacterial activities of rifampicin, rifabutin and KRM-1648 and rpoB mutations of Mycobacterium tuberculosis. *J Antimicrob Chemother* 1998;42(5):621–628.

224. Park YK, Kim BJ, Ryu S, et al. Cross-resistance between rifampicin and KRM-1648 is associated with specific rpoB alleles in Mycobacterium tuberculosis. *Int J Tuberc Lung Dis* 2002;6(2):166–170.

225. Piddock LJ, Williams KJ, Ricci V. Accumulation of rifampicin by *Mycobacterium aurum, Mycobacterium smegmatis* and *Mycobacterium tuberculosis. J Antimicrob Chemother* 2000;45(2):159–165.

226. Iseman MD. Treatment of multidrug-resistant tuberculosis. *New Engl J Med* 1993;329(11):784–791.

227. Luna-Herrera J, Reddy V, Daneluzzi D, et al. Antituberculosis activity of clarithromycin. *Antimicrob Agents Chemother* 1995;39(12):2692–2695.

228. Truffot-Pernot C, Lounis N, Grosset JH, et al. Clarithromycin is inactive against *Mycobacterium tuberculosis. Antimicrob Agents Chemother* 1995;39(12):2827–2828.

229. Rastogi N, Goh KS, Bryskier A. Activities of roxithromycin used alone and in combination with ethambutol, rifampin, amikacin, ofloxacin, and clofazimine against Mycobacterium avium complex. *Antimicrob Agents Chemother* 1994;38(6):1433–1438.

230. Bonnet M, Van de Auwera P. In vitro and in vivo intraleukocytic accumulation of azithromycin (CP-62, 993) and its influence on ex vivo leukocyte chemiluminescence. *Antimicrob Agents Chemother* 1992;36(6):1302–1309.

231. Costa P, Desclaux d-F, Gouby A, et al. Disposition of roxithromycin in the epididymis after repeated oral administration. *J Antimicrob Chemother* 1992;30(2):197–201.

232. Fraschini F, Scaglione F, Pintucci G, et al. The diffusion of clarithromycin and roxithromycin into nasal mucosa, tonsil and lung in humans. *J Antimicrob Chemother* 1991;27(Suppl A):61–65.

233. Nilsen OG. Pharmacokinetics of macrolides. Comparison of plasma, tissue and free concentrations with special reference to roxithromycin. *Infection* 1995;23(Suppl 1):S5–S9.

234. Zhanel GG, Walters M, Noreddin A, et al. The ketolides: a critical review. *Drugs* 2002;62(12):1771–1804.

235. Douthwaite S, Champney WS. Structures of ketolides and macrolides determine their mode of interaction with the ribosomal target site. *J Antimicrob Chemother* 2001;48(90002):1–8.

236. Leclercq R. Overcoming antimicrobial resistance: profile of a new ketolide antibacterial, telithromycin. *J Antimicrob Chemother* 2001;48(Suppl T1):9–23.

237. Capobianco JO, Cao Z, Shortridge VD, et al. Studies of the novel ketolide ABT-773: transport, binding to ribosomes, and inhibition of protein synthesis in Streptococcus pneumoniae. *Antimicrob Agents Chemother* 2000;44(6):1562–1567.

238. Rosato A, Vicarini H, Bonnefoy A, et al. A new ketolide, HMR3004, active against streptococci inducibly resistant to erythromycin. *Antimicrob Agents Chemother* 1998; 42(6):1392–1396.

239. Yang SC, Hsueh PR, Lai HC, et al. High prevalence of antimicrobial resistance in rapidly growing mycobacteria in Taiwan. *Antimicrob Agents Chemother* 2003;47(6):1958–1962.

240. Rastogi N, Goh KS, Berchel M, et al. In vitro activities of the ketolides telithromycin (HMR 3647) and HMR 3004 compared to those of clarithromycin against slowly growing mycobacteria at pHs 6.8 and 7.4. *Antimicrob Agents Chemother* 2000;44(10):2848–2852.

241. Fernandez-Roblas R, Esteban J, Cabria F, et al. In vitro susceptibilities of rapidly growing mycobacteria to telithromycin (HMR 3647) and seven other antimicrobials. *Antimicrob Agents Chemother* 2000;44(1):181–182.

242. Cynamon MH, Carter JL, Shoen CM. Activity of ABT-773 against Mycobacterium avium complex in the beige mouse model. *Antimicrob Agents Chemother* 2000;44(10):2895–2896.

243. Consigny S, Bentoucha A, Bonnafous P, et al. Bactericidal activities of HMR 3647, moxifloxacin, and rifapentine against Mycobacterium leprae in mice. *Antimicrob Agents Chemother* 2000;44(10):2919–2921.

244. Bermudez LE, Inderlied CB, Kolonoski P, et al. Telithromycin is active against Mycobacterium avium in mice despite lacking significant activity in standard in vitro and macrophage assays and is associated with low frequency of resistance during treatment. *Antimicrob Agents Chemother* 2001;45(8):2210–2214.

245. Douthwaite S, Aagaard C. Erythromycin binding is reduced in ribosomes with conformational alterations in the 23 S rRNA peptidyl transferase loop. *J Mol Biol* 1993;232(3):725–731.

246. Zhanel GG, Dueck M, Hoban DJ, et al. Review of macrolides and ketolides: focus on respiratory tract infections. *Drugs* 2001;61(4):443–498.

247. Weisblum B. Erythromycin resistance by ribosome modification. *Antimicrob Agents Chemother* 1995;39(3): 577–585.

248. Roberts MC, Sutcliffe J, Courvalin P, et al. Nomenclature for macrolide and macrolide-lincosamide-streptogramin B resistance determinants. *Antimicrob Agents Chemother* 1999;43(12):2823–2830.

249. Meier A, Kirschner P, Springer B, et al. Identification of mutations in 23S rRNA gene of clarithromycin-resistant Mycobacterium intracellulare. *Antimicrob Agents Chemother* 1994;38(2):381–384.

250. Nash KA, Inderlied CB. Genetic basis of macrolide resistance in Mycobacterium avium. *Antimicrob Agents Chemother* 1995;39(12):2625–2630.

251. Doucet-Populaire F, Capobianco JO, Zakula D, et al. Molecular basis of clarithromycin activity against *Mycobacterium avium* and *Mycobacterium smegmatis. J Antimicrob Chemother* 1998;41(2):179–187.

252. Debets-Ossenkopp YJ, Sparrius M, Kusters JG, et al. Mechanism of clarithromycin resistance in clinical isolates of *Helicobacter pylori. FEMS Microbiol Lett* 1996;142(1):37–42.

253. Stone GG, Shortridge D, Flamm RK, et al. Identification of a 23S rRNA gene mutation in clarithromycin-resistant *Helicobacter pylori. Helicobacter* 1996;1(4): 227–228.

254. Versalovic J, Shortridge D, Kibler K, et al. Mutations in 23S rRNA are associated with clarithromycin resistance in *Helicobacter pylori. Antimicrob Agents Chemother* 1996;40(2):477–480.

255. Nash KA, Brown-Elliott BA, Wallace RJ Jr. A novel gene, erm(41), confers inducible macrolide resistance to clinical isolates of Mycobacterium abscessus but is absent from Mycobacterium chelonae. *Antimicrob Agents Chemother* 2009;53(4):1367–1376.

256. Nash KA. Mycobacterial factors that effect susceptibility to macrolides. Paper presented at: 103rd General Meeting of the American Society for Microbiology; May 18–22, 2003; Washington, DC.

257. Maus CE, Plikaytis BB, Shinnick TM. Mutation of tlyA confers capreomycin resistance in Mycobacterium tuberculosis. *Antimicrob Agents Chemother* 2005;49(2): 571–577.

258. Rhienberger H-J, Giegenmuller U, Gnirke A, et al. Allosteric three-site model for the ribosomal elongation cycle. In: Hill WE, Dahlberg A, Garrett RA, et al, eds. *The ribosome: structure, function and evolution.* Washington, DC: American Society for Microbiology, 1990:318–330.

259. Shaila MS, Gopinathan KP, Ramakrishnan T. Protein synthesis in Mycobacterium tuberculosis H37Rv and the effect of streptomycin in streptomycin-susceptible and -resistant strains. *Antimicrob Agents Chemother* 1971; 4:205–213.

260. Yamada T, Nagata A, Ono Y, et al. Alteration of ribosomes and RNA polymerase in drug-resistant clinical isolates of *Mycobacterium tuberculosis*. *Antimicrob Agents Chemother* 1985;27(6):921–924.

261. Yamada T. The role of ribosomes in the sensitivity of mycobacteria to tuberactinomycin. *Microbiol Immunol* 1987;31(2):179–181.

262. Verbist L, Gyselen A. Capreomycin susceptibility of strains resistant to streptomycin and/or viomycin. *Am Rev Respir Dis* 1964;90:640–641.

263. Böttger EC. Resistance to drugs targeting protein synthesis in mycobacteria. *Trends Microbiol* 1994;2(10):416–421.

264. Maus CE, Plikaytis BB, Shinnick TM. Molecular analysis of cross-resistance to capreomycin, kanamycin, amikacin, and viomycin in Mycobacterium tuberculosis. *Antimicrob Agents Chemother* 2005;49(8):3192–3197.

265. Jugheli L, Bzekalava N, de Rijk P, et al. High level of cross-resistance between kanamycin, amikacin, and capreomycin among Mycobacterium tuberculosis isolates from Georgia and a close relation with mutations in the rrs gene. *Antimicrob Agents Chemother* 2009;53(12): 5064–5068.

266. Dubovsky H. Correspondence with a pioneer, Jurgen Lehmann (1898–1989), producer of the first effective antituberculosis specific. *S Afr Med J* 1991;79(1):48–50.

267. Heifets L, Lindholm-Levy P. Comparison of bactericidal activities of streptomycin, amikacin, kanamycin, and capreomycin against *Mycobacterium avium* and *M. tuberculosis*. *Antimicrob Agents Chemother* 1989;33: 1298–1301.

268. Hausner T-P, Geigenmuller U, Nierhaus KH. The allosteric three-site model for the ribosomal elongation cycle. *J Biol Chem* 1988;263:13103–13111.

269. Yamada T, Masuda K, Shoji K, et al. Analysis of ribosomes from viomycin-sensitive and -resistant strains of Mycobacterium smegmatis. *J Bacteriol* 1972;112:1–6.

270. Yamada T, Mizuguchi Y, Nierhaus KH, et al. Resistance to viomycin conferred by RNA of either ribosomal subunit. *Nature* 1978;275(5679):460–461.

271. Choi EC, Misumi M, Nishimura T, et al. Viomycin resistance: alterations of either ribosomal subunit affect the binding of the antibiotic to the pair subunit and the entire ribosome becomes resistant to the drug. *Biochem Biophys Res Commun* 1979;87(3):904–910.

272. Mizuguchi Y, Suga K, Yamada T. Interaction between 30 S ribosomal components in a viomycin resistant mutant of Mycobacterium smegmatis. *Microbiol Immunol* 1979;23(7):595–604.

273. Mizuguchi Y, Suga K, Yamada T. Interactions between viomycin resistance and streptomycin resistance on ribosomes of Mycobacterium smegmatis. *Microbiol Immunol* 1979;23(7):581–594.

274. Finken M, Kirschner P, Meier A, et al. Molecular basis of streptomycin resistance in Mycobacterium tuberculosis: alterations of the ribosomal protein S12 gene and point mutations within a functional 16S ribosomal RNA pseudoknot. *Mol Microbiol* 1993;9(6):1239–1246.

275. Nair J, Rouse DA, Bai GH, et al. The rpsL gene and streptomycin resistance in single and multiple drug-resistant strains of Mycobacterium tuberculosis. *Mol Microbiol* 1993;10(3):521–527.

276. Honore N, Cole ST. Streptomycin resistance in mycobacteria. *Antimicrob Agents Chemother* 1994;38(2): 238–242.

277. Meier A, Kirschner P, Bange FC, et al. Genetic alterations in streptomycin-resistant Mycobacterium tuberculosis: mapping of mutations conferring resistance. *Antimicrob Agents Chemother* 1994;38(2):228–233.

278. Prammananan T, Sander P, Brown BA, et al. A single 16S ribosomal RNA substitution is responsible for resistance to amikacin and other 2-deoxystreptamine aminoglycosides in Mycobacterium abscessus and Mycobacterium chelonae. *J Infect Dis* 1998;177(6): 1573–1581.

279. Kenney TJ, Churchward G. Cloning and sequence analysis of the rpsL and rpsG genes of Mycobacterium smegmatis and characterization of mutations causing resistance to streptomycin. *J Bacteriol* 1994;176(19): 6153–6156.

280. Cooksey RC, Morlock GP, McQueen A, et al. Characterization of streptomycin resistance mechanisms among Mycobacterium tuberculosis isolates from patients in New York City. *Antimicrob Agents Chemother* 1996;40(5): 1186–1188.

281. Sreevatsan S, Pan X, Stockbauer KE, et al. Characterization of rpsL and rrs mutations in streptomycin-resistant Mycobacterium tuberculosis isolates from diverse geographic localities. *Antimicrob Agents Chemother* 1996; 40(4):1024–1026.

282. Springer B, Kidan YG, Prammananan T, et al. Mechanisms of streptomycin resistance: selection of mutations in the 16S rRNA gene conferring resistance. *Antimicrob Agents Chemother* 2001;45(10):2877–2884.

283. Nachamkin I, Kang C, Weinstein MP. Detection of resistance to isoniazid, rifampin, and streptomycin in clinical isolates of Mycobacterium tuberculosis by molecular methods. *Clin Infect Dis* 1997;24(5):894–900.

284. Brimacombe R, Greuer B, Mitchell P, et al. Three-dimensional structure and function of *Escherichia coli* 16S and 23S rRNA as studied by cross-linking techniques. In: Hill WE, Dahlberg A, Garrett RA, et al, eds. *The ribosome: structure, function and evolution*. Washington, DC: American Society for Microbiology, 1990:73–92.

285. Victor TC, van Rie A, Jordaan AM, et al. Sequence polymorphism in the rrs gene of Mycobacterium tuberculosis is deeply rooted within an evolutionary clade and is not associated with streptomycin resistance. *J Clin Microbiol* 2001;39(11):4184–4186.

286. Spies FS, da Silva PE, Ribeiro MO, et al. Identification of mutations related to streptomycin resistance in clinical isolates of Mycobacterium tuberculosis and possible involvement of efflux mechanism. *Antimicrob Agents Chemother* 2008;52(8):2947–2949.

287. Meier A, Sander P, Schaper KJ, et al. Correlation of molecular resistance mechanisms and phenotypic resistance levels in streptomycin-resistant Mycobacterium tuberculosis. *Antimicrob Agents Chemother* 1996;40(11): 2452–2454.

288. Cundliffe E. Recognition sites for antibiotics within rRNA. In: Hill WE, Dahlberg A, Garrett RA, et al, eds. *The ribosome: structure, function and evolution*. Washington, DC: American Society for Microbiology, 1990:479–490.

289. Shaw KJ, Rather PN, Hare RS, et al. Molecular genetics of aminoglycoside resistance genes and familial relationships of the aminoglycoside-modifying enzymes. *Microbiol Rev* 1993;57:138–163.

290. Hull SI, Wallace RJ Jr, Bobey DG, et al. Presence of aminoglycoside acetyltransferase and plasmids in *Mycobacterium fortuitum*. Lack of correlation with intrinsic aminoglycoside resistance. *Am Rev Respir Dis* 1984;129(4):614–618.

291. Udou T, Mizuguchi Y, Wallace RJ Jr. Patterns and distribution of aminoglycoside-acetylating enzymes in rapidly growing mycobacteria. *Am Rev Respir Dis* 1987; 136(2):338–343.

292. Wallace RJ Jr, Hull SI, Bobey DG, et al. Mutational resistance as the mechanism of acquired drug resistance to aminoglycosides and antibacterial agents in *Mycobacterium fortuitum* and *Mycobacterium chelonei*. Evidence is based on plasmid analysis, mutational frequencies, and aminoglycoside-modifying enzyme assays. *Am Rev Respir Dis* 1985;132(2):409–416.

293. Ainsa JA, Perez E, Pelicic V, et al. Aminoglycoside 2′-N-acetyltransferase genes are universally present in mycobacteria: characterization of the aac(2′)-Ic gene from Mycobacterium tuberculosis and the aac(2′)-Id gene from Mycobacterium smegmatis. *Mol Microbiol* 1997;24(2):431–441.

294. Kilburn JO, Greenberg J. Effect of ethambutol on the viable cell count in Mycobacterium smegmatis. *Antimicrob Agents Chemother* 1977;11:534–540.

295. Takayama K, Armstrong EL, Kunugi KA, et al. Inhibition by ethambutol of mycolic acid transfer into the cell wall of Mycobacterium smegmatis. *Antimicrob Agents Chemother* 1979;16:240–242.

296. Poso H, Paulin L, Brander E. Specific inhibition of spermidine synthase from Mycobacteria by ethambutol. *Lancet* 1983;2:1418.

297. Paulin LG, Brander EE, Poso HJ. Specific inhibition of spermidine synthesis in Mycobacteria spp. by the dextro isomer of ethambutol. *Antimicrob Agents Chemother* 1985;28:157–159.

298. Kilburn JO, Takayama K. Effects of ethambutol on accumulation and secretion of trehalose mycolates and free mycolic acid in Mycobacterium smegmatis. *Antimicrob Agents Chemother* 1981;20:401–404.

299. Takayama K, Kilburn JO. Inhibition of synthesis of arabinogalactan by ethambutol in *Mycobacterium smegmatis*. *Antimicrob Agents Chemother* 1989;33:1493–1499.

300. Deng L, Mikusova K, Robuck KG, et al. Recognition of multiple effects of ethambutol on metabolism of mycobacterial cell envelope. *Antimicrob Agents Chemother* 1995;39(3):694–701.

301. Wolucka BA, McNeil MR, de Hoffmann E, et al. Recognition of the lipid intermediate for arabinogalactan/arabinomannan biosynthesis and its relation to the mode of action of ethambutol on mycobacteria. *J Biol Chem* 1994;269(37):23328–23335.

302. Lee RE, Mikusova K, Brennan PJ, et al. Synthesis of the mycobacterial arabinose donor β-D-arabinofuranosyl-1-monophosphoryldecaprenol, development of a basic arabinosyl-transferase assay, and identification of ethambutol as an arabinosyl transferase inhibitor. *J Am Chem Soc* 1995;117:11829–11832.

303. Hoffner SE, Kallenius G, Beezer AE, et al. Studies on the mechanisms of the synergistic effects of ethambutol and other antibacterial drugs on *Mycobacterium avium* complex. *Acta Leprol* 1989;7(Suppl 1):195–199.

304. Rastogi N, Barrow WW. Cell envelope constituents and the multifaceted nature of *Mycobacterium avium* pathogenicity and drug resistance. *Res Microbiol* 1993; 145(3):243–252.

305. Belanger AE, Besra GS, Ford ME, et al. The embAB genes of Mycobacterium avium encode an arabinosyl transferase involved in cell wall arabinan biosynthesis that is the target for the antimycobacterial drug ethambutol. *Proc Natl Acad Sci USA* 1996;93(21): 11919–11924.

306. Telenti A, Philipp WJ, Sreevatsan S, et al. The emb operon, a gene cluster of Mycobacterium tuberculosis involved in resistance to ethambutol. *Nature Med* 1997;3(5):567–570.

307. Sreevatsan S, Stockbauer KE, Pan X, et al. Ethambutol resistance in Mycobacterium tuberculosis: critical role of embB mutations. *Antimicrob Agents Chemother* 1997;41(8):1677–1681.

308. Ramaswamy SV, Amin AG, Goksel S, et al. Molecular genetic analysis of nucleotide polymorphisms associated with ethambutol resistance in human isolates of Mycobacterium tuberculosis. *Antimicrob Agents Chemother* 2000;44(2):326–336.

309. Alcaide F, Pfyffer GE, Telenti A. Role of embB in natural and acquired resistance to ethambutol in mycobacteria. *Antimicrob Agents Chemother* 1997;41(10):2270–2273.

310. Mokrousov I, Otten T, Vyshnevskiy B, et al. Detection of embB306 mutations in ethambutol-susceptible clinical isolates of Mycobacterium tuberculosis from Northwestern Russia: implications for genotypic resistance testing. *J Clin Microbiol* 2002;40(10):3810–3813.

311. Tsukamura M. Resistance pattern of *Mycobacterium tuberculosis* and *Mycobacterium bovis* to ethambutol. *Acta Tuberc Scand* 1965;46:89–92.

312. Heifets LB, Iseman MD, Crowle AJ, et al. Pyrazinamide is not active in vitro against Mycobacterium avium complex. *Am Rev Respir Dis* 1986;134(6):1287–1288.

313. Lowrie DD. The macrophage and mycobacterial infections. *Trans R Soc Trop Med Hyg* 1983;77:646–655.

314. McClatchy JK, Tsang AY, Cernich MS. Use of pyrazinamidase activity in Mycobacterium tuberculosis as a rapid method for determination of pyrazinamide susceptibility. *Antimicrob Agents Chemother* 1981;20: 556–557.

315. Butler WR, Kilburn JO. Susceptibility of *Mycobacterium tuberculosis* to pyrazinamide and its relationship to pyrazinamidase activity. *Antimicrob Agents Chemother* 1983;24(4):600–601.

316. Scorpio A, Zhang Y. Mutations in pncA, a gene encoding pyrazinamidase/nicotinamidase, cause resistance to the antituberculous drug pyrazinamide in tubercle bacillus. *Nature Med* 1996;2(6):662–667.

317. Tarnok I, Pechmann H, Krallmann-Wenzel U, et al. Nikotinamidase und die sogenannte Pyrazinamidase in Mycobakterien; gekoppeltes Auftreten der beiden Enzymaktivitaten. *Zentralbl Bakteriol [Orig A]* 1979;244 (2–3):302–308.

318. Speirs RJ, Welch JT, Cynamon MH. Activity of *n*-propyl pyrazinoate against pyrazinamide-resistant *Mycobacterium tuberculosis*: investigations into mechanism of action of and mechanism of resistance to pyrazinamide. *Antimicrob Agents Chemother* 1995;39(6):1269–1271.

319. Zhang Y, Scorpio A, Nikaido H, et al. Role of acid pH and deficient efflux of pyrazinoic acid in unique susceptibility of Mycobacterium tuberculosis to pyrazinamide. *J Bacteriol* 1999;181(7):2044–2049.

320. Zhang Y, Wade MM, Scorpio A, et al. Mode of action of pyrazinamide: disruption of Mycobacterium tuberculosis membrane transport and energetics by pyrazinoic acid. *J Antimicrob Chemother* 2003;52(5):790–795.

321. Scorpio A, Collins D, Whipple D, et al. Rapid differentiation of bovine and human tubercle bacilli based on a characteristic mutation in the bovine pyrazinamidase gene. *J Clin Microbiol* 1997;35(1):106–110.

322. Wallace RJ Jr, Griffith DE. Antimycobacterial agents. In: Mandell GL, Bennett JE, Dolin R, eds. *Principles and practice of infectious diseases.* Vol 1. 7th ed. Philadelphia: Churchill Livingstone Elsevier, 2010:533–548.

323. Berning SE. The role of fluoroquinolones in tuberculosis today. *Drugs* 2001;61(1):9–18.

324. Zhanel GG, Noreddin AM. Pharmacokinetics and pharmacodynamics of the new fluoroquinolones: focus on respiratory infections. *Curr Opin Pharmacol* 2001;1(5):459–463.

325. Cambau E, Sougakoff W, Besson M, et al. Selection of a gyrA mutant of *Mycobacterium tuberculosis* resistant to fluoroquinolones during treatment with ofloxacin. *J Infect Dis* 1994;170(2):479–483.

326. Cambau E, Sougakoff W, Jarlier V. Amplification and nucleotide sequence of the quinolone resistance-determining region in the gyrA gene of mycobacteria. *FEMS Microbiol Lett* 1994;116(1):49–54.

327. Revel V, Cambau E, Jarlier V, et al. Characterization of mutations in *Mycobacterium smegmatis* involved in resistance to fluoroquinolones. *Antimicrob Agents Chemother* 1994;38(9):1991–1996.

328. Takiff HE, Salazar L, Guerrero C, et al. Cloning and nucleotide sequence of *Mycobacterium tuberculosis* gyrA and gyrB genes and detection of quinolone resistance mutations. *Antimicrob Agents Chemother* 1994;38(4): 773–780.

329. Siddiqi N, Shamim M, Hussain S, et al. Molecular characterization of multidrug-resistant isolates of Mycobacterium tuberculosis from patients in North India. *Antimicrob Agents Chemother* 2002;46(2):443–450.

330. Guillemin I, Jarlier V, Cambau E. Correlation between quinolone susceptibility patterns and sequences in the A and B subunits of DNA gyrase in mycobacteria. *Antimicrob Agents Chemother* 1998;42(8):2084–2088.

331. Wang JY, Lee LN, Lai HC, et al. Fluoroquinolone resistance in Mycobacterium tuberculosis isolates: associated genetic mutations and relationship to antimicrobial exposure. *J Antimicrob Chemother* 2007;59(5):860–865.

332. Lee AS, Tang LL, Lim IH, et al. Characterization of pyrazinamide and ofloxacin resistance among drug resistant *Mycobacterium tuberculosis* isolates from Singapore. *Int J Infect Dis* 2002;6(1):48–51.

333. Cheng AF, Yew WW, Chan EW, et al. Multiplex PCR amplimer conformation analysis for rapid detection of gyrA mutations in fluoroquinolone-resistant Mycobacterium tuberculosis clinical isolates. *Antimicrob Agents Chemother* 2004;48(2):596–601.

334. Howard BM, Pinney RJ, Smith JT. Function of the SOS process in repair of DNA damage induced by modern 4-quinolones. *J Pharm Pharmacol* 1993;45(7):658–662.

335. Aeschlimann JR. The role of multidrug efflux pumps in the antibiotic resistance of *Pseudomonas aeruginosa* and other gram-negative bacteria. Insights from the Society of Infectious Diseases Pharmacists. *Pharmacother* 2003;23(7):916–924.

336. Sander P, De Rossi E, Boddinghaus B, et al. Contribution of the multidrug efflux pump LfrA to innate mycobacterial drug resistance. *FEMS Microbiol Lett* 2000;193(1):19–23.

337. Liu J, Takiff HE, Nikaido H. Active efflux of fluoroquinolones in *Mycobacterium smegmatis* mediated by LfrA, a multidrug efflux pump. *J Bacteriol* 1996;178(13): 3791–3795.

338. Drlica K, Malik M. Fluoroquinolones: action and resistance. *Curr Top Med Chem* 2003;3(3):249–282.

339. Alcala L, Ruiz-Serrano MJ, Perez-Fernandez Turegano C, et al. In vitro activities of linezolid against clinical isolates of *Mycobacterium tuberculosis* that are susceptible or resistant to first-line antituberculous drugs. *Antimicrob Agents Chemother* 2003;47(1):416–417.

340. Braback M, Riesbeck K, Forsgren A. Susceptibilities of *Mycobacterium marinum* to gatifloxacin, gemifloxacin, levofloxacin, linezolid, moxifloxacin, telithromycin, and quinupristin-dalfopristin (Synercid) compared to its susceptibilities to reference macrolides and quinolones. *Antimicrob Agents Chemother* 2002;46(4):1114–1116.

341. Brickner SJ, Hutchinson DK, Barbachyn MR, et al. Synthesis and antibacterial activity of U-100592 and U-100766, two oxazolidinone antibacterial agents for the potential treatment of multidrug-resistant gram-positive bacterial infections. *J Med Chem* 1996;39(3): 673–679.

342. Brown-Elliott BA, Crist CJ, Mann LB, et al. In vitro activity of linezolid against slowly growing nontuberculous mycobacteria. *Antimicrob Agents Chemother* 2003; 47(5):1736–1738.

343. Rodriguez JC, Ruiz M, Lopez M, et al. In vitro activity of moxifloxacin, levofloxacin, gatifloxacin and linezolid against *Mycobacterium tuberculosis*. *Int J Antimicrob Agents* 2002;20(6):464–467.

344. Wallace RJ Jr, Brown-Elliott BA, Ward SC, et al. Activities of linezolid against rapidly growing mycobacteria. *Antimicrob Agents Chemother* 2001;45(3):764–767.

345. Rodriguez Diaz JC, Ruiz M, Lopez M, Royo G. Synergic activity of fluoroquinolones and linezolid against *Mycobacterium tuberculosis*. *Int J Antimicrob Agents* 2003;21(4): 354–356.

346. Williams KN, Stover CK, Zhu T, et al. Promising antituberculosis activity of the oxazolidinone PNU-100480 relative to that of linezolid in a murine model. *Antimicrob Agents Chemother* 2009;53(4):1314–1319.

347. Cynamon MH, Klemens SP, Sharpe CA, et al. Activities of several novel oxazolidinones against *Mycobacterium tuberculosis* in a murine model. *Antimicrob Agents Chemother* 1999;43(5):1189–1191.

348. Park IN, Hong SB, Oh YM, et al. Efficacy and tolerability of daily-half dose linezolid in patients with intractable multidrug-resistant tuberculosis. *J Antimicrob Chemother* 2006;58(3):701–704.

349. Yew WW, Chau CH, Wen KH. Linezolid in the treatment of "difficult" multidrug-resistant tuberculosis. *Int J Tuberc Lung Dis* 2008;12(3):345–346.

350. Brown-Elliott BA, Wallace RJ Jr, Blinkhorn R, et al. Successful treatment of disseminated *Mycobacterium chelonae* infection with linezolid. *Clin Infect Dis* 2001;33(8):1433–1434.

351. Aoki H, Ke L, Poppe SM, et al. Oxazolidinone antibiotics target the P site on *Escherichia coli* ribosomes. *Antimicrob Agents Chemother* 2002;46(4):1080–1085.

352. Colca JR, McDonald WG, Waldon DJ, et al. Cross-linking in the living cell locates the site of action of oxazolidinone antibiotics. *J Biol Chem* 2003;278(24): 21972–21979.

353. Patel U, Yan YP, Hobbs FW Jr, et al. Oxazolidinones mechanism of action: inhibition of the first peptide bond formation. *J Biol Chem* 2001;276(40):37199–37205.

354. Livermore DM. Linezolid in vitro: mechanism and antibacterial spectrum. *J Antimicrob Chemother* 2003;51 (Suppl 2):ii9–ii16.

355. Kloss P, Xiong L, Shinabarger DL, et al. Resistance mutations in 23 S rRNA identify the site of action of the protein synthesis inhibitor linezolid in the ribosomal peptidyl transferase center. *J Mol Biol* 1999;294(1): 93–101.

356. Shinabarger DL, Marotti KR, Murray RW, et al. Mechanism of action of oxazolidinones: effects of linezolid and eperezolid on translation reactions. *Antimicrob Agents Chemother* 1997;41(10):2132–2136.

357. Hedgecock LW. Antagonism of the inhibitory action of aminosalicylic acid on *Mycobacterium tuberculosis* by methionine, biotin and certain fatty acids, amino acids and purines. *J Bacteriol* 1956;72:839–846.

358. Ratledge C, Brown KA. Inhibition of mycobactin formation in *Mycobacterium smegmatis* by p-aminosalicylate. A new proposal for the mode of action of p-aminosalicylate. *Am Rev Respir Dis* 1972;106:774–776.

359. Snow GA. Mycobactins: iron-chelating growth factors from mycobacteria. *Bacteriol Rev* 1970;34:99–125.

360. Brown KA, Ratledge C. The effect of p-aminosalicylic acid on iron transport and assimilation in mycobacteria. *Biochim Biophys Acta* 1975;385:207–220.

361. Brown KA, Ratledge C. Iron transport in Mycobacterium smegmatis: ferrimycobactin reductase (NAD(P)H: ferrimycobactin oxidoreductase), the enzyme releasing iron from its carrier. *FEBS Lett* 1975;53:262–266.

362. Kuntz E. Die heutige Bedeutung der PAS fur die Basis-Behandlung der Lungentuberkulos. Klinische Ergebnisse bei 20000 iv. PAS-streptomycin-INH infusionen. *Prax Pneumol* 1965;19:610–615.

363. David HL, Takayama K, Goldman DS. Susceptibility of mycobacterial D-alanyl-D-alanine synthetase to D-cycloserine. *Am Rev Respir Dis* 1969;100:579–582.

364. Hawkins JE, McClean VR. Comparative studies of cycloserine inhibition of mycobacteria. *Am Rev Respir Dis* 1966;93:594–602.

365. Zygmunt WA. Antagonism of D-cycloserine inhibition of mycobacterial growth by D-alaine. *J Bacteriol* 1963;85:1217–1220.

366. Caceres NE, Harris NB, Wellehan JF, et al. Overexpression of the D-alanine racemase gene confers resistance to D-cycloserine in *Mycobacterium smegmatis*. *J Bacteriol* 1997;179(16):5046–5055.

367. Chacon O, Feng Z, Harris NB, et al. *Mycobacterium smegmatis* D-alanine racemase mutants are not dependent on D-alanine for growth. *Antimicrob Agents Chemother* 2002;46(1):47–54.

368. Peteroy M, Severin A, Zhao F, et al. Characterization of a *Mycobacterium smegmatis* mutant that is simultaneously resistant to D-cycloserine and vancomycin. *Antimicrol Agents Chemother* 2000;44(6):1701–1704.

369. Neuhaus FC, Lynch JL. The enzymatic synthesis of D-alanyl-D-alanine. 3. On the inhibition of D-alanyl-D-alanine synthetase by the antibiotic D-cycloserine. *Biochemistry* 1965;3:471–480.

370. Strominger JL, Threnn RH, Scott SS. Oxamycin, a competitive antagonist of the incorporation of D-alanine into a uridine nucleotide in *Staphylococcus aureus*. *J Am Chem Soc* 1959;81:3803–3804.

371. Winder FG, Collins PB, Whelan D. Effects of ethionamide and isoxyl on mycolic acid synthesis in *Mycobacterium tuberculosis* BCG. *J Gen Microbiol* 1971;66:379–380.

372. Baulard AR, Betts JC, Engohang-Ndong J, et al. Activation of the pro-drug ethionamide is regulated in mycobacteria. *J Biol Chem* 2000;275(36):28326–28331.

373. DeBarber AE, Mdluli K, Bosman M, et al. Ethionamide activation and sensitivity in multidrug-resistant *Mycobacterium tuberculosis*. *Proc Nat Acad Sci USA* 2000;97(17):9677–9682.

374. Zaunbrecher MA, Sikes RD Jr, Metchock B, et al. Overexpression of the chromosomally encoded aminoglycoside acetyltransferase eis confers kanamycin resistance in Mycobacterium tuberculosis. *Proc Natl Acad Sci USA* 2009;106(47):20004–20009.

375. Chen W, Biswas T, Porter VR, et al. Unusual regioversatility of acetyltransferase Eis, a cause of drug resistance in XDR-TB. *Proc Natl Acad Sci USA* 2011;108(24):9804–9808.

376. Johansen SK, Maus CE, Plikaytis BB, et al. Capreomycin binds across the ribosomal subunit interface using tlyA-encoded 2′-O-methylations in 16S and 23S rRNAs. *Mol Cell* 2006;23(2):173–182.

377. De Rossi E, Ainsa JA, Riccardi G. Role of mycobacterial efflux transporters in drug resistance: an unresolved question. *FEMS Microbiol Rev* 2006;30(1):36–52.

378. Ramon-Garcia S, Martin C, Ainsa JA, et al. Characterization of tetracycline resistance mediated by the efflux pump Tap from Mycobacterium fortuitum. *J Antimicrob Chemother* 2006;57(2):252–259.

379. Srivastava S, Musuka S, Sherman C, et al. Efflux-pump-derived multiple drug resistance to ethambutol monotherapy in Mycobacterium tuberculosis and the pharmacokinetics and pharmacodynamics of ethambutol. *J Infect Dis* 2010;201(8):1225–1231.

380. Balganesh M, Dinesh N, Sharma S, et al. Efflux pumps of Mycobacterium tuberculosis play a significant role in antituberculosis activity of potential drug candidates. *Antimicrob Agents Chemother* 2012;56(5):2643–2651.

381. Frieden TR, Sterling T, Pablos-Mendez A, et al. The emergence of drug-resistant tuberculosis in New York City. *N Engl J Med* 1993;328(8):521–526.

382. Jassal M, Bishai WR. Extensively drug-resistant tuberculosis. *Lancet Infect Dis* 2009;9(1):19–30.

383. Centers for Disease Control and Prevention. Extensively drug-resistant tuberculosis—United States, 1993-2006. *MMWR Morb Mortal Wkly Rep* 2007;56(11):250–253.

384. World Health Organization. *Totally drug-resistant TB: a WHO consultation on the diagnostic definition and treatment options*. Geneva: WHO, 2012.

385. Zumla A, Abubakar I, Raviglione M, et al. Drug-resistant tuberculosis—current dilemmas, unanswered questions, challenges, and priority needs. *J Infect Dis* 2012;205(Suppl 2):S228–S240.

386. Caminero JA, Sotgiu G, Zumla A, et al. Best drug treatment for multidrug-resistant and extensively drug-resistant tuberculosis. *Lancet Infect Dis* 2010;10(9):621–629.

387. Gordon SM, Horsburgh CR Jr, Peloquin CA, et al. Low serum levels of oral antimycobacterial agents in patients with disseminated *Mycobacterium avium* complex disease. *J Infect Dis* 1993;168(6):1559–1562.

388. Peloquin CA, MacPhee AA, Berning SE. Malabsorption of antimycobacterial medications. *N Engl J Med* 1993;329(15):1122–1123.

389. Peloquin CA. Pharmacology of the antimycobacterial drugs. *Med Clin North Am* 1993;77(6):1253–1262.

390. Holdiness MR. Chromatographic analysis of antituberculosis drugs in biological samples. *J Chromatog* 1985;340:321–359.

391. Holdiness MR. Clinical pharmacokinetics of the antituberculosis drugs. *Clin Pharmacokinet* 1984;9:511–544.

392. Peloquin CA. Therapeutic drug monitoring in the treatment of tuberculosis. *Drugs* 2002;62(15):2169–2183.

393. McClatchy JK. Antimycobacterial drugs: mechanisms of action, drug resistance, susceptibility testing, and assays of activity in biological fluids. In: Lorian V, ed. *Antibiotics in laboratory medicine.* 2nd ed. Baltimore: Williams & Wilkins, 1986:181–222.

394. Lunde PKM, Frislid K, Hansteen V. Disease and acetylation polymorphism. *Clin Pharmacokinet* 1977;2:182–197.

395. Gangadharam PRJ. Isoniazid, rifampin, and hepatotoxicity. *Am Rev Respir Dis* 1986;133:963–965.

396. Singapore Tuberculosis Service, Council BMR. Controlled trial of intermittent regimen of rifampicin plus isoniazid for pulmonary tuberculosis in Singapore: the results up to 30 months. *Am Rev Respir Dis* 1977;116:807–820.

397. El-Sayed YM, Islam SI. Acetylation phenotyping of isoniazid using a simple and accurate high-performance liquid chromatography. *J Clin Phar Ther* 1989;14:197–205.

398. Hanson A, Melander A, Wahlin-Boll E. Acetylator phenotyping: a comparison of the isoniazid and dapsone tests. *Eur J Clin Pharmacol* 1981;20:233–234.

399. Hutchings A, Routledge PA. A simple method for determining acetylator phenotype using isoniazid. *Br J Clin Pharmacol* 1986;22:343–345.

400. Guillaumont M, Leclercq M, Forbert Y, et al. Determination of rifampicin, desacetylrifampicin, isoniazid and acetylisoniazid by high-performance liquid chromatography; application to human serum extracts, polymorphonucleocytes and alveolar macrophages. *J Chromatogr* 1982;232:369–376.

401. Holdiness MR. High pressure liquid chromatographic determination of isoniazid and acetyisoniazid in human plasma. *J Liq Chromatogr* 1982;5:707–714.

402. Hutchings A, Monie RD, Spragg B, et al. High performance liquid chromatographic analysis of isoniazid and acetyisoniazid in biological fluids. *J Chromatogr* 1983;227:385–390.

403. Kimerling ME, Phillips P, Patterson P, et al. Low serum antimycobacterial drug levels in non-HIV-infected tuberculosis patients. *Chest* 1998;113(5):1178–1183.

404. Peloquin CA, Jaresko GS, Yong CL, et al. Population pharmacokinetic modeling of isoniazid, rifampin, and pyrazinamide. *Antimicrob Agents Chemother* 1997;41(12):2670–2679.

405. Moulin MA, Albessard F, Lacotte J, et al. Hydrophilic ion-pair reversed-phase high- performance liquid chromatography for the simultaneous assay of isoniazid and acetylisoniazid in serum: a microscale procedure. *J Chromatogr* 1981;226:250–254.

406. Saxena SJ, Stewart JT, Honigsberg IL, et al. Liquid chromatography in pharmaceutical analysis. VIII. Determination of isoniazid and acetyl derivative in plasma and urine samples. *J Pharmaceut Sci* 1977;6:813–816.

407. Kenny MT, Strates B. Metabolism and pharmacokinetics of the antibiotic rifampin. *Drug Metab Rev* 1981;12:159–218.

408. Cocchiara G, Benedetti MS, Vicario GP, et al. Urinary metabolites of rifabutin, a new antimycobacterial agent, in human volunteers. *Xenobiotica* 1989;19:769–780.

409. Ratti B, Parenti RR, Toselli A, et al. Quantitative assay of rifampicin and its main metabolite 25-desacetyl-rifampicin in human plasma by reversed-phase high-performance liquid chromatography. *J Chromatogr* 1981;225:526–531.

410. Ishii M, Ogata H. Determination of rifampicin and its main metabolites in human plasma by high-performance liquid chromatography. *J Chromatogr* 1988;426:412–416.

411. Peets EA, Sweeney WM, Place VA, et al. The absorption, excretion and metabolic fate of ethambutol in man. *Am Rev Respir Dis* 1964;88:51–58.

412. Gundert-Remy U, Klett M, Weber E. Concentration of ethambutol in cerebrospinal fluid in man as a function of the non-protein-bound drug fraction in serum. *Eur J Clin Pharmacol* 1973;6:133–136.

413. Strauss I, Erhardt F. Ethambutol absorption, excretion and dosage in patients with renal tuberculosis. *Chemother* 1970;15:148-157.

414. Holdiness MR, Israili ZH, Justice JB. Gas chromatographic-mass spectrophotometric determination of ethambutol in human plasma. *J Chromatogr* 1981;224:415–422.

415. Lee CC, Varughese A. Disposition kinetics of ethambutol in nephrectomized dogs. *J Pharma Sci* 1984;73:787–789.

416. Lee CS, Benet LZ. Gas-liquid chromatographic determination of ethambutol in plasma and urine of man and monkey. *J Chromatogr* 1976;128:188–192.

417. Ohya K, Shintani S, Sano M. Determination of ethambutol in plasma using selected ion monitoring. *J Chromatogr* 1980;221:293–299.

418. Yamamoto T, Moriwaki Y, Takahashi S, et al. Study of the metabolism of pyrazinamide using a high-performance liquid chromatographic analysis of urine samples. *Anal Biochem* 1987;160:346–349.

419. Yamamoto T, Moriwaki Y, Takahashi S, et al. Rapid and simultaneous determination of pyrazinamide and its major metabolites in human plasma by high-performance liquid chromatography. *J Chromatogr* 1987;413:342–346.

420. Woo J, Wong CL, Teoh R, et al. Liquid chromatographic assay for the simultaneous determination of pyrazinamide and rifampicin in serum samples from patients with tuberculous meningitis. *J Chromatogr* 1987;420:73–80.

421. Donald PR, Seifart H. Cerebrospinal fluid pyrazinamide de concentrations in children with tuberculous meningitis. *Pediatr Infect Dis J* 1988;7(7):469–471.

422. Jenner PJ, Ellard GA, Gruer PJK, et al. A comparison of the blood levels and urinary excretion of ethionamide and prothionamide in man. *J Antimicrob Chemother* 1984;13:267–277.

423. Brendel E, Meineke I, Stuwe E, et al. Stability of 5-aminosalicylic acid and 5-acetylaminosalicylic acid in plasma. *J Chromatogr* 1988;432:358–362.

424. Brendel E, Meineke I, Witsch D, et al. Simultaneous determination of 5-aminosalicylic acid and 5-acetylaminosalicylic acid by high-performance liquid chromatography. *J Chromatogr* 1987;385:299–304.

425. Lee EJD, Ang SB. Simple and sensitive high-performance liquid chromatographic assay for 5-aminosalicylic acid and acetyl-5-aminosalicylic acid in serum. *J Chromatogr* 1987;413:300–304.

426. Honigberg IL, Stewart JT, Clark TC, et al. Non-extractive fluorometric measurement of p-aminosalicylic acid in plasma by ion-pairing techniques and high-performance chromatography. *J Chromatogr* 1980;181:266–271.

427. Huang WL, Chi TL, Wu MH, et al. Performance assessment of the GenoType MTBDRsl test and DNA sequencing for detection of second-line and ethambutol drug resistance among patients infected with multidrug-resistant Mycobacterium tuberculosis. *J Clin Microbiol* 2011;49(7):2502–2508.

428. Amsden GM. Tables of antimicrobial agent pharmacology. In: Mandell GL, Bennett JE, Dolin R, eds. *Principles and practice of infectious diseases*. Vol 1. 7th ed. Philadelphia: Churchill Livingstone Elsevier, 2010:705–761.

429. Mitnick CD, McGee B, Peloquin CA. Tuberculosis pharmacotherapy: strategies to optimize patient care. *Expert Opin Pharmacother* 2009;10(3):381–401.

430. Woods GL, Lin SY, Desmond EP. Susceptibility test methods: mycobacteria, Nocardia, and other actinomycetes. In: *Manual of clinical microbiology*. Vol 1. 10th ed. Washington, DC: ASM Press, 2011:1215–1238.

431. Stover CK, Warrener P, VanDevanter DR, et al. A small-molecule nitroimidazopyran drug candidate for the treatment of tuberculosis. *Nature* 2000;405(6789):962–966.

432. Feuerriegel S, Koser CU, Bau D, et al. Impact of Fgd1 and ddn diversity in Mycobacterium tuberculosis complex on in vitro susceptibility to PA-824. *Antimicrob Agents Chemother* 2011;55(12):5718–5722.

433. Matsumoto M, Hashizume H, Tomishige T, et al. OPC-67683, a nitro-dihydro-imidazooxazole derivative with promising action against tuberculosis in vitro and in mice. *PLoS Med* 2006;3(11):e466.

434. Igarashi M, Nakagawa N, Doi N, et al. Caprazamycin B, a novel anti-tuberculosis antibiotic, from Streptomyces sp. *J Antibiot (Tokyo)* 2003;56(6):580–583.

435. Hirano S, Ichikawa S, Matsuda A. Structure-activity relationship of truncated analogs of caprazamycins as potential anti-tuberculosis agents. *Bioorg Med Chem* 2008;16(9):5123–5133.

436. Disratthakit A, Doi N. In vitro activities of DC-159a, a novel fluoroquinolone, against Mycobacterium species. *Antimicrob Agents Chemother* 2010;54(6):2684–2686.

437. Sekiguchi J, Disratthakit A, Maeda S, et al. Characteristic resistance mechanism of Mycobacterium tuberculosis to DC-159a, a new respiratory quinolone. *Antimicrob Agents Chemother* 2011;55(8):3958–3960.

438. Bogatcheva E, Hanrahan C, Chen P, et al. Discovery of dipiperidines as new antitubercular agents. *Bioorg Med Chem Lett* 2010;20(1):201–205.

439. Bogatcheva E, Hanrahan C, Nikonenko B, et al. Identification of SQ609 as a lead compound from a library of dipiperidines. *Bioorg Med Chem Lett* 2011;21(18):5353–5357.

440. Villemagne B, Crauste C, Flipo M, et al. Tuberculosis: the drug development pipeline at a glance. *Eur J Med Chem* 2012;51:1–16.

441. Protopopova M, Hanrahan C, Nikonenko B, et al. Identification of a new antitubercular drug candidate, SQ109, from a combinatorial library of 1,2-ethylenediamines. *J Antimicrob Chemother* 2005;56(5):968–974.

442. Tahlan K, Wilson R, Kastrinsky DB, et al. SQ109 targets MmpL3, a membrane transporter of trehalose monomycolate involved in mycolic acid donation to the cell wall core of Mycobacterium tuberculosis. *Antimicrob Agents Chemother* 2012;56(4):1797–1809.

443. Reddy VM, Einck L, Nacy CA. In vitro antimycobacterial activities of capuramycin analogues. *Antimicrob Agents Chemother* 2008;52(2):719–721.

444. Bogatcheva E, Dubuisson T, Protopopova M, et al. Chemical modification of capuramycins to enhance antibacterial activity. *J Antimicrob Chemother* 2011;66(3):578–587.

445. Murakami R, Fujita Y, Kizuka M, et al. A-102395, a new inhibitor of bacterial translocase I, produced by Amycolatopsis sp. SANK 60206. *J Antibiot (Tokyo)* 2007;60(11):690–695.

446. Alffenaar JW, van der Laan T, Simons S, et al. Susceptibility of clinical Mycobacterium tuberculosis isolates to a potentially less toxic derivate of linezolid, PNU-100480. *Antimicrob Agents Chemother* 2011;55(3):1287–1289.

447. Andries K, Verhasselt P, Guillemont J, et al. A diarylquinoline drug active on the ATP synthase of Mycobacterium tuberculosis. *Science* 2005;307(5707):223–227.

448. Huitric E, Verhasselt P, Andries K, et al. In vitro antimycobacterial spectrum of a diarylquinoline ATP synthase inhibitor. *Antimicrob Agents Chemother* 2007;51(11):4202–4204.

449. La Rosa V, Poce G, Canseco JO, et al. MmpL3 is the cellular target of the antitubercular pyrrole derivative BM212. *Antimicrob Agents Chemother* 2012;56(1):324–331.

450. Deidda D, Lampis G, Fioravanti R, et al. Bactericidal activities of the pyrrole derivative BM212 against multidrug-resistant and intramacrophagic Mycobacterium tuberculosis strains. *Antimicrob Agents Chemother* 1998;42(11):3035–3037.

451. Biava M, Porretta GC, Deidda D, et al. Antimycobacterial compounds. New pyrrole derivatives of BM212. *Bioorg Med Chem* 2004;12(6):1453–1458.

452. Chambers HF, Turner J, Schecter GF, et al. Imipenem for treatment of tuberculosis in mice and humans. *Antimicrob Agents Chemother* 2005;49(7):2816–2821.

453. Watt B, Edwards JR, Rayner A, et al. In vitro activity of meropenem and imipenem against mycobacteria: development of a daily antibiotic dosing schedule. *Tuber Lung Dis* 1992;73(3):134–136.

454. Brown BA, Wallace RJ Jr, Onyi GO. Activities of clarithromycin against eight slowly growing species of nontuberculous mycobacteria, determined by using a broth microdilution MIC system. *Antimicrob Agents Chemother* 1992;36(9):1987–1990.

455. Wallace RJ Jr, Brown BA, Onyi GO. Susceptibilities of Mycobacterium fortuitum biovar. fortuitum and the two subgroups of Mycobacterium chelonae to imipenem, cefmetazole, cefoxitin, and amoxicillin-clavulanic acid. *Antimicrob Agents Chemother* 1991;35(4):773–775.

456. Good RC, Silcox VA, Kilburn JO, et al. Identification and drug susceptibility test results for Mycobacterium spp. *Clin Microbiol Newsltr* 1985;7(18):133–136.

457. Collins CH, Uttley AH. In-vitro activity of seventeen antimicrobial compounds against seven species of mycobacteria. *J Antimicrob Chemother* 1988;22(6):857–861.

458. Khardori N, Rolston K, Rosenbaum B, et al. Comparative in-vitro activity of twenty antimicrobial agents against clinical isolates of Mycobacterium avium complex. *J Antimicrob Chemother* 1989;24:667–673.

459. Cynamon MH, Palmer GS, Sorg TB. Comparative in vitro activities of ampicillin, BMY 28142, and imipenem against Mycobacterium avium complex. *Diag Microbiol Infect Dis* 1987;6(2):151–155.

460. Naik S, Ruck R. In vitro activities of several new macrolide antibiotics against Mycobacterium avium complex. *Antimicrob Agents Chemother* 1989;33:1614–1616.

461. Woodley CL, Kilburn JO. In vitro susceptibility of Mycobacterium avium complex and Mycobacterium tuberculosis strains to a spiro-piperidyl rifamycin. *Am Rev Respir Dis* 1982;126:586–587.

462. Salfinger M, Stool EW, Pito D, et al. Comparison of three methods for recovery of Mycobacterium avium complex from blood specimens. *J Clin Microbiol* 1988;26(6):1225–1226.

463. Collins CH, Uttley AH. In-vitro susceptibility of mycobacteria to ciprofloxacin. *J Antimicrob Chemother* 1985;16(5):575–580.

464. Rodriguez Diaz JC, Lopez M, Ruiz M, Royo G. In vitro activity of new fluoroquinolones and linezolid against non-tuberculous mycobacteria. *Int J Antimicrob Agents* 2003;21(6):585–588.

465. Davis CEJ, Carpenter JL, Trevino S, et al. In vitro susceptibility of *Mycobacterium avium* complex to antibacterial agents. *Diag Microbiol Infect Dis* 1987;8(3):149–155.

466. Leysen DC, Haemers A, Pattyn SR. Mycobacteria and the new quinolones. *Antimicrob Agents Chemother* 1989;33(1):1–5.

467. Ernst F, van der Auwera P. In-vitro activity of fleroxacin (Ro 23-6240), a new fluoro-quinolone, and other agents, against mycobacterium spp. *J Antimicrob Chemother* 1988;21(4):501–504.

468. Ausina V, Condom MJ, Mirelis B, et al. In vitro activity of clofazimine against rapidly growing nonchromogenic mycobacteria. *Antimicrob Agents Chemother* 1986;29(5):951–952.

469. Tomioka H, Saito H, Sato K. Comparative antimycobacterial activities of the newly synthesized quinolone AM-1155, sparfloxacin, and ofloxacin. *Antimicrob Agents Chemother* 1993;37(6):1259–1263.

470. Bernard EM, Edwards FF, Kiehn TE, et al. Activities of antimicrobial agents against clinical isolates of *Mycobacterium haemophilum*. *Antimicrob Agents Chemother* 1993;37:2323–2326.

471. Fenlon CH, Cynamon MH. Comparative in vitro activities of ciprofloxacin and other 4-quinolones against *Mycobacterium tuberculosis* and *Mycobacterium intracellulare*. *Antimicrob Agents Chemother* 1986;29(3): 386–388.

472. Haneishi T, Nakajima M, Shiraishi A, et al. Antimycobacterial activities in vitro and in vivo and pharmacokinetics of dihydromycoplanecin A. *Antimicrob Agents Chemother* 1988;32(1):125–127.

473. Cynamon MH. Comparative in vitro activities of MDL 473, rifampin, and ansamycin against *Mycobacterium intracellulare*. *Antimicrob Agents Chemother* 1985;28(3):440–441.

474. Garcia-Rodriguez JA, Gomez G-AC. In-vitro activities of quinolones against mycobacteria. *J Antimicrob Chemother* 1993;32(6):797–808.

475. Wallace RJ Jr, Dunbar D, Brown BA, et al. Rifampin-resistant *Mycobacterium kansasii*. *Clin Infect Dis* 1994;18(5):736–743.

476. Wallace RJ Jr, Wiss K. Susceptibility of *Mycobacterium marinum* to tetracyclines and aminoglycosides. *Antimicrob Agents Chemother* 1981;20:610–612.

477. Heifets LB, Iseman MD. Determination of in vitro susceptibility of mycobacteria to ansamycin. *Am Rev Respir Dis* 1985;132(3):710–711.

478. Yew WW, Piddock LJ, Li MS, et al. In-vitro activity of quinolones and macrolides against mycobacteria. *J Antimicrob Chemother* 1994;34(3):343–351.

479. Juréen P, Ängeby K, Sturegård E, et al. Wild-type MIC distributions for aminoglycoside and cyclic polypeptide antibiotics used for treatment of Mycobacterium tuberculosis infections. *J Clin Microbiol* 2010;48(5):1853–1858.

480. Byrne SK, Crawford CE, Geddes GL, et al. In vitro susceptibilities of *Mycobacterium tuberculosis* to 10 antimicrobial agents. *Antimicrob Agents Chemother* 1988;32(9): 1441–1442.

481. Gorzynski EA, Gutman SE, Allen W. Comparative antimycobacterial activities of difloxacin, temafloxacin, enoxacin, pefloxacin, reference fluoroquinolones, and a new macrolide, clarithromycin. *Antimicrob Agents Chemother* 1989;33(4):591–592.

482. Alvirez-Freites EJ, Carter JL, Cynamon MH. In vitro and in vivo activities of gatifloxacin against *Mycobacterium tuberculosis*. *Antimicrob Agents Chemother* 2002;46(4):1022–1025.

483. Ängeby KA, Juréen P, Giske CG, et al. Wild-type MIC distributions of four fluoroquinolones active against Mycobacterium tuberculosis in relation to current critical concentrations and available pharmacokinetic and pharmacodynamic data. *J Antimicrob Chemother* 2010;65(5):946–952.

484. Inderlied C, Nash KA. Microbiology and in vitro susceptibility testing. In: Benson C, Korvick J, eds. *Mycobacterium avium complex infection: progress in research and treatment*. New York: Marcel Dekker, 1995: 109–140.

485. Artsimovitch I, Vassylyev DG. Is it easy to stop RNA polymerase? *Cell Cycle* 2006;5(4):399–404.

486. Metushi IG, Cai P, Zhu X, et al. A fresh look at the mechanism of isoniazid-induced hepatotoxicity. *Clin Pharmacol Ther* 2011;89(6):911–914.

Chapter 6

Antifungal Drugs: Mechanisms of Action, Drug Resistance, Susceptibility Testing, and Assays of Activity in Biologic Fluids

George R. Thompson III and Thomas F. Patterson

The number of agents available to treat fungal infections has increased by 30% since the year 2000 and several more agents are currently in various stages of clinical development. The greater number of medications now available allows for therapeutic choices; however, differences in antifungal spectrum of activity, bioavailability, formulation, drug interactions, and side effects necessitate a detailed knowledge of each drug class (1).

Despite these advances in antifungal therapy, mortality remains high especially in severely immunocompromised patients. The number of those at risk continues to increase with the greater number of solid organ and bone marrow transplant patients, the use of corticosteroids and other immune-modulating drugs such as tumor necrosis factor alpha (TNF-α) inhibitors, and the epidemic of infection with HIV.

In this chapter, we will review currently available antifungal agents, both systemic and topical (Table 6.1). We will discuss their spectrum, potency, mechanism of action, clinical indications for use, and summarize pharmacokinetic and pharmacodynamic parameters. Furthermore, we will discuss the mechanisms of resistance to the various classes of antifungal agents and the in vitro methods for determining the susceptibility and resistance of fungi to currently available agents. Finally, we will provide an overview of the methods for measuring the concentration of antifungal agents in clinical samples and, where appropriate, discuss the indication for performing such analysis.

POLYENES

Amphotericin B (AmB), natamycin, and nystatin are the currently available polyenes, although differing safety profiles have limited natamycin and nystatin to topical use (2). Polyenes possess a large lactone ring, with a lipophilic chain containing three to seven double bonds and a flexible hydrophilic portion bearing several hydroxyl groups. AmB contains seven conjugated double bonds and may be inactivated by heat, light, and extremes of pH (3). Additionally, AmB is poorly soluble and is not absorbed following oral or intramusclar delivery.

The polyenes bind to ergosterol present within the fungal cell wall membrane. This process disrupts cell wall permeability with the subsequent efflux of potassium and intracellular molecules, causing fungal death due to osmotic instability (4). There is also evidence that AmB acts as a proinflammatory agent and further serves to stimulate innate host immunity. This process involves the interaction of AmB with toll-like receptor 2 (TLR-2), the CD14 receptor, and by stimulating the release of cytokines, chemokines, and other immunologic mediators (5). It has been suggested that AmB may interact with host humoral immunity following the observation of synergistic activity of AmB and antibodies directed at heat shock protein 90 (hsp90), although further confirmatory data is needed (4). These secondary mechanims serve to increase the cascade of oxidative reactions, allowing for the rapid fungicidal activity of AmB formulations.

Table 6.1

Systemic and Topical Antifungal Agents in Use and in Development			
Antifungal Agents	**Route**	**Mechanism of Action**	**Comments**
Allylamines			
Naftifine	Topical	Inhibition of squalene epoxidase	Terbinafine has very broad-spectrum activity and acts synergistically with other antifungals
Terbinafine	Oral, topical		
Antimetabolite			
Flucytosine	Oral	Inhibition of DNA and RNA synthesis	Used in combination with ampho-tericin B and fluconazole; toxicity and secondary resistance are problems
Imidazoles			
Ketoconazole, bifonazole, clotrimazole, econazole, miconazole, oxiconazole, sulconazole, terconazole, tioconazole	Oral, topical	Inhibits lanosterol 14-α-demethylase cytochrome P450–dependent enzymes	Ketoconazole has modest broad-spectrum activity and toxicity problems
Triazoles			
Fluconazole	Oral, IV	Same as imidazoles but more specific binding to target	Limited spectrum (yeasts); good central nervous system penetra-tion; good in vivo activity; primary and secondary resistance seen with *C. krusei* and *C. glabrata*, respectively
Itraconazole	Oral	Same as imidazoles but more specific binding to target enzyme	Broad-spectrum activity; erratic absorption; toxicity and drug interactions are problems
Voriconazole	Oral, IV	Same as imidazoles but more specific binding to target enzyme	Broad spectrum including yeasts and molds; active vs. *C. krusei*; many drug interactions
Posaconazole	Oral	Same as imidazoles but more specific binding to enzyme	Broad spectrum including activity vs. Zygomycetes
Ravuconazole	Oral, IV	Same as imidazoles but more specific binding to target enzyme	Investigational; broad spectrum including yeasts and molds
Isavuconazole	Oral, IV	Same as imidazoles but more specific binding to target enzyme	Investigational, broad spectrum including activity vs. Zygomycetes
Echinocandins			
Caspofungin	IV	Inhibition of fungal cell wall glucan synthesis	Fungicidal activity against *Candida*
Micafungin	IV		
Anidulafungin	IV		

(Continued)

Table 6.1 *(Continued)*

Systemic and Topical Antifungal Agents in Use and in Development[a]			
Antifungal Agents	**Route**	**Mechanism of Action**	**Comments**
Polyenes			
Amphotericin B	IV, topical	Binds to ergosterol, causing direct oxidative membrane damage	Established agent; broad spectrum; toxic
Lipid formulations (amphotericin B lipid complex or colloidal dispersion, liposomal amphotericin B)	IV	Same as amphotericin B	Broad spectrum; less toxic, expensive
Nystatin	Oral suspension, topical	Same as amphotericin B	Liposomal formulation (IV) under investigation
Natamycin	Topical		Typically used as adjunctive therapy for fungal keratitis
Chitin synthesis inhibitor			
Nikkomycin Z	IV	Inhibition of fungal cell wall chitin synthesis	Investigational agent; possibly useful in combination with other antifungals
Other			
Amorolfine	Topical	Miscellaneous, varied	
Butenafine HCl	Topical		
Ciclopirox olamine	Topical		
Griseofulvin	Oral		
Haloprogin	Topical		
Tolnaftate	Topical		
Undecylenate	Topical		

The spectrum of activity of AmB is broad and includes most strains of *Candida*, *Cryptococcus neoformans*, *Aspergillus* spp, the *Mucorales*, *Blastomyces dermatitidis*, *Coccidioides* spp, *Histoplasma capsulatum*, and *Paracoccidioides brasiliensis*. *Candida lusitaniae*, *Aspergillus terreus*, *Fusarium* spp, *Pseudallescheria boydii*, *Scedosporium* spp, and *Trichosporon asahii* and certain dematiaceous fungi may be resistant to AmB (6–9).

When AmB resistance occurs, it is generally attributed to reductions in ergosterol biosynthesis or the synthesis of alternative sterols with a reduced affinity for AMB. However, decreased susceptibility to oxidative damage secondary to increased catalase activity has also been described and may play a secondary role in polyene resistance (10).

Conventional amphotericin B deoxycholate (AmB-d) has been the mainstay of antifungal therapy prior to the development of other antifungal classes; yet the nephrotoxicity of AmB-d was one of the predominant forces driving the pursuit of alternative agents with a diminished side effect profile. Lipid formulations of AmB have subsequently been developed and in most instances have replaced AmB-d (11). The lipid-based formulations of AmB include amphotericin B lipid complex (ABLC), liposomal amphotericin B (L-AmB), and amphotericin B cholesteryl sulfate complex (ABCD) and exhibit a lower incidence of nephrotoxicity than that of AmB-d (12), although the safety profile of ABCD has limited its clinical use.

AmB must be administered parenterally because of its poor solubility and poor absorption when administered orally. It is widely distributed in various tissues and organs, including liver, spleen, bone marrow, kidney, and lung (13). Despite negligible concentration in cerebrospinal fluid (CSF), AmB formulations are effective in treating fungal infections of the central nervous system (CNS). In the past, intrathecal administration of AmB-d was used to treat meningeal infection (14,15); however, this practice is seldom used due to the difficulty of administration, poor patient tolerability, availability of alternative agents, and diminishing physician familiarity with this technique. The tissue distribution of the lipid formulations is similar to that of AmB-d; however, urinary excretion of lipid drugs is lower than that of AmB-d (16). All currently available formulations are highly protein bound (>95%, primarily to albumin) and have long half-lives.

AmB displays concentration-dependent fungicidal activity against many fungi with an optimal maximal concentration-to-mean inhibitory concentration (C_{max}-to-MIC) ratio of 4–8:1 and a postantifungal effect of up to 12 hours (17). These findings suggest the peak serum level-to-MIC ratio is the best pharmacologic predictor of outcomes with polyene therapy. Drug levels are infrequently measured nor are necessary and are typically necessary only in the research setting (18).

AmB exhibits poor CSF levels (<5% of concurrent serum concentration); however, this agent remains the treatment of choice for cryptococcal meningitis (19). AmB formulations also have low vitreous penetration (0% to 38%) and intraocular injections may be required to achieve appropriate levels during therapy of deep ophthalmologic fungal infections including candidal endophthalmitis (20,21). The exact route of elimination of AmB is not known and despite the well-known nephrotoxicity, dosing need not be adjusted in patients with a decreased glomerular filtration rate (GFR).

AmB formulations are currently used primarily in the treatment of invasive cryptococcosis and moderate to severe infections with the endemic fungi (*Histoplasma, Coccidioides, Blastomyces*, etc.). Its use in the treatment of candidiasis and aspergillosis has been largely supplanted by other agents following landmark clinical trials (22,23). L-AmB is also commonly used in the treatment of febrile neutropenia refractory to broad-spectrum antibacterial agents (24). Histoplasmosis and cryptococcosis remain the only infections for which a lipid formulation of AmB (L-AmB) has demonstrated greater efficacy than the conventional form (25,26).

AmB formulations were previously the preferred first-line agent during the treatment of invasive aspergillosis (IA); however, a greater therapeutic response and survival have been demonstrated when voriconazole is administered in this setting—relegating AmB to second-line or salvage

therapy during the treatment of IA (27). AmB does remain the agent of choice when *Mucorales* are encountered. In fact, a delay in the prescribing of an AmB formulation in patients infected with an agent of mucormycosis resulted in a twofold greater risk of death (28). Discriminating between invasive mucormycosis and aspergillosis is difficult, but the differences in the choice of antifungal agents and outcomes mandate an aggressive diagnostic strategy and prompt initiation of antifungal agents.

In attempts to avoid the potential nephrotoxicity of systemic administration and to deliver higher local concentrations, different formulations of AmB have been given via the inhalational route. AmB-d is often difficult to effectively administer in an aerosol form due to foaming caused by the solubilizing agent and the detergent-like effects are thought to possibly affect alveolar surfactant (28–31). Thus, lipid preparations are preferred for inhalation delivery. Aerosol delivery has been found effective in the prevention of pulmonary fungal infections in lung transplantation and in bone marrow transplant recipients, although data supporting its efficacy in other settings is limited (29).

Intravenous (IV) infusion of AmB-d is associated with reactions such as fever, chills, rigors, myalgias, bronchospasm, nausea and vomiting, tachycardia, tachypnea, and hypertension (32). These events are less likely to occur when one of the lipid formulations is used; however, ABCD has been associated with the development of dyspnea and hypoxia and L-AmB has been associated with back pain during infusion (20). AmB has been associated with acute kidney injury and nephrotoxicity in many studies and is a well-known potential complication of therapy occurring in up to 30% of patients. This toxicity is thought secondary to vascular smooth muscle dysfunction with resultant vasoconstriction and ischemia (33). For this reason, most advocate ensuring adequate volume status prior to administration. Lipid preparations of AmB have a lower incidence of renal toxicity, and studies have shown that when AmB-d is replaced by a lipid formulation after the development of creatinine elevation, renal function stabilizes or improves in a significant proportion of patients (34).

The avoidance of AmB-d and use of a lipid formulation has been met with skepticism by some due to the price difference in compounds. The reduction in hospital days when toxicity is avoided has proven the lipid formulations more cost-effective than AmB (34).

TRIAZOLES

The antifungal azoles include the imidazoles and the triazoles, which differ in terms of their chemical structure. Among the imidazoles (two nitrogens in the azole ring), only ketoconazole has systemic activity, and this agent has been replaced by more efficacious and less toxic alternatives and thus will not be discussed in this chapter. The triazoles (three nitrogens in the azole ring) all have systemic activity and include fluconazole, itraconazole, voriconazole, and posaconazole. An additional triazole, isavuconazole, is currently in phase III clinical trials.

The triazoles also exert their effects within the fungal cell membrane. The inhibition of cytochrome P450 (CYP)–dependent 14-α-demethylase prevents the conversion of lanosterol to ergosterol. This mechanism results in the accumulation of toxic methylsterols and resultant inhibition of fungal cell growth and replication (Fig. 6.1). This class of agents has demonstrated both species- and strain-dependent fungistatic or fungicidal activity in vitro (35). Generally, these agents exhibit fungistatic activity against yeasts such as *Candida* and *Cryptococcus*; however, voriconazole appears to be fungicidal against *Aspergillus* spp. The area under the curve-to-MIC ratio (AUC/MIC) is the primary predictor of drug efficacy (36).

The indirect immunomodulatory effects are poorly understood due to the complex interaction of triazoles and phagocytic cells. Evidence suggests that ergosterol depletion increases fungal cell vulnerability to phagocytic oxidative damage (37) and voriconazole has been shown to induce the expression of TLR-2, nuclear factor-κB (NF-κB), and TNF-α (4).

Azoles differ in their affinity for the 14-α-demethylase enzyme and this difference is largely responsible for their varying antifungal potency and spectrum of activity. Cross-inhibition of several human CYP-dependent enzymes (3A4, 2C9, and 2C19) is responsible for the majority of the clinical side effects and drug interaction profiles that have been described with this class (38–41).

Itraconazole and posaconazole act primarily as inhibitors of 3A4 and 2C9 with little effect on 2C19. However, voriconazole acts as both an inhibitor and a substrate on all three isoenzymes, providing ample opportunity for drug–drug interactions due to this frequently shared metabolic pathway (41).

Comprehensive lists of triazole drug interactions can be found elsewhere (42). Briefly, caution should be used when these agents are concurrently administered with most HMG-CoA reductase inhibitors, benzodiazepines, phenytoin, carbamazepine, cyclosporine, tacrolimus, sirolimus, methylprednisolone, buspirone, alfentanil; the dihydropyridine calcium channel blockers verapamil and diltiazem; the sulfonylureas, rifampin,

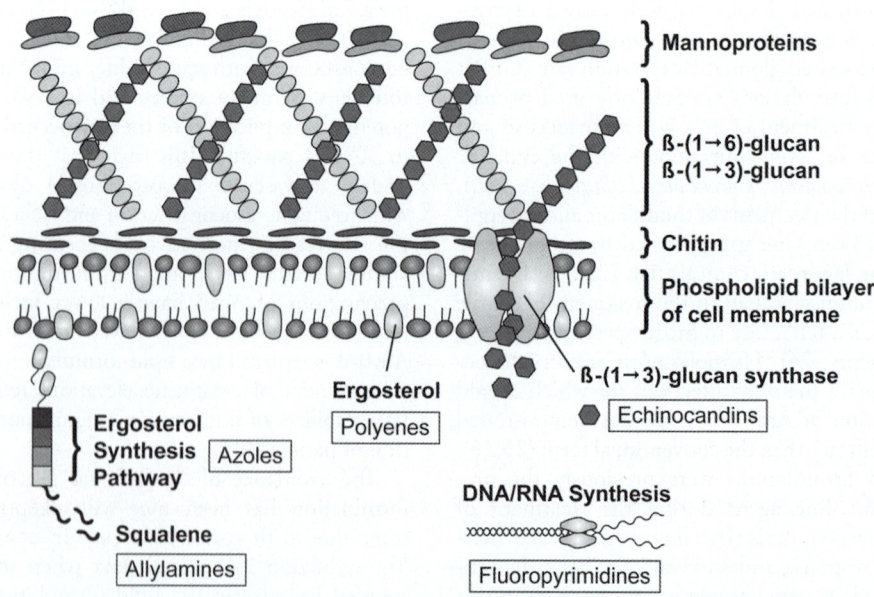

Figure 6.1 ■ **Targets of systemic antifungal agents.** (See Color Plate in the front of the book.)

rifabutin, vincristine, busulfan, docetaxel, trimetrexate; and the protease inhibitors ritonavir, indinavir, and saquinavir (43–49).

The triazoles have also been associated with QTc prolongation (50) and coadministration with other agents known to have similar effects (cisapride, terfenadine, astemizole, mizolastine, dofetilide, quinidine, and pimozide, among others) should be avoided (51–53). The triazoles are additionally embryotoxic and teratogenic and are secreted into breast milk and thus, administration should be avoided during pregnancy or while lactating (50,54,55).

Fluconazole

Fluconazole remains one of the most frequently prescribed triazoles due to its excellent bioavailability, tolerability, and side effect profile. More than 80% of ingested drug is found in the circulation, protein binding is low (approximately 10%), and 60% to 70% is excreted unchanged in the urine (56). Oral absorption remains unchanged in patients receiving acid suppressive therapy (proton pump inhibitors or H_2-blockers) (57).

Fluconazole is a water-soluble compound with excellent tissue penetration and is available in both oral and IV formulations. CSF levels are 50% to 70% of matched serum levels, and levels reported in saliva, sputum, and other sites are well within therapeutic ranges (58,59). The half-life is 27 to 34 hours in the presence of normal renal function, allowing once-daily dosing and it exhibits linear pharmacokinetics that are independent of doses and formulation. In patients with diminished creatinine clearance (CrCl), the normal dose should be reduced by 50% (38). Fluconazole exhibits concentration-independent fungistatic activity against *Candida* and *Cryptococcus neoformans* (60,61). The AUC/MIC ratio appears to be the most predictive pharmacodynamic parameter for fluconazole (62). Fluconazole serum levels are rarely necessary in clinical practice due to its predictable oral absorption and pharmacokinetic profile.

Fluconazole is active against most *Candida* spp with the exception of *Candida krusei*, which is intrinsically resistant to fluconazole (63). *Candida glabrata* is significantly less susceptible to fluconazole than *Candida albicans*, although wild-type isolates have MICs that extend to an MIC of more than 64 μg/mL. Previously, *Candida glabrata* strains were considered susceptible-dose dependent (S-DD at an MIC of 16 to 32 μg/mL), with roughly 10% exhibiting high-level resistance (MIC, more than 64 μg/mL) (21,64). A recent

Clinical and Laboratory Standards Institute (CLSI) reclassification has resulted in the breakpoint for susceptible *Candida glabrata* being eliminated and strains considered S-DD at an MIC of less than or equal to 32 μg/mL. Fluconazole is active against most species of *Candida*, *Cryptococcus neoformans*, dermatophytes, *Trichosporon* spp, *H. capsulatum*, *Coccidioides immitis*, and *P. brasiliensis* (65,66). Only limited activity is seen against *B. dermatitidis* and resistance may develop when fluconazole is used to treat histoplasmosis (67). Fluconazole has no useful activity against molds including *Aspergillus* spp, *Fusarium* spp, or *Mucorales* (68).

Fluconazole has an important role in the treatment of candidiasis, cryptococcosis, and coccidioidomycosis (14,69,70). Fluconazole is used as primary therapy for candidemia and mucosal candidiasis, as well as prophylaxis in selected high-risk populations who are at lower risk for molds like *Aspergillus* (69). Patients with oropharyngeal candidiasis (OPC) are typically prescribed 100 mg/day for 7 to 14 days (21). Newer data suggests a one-time dose of 750 mg for the treatment of OPC with equivalent relapse rates to standard therapy (71). Patients with frequent relapse should remain on chronic suppressive fluconazole until immune reconstitution has been documented.

It is also used in maintenance therapy of cryptococcal meningitis in patients with AIDS (14,72). Following induction therapy with AmB and flucytosine, fluconazole is prescribed as an initial dose of 400 mg for 10 weeks followed by 200 mg weekly pending immune reconstitution (19). Although recent data has accrued regarding the use of high-dose fluconazole monotherapy during the induction course of cryptococcal meningitis, this practice should be used only in resource-limited settings and not when AmB is available (73).

Fluconazole is also the agent of choice in the treatment of disseminated coccidioidomycosis including meningitis. In these cases, high-dose fluconazole (up to 2 g daily) is often necessary (74). Similarly, other endemic mycoses respond favorable to fluconazole and this agent is considered second line during treatment of histoplasmosis and sporotrichosis (75,76).

Fluconazole has also been used for prophylaxis in those at high risk of invasive fungal infections. Initiation of 400 mg/day of fluconazole for the first 75 days following bone marrow transplantation (BMT) has been found effective in reducing cases of candidemia (77). Preemptive therapy in other settings, including within intensive care unit (ICU), remains controversial. The high incidence of invasive candidiasis within this setting (1% to 2% of all patients) makes prophylaxis an attractive option; however, the largest randomized, multicenter, blinded clinical trial comparing empiric fluconazole therapy to placebo in ICU patients with several risk factors for invasive candidiasis showed no clear benefit to fluconazole therapy (78).

Drug–drug interactions are less commonly observed with fluconazole than other triazole compounds, although caution remains necessary due to increases in the serum levels of phenytoin, glipizide, glyburide, warfarin, rifabutin, and cyclosporine. Fluconazole levels are reduced in the presence of rifampin (38).

Fluconazole is well tolerated by most patients, even if chronic therapy is necessary (79). Headache, alopecia, and anorexia are the side effects most common (10%), with transaminase elevation seen in fewer than 10%. Severe side effects such as exfoliative dermatitis and liver failure are very uncommon (38).

Itraconazole

Itraconazole is a lipophilic triazole currently available as both capsules and an oral solution suspended in hydroxypropyl-β-cyclodextrin (HP-β-CD) (39). The IV preparation of itraconazole is no longer commercially available.

The IV formulation provides optimal bioavailability with peak plasma levels obtained within 1 hour of administration. The HP-β-CD carrier is cleared renally and caution is recommended when administering the IV formulation to patients with impaired renal function (80). Itraconazole exhibits poor penetration into the CNS and a P-glycoprotein efflux mechanism has been found in mice to actively transport itraconazole out of the brain (81). The high protein binding (less than 1% available as free drug) and lipophilic nature of itraconazole also results in high concentrations in fatty tissues and purulent exudates (82).

Itraconazole exhibits concentration-independent fungistatic activity against *Candida* spp and *Cryptococcus neoformans* (83). In contrast, itraconazole has been shown to exert a time- and concentration-dependent fungicidal effect against *Aspergillus* spp (84).

The antifungal activity of itraconazole is broad and includes *Candida* spp, *Cryptococcus* spp, *Aspergillus* spp, dermatophytes, dematiaceous molds, *Pseudallescheria boydii*, *Penicillium marneffei*, *B. dermatitidis*, *Coccidioides immitis*, *H. capsulatum*, *Paracoccidioides brasiliensis*, and *Sporothrix schenckii*

(Table 6.2). Itraconazole has activity against some, but not all, fluconazole-resistant strains of *Candida krusei* and *Candida glabrata*. Although rare, strains of *Aspergillus fumigatus* that are resistant to itraconazole have been reported and may be increasing in some regions (85,86). *Mucorales*, most strains of *Fusarium*, and *Scedosporium prolificans* are resistant to itraconazole (35).

Absorption of itraconazole capsules is erratic and requires an acidic gastric pH and administration with food. Itraconazole solution allows for greater oral bioavailability and the AUC and peak concentrations are both increased by 30% when itraconazole solution is taken in the fasting state (87,88). The cyclodextrin carrier has minimal absorption and no systemic side effects have been attributed to its use in the oral formulation (89). With once-daily dosing, steady state is reached in 7 to 14 days, although oral loading (200 mg three times daily for 3 days) allows for more rapid attainment of therapeutic serum levels (90).

Itraconazole is extensively metabolized by the liver and its major metabolite, hydroxyitraconazole, also possesses antifungal activity similar to that of the parent drug. Despite similar antifungal efficacy, hydroxyitraconazole is not measured during serum drug level determination by high-performance liquid chromatography (HPLC) and ultra-performance liquid chromatography with mass spectrometry (UPLC/MS) is instead required. The active metabolite is detected by bioassay (91).

The development of newer and more effective antifungal agents (i.e., voriconazole) has relegated itraconazole to second-line therapy during the treatment of IA. Itraconazole is thus licensed in the United States only for salvage therapy of IA and allergic bronchopulmonary aspergillosis (27).

Itraconazole remains the drug of choice for those with mild to moderate infection caused by histoplasmosis and is the mainstay of secondary prophylaxis in HIV patients with a history of histoplasmosis prior to immune reconstitution with antiretrovirals (75).

It is also useful for lymphocutaneous sporotrichosis and non–life-threatening, nonmeningeal forms of histoplasmosis, paracoccidioidomycosis, and blastomycosis (75,76,92–94), and nonmeningeal coccidioidomycosis and is the preferred agent for osseous manifestations of coccidioidomycosis (95). Additionally, itraconazole has been used for maintenance treatment of cryptococcal meningitis (14) and for some forms of phaeohyphomycosis (96). It has no activity against *Fusarium* spp, *Mucorales*, or *S. prolificans* (35).

Table 6.2

Antifungal Spectrum of Activity Against Common Molds and Yeast

Organism	AMB	FLU	ITR	POS	VOR	ANI	MFG	CAS	5FC
Aspergillus fumigatus	+	−	+	+	+	+	+	+	−
Aspergillus flavus	+/−	−	+	+	+	+	+	+	−
Aspergillus terreus	−	−	+	+	+	+	+	+	−
Aspergillus niger	+	−	+/−	+	+	+	+	+	−
Aspergillus nidulans	+	−	+/−	+	+	+	+	+	−
Candida albicans	+	+	+	+	+	+	+	+	+
Candida glabrata	+	+/−	+/−	+/−	+/−	+	+	+	+
Candida krusei	+	−	+/−	+	+	+	+	+	+/−
Candida tropicalis	+	+	+	+	+	+	+	+	+
Candida parapsilosis	+	+	+	+	+	+/−	+/−	+/−	+
Candida guillermondii	+	+	+	+	+	−	−	−	+
Candida lusitaniae	−	+	+	+	+	+	+	+	+
Cryptococcus spp	+	+	+	+	+	−	−	−	+
Blastomyces	+	+	+	+	+	+/−	+/−	+/−	−
Histoplasma	+	+/−	+	+	+	+/−	+/−	+/−	−
Coccidioides	+	+	+	+	+	−	−	−	−
Sporothrix	+	−	+	+/−	−	+/−	+/−	+/−	−
Fusarium spp	+/−	−	−	+	+	−	−	−	−
Phaeohyphomycoses[a]	+	−	+	+	+	+	+	+	−
Pichia spp	+	+	+/−	+	+	+	+	+	+
Saccharomyces spp	+	+	+	+	+	+	+	+	+
Scedosporium apiospermum	+/−	−	+/−	+	+	−	−	−	−
Scedosporium prolificans	−	−	−	+/−	+/−	−	−	−	−
Trichosporon spp	+/−	+	+	+	+	−	−	−	+
Mucorales	+/−	−	−	+	−	−	−	−	−

[a]Infection requires debridement in almost all circumstances.
AMB, amphotericin; FLU, fluconazole; ITR, itraconazole; POS, posaconazole; VOR, voriconazole; ANI, anidulafungin; MFG, micafungin; CAS, caspofungin; 5FC, flucytosine. (+) implies antifungal activity against isolates, (−) implies no or limited activity against isolate, (+/−) implies variable activity against isolates.
Modified from Dodds Ashley ES, Lewis R, Lewis JS, et al. Pharmacology of systemic antifungal agents. *Clin Infect Dis* 2006;43(Suppl 1):S28–S39; Enache-Angoulvant A, Hennequin C. Invasive *Saccharomyces* infection: a comprehensive review. *Clin Infect Dis* 2005;41(11):1559–1568; da Matta VL, de Souza Carvalho Melhem M, Colombo AL, et al. Antifungal drug susceptibility profile of *Pichia anomala* isolates from patients presenting with nosocomial fungemia. *Antimicrob Agents Chemother* 2007;51(4):1573–1576; Paphitou NI, Ostrosky-Zeichner L, Paetznick VL, et al. In vitro antifungal susceptibilities of *Trichosporon* species. *Antimicrob Agents Chemother* 2002;46(4):1144–1146.

The recommended dosage of oral itraconazole in adults is 400 mg/day (capsules) and 2.5 mg/kg twice daily (HP-β-CD solution) (27). However, steady-state levels can be more rapidly attained when administered as 200 mg three times daily for 3 days and then 200 mg twice daily for the duration of therapy. Considerable concern remains regarding adequate oral absorption and oral itraconazole is not recommended in seriously ill or patients with life-threatening disease. Dose adjustment is not indicated when the oral formulations of itraconazole is used in patients with renal insufficiency or those receiving hemodialysis/continuous ambulatory peritoneal dialysis (CAPD). The half-life of itraconazole is prolonged in patients with hepatic dysfunction and drug dose adjustment, liver function testing, and drug interactions should be carefully assessed (97).

Side effects due to itraconazole may occur including gastrointestinal intolerance, hypokalemia, edema, rash, and elevated transaminases (39). Severe hepatotoxicity is rare (98). In contrast to fluconazole, drug interactions are relatively common with itraconazole because of the inhibition of the oxidative metabolism of agents that are metabolized by hepatic cytochrome P450 enzymes (39,42).

Itraconazole is usually well tolerated, although adverse reactions have been observed in up to 39% of patients and dose-limited toxicity requiring discontinuation of therapy can occur. The most frequent side effects include nausea and vomiting (<10%), hypertriglyceridemia (9%), hypokalemia (6%), liver enzyme elevations (5%), skin rashes/pruritus (2%), headache and dizziness (<2%), and pedal edema (1%) (99). Gastrointestinal intolerance (46%) is exceedingly common with the oral HP-β-CD solution at doses greater than 400 mg per day, with vomiting as the most frequent complaint (100). The myocardial depressant effects of itraconazole are also well known and cases of congestive heart failure have been reported (101).

Posaconazole

Posaconazole is a lipophilic second-generation antifungal triazole with a similar molecular structure to that of itraconazole. However, posaconazole's improved spectrum of activity also exhibits efficacy against *Mucorales* and has enhanced activity against *Aspergillus* spp compared to itraconazole (102).

Posaconazole is insoluble in water and an IV formulation is currently in phase III clinical trials while a solid oral formulation is also currently in development. It is currently administered as a cherry-flavored suspension using polysorbate 80 as the emulsifying agent (103). Optimal dosing of posaconazole is obtained when given as two to four divided doses administered with food or a liquid nutritional supplement (104,105). Although initial studies suggested gastric acidity did not affect posaconazole absorption subsequent work has shown H_2-receptor antagonists and proton pump inhibitors may decrease posaconazole serum levels and coadministration should be avoided (54,103,106,107).

Posaconazole has demonstrated dose-dependent pharmacokinetics with saturable absorption above 800 mg per day. Oral loading is thus not possible and steady state is reached only after 7 to 10 days of therapy (108). This prolonged time required to reach steady-state levels also impacts enthusiasm for the use of posaconazole as primary therapy for invasive fungal infections. Posaconazole has a large volume of distribution, despite its high protein binding, and a half-life of approximately 24 hours.

Peak serum concentrations have shown considerable interpatient variability for reasons that remain unclear. Some have proposed genetic polymorphisms within P-glycoprotein play a role as posaconazole is both a substrate and inhibitor, but this remains unproven (109). Glucuronidation plays a minor role in posaconazole metabolism and single-nucleotide polymorphisms within *UGT* (uridine diphosphate-glucuronosyltransferase) have been proposed to account for these differences but confirmatory studies have not been performed (110). This unpredictable variation in serum posaconazole levels has heightened interest and the necessity of therapeutic drug monitoring (TDM).

Posaconazole is hepatically metabolized and, as discussed earlier, undergoes minimal glucuronidation. Renal clearance plays a minor role in the clearance of posaconazole, which is predominantly eliminated fecally.

Oral posaconazole has proven effective in the prevention of proven or probable IA in neutropenic patients with acute myelogenous leukemia (AML) and in hematopoietic stem cell transplant recipients with graft-versus-host disease (GVHD) (111,112). The efficacy and safety of posaconazole in the treatment of invasive fungal infections has also been assessed, and although this study predates the widespread use of echinocandins and voriconazole, the observed efficacy allows for its use during salvage therapy (113).

Currently, 200 mg three times daily is recommended for prophylaxis, and 800 mg divided in two or four doses is recommended in the salvage setting. Patients not tolerating food should be given a liquid nutritional supplement in attempts to increase drug absorption (109). Pediatric dosing schedules have yet to be definitively established yet retrospective data has demonstrated the safety and efficacy in this population (27,114). Dose adjustment by age, sex, race, and hepatic or renal insufficiency is not necessary given the minimal glucuronidation and renal clearance of posaconazole (115).

Posaconazole is typically well tolerated and infrequently requires discontinuation due to adverse drug events. The most frequent side effects of posaconazole therapy are gastrointestinal (14%), with transaminase elevation and hyperbilirubinemia occurring in 3% (112). However, in one trial, more serious adverse events were reported in patients treated with posaconazole than with fluconazole. Three cardiac events were reported among those possibly related to posaconazole treatment including decreased ejection fraction, QTc prolongation, and torsades de pointes (111). Nevertheless, for most patients, posaconazole is well tolerated and even long-term therapy (>6 months) is frequently without toxicity (116).

Posaconazole is not significantly metabolized through the cytochrome P450 system and serum levels are unlikely to be increased by concomitant administration of P450 inhibitors. Posaconazole is known to decrease the metabolism of other medications metabolized through these pathways and caution should be taken with coadministration.

Voriconazole

Voriconazole is a low-molecular-weight water-soluble extended-spectrum triazole with a chemical structure similar to fluconazole. Available in both oral and IV formulations, the latter is dependent on sulfobutyl ether β-cyclodextrin (SBECD) for solubility (117). The oral formulation of voriconazole is well absorbed with a bioavailability of more than 90% (118,119). Steady-state plasma levels range from 2 to 3 μg/mL following oral administration and 3 to 6 μg/mL after IV infusion. When 3 to 6 mg/kg of daily voriconazole is administered, steady-state levels are reached in 5 to 6 days. However, if oral or IV loading is given, steady state can be reached within 1 day (120).

Voriconazole is 58% protein-bound and has excellent penetration into the CNS as well as other tissues (121,122). It is metabolized in the liver via the cytochrome P450 enzyme family and less than 5% of voriconazole is excreted unchanged in urine (41,117).

Although voriconazole in children has demonstrated linear pharmacokinetics, in adults, nonlinear metabolism is observed, likely secondary to saturable metabolic enzymes required for drug clearance (120). Interpatient serum concentration differences have been attributed to polymorphisms within CYP2C19, the major metabolic pathway for voriconazole (117). Up to 20% of non–Indian Asians have low CYP2C19 activity and voriconazole serum levels are thus up to four times higher than those found in White or Black populations in which the "poor metabolizer" status is uncommon (123). The unpredictability of patient enzymatic activity has generated an increased interest in the routine use of voriconazole TDM.

For IV administration, 6 mg/kg twice daily on day 1, followed by 4 mg/kg IV twice daily for the duration of therapy is recommended. The oral dosages in adults are also weight based. For those weighing greater than 40 kg, 400 mg twice daily on day 1, followed by 200 mg twice daily until completion of therapy is suggested, whereas those weighing less than 40 kg should receive 200 mg twice daily for 1 day followed by 100 mg twice daily (123). Pediatric patients are known to hypermetabolize voriconazole and for this reason an IV dose of 7 mg/kg twice daily and oral dosing of 200 mg twice daily without loading is recommended (55). In patients with liver dysfunction, standard loading doses should be given, but the maintenance dose reduced by 50%. The safety of voriconazole use in severe liver disease remains uncertain. No dosage adjustment is required if oral drug is given to patients with renal insufficiency. However, the presence of a cyclodextrin vehicle within the IV formulation has caused concerns about vehicle accumulation in renal insufficiency or dialysis dependence and IV administration is best avoided in patients with a CrCl less than 50 mL (117).

Voriconazole exhibits concentration-independent fungistatic activity against *Candida* spp and *Cryptococcus neoformans* with no apparent post–antifungal effect (124). Recent in vivo studies of disseminated *Candida albicans* infection indicate that an AUC/MIC ratio of 20 to 25:1 predicts treatment success (125). In contrast, voriconazole appears to exert a dose-dependent fungicidal effect on *Aspergillus* based on both time-kill studies (126) and clearance of fungal burden in target organs of animal models of IA (127).

Voriconazole has a broad spectrum of activity that includes *Candida* spp, *Cryptococcus neoformans*, *Trichosporon* spp, *Aspergillus* spp, *Fusarium* spp, and other hyaline molds, dematiaceous fungi, and the endemic fungi. The anticandidal activity of voriconazole encompasses *Candida krusei* and most, but not all, strains of *Candida albicans*. Although activity of voriconazole in vitro against *Candida glabrata* can be demonstrated, the high MICs seen with wild-type *Candida glabrata* against voriconazole has resulted in no susceptible breakpoints for voriconazole against *Candida glabrata* in recent CLSI guidance (128,129). Voriconazole is also active against some fungi that are resistant to AmB, including *A. terreus* and *P. boydii* (130,131). Voriconazole exhibits a broad spectrum of activity against molds with the exception of agents of mucormycosis (117), and in fact, *Mucorales* have been proven more virulent if exposed to voriconazole (132).

Voriconazole is approved for the primary treatment of IA (22,133) and for treatment of infections due to *P. boydii* (*Scedosporium apiospermum*) and *Fusarium* spp in patients intolerant of, or with infections refractory to, other antifungal agents (134). Importantly, voriconazole was shown to be more effective than AmB (53% vs. 32% complete or partial response at week 12 of treatment and 71% vs. 58% survival, respectively) for primary treatment of IA (23). Voriconazole has also been shown to have good efficacy in the treatment of various forms of candidiasis (135,136). It has not been approved for empirical treatment of febrile, neutropenic patients despite documented efficacy in the treatment of IA and in the prevention of breakthrough fungal infections in this same patient population (137).

Typically well tolerated, the side effect profile of voriconazole is similar to other triazoles with a few notable exceptions. The majority of those experiencing a reported adverse reaction to voriconazole describe abnormal vision (up to 23%) that is transient, infusion related, and without long-term sequelae (138). This unique effect typically occurs 30 minutes after infusion and abates 30 minutes after onset.

Other well-known effects of voriconazole therapy include skin rash and transaminase elevation in 10% to 20% of recipients (133). Baseline evaluation of hepatic function has been recommended before and during treatment, and rare cases of hepatic failure during voriconazole use have been reported (139). Elevated voriconazole serum levels have been attributed to the majority of side effects

encountered in clinical practice, and higher levels (>5.5 mg/L), although associated with favorable outcomes, have also been suggested responsible for the uncommon potential side effects of encephalopathy or hallucinations (140–142).

Therapeutic Drug Monitoring for Azole Antifungals

Commercial assays are available for monitoring the serum concentrations of all currently available triazoles; however, at this time, existing guidelines recommend only itraconazole TDM (75,143,144). A strong argument can also be made for routine TDM of both posaconazole and voriconazole as well.

Itraconazole levels should be drawn after steady state is reached to ensure therapeutic levels (>1 µg/mL). Fluconazole levels are infrequently monitored due to the excellent bioavailability of this agent. However, clinical circumstances may dictate drug monitoring when therapeutic levels are uncertain (i.e., concurrent use of rifampin, rifampicin, etc.).

The extended-spectrum triazoles, posaconazole and voriconazole, have received increased attention due to their erratic absorption (posaconazole), or concerns for toxicity and the interpatient variability of serum levels (voriconazole). No guidelines exist for posaconazole TDM; however, past evidence supports a relationship between posaconazole serum drug level and efficacy (145). TDM should also be considered when drug interactions are of concern, such as the aforementioned potential for acid-suppressive agents to reduce absorption, although goal levels remain to be determined. Most experts suggest target trough concentrations greater than or equal to 0.5 µg/mL when given for antifungal prophylaxis. The interpatient variability of voriconazole also warrants consideration of TDM during use. Low concentrations (<1 mg/L) are more common in those receiving oral therapy and failure rates have been associated with low serum drug levels (133). Conversely, levels greater than 5.5 mg/L have been associated with encephalopathy without an improvement in efficacy (140). However, the frequency with which to monitor these newer triazoles remains to be determined.

ECHINOCANDINS

Echinocandins (caspofungin, micafungin, anidulafungin) are semisynthetic lipopeptides that inhibit the synthesis of β-1,3 glucan, an important constituent of the fungal cell wall (see Fig. 6.1), by inhibiting the activity of glucan synthase. The glucans are important in maintaining the osmotic integrity of the fungal cell and play a key role in cell division and cell growth (1,146). Disruption of β-1,3 glucan synthesis thus impairs cell wall integrity and leads to osmotic lysis (147).

The echinocandins are currently available only in IV formulations. The echinocandins exhibit dose-dependent linear pharmacokinetics and are highly (more than 95%) protein bound (148–150). They are broadly distributed to all major organs, including the brain (151), although concentrations in CSF are low (152). Metabolism occurs in the liver by a cytochrome P450 independent mechanism and the inactive metabolites are excreted in the feces and urine; less than 2% of a dose is excreted in the urine in active form (153,154).

Both in vitro and in vivo studies in *Candida* spp have shown a concentration-dependent fungicidal effect that is optimized at a peak-to-MIC ratio of approximately 8:1 (18,155) and a postantifungal effect of up to 12 hours (156). In contrast, activity against *Aspergillus* spp is neither classically fungistatic nor fungicidal, with activity localized to the growing hyphal tips and branch points with resultant inhibition of growth and angioinvasion but only a modest effect on the fungal burden in tissues (157–159).

TDM of echinocandins is almost never required and not recommended. Administered as standard doses, this class of antifungals has recently received attention for dosing strategies that may be needed in those with morbid obesity, although definitive recommendations have not been made (160,161).

Multiple in vitro studies have confirmed a paradoxical effect of the echinocandins. In this circumstance above a certain concentration of drug decreased antifungal activity is observed. The exact mechanism responsible for this phenomenon has not been fully elucidated, although studies have shown the involvement of the protein kinase C cell wall integrity pathway and an increase in cell wall chitin content as potential mechanisms responsible for this phenomenon (162). The clinical significance of these in vitro findings remains uncertain (163) and higher echinocandin doses have been evaluated in prospective trials and outcomes are no different from those at standard dosing (164).

Echinocandins have poor oral absorption and current agents are available only in the

IV formulation. Echinocandins are highly protein bound (anidulafungin 98%, caspofungin 96%, and micafungin 99.8%) and have a half-life of 40 hours, 10.6 hours, and 11 to 17 hours, respectively (80). Their vitreal and CSF penetration is negligible and this point is of clinical significance during the treatment of candidemia if endophthalmitis is also observed (165).

Caspofungin was the first available agent of this class and is metabolized by both hepatic hydrolysis and *N*-acetylation. Inactive metabolites are subsequently eliminated in the urine. Severe hepatic dysfunction thus mandates caspofungin dose reduction (20). Caspofungin has several drug interactions with agents metabolized through the cytochrome P450 system and serum levels are reduced in the presence of rifampin and may increase levels of sirolimus, nifedipine, and cyclosporine (20). Micafungin is metabolized by nonoxidative metabolism within the liver and anidulafungin undergoes nonenzymatic degradation within the kidney. Both agents are eliminated in feces. These agents therefore do not require dosage adjustment with hepatic impairment (20).

Their clinical use is primarily limited to *Candida* spp and *Aspergillus* spp and they lack activity against *Mucorales*, *Cryptococcus* spp, and other clinically important molds (Table 6.1). Although activity is observed against all *Candida* spp, the mean inhibitory concentrations (MICs) are elevated (>1 μg/mL) when *Candida parapsilosis* and *Candida guilliermondii* are encountered. Susceptibility differences between the different agents in this class are minimal (166). Recent changes in CLSI breakpoints recognize that although clinical activity of the echinocandins is good even with higher MICs, mutations in the target *FKS1/2* gene are likely present with MICs over 0.25 μg/mL for most species with higher breakpoints for *C. parapsilosis* and *C. guilliermondii*. Echinocandins also have immunomodulatory effects. By exposing β-glucan by the disruption of fungal cell wall mannoproteins, additional antigens are exposed for antibody deposition and fungal recognition by the host immune system, which may add activity against organisms such as molds like *Mucorales* and *Fusarium* for which they have minimal intrinsic activity (167).

In addition to activity against *Candida* and *Aspergillus* spp, the echinocandins have moderate activity against dematiaceous fungi (168,169) and low activity against the endemic dimorphic pathogens (169,170). They are inactive against *Fusarium* and other hyalohyphomycetes, *Cryptococcus neoformans*, *Trichosporum* spp, and

Mucorales (150,171). Primary resistance to echinocandins appears to be uncommon in *Candida albicans* and *Aspergillus* spp and notably, echinocandins are active against fluconazole-resistant strains of *Candida* spp (32,172,173).

The increased incidence of triazole-resistant *Candida* spp and the fungicidal activity of the echinocandins (caspofungin, micafungin, and anidulafungin) have prompted some authorities to recommend these agents as first-line therapy for invasive candidiasis and recent meta-analysis has shown improved outcomes in those who receive echinocandins as first-line therapy (174). Additionally, their proven efficacy, infrequency of side effects, and favorable drug interaction profiles make them attractive options over other available antifungals (32,164,175,176).

Comparative trials have found the echinocandins equally efficacious and better tolerated than AmB in the treatment of candidemia (32). In one such trial, caspofungin (70 mg loading dose followed by 50 mg daily) was compared to AmB-d (0.6 to 1 mg/kg) in the treatment of invasive candidiasis. Although *C. albicans* was more common in the AmB arm, modified intention to treat analysis revealed similar survival in each group, with a trend toward increased survival and a statistically significant decrease in drug side effects in those receiving caspofungin (32).

Similarly, micafungin (100 mg IV daily) has been compared to L-AmB 3 mg/kg IV daily in an international, double-blind trial. In this study assigning patients to 14 days of IV treatment, successful treatment was equivalent in each group. However, there were fewer treatment-related adverse events with micafungin than there were with liposomal amphotericin (175).

Only one comparative trial of different echinocandins has been performed in invasive candidiasis. In this trial, patients were enrolled to one of three treatment groups: micafungin 100 mg/day IV daily, micafungin 150 mg IV daily, or caspofungin 70 mg IV loading dose followed by 50 mg IV daily. No differences were found between treatment groups including microbiologic failure or all-cause mortality (164). Although this trial found that higher doses of an echinocandin may not equate to a greater therapeutic response, no increase in toxicity was seen with higher doses nor was a paradoxical effect observed.

Anidulafungin has been compared with fluconazole for the treatment of invasive candidiasis and treatment was successful in 75.6% of patients treated with anidulafungin, as compared with 60.2% of those treated with fluconazole. Survival was improved with anidulafungin but was not statistically significant compared to the fluconazole arm (176).

Collectively, these trials have shown a high level of efficacy and low toxicity for the echinocandins. This class has since become "first-line" therapy in the treatment of candidiasis in most medical centers pending species identification and documented clinical improvement in the patient. After clinical improvement is obtained or the absence of fluconazole resistance documented, therapy is often changed to a triazole such as fluconazole (69). As noted earlier, CNS and intraocular infections should not be treated with echinocandin monotherapy due to their poor penetration into these sites.

Although clinical trials have been primarily limited to patients with candidemia, observational data has shown efficacy in candidal osteomyelitis, peritoneal infections, and abdominal abscesses (177). Additional retrospective data has also shown echinocandins may play a role in the treatment of infective endocarditis caused by *Candida* spp (178).

The echinocandins have also been found efficacious in the treatment of IA, although they are fungistatic against this genus. The known toxicity of AmB and its different formulations and the potential for voriconazole-induced drug–drug interactions or toxicity has increased interest in the echinocandins for use during treatment of IA (179).

Caspofungin as a potential first-line agent for IA has been evaluated in limited settings but data is not sufficient to recommend caspofungin or any of the echinocandins for first-line therapy in the treatment of IA. Thus, these agents are currently recommended in the treatment of IA only in those patients refractory to or intolerant of other agents (27,179). In vitro studies and limited clinical data have also shown the potential role for combination therapy (an echinocandin plus AmB or an azole) and a prospective trial of anidulafungin and voriconazole has been completed, with results suggesting benefit in subpopulations of patients but not in the entire population studied, although at the present time, full publication of the trial data has not occurred.

The side-effect profile of the echinocandins is very favorable and these agents are typically well tolerated. The most frequently reported adverse effects include increased liver transaminases, gastrointestinal upset, and headache (32,153).

An infusion-related reaction has been described if rapid administration is given with tachycardia, hypotension, and/or thrombophlebitis. Drug interactions are rare; however, concomitant administration of caspofungin and cyclosporine is not recommended, yet reports have shown it may be safe to do so in selected cases (180,181). Cyclosporine has been noted to increase the AUC of caspofungin by approximately 35%, but these alterations are not sufficient to suggest dosage modifications (150). The authors do not typically make dose adjustments of the echinocandins in any of these situations.

ANTIMETABOLITES

Flucytosine

Flucytosine (5-FC) is a water-soluble, synthetic, fluorinated pyrimidine analogue that exerts antifungal activity by interfering with the synthesis of DNA, RNA, and proteins in the fungal cell. In vivo, 5-FC is taken up into the cell by a fungus-specific cytosine permease and deaminated in the cytoplasm to 5-fluorouracil (5-FU) by cytosine deaminase. 5-FU is further converted to 5-fluorodeoxyuridylic acid, which interferes with DNA synthesis. Mammalian cells lack cytosine deaminase, allowing for a selective inhibition of fungal organisms (see Fig. 6.1) (182). This agent may be either fungistatic or fungicidal, depending on both fungal species and strain.

5-FC is available in an oral formulation with excellent bioavailability. Unfortunately, the IV formulation is no longer widely available. High concentrations of 5-FC may be achieved in serum, CSF, and other body fluids (183). In vitro pharmacodynamic studies have determined that 5-FC exhibits concentration-independent fungistatic activity against *Candida* spp that is optimized at concentrations four times the MIC (184). Furthermore, 5-FC exerts a significant post–antifungal effect of 2.5 to 4 hours against *Candida* spp (184). These findings have been confirmed in vivo by Andes and van Ogtrop (185), who showed that time above the MIC was the pharmacodynamic parameter that correlated best with outcome in 5-FC treatment of murine candidiasis. Maximum efficacy was seen when 5-FC blood levels exceeded the MIC for only 20% to 25% of the dosing interval (185). The later observation may be accounted for by the post–antifungal effect of 5-FC.

5-FC has excellent oral bioavailability with over 80% to 90% absorption. Peak serum levels occur 1 to 2 hours after ingestion (30 to 45 μg/mL) of a single dose. The volume of distribution (Vd) of 5-FC is 0.6 to 0.9, yet bone, peritoneal, and synovial fluid 5-FC levels have been demonstrated and urinary levels are several folds higher than concurrent serum levels. Greater than 95% of 5-FC is eliminated unchanged in the urine. 5-FC is typically administered by mouth at 100 mg/kg/day divided in four doses (80) and that that dose is usually well tolerated without the need to adjust the dose based on drug levels.

Activity has been observed against most fungal pathogens including *Candida*, *Cryptococcus*, *Cladosporium*, *Phialophora*, and *Saccharomyces* spp. However, *Aspergillus* spp, *Mucorales*, dermatophytes, and the endemic mycoses are all resistant to 5-FC (1). Additionally, resistance commonly develops when 5-FC is used as monotherapy even in susceptible organisms and it should not be used as such except during the treatment of chromoblastomycoses or during the treatment of localized candidal infections when alternative agents are unavailable or contraindicated.

5-FC is primarily used only in the treatment of cryptococcus (combined with AmB) and chromoblastomycosis. Despite concerns for additive toxicity, the synergistic effects of dual therapy in *Cryptococcus* allow for more rapid CSF clearance (186).

Peak plasma levels of 40 μg/mL easily exceed the MICs of most *Candida* spp and *Cryptococcus neoformans* (187,188) and provide optimal antifungal activity while minimizing hematologic adverse effects (189). The marrow suppressive effects are more common if blood levels exceed 100 to 125 μg/mL (190). In the presence of prolonged therapy (>7 days) or with alterations in renal function, serum drug monitoring can be considered but at the lower doses typically recommended for use, drug level monitoring is not frequently necessary. Other less common side effects such as abdominal pain or diarrhea are frequently indirect markers of elevated 5-FC levels and therapy is typically stopped in these circumstances. Rash and hepatic transaminase elevation have also been reported with liver abnormalities frequently observed (183). 5-FC is teratogenic and should not be administered during pregnancy.

Allylamines

The allylamine class of antifungal agents is composed of terbinafine and naftifine. Only terbinafine has systemic activity. Both terbinafine and naftifine inhibit the enzyme squalene epoxidase, which results in the accumulation of squalene and blocks the synthesis of ergosterol (191). The accumulation of high concentrations of squalene results in increased membrane permeability and, ultimately, cell death.

Terbinafine

Terbinafine is a lipophilic antifungal agent that is available in oral and topical formulations (192). Terbinafine has a broad spectrum of activity that includes dermatophytes, *Candida* spp, *Malassezia furfur*, *Aspergillus* spp, *Cryptococcus neoformans*, *Trichosporon* spp, *S. schenckii*, and *P. marneffei* (193–196).

Terbinafine is well absorbed orally and is concentrated in fatty tissues, skin, hair, and nails but low serum levels of drug are found (197). Low toxicity and good efficacy in the treatment of virtually all dermatomycoses, including onychomycosis, is seen with terbinafine (198,199). The combination of terbinafine and fluconazole has shown efficacy in the treatment of fluconazole-resistant *Candida* spp yet with the recent availability of alternative antifungals, other agents are typically chosen (200). Terbinafine also has shown clinical efficacy in cases of sporotrichosis, aspergillosis, and chromoblastomycosis (201).

It is an inhibitor of CYP2D6, but this generally results in less important drug–drug interactions than inhibitors of CYP3A4. The most commonly reported side effects include gastrointestinal upset and cutaneous reactions (202). Reversible agranulocytosis has also been reported but is rare (203,204). Hepatic dysfunction and even fulminant hepatic failure are uncommon but have been reported during terbinafine administration and for this reason, terbinafine is not recommended in those with underlying liver disease (202).

Griseofulvin

Griseofulvin is a long-standing oral agent used for the treatment of dermatomycoses. Its mechanism of action is thought to involve interaction with microtubules within the fungal cell and inhibition of mitosis (205,206).

Griseofulvin is active against most dermatophytes; however, alternative agents, such as itraconazole and terbinafine, appear to be more potent and exhibit greater efficacy in prospective clinical trials (207–210).

Griseofulvin is best absorbed orally when administered in an ultramicrocrystalline form with an accompanying meal. It is deposited primarily in keratin precursor cells. Administration of griseofulvin is associated with a number of mild side effects including nausea, diarrhea, headache, cutaneous disruptions, hepatotoxicity, and neurologic complaints (211).

ANTIFUNGAL AGENTS FOR TOPICAL USE

There are numerous topical antifungal preparations available for the treatment of superficial cutaneous and mucosal fungal infections. The available preparations encompass a wide variety of antifungal classes including polyenes (AmB, nystatin, and natamycin), allylamines (naftifine and terbinafine), and numerous imidazoles and other miscellaneous agents. Preparations for use in cutaneous disease and onychomycosis include creams, lotions, ointments, powders, and sprays, whereas suspensions, tablets, troches, and suppositories are used for treatment of various forms of mucosal candidiasis (69,212,213).

The selection of topical versus systemic therapy for cutaneous or mucosal fungal infections depends on the status of the host and the type and extent of the infection. The refractory nature of infections such as onychomycosis or tinea capitis usually mandates long-term systemic therapy, whereas most cutaneous dermatophytic infections and oral or vaginal thrush respond favorably to topical therapy. Systemic agents are generally recommended for chronic, recurrent oral or vaginal candidiasis and for candidal esophagitis (69,213).

ANTIFUNGAL AGENTS UNDER DEVELOPMENT

Currently, several different antifungal agents are under active development, including those with established modes of action as well as novel new classes of antifungal agents (Table 6.1). These include a novel triazole agent (isavuconazole), IV and tablet posaconazole formulations, oral echinocandins, a chitin synthase inhibitor (nikkomycin Z), and agents with new mechanisms of action such as blocking critical or unique fungal cell pathways, such as elongation factor, fungal gene methylation, chitin synthesis, and others. The mechanisms of action and spectra of activity of the novel triazoles and the echinocandins are essentially the same as currently available agents. In each case, the newer agents in the respective classes offer the potential of fewer toxicities and drug interactions, more favorable pharmacokinetic and pharmacodynamic properties, and possible improved activity against selected refractory pathogens. Nikkomycin Z, which inhibits chitin synthesis in the fungal cell wall, provides another novel mode of action that may act in concert with other inhibitors of cell wall or cell membrane synthesis. The introduction of several of these new agents such as isavuconazole, which is in active clinical development and the new formulations of posaconazole, should augment our available antifungal resources. The development of agents with novel modes of action is both necessary and promising for future antifungal therapy.

MECHANISMS OF RESISTANCE TO ANTIFUNGAL AGENTS

Resistance to antimicrobial agents is an issue of concern worldwide with important implications for morbidity, mortality, and the costs of health care. Although much attention has been focused on antibacterial resistance (214), innate or acquired resistance to antifungal agents is now recognized among several pathogenic fungi (215,219). This recognition has spurred the development of new antifungal agents as well as intensive efforts to define the molecular mechanisms of resistance to various agents (Table 6.3).

The extensive utilization of fluconazole has been coupled with increasing reports of azole resistance (216,217) and some of the most elegant investigations of antifungal resistance mechanisms have involved the azole class of antifungals and *Candida* spp (218). In this section, we will review what is known of the molecular and cellular mechanisms of resistance to antifungal agents as well as the clinical factors that may result in resistance to antifungal therapy.

Molecular and Cellular Mechanisms of Resistance to Antifungal Agents

Most fungal infections are caused by *Candida* spp and most of our understanding of the mechanisms of resistance comes from studies of *Candida albicans* and other species of *Candida* (218–220). Although *Aspergillus* spp and *Cryptococcus neoformans* constitute a significant proportion of opportunistic mycoses, fewer studies have been performed on these organisms and little information on antifungal resistance mechanisms is available for other opportunistic fungal pathogens (68).

Although there are many parallels that exist between antibacterial resistance mechanisms and antifungal resistance mechanisms (191), there are no data to suggest that destruction or modification of antifungal agents is an important component of antifungal resistance. Likewise, it does not appear that fungi can employ the genetic exchange mechanisms that allow rapid transmission of antimicrobial resistance in bacteria. On the other hand, it is apparent that multidrug efflux pumps, target alterations, and reduced access to targets are important mechanisms of resistance to antifungal agents, just as they are important in antibacterial resistance (220,221). In contrast to the rapid emergence of high-level antimicrobial resistance that occurs among bacteria, antifungal resistance usually develops slowly and involves the emergence of intrinsically resistant species or a gradual, stepwise alteration of cellular structures or functions that results in resistance to an agent to which there has been prior exposure (221,222).

Polyenes

Resistance to AmB remains uncommon despite extensive utilization over more than 40 years. Among the *Candida* spp, decreased susceptibility to AmB has been reported in *C. lusitaniae*, *C. glabrata*, *C. krusei*, and *C. guilliermondii* (219,223–226). Although primary resistance to AmB is seen chiefly among *C. lusitaniae*, *C. krusei*, and *C. guilliermondii* (68,227,228). Most reports of AmB resistance in *Candida* spp appear to be secondary to AmB exposure during treatment (219,223).

Most isolates of *Aspergillus* spp appear susceptible to AmB; however, *A. terreus* seems to be resistant to AmB both in vitro and in vivo (229,230). Similarly, some of the "cryptic" strains of *Aspergillus* such as *Aspergillus lentulus* and others such as *Aspergillus calidoustus* may show decreased amphotericin susceptibility. Primary resistance to AmB among *C. neoformans* has not been reported while secondary resistance appears rare (187,231,232).

Our understanding of the mechanism of resistance to AmB stems largely from studies of mutants of *Candida* spp and *Cryptococcus neoformans* derived from sequential passage in varying concentrations of AmB (233) and from characterization of serial isolates from patients failing AmB therapy (218,223,231,234–238). The mechanism of AmB resistance appears to be from a qualitative or quantitative alteration in the sterol content of cells (239,240), defense mechanisms against

Table 6.3

Mechanisms Involved in the Development of Resistance to Antifungal Agents in Pathogenic Fungi

Fungus	Amphotericin B	Flucytosine	Itraconazole/Voriconazole	Fluconazole	Echinocandins
Aspergillus fumigatus			Altered target enzyme, 14-α-demethylase Decreased azole accumulation (TR/L98H) promotor mutation, HapE transcription factor mutations		Mutation in *FKS1/2* genes
Candida albicans	Decrease in ergosterol Replacement of polyene-binding sterols Masking of ergosterol	Loss of permease activity Loss of cytosine deaminase activity Loss of uracil phosphoribosyl-transferase activity		Overexpression or mutation of 14-α-demethylase Overexpression of efflux pumps, *CDR* and *MDR* genes	
Candida glabrata	Alteration or decrease in ergosterol content	Loss of permease activity		Overexpression of efflux pumps (*CgCDR* genes)	Mutation in *FKS1/2* genes
Candida krusei	Alteration or decrease in ergosterol content			Active efflux Reduced affinity for target enzyme, 14-α-demethylase	Mutation in *FKS1/2* genes
Candida lusitaniae	Alteration or decrease in ergosterol content Production of modified sterols				
Cryptococcus neoformans	Defects in sterol synthesis Decreased ergosterol Production of modified sterols			Alterations in target enzyme Overexpression of MDR efflux pump	

oxidative damage (241), defects in ergosterol bio-synthetic genes (242), and alterations in the sterol-to-phospholipid ratio (239).

Ergosterol is the primary sterol target for AmB in the fungal cell membrane and resistant yeast containing an altered sterol content bind lesser amounts of AmB than do susceptible cells. Accordingly, mutants of *Candida* spp and *Cryptococcus neoformans* resistant to AmB have been shown to have a reduced total ergosterol content (231,235), replacement of polyene-binding sterols (ergosterol) by ones that bind polyenes less well (fecosterol) (231,243), or masking of ergosterol in the cell membrane so that binding with polyenes is hindered by steric or thermodynamic factors (191,244). One or more of these factors may account for decreased susceptibility to AmB. This resistance is often specific for AmB, but cross-resistance to azoles has also been reported and (5,6)-desaturase (Erg3p) mutants identified as causal in isolates with resistance to both classes (223,245). The molecular mechanisms of AmB resistance in *Candida* and *Cryptococcus neoformans* have not been determined; however, sterol analyses of resistant isolates suggest that they are defective in *erg2* or *erg3*, genes encoding for the C-8 sterol isomerase and C-5 sterol desaturase enzymes, respectively (218).

Azoles

The excellent safety profile of fluconazole has led to extensive utilization of this agent worldwide. Concomitant with this utilization reports of emerging resistance to fluconazole and other azoles have appeared (246). Despite these reports, primary resistance to fluconazole is unusual among most species of *Candida* causing bloodstream infections (216). Among the five most common species of *Candida* isolated from blood (*C. albicans*, *C. glabrata*, *C. parapsilosis*, *C. tropicalis*, and *C. krusei*), the overall frequency of high-level resistance (previously reported as an MIC >64 μg/mL) to fluconazole is less than 3%. Resistance is uncommon among bloodstream infections of *C. albicans* (0% to 7%) (216,247), *C. parapsilosis* (0% to 4%), and *C. tropicalis* (0% to 6%), whereas approximately 12% or more of *C. glabrata* isolates exhibit primary resistance to this agent (247,248). *C. krusei* is considered intrinsically resistant to fluconazole and MICs are usually more than 32 μg/mL for this species (36,249). Notably, the frequency of resistance to fluconazole among bloodstream infection isolates of *Candida* spp has not increased

substantially after more than two decades of utilization worldwide (216,247,250).

The new triazoles (posaconazole and voriconazole) exhibit more potent activity against *Candida* spp than that of fluconazole, including activity against *C. krusei* and some fluconazole-resistant strains of *Candida* (251–255). Isolates of *C.glabrata* for which fluconazole MICs are less than 16 μg/mL typically have MICs less than 1 μg/mL to voriconazole and posaconazole (129,256,257); however, those isolates with higher fluconazole MICs tend to be less susceptible to the new triazoles with MICs more than 2 μg/mL (129,256). Recent breakpoints for voriconazole do not include a susceptible category for voriconazole for *C. glabrata* and posaconazole breakpoints have not yet been established. In general, among *Candida* isolates, there is a strong positive correlation between fluconazole MICs and those of voriconazole and posaconazole, suggesting significance cross-resistance, especially for some species such as *C. glabrata* (129,254).

Similar to *Candida* spp, primary resistance to fluconazole is uncommon among isolates of *Cryptococcus neoformans* (187,258,259), although secondary resistance has been described among individuals with AIDS and relapsing cryptococcal meningitis (260). Despite these reports, the susceptibility profile of this organism to fluconazole has remained unchanged over the past 30 years (187,260).

Although *Aspergillus* spp are intrinsically resistant to fluconazole, most isolates appear susceptible to itraconazole and the new triazoles (261). MICs greater than 1 μg/mL for these azoles are unusual among clinical isolates of *Aspergillus*, although the incidence may be increasing in certain regions due to environmental use of triazole fungicides (262,263). In contrast to *Candida*, cross-resistance between itraconazole and the new triazoles is not complete: cross-resistance between itraconazole and posaconazole, but not voriconazole, has been observed in some strains (264).

The mechanism of azole resistance in *Candida* has been extensively evaluated for fluconazole and *C. albicans* (218,221). Resistance can result from a modification in the quality or quantity of the target enzyme, reduced access of the drug to the target, or some combination of these mechanisms. In the first instance, point mutations in the gene (*ERG11*) encoding for the target enzyme, 14-α-demethylase, leads to an altered target with decreased affinity for azoles. Overexpression of *ERG11* results in the production of high concentrations of the target enzyme, creating the need for higher intracellular azole concentrations to inhibit increased available substrate. Loss of allelic variation in the *ERG11* promoter may also result in a resistant strain that is homozygous for the mutated gene (265).

The second major mechanism involves active efflux of azole antifungal agents out of the cell through the action of two types of multidrug efflux transporters: the major facilitators (encoded by *MDR* genes) and those of the ATP-binding cassette superfamily (encoded by *CDR* genes) (219). Upregulation of the *MDR1* gene leads to fluconazole resistance, whereas upregulation of *CDR* genes leads to resistance to multiple azoles (221,266–269). Evidence that these mechanisms may act individually, sequentially, and in concert has been derived by studying serial isolates of *C. albicans* from AIDS patients with OPC (270–272).

It appears that the mechanisms of resistance to azoles in *C. glabrata* involve upregulation of *CDR1* genes, resulting in resistance to multiple azoles (266). Azole resistance in *C. krusei* appears to be mediated by reduced susceptibility of the target enzyme to inhibition by fluconazole and itraconazole (63). This does not seem to be the case with the new triazoles, given their potent aforementioned activity against *C. krusei*.

In *Aspergillus*, the azole target cyp51A is an established "hot spot" for mutations that confer phenotypic triazole resistance (273). A substitution of leucine 98 for histidine in the *cyp51A* gene, together with two copies of a 34-bp sequence in tandem in the gene promoter (TR/L98H), was found to be the dominant resistance mechanism. Recently, a mutation in the transcription factor complex subunit HapE has also been reported (274) and with the advent of whole genome sequencing, other mechanisms are likely to be seen in the near future.

The *C. neoformans* isolates that have developed secondary resistance to fluconazole have been shown to have an altered target enzyme or overexpression of MDR efflux pumps (275,276). The latter mechanism, termed heteroresistance, is intrinsic in all cryptococcal isolates and is easily induced in vitro (277).

Echinocandins

Caspofungin, anidulafungin, and micafungin all exhibit potent fungicidal activity against most species of *Candida*, including azole-resistant strains (18,278,279). Isolates for which echinocandin MICs exceed 1 μg/mL rarely occur outside

of *C. parapsilosis* and *C. guilliermondii*; however, recent evidence has suggested the incidence of echinocandins resistance in *C. glabrata* may be increasing (216). Efforts to produce laboratory mutants of *Candida* spp with reduced susceptibility to caspofungin have demonstrated that the frequency of these mutants is extremely low (1 in 10^8 cells), suggesting a low potential for the emergence of resistance in the clinical setting (280,281); however, the development of resistance despite continuous receipt of an echinocandins has been reported (282). Likewise, isolates of *Aspergillus* spp from clinical sources with reduced susceptibility to echinocandins have been observed, although this appears an uncommon occurrence (171,283).

Studies of laboratory-derived mutants of *C. albicans* with reduced in vitro and in vivo susceptibility to the echinocandins have documented point mutations in the *FKS1* and *FKS2* genes encoding for the glucan-synthesis enzyme complex (282,284,285). These mutant strains demonstrate an increased 50% inhibitory concentration (IC_{50}) for inhibition of the glucan synthesis enzyme complex and reduced susceptibility to all echinocandins in vitro and in vivo in animal models (280,281,286). These strains remain susceptible to polyenes and azole antifungal agents, although multidrug resistance to both echinocandins and azoles has been reported with *C. glabrata*. *FKS* genes are similarly essential in *Aspergillus* spp (287), and increased expression of the *FKS* gene has been observed in a resistant isolate (283), whereas other strains have been found to have mutations in the *ECM33* gene (*AfuEcm33*), encoding cell wall proteins important for fungal cell wall organization (288,289). Although there are limited data currently, these observations suggest that while mutations in the hot spot regions of the *FKS* gene is the predominant resistance mechanism in *Candida*, it is possible that mechanisms outside the target gene may be more important in *Aspergillus*.

Flucytosine

Despite reports in the older literature of a higher frequency of primary resistance to 5-FC among *Candida* spp and *Cryptococcus neoformans* (290,291), more recent studies using validated, standardized test methods indicate that primary resistance is actually uncommon among bloodstream infection isolates of both *Candida* spp and *Cryptococcus* (187,188). Secondary resistance to 5-FC, on the other hand, is well documented to occur among both *Candida* spp and *Cryptococcus neoformans* during monotherapy with this agent (292).

Resistance to 5-FC may develop from decreased uptake (loss of permease activity) or by loss of enzymatic activity required for the conversion of 5-FC to 5-FU (cytosine deaminase) and 5-fluorouridylic acid (FUMP pyrophosphorylase) (292,293). Of these possible mechanisms, the most important appear to be the loss of cytosine deaminase activity or the loss of UMP pyrophosphorylase activity. Uracil phosphoribosyltransferase, another enzyme in the primidine salvage pathway, is also important in the formation of FUMP and loss of its activity is sufficient to confer resistance to 5-FC (293).

Allylamines

Allylamine resistance has been infrequently reported despite clinical failures in close to 25% of patients treated with these agents (191). Laboratory-created resistant isolates have been found to carry extra copies of the *ERG1* gene (294) or single base pair exchanges in the *ERG1* gene coding for squalene epoxidase, the target of terbinafine (295). Subsequently, clinical isolates with amino acid substitutions within the *ERG1* gene have also been reported (296,297). Sanglard et al. (267) have reported that the CDR1 multidrug efflux pump can use terbinafine as a substrate, thus the possibility of efflux-mediated resistance to allylamines exists.

Clinical Factors Contributing to Antifungal Resistance

Fungal infections may fail to respond to appropriate antifungal therapy, thereby demonstrating "clinical resistance," despite the fact that the drug employed is active against the infecting organism. The interaction of the host, the drug, and the fungus is complex and clinical outcomes are influenced by a number of interactions (298).

During treatment of invasive fungal infections, the immune status of the host is the most important factor in determining outcomes. The presence of neutrophils, utilization of immunomodulating drugs, concomitant infections (e.g., HIV), surgical procedures, age, and nutritional status all may be more important than the ability, or lack thereof, of antifungal agents to inhibit or kill the infecting organism. Likewise, the site and severity of infection plays a critical role in the pharmacokinetic/pharmacodynamic interactions during antifungal therapy. The presence of a foreign body, such as a catheter, prosthetic valve, or vascular graft material, may allow an otherwise susceptible organism

to cause an infection that is recalcitrant to therapy with an otherwise active agent. Finally, an antifungal agent cannot act if the patient does not take it in the prescribed manner. Noncompliance is a major cause of apparent "resistance" to antifungal therapy and additionally may contribute to the development of resistant strains.

The absorption, distribution, and metabolism of an antifungal agent all contribute to the effectiveness of the drug at the site of infection. Insufficient (too low) dosing practices may influence both therapeutic efficacy and the potential for resistance development (299). The ability of an antifungal agent to exhibit fungicidal activity versus fungistatic activity may be especially important in severe infections, in infections where the organism burden is high, and in the neutropenic host (64,300). Drug–drug interactions may also affect the activity of an antifungal agent: drugs that are metabolized by the cytochrome P450 enzyme system, such as rifamycin, may dramatically decrease the achievable concentrations of azole antifungal agents such as itraconazole and voriconazole (301).

Fungal properties, aside from the expression of known resistance factors, may also impact the clinical success or failure of antifungal therapy. The different morphologic forms of fungi (e.g., blastospore, hypha, pseudohypha, conidia, chlamydospore) may all have different susceptibilities to various antifungal agents (302,303). Phenotypic switching in *Candida* has been shown to have a dramatic impact on the susceptibility of various species to polyenes and azoles (223,304). Finally, the rate of growth of a fungus and whether or not it is growing in a planktonic or biofilm form can determine whether it will require low or high concentrations of an antifungal to inhibit growth (305,306). *Candida* spp are increasingly resistant to antifungals when grown in a biofilm compared to those grown in solution (307).

CONCLUSION

The incidence of infection with invasive mycoses continues to rise with the increasing immunosuppressed patient population. The recently expanded antifungal armamentarium offers the potential for more effective and less toxic therapy and these agents offer distinct pharmacologic profiles and indications for use. An understanding of the differing spectrum of activity, pharmacokinetics/pharmacodynamics, and dosing regimens enables the clinician to provide patients the best chance of favorable outcomes.

ANTIFUNGAL SUSCEPTIBILITY TESTING

The increasing number and diversity of invasive infections, expanding utilization of new and established antifungal agents, and recognition of antifungal resistance as an important clinical problem have contributed to the need for reproducible, clinically relevant antifungal susceptibility testing, especially for yeasts, but also for the filamentous fungi (298).

Rationale for Antifungal Susceptibility Testing

The central objective of all in vitro susceptibility testing is to help predict the likely impact of administration of the tested agent on the outcome of disease caused by the tested organism or similar organisms. As such, in vitro susceptibility tests of antifungal agents are performed for the same reasons as tests of antibacterial agents: (a) to provide a reliable estimate of the relative activities of antimicrobial agents, (b) to correlate with in vivo activity and predict the outcome of the therapy, (c) to provide a means by which to survey the development of resistance among a normally susceptible population of organisms, and (d) to predict the therapeutic potential of newly developed investigational agents. In the clinical microbiology/mycology laboratory, the focus of testing is on a specific isolate from an individual patient. In drug discovery, the focus of testing may be on the selection of the most potent of a series of compounds for further development. In antimicrobial resistance surveillance, the issue may be the tendency of resistance to emerge in initially susceptible isolates or species and to establish local, regional, or national patterns of resistance. In each of these settings, it is necessary to remember that outcome prediction is difficult and dependent on complex and dynamic biologic system and may substantially differ from results obtained in an artificial and well-defined matrix (antimicrobial susceptibility test). Decades of experience with antibacterial susceptibility testing confirms the limited degree of in vitro–in vivo correlation that can be achieved. The in vitro susceptibility of *Enterococcus* to trimethoprim-sulfamethoxazole and in vivo resistance to this combination is illustrative of this fact (308,309). In vitro susceptibility does not always predict successful therapy (298).

Development of Standardized Methods

At the present time, the state-of-the-art method for susceptibility testing of yeasts is comparable with that of bacteria (298). The CLSI Subcommittee on Antifungal Susceptibility Testing has developed and published approved methods for broth dilution testing of yeasts (310) and for disk diffusion testing of yeasts against fluconazole (311). These methods are reproducible, accurate, and available for use in clinical laboratories (312,313). Standardized methods have also been developed for broth dilution testing of filamentous fungi (314) but require further refinement and studies to establish the in vivo correlation with the in vitro data.

Standardized Broth Dilution Methods for Yeasts

In the United States, the National Committee for Clinical Laboratory Standards (NCCLS) (now CLSI) Subcommittee on Antifungal Susceptibility Testing was established in 1982 and focused on the key in vitro testing variables of inoculum preparation and size, medium composition, temperature and duration of incubation, and MIC end point determination in an effort to develop a standardized approach to antifungal susceptibility testing of yeasts (*Candida* spp and *Cryptococcus neoformans*) using a broth dilution format (315–319). As a result of these collaborative studies, consensus within the subcommittee was achieved on all of the variables, leading to the publication of a proposed broth macrodilution method, *M27-P*, in 1992 (320). This document was revised and published in 1995 as NCCLS document *M27-T* (tentative standard), which described the broth microdilution method and provided reference MIC ranges for two quality control (QC) strains for the available antifungal agents. In 1997, the subcommittee established interpretive MIC breakpoints for three antifungal agents (fluconazole, itraconazole, and 5-FC) (321) and the NCCLS-approved standard M27-A was published. Since then, the subcommittee has developed 24- and 48-hour reference QC MIC ranges for microdilution testing of both established (AmB, 5-FC, fluconazole, itraconazole, and ketoconazole) and newly introduced (voriconazole and posaconazole) agents (322). The results of these studies are included in the second edition of NCCLS document M27, *M27-A2*, published in 2002 (323). Since this time, the M27-A3 document was published in 2008 with the addition of caspofungin, micafungin, and anidulafungin susceptibility recommendations (324).

Adherence to the NCCLS M27-A3 method provides excellent intralaboratory and interlaboratory reproducibility and utilization of the recommended QC isolates will further ensure reliable test performance (324). The most recently published CLSI guidelines established revised breakpoints for fluconazole and voriconazole along with the echinocandins, which are species specific (Tables 6.4 and 6.5). These revised breakpoints recognize the wild-type distributions of *Candida* species against both azoles (fluconazole and voriconazole) and the echinocandins along with predicted pharmacokinetic and pharmacodynamic parameters of the drugs. These have generally resulted in much lower breakpoints for most species.

Standardized Disk Diffusion Methods for Yeasts and Nondermatophyte Filamentous Fungi

Disk diffusion testing has served as a simple, rapid, and cost-effective alternative to broth dilution testing of antibacterial agents for many years (311,325). Disk diffusion testing of antifungal

Table 6.4

New Clinical and Laboratory Standards Institute Breakpoints for *Candida* spp					
		Clinical Breakpoint (μg/mL)			
***Candida* spp**	**Antifungal Agent**	**S**	**S-DD**	**I**	**R**
C. albicans	Amphotericin B				
	Flucytosine				
	Fluconazole	<2	4		≥8
	Itraconazole	≤0.12	0.25–0.5		≥1
	Voriconazole	≤0.12		0.25–0.5	≥1
C. glabrata	Amphotericin B				
	Flucytosine				
	Fluconazole		≤32		≥64
	Itraconazole				
	Voriconazole				
C. parapsilosis	Amphotericin B				
	Flucytosine				
	Fluconazole	<2	4		≥8
	Itraconazole				
	Voriconazole	≤0.12		0.25–0.5	≥1
C. tropicalis	Amphotericin B				
	Flucytosine				
	Fluconazole	<2	4		≥8
	Itraconazole				
	Voriconazole	≤0.12		0.25–0.5	≥1
C. krusei	Amphotericin B				
	Flucytosine				
	Fluconazole				
	Itraconazole				
	Voriconazole	≤0.5		1	≥2

Table 6.5

Proposed Clinica and Laboratory Standards Institute Breakpoints for Echinocandins				
		MIC Breakpoint		
Agent	**Species**	**S**	**I**	**R**
Anidulafungin	C. albicans	≤0.25	0.5	≥1
	C. glabrata	≤0.12	0.25	≥0.5
	C. tropicalis	≤0.25	0.5	≥1
	C. parapsilosis	≤2	4	≥8
	C. krusei	≤0.25	0.5	≥1
Caspofungin	C. albicans	≤0.25	0.5	≥1
	C. glabrata	≤0.12	0.25	≥0.5
	C. tropicalis	≤0.25	0.5	≥1
	C. parapsilosis	≤2	4	≥8
	C. krusei	≤0.25	0.5	≥1
Micafungin	C. albicans	≤0.25	0.5	≥1
	C. glabrata	≤0.06	0.12	≥0.25
	C. tropicalis	≤0.25	0.5	≥1
	C. parapsilosis	≤2	4	≥8
	C. krusei	≤0.25	0.5	≥1

agents has been slow to develop; however, early studies with fluconazole disks showed promise for testing *Candida* spp (326,327). Further development of this method has documented the precision and accuracy of the fluconazole disk diffusion test and has established QC zone diameter limits for both fluconazole and voriconazole when tested against *Candida* spp (328).

The NCCLS M44-A method uses Mueller-Hinton agar supplemented with 2% glucose and 0.5 µg/mL of methylene blue (311,312,329). The increased glucose and the methylene blue supplementation provides improved growth and sharper zones surrounding the fluconazole and voriconazole disks (312). This method employs an inoculum suspension adjusted to the turbidity of 0.5 McFarland Standard and 24-hour incubation at 35°C. The zone diameters surrounding the 25-µg fluconazole disks and the 1-µg voriconazole disks are read using reflected light and measured to the nearest whole millimeter at the point at which there is prominent reduction in growth. Pinpoint microcolonies at the zone edge or large colonies within a zone are ignored.

This method provides qualitative susceptibility results 24 hours sooner than the standard NCCLS M27-A2 MIC method for yeasts (330). The disk test results correlate well with reference MICs for both fluconazole and voriconazole and have allowed the establishment of zone interpretive criteria (breakpoints) for fluconazole and QC parameters for both fluconazole and voriconazole. The use of supplemented Mueller-Hinton agar in lieu of RPMI 1640 medium should make antifungal susceptibility testing available to a larger number of clinical laboratories at reduced cost. Since publication of the initial M44-A document, an update has been released (M44-A2) with zone diameter interpretive standards added for caspofungin, voriconazole, and posaconazole (311).

Similarly, the CLSI has developed a reference method for disk diffusion antifungal susceptibility testing of nondermatophyte filamentous fungi (325,331). These documents provide guidelines for testing the susceptibility of opportunistic molds to triazoles, AmB, and caspofungin and more recent publications have proposed QC and reference zone diameter limits for three strains selected as QC isolates (*A. fumigatus* ATCC MYA-3626, *Paecilomyces variotii* ATCC MYA-3630, and *C. krusei* ATCC 6258). These QC would assist in monitoring the performance of in vitro antifungal disk diffusion susceptibility testing by the CLSI M51-A and alternative methods (332). Additional studies are ongoing to further clarify testing condition with other echinocandins by this methodology (333).

Standardized Broth Dilution Methods for Filamentous Fungi

Serious infections due to filamentous fungi (molds), especially those due to *Aspergillus* spp, continue to increase and improving outcomes for these infections is an area of ongoing need. Given the increasing array of antifungal agents with systemic activity against the filamentous fungi, it is recognized that antifungal susceptibility testing of those opportunistic pathogens may be important in guiding the selection of antifungal agents for treatment of invasive disease. This is especially true for the newer triazoles (posaconazole and voriconazole) and echinocandins (caspofungin, micafungin, and anidulafungin) agents, all of which have varying degrees of activity against the opportunistic molds (171,334). Based on the achievements in standardizing in vitro susceptibility testing of yeasts, the CLSI antifungal subcommittee proceeded to develop a standardized method for the broth dilution testing of molds, NCCLS M38-A (335). The CLSI subcommittee used the M27-A2 microdilution method as a template for the development of the method for filamentous fungi. The approved method, M38-A, is applicable for testing *Aspergillus* spp, *Fusarium* spp, *P. boydii*, and *Mucorales*, and efforts remain ongoing to validate these methods for other agents (336). These guidelines were updated in 2008 with the publication of CLSI M38-A2 and provide MIC and minimum effective concentration (MEC) recommendations for the echinocandins, ciclopirox, griseofulvin, and terbinafine (314).

Progress and New Developments in Antifungal Susceptibility Testing

The availability of the M27 reference method for broth dilution testing of yeasts paved the way for the development of the reference method for filamentous fungi and was a necessary precursor to the disk diffusion methods. In addition, the M27 method has served as a cornerstone for the evaluation of new and improved methods for performing antifungal testing in the clinical laboratory and has facilitated the performance of large-scale national and international surveillance studies of the in vitro susceptibility of *Candida* spp and

other fungi to both established and investigational antifungal agents (171,187,216,337–339). These studies have allowed broad MIC distribution profiles for clinical isolates to be generated and are immensely helpful to clinicians in determining initial antifungal agents prior to isolate specific susceptibility results returning and for identifying isolates to be used in the characterization of resistance mechanisms (187,316,340). Finally, the standardization of antifungal susceptibility testing has made it possible to conduct nationwide studies of laboratory proficiency and to begin to establish the clinical relevance of antifungal susceptibility testing (341–343).

New Test Development

The purpose of reference methods for antimicrobial susceptibility testing is to encourage standardization of the process and improve reproducibility among laboratories; however, reference methods may not be ideal for individual clinical laboratories. Other methods currently used include a microdilution format read spectrophotometrically or colorimetrically (344–348).

In addition, novel breakpoint methods including culture on a porous aluminum oxide (PAO) support combined with microscopy (349) and flow cytometry (350,351) have been applied with varying degrees of success. The advent of whole-genome sequencing and rapidly decreasing costs for this method may in the future be the backbone behind susceptibility testing; however, the molecular changes responsible for phenotypic resistance in yeasts/molds remain incompletely defined and substantial work is needed in this area before genetic sequencing will replace in vitro susceptibility testing.

The utilization of colorimetric growth indicators has been applied to the microdilution method in an effort to provide improved ease and precision of MIC end point determination and possibly provide a more rapid means of testing clinically important fungi. Colorimetric determination of residual glucose (352,353), pH indicator dyes (354), and various tetrazolium salt methods (355,356) have all shown promise and are currently used in the Vitek 2 system employed in a large number of clinical laboratories (357–359). The use of the oxidation reduction indicator alamarBlue (AccuMed International Inc, Chicago, IL) is one of the best studied and most widely used approaches (360–362). In broth media, fungal growth causes the alamarBlue indicator to change from blue to pink. In an alamarBlue-containing system, the MIC for an antifungal agent is recorded as the first well to show a change from pink (growth) to purple or blue (growth inhibition). The alamarBlue indicator has been incorporated into a commercially available broth microdilution system, the Sensititre YeastOne colormetric antifungal plate (TREK Diagnostics Systems, Westlake, OH). The YeastOne system has been shown to perform comparably to the CLSI reference method (362–364) and is approved by the U.S. Food and Drug Administration for in vitro susceptibility testing of yeasts.

The use of spectrophotometry has long been employed to measure the growth of microbes in a broth system. Spectrophotometric determination of fungal growth in the presence and absence of antifungal agents has been utilized to provide a more precise and objective means of MIC end point reading, especially for the azole class of antifungal agents (348,365,366).

In many clinical settings, determination of precise MICs using a full-range dilution series is not necessary. Testing of the clinical isolate against one or two antimicrobial drug concentrations that distinguish susceptible from resistant strains, so-called "breakpoint testing," is often all that is necessary to allow the selection of optimal antifungal therapy (367). The agar-based methods for antifungal susceptibility testing include the previously mentioned disk diffusion method (NCCLS M44), the Etest stable agar gradient method (368–373), and the semisolid agar dilution method (374). The Etest method (AB Biodisk, Solna, Sweden) has been widely employed as a means of producing an accurate, reproducible, and quantitative MIC result using an agar diffusion format (369). This method is based on the diffusion of a continuous concentration gradient of an antimicrobial agent from a plastic strip into an agar medium. When an Etest strip is placed on an agar plate inoculated with a test organism and incubated for 24 to 48 hours, an ellipse of growth inhibition occurs and the intersection of the ellipse with the numeric scale on the strip allows the reading of the MIC. This test method has been extensively studied for utilization in antibacterial testing and is comparable with the reference broth and agar dilution MIC methods. The Etest is also applicable to antifungal susceptibility testing. Numerous studies demonstrate the usefulness of Etest for determining the in vitro susceptibility of both yeasts and molds to a variety of antifungal agents including AmB, 5-FC, ketoconazole, itraconazole, voriconazole, posaconazole, and caspofungin. MICs determined by Etest generally agree quite

well with those determined by the NCCLS reference method (312); however, this agreement may vary, depending on the antifungal agent tested, the choice of agar medium, and the organism species (372). The use of RPMI agar supplemented with 2% glucose works well for most organisms and antifungal agents, yet decreased agreement has been reported for fluconazole and itraconazole tested against *Candida glabrata* and *Candida tropicalis* (330,375). The use of Mueller-Hinton agar supplemented with glucose and methylene blue has been shown to improve the overall agreement of Etest MICs with the reference method when testing *Candida glabrata* against fluconazole and voriconazole (375). Of major importance is the fact that Etest is the most sensitive and reliable method for detecting decreased susceptibility to AmB among isolates of *Candida* spp and *Cryptococcus neoformans* (376–379).

A semisolid agar dilution method was proposed by Provine and Hadley (374) to serve as a rapid, breakpoint screening test to detect isolates of *Candida* spp with decreased susceptibility to fluconazole. The method employs heart infusion broth with 0.5% agar and without glucose. The organism is inoculated into the system by stabbing the agar and the resulting conditions are considered to mimic more closely the growth conditions of infected tissue (374). This simple method provides good categorical agreement with the M27 reference method, although the number of isolates tested to date is limited.

Flow cytometric methods have been employed with good success in testing *Candida* spp against fluconazole and AmB (351,380). This approach uses a standard flow cytometer and fluorescent DNA binding dyes to detect fungal cell damage following exposure to an antifungal agent. The method produces results within 6 hours that agree very well with MICs determined by the M27 reference method.

Surveillance and New Drug Evaluation

One of the important offshoots of the standardization process has been the ability to conduct active surveillance of resistance to antifungal agents (187,216). Meaningful large-scale studies of antifungal susceptibility and resistance conducted over time would not be possible without a standardized microdilution method for performing the in vitro studies and several such studies have now been published. Furthermore, studies analyzing resistance trends to commonly utilized antifungal agents and comparative analyses of licensed and established antifungal agents have provided large amounts of useful data and have been greatly facilitated by a standardized microdilution method. As new antifungal agents are evaluated in clinical trials, in vitro susceptibility testing of clinical isolates utilizing a reference method will be essential and allow further establishment of in vitro/in vivo correlations.

Proficiency Testing

The participation of clinical laboratories in proficiency testing programs is considered an important step in ensuring quality and standardization in the performance of antimicrobial susceptibility testing (381). Prior to the publication of NCCLS document M27-A, little was known of the proficiency of clinical laboratories in performing antifungal susceptibility testing aside from those laboratories actively engaged in NCCLS-conducted studies. Following the publication in 1997 of the NCCLS M27-A reference method for testing yeasts, the College of American Pathologists initiated a proficiency-testing program for antifungal susceptibility testing, and following this, the number of participants has continued to increase and laboratory performance has steadily improved (382). This program provides important information regarding the performance of antifungal susceptibility testing in the United States and indicates a level of performance that is on par with that of antibacterial testing.

Global Standardization

Subsequent to the development of the NCCLS M27-A method for broth microdilution testing of yeasts, a similar method has been developed under the auspices of the Subcommittee on Antifungal Susceptibility Testing (AFST) of the European Committee on Antibiotic Susceptibility Testing (EUCAST) and periodically updated with technical notes on specific antifungal compounds (383–388). This method is very similar to the NCCLS M27-A2 method and employs a higher inoculum (10^5 CFU/mL), RPMI 1640 medium supplemented with additional glucose (2%), and spectrophotometric readings of MIC end points following incubation at 35°C to 37°C for 24 hours (389). The efforts of the EUCAST-AFST subcommittee have stimulated a collaboration with the CLSI subcommittee and recent multicenter studies have documented good intralaboratory reproducibility of the EUCAST method (390) and good agreement between the EUCAST and CLSI microdilution methods (391). In addition, global surveillance programs such as the ARTEMIS global antifungal program for disk testing and MIC testing, the European Confederation of Medical Mycology survey of candidemia, and the SENTRY antifungal surveillance program promote the use of standardized disk and broth dilution MIC methods and provide useful and consistent antifungal susceptibility data from a broad network of hospitals and laboratories on an international scale.

Clinical Relevance of Antifungal Susceptibility Test Results

In order to be useful clinically, in vitro susceptibility testing of antimicrobial agents should reliably predict the in vivo response to therapy in human infections (Table 6.6). However, the in vitro susceptibility of an infecting organism to the antimicrobial agent is only one of several factors that may influence the likelihood that therapy for an infection will be successful (298). Factors related to the host immune response and/or the status of the current underlying disease, drug pharmacokinetics and pharmacodynamics, drug interactions, proper patient management, and factors related to the virulence of the infecting organism and its interaction with both the host and the antimicrobial agent administered all influence the outcome of treatment of an infectious episode (298,321). In order to appreciate the clinical value of antifungal susceptibility testing, one must understand that after more than 30 years of study, in vitro susceptibility testing can be said to predict the outcome of *bacterial* infections with an accuracy that has been summarized as the "90–60 rule" (298): infections due to susceptible isolates respond to therapy approximately 90% of the time, whereas infections due to resistant isolates respond approximately 60% of the time. There is now a considerable body of data indicating that standardized antifungal susceptibility testing (NCCLS M27-A3) for selected organism–drug combinations (most notably *Candida* spp and azole antifungal agents) provides results that have a predictive utility consistent with the 90–60 rule. The EUCAST breakpoints are significantly lower than those initially reported from the CLSI due in part to the fact that more cases of candidemia than OPC were used to calculate initial CLSI breakpoint values. Recent CLSI guidance more closely correlates with the EUCAST breakpoints. In addition, it is clear that breakpoints should ideally not cross the breakpoint

Table 6.6

Recommendations for Studies of Fungal Isolates in the Clinical Laboratory

Clinical Setting	Recommendation
Routine	• Species level identification of all *Candida* isolates from deep sites (e.g., blood, normally sterile fluids, tissues, abscesses) • Species level identification of *Aspergillus*, genus level for all other molds • Routine antifungal testing of fluconazole against *Candida glabrata* isolated from deep sites (with correlation seen for other azole antifungals) • Routine testing of fluconazole and flucytosine against other species of *Candida* may be helpful but susceptibility usually predictable
Oropharyngeal candidiasis	• Determination of susceptibility not routinely necessary • Susceptibility testing may be useful for patients unresponsive to azole therapy
Invasive disease with clinical failure of initial therapy	• Consider susceptibility testing as an adjunct *Candida* spp and amphotericin B, flucytosine, fluconazole, voriconazole, caspofungin *Cryptococcus neoformans* and fluconazole, flucytosine, or amphotericin B *Histoplasma capsulatum* and fluconazole • Consultation with an experienced microbiologist recommended
Infection with species with high rates of intrinsic or acquired resistance	• Susceptibility testing not necessary when intrinsic resistance is known *Candida krusei* and fluconazole *Aspergillus terreus* and amphotericin B Select therapy based on literature • When high rates of acquired resistance, monitor closely for signs of failure and perform susceptibility testing *C. glabrata* and fluconazole, AmB, or echinocandins *C. krusei* and amphotericin B *Candida lusitaniae* and amphotericin B *Candida* spp and flucytosine
New treatment options (e.g., caspofungin, voriconazole) or unusual organisms	• Select therapy based on published consensus guidelines and review of survey data on the organism–drug combination in question • Susceptibility testing may be helpful when patient is not responding to what should effective therapy
Patients who respond to therapy despite being infected with an organism later found to be resistant	• Best approach not clear • Take into account severity of infection, patient immune status, consequences of recurrent infection, etc. • Consider alternative therapy for infections with isolates that appear to be highly resistant to therapy selected
Mold infections	• Susceptibility testing not recommended as a routine • Interpretive criteria have not been established for any agents • Identification to genus and species desirable
Selection of susceptibility testing methods	• Standardized methods • NCCLS broth-based methods Yeasts; M27-S4 Molds; M38-A • CLSI agar-based methods Disk diffusion; yeasts M44-A • EUCAST broth-based method Yeasts • Other Etest, numerous agents, yeasts, and molds

NCCLS, National Committee for Clinical Laboratory Standards; CLSI, Clinical and Laboratory Standards Institute; EUCAST, European Committee for Antimicrobial Susceptibility Testing.

for a wild-type population (i.e., the epidemiologic cutoff value or ECV) of a species. Theoretically, the ECV establishes the 95% breakpoint where isolates in a given species will not exhibit any resistance mechanisms and thus be more likely to be nonresponders in a clinical setting (392). Thus, the most recent CLSI breakpoint guidance establishes breakpoints for individual *Candida* species for both azoles (fluconazole and voriconazole) and the echinocandins (anidulafungin, caspofungin, and micafungin). In most cases, these breakpoints are significantly lower than those recommended in early documents and are based on predicted pharmacokinetic/pharmacodynamic parameters of the agents, wild-type distributions of the MICs and clinical/in vivo responses to the agents.

Of note in the new CLSI breakpoints are changes in *C. glabrata* susceptibility. Due to the wide distribution of wild-type *C. glabrata* MICs against both voriconazole and fluconazole and the potential for clinical resistance, breakpoints for fully susceptible *C. glabrata* have been eliminated for those agents. Fluconazole is reported as S-DD at an MIC of 32 or less and resistance at 64 or greater, whereas no susceptibility for voriconazole is recommended. Similarly, the breakpoints for full echinocandin susceptibility against *C. glabrata* for micafungin is now 0.06 µg/mL and for caspofungin/anidulafungin 0.12 µg/mL (due to differences in protein binding), with the recognition that isolates with higher MICs have a significant likelihood of harboring hot spot mutations in the target *FSK1/2* genes.

Antifungal susceptibility testing is now increasingly and appropriately utilized as a routine adjunct to the treatment of fungal infections and guidelines for the utilization of antifungal testing, and other laboratory studies, have been developed (298). Selective application of antifungal susceptibility testing, coupled with broader identification of fungi to the species level, has proven useful especially in difficult-to-manage fungal infections. Future efforts will be dedicated to the further validation of interpretive breakpoints for established antifungal agents and developing them for newly introduced systemically active agents. In addition, procedures must be further refined for testing non-*Candida* yeasts (e.g., *Trichosporon* spp) and molds.

QUANTITATION OF ANTIFUNGAL AGENTS IN BIOLOGIC FLUIDS

The determination of antifungal drug concentrations in serum, CSF, and other body fluids may provide clinicians with information that can be maximized to increase the probability of favorable patient outcomes. Numerous methods are available to determine drug levels in body fluids including microbiologic bioassay, gas–liquid chromatography, HPLC, UPLC/MS, fluorometry, spectrophotometry, thin-layer chromatography, and others. Physicochemical assay methods are more sensitive, specific, rapid, and less labor-intensive than bioassay methods. They are also capable of separating the parent compound from a biologically active metabolite, whereas bioassays are typically unable to do this (393–395).

Bioassay methods are available for several of the systemically active antifungal agents. Bioassays have some advantages over physicochemical assays in that they do not require initial extraction steps or specialized instrumentation. In addition, bioassays evaluate the biologic activity of the antifungal agent, as well as any active metabolites, in the body fluid, whereas physiochemical determinations do not necessarily indicate biologically active drugs (343,393). The easiest and most practical bioassays to perform in the clinical laboratory are agar diffusion assays. AmB levels in body fluids are often determined by using an agar diffusion bioassay method. Briefly, molten agar is seeded with a standardized suspension of *P. variotii* (ATCC 36257), poured into 150-mL Petri dishes, and allowed to solidify on a level surface. Known concentrations of the antifungal agent to be tested, as well as the patient's serum, are placed into wells cut from the agar and allowed to diffuse into the medium. The plates are incubated at 30°C for 24 to 48 hours, and the zones of inhibition around the reservoirs are measured to the nearest millimeter. A standard curve is plotted on semilogarithmic paper using the known concentrations of the drug and the corresponding zones of inhibition. Once the standard curve has been constructed, the drug levels in the patient's body fluid may be determined by plotting the zone of inhibition on the standard curve. To ensure intralaboratory reproducibility, internal standards of known concentrations should be included with each assay.

AmB concentrations may be determined in the presence of 5-FC by substituting a 5-FC–resistant strain of *Chrysosporium pruinosum* (ATCC 36374) for *P. variotii*. The medium may also be supplemented with the 5-FC antagonist cytosine (10 µg/mL). These measures prevent the 5-FC from interfering with the determination of the AmB concentration.

5-FC concentrations in body fluids are determined in the same manner as those of AmB except that *Saccharomyces cerevisiae* (ATCC 36375) is substituted for *P. variotii* and yeast morphology agar is used instead of antibiotic medium 12. To assay for 5-FC in the presence of AmB, the latter is inactivated by heating the sample for 30 minutes at 90°C. Once the serum has been heated and the AmB inactivated, the sample may be assayed to determine the concentration of 5-FC present.

Microbiologic bioassays are also available to determine the concentrations of itraconazole, posaconazole, voriconazole, and the echinocandins in serum, plasma, or CSF (396). Importantly, the bioassay for itraconazole reflects the activity of both itraconazole and the hydroxylated metabolite, hydroxyitraconazole (393). The antifungal activity of these metabolites is unclear with a *Candida kefyr* isolate demonstrating twofold less activity of itraconazole than to hydroxyitraconazole (393), whereas other studies have shown a twofold difference in the opposite direction with itraconazole more active than hydroxyitraconazole (differences of only two dilutions fall well within the range of normal replicate variability) (397,398).

These findings have obvious implications in the interpretation of bioassay results for itraconazole and will be highly discrepant when compared with itraconazole concentrations determined by physiochemical methods unless the physiochemical determination of hydroxyitraconazole is also taken into account such as with UPLC/MS (396). In contrast, metabolism of voriconazole results in inactive metabolites and an excellent correlation between bioassay

and HPLC determinations of voriconazole and posaconazole in serum has been reported (394,399).

CONCLUSION

In response to the challenge of invasive mycoses and the development of resistance by several of the non-albicans *Candida* species, the number of systemically active agents has increased over the past several years. As a result of this challenge, greater understanding of the mechanism of action of these agents as well as the capability of fungal pathogens to demonstrate resistance is needed. Antifungal susceptibility testing has undergone continued standardized refinement; it is generally considered to play a significant role in the clinical management of invasive mycoses. Guidelines for the role of antifungal susceptibility testing have been clearly codified and structured. Although significant progress has been made in these areas, additional efforts are needed to optimize testing methods for newly developed antifungal compounds and for testing pathogens other than *Candida*. Ongoing national and international investigations and collaborations targeted to address these several issues will serve to refine and improve the management of invasive fungal infections.

ACKNOWLEDGEMENTS

The authors thank Drs. Michael Pfaller, Daniel J. Diekema, and Michael G. Rinaldi for the content of this chapter's previous edition, which has been included in part within this update.

REFERENCES

1. Thompson GR 3rd, Cadena J, Patterson TF. Overview of antifungal agents. *Clin Chest Med* 2009;30(2):203–215, v.
2. Ellis D. Amphotericin B: spectrum and resistance. *J Antimicrob Chemother* 2002;49(Suppl 1):7–10.
3. Amphotericin B [package insert]. Big Flats, NY: X-Gen Pharmaceuticals; 2009.
4. Ben-Ami R, Lewis RE, Kontoyiannis DP. Immunocompromised hosts: immunopharmacology of modern antifungals. *Clin Infect Dis* 2008;47(2):226–235.
5. Bellocchio S, Gaziano R, Bozza S, et al. Liposomal amphotericin B activates antifungal resistance with reduced toxicity by diverting toll-like receptor signalling from TLR-2 to TLR-4. *J Antimicrob Chemother* 2005;55(2):214–222.
6. Steinbach WJ, Benjamin DK Jr, Kontoyiannis DP, et al. Infections due to *Aspergillus terreus*: a multicenter retrospective analysis of 83 cases. *Clin Infect Dis* 2004;39(2):192–198.
7. Nucci M, Anaissie E. Fusarium infections in immunocompromised patients. *Clin Microbiol Rev* 2007;20(4):695–704.
8. Meletiadis J, Meis JF, Mouton JW, et al. In vitro activities of new and conventional antifungal agents against clinical *Scedosporium* isolates. *Antimicrob Agents Chemother* 2002;46(1):62–68.
9. Kontoyiannis DP, Lewis RE. Antifungal drug resistance of pathogenic fungi. *Lancet* 2002;359(9312):1135–1144.
10. Blum G, Perkhofer S, Haas H, et al. Potential basis for amphotericin B resistance in *Aspergillus terreus*. *Antimicrob Agents Chemother* 2008;52(4):1553–1555.
11. White MH, Anaissie EJ, Kusne S, et al. Amphotericin B colloidal dispersion vs. amphotericin B as therapy for invasive aspergillosis. *Clin Infect Dis* 1997;24(4):635–642.
12. Mistro S, Maciel Ide M, de Menezes RG, et al. Does lipid emulsion reduce amphotericin B nephrotoxicity?

A systematic review and meta-analysis. *Clin Infect Dis* 2012;54(12):1774–1777.

13. Collette N, van der Auwera P, Lopez AP, et al. Tissue concentrations and bioactivity of amphotericin B in cancer patients treated with amphotericin B-deoxycholate. *Antimicrob Agents Chemother* 1989;33(3):362–368.

14. Perfect JR, Dismukes WE, Dromer F, et al. Clinical practice guidelines for the management of cryptococcal disease: 2010 update by the Infectious Diseases Society of America. *Clin Infect Dis* 2010;50(3):291–322.

15. Stevens DA, Shatsky SA. Intrathecal amphotericin in the management of coccidioidal meningitis. *Semin Respir Infect* 2001;16(4):263–269.

16. Bekersky I, Fielding RM, Dressler DE, et al. Pharmacokinetics, excretion, and mass balance of liposomal amphotericin B (AmBisome) and amphotericin B deoxycholate in humans. *Antimicrob Agents Chemother* 2002;46(3):828–833.

17. Wiederhold NP, Tam VH, Chi J, et al. Pharmacodynamic activity of amphotericin B deoxycholate is associated with peak plasma concentrations in a neutropenic murine model of invasive pulmonary aspergillosis. *Antimicrob Agents Chemother* 2006;50(2):469–473.

18. Andes D. In vivo pharmacodynamics of antifungal drugs in treatment of candidiasis. *Antimicrob Agents Chemother* 2003;47(4):1179–1186.

19. Saag MS, Graybill RJ, Larsen RA, et al. Practice guidelines for the management of cryptococcal disease. Infectious Diseases Society of America. *Clin Infect Dis* 2000;30(4):710–718.

20. Dodds Ashley ES, Lewis R, Lewis JS, et al. Pharmacology of systemic antifungal agents. *Clin Infect Dis* 2006;43(Suppl 1):S28–S39.

21. Pappas PG, Rex JH, Sobel JD, et al. Guidelines for treatment of candidiasis. *Clin Infect Dis* 2004;38(2):161–189.

22. Rex JH, Bennett JE, Sugar AM, et al. A randomized trial comparing fluconazole with amphotericin B for the treatment of candidemia in patients without neutropenia. Candidemia Study Group and the National Institute. *N Engl J Med* 1994;331(20):1325–1330.

23. Herbrecht R, Denning DW, Patterson TF, et al. Voriconazole versus amphotericin B for primary therapy of invasive aspergillosis. *N Engl J Med* 2002;347(6):408–415.

24. Freifeld AG, Bow EJ, Sepkowitz KA, et al. Clinical practice guideline for the use of antimicrobial agents in neutropenic patients with cancer: 2010 update by the Infectious Diseases Society of America. *Clin Infect Dis* 2011;52(4):427–431.

25. Johnson PC, Wheat LJ, Cloud GA, et al. Safety and efficacy of liposomal amphotericin B compared with conventional amphotericin B for induction therapy of histoplasmosis in patients with AIDS. *Ann Intern Med* 2002;137(2):105–109.

26. Sun HY, Alexander BD, Lortholary O, et al. Lipid formulations of amphotericin B significantly improve outcome in solid organ transplant recipients with central nervous system cryptococcosis. *Clin Infect Dis* 2009;49(11):1721–1728.

27. Walsh TJ, Anaissie EJ, Denning DW, et al. Treatment of aspergillosis: clinical practice guidelines of the Infectious Diseases Society of America. *Clin Infect Dis* 2008;46(3):327–360.

28. Chamilos G, Lewis RE, Kontoyiannis DP. Delaying amphotericin B-based frontline therapy significantly increases mortality among patients with hematologic malignancy who have zygomycosis. *Clin Infect Dis* 2008;47(4):503–509.

29. Borro JM, Sole A, de la Torre M, et al. Efficiency and safety of inhaled amphotericin B lipid complex (abelcet) in the prophylaxis of invasive fungal infections following lung transplantation. *Transplant Proc* 2008;40(9):3090–3093.

30. Slobbe L, Boersma E, Rijnders BJ. Tolerability of prophylactic aerosolized liposomal amphotericin-B and impact on pulmonary function: data from a randomized placebo-controlled trial. *Pulm Pharmacol Ther* 2008;21(6):855–859.

31. Rijnders BJ, Cornelissen JJ, Slobbe L, et al. Aerosolized liposomal amphotericin B for the prevention of invasive pulmonary aspergillosis during prolonged neutropenia: a randomized, placebo-controlled trial. *Clin Infect Dis* 2008;46(9):1401–1408.

32. Mora-Duarte J, Betts R, Rotstein C, et al. Comparison of caspofungin and amphotericin B for invasive candidiasis. *N Engl J Med* 2002;347(25):2020–2029.

33. Saliba F, Dupont B. Renal impairment and amphotericin B formulations in patients with invasive fungal infections. *Med Mycol* 2008;46(2):97–112.

34. Kleinberg M. What is the current and future status of conventional amphotericin B? *Int J Antimicrob Agents* 2006;27(Suppl 1):12–16.

35. Johnson EM, Szekely A, Warnock DW. In-vitro activity of voriconazole, itraconazole and amphotericin B against filamentous fungi. *J Antimicrob Chemother* 1998;42(6):741–745.

36. Hope WW, Billaud EM, Lestner J, et al. Therapeutic drug monitoring for triazoles. *Curr Opin Infect Dis* 2008;21(6):580–586.

37. Shimokawa O, Nakayama H. Increased sensitivity of *Candida albicans* cells accumulating 14 alpha-methylated sterols to active oxygen: possible relevance to in vivo efficacies of azole antifungal agents. *Antimicrob Agents Chemother* 1992;36(8):1626–1629.

38. Fluconazole [package insert]. New York: Pfizer Laboratories; 2004.

39. Itraconazole [package insert]. (Sempera) product monograph. Neuss, Germany: Janssen-Cilag GmbH; 2003.

40. Posaconazole [package insert]. Kenilworth, NJ: Schering Corporation; 2006.

41. Voriconazole [package insert]. New York: Pfizer Inc; 2002.

42. Gubbins PO, Heldenbrand S. Clinically relevant drug interactions of current antifungal agents. *Mycoses* 2010;53(2):95–113.

43. Kramer MR, Marshall SE, Denning DW, et al. Cyclosporine and itraconazole interaction in heart and lung transplant recipients. *Ann Intern Med* 1990;113(4):327–329.

44. Varis T, Kaukonen KM, Kivisto KT, et al. Plasma concentrations and effects of oral methylprednisolone are considerably increased by itraconazole. *Clin Pharmacol Ther* 1998;64(4):363–368.

45. Tucker RM, Denning DW, Hanson LH, et al. Interaction of azoles with rifampin, phenytoin, and carbamazepine: in vitro and clinical observations. *Clin Infect Dis* 1992;14(1):165–174.

46. Kivisto KT, Lamberg TS, Kantola T, et al. Plasma buspirone concentrations are greatly increased by erythromycin and itraconazole. *Clin Pharmacol Ther* 1997;62(3):348–354.

47. Engels FK, Ten Tije AJ, Baker SD, et al. Effect of cytochrome P450 3A4 inhibition on the pharmacokinetics of docetaxel. *Clin Pharmacol Ther* 2004;75(5):448–454.

48. Grub S, Bryson H, Goggin T, et al. The interaction of saquinavir (soft gelatin capsule) with ketoconazole, erythromycin and rifampicin: comparison of the effect in healthy volunteers and in HIV-infected patients. *Eur J Clin Pharmacol* 2001;57(2):115–121.

49. Jeng MR, Feusner J. Itraconazole-enhanced vincristine neurotoxicity in a child with acute lymphoblastic leukemia. *Pediatr Hematol Oncol* 2001;18(2):137–142.
50. Itraconazole [package insert]. (Sempera) product monograph. Neuss, Germany: Janssen-Cilag GmbH; 2003.
51. Kaukonen KM, Olkkola KT, Neuvonen PJ. Itraconazole increases plasma concentrations of quinidine. *Clin Pharmacol Ther* 1997;62(5):510–517.
52. Lefebvre RA, Van Peer A, Woestenborghs R. Influence of itraconazole on the pharmacokinetics and electrocardiographic effects of astemizole. *Br J Clin Pharmacol* 1997;43(3):319–322.
53. Honig PK, Wortham DC, Hull R, et al. Itraconazole affects single-dose terfenadine pharmacokinetics and cardiac repolarization pharmacodynamics. *J Clin Pharmacol* 1993;33(12):1201–1206.
54. Posaconazole [package insert]. Kenilworth, NJ: Schering Corporation; 2006.
55. Voriconazole (V-fend) [package insert]. Summary of Product Characteristics SAahemou.
56. DeMuria D, Forrest A, Rich J, et al. Pharmacokinetics and bioavailability of fluconazole in patients with AIDS. *Antimicrob Agents Chemother* 1993;37(10):2187–2192.
57. Blum RA, D'Andrea DT, Florentino BM, et al. Increased gastric pH and the bioavailability of fluconazole and ketoconazole. *Ann Intern Med* 1991;1149(9):755.
58. Arndt CA, Walsh TJ, McCully CL, et al. Fluconazole penetration into cerebrospinal fluid: implications for treating fungal infections of the central nervous system. *J Infect Dis* 1988;157(1):178–180.
59. Savani DV, Perfect JR, Cobo LM, et al. Penetration of new azole compounds into the eye and efficacy in experimental *Candida* endophthalmitis. *Antimicrob Agents Chemother* 1987;31(1):6–10.
60. Andes D, van Ogtrop M. Characterization and quantitation of the pharmacodynamics of fluconazole in a neutropenic murine disseminated candidiasis infection model. *Antimicrob Agents Chemother* 1999;43(9):2116–2120.
61. Klepser ME, Wolfe EJ, Pfaller MA. Antifungal pharmacodynamic characteristics of fluconazole and amphotericin B against *Cryptococcus neoformans*. *J Antimicrob Chemother* 1998;41(3):397–401.
62. Louie A, Drusano GL, Banerjee P, et al. Pharmacodynamics of fluconazole in a murine model of systemic candidiasis. *Antimicrob Agents Chemother* 1998;42(5):1105–1109.
63. Orozco AS, Higginbotham LM, Hitchcock CA, et al. Mechanism of fluconazole resistance in *Candida krusei*. *Antimicrob Agents Chemother* 1998;42(10):2645–2649.
64. Baddley JW, Patel M, Bhavnani SM, et al. Association of fluconazole pharmacodynamics with mortality in patients with candidemia. *Antimicrob Agents Chemother* 2008;52(9):3022–3028.
65. Lortholary O, Denning DW, Dupont B. Endemic mycoses: a treatment update. *J Antimicrob Chemother* 1999;43(3):321–331.
66. Zonios DI, Bennett JE. Update on azole antifungals. *Semin Respir Crit Care* 2008;29(2):198–210.
67. Wheat J, Marichal P, Vanden Bossche H, et al. Hypothesis on the mechanism of resistance to fluconazole in *Histoplasma capsulatum*. *Antimicrob Agents Chemother* 1997;41(2):410–414.
68. Perea S, Patterson TF. Antifungal resistance in pathogenic fungi. *Clin Infect Dis* 2002;35(9):1073–1080.
69. Pappas PG, Kauffman CA, Andes D, et al. Clinical practice guidelines for the management of candidiasis: 2009 update by the Infectious Diseases Society of America. *Clin Infect Dis* 2009;48(5):503–535.
70. Galgiani JN, Ampel NM, Blair JE, et al. Coccidioidomycosis. *Clin Infect Dis* 2005;41(9):1217–1223.
71. Hamza OJ, Matee MI, Bruggemann RJ, et al. Single-dose fluconazole versus standard 2-week therapy for oropharyngeal candidiasis in HIV-infected patients: a randomized, double-blind, double-dummy trial. *Clin Infect Dis* 2008;47(10):1270–1276.
72. Saag MS, Cloud GA, Graybill JR, et al. A comparison of itraconazole versus fluconazole as maintenance therapy for AIDS-associated cryptococcal meningitis. National Institute of Allergy and Infectious Diseases Mycoses Study Group. *Clin Infect Dis* 1999;28(2):291–296.
73. Longley N, Muzoora C, Taseera K, et al. Dose response effect of high-dose fluconazole for HIV-associated cryptococcal meningitis in southwestern Uganda. *Clin Infect Dis* 2008;47(12):1556–1561.
74. Johnson RH, Einstein HE. Coccidioidal meningitis. *Clin Infect Dis* 2006;42(1):103–107.
75. Wheat LJ, Freifeld AG, Kleiman MB, et al. Clinical practice guidelines for the management of patients with histoplasmosis: 2007 update by the Infectious Diseases Society of America. *Clin Infect Dis* 2007;45(7):807–825.
76. Kauffman CA, Bustamante B, Chapman SW, et al. Clinical practice guidelines for the management of sporotrichosis: 2007 update by the Infectious Diseases Society of America. *Clin Infect Dis* 2007;45(10):1255–1265.
77. Slavin MA, Osborne B, Adams R, et al. Efficacy and safety of fluconazole prophylaxis for fungal infections after marrow transplantation—a prospective, randomized, double-blind study. *J Infect Dis* 1995;171(6):1545–1552.
78. Schuster MG, Edwards JE Jr, Sobel JD, et al. Empirical fluconazole versus placebo for intensive care unit patients: a randomized trial. *Ann Intern Med* 2008;149(2):83–90.
79. Stevens DA, Diaz M, Negroni R, et al. Safety evaluation of chronic fluconazole therapy. Fluconazole Pan-American Study Group. *Chemotherapy* 1997;43(5):371–377.
80. Dodds Ashley ES, Lewis R, Lewis JS, et al. Pharmacology of systemic antifungal agents. *Clin Infect Dis* 2006;43(Suppl 1):S28–S39.
81. Miyama T, Takanaga H, Matsuo H, et al. P-glycoprotein-mediated transport of itraconazole across the blood-brain barrier. *Antimicrob Agents Chemother* 1998;42(7):1738–1744.
82. Sheehan DJ, Hitchcock CA, Sibley CM. Current and emerging azole antifungal agents. *Clin Microbiol Rev* 1999;12(1):40–79.
83. Groll AH, Kolve H. Antifungal agents: in vitro susceptibility testing, pharmacodynamics, and prospects for combination therapy. *Eur J Clin Microbiol Infect Dis* 2004;23(4):256–270.
84. Manavathu EK, Cutright JL, Chandrasekar PH. Organism-dependent fungicidal activities of azoles. *Antimicrob Agents Chemother* 1998;42(11):3018–3021.
85. Verweij PE, Mellado E, Melchers WJ. Multiple-triazole-resistant aspergillosis. *N Engl J Med* 2007;356(14):1481–1483.
86. Verweij PE, Voss A, Meis JF. Resistance of *Aspergillus fumigatus* to itraconazole. *Scand J Infect Dis* 1998;30(6):642–643.
87. Barone JA, Moskovitz BL, Guarnieri J, et al. Enhanced bioavailability of itraconazole in hydroxypropyl-beta-cyclodextrin versus capsules in healthy volunteers. *Antimicrob Agents Chemother* 1998;42(7):1862–1865.
88. Van de Velde VJ, Van Peer AP, Heykants JJ, et al. Effect of food on the pharmacokinetics of a new hydroxypropyl-beta-cyclodextrin formulation of itraconazole. *Pharmacology* 1996;16(3):424–428.

89. Stevens DA. Itraconazole in cyclodextrin solution. *Pharmacotherapy* 1999;19(5):603–611.

90. Como JA, Dismukes WE. Oral azole drugs as systemic antifungal therapy. *N Engl J Med* 1994;330(4):263–272.

91. Warnock DW, Turner A, Burke J. Comparison of high performance liquid chromatographic and microbiological methods for determination of itraconazole. *J Antimicrob Chemother* 1988;21(1):93–100.

92. Limper AH, Knox KS, Sarosi GA, et al. An official American Thoracic Society statement: treatment of fungal infections in adult pulmonary and critical care patients. *Am J Respir Crit Care Med* 2011;183(1):96–128.

93. Chapman SW, Dismukes WE, Proia LA, et al. Clinical practice guidelines for the management of blastomycosis: 2008 update by the Infectious Diseases Society of America. *Clin Infect Dis* 2008;46(12):1801–1812.

94. Restrepo A, Benard G, de Castro CC, et al. Pulmonary paracoccidioidomycosis. *Semin Respir Crit Care Med* 2008; 29(2):182–197.

95. Galgiani JN, Catanzaro A, Cloud GA, et al. Comparison of oral fluconazole and itraconazole for progressive, nonmeningeal coccidioidomycosis. A randomized, double-blind trial. Mycoses Study Group. *Ann Intern Med* 2000; 133(9):676–686.

96. Revankar SG. Phaeohyphomycosis. *Infect Dis Clin North Am* 2006;20(3):609–620.

97. De Beule K, Van Gestel J. Pharmacology of itraconazole. *Drugs* 2001;61(Suppl 1):27–37.

98. Sharkey PK, Rinaldi MG, Dunn JF, et al. High-dose itraconazole in the treatment of severe mycoses. *Antimicrob Agents Chemother* 1991;35(4):707–713.

99. Tucker RM, Haq Y, Denning DW, et al. Adverse events associated with itraconazole in 189 patients on chronic therapy. *J Antimicrob Chemother* 1990;26(4):561–566.

100. Glasmacher A, Hahn C, Molitor E, et al. Itraconazole through concentrations in antifungal prophylaxis with six different dosing regimens using hydroxypropyl-beta-cyclodextrin oral solution or coated-pellet capsules. *Mycoses* 1999;42(11–12):591–600.

101. Ahmad SR, Singer SJ, Leissa BG. Congestive heart failure associated with itraconazole. *Lancet* 2001;357(9270): 1766–1767.

102. Manavathu EK, Cutright JL, Loebenberg D, et al. A comparative study of the in vitro susceptibilities of clinical and laboratory-selected resistant isolates of *Aspergillus* spp. to amphotericin B, itraconazole, voriconazole and posaconazole (SCH 56592). *J Antimicrob Chemother* 2000;46(2):229–234.

103. Nagappan V, Deresinski S. Reviews of anti-infective agents: posaconazole: a broad-spectrum triazole antifungal agent. *Clin Infect Dis* 2007;45(12):1610–1617.

104. Courtney R, Wexler D, Radwanski E, et al. Effect of food on the relative bioavailability of two oral formulations of posaconazole in healthy adults. *Br J Clin Pharmacol* 2004;57(2):218–222.

105. Ezzet F, Wexler D, Courtney R, et al. Oral bioavailability of posaconazole in fasted healthy subjects: comparison between three regimens and basis for clinical dosage recommendations. *Clin Pharmacokinet* 2005;44(2):211–220.

106. Jain R, Pottinger P. The effect of gastric acid on the absorption of posaconazole. *Clin Infect Dis* 2008;46(10): 1627; author reply 1627–1628.

107. Krishna G, Ma L, Malavade D, et al. Effect of gastric pH, dosing regimen and prandial state, food and meal timing relative to dose, and gastrointestinal motility on absorption and pharmacokinetics of the antifungal posaconazole. In: 18th European Congress of Clinical

Microbiology and Infectious Diseases; March. Barcelona, Spain. 2008:P1264.

108. Courtney R, Pai S, Laughlin M, et al. Pharmacokinetics, safety, and tolerability of oral posaconazole administered in single and multiple doses in healthy adults. *Antimicrob Agents Chemother* 2003;47(9):2788–2795.

109. Sansone-Parsons A, Krishna G, Calzetta A, et al. Effect of a nutritional supplement on posaconazole pharmacokinetics following oral administration to healthy volunteers. *Antimicrob Agents Chemother* 2006;50(5): 1881–1883.

110. Meletiadis J, Chanock S, Walsh TJ. Human pharmacogenomic variations and their implications for antifungal efficacy. *Clin Microbiol Rev* 2006;19(4):763–787.

111. Cornely OA, Maertens J, Winston DJ, et al. Posaconazole vs. fluconazole or itraconazole prophylaxis in patients with neutropenia. *N Engl J Med* 2007;356(4): 348–359.

112. Ullmann AJ, Lipton JH, Vesole DH, et al. Posaconazole or fluconazole for prophylaxis in severe graft-versus-host disease. *N Engl J Med* 2007;356(4):335–347.

113. Walsh TJ, Raad I, Patterson TF, et al. Treatment of invasive aspergillosis with posaconazole in patients who are refractory to or intolerant of conventional therapy: an externally controlled trial. *Clin Infect Dis* 2007; 44(1):2–12.

114. Lehrnbecher T, Attarbaschi A, Duerken M, et al. Posaconazole salvage treatment in paediatric patients: a multicentre survey. *Eur J Clin Microbiol Infect Dis* 2010; 29(8):1043–1045.

115. Courtney R, Sansone A, Smith W, et al. Posaconazole pharmacokinetics, safety, and tolerability in subjects with varying degrees of chronic renal disease. *J Clin Pharmacol* 2005;45(2):185–192.

116. Raad II, Graybill JR, Bustamante AB, et al. Safety of long-term oral posaconazole use in the treatment of refractory invasive fungal infections. *Clin Infect Dis* 2006; 42(12):1726–1734.

117. Johnson LB, Kauffman CA. Voriconazole: a new triazole antifungal agent. *Clin Infect Dis* 2003;36(5): 630–637.

118. Purkins L, Wood N, Kleinermans D, et al. Effect of food on the pharmacokinetics of multiple-dose oral voriconazole. *Br J Clin Pharmacol* 2003;56(Suppl 1):17–23.

119. Thompson GR 3rd, Lewis JS 2nd. Pharmacology and clinical use of voriconazole. *Expert Opin Drug Metab Toxicol* 2010;6(1):83–94.

120. Purkins L, Wood N, Ghahramani P, et al. Pharmacokinetics and safety of voriconazole following intravenous-to oral-dose escalation regimens. *Antimicrob Agents Chemother* 2002;46(8):2546–2553.

121. Hariprasad SM, Mieler WF, Holz ER, et al. Determination of vitreous, aqueous, and plasma concentration of orally administered voriconazole in humans. *Arch Ophthalmol* 2004;122(1):42–47.

122. Nierenberg NE, Thompson GR, Lewis JS, et al. Voriconazole use and pharmacokinetics in combination with interferon-gamma for refractory cryptococcal meningitis in a patient receiving low-dose ritonavir. *Med Mycol* 2010;48(3):532–536.

123. Ikeda Y, Umemura K, Kondo K, et al. Pharmacokinetics of voriconazole and cytochrome P450 2C19 genetic status. *Clin Pharmacol Ther* 2004;75(6):587–588.

124. Klepser ME, Malone D, Lewis RE, et al. Evaluation of voriconazole pharmacodynamics using time-kill methodology. *Antimicrob Agents Chemother* 2000;44(7): 1917–1920.

125. Andes D, Marchillo K, Stamstad T, et al. In vivo pharmacokinetics and pharmacodynamics of a new triazole, voriconazole, in a murine candidiasis model. *Antimicrob Agents Chemother* 2003;47(10):3165–3169.

126. Krishnan S, Manavathu EK, Chandrasekar PH. A comparative study of fungicidal activities of voriconazole and amphotericin B against hyphae of *Aspergillus fumigatus*. *J Antimicrob Chemother* 2005;55(6):914–920.

127. Kirkpatrick WR, McAtee RK, Fothergill AW, et al. Efficacy of voriconazole in a guinea pig model of disseminated invasive aspergillosis. *Antimicrob Agents Chemother* 2000;44(10):2865–2868.

128. Nguyen MH, Yu CY. Voriconazole against fluconazole-susceptible and resistant *Candida* isolates: in-vitro efficacy compared with that of itraconazole and ketoconazole. *J Antimicrob Chemother* 1998;42(2):253–256.

129. Pfaller MA, Messer SA, Hollis RJ, et al. In vitro activities of ravuconazole and voriconazole compared with those of four approved systemic antifungal agents against 6,970 clinical isolates of *Candida* spp. *Antimicrob Agents Chemother* 2002;46(6):1723–1727.

130. Sutton DA, Sanche SE, Revankar SG, et al. In vitro amphotericin B resistance in clinical isolates of *Aspergillus terreus*, with a head-to-head comparison to voriconazole. *J Clin Microbiol* 1999;37(7):2343–2345.

131. Cuenca-Estrella M, Ruiz-Diez B, Martinez-Suarez JV, et al. Comparative in-vitro activity of voriconazole (UK-109,496) and six other antifungal agents against clinical isolates of *Scedosporium prolificans* and *Scedosporium apiospermum*. *J Antimicrob Chemother* 1999;43(1):149–151.

132. Lamaris GA, Ben-Ami R, Lewis RE, et al. Increased virulence of Zygomycetes organisms following exposure to voriconazole: a study involving fly and murine models of zygomycosis. *J Infect Dis* 2009;199(9):1399–1406.

133. Denning DW, Ribaud P, Milpied N, et al. Efficacy and safety of voriconazole in the treatment of acute invasive aspergillosis. *Clin Infect Dis* 2002;34(5):536–571.

134. Perfect JR, Marr KA, Walsh TJ, et al. Voriconazole treatment for less-common, emerging, or refractory fungal infections. *Clin Infect Dis* 2003;36(9):1122–1131.

135. Kullberg BJ, Sobel JD, Ruhnke M, et al. Voriconazole versus a regimen of amphotericin B followed by fluconazole for candidaemia in non-neutropenic patients: a randomised non-inferiority trial. *Lancet* 2005;366(9495):1435–1442.

136. Ally R, Schurmann D, Kreisel W, et al. A randomized, double-blind, double-dummy, multicenter trial of voriconazole and fluconazole in the treatment of esophageal candidiasis in immunocompromised patients. *Clin Infect Dis* 2001;33(9):1447–1454.

137. Walsh TJ, Pappas P, Winston DJ, et al. Voriconazole compared with liposomal amphotericin B for empirical antifungal therapy in patients with neutropenia and persistent fever. *N Engl J Med* 2002;346(4):225–234.

138. Kinoshita J, Iwata N, Ohba M, et al. Mechanism of voriconazole-induced transient visual disturbance: reversible dysfunction of retinal ON-bipolar cells in monkeys. *Invest Ophthalmol Vis Sci* 2011;52(8):5058–5063.

139. Scherpbier HJ, Hilhorst MI, Kuijpers TW. Liver failure in a child receiving highly active antiretroviral therapy and voriconazole. *Clin Infect Dis* 2003;37(6):828–830.

140. Pascual A, Calandra T, Bolay S, et al. Voriconazole therapeutic drug monitoring in patients with invasive mycoses improves efficacy and safety outcomes. *Clin Infect Dis* 2008;46(2):201–211.

141. Lewis RE. What is the "therapeutic range" for voriconazole? *Clin Infect Dis* 2008;46(2):212–214.

142. Zonios DI, Gea-Banacloche J, Childs R, et al. Hallucinations during voriconazole therapy. *Clin Infect Dis* 2008;47(1):e7–e10.

143. Chapman SW, Bradsher RW Jr, Campbell GD Jr, et al. Practice guidelines for the management of patients with blastomycosis. Infectious Diseases Society of America. *Clin Infect Dis* 2000;30(4):679–683.

144. Kauffman CA, Hajjeh R, Chapman SW. Practice guidelines for the management of patients with sporotrichosis. For the Mycoses Study Group. Infectious Diseases Society of America. *Clin Infect Dis* 2000;30(4):684–687.

145. Goodwin ML, Drew RH. Antifungal serum concentration monitoring: an update. *J Antimicrob Chemother* 2008;61(1):17–25.

146. Onishi J, Meinz M, Thompson J, et al. Discovery of novel antifungal (1,3)-beta-D-glucan synthase inhibitors. *Antimicrob Agents Chemother* 2000;44(2):368–377.

147. Cappelletty D, Eiselstein-McKitrick K. The echinocandins. *Pharmacotherapy* 2007;27(3):369–388.

148. Abe F, Ueyama J, Kawasumi N, et al. Role of plasma proteins in pharmacokinetics of micafungin, an antifungal antibiotic, in analbuminemic rats. *Antimicrob Agents Chemother* 2008;52(9):3454–3456.

149. Andes D, Diekema DJ, Pfaller MA, et al. In vivo comparison of the pharmacodynamic targets for echinocandin drugs against *Candida* species. *Antimicrob Agents Chemother* 2010;54(6):2497–2506.

150. Deresinski SC, Stevens DA. Caspofungin. *Clin Infect Dis* 2003;36(11):1445–1457.

151. Lat A, Thompson GR 3rd, Rinaldi MG, et al. Micafungin concentrations from brain tissue and pancreatic pseudocyst fluid. *Antimicrob Agents Chemother* 2010;54(2):943–944.

152. Kethireddy S, Andes D. CNS pharmacokinetics of antifungal agents. *Expert Opin Drug Metab Toxicol* 2007;3(4):573–581.

153. Keating GM, Jarvis B. Caspofungin. *Drugs* 2001;61(8):1121–1129; discussion 30–31.

154. Chandrasekar PH, Sobel JD. Micafungin: a new echinocandin. *Clin Infect Dis* 2006;42(8):1171–1178.

155. Andes D, Diekema DJ, Pfaller MA, et al. In vivo pharmacodynamic characterization of anidulafungin in a neutropenic murine candidiasis model. *Antimicrob Agents Chemother* 2008;52(2):539–550.

156. Ernst EJ, Klepser ME, Pfaller MA. Postantifungal effects of echinocandin, azole, and polyene antifungal agents against *Candida albicans* and *Cryptococcus neoformans*. *Antimicrob Agents Chemother* 2000;44(4):1108–1111.

157. Bowman JC, Hicks PS, Kurtz MB, et al. The antifungal echinocandin caspofungin acetate kills growing cells of *Aspergillus fumigatus* in vitro. *Antimicrob Agents Chemother* 2002;46(9):3001–3012.

158. Petraitiene R, Petraitis V, Groll AH, et al. Antifungal efficacy of caspofungin (MK-0991) in experimental pulmonary aspergillosis in persistently neutropenic rabbits: pharmacokinetics, drug disposition, and relationship to galactomannan antigenemia. *Antimicrob Agents Chemother* 2002;46(1):12–23.

159. Petraitis V, Petraitiene R, Groll AH, et al. Comparative antifungal activities and plasma pharmacokinetics of micafungin (FK463) against disseminated candidiasis and invasive pulmonary aspergillosis in persistently neutropenic rabbits. *Antimicrob Agents Chemother* 2002;46(6):1857–1869.

160. Ryan DM, Lupinacci RJ, Kartsonis NA. Efficacy and safety of caspofungin in obese patients. *Med Mycol* 2011; 49(7):748–754.

161. Hall RG, Swancutt MA, Gumbo T. Fractal geometry and the pharmacometrics of micafungin in overweight, obese, and extremely obese people. *Antimicrob Agents Chemother* 2011;55(11):5107–5112.

162. Wiederhold NP. Paradoxical echinocandin activity: a limited in vitro phenomenon? *Med Mycol* 2009; 47(Suppl 1):S369–S375.

163. Wiederhold NP. Attenuation of echinocandin activity at elevated concentrations: a review of the paradoxical effect. *Curr Opin Infect Dis* 2007;20(6):574–578.

164. Pappas PG, Rotstein CM, Betts RF, et al. Micafungin versus caspofungin for treatment of candidemia and other forms of invasive candidiasis. *Clin Infect Dis* 2007; 45(7):883–893.

165. Riddell J, Comer GM, Kauffman CA. Treatment of endogenous fungal endophthalmitis: focus on new antifungal agents. *Clin Infect Dis* 2011;52(5):648–653.

166. Pfaller MA, Diekema DJ, Ostrosky-Zeichner L, et al. Correlation of MIC with outcome for *Candida* species tested against caspofungin, anidulafungin, and micafungin: analysis and proposal for interpretive MIC breakpoints. *J Clin Microbiol* 2008;46(8): 2620–2629.

167. Lamaris GA, Lewis RE, Chamilos G, et al. Caspofungin-mediated beta-glucan unmasking and enhancement of human polymorphonuclear neutrophil activity against *Aspergillus* and non-*Aspergillus* hyphae. *J Infect Dis* 2008; 198(2):186–192.

168. Nakai T, Uno J, Otomo K, et al. In vitro activity of FK463, a novel lipopeptide antifungal agent, against a variety of clinically important molds. *Chemotherapy* 2002; 48(2):78–81.

169. Espinel-Ingroff A. Comparison of in vitro activities of the new triazole SCH56592 and the echinocandins MK-0991 (L-743,872) and LY303366 against opportunistic filamentous and dimorphic fungi and yeasts. *J Clin Microbiol* 1998;36(10):2950–2956.

170. Ramani R, Chaturvedi V. Antifungal susceptibility profiles of *Coccidioides immitis* and *Coccidioides posadasii* from endemic and non-endemic areas. *Mycopathologica* 2007;163(6):315–319.

171. Diekema DJ, Messer SA, Hollis RJ, et al. Activities of caspofungin, itraconazole, posaconazole, ravuconazole, voriconazole, and amphotericin B against 448 recent clinical isolates of filamentous fungi. *J Clin Microbiol* 2003;41(8):3623–3626.

172. Messer SA, Diekema DJ, Boyken L, et al. Activities of micafungin against 315 invasive clinical isolates of fluconazole-resistant *Candida* spp. *J Clin Microbiol* 2006; 44(2):324–326.

173. Pfaller MA, Boyken L, Hollis RJ, et al. In vitro susceptibility of invasive isolates of *Candida* spp. to anidulafungin, caspofungin, and micafungin: six years of global surveillance. *J Clin Microbiol* 2008;46(1):150–156.

174. Andes DR, Safdar N, Baddley JW, et al. Impact of treatment strategy on outcomes in patients with candidemia and other forms of invasive candidiasis: a patient-level quantitative review of randomized trials. *Clin Infect Dis* 2012;54(8):1110–1122.

175. Kuse ER, Chetchotisakd P, da Cunha CA, et al. Micafungin versus liposomal amphotericin B for candidaemia and invasive candidosis: a phase III randomised double-blind trial. *Lancet* 2007;369(9572):1519–1527.

176. Reboli AC, Rotstein C, Pappas PG, et al. Anidulafungin versus fluconazole for invasive candidiasis. *N Engl J Med* 2007;356(24):2472–2482.

177. Cornely OA, Lasso M, Betts R, et al. Caspofungin for the treatment of less common forms of invasive candidiasis. *J Antimicrob Chemother* 2007;60(2):363–369.

178. Baddley JW, Benjamin DK Jr, Patel M, et al. *Candida* infective endocarditis. *Eur J Clin Microbiol Infect Dis* 2008;27(7):519–529.

179. Heinz WJ, Einsele H. Caspofungin for treatment of invasive *Aspergillus* infections. *Mycoses* 2008;51(Suppl 1): 47–57.

180. Marr KA, Hachem R, Papanicolaou G, et al. Retrospective study of the hepatic safety profile of patients concomitantly treated with caspofungin and cyclosporin A. *Transplant Infect Dis* 2004;6(3):110–116.

181. Sable CA, Nguyen BY, Chodakewitz JA, et al. Safety and tolerability of caspofungin acetate in the treatment of fungal infections. *Transpl Infect Dis* 2002;4(1):25–30.

182. Polak A, Scholer HJ. Mode of action of 5-fluorocytosine and mechanisms of resistance. *Chemotherapy* 1975;21(3–4):113–130.

183. Vermes A, Guchelaar HJ, Dankert J. Flucytosine: a review of its pharmacology, clinical indications, pharmacokinetics, toxicity and drug interactions. *J Antimicrob Chemother* 2000;46(2):171–179.

184. Lewis RE, Klepser ME, Pfaller MA. In vitro pharmacodynamic characteristics of flucytosine determined by time-kill methods. *Diagn Microbiol Infect Dis* 2000;36(2):101–105.

185. Andes D, van Ogtrop M. In vivo characterization of the pharmacodynamics of flucytosine in a neutropenic murine disseminated candidiasis model. *Antimicrob Agents Chemother* 2000;44(4):938–942.

186. Brouwer AE, Rajanuwong A, Chierakul W, et al. Combination antifungal therapies for HIV-associated cryptococcal meningitis: a randomised trial. *Lancet* 2004; 363(9423):1764–1767.

187. Brandt ME, Pfaller MA, Hajjeh RA, et al. Trends in antifungal drug susceptibility of *Cryptococcus neoformans* isolates in the United States: 1992 to 1994 and 1996 to 1998. *Antimicrob Agents Chemother* 2001;45(11):3065–3069.

188. Pfaller MA, Messer SA, Boyken L, et al. In vitro activities of 5-fluorocytosine against 8,803 clinical isolates of *Candida* spp.: global assessment of primary resistance using National Committee for Clinical Laboratory Standards susceptibility testing methods. *Antimicrob Agents Chemother* 2002;46(11):3518–3521.

189. Vermes A, van Der Sijs H, Guchelaar HJ. Flucytosine: correlation between toxicity and pharmacokinetic parameters. *Chemotherapy* 2000;46(2):86–94.

190. Stamm AM, Diasio RB, Dismukes WE, et al. Toxicity of amphotericin B plus flucytosine in 194 patients with cryptococcal meningitis. *Am J Med* 1987;83(2):236–242.

191. Ghannoum MA, Rice LB. Antifungal agents: mode of action, mechanisms of resistance, and correlation of these mechanisms with bacterial resistance. *Clin Microbiol Rev* 1999;12(4):501–517.

192. Krishnan-Natesan S. Terbinafine: a pharmacological and clinical review. *Expert Opin Pharmacother* 2009;10(16):2723–2733.

193. Jessup CJ, Ryder NS, Ghannoum MA. An evaluation of the in vitro activity of terbinafine. *Med Mycol* 2000;38(2):155–159.

194. McGinnis MR, Pasarell L. In vitro evaluation of terbinafine and itraconazole against dematiaceous fungi. *Med Mycol* 1998;36(4):243–246.

195. McGinnis MR, Nordoff NG, Ryder NS, et al. In vitro comparison of terbinafine and itraconazole against Penicillium marneffei. *Antimicrob Agents Chemother* 2000; 44(5):1407–1408.

196. Ryder NS. Activity of terbinafine against serious fungal pathogens. *Mycoses* 1999;42(Suppl 2):115–119.

197. Gupta AK, Shear NH. Terbinafine: an update. *J Am Acad Dermatol* 1997;37(6):979–988.

198. Faergemann J, Anderson C, Hersle K, et al. Double-blind, parallel-group comparison of terbinafine and griseofulvin in the treatment of toenail onychomycosis. *J Am Acad Dermatol* 1995;32(5 Pt 1):750–753.

199. Hofmann H, Brautigam M, Weidinger G, et al. Treatment of toenail onychomycosis. A randomized, double-blind study with terbinafine and griseofulvin. LAGOS II Study Group. *Arch Dermatol* 1995;131(8):919–922.

200. Ghannoum MA, Elewski B. Successful treatment of fluconazole-resistant oropharyngeal candidiasis by a combination of fluconazole and terbinafine. *Clin Diagn Lab Immunol* 1999;6(6):921–923.

201. Esterre P, Inzan CK, Ramarcel ER, et al. Treatment of chromomycosis with terbinafine: preliminary results of an open pilot study. *Br J Dermatol* 1996;134(Suppl 46): 33–36; discussion 40.

202. Terbinafine [package insert]. East Hanover, NJ: Novartis Pharmaceuticals Corporation; 2012.

203. Hall M, Monka C, Krupp P, et al. Safety of oral terbinafine: results of a postmarketing surveillance study in 25,884 patients. *Arch Dermatol* 1997;133(10):1213–1219.

204. Ornstein DL, Ely P. Reversible agranulocytosis associated with oral terbinafine for onychomycosis. *J Am Acad Dermatol* 1998;39(6):1023–1024.

205. De Carli L, Larizza L. Griseofulvin. *Mutat Res* 1988; 195(2):91–126.

206. Balfour JA, Faulds D. Terbinafine. A review of its pharmacodynamic and pharmacokinetic properties, and therapeutic potential in superficial mycoses. *Drugs* 1992; 43(2):259–284.

207. Fleece D, Gaughan JP, Aronoff SC. Griseofulvin versus terbinafine in the treatment of tinea capitis: a meta-analysis of randomized, clinical trials. *Pediatrics* 2004; 114(5):1312–1315.

208. Gonzalez U, Seaton T, Bergus G, et al. Systemic antifungal therapy for tinea capitis in children. *Cochrane Database Syst Rev* 2007;(4):CD004685.

209. Elewski BE, Caceres HW, DeLeon L, et al. Terbinafine hydrochloride oral granules versus oral griseofulvin suspension in children with tinea capitis: results of two randomized, investigator-blinded, multicenter, international, controlled trials. *J Am Acad Dermatol* 2008; 59(1):41–45.

210. Lipozencic J, Skerlev M, Orofino-Costa R, et al. A randomized, double-blind, parallel-group, duration-finding study of oral terbinafine and open-label, high-dose griseofulvin in children with tinea capitis due to *Microsporum* species. *Br J Dermatol* 2002;146(5):816–823.

211. Griseofulvin [package insert]. Lincoln, NE: Novartis Pharmaceuticals Corporation; 2009.

212. Darouiche RO. Oropharyngeal and esophageal candidiasis in immunocompromised patients: treatment issues. *Clin Infect Dis* 1998;26(2):259–272; quiz 73–74.

213. Kaplan JE, Benson C, Holmes KH, et al. Guidelines for prevention and treatment of opportunistic infections in HIV-infected adults and adolescents: recommendations from CDC, the National Institutes of Health, and the HIV Medicine Association of the Infectious Diseases Society of America. *MMWR Recomm Rep* 2009;58(RR-4):1–207; quiz CE1–CE4.

214. Boucher HW, Talbot GH, Bradley JS, et al. Bad bugs, no drugs: no ESKAPE! An update from the Infectious Diseases Society of America. *Clin Infect Dis* 2009;48(1):1–12.

215. Johnson EM. Issues in antifungal susceptibility testing. *J Antimicrob Chemother* 2008;61(Suppl 1):i13–i18.

216. Cleveland AA, Farley MM, Harrison LH, et al. Changes in incidence and antifungal drug resistance in candidemia: results from population-based laboratory surveillance in Atlanta and Baltimore, 2008-2011. *Clin Infect Dis* 2012;55(10):1352–1361.

217. Pfaller MA, Castanheira M, Lockhart SR, et al. Frequency of decreased susceptibility and resistance to echinocandins among fluconazole-resistant bloodstream isolates of *Candida glabrata*. *J Clin Microbiol* 2012; 50(4):1199–1203.

218. White TC, Marr KA, Bowden RA. Clinical, cellular, and molecular factors that contribute to antifungal drug resistance. *Clin Microbiol Rev* 1998;11(2):382–402.

219. Sanglard D, Odds FC. Resistance of *Candida* species to antifungal agents: molecular mechanisms and clinical consequences. *Lancet Infect Dis* 2002;2(2):73–85.

220. Cannon RD, Lamping E, Holmes AR, et al. Efflux-mediated antifungal drug resistance. *Clin Microbiol Rev* 2009;22(2):291–321, Table of Contents.

221. White TC. Increased mRNA levels of ERG16, CDR, and MDR1 correlate with increases in azole resistance in *Candida albicans* isolates from a patient infected with human immunodeficiency virus. *Antimicrob Agents Chemother* 1997;41(7):1482–1487.

222. Franz R, Kelly SL, Lamb DC, et al. Multiple molecular mechanisms contribute to a stepwise development of fluconazole resistance in clinical *Candida albicans* strains. *Antimicrob Agents Chemother* 1998;42(12):3065–3072.

223. Favel A, Michel-Nguyen A, Peyron F, et al. Colony morphology switching of Candida lusitaniae and acquisition of multidrug resistance during treatment of a renal infection in a newborn: case report and review of the literature. *Diagnostic Microbiol Infect Dis* 2003; 47(1):331–339.

224. Kanafani ZA, Perfect JR. Antimicrobial resistance: resistance to antifungal agents: mechanisms and clinical impact. *Clin Infect Dis* 2008;46(1):46–48.

225. Rex JH, Cooper CR Jr, Merz WG, et al. Detection of amphotericin B-resistant *Candida* isolates in a broth-based system. *Antimicrob Agents Chemother* 1995;39(4): 906–909.

226. Blignaut E, Molepo J, Pujol C, et al. Clade-related amphotericin B resistance among South African *Candida albicans* isolates. *Diagn Microbiol Infect Dis* 2005; 53(1):29–231.

227. Pfaller MA, Diekema DJ, Gibbs DL, et al. *Candida krusei*, a multidrug-resistant opportunistic fungal pathogen: geographic and temporal trends from the ARTEMIS DISK Antifungal Surveillance Program, 2001 to 2005. *J Clin Microbiol* 2008;46(2):515–521.

228. Pfaller MA, Diekema DJ, Messer SA, et al. In vitro activities of voriconazole, posaconazole, and four licensed systemic antifungal agents against *Candida* species infrequently isolated from blood. *J Clin Microbiol* 2003;41(1):78–83.

229. Escribano P, Pelaez T, Recio S, et al. Characterization of clinical strains of *Aspergillus terreus* complex: molecular identification and antifungal susceptibility to azoles

and amphotericin B. *Clin Microbiol Infect* 2012;18(2): E24–E26.

230. Lass-Florl C, Alastruey-Izquierdo A, Cuenca-Estrella M, et al. In vitro activities of various antifungal drugs against *Aspergillus terreus*: global assessment using the methodology of the European Committee on Antimicrobial Susceptibility testing. *Antimicrob Agents Chemother* 2009;53(2):794–795.

231. Kelly SL, Lamb DC, Taylor M, et al. Resistance to amphotericin B associated with defective sterol delta 8—>7 isomerase in a *Cryptococcus neoformans* strain from an AIDS patient. *FEMS Microbiol Lett* 1994;122(1–2):39–42.

232. Witt MD, Lewis RJ, Larsen RA, et al. Identification of patients with acute AIDS-associated cryptococcal meningitis who can be effectively treated with fluconazole: the role of antifungal susceptibility testing. *Clin Infect Dis* 1996;22(2):322–328.

233. Athar MA, Winner HI. The development of resistance by *Candida* species to polyene antibiotics in vitro. *J Med Microbiol* 1971;4(4):505–517.

234. Dick JD, Rosengard BR, Merz WG, et al. Fatal disseminated candidiasis due to amphotericin-B-resistant *Candida guilliermondii. Ann Intern Med* 1985;102(1):67–68.

235. Dick JD, Merz WG, Saral R. Incidence of polyene-resistant yeasts recovered from clinical specimens. *Antimicrob Agents Chemother* 1980;18(1):158–163.

236. Powderly WG, Kobayashi GS, Herzig GP, et al. Amphotericin B-resistant yeast infection in severely immuno-compromised patients. *Am J Med* 1988;84(5):826–832.

237. Safe LM, Safe SH, Subden RE, et al. Sterol content and polyene antibiotic resistance in isolates of *Candida krusei, Candida parakrusei*, and *Candida tropicalis. Can J Microbiol* 1977;23(4):398–401.

238. Yoon SA, Vazquez JA, Steffan PE, et al. High-frequency, in vitro reversible switching of *Candida lusitaniae* clinical isolates from amphotericin B susceptibility to resistance. *Antimicrob Agents Chemother* 1999;43(4):836–845.

239. Hitchcock CA, Barrett-Bee KJ, Russell NJ. The lipid composition and permeability to azole of an azole- and polyene-resistant mutant of *Candida albicans. J Med Vet Mycol* 1987.

240. Subden RE, Safe L, Morris DC, et al Eburicol, lichesterol, ergosterol, and obtusifoliol from polyene antibiotic-resistant mutants of *Candida albicans. Can J Microbiol* 1977;23(6):751–754.

241. Sokol-Anderson M, Sligh JE Jr, Elberg S, et al. Role of cell defense against oxidative damage in the resistance of *Candida albicans* to the killing effect of amphotericin B. *Antimicrob Agents Chemother* 1988;32(5):702–705.

242. Nolte FS, Parkinson T, Falconer DJ, et al. Isolation and characterization of fluconazole- and amphotericin B-resistant *Candida albicans* from blood of two patients with leukemia. *Antimicrob Agents Chemother* 1997;41(1): 196–199.

243. Fryberg M, Oehlschlager AC, Unrau AM. Sterol biosynthesis in antibiotic-resistant yeast: nystatin. *Arch Biochem Biophys* 1974;160(1):83–89.

244. Gale EF, Johnson AM, Kerridge D, et al. Factors affecting the changes in amphotericin sensitivity of *Candida albicans* during growth. *J Gen Microbiol* 1975;87(1): 20–36.

245. Morio F, Pagniez F, Lacroix C, et al. Amino acid substitutions in the *Candida albicans* sterol Δ5,6-desaturase (Erg3p) confer azole resistance: characterization of two novel mutants with impaired virulence. *J Antimicrob Chemother* 2012;67(9):2131–2138.

246. Akins RA. An update on antifungal targets and mechanisms of resistance in *Candida albicans. Med Mycol* 2005;43(4):285–318.

247. Pfaller MA, Diekema DJ. Twelve years of fluconazole in clinical practice: global trends in species distribution and fluconazole susceptibility of bloodstream isolates of *Candida. Clin Microbiol Infect* 2004;10(Suppl 1):11–23.

248. Lockhart SR, Iqbal N, Cleveland AA, et al. Species identification and antifungal susceptibility testing of *Candida* bloodstream isolates from population-based surveillance studies in two U.S. cities from 2008 to 2011. *J Clin Microbiol* 2012;50(11):3435–3442.

249. Fukuoka T, Johnston DA, Winslow CA, et al. Genetic basis for differential activities of fluconazole and voriconazole against *Candida krusei. Antimicrob Agents Chemother* 2003;47(4):1213–1219.

250. Sipsas NV, Lewis RE, Tarrand J, et al. Candidemia in patients with hematologic malignancies in the era of new antifungal agents (2001-2007): stable incidence but changing epidemiology of a still frequently lethal infection. *Cancer* 2009;115(20):4745–4752.

251. Ghannoum MA, Okogbule-Wonodi I, Bhat N, et al. Antifungal activity of voriconazole (UK-109,496), fluconazole and amphotericin B against hematogenous *Candida krusei* infection in neutropenic guinea pig model. *J Chemother* 1999;11(1):34–39.

252. Cuenca-Estrella M, Diaz-Guerra TM, Mellado E, et al. Comparative in vitro activity of voriconazole and itraconazole against fluconazole-susceptible and fluconazole-resistant clinical isolates of *Candida* species from Spain. *Eur J Clin Microbiol Infect Dis* 1999;18(6): 432–435.

253. Ostrosky-Zeichner L, Oude Lashof AM, Kullberg BJ, et al. Voriconazole salvage treatment of invasive candidiasis. *Eur J Clin Microbiol Infect Dis* 2003;22(11): 651–655.

254. Pfaller MA, Diekema DJ, Jones RN, et al. Trends in antifungal susceptibility of *Candida* spp. isolated from pediatric and adult patients with bloodstream infections: SENTRY Antimicrobial Surveillance Program, 1997 to 2000. *J Clin Microbiol* 2002;40(3):852–856.

255. Majithiya J, Sharp A, Parmar A, et al. Efficacy of isavuconazole, voriconazole and fluconazole in temporarily neutropenic murine models of disseminated *Candida tropicalis* and *Candida krusei. J Antimicrob Chemother* 2009;63(1):161–166.

256. Pfaller MA, Messer SA, Boyken L, et al. In vitro activities of voriconazole, posaconazole, and fluconazole against 4,169 clinical isolates of *Candida* spp. and *Cryptococcus neoformans* collected during 2001 and 2002 in the ARTEMIS global antifungal surveillance program. *Diagn Microbiol Infect Dis* 2004;48(3):201–205.

257. Spreghini E, Maida CM, Tomassetti S, et al. Posaconazole against *Candida glabrata* isolates with various susceptibilities to fluconazole. *Antimicrob Agents Chemother* 2008;52(6):1929–1933.

258. Espinel-Ingroff A, Aller AI, Canton E, et al. *Cryptococcus neoformans-Cryptococcus gattii* species complex: an international study of wild-type susceptibility endpoint distributions and epidemiological cutoff values for fluconazole, itraconazole, posaconazole, and voriconazole. *Antimicrob Agents Chemother* 2012;56(11):5898–5906.

259. Thompson GR 3rd, Wiederhold NP, Fothergill AW, et al. Antifungal susceptibilities among different serotypes of *Cryptococcus gattii* and *Cryptococcus neoformans. Antimicrob Agents Chemother* 2009;53(1):309–311.

260. Casadevall A, Spitzer ED, Webb D, et al. Suscepti-bilities of serial *Cryptococcus neoformans* isolates from patients with recurrent cryptococcal meningitis to amphotericin B and fluconazole. *Antimicrob Agents Chemother* 1993;37(6):1383–1386.

261. Baddley JW, Marr KA, Andes DR, et al. Patterns of sus-ceptibility of *Aspergillus* isolates recovered from patients enrolled in the Transplant-Associated Infection Surveil-lance Network. *J Clin Microbiol* 2009;47(10):3271–3275.

262. Verweij PE, Kema GH, Zwaan B, et al. Triazole fungi-cides and the selection of resistance to medical triazoles in the opportunistic mould *Aspergillus fumigatus*. *Pest Manag Sci* 2012.

263. Snelders E, Camps SM, Karawajczyk A, et al. Triazole fungicides can induce cross-resistance to medical triazoles in *Aspergillus fumigatus*. *PLoS One* 2012;7(3):e31801.

264. Mosquera J, Denning DW. Azole cross-resistance in *As-pergillus fumigatus*. *Antimicrob Agents Chemother* 2002; 46(2):556–557.

265. White TC. The presence of an R467K amino acid sub-stitution and loss of allelic variation correlate with an azole-resistant lanosterol 14alpha demethylase in *Can-dida albicans*. *Antimicrob Agents Chemother* 1997;47(7): 1488–1494.

266. Sanglard D, Ischer F, Calabrese D, et al. The ATP binding cassette transporter gene CgCDR1 from *Candida glabrata* is involved in the resistance of clinical isolates to azole antifungal agents. *Antimicrob Agents Chemother* 1999; 43(11):2753–2765.

267. Sanglard D, Ischer F, Monod M, et al. Cloning of *Can-dida albicans* genes conferring resistance to azole antifungal agents: characterization of CDR2, a new multidrug ABC transporter gene. *Microbiology* 1997;143(Pt 2):405–416.

268. Sanglard D, Kuchler K, Ischer F, et al. Mechanisms of resistance to azole antifungal agents in *Candida albi-cans* isolates from AIDS patients involve specific mul-tidrug transporters. *Antimicrob Agents Chemother* 1995; 39(11):2378–2386.

269. MacCallum DM, Coste A, Ischer F, et al. Genetic dissection of azole resistance mechanisms in *Candida albicans* and their validation in a mouse model of dis-seminated infection. *Antimicrob Agents Chemother* 2010; 54(4):1476–1483.

270. Lopez-Ribot JL, McAtee RK, Lee LN, et al. Distinct patterns of gene expression associated with development of fluconazole resistance in serial *Candida albicans* iso-lates from human immunodeficiency virus-infected pa-tients with oropharyngeal candidiasis. *Antimicrob Agents Chemother* 1998;42(11):2932–2937.

271. Lopez-Ribot JL, McAtee RK, Perea S, et al. Multiple resistant phenotypes of *Candida albicans* coexist during episodes of oropharyngeal candidiasis in human immu-nodeficiency virus-infected patients. *Antimicrob Agents Chemother* 1999;43(7):1621–1630.

272. Redding S, Smith J, Farinacci G, et al. Resistance of *Candida albicans* to fluconazole during treatment of oropharyngeal candidiasis in a patient with AIDS: doc-umentation by in vitro susceptibility testing and DNA subtype analysis. *Clin Infect Dis* 1994;18(2):240–242.

273. Snelders E, van der Lee HA, Kuijpers J, et al. Emergence of azole resistance in *Aspergillus fumigatus* and spread of a single resistance mechanism. *PLoS Med* 2008;5(11):e219.

274. Camps SM, Dutilh BE, Arendrup MC, et al. Discovery of a hapE mutation that causes azole resistance in *Asper-gillus fumigatus* through whole genome sequencing and sexual crossing. *PLoS One* 2012;7(11):e50034.

275. Joseph-Horne T, Hollomon D, Loeffler RS, et al. Cross-resistance to polyene and azole drugs in *Cryptococcus neoformans*. *Antimicrob Agents Chemother* 1995;39(7): 1526–1529.

276. Lamb DC, Corran A, Baldwin BC, et al. Resist-ant P45051A1 activity in azole antifungal tolerant *Cryptococcus neoformans* from AIDS patients. *FEBS Lett* 1995;368(2):326–330.

277. Sionov E, Chang YC, Garraffo HM, et al. Heterore-sistance to fluconazole in *Cryptococcus neoformans* is in-trinsic and associated with virulence. *Antimicrob Agents Chemother* 2009;53(7):2804–2815.

278. Pfaller MA, Messer SA, Boyken L, et al. Caspofungin activity against clinical isolates of fluconazole-resistant *Candida*. *J Clin Microbiol* 2003;41(12):5729–5731.

279. Pfaller MA, Diekema DJ, Messer SA, et al. In vitro activ-ities of caspofungin compared with those of fluconazole and itraconazole against 3,959 clinical isolates of *Can-dida* spp., including 157 fluconazole-resistant isolates. *Antimicrob Agents Chemother* 2003;47(3):1068–1071.

280. Kurtz MB, Abruzzo G, Flattery A, et al. Characteriza-tion of echinocandin-resistant mutants of *Candida albicans*: genetic, biochemical, and virulence studies. *Infect Immun* 1996;64(8):3244–3251.

281. Douglas CM, D'Ippolito JA, Shei GJ, et al. Identifica-tion of the FKS1 gene of *Candida albicans* as the es-sential target of 1,3-beta-D-glucan synthase inhibitors. *Antimicrob Agents Chemother* 1997;41(11):2471–2479.

282. Thompson GR 3rd, Wiederhold NP, Vallor AC, et al. Development of caspofungin resistance follow-ing prolonged therapy for invasive candidiasis second-ary to *Candida glabrata* infection. *Antimicrob Agents Chemother* 2008;52(10):3783–3785.

283. Arendrup MC, Perkhofer S, Howard SJ, et al. Establish-ing in vitro-in vivo correlations for *Aspergillus fumigatus*: the challenge of azoles versus echinocandins. *Antimicrob Agents Chemother* 2008;52(10):3504–3511.

284. Kahn JN, Garcia-Effron G, Hsu MJ, et al. Acquired echinocandin resistance in a *Candida krusei* isolate due to modification of glucan synthase. *Antimicrob Agents Chemother* 2007;51(5):1876–1878.

285. Park S, Kelly R, Kahn JN, et al. Specific substitutions in the echinocandin target Fks1p account for reduced susceptibility of rare laboratory and clinical *Candida* sp. isolates. *Antimicrob Agents Chemother* 2005;49(8): 3264–3273.

286. Katiyar S, Pfaller M, Edlind T. *Candida albicans* and *Candida glabrata* clinical isolates exhibiting re-duced echinocandin susceptibility. *Antimicrob Agents Chemother* 2006;50(8):2892–2894.

287. Beauvais A, Bruneau JM, Mol PC, et al. Glucan synthase complex of *Aspergillus fumigatus*. *J Bacteriol* 2001;183(7): 2273–2279.

288. Gardiner RE, Souteropoulos P, Park S, et al. Char-acterization of *Aspergillus fumigatus* mutants with re-duced susceptibility to caspofungin. *Med Mycol* 2005; 43(Suppl 1):S299–S305.

289. Romano J, Nimrod G, Ben-Tal N, et al. Disruption of the *Aspergillus fumigatus* ECM33 homologue re-sults in rapid conidial germination, antifungal resist-ance and hypervirulence. *Microbiology* 2006;152(Pt 7): 1919–1928.

290. Stiller RL, Bennett JE, Scholer HJ, et al. Susceptibil-ity to 5-fluorocytosine and prevalence of serotype in 402 *Candida albicans* isolates from the United States. *Antimicrob Agents Chemother* 1982;22(3):482–487.

291. Defever KS, Whelan WL, Rogers AL, et al. *Candida albicans* resistance to 5-fluorocytosine: frequency of partially resistant strains among clinical isolates. *Antimicrob Agents Chemother* 1982;22(5):810–815.

292. Whelan WL. The genetic basis of resistance to 5-fluorocytosine in *Candida* species and *Cryptococcus neoformans*. *Cerit Rev Microbiol* 1987;15(1):45–56.

293. Whelan WL, Kerridge D. Decreased activity of UMP pyrophosphorylase associated with resistance to 5-fluorocytosine in *Candida albicans*. *Antimicrob Agents Chemother* 1984;26(4):570–574.

294. Liu W, May GS, Lionakis MS, et al. Extra copies of the *Aspergillus fumigatus* squalene epoxidase gene confer resistance to terbinafine: genetic approach to studying gene dose-dependent resistance to antifungals in *A. fumigatus*. *Antimicrob Agents Chemother* 2004;48(7):2490–2496.

295. Leber R, Fuchsbichler S, Klobucnikova V, et al. Molecular mechanism of terbinafine resistance in *Saccharomyces cerevisiae*. *Antimicrob Agents Chemother* 2003;47(12):3890–3900.

296. Osborne CS, Leitner I, Hofbauer B, et al. Biological, biochemical, and molecular characterization of a new clinical *Trichophyton rubrum* isolate resistant to terbinafine. *Antimicrob Agents Chemother*

297. Osborne CS, Leitner I, Favre B, et al. Amino acid substitution in *Trichophyton rubrum* squalene epoxidase associated with resistance to terbinafine. *Antimicrob Agents Chemother* 2005;49(7):2840–2844.

298. Rex JH, Pfaller MA. Has antifungal susceptibility testing come of age? *Clin Infect Dis* 2002;35(8):982–989.

299. Pittrow L, Penk A. Special pharmacokinetics of fluconazole in septic, obese and burn patients. *Mycoses* 1999;42(Suppl 2):87–90.

300. Pfaller MA, Sheehan DJ, Rex JH. Determination of fungicidal activities against yeasts and molds: lessons learned from bactericidal testing and the need for standardization. *Clin Microbiol Rev* 2004;17(2):268–280.

301. Lat A, Thompson GR 3rd. Update on the optimal use of voriconazole for invasive fungal infections. *Infect Drug Resist* 2011;4:43–53.

302. Fernandez-Torres B, Inza I, Guarro J. Comparison of in vitro antifungal susceptibilities of conidia and hyphae of dermatophytes with thick-wall macroconidia. *Antimicrob Agents Chemother* 2003;47(10):3371–3372.

303. Perkhofer S, Jost D, Dierich MP, et al. Susceptibility testing of anidulafungin and voriconazole alone and in combination against conidia and hyphae of *Aspergillus* spp. under hypoxic conditions. *Antimicrob Agents Chemother* 2008;52(5):1873–1875.

304. Vargas K, Messer SA, Pfaller M, et al. Elevated phenotypic switching and drug resistance of *Candida albicans* from human immunodeficiency virus-positive individuals prior to first thrush episode. *J Clin Microbiol* 2000;38(10):3595–3607.

305. Al-Fattani MA, Douglas LJ. Biofilm matrix of *Candida albicans* and *Candida tropicalis*: chemical composition and role in drug resistance. *J Med Microbiol* 2006;55(Pt 8):999–1008.

306. Baillie GS, Douglas LJ. Matrix polymers of *Candida* biofilms and their possible role in biofilm resistance to antifungal agents. *J Antimicrob Chemother* 2000;46(3):397–403.

307. Chandra J, Kuhn DM, Mukherjee PK, et al. Biofilm formation by the fungal pathogen *Candida albicans*: development, architecture, and drug resistance. *J Bacteriol* 2001;183(13):5385–5395.

308. Chenoweth CE, Robinson KA, Schaberg DR. Efficacy of ampicillin versus trimethoprim-sulfamethoxazole in a mouse model of lethal enterococcal peritonitis. *Antimicrob Agents Chemother* 1990;34(9):1800–1802.

309. Grayson ML, Thauvin-Eliopoulos C, Eliopoulos GM, et al. Failure of trimethoprim-sulfamethoxazole therapy in experimental enterococcal endocarditis. *Antimicrob Agents Chemother* 1990;34(9):1792–1794.

310. Clinical and Laboratory Standards Institute. *Reference method for broth dilution antifungal susceptibility testing of yeasts; approved standard.* Wayne, PA: Clinical and Laboratory Standards Institute, 2008. CLSI document M27-A3.

311. Clinical and Laboratory Standards Institute. *Method for antifungal disk diffusion susceptibility testing of yeasts; approved standard.* Wayne, PA: Clinical and Laboratory Standards Institute, 2008. CLSI document M44-A2.

312. Barry AL, Pfaller MA, Rennie RP, et al. Precision and accuracy of fluconazole susceptibility testing by broth microdilution, Etest, and disk diffusion methods. *Antimicrob Agents Chemother* 2002;46(6):1781–1784.

313. Pfaller MA, Diekema DJ, Sheehan DJ. Interpretive breakpoints for fluconazole and *Candida* revisited: a blueprint for the future of antifungal susceptibility testing. *Clin Microbiol Rev* 2006;19(2):435–447.

314. Clinical and Laboratory Standards Institute. *Reference method for broth dilution antifungal susceptibility testing of filamentous fungi; approved standard.* Wayne, PA: Clinical and Laboratory Standards Institute, 2008. CLSI document M38-A2.

315. Fromtling RA, Galgiani JN, Pfaller MA, et al. Multicenter evaluation of a broth macrodilution antifungal susceptibility test for yeasts. *Antimicrob Agents Chemother* 1993;37(1):39–45

316. Pfaller MA, Diekema DJ. Progress in antifungal susceptibility testing of *Candida* spp. by use of Clinical and Laboratory Standards Institute broth microdilution methods, 2010 to 2012. *J Clin Microbiol* 2012;50(9):2846–2856.

317. Pfaller MA, Castanheira M, Messer SA, et al. Echinocandin and triazole antifungal susceptibility profiles for *Candida* spp., *Cryptococcus neoformans*, and *Aspergillus fumigatus*: application of new CLSI clinical breakpoints and epidemiologic cutoff values to characterize resistance in the SENTRY Antimicrobial Surveillance Program (2009). *Diagn Microbiol Infect Dis* 2011;69(1):45–50.

318. Pfaller MA, Rinaldi MG, Galgiani JN, et al. Collaborative investigation of variables in susceptibility testing of yeasts. *Antimicrob Agents Chemother* 1990;34(9):1648–1654.

319. Pfaller MA, Burmeister L, Bartlett MS, et al. Multicenter evaluation of four methods of yeast inoculum preparation. *J Clin Microbiol* 1988;26(8):1437–1441.

320. National Committee for Clinical Laboratory Standards. *Reference method for broth dilution susceptibility testing of yeasts: proposed standard.* Villanova, PA: National Committee for Clinical Laboratory Standards, 1992. NCCLS document M27-P.

321. Rex JH, Pfaller MA, Galgiani JN, et al. Development of interpretive breakpoints for antifungal susceptibility testing: conceptual framework and analysis of in vitro-in vivo correlation data for fluconazole, itraconazole, and *Candida* infections. Subcommittee on Antifungal Susceptibility Testing of the National Committee for Clinical Laboratory Standards. *Clin Infect Dis* 1997;24(2):235–247.

322. Barry AL, Pfaller MA, Brown SD, et al. Quality control limits for broth microdilution susceptibility tests of ten antifungal agents. *J Clin Microbiol* 2000;38(9):3457–3459.

323. National Committee for Clinical Laboratory Standards. *Reference method for broth dilution antifungal susceptibility testing of yeasts.* Wayne, PA: National Committee for Clinical Laboratory Standards, 2002. NCCLS document M27-A2.

324. Hata K, Kimura J, Miki H, et al. Efficacy of ER-30346, a novel oral triazole antifungal agent, in experimental models of aspergillosis, candidiasis, and cryptococcosis. *Antimicrob Agents Chemother* 1996;40(10):2243–2247.

325. Clinical and Laboratory Standards Institute. *Reference method for broth dilution antifungal susceptibility testing of filamentous fungi; approved standard, 2nd ed.* CLSI document M38-A2. Wayne, PA: Clinical and Laboratory Standards Institute, 2008.

326. Liebowitz LD, Ashbee HR, Evans EG, et al. A two year global evaluation of the susceptibility of *Candida* species to fluconazole by disk diffusion. *Diagn Microbiol Infect Dis* 2001;40(1–2):27–33.

327. Bille J, Glauser MP. Evaluation of the susceptibility of pathogenic *Candida* species to fluconazole. Fluconazole Global Susceptibility Study Group. *Eur J Clin Microbiol Infect Dis* 1997;16(12):924–928.

328. Pfaller MA, Diekema DJ, Rinaldi MG, et al. Results from the ARTEMIS DISK Global Antifungal Surveillance Study: a 6.5-year analysis of susceptibilities of *Candida* and other yeast species to fluconazole and voriconazole by standardized disk diffusion testing. *J Clin Microbiol* 2005;43(12):5848–5859.

329. Barry A, Bille J, Brown S, et al. Quality control limits for fluconazole disk susceptibility tests on Mueller-Hinton agar with glucose and methylene blue. *J Clin Microbiol* 2003;41(7):3410–3412.

330. Pfaller MA, Diekema DJ, Messer SA, et al. Activities of fluconazole and voriconazole against 1,586 recent clinical isolates of *Candida* species determined by Broth microdilution, disk diffusion, and Etest methods: report from the ARTEMIS Global Antifungal Susceptibility Program, 2001. *J Clin Microbiol* 2003;41(4):1440–1446.

331. Clinical and Laboratory Standards Institute. *Method for antifungal disk diffusion susceptibility testing of yeasts; approved guideline, 2nd ed.* CLSI document M44-A2. Wayne, PA: Clinical and Laboratory Standards Institute, 2009.

332. Espinel-Ingroff A, Canton E, Fothergill A, et al. Quality control guidelines for amphotericin B, Itraconazole, posaconazole, and voriconazole disk diffusion susceptibility tests with nonsupplemented Mueller-Hinton Agar (CLSI M51-A document) for nondermatophyte Filamentous Fungi. *J Clin Microbiol* 2011;49(7):2568–2571.

333. Martos AI, Martin-Mazuelos E, Romero A, et al. Evaluation of disk diffusion method compared to broth microdilution for antifungal susceptibility testing of 3 echinocandins against *Aspergillus* spp. *Diagn Microbiol Infect Dis* 2012;73(1):53–56.

334. Espinel-Ingroff A, Boyle K, Sheehan DJ. In vitro antifungal activities of voriconazole and reference agents as determined by NCCLS methods: review of the literature. *Mycopathologia* 2001;150(3):101–115.

335. National Committee for Clinical Laboratory Standards. *Reference method for broth dilution antifungal susceptibility testing of filamentous fungi; approved standard.* Wayne, PA: National Committee for Clinical Laboratory Standards, 2002. NCCLS document M38-A.

336. Ghannoum MA, Arthington-Skaggs B, Chaturvedi V, et al. Interlaboratory study of quality control isolates for a broth microdilution method (modified CLSI M38-A) for testing susceptibilities of dermatophytes to antifungals. *J Clin Microbiol* 2006;44(12):4353–4356.

337. Chen YC, Chang SC, Luh KT, et al. Stable susceptibility of *Candida* blood isolates to fluconazole despite increasing use during the past 10 years. *J Antimicrob Chemother* 2003;52(1):71–77.

338. Pfaller M, Neofytos D, Diekema D, et al. Epidemiology and outcomes of candidemia in 3648 patients: data from the Prospective Antifungal Therapy (PATH Alliance®) registry, 2004-2008. *Diagn Microbiol Infect Dis* 2012;74(4):323–331.

339. Lepak A, Castanheira M, Diekema D, et al. Optimizing echinocandin dosing and susceptibility breakpoint determination via in vivo pharmacodynamic evaluation against *Candida glabrata* with and without fks mutations. *Antimicrob Agents Chemother* 2012;56(11):5875–5882.

340. Canton E, Peman J, Quindos G, et al. Prospective multicenter study of the epidemiology, molecular identification, and antifungal susceptibility of *Candida parapsilosis*, *Candida orthopsilosis*, and *Candida metapsilosis* isolated from patients with candidemia. *Antimicrob Agents Chemother* 2011;55(12):5590–5596.

341. Ramani R, Chaturvedi V. Proficiency testing program for clinical laboratories performing antifungal susceptibility testing of pathogenic yeast species. *J Clin Microbiol* 2003;41(3):1143–1146.

342. Ranque S, Lachaud L, Gari-Toussaint M, et al. Interlaboratory reproducibility of Etest amphotericin B and caspofungin yeast susceptibility testing and comparison with the CLSI method. *J Clin Microbiol* 2012;50(7):2305–2309.

343. Odds FC, Motyl M, Andrade R, et al. Interlaboratory comparison of results of susceptibility testing with caspofungin against *Candida* and *Aspergillus* species. *J Clin Microbiol* 2004;42(8):3475–3482.

344. Canton E, Peman J, Hervas D, et al. Comparison of three statistical methods for establishing tentative wild-type population and epidemiological cutoff values for echinocandins, amphotericin B, flucytosine, and six *Candida* species as determined by the colorimetric Sensititre YeastOne method. *J Clin Microbiol* 2012;50(12):3921–3926.

345. Pfaller MA, Chaturvedi V, Diekema DJ, et al. Comparison of the Sensititre YeastOne colorimetric antifungal panel with CLSI microdilution for antifungal susceptibility testing of the echinocandins against *Candida* spp., using new clinical breakpoints and epidemiological cutoff values. *Diagn Microbiol Infect Dis* 2012;73(4):365–368.

346. Radetsky M, Wheeler RC, Roe MH, et al. Microtiter broth dilution method for yeast susceptibility testing with validation by clinical outcome. *J Clin Microbiol* 1986;24(4):600–606.

347. Nett JE, Cain MT, Crawford K, et al. Optimizing a *Candida* biofilm microtiter plate model for measurement of antifungal susceptibility by tetrazolium salt assay. *J Clin Microbiol* 2011;49(4):1426–1433.

348. Cuenca-Estrella M, Moore CB, Barchiesi F, et al. Multicenter evaluation of the reproducibility of the proposed antifungal susceptibility testing method for fermentative yeasts of the Antifungal Susceptibility Testing Subcommittee of the European Committee on Antimicrobial Susceptibility Testing (AFST-EUCAST). *Clin Microbiol Infect* 2003;9(6):467–474.

349. Ingham CJ, Boonstra S, Levels S, et al. Rapid susceptibility testing and microcolony analysis of *Candida* spp. cultured and imaged on porous aluminum oxide. *PLoS One* 2012;7(3):e33818.

350. Rudensky B, Broide E, Berko N, et al. Direct fluconazole susceptibility testing of positive *Candida* blood cultures by flow cytometry. *Mycoses* 2008;51(3):200–204.

351. Ramani R, Chaturvedi V. Flow cytometry antifungal susceptibility testing of pathogenic yeasts other than *Candida albicans* and comparison with the NCCLS broth microdilution test. *Antimicrob Agents Chemother* 2000;44(10):2752–2758.

352. Li RK, Elie CM, Clayton GE, et al. Comparison of a new colorimetric assay with the NCCLS broth microdilution method (M-27A) for antifungal drug MIC determination. *J Clin Microbiol* 2000;38(6):2334–2338.

353. Riesselman MH, Hazen KC, Cutler JE. Determination of antifungal MICs by a rapid susceptibility assay. *J Clin Microbiol* 2000;38(1):333–340.

354. Fournier C, Gaspar A, Boillot F, et al. Evaluation of a broth microdilution antifungal susceptibility test with a pH indicator: comparison with the broth macrodilution procedures. *J Antimicrob Chemother* 1995;35(3):373–380.

355. Hawser SP, Norris H, Jessup CJ, et al. Comparison of a 2,3-bis(2-methoxy-4-nitro-5-sulfophenyl)-5-[(phenylamino)carbonyl]-2H-tetrazolium hydroxide (XTT) colorimetric method with the standardized National Committee for Clinical Laboratory Standards method of testing clinical yeast isolates for susceptibility to antifungal agents. *J Clin Microbiol* 1998;36(5):1450–1452.

356. Jahn B, Martin E, Stueben A, et al. Susceptibility testing of *Candida albicans* and *Aspergillus* species by a simple microtiter menadione-augmented 3-(4,5-dimethyl-2-t hiazolyl)-2,5-diphenyl-2H-tetrazolium bromide assay. *J Clin Microbiol* 1995;33(3):661–667.

357. Borghi E, Iatta R, Sciota R, et al. Comparative evaluation of the Vitek 2 yeast susceptibility test and CLSI broth microdilution reference method for testing antifungal susceptibility of invasive fungal isolates in Italy: the GISIA3 study. *J Clin Microbiol* 2010;48(9):3153–3157.

358. Peterson JF, Pfaller MA, Diekema DJ, et al. Multicenter comparison of the Vitek 2 antifungal susceptibility test with the CLSI broth microdilution reference method for testing caspofungin, micafungin, and posaconazole against *Candida* spp. *J Clin Microbiol* 2011;49(5):1765–1771.

359. Pfaller MA, Diekema DJ, Procop GW, et al. Multicenter comparison of the VITEK 2 yeast susceptibility test with the CLSI broth microdilution reference method for testing fluconazole against *Candida* spp. *J Clin Microbiol* 2007;45(3):796–802.

360. Jahn B, Stuben A, Bhakdi S. Colorimetric susceptibility testing for *Aspergillus fumigatus*: comparison of menadione-augmented 3-(4,5-dimethyl-2-thiazolyl)-2,5-diphenyl-2H-tetrazolium bromide and Alamar blue tests. *J Clin Microbiol* 1996;34(8):2039–2041.

361. Espinel-Ingroff A, Pfaller M, Messer SA, et al. Multicenter comparison of the Sensititre YeastOne colorimetric antifungal panel with the NCCLS M27-A2 reference method for testing new antifungal agents against clinical isolates of *Candida* spp. *J Clin Microbiol* 2004;42(2):718–721.

362. Espinel-Ingroff A, Pfaller M, Messer SA, et al. Multicenter comparison of the sensititre YeastOne Colorimetric Antifungal Panel with the National Committee for Clinical Laboratory standards M27-A reference method for testing clinical isolates of common and emerging *Candida* spp., *Cryptococcus* spp., and other yeasts and yeast-like organisms. *J Clin Microbiol* 1999;37(3):591–595.

363. Castro C, Serrano MC, Flores B, et al. Comparison of the Sensititre YeastOne colorimetric antifungal panel with a modified NCCLS M38-A method to determine the activity of voriconazole against clinical isolates of *Aspergillus* spp. *J Clin Microbiol* 2004;42(9):4358–4380.

364. Morace G, Amato G, Bistoni F, et al. Multicenter comparative evaluation of six commercial systems and the National Committee for Clinical Laboratory Standards m27-a broth microdilution method for fluconazole susceptibility testing of *Candida* species. *J Clin Microbiol* 2002;40(8):2953–2958.

365. Anaissie E, Paetznick V, Bodey GP. Fluconazole susceptibility testing of *Candida albicans*: microtiter method that is independent of inoculum size, temperature, and time of reading. *Antimicrob Agents Chemother* 1991;35(8):1641–1646.

366. Pfaller MA, Messer SA, Coffmann S. Comparison of visual and spectrophotometric methods of MIC endpoint determinations by using broth microdilution methods to test five antifungal agents, including the new triazole D0870. *J Clin Microbiol* 1995;33(5):1094–1097.

367. Arendrup MC, Park S, Brown S, et al. Evaluation of CLSI M44-A2 disk diffusion and associated breakpoint testing of caspofungin and micafungin using a well-characterized panel of wild-type and fks hot spot mutant *Candida* isolates. *Antimicrob Agents Chemother* 2011;55(5):1891–1895.

368. Colombo AL, Barchiesi F, McGough DA, et al. Comparison of Etest and National Committee for Clinical Laboratory Standards broth macrodilution method for azole antifungal susceptibility testing. *J Clin Microbiol* 1995;33(3):535–540.

369. Pfaller MA, Messer SA, Bolmstrom A, et al. Multisite reproducibility of the Etest MIC method for antifungal susceptibility testing of yeast isolates. *J Clin Microbiol* 1996;34(7):1691–1693.

370. Pfaller MA, Messer SA, Houston A, et al. Evaluation of the Etest method for determining voriconazole susceptibilities of 312 clinical isolates of *Candida* species by using three different agar media. *J Clin Microbiol* 2000;38(10):3715–3717.

371. Pfaller MA, Messer SA, Mills K, et al. Evaluation of Etest method for determining posaconazole MICs for 314 clinical isolates of *Candida* species. *J Clin Microbiol* 2001;39(11):3952–3954.

372. Espinel-Ingroff A, Pfaller M, Erwin ME, et al. Interlaboratory evaluation of Etest method for testing antifungal susceptibilities of pathogenic yeasts to five antifungal agents by using Casitone agar and solidified RPMI 1640 medium with 2% glucose. *J Clin Microbiol* 1996;34(4):848–852.

373. Espinel-Ingroff A. Etest for antifungal susceptibility testing of yeasts. *Diagnostic Microbiol Infect Dis* 1994;19(4):217–220.

374. Provine H, Hadley S. Preliminary evaluation of a semisolid agar antifungal susceptibility test for yeasts and molds. *J Clin Microbiol* 2000;38(2):537–541.

375. Pfaller MA, Diekema DJ, Boyken L, et al. Evaluation of the Etest and disk diffusion methods for determining susceptibilities of 235 bloodstream isolates of *Candida glabrata* to fluconazole and voriconazole. *J Clin Microbiol* 2003;41(5):1875–1880.

376. Clancy CJ, Nguyen MH. Correlation between in vitro susceptibility determined by E test and response to therapy with amphotericin B: results from a multicenter prospective study of candidemia. *Antimicrob Agents Chemother* 1999;43(5):1289–1290.

377. Law D, Moore CB, Denning DW. Amphotericin B resistance testing of *Candida* spp.: a comparison of methods. *J Antimicrob Chemother* 1997;40(1):109–112.

378. Lozano-Chiu M, Paetznick VL, Ghannoum MA, et al. Detection of resistance to amphotericin B among *Cryptococcus neoformans* clinical isolates: performances of three different media assessed by using E-test and National Committee for Clinical Laboratory Standards M27-A methodologies. *J Clin Microbiol* 1998;36(10):2817–2822.

379. Wanger A, Mills K, Nelson PW, et al. Comparison of Etest and National Committee for Clinical Laboratory Standards broth macrodilution method for antifungal susceptibility testing: enhanced ability to detect amphotericin B-resistant *Candida* isolates. *Antimicrob Agents Chemother* 1995;39(11):2520–2522.

380. Chaturvedi V, Ramani R, Pfaller MA. Collaborative study of the NCCLS and flow cytometry methods for antifungal susceptibility testing of *Candida albicans*. *J Clin Microbiol* 2004;42(5):2249–2251.

381. Pfaller MA, Jones RN. Performance accuracy of antibacterial and antifungal susceptibility test methods: report from the College of American Pathologists Microbiology Surveys Program (2001-2003). *Arch Pathol Lab Med* 2006;130(6):767–778.

382. Pfaller MA, Yu WL. Antifungal susceptibility testing. New technology and clinical applications. *Infect Dis Clin North Am* 2001;15(4):1227–1261.

383. Arendrup MC, Cuenca-Estrella M, Lass-Florl C, et al. EUCAST technical note on the EUCAST definitive document EDef 7.2: method for the determination of broth dilution minimum inhibitory concentrations of antifungal agents for yeasts EDef 7.2 (EUCAST-AFST). *Clin Microbiol Infect* 2012;18(7):E246–E247.

384. Lass-Florl C, Arendrup MC, Rodriguez-Tudela JL, et al. EUCAST technical note on Amphotericin B. *Clin Microbiol Infect* 2011;17(12):E27–E29.

385. Arendrup MC, Cuenca-Estrella M, Donnelly JP, et al. EUCAST technical note on posaconazole. *Clin Microbiol Infect* 2011;17(11):E16–E17.

386. Arendrup MC, Rodriguez-Tudela JL, Lass-Florl C, et al. EUCAST technical note on anidulafungin. *Clin Microbiol Infect* 2011;17(11):E18–E20.

387. Subcommittee on Antifungal Susceptibility Testing of the ESCMID European Committee for Antimicrobial Susceptibility Testing. EUCAST technical note on voriconazole. *Clin Microbiol Infect* 2008;14(10):985–987.

388. European Committee on Antimicrobial Susceptibility Testing-Subcommittee on Antifungal Susceptibility Testing. EUCAST technical note on fluconazole. *Clin Microbiol Infect* 2008;14(2):193–195.

389. Subcommittee on Antifungal Susceptibility Testing of the ESCMID European Committee for Antimicrobial Susceptibility Testing. EUCAST definitive document EDef 7.1: method for the determination of broth dilution MICs of antifungal agents for fermentative yeasts. *Clin Microbiol Infect* 2008;14(4):398–405.

390. Cuenca-Estrella M, Arendrup MC, Chryssanthou E, et al. Multicentre determination of quality control strains and quality control ranges for antifungal susceptibility testing of yeasts and filamentous fungi using the methods of the Antifungal Susceptibility Testing Subcommittee of the European Committee on Antimicrobial Susceptibility Testing (AFST-EUCAST). *Clin Microbiol Infect* 2007;13(10):1018–1022.

391. Cuenca-Estrella M, Lee-Yang W, Ciblak MA, et al. Comparative evaluation of NCCLS M27-A and EUCAST broth microdilution procedures for antifungal susceptibility testing of candida species. *Antimicrob Agents Chemother* 2002;46(11):3644–3647.

392. Pfaller MA. Antifungal drug resistance: mechanisms, epidemiology, and consequences for treatment. *Am J Med* 2012;125(Suppl 1):S3–S13.

393. Hostetler JS, Heykants J, Clemons KV, et al. Discrepancies in bioassay and chromatography determinations explained by metabolism of itraconazole to hydroxyitraconazole: studies of interpatient variations in concentrations. *Antimicrob Agents Chemother* 1993; 37(10):2224–2227.

394. Perea S, Pennick GJ, Modak A, et al. Comparison of high-performance liquid chromatographic and microbiological methods for determination of voriconazole levels in plasma. *Antimicrob Agents Chemother* 2000;44(5):1209–1213.

395. Cleary JD, Chapman SW, Hardin TC, et al. Amphotericin B enzyme-linked immunoassay for clinical use: comparison with bioassay and HPLC. *Ann Pharmacother* 1997;31(1):39–44.

396. Decosterd LA, Rochat B, Pesse B, et al. Multiplex ultra-performance liquid chromatography-tandem mass spectrometry method for simultaneous quantification in human plasma of fluconazole, itraconazole, hydroxyitraconazole, posaconazole, voriconazole, voriconazole-N-oxide, anidulafungin, and caspofungin. *Antimicrob Agents Chemother* 2010;54(12):5303–5315.

397. Mikami Y, Sakamoto T, Yazawa K, et al. Comparison of in vitro antifungal activity of itraconazole and hydroxy-itraconazole by colorimetric MTT assay. *Mycoses* 1994;37(1–2):27–33.

398. Odds FC, Bossche HV. Antifungal activity of itraconazole compared with hydroxy-itraconazole in vitro. *J Antimicrob Chemother* 2000;45(3):371–373.

399. Cendejas-Bueno E, Forastiero A, Rodriguez-Tudela JL, et al. HPLC/UV or bioassay: two valid methods for posaconazole quantification in human serum samples. *Clin Microbiol Infect* 2012;18(12):1229–1235.

400. Enache-Angoulvant A, Hennequin C. Invasive *Saccharomyces* infection: a comprehensive review. *Clin Infect Dis* 2005;41(11):1559–1568.

401. da Matta VL, de Souza Carvalho Melhem M, Colombo AL, et al. Antifungal drug susceptibility profile of *Pichia anomala* isolates from patients presenting with nosocomial fungemia. *Antimicrob Agents Chemother* 2007;51(4):1573–1576.

402. Paphitou NI, Ostrosky-Zeichner L, Paetznick VL, et al. In vitro antifungal susceptibilities of *Trichosporon* species. *Antimicrob Agents Chemother* 2002;46(4): 1144–1146.

Chapter 7

Antimicrobial Susceptibility Testing for Some Atypical Microorganisms (*Chlamydia, Mycoplasma, Rickettsia, Ehrlichia, Coxiella*, and Spirochetes)

Jean-Marc Rolain

This chapter discusses susceptibility testing for fastidious organisms, including mycoplasmas (1), *Borrelia burgdorferi* (2), *Leptospira*, and those that cannot be cultured without the use of animals or tissue culture (*Chlamydia, Rickettsia, Ehrlichia,* and *Coxiella burnetii*). The special testing requirements using cells make it very difficult for all but research laboratories to perform susceptibility testing of these organisms. Thus, the susceptibility testing that has been done has been somewhat limited in terms of both the number of isolates tested and the number of different antiinfective agents evaluated. Furthermore, frequently, only well-characterized laboratory strains have been tested rather than recent clinical isolates.

Nonetheless, continual progress is being made in the use of tissue culture for some of these highly fastidious agents, such as *Treponema pallidum* (3), and it should soon be possible to carry out more extensive studies. Expanding the range of studies will certainly be important, because resistance will continue to remain unconfirmed if testing is not carried out (4). This will be true even if resistance is suspected from observations of patients, as was true in the case of a *T. pallidum* infection (135).

The complexity of the methods needed to propagate these organisms argues for an attempt to standardize the methods used for susceptibility testing. In the case of chlamydiae, standardization should be possible, but despite the many different techniques used for the testing of chlamydiae, the results obtained have been remarkably consistent (6).

Nonetheless, greater uniformity of testing techniques would make it easier to compare results obtained in different laboratories. European guidelines for susceptibility testing of intracellular and cell-associated pathogens have been recently published and should be used by laboratories to allow comparison of the results obtained (7).

Since the previous publication of this chapter, new information has been published on the susceptibility of chlamydiae, mycoplasmas, and rickettsiae, especially by the use of new quantitative real-time polymerase chain reaction (PCR) methods. Moreover, recent breakthroughs have occurred leading to the development of new axenic culture for intracellular bacteria including *Tropheryma whipplei* and *Coxiella burnetii* that will open the way in the future for development of new axenic media for these intracellular bacteria to facilitate antibiotic susceptibility testing (8). Resistance to antimicrobials has been infrequent among the organisms considered in this chapter, although resistance of genital mycoplasmas to tetracycline has been reported (9), as well as resistance of *Chlamydia trachomatis* to erythromycin and tetracycline (10,11).

CHLAMYDIAE

Chlamydiae are obligate intracellular bacteria that undergo a complex growth cycle. Three human pathogens, *C. trachomatis* (4), *Chlamydia psittaci* (12), and *Chlamydia pneumoniae* (TWAR) (13), occur in this genus of obligate, intracellular parasites. *C. trachomatis* is a major human pathogen and is probably the most prevalent sexually transmitted pathogen in the United States (14), *C. psittaci* is a mainly animal pathogen that occasionally causes pneumonia in humans (15), and *C. pneumoniae* is an important cause of community-acquired respiratory infections and is responsible for an average of 10% of cases of pneumonia and 5% of cases of bronchitis and sinusitis. Although many research groups perform antimicrobial susceptibility testing of *Chlamydia* organisms, there is not a standardized methodology or a uniformly accepted interpretation of results. The techniques used for susceptibility testing of these organisms is similar and involve inoculating cell monolayers with the bacteria and incubating them in the presence of serial dilutions of antibiotic (16). However, detection of bacteria varied from enumeration of bacterial inclusions after staining (Giemsa or immunofluorescence) to quantification using reverse transcriptase-polymerase chain reaction (RT-PCR) (17) or flow cytometry (18). Because of the importance of these pathogens in human disease, susceptibility testing of *Chlamydia* has been extensive (Table 7.1)

Cell Lines and Organism

A number of different cell lines have been used to propagate *C. trachomatis*, including McCoy, HeLa 229, and BHK-21 (clone 13). According to a recent study, it seems that the recommended cell line for susceptibility testing for *C. trachomatis* should be the McCoy line, and Hep-2 should be used for *C. pneumoniae*. To render these cells more susceptible to infection, a variety of treatments have been employed, including cycloheximide, diethylaminoethyl (DEAE)-dextran, 5-iodo-2-deoxyuridine, cytochalasin B, and irradiation. However, there is general agreement that the treatment of choice is cycloheximide. Cycloheximide is used at a concentration of 0.5 to 2.0 g/mL. Each lot should be tested for potency by dose-response curve analysis because this varies, and the optimum concentration for any lot can be determined only by experimentation. An acceptable growth medium is Minimum Essential Eagle Medium (EMEM) supplemented with 2 mmol/L glutamine, 4.4% (wt/vol) sodium bicarbonate, and 10% (vol/vol) fetal bovine serum (19).

McCoy cells should undergo at least two passages in an antibiotic-free medium to ensure that all traces of antibiotic in the growth medium have been removed. Some investigators carry out 10 to 15 passages in antibiotic-free medium before using the cells for susceptibility testing (4,19). When microdilution plates are used, the cells are seeded at a concentration of 3×10^5 cells per well, and the plates are incubated for 48 to 72 hours, at the end of which time the cells should have formed a subconfluent monolayer (4).

Despite the widespread use of HeLa and McCoy cells for susceptibility studies with *C. trachomatis*, these cells may not provide a relevant in vitro environment for such testing. This was demonstrated in a publication by Wyrick et al. (20), who showed that the minimal inhibitory concentration (MIC) for azithromycin was substantially lower with polarized human endometrial gland epithelial cells than with similar nonpolarized cells (0.125 g/mL and 0.5 g/mL, respectively). This was later confirmed by Paul et al. (21). However, the use of such cells is still not practical for most laboratories, and further work will have to be done to determine whether the extra effort of employing such cell systems is going to yield results that are more clinically relevant.

Chlamydial organisms should undergo at least one passage in antibiotic-free tissue culture cells, and sufficiently high-titered pools should be developed so that 10^2 to 10^3 inclusion-forming units (IFU) per coverslip are achieved. Because relatively little variation in susceptibility has been seen among different clinical isolates, investigators either have used well-characterized laboratory isolates (19) or recent clinical isolates (22–25). The latter are preferable if an attempt is being made to detect whether resistance is developing in current clinical isolates.

Antimicrobial Susceptibility Testing

Some workers prefer 1-dram shell vials, as opposed to microdilution plates, because the larger surface area of the coverslips (diameters vary from 10 to 12 mm) used with the vials makes it somewhat easier to detect low numbers of inclusions. The larger area provides greater assurance that a valid end point (MIC) will be obtained. On the other hand, if one uses high-titered pools of chlamydiae so that 10^2 to 10^3 IFU per coverslip are achieved, there is no reason why microdilution plates with 96 wells cannot be used (4,26). An alternative is to use 24-well plates with wells of a 13-mm diameter, which effectively circumvents the problem of too small a surface area (27). Probably, perfectly

Table 7.1

Antimicrobial Susceptibility of *Chlamydia trachomatis* and *Chlamydia pneumoniae*

Drug	C. trachomatis MIC (µg/mL)	References	C. pneumoniae MIC (µg/mL)	References
Aminoglycosides				
Gentamicin	500	(145)	ND	ND
Kanamycin	>100	(146)	ND	ND
Spectinomycin	250	(147)	ND	ND
Trospectomycin	3.5–12.5	(147)	10–20	(16)
Cephalosporins				
Cefamandole	256–1,024	(148)	ND	ND
Cefoperazone	16–32	(149)	ND	ND
Cefotaxime	≥64	(150)	ND	ND
Cefoxitin	1,024–2,048	(148)	ND	ND
Cefsulodin	≥128	(149)	ND	ND
Ceftriaxone	8–16	(151)	ND	ND
Cephalothin	16	(151)	ND	ND
Moxalactam	≥128	(149)	ND	ND
Macrolides				
Azithromycin	0.03–1 (azi)	(152,153)	0.06–1	(152,154)
Clarithromycin	0.002–0.008	(155)	0.004–0.25	(156)
Erythromycin	0.1–1	(145)	0.01–0.25	(153)
Josamycin	0.032	(39)	0.25	(156)
Roxithromycin	≤0.125	(157,158)	0.125–0.25	(28)
Telithromycin	ND	ND	0.031–0.25	(159)
Cethromycin	ND	ND	0.016–0.031	(160)
Penicillins				
Amoxicillin	2->4	(145)	ND	ND
Ampicillin	0.5–50	(161)	>100	(16)
Penicillin	1–10	(161)	>500	(162)
Piperacillin	≥4,096	(148)	ND	ND
Ticarcillin	>960	(30)	ND	ND
Quinolones				
Ciprofloxacin	0.5–2	(163,37)	0.25–4 (cip)	(163)
Difloxacin	0.125–0.25	(37)	ND	ND
Enoxacin	3.13–6.25	(164)	ND	ND
Fleroxacin	3.13–6.25	(164)	2–8	(67)
Garenoxacin	0.007–0.03	(129)	0.015–0.03	(129,165)
Gatifloxacin	0.06–0.25	(166)	0.06–0.25	(166,167)
Gemifloxacin	ND	ND	0.06–0.25	(167)
Grepafloxacin	0.06–0.125	(159)	0.06–0.5	(163,167)
Levofloxacin	0.25–0.5	(163)	0.25–1	(163,167)

(Continued)

Table 7.1 (Continued)

Antimicrobial Susceptibility of *Chlamydia trachomatis* and *Chlamydia pneumoniae*

Drug	C. trachomatis MIC (μg/mL)	References	C. pneumoniae MIC (μg/mL)	References
Moxifloxacin	0.06–0.125	(163)	0.125–1	(163,167)
Nalidixic acid	>50	(168)	ND	ND
Norfloxacin	8≥16	(169)	ND	ND
Ofloxacin	1	(19,158)	0.5–2	(67,170)
Pefloxacin	4	(39)	ND	ND
Sparfloxacin	0.03–0.06	(163,171)	0.06–0.5	(163,170)
Temafloxacin	0.125–0.25	(169)	0.125–4	(172)
Trovafloxacin	0.031–1	(173)	0.5–1	(172)
Tetracyclines				
Chlortetracycline	0.125–2.5	(174)	ND	ND
Doxycycline	0.012–0.025	(168)	0.05–0.5	(172,175)
Minocycline	0.025–0.05	(164)	0.0075–0.015	(176)
Tetracycline	0.3	(19)	0.05–1	(28,86)
Sulfamethoxazole	50	(146)	>500	(28)
Miscellaneous				
Chloramphenicol	2–4	(38)	ND	ND
Clindamycin	2–16	(177)	ND	ND
Imipenem	32	(149)	ND	ND
Metronidazole	>5,000	(145)	ND	ND
Rifampin	0.005–0.25	(178)	0.005–0.031	(162,179)
Trimethoprim	>100	(146)	>400	(40)
Cotrimoxazole	0.03/0.6–32/640	(26)	>400	(40)
Vancomycin	1.000	(180)	ND	ND

ND, not determined.

valid results can be obtained with microdilution plates, and if larger numbers of clinical isolates are to be tested or if larger numbers of compounds are to be evaluated, then the use of microdilution plates (or plates with at least 24 wells) is the only practical alternative.

Recommended Technique: Microdilution Plate Method

Prior to inoculation, the monolayers are exposed to DEAE-dextran at a concentration of 30 g/mL for 10 to 30 minutes (4,28). Each of the 24-well plates is inoculated with an inoculum of chlamydiae that yields 5×10^3 IFU/mL. The infectious inoculum (0.1 mL) is centrifuged onto the monolayer at 1,200 g for 60 minutes at room temperature. This centrifugation step is essential to infect cells with all *C. trachomatis* strains other than those that cause lymphogranuloma venereum. After centrifugation, the growth medium is removed and replaced with EMEM supplemented with glucose (5 mg/L), cycloheximide (generally 1 mg/L), 3% fetal bovine serum, and serial twofold dilutions of each antibiotic to be tested (19). All tests are performed in triplicate. The plates are then incubated at 35°C in a CO_2 incubator for 48 to 72 hours. Then the coverslips are removed from the wells, fixed in absolute methanol-acetone, and stained (4,28).

Detection of Inclusions

Most investigators who have done susceptibility testing of *C. trachomatis* have used iodine staining for the detection of inclusions (6). One of the major disadvantages of this stain is that the inclusions may not be detected if they are particularly small or aberrant in shape. Aberrantly shaped inclusions are particularly common when *C. trachomatis* is cultured in the presence of β-lactam antibiotics (29). Giemsa staining has also been used, but it is evident that either direct or indirect fluorescent staining of the monolayers is the most sensitive method for detecting chlamydial antigen in cell monolayers (4,19,29). Initially, fluorescent staining for susceptibility testing used an indirect fluorescent antibody technique employing a polyclonal antibody raised in a rabbit against the same serovar E strain used in the susceptibility studies (30). However, with the availability of fluorescein-conjugated monoclonal antibodies (Syva, Palo Alto, CA; Ortho Clinical Diagnostics, Raritan, NJ; or Kallestad, Chaska, MN) to *C. trachomatis*, direct fluorescent staining has become the method of choice for detecting chlamydial antigen in tissue culture (4,22–24,26,31–37). In using fluorescent stains, the manufacturers' directions should be followed. When Giemsa staining and direct immunofluorescent (using the Syva monoclonal antibody) techniques were compared, it was evident that the MICs obtainable with the monoclonal antibody were about two times higher than those obtained with Giemsa staining (29). Enzyme-linked immunosorbent assays (ELISA) have also been used to detect chlamydial antigen, and these yield MIC values comparable to those obtained with the immunofluorescent method (38). A commercially available enzyme immunoassay (Chlamydiazyme; Abbott Laboratories, North Chicago, IL) has also been used to detect antigen, and the results were similar to those obtained using a genus-specific monoclonal antibody (Ortho Clinical Diagnostics) in an immunoperoxidase test (39).

The MIC is defined as the lowest concentration of antibiotic that completely inhibits inclusion formation after 48 to 72 hours of incubation, and the minimal bactericidal concentration (MBC) is defined as the lowest concentration of antibiotic that completely inhibits the development of inclusions when the cells are disrupted at 48 to 72 hours and passed into tissue culture medium that is free of antibiotics.

Other Assays

Antibiotic susceptibility testing for *Chlamydia* has also been performed using flow cytometry (18).

In this assay, evaluation of antibiotic activity was done at the 25-hour time point, and cells were best permeabilized using the Ortho/Permeafix treatment. The mean fluorescence intensity (MFI) of cells was determined by this method after staining of chlamydial inclusions with an anti-*Chlamydia* fluorescent monoclonal antibody. Calculation of the inhibitory concentration 50 (IC_{50}), defined as the antibiotic concentration required to reduce the drug-free control MFI by 50%, by flow cytometry allowed a more objective and precise evaluation of antibiotic activity than MIC (18).

Finally, an RT-PCR–based method has been developed for antimicrobial susceptibility testing of *C. pneumoniae* (40) and *C. trachomatis* (17). The results obtained in these studies were in the range previously reported using immunofluorescent staining, and the MICs obtained by RT-PCR were consistently higher (17,40). The advantage of the RT-PCR technique over ordinary PCR methods is that only viable organisms will produce RNA.

Results of Susceptibility Testing

Table 7.1 presents the results of MICs of antimicrobial agents against *C. trachomatis* and *C. pneumoniae* indicating the intense interest in antimicrobials with activity against these important human pathogens. In Table 7.1, as in all subsequent tables, a range is given for the MIC values, except in those instances when so few isolates were studied that only a single MIC value is available. Aminoglycosides are without any activity and can therefore be incorporated into tissue culture media used for the isolation of this organism. β-Lactamine compounds, chloramphenicol, clindamycin, imipenem, metronidazole, and vancomycin are not active against *Chlamydia*. The β-lactams result in the formation of aberrant inclusions but lack significant activity. Susceptibility of *C. pneumoniae* is similar to that of *C. trachomatis*, except that *C. pneumoniae* is resistant to sulfonamides. The most active agents against *Chlamydia* are the macrolides, tetracyclines, rifampin, and fluoroquinolones. However, rifampin is not used clinically because resistance develops rapidly in vitro (41).

Antimicrobial Resistance

The development of significant resistance to currently used antimicrobials has not been a problem in human isolates, although relative resistance to sulfonamides, erythromycin, rifamycins, and fluoroquinolones has been reported for *C. trachomatis* (10,11,42,43), arguing for the continued surveillance of current clinical isolates. One potential explanation for the lack of resistance by chlamydiae is their unique life cycle (5). However, resistance to tetracycline in swine *Chlamydia suis* has been reported in the Midwestern United States (44,45). Despite the lack of evidence for frequent resistance in chlamydiae in human isolates, it is clearly possible to induce resistance in the laboratory by serial passages of organisms in subinhibitory concentrations of antimicrobials (46).

MYCOPLASMAS

Disease in humans is associated with at least four *Mycoplasma* species: respiratory infections with *Mycoplasma pneumoniae* and urogenital infections with *Mycoplasma hominis*, *Mycoplasma genitalium*, and *Ureaplasma urealyticum*. Finally, *Mycoplasma fermentans* has been isolated from patients with AIDS, and there has been conjecture about the possible role of these mycoplasmas as cofactors in the disease caused by HIV. *M. fermentans* has also been detected in some cases of fatal respiratory distress in immunocompetent adults (47).

The main structural characteristic of mycoplasmas is their lack of a cell wall, which makes them naturally resistant to β-lactams and all antibiotics that target the cell wall, including glycopeptides and polymyxins and agents that interfere with the synthesis of folic acid (9).

The techniques for isolating and identifying these agents are well known (48), but the techniques for performing antimicrobial susceptibility studies are less well defined (1). Both the agar dilution (49) and broth dilution (50) methods have their proponents. The two methods may yield quite disparate results for certain antibiotics, and so it is always important to consider the method used when evaluating the results of susceptibility studies (51).

A particular problem with each is that there is some drift of end points with time (a progressive increase in MIC values with prolonged incubation), as long incubation times are required for most mycoplasmas because of their slow growth. One of the probable reasons for the phenomenon of drift is that antibiotic inactivation occurs during incubation.

One advantage of the agar method is that in a mixture of sensitive and resistant strains, the two types of strains can be differentiated. With the broth method, differentiation is impossible

without the cloning of isolates (49). On the other hand, from a purely clinical standpoint, it is probably of little importance to detect a mixture of resistant and susceptible strains, although it could be of considerable research interest (52).

Tanner et al. (53) adapted commercially available Sensititre broth microdilution plates for the susceptibility testing of *Mycoplasma hyopneumoniae*, and this technique was also successfully employed by Poulin et al. (54) for testing AIDS-associated mycoplasmas. The technique yields results comparable to those obtained with the macrodilution method.

Limb et al. (55) have utilized the measurement of ATP bioluminescence for the susceptibility testing of mycoplasmas. Using this technique, they were able to demonstrate good correlation with conventional methods and could achieve results within 6 hours.

Media and Organisms

Actively growing broth cultures are frozen at −70°C. A suitable medium for *M. pneumoniae*, *M. fermentans*, *Mycoplasma incognitus*, and *M. genitalium* is SP-4 medium (56), and a suitable medium for both of the genital mycoplasmas is 10-B broth. 10-B broth is usually made with penicillin, which should be omitted in susceptibility testing. Commercially prepared 10-B broth, as well as other specialized media for the isolation and propagation of mycoplasmas, may be obtained from commercial sources (e.g., Regional Media Laboratories, Lenexa, KS) and can be ordered without antibiotics for susceptibility testing.

For the culture of *M. hominis*, arginine, rather than urea, is incorporated into the medium (48). An aliquot of the culture is thawed, and serial dilutions are carried out to determine how many color changing units (CCUs) are present per milliliter. One CCU is the minimum inoculum required to produce enough growth to cause a color change in the phenol red indicator.

Antimicrobial Susceptibility Testing

The authors favor the broth dilution technique because it can be carried out in microdilution plates, allowing relatively large numbers of isolates to be tested against a reasonable number of different antimicrobials (57). Furthermore, the technique is adaptable for a variety of mycoplasmas, and when tests are carried out in triplicate, very good reproducibility is noted (57,58).

In the case of *U. urealyticum*, there has been good agreement noted between the more laborious tube dilution technique and the microdilution technique (59). Furthermore, both the MIC and the MBC can be determined using the broth dilution technique, whereas only the MIC can be determined using the agar dilution technique. Finally, the antibiotic broth dilution technique is really just an adaptation of the metabolic inhibition test (48), which has been used for identifying and serotyping mycoplasmas as well as for serodiagnosis. For this reason, laboratories may already be familiar with the basic components of the broth dilution technique.

The metabolic inhibition technique depends on the presence of either antibodies or, in the case of susceptibility testing, antimicrobials inhibiting the growth of the mycoplasmas. Inhibition of growth is detected by the lack of color change of a pH indicator, generally phenol red. Suitable substrates are included in the growth medium for the varying mycoplasmas: glucose in the case of *M. pneumoniae*, arginine for *M. hominis*, and urea for *U. urealyticum*.

Recommended Technique: Broth Dilution Technique

The broth dilution method is performed in 96-well plates with a volume of 200 μL in each well. Each stock antibiotic is added in a volume of 0.025 mL to a well of a microdilution plate, generally in triplicate (1,57). An aliquot of a previously frozen (−70°C), actively growing broth culture is thawed on the day of the assay and added to 50 mL of the appropriate broth medium (SP-4 for *M. pneumoniae* and 10-B broth for *M. hominis* and *U. urealyticum*) for each antibiotic to be tested. The stock culture is diluted to yield 10^3 to 10^4 organisms per microdilution well. To further establish how many CCUs have been added to each well, 10-fold dilutions of the inoculum are made to verify that at least 10^3 CCUs but no more than 10^5 CCUs have been added to each well. Inoculated broths are incubated for 2 hours at 37°C before these broths are added to the microdilution plates. Mycoplasma suspensions are added in 0.175-mL aliquots to each well containing antibiotics. The plates are sealed in plastic bags containing sterile gauze moistened with distilled water and are incubated at 35°C to 37°C under atmospheric conditions.

Three controls are included: (a) a broth control with no mycoplasmas, (b) a drug control consisting of the maximum drug concentration tested in broth alone, and (c) a mycoplasma control consisting of the mycoplasma suspension alone in a total of 0.2 mL of broth. Plates are examined after 17 to 20 hours of incubation and once daily until growth is noted in the mycoplasma control well. The MIC will be generally available for *U. urealyticum* at 24 hours, for *M. hominis* at 48 hours, and for *M. pneumoniae* after 5 or more days.

Determination of Minimal Inhibitory Concentration and Minimal Bactericidal Concentration

With SP-4 medium and 10-B broth, growth of *U. urealyticum* sufficient for determination of the MIC occurs overnight. Comparable times are 24 to 48 hours for *M. hominis* and 3 to 5 days for *M. pneumoniae*. Often, investigators determine both initial and final MICs (57); the initial MIC is the minimum amount of antibiotic required to inhibit any color change of the broth when the control well (containing organisms but no antibiotic) first shows a color change, and the final MIC is the minimum concentration of antibiotic that prevents a color change over a period of 2 consecutive days. The final MIC is employed with mycoplasmas because of their slow growth characteristics, which result in the drift of the MIC. In fact, the final MIC may be as much as eight times higher than the initial MIC for some antimicrobials (57).

It is also possible to determine the MBC, by diluting the broth from wells showing no color change in antibiotic-free medium. Generally, this is a 20-fold dilution, which is usually sufficient to dilute the antibiotic to a level below the antibiotic's MIC value (1), but hopefully not to a point where organisms can no longer be detected. An alternate method avoids these possible pitfalls by filtering the broth from wells with no color change through a filter with a pore size of 220 nm, washing the filter free of residual antibiotic, and culturing the filter (60). Using the latter technique, Taylor-Robinson and Furr (60) were able to show that the macrolide rosaramicin acted in a purely mycoplasmastatic fashion on some ureaplasmas.

In the case of ureaplasmas, there is a self-sterilizing effect, so that by 24 hours, there is often a precipitous fall in the number of organisms (1). Because Taylor-Robinson and Furr (60) showed that there is no change in the MIC values for these organisms between 5 and 25 hours, subculturing for the determination of MBC values can be done as early as 5 hours, which avoids any problems that may be caused by the self-sterilizing phenomenon (1).

Results of Susceptibility Testing

The results of susceptibility testing on mycoplasmas are summarized in Tables 7.2 and 7.3. Mycoplasmas lack peptidoglycan and penicillin-binding proteins and thus are naturally resistant to β-lactam antibiotics. Moreover, they are also resistant to rifampin, owing to the particular structure of their RNA polymerase, and also to polymyxins, nalidixic acid, sulfonamides, and trimethoprim. Tetracyclines, erythromycin, clindamycin, chloramphenicol, aminoglycosides, and

fluoroquinolones have been shown to have activity against one or more mycoplasmal species (61).

Mycoplasma pneumoniae

Erythromycin and tetracyclines are usually active against *M. pneumoniae*. Resistance to erythromycin has now been described (62,63), although resistance to tetracycline has not been documented (64). Azithromycin and telithromycin are more active against *M. pneumoniae* in vitro than erythromycin, clarithromycin, or roxithromycin (32,65,66). Fluoroquinolone compounds are also active against *M. pneumoniae*, but in vitro studies have shown that they are not as effective as macrolides (67–69). Clinical strains with acquired

Table 7.2

Antimicrobial Susceptibility of *Mycoplasma pneumoniae*

Drug	MIC (μg/mL)	References
Aminoglycosides		
Gentamicin	0.3–0.8	(181)
Kanamycin	3.1–6.3	(181)
Streptomycin	0.15–0.2	(181)
Macrolides		
Azithromycin	0.008–0.12	(61,66,182,183)
Clarithromycin	0.015–0.06	(65,66,182)
Erythromycin	0.03–0.12	(182,184)
Josamycin	0.03–0.12	(66,182,184)
Roxithromycin	0.06–0.25	(182,185)
Telithromycin	0.008–0.06	(182,185)
Quinolones		
Ciprofloxacin	0.5–4	(50,186,187)
Gatifloxacin	0.25–1	(187)
Grepafloxacin	0.06–0.25	(187)
Levofloxacin	0.06–2	(50,187)
Moxifloxacin	0.016–0.125	(50,187)
Ofloxacin	1	(188)
Sparfloxacin	0.125–0.25	(50,187)
Trovafloxacin	0.12–0.5	(187)
Tetracyclines		
Chloramphenicol	0.8–2.4	(50,181)
Doxycycline	0.016–0.5	(189)
Minocycline	0.25–1	(187)
Tetracycline	0.5–2	(187)

Table 7.3

Antimicrobial Susceptibility of *Mycoplasma hominis* and *Ureaplasma urealyticum*				
	M. hominis		**U. urealyticum**	
Drug	**MIC (μg/mL)**	**References**	**MIC (μg/mL)**	**References**
Macrolides				
Azithromycin	16–32	(182)	0.125–4	(50,182)
Clarithromycin	>32	(182)	≤0.06–2	(50,182)
Erythromycin	>32	(182)	0.125–8	(50,182)
Josamycin	0.25–0.5	(182)	0.5–2	(182)
Roxithromycin	>32	(182)	1–4	(182)
Telithromycin	16–32	(182)	0.06–0.25	(182)
Quinolones				
Ciprofloxacin	0.016–1	(50,182)	1–16	(50)
Gatifloxacin	0.06–0.25	(182)	1–2	(182)
Levofloxacin	0.016–2	(50,182)	0.25–2	(50,182)
Moxifloxacin	≤0.008–0.06	(94,182)	0.03–1	(50,182)
Ofloxacin	0.5–1	(190)	1–4	(182,190)
Sparfloxacin	≤0.008–0.125	(50,182)	0.06–2	(50,182)
Trovafloxacin	0.015–0.125	(182)	0.06–5	(190)
Tetracyclines				
Doxycycline	0.03–2	(192)	1–2	(192)
Minocycline	0.06–0.5[a]	(182)	0.06–0.5	(182)
Tetracycline	0.5–4[a]	(182)	0.5–4	(182)
Chloramphenicol	4–25	(191)	NA	

[a]Tetracycline-susceptible strains (resistant strains had MICs >32 μg/mL).

resistance to macrolides have recently emerged worldwide with resistances to erythromycin and azithromycin mainly due to mutations in 23S rRNA (64).

Mycoplasma hominis

M. hominis is usually naturally susceptible to tetracyclines but tetracycline-resistant isolates containing DNA sequences homologous to the streptococcal determinant *tetM* have been reported (52). It has been convincingly demonstrated that *tetM* is not a plasmid and that it is present in both species of genital mycoplasmas. Resistance to tetracycline in vitro is associated with failure of tetracycline treatment to eradicate *M. hominis* (9). A recent study from Germany has shown that the prevalence of resistance to tetracyclines and fluoroquinolones has increased between 1989 and 2004,

but doxycycline still remains the drug of choice for the treatment (70). The new glycylcyclines have been shown to be active in vitro against *M. hominis* strains resistant to other tetracyclines. Because of this emerging resistance, it is proving to be increasingly difficult to devise suitable antimicrobial regimens for the effective therapy of genital mycoplasma infections (9,71–73). Clindamycin can be used for the treatment of *M. hominis* infections resistant to tetracyclines, and erythromycin or quinolones can be used for tetracycline-resistant *U. urealyticum* infections (9,39). Usually, fluoroquinolone compounds are active against *M. hominis*, but resistance to fluoroquinolones has been reported and is associated with mutations in DNA gyrase (74). A fatal case of a disseminated infection with clindamycin and ciprofloxacin-resistant *M. hominis* has been recently reported in Germany (75). *M. hominis* is resistant to erythromycin, roxithromycin, azithromycin, and clarithromycin but remains susceptible to josamycin (Table 7.3).

Ureaplasma urealyticum

Tetracyclines and fluoroquinolone compounds are active against *U. urealyticum*. Erythromycin is generally active against ureaplasmas, but resistance has been noted (14) and is associated with specific mutations in the 23S rRNA gene (76).

RICKETTSIA

All members of the genus *Rickettsia* are obligate, gram-negative, intracellular bacteria. The genus comprises typhus group rickettsiae, which include *Rickettsia prowazekii*, the agent of epidemic typhus, and *Rickettsia typhi*, the agent of murine typhus; *Orientia tsutsugamushi*, the agent of scrub typhus (77); and spotted fever group (SFG) rickettsiae. The number of recognized SFG rickettsioses has recently increased. The six SFG rickettsioses previously described are Rocky Mountain spotted fever, caused by *Rickettsia rickettsii*; Mediterranean spotted fever, caused by *Rickettsia conorii* subsp *conorii*; Siberian tick typhus, caused by *Rickettsia sibirica* subsp *sibirica*; Israeli spotted fever, caused by *R. conorii* subsp *israelensis* (77); Queensland tick typhus, caused by *Rickettsia australis*; and rickettsialpox, caused by *Rickettsia akari*. Since 1984, 12 new SFG rickettsiosis have been described (77): the Japanese or Oriental spotted fever, caused by *Rickettsia japonica* and described in 1984; Flinders Island spotted fever, caused by *Rickettsia honei* and described in 1991; Astrakhan fever, caused by *R. conorii* subsp *caspia* and reported in 1991; African tick-bite fever, caused by *Rickettsia africae* and described in 1992; a new spotted fever due to *Rickettsia mongolitimonae*, reported in France in 1996; *Rickettsia slovaca* infection, reported in 1997; *Rickettsia helvetica* infection, described in 2000; flea-borne rickettsioses, caused by *Rickettsia felis* and reported in 2001; *Rickettsia aeschlimannii* infection, reported in 2001; *Rickettsia heilongjiangensis* infection; *Rickettsia parkeri* infection, reported in 2003; *Rickettsia massiliae*; and *Rickettsia marmionii* (77).

All of the members of the genus *Rickettsia* are obligate intracellular pathogens and, therefore, require either animal models, embryonated eggs, or tissue culture for susceptibility assays (78). It would appear that, of the in vitro techniques now available, the plaque assay and a colorimetric assay (78) are the most practical for evaluating antiinfectives for this group of organisms. However, because of the technical difficulties in working with these agents, susceptibility testing will probably be confined to relatively few laboratories. Furthermore, it is evident that when in vivo techniques, such as suppression of lethality in chicken embryos, are compared with in vitro techniques, such as the plaque assay, the results may be somewhat discrepant (79). The two assays (plaque assay and colorimetric assay) depend on the induction of cytopathic effects and plaque formation in cell cultures by the rickettsiae, but some rickettsiae do not normally cause cytopathic effects in primary cultures (80,81). Recently, Ives et al. (82,83) described a new assay that uses immunofluorescent staining, which avoids the problem of a lack of cytopathic effects. Very recently, we have developed a new quantitative PCR DNA assay using the LightCycler system for the evaluation of antibiotic susceptibilities of three rickettsial species, including *R. felis*, a rickettsial species that does not induce plaque in cell cultures (81).

Cell Lines and Organisms

Organisms used for these studies are laboratory strains. For example, in the case of *R. rickettsii*, the Sheila Smith strain is used (78), and for *R. conorii*, the American Type Culture Collection VR 141 Moroccan strain is used (84). Only a few studies on in vitro antibiotic susceptibilities of SFG rickettsiae other than *R. conorii*, *R. rickettsii*, and *R. akari* are available. We recently reported an extensive study that investigated the reaction of 27 rickettsiae to 13 antimicrobials (Table 7.4) (80).

Antimicrobial Susceptibility Testing

Reference Method: Plaque Assay

Vero cell monolayers seeded 24 hours before use in round, plastic, tissue culture Petri dishes (60 mm; Corning Glass Works, Corning, NY) are infected with 1 mL of a solution containing 4×10^3 plaque-forming units (PFU) of the desired rickettsial strain (78). After 1 hour of incubation at room temperature (22°C), the plates are overlaid with 4 mL of a medium containing Minimum Essential Eagle Medium (Gibco Laboratories, Grand Island, NY), 2% newborn calf serum, 2% (*N*-[2-hydroxyethyl]) piperazine-*N'*-[2-ethanesulfonic acid]) (HEPES, Sigma-Aldrich, St. Louis, MO), and 0.5% agar. The antibiotic solutions are added to the medium

Table 7.4

Antimicrobial Susceptibility of *Rickettsia*[a]

Strain	Doxy	Thiam	Rifam	Ery	Clar	Josa	Prist	Cip	Ofl	Pef
R. prowazekii	0.06	2	0.06	0.125	0.5	0.5	4	0.5	1	1
R. typhi	0.125	1	0.25	0.5	1	1	2	1	1	1
R. akari	0.06	1	0.25	8	2	1	4	0.5	0.5	1
R. conorii Seven	0.06–0.125	1–2	0.125	8	1	0.5	1–2	0.5	1	0.5–1
R. conorii strain Moroccan	0.06–0.125	1–2	0.25	4	2	1	2	0.25	1	0.5–1
R. conorii serotype Israeli	0.06	1	0.5	4	1	0.5	1	0.5	1	1
R. conorii serotype Astrakhan	0.06	0.5	0.03	8	0.5	0.5	2	0.5	0.5	0.5
R. sibirica	0.06	0.5	0.06	2	2	1	2	0.5	1	1
R. australis	0.06	2	0.125	8	4	0.5	2	0.5	1	1
R. japonica	0.125	1	0.25	8	1	1	8	0.5	1	1
R. honei	0.06	2	0.5	4	1	0.5	2	0.5	1	1
R. africae	0.125	1	0.125	8	2	0.5	2	0.5	1	1
R. "mongolitimonae"	0.125	1	0.125	8	4	1	2	0.5	1	1
R. slovaca	0.06	1	0.5	2	0.5	1	1	0.5	1	1
R. felis	0.06–0.125	1–2	0.06–0.25	16	ND	ND	ND	0.05–1	0.05–1	ND
R. bellii	0.125	0.5	0.06	4	4	1	2	0.5	0.5	1
R. canada	0.06	1	0.125	4	1	1	2	0.5	0.5	1
R. helvetica	0.125	1	0.06	2	1	0.5	2	0.25	0.5	1
R. parkeri	0.25	4	0.25	4	1	0.5	2	0.25	0.25	0.5
Thai tick typhus rickettsia	0.06	2	0.125	8	1	1	4	0.5	2	1
Strain Bar29	0.06	1	2	4	2	0.5	4	0.25	0.5	0.5
R. massiliae	0.06	1	2	2	1	1	1	0.25	0.5	0.5
R. aeschlimannii	0.06	1	2	8	1	0.5	2	0.5	0.5	1
R. montana	0.125	2	2	8	1	2	4	1	1	1
R. rhipicephali	0.25	1	2	4	1	1	2	1	1	1

[a]Susceptibility is given in terms of MIC (µg/mL).
Clar, clarithromycin; Cip, ciprofloxacin; Doxy, doxycycline; Ery, erythromycin; Josa, josamycin; ND, not determined; Ofl, ofloxacin; Pef, pefloxacin; Prist, pristinamycin; Rifam, rifampin; Thiam, thiamphenicol.

to obtain the desired final concentrations (an antibiotic-free control plate is also included), and the plates are incubated for 4 to 7 days at 35°C in a CO_2 incubator. All antibiotics are assayed in triplicate, at a minimum. After incubation, the monolayers are fixed with 4% formaldehyde and stained with 1% crystal violet in 20% ethanol. The MIC is the lowest concentration of the agent tested causing complete inhibition of plaque formation, compared with the drug-free controls. Plates may then be photographed to obtain a permanent record of the results. The major problem with this technique is that some rickettsial strains may not induce the formation of plaques in cell cultures. In this case, several passages in various cell lines may allow selection of variants able to produce plaques.

Rickettsiacidal activity can be determined from this assay by staining surviving cells with either Gimenez or immunofluorescent stain (79).

The minimal concentration of antibiotic that completely sterilizes the monolayer is defined as the minimum rickettsiacidal concentration.

Dye-Uptake Assay

Flat-bottomed microdilution plates are seeded with 1.5×10^4 Vero cells (suspended in a solution of EMEM, 5% newborn calf serum, and 2 mmol/L L-glutamine) per well and subsequently infected with varying concentrations of a suspension of *Rickettsia* organisms (78). The Vero cell suspension (100 μL) is added to each well. The infectious inoculum is added to individual wells in a final volume of 50 μL. For each 96-well plate, the first horizontal row of 8 wells contains no rickettsiae, the second horizontal row is inoculated with 2,000 PFU, the third horizontal row with 200 PFU, and the fourth with 20 PFU (Fig. 7.1).

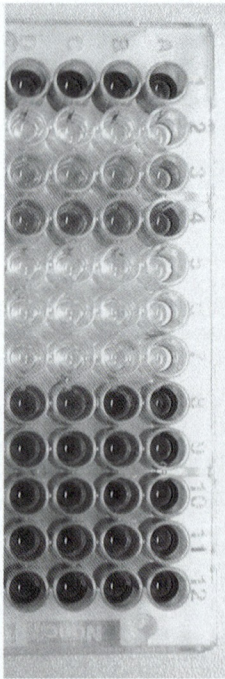

Dye uptake assay

Noninfected cells optical density (OD) = 1

Infected cells with 2000 PFU OD = 0

Infected cells with 200 PFU OD = 0

Infected cells with 20 PFU OD = 0

Doxycycline 0.015 μg/ml DO = 0

Doxycycline 0.03 μg/ml DO = 0

Doxycycline 0.06 μg/ml DO = 0

Doxycycline 0.125 μg/ml DO = 0.89 MIC

Doxycycline 0.25 μg/ml DO = 0.95

Doxycycline 0.5 μg/ml DO = 1

Doxycycline 1 μg/ml DO = 1

Noninfected cells

Figure 7.1 ■ Dye-uptake assay for *Rickettsia conorii*. The MIC is considered to be any OD value that falls between the mean OD of the wells containing 20 PFU and the mean OD of the control wells containing only Vero cells. In this example, the doxycycline MIC = 0.125 μg/mL.

Two antibiotics are tested per plate, four concentrations of each antibiotic are tested, and each concentration of antibiotic is replicated 12 times; that is, each row contains the same antibiotic at the same concentration. Antibiotics are added in 50-μL volumes. Incubation is then carried out at 36°C for 4 days in a CO_2 incubator.

After this, the medium is removed, 50 μL of neutral red dye (0.15% in saline, pH 5.5; Sigma Chemical Co, St. Louis, MO) is added to each well, and the plate is incubated for 60 minutes at 36°C. Unincorporated dye is then washed (three washes) from the cells using phosphate-buffered saline (pH 6.5). Incorporated dye is removed from the well using 100 μL of phosphate-ethanol buffer (10% ethanol in phosphate-buffered saline, adjusted to pH 4.2).

Finally, the optical density (OD) of the solution is read at 492 nm with a multichannel spectrophotometer designed for use with microdilution plates (EIA Autoreader, model EL310; BioTek Instruments, Winooski, VT). The mean OD of the control wells (containing only Vero cells) is assigned a value of 1, and the mean OD of the wells containing 2,000 PFU is assigned a value of 0 (Fig. 7.1). The MIC is considered to be any OD value that falls between the mean OD of the wells containing 20 PFU and the mean OD of the control wells containing only Vero cells.

This assay is an adaptation of an assay used to determine the efficacy of agents against herpes viruses (85) and is dependent on the fact that intact cells take up neutral red dye. Hence, wells that contain fewer cells take up less neutral red and yield lower OD values. This test is, therefore, a derivative of the plaque assay but has the advantage of using microdilution technology as well as an automated means of reading the plates.

Other Assays

Immunofluorescence Assay. More recently, an immunofluorescence assay was described by Ives (83). In this model, Vero cells cultured in wells of chamber culture microscope slides were infected with rickettsiae. After incubation of cultures for 3 hours at 37°C in a 5% CO_2 atmosphere, cell supernatants were replaced by new medium containing various concentrations of the antibiotics to be tested. Drug-free cultures served as controls. Cell culture monolayers were then fixed with methanol and stained using an immunofluorescence assay to reveal the presence of immunofluorescent foci (clusters of rickettsiae) in 25 random fields for

each well. The minimal antibiotic concentration allowing complete inhibition of foci formation as compared with the drug-free controls was recorded as the MIC.

LightCycler Polymerase Chain Reaction Assay. Cells cultured in 24-well plates were infected with rickettsiae and incubated for 7 days at 37°C in a 5% CO_2 atmosphere with medium containing various concentrations of the antibiotics to be tested. Wells were harvested each day for 7 days and stored at −20°C before the PCR assay. Real-time PCR was performed on LightCycler instrumentation (Roche Biochemicals, Mannheim, Germany) (86). The specificity of amplification can be confirmed by melting curve analysis. Single melting peaks can be generated by depicting the negative derivative of fluorescence versus temperature (−dF/dT) over the course of a gradual PCR product melt.

Extraction of DNA. After thawing, harvested tubes were centrifuged at 5,000 rpm for 10 minutes, supernatant was discarded, and pellet was washed twice with sterile distilled water and finally resuspended with 200 μL of sterile distilled water. Extraction of the DNA was performed using Chelex (biotechnology-grade chelating resin, Chelex 100, Bio-Rad, Richmond, CA) at 20% in sterile water. Briefly, 500 μL of Chelex was added to each tube, then the tubes were vortex-mixed and placed in a boiling water bath for 30 minutes. The tubes were then centrifuged at 14,000 rpm for 10 minutes, and supernatant was harvested and stored in sterile tubes at 4°C before use.

Polymerase Chain Reaction Master Mix. Master mixes were prepared by following the manufacturer's instructions, using the primers CS877F (5′-GGG GGC CTG CTC ACG GCG G-3′) and CS1258R (5′-ATT GCA AAA AGT ACA GTG AAC A-3′) of the citrate synthase gene. The 20-μL sample volume in each glass capillary contained the following: for all single experiments, 2 μL of LightCycler DNA Master SYBR Green (Roche Biochemicals, Mannheim, Germany), 2.4 μL of $MgCl_2$ at 4 mM, 1 μL of each primer at 0.5 μM, 11.6 μL of sterile distilled water, and 2 μL of DNA.

Polymerase Chain Reaction Cycling and Melting Curve Conditions. After one-pulse centrifugation to allow mixing and to drive the mix into the distal end of each tube, glass capillaries were placed in the LightCycler instrument. The amplification program included an initial denaturation step consisting of 1 cycle at 95°C for 120 seconds and 40 cycles of denaturation at 95°C for 15 seconds, annealing at 54°C for 8 seconds, and extension at 72°C for 15 seconds, with fluorescence acquisition at 54°C in single mode. Melting curve analysis was done at 45°C to 90°C (temperature transition, 20°C per second), with stepwise fluorescence acquisition by real-time measurement of fluorescence directly in the clear glass capillary tubes. Sequence-specific standard curves were generated using 10-fold serial dilutions (10^5 to 10^6 copies) of a standard bacterial concentration of *Rickettsia* organisms. The number of copies of each sample transcript was then calculated from a standard curve using the LightCycler software. The MIC was defined as the first antibiotic concentration allowing the inhibition of growth of bacteria as compared with the number of DNA copies at day 0. Experiments were made twice in duplicate. This technique is specific, reproducible, easy to perform, and rapid. It can also be used to measure the number of DNA copies at any time, and we were able to perform for the first time a kinetic of the growth of *Rickettsia* organisms even if the bacteria did not lead to plaque in vitro in cell cultures.

Results of Susceptibility Testing

The results of susceptibility testing of *Rickettsia* species are presented in Table 7.4. Sensitivities to amoxicillin (MICs from 128 to 256 µg/mL), gentamicin (MICs from 4 to 16 µg/mL), and co-trimoxazole were poor (80,81). Doxycycline was the most effective antibiotic against all strains tested, with MICs ranging from 0.06 to 0.25 µg/mL. The MICs of thiamphenicol ranged from 0.5 to 4 µg/mL, and the MICs for fluoroquinolone compounds ranged from 0.25 to 2 µg/mL. Among the macrolide compounds, josamycin was the most effective antibiotic, with MICs ranging from 0.5 to 1 µg/mL. Typhus group rickettsiae were susceptible to erythromycin (MICs from 0.125 to 0.5 µg/mL), whereas SFG rickettsiae were not (MICs from 2 to 8 µg/mL), and this difference is likely due to mutations in L22 ribosomal protein for SFG rickettsiae (87). Recently, we demonstrated that the new ketolide compound telithromycin was very effective against typhus group rickettsiae and SFG rickettsiae, with MICs ranging from 0.5 to 1 µg/mL (97). Susceptibilities to rifampin varied: typhus group rickettsiae

and most SFG rickettsiae were susceptible (MICs from 0.03 to 1 µg/mL), but a cluster including *R. massiliae*, *Rickettsia montana*, *Rickettsia rhipicephali*, *R. aeschlimannii*, and strain Bar 29 were more resistant (MICs from 2 to 4 µg/mL). This relative resistance to rifampin was linked to natural mutations in the *rpoB* gene (88).

EHRLICHIA

Ehrlichioses are emerging infectious diseases caused by obligate, gram-negative, intracellular bacteria belonging to the *Proteobacteria* α subgroup (89). The genus *Ehrlichia* is divided into three genogroups: the group *Neorickettsia*, with *Neorickettsia sennetsu*, *Neorickettsia risticii*, and *Neorickettsia helminthoeca*; the group *Ehrlichia*, with *Ehrlichia canis*, *Ehrlichia chaffeensis*, *Ehrlichia rumitantium*, *Ehrlichia muris*, and *Ehrlichia ewingii*; and the group *Anaplasma* with *Anaplasma platys*, *Anaplasma marginale*, and *Anaplasma phagocytophilum* (89,90).

They are responsible for human and animal diseases. *E. chaffeensis* is the agent of human monocytic ehrlichiosis (HME); *A. phagocytophilum*, the agent of human granulocytic ehrlichiosis (HGE); and *E. canis*, the agent of canine ehrlichiosis. In vitro and in vivo antibiotic susceptibility studies have been carried out on various species of *Ehrlichia*. All have found that doxycycline and rifampin are highly effective against ehrlichiae, and thus they are currently preferred for treating animal and in human ehrlichiosis.

Antimicrobial Susceptibility Testing

Animal Models

N. sennetsu was first isolated in mice, and subsequently, infections in mice have been used as a model for Sennetsu fever. Although the growth of *N. sennetsu* in mice is much slower than the growth of other rickettsiae, treatment of mice with cyclophosphamide prior to inoculation has been found to enhance the growth of *N. sennetsu* (91), and this technique has been used for the preparation of antigen in mice. The first study of antibiotic susceptibility in mice for *N. sennetsu* has shown that erythromycin, sulfisoxazole, penicillin, streptomycin, polymyxin B, bacitracin, and chloramphenicol were ineffective even at high concentrations (92). Chlortetracycline was more effective than oxytetracycline and tetracycline. Further studies have evaluated the effect of tetracycline therapy on spleen size as a percentage of body weight and on the splenic infectious burden in mice infected with *N. sennetsu* (93,94). In mice, in which tetracycline therapy was initiated at the same time as inoculation, there were no detectable ehrlichiae in the spleen (93). Therefore, it would appear that the time of initiation of treatment may be important in controlling the course of infection with *N. sennetsu* and that delayed therapy may allow the development of chronic infections.

Cell Culture Model

The susceptibility of *Ehrlichia* species to various antibiotics has been tested using ehrlichiae-infected contact-inhibition-growth cell lines incubated for 48 to 72 hours in the antibiotic concerned. Thereafter, the antibiotic-containing media is removed, and ehrlichiae-infected cells are incubated with antibiotic-free media for at least 3 more days. The number of ehrlichiae-infected cells is counted every day, and an antibiotic is considered ineffective if the number of ehrlichiae-infected cells after exposure to the antibiotic is similar to that of noninfected control cells. If the number of ehrlichiae-infected cells is found to decrease during incubation with an antibiotic, the antibiotic is regarded as being bactericidal. Antibiotics are considered bacteriostatic if there is no increase or decrease in ehrlichiae-infected cells when the antibiotic is present but the number of infected cells increases when antibiotic-free media is provided.

Results of Susceptibility Testing

Results of susceptibility testing for *A. phagocytophilum*, *E. canis*, and *E. chaffeensis* using the Diff-Quick assay are presented in Table 7.5. The in vitro susceptibility of *N. sennetsu* Miyayama strain to eight antibiotics was determined using Diff-Quick staining of infected P388D1 cells over a 5-day period (95). In this study, it was also demonstrated that Diff-Quick staining was as reliable as immunofluorescence assay for detecting infected cells. It was found that *N. sennetsu* was not susceptible to penicillin, gentamicin, co-trimoxazole, erythromycin, and chloramphenicol, whereas rifampin, doxycycline, and ciprofloxacin were effective, with MICs of 0.5, 0.125, and 0.125 μg/mL, respectively.

The in vitro antibiotic susceptibility of *E. chaffeensis* was studied recently (96,97) by means of

Table 7.5

MICs (μg/mL) of Antibiotics against *Anaplasma phagocytophilum*, *Ehrlichia canis*, and *Ehrlichia chaffeensis* as Determined Using the Diff-Quick Assay

Antibiotic	A. phagocytophilum		E. chaffeensis		E. canis	
	Klein et al. (99) (M, NY, W)	Horowitz et al. (98) (6 strains NY)	Maurin et al. (100) (Webster, W)	Brouqui et al. (193)	Brouqui et al. (96) (Atlanta)	Rolain et al. (97) (Atlanta)
Gentamicin	50	Amiklin >16	Amiklin >64	>100	>32	ND
Ceftriaxone	>64	>64	>128	ND	ND	ND
Amoxicillin	>32	>32	>128	1000	ND	ND
Ofloxacin	2	<2	ND	ND	ND	ND
Ciprofloxacin	2	ND	ND	Pefloxacin >2	>2[a]	ND
Levofloxacin	ND	<1	0.5	ND	ND	ND
Rifampin	0.5	<0.125	0.03	0.03	0.125	ND
Doxycycline	0.25	<0.125	0.03	0.03	<0.5	ND
Co-trimoxazole	>16	ND	50	>4	>4	ND
Chloramphenicol	>32	>16	2–8[a]	>4	>4	ND
Telithromycin	ND	ND	ND	ND	ND	>1
Erythromycin	>8	>8	>16	>4	>8	ND

[a]MIC = 2–8 μg/mL according to strains tested.
M, Minnesota; ND, not done; NY, New York; W, Wisconsin.

a microplate colorimetric assay using ehrlichiae-infected DH82 cell culture. The percentage of infected cells was determined each day by Diff-Quick staining, which has been found to stain only viable organisms. On the third day of incubation, the antibiotic-containing medium was removed and replaced with antibiotic-free medium. Using these methods, it was found that *E. chaffeensis* was sensitive to 0.5 µg/mL of doxycycline and 0.125 µg/mL of rifampin. Chloramphenicol, co-trimoxazole, erythromycin, telithromycin penicillin, gentamicin, and ciprofloxacin were not effective against *E. chaffeensis*.

The HGE agent is sensitive to doxycycline, ofloxacin, ciprofloxacin, and trovafloxacin but is resistant to clindamycin, co-trimoxazole, erythromycin, azithromycin, ampicillin, ceftriaxone, and imipenem (98–100). Chloramphenicol and aminoglycosides only display a poor bacteriostatic activity and are never bactericidal (99). Fluoroquinolones are more active in vitro against *A. phagocytophilum* than against *E. chaffeensis* and *E. canis* (Table 7.5).

Fluoroquinolones might represent a potential therapeutic alternative to tetracycline for HGE, but they have not received U.S. Food and Drug Administration (FDA) approval for use in children and pregnant women. Moreover, a *Gyr* A–mediated resistance in the related species *E. canis* and *E. chaffeensis* has recently been described and can explain this difference (101).

Recently, an evaluation of antibiotic susceptibilities against *E. canis*, *E. chaffeensis*, and *A. phagocytophilum* has been performed using a new real-time PCR assay (102). Although doxycycline and rifampin were highly active against the three species, there was a heterogeneity of susceptibility for fluoroquinolones. Interestingly, macrolide compounds and telithromycin were not effective because of numerous point mutations in their 23S RNA genes (102). A new real-time PCR assay for antibiotic susceptibility testing has been also developed and tested for 18 *O. tsutsugamushi* fresh isolates that demonstrates an intrinsic heterogeneity of susceptibility against fluoroquinolone compounds due to a point mutation in their quinolone resistance-determining region (QRDR) domain (103).

COXIELLA BURNETII

C. burnetii, the agent of Q fever, is an obligate, intracellular bacterium that multiplies within acidic vacuoles of eukaryotic cells (104). *C. burnetii* is classified in the family of Rickettsiaceae, where it belongs to the *Proteobacteria* γ subgroup based on 16S-rRNA sequence analysis (105). *C. burnetii* is a bioterrorism agent that is resistant to heat and drying and can survive in the environment for months. It is also highly infectious by the aerosol route. Owing to these features, Q fever has been investigated and developed as a bioweapon. If used, it would not generate mass fatalities but rather act as an incapacitating agent (106,107). Acute Q fever is the primary infection, and in specific hosts, it may become chronic (108). A few patients (~0.7%) suffer from chronic Q fever, which in most cases corresponds to chronic endocarditis, especially in patients with previous cardiac valve defects and/or with a cardiac valve prosthesis, in immunocompromised patients, and in pregnant women (105).

Antimicrobial Susceptibility Testing and Results

Antibiotic susceptibility testing of *C. burnetii* was difficult because this organism is an obligate, intracellular bacterium. Previously, three models of infection have been previously developed: animals, chick embryos, and cell culture. Since the previous version of this chapter, quantitative real-time PCR assay have been developed for antibiotic susceptibility testing of *C. burnetii* (109,110) that have led to the possibility to test new isolates and compounds, including doxycycline-resistant isolates (110,111). Moreover, an axenic medium has been recently described for the culture of *C. burnetii* (112,113) that will probably facilitate genetic manipulation and susceptibility testing of this bacterium in the future. The method that has been mostly used to test antibiotic susceptibility of *C. burnetii* is based on cell culture models. Torres and Raoult (118) have developed a shell vial assay with human embryonic lung (HEL) cells for assessment of the bacteriostatic effect of antibiotics, but quantitative real-time PCR could now be used routinely to assess susceptibility to antibiotics from clinical isolates (111).

Recommended Technique: The Shell Vial Assay

In this model, HEL fibroblast cells are grown in shell vials at 37°C in a 5% CO_2 atmosphere. Cell monolayers are infected with a *C. burnetii* inoculum previously determined to induce 30% to 50% infection of HEL cells after 6 days of incubation in the absence of antimicrobial agents, as revealed by an immunofluorescence technique with anti–*C. burnetii* polyclonal antibodies. The percentage

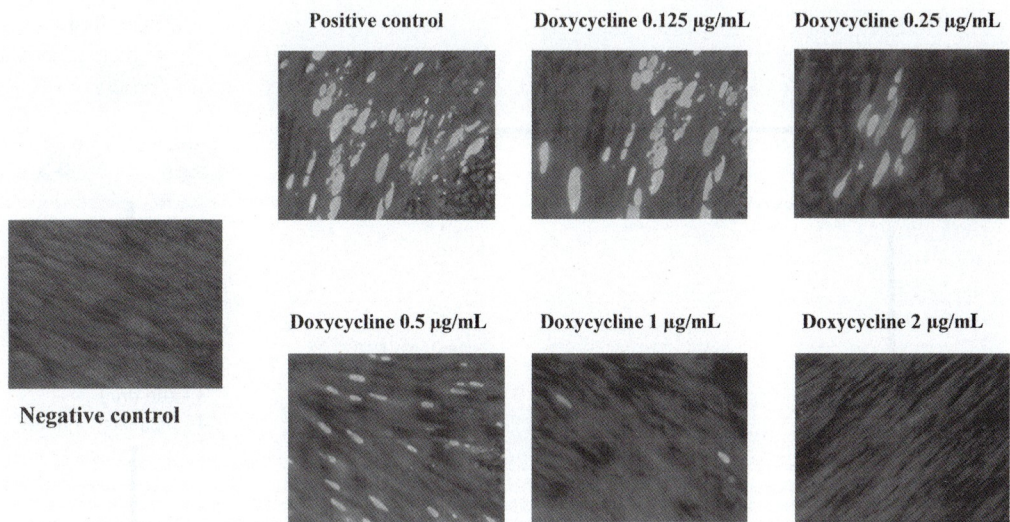

Figure 7.2 ■ Shell vial assay for *Coxiella burnetii*. MICs correspond to the minimum antimicrobial concentration allowing complete inhibition of growth (i.e., 0% infected cells after the 6-day incubation period). In this example, the doxycycline MIC = 2 µg/mL.

of infected cells in antimicrobial-containing cultures is determined after the same incubation time using the same immunofluorescence procedure. MICs correspond to the minimum antimicrobial concentration allowing complete inhibition of growth, that is, 0% infected cells after the 6-day incubation period (Fig. 7.2).

Amikacin and amoxicillin were not effective; ceftriaxone and fusidic acid were inconsistently active (118), whereas co-trimoxazole, rifampin, doxycycline, tigecycline, clarithromycin, and the quinolones were bacteriostatic (114–116). There was a heterogeneity of susceptibility to erythromycin of the strains tested (117,118). *C. burnetii* can establish a persistent infection in several cell lines, including L929 mouse fibroblasts and J774 or P388D1 murine macrophage-like cells (119). Infected cells can be maintained in continuous cultures for months (120). Raoult et al., using P388D1 and L929 cells, showed that pefloxacin, rifampin, and doxycycline (121) as well as clarithromycin (115) were bacteriostatic against *C. burnetii*. A real-time quantitative PCR assay was recently used for antibiotic susceptibility testing on *C. burnetii* and proved to be more specific and sensitive than the shell vial assay (109,110). Moreover, this technique was recently used to evaluate susceptibility to antibiotics against 13 new isolates to demonstrate that telithromycin compound was effective (111). This has led also to the description of the first doxycycline-resistant

human isolate from a German patient (111) for which whole genome sequence has been recently published (122).

An original model of killing assay has been developed by Maurin to assess the bactericidal activity of antibiotics against *C. burnetii* (123). The bactericidal activity of antibiotics in this technique is directly evaluated by titration of residual viable bacteria in persistently infected P388D1 cell cultures (Fig. 7.3). On the first day of the experiment, P388D1 cells infected with *C. burnetii* were harvested from a 150-cm² culture flask and seeded into 25-cm² flasks so that each flask received the same primary inoculum. Antibiotics were added to some of the flasks, and all the flasks, with or without antibiotics, were incubated for 24 hours at 37°C. Then cells were lysed, and 10-fold serial dilutions of cell lysates were distributed into shell vials containing uninfected HEL cells (124). After 6 days of incubation, *C. burnetii* were stained by indirect immunofluorescence in the shell vials. It was demonstrated that doxycycline, pefloxacin, and rifampin did not show any significant bactericidal activity. The lack of bactericidal activity was related to inactivation by the low pH of the phagolysosomes in which *C. burnetii* survives. Raoult demonstrated that the addition of a lysosomotropic alkalinizing agent, chloroquine, to antibiotics improved the activities of doxycycline and pefloxacin, which then became bactericidal (123).

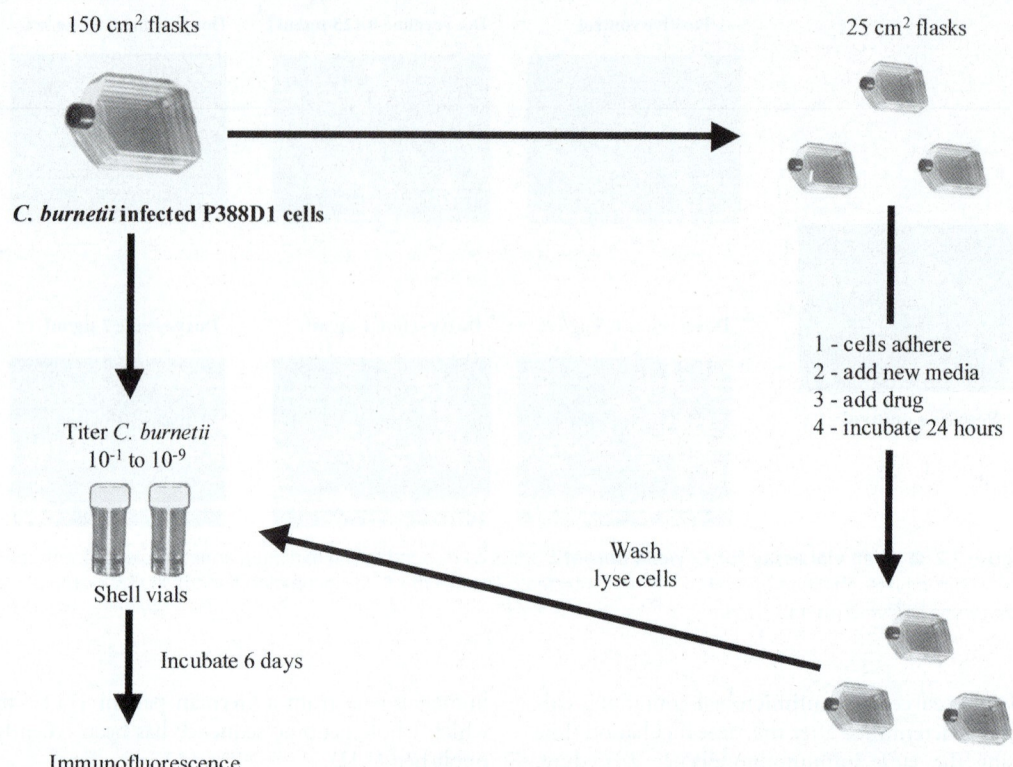

150 cm² flasks

25 cm² flasks

C. burnetii infected P388D1 cells

1 - cells adhere
2 - add new media
3 - add drug
4 - incubate 24 hours

Titer *C. burnetii*
10^{-1} to 10^{-9}

Wash
lyse cells

Shell vials

Incubate 6 days

Immunofluorescence

Figure 7.3 ■ Intracellular *Coxiella burnetii* killing assay.

SPIROCHETES

There are several pathogens of major importance in this group, including the leptospires, *Borrelia* species (including *B. burgdorferi*, the etiologic agent of Lyme disease), and *Treponema* species (including *T. pallidum*, the etiologic agent of syphilis). Whereas *B. burgdorferi* can be grown in a cell-free system (2,125), *T. pallidum* requires tissue culture for propagation (126). Because of the complexities of working with *T. pallidum*, as well as the fact that it is rarely isolated from clinical material, susceptibility testing for *T. pallidum* will have to be carried out in specialized research laboratories whose personnel have both the interest and the competence to work with this fastidious organism.

Borrelia burgdorferi

Antimicrobial Susceptibility Testing

A modified Kelly bovine serum medium has been developed that will support the growth of laboratory-adapted strains of this organism as well as fresh clinical isolates (2). The in vitro susceptibility tests use macro- or microdilution methods and standard Barbour-Stoenner-Kelly (BSK) medium (127). Using this medium, a tube dilution susceptibility test has been developed that yields both MIC and MBC values. The MIC was defined by Berger et al. (2) as the minimum concentration of antibiotic that did not allow the spirochete to multiply, whereas Preac-Mursic et al. (128) defined the MIC as the minimum concentration that prevented growth altogether. The MBC was also determined by Berger et al. (2) by subculturing all tubes that showed inhibition of growth of the spirochete into tubes containing antibiotic-free Kelly bovine serum medium. The minimum antibiotic concentration that yielded no organisms on subculture was defined as the MBC. From these definitions of MIC and MBC, it would appear that what Preac-Mursic et al. (128) defined as the MIC was what Berger et al. (2) defined as the MBC. This indeed seems to be confirmed by the results obtained by the two groups. Thus, the MBCs obtained by Berger et al. (2) for penicillin G ranged from 0.08 to 2.5 units/mL and were comparable to the range of MICs (0.06 to 3.0 g/mL) obtained by Preac-Mursic et al. (128).

Tube Dilution Technique

The procedure developed by Berger et al. (2) is described here. In this technique, a serum-free Kelly medium is used. This medium is prepared as follows: 5 g of neopeptone (Difco Laboratories, Detroit, MI) is dissolved in 50 mL of boiling water, and after the solution cools to 37°C, the mixture is filtered through a no. 42 Whatman filter (Whatman Ltd., Maidstone, England). Bovine serum albumin (40 g) (fraction V, no. A2152; Sigma Chemical Co, St. Louis, MO) is dissolved in 200 mL of distilled water, filtered through a coarse filter, and then filtered through Whatman no. 42 paper. Next, the albumin and neopeptone solutions are added to sufficient distilled water to make a total of 900 mL.

The remaining ingredients of modified Kelly medium are as follows: 100 mL of CMRL 1066 medium with glutamine and without sodium bicarbonate (10; Gibco Laboratories, Grand Island, NY), 6.0 g of HEPES (Sigma Chemical Co, St. Louis, MO), 0.7 g of sodium citrate, 5.0 g of glucose, 0.8 g of sodium pyruvate, 0.4 g of N-acetylglucosamine, 2.2 g of sodium bicarbonate, and 1.25 g of yeastolate (Difco Laboratories, Detroit, MI). This solution is adjusted to pH 7.2 with 5.0 mol/L NaOH; after which, 200 mL of a warm 7% solution of gelatin is added. Finally, the medium is sterilized by passing it through a 0.2-m filter (Nalgene sterilization filter unit type LS; Nalge Co, Rochester, NY).

B. burgdorferi, including laboratory-adapted strains, readily grow in modified Kelly medium; by 72 hours, counts as high as 6×10^6 spirochetes can be achieved. Fresh human isolates tend to clump when they grow, which is not as true for the laboratory-adapted strains. Incubation is carried out at 32°C to 33°C, and cell counts are carried out by performing serial 10-fold dilutions to 1:1,000 and examining 6 µL on a slide by dark-field microscopy. Slides are prepared by covering the sample gently with a coverslip ringed with petrolatum.

Susceptibility testing is carried out in 13 × 100-mm test tubes prepared with 5 mL of modified Kelly medium, 1 mL of antibiotic solution containing seven times the final desired antibiotic concentration, and 1.0 mL of spirochetes at a concentration of 7×10^5/mL. The MIC is determined after 72 hours of incubation and is defined as the antibiotic concentration in which more than 90% of the spirochetes are motile (as determined by examination under dark-field microscopy, as described previously) and yet the number of spirochetes is not greater than the original inoculum. The MBC is determined by transferring 50 µL from all tubes showing no growth at 72 hours to 7.0 mL of modified Kelly medium. These tubes are subsequently examined at 11 days by removing 10 µL and viewing this under a dark-field microscope. The MBC is defined as the concentration of antibiotic that prevents growth. It should be noted, however, that the developers of this technique found that the MBC determinations were not reproducible (2).

Dever et al. (127) adapted the macrodilution method to a microdilution method using microtiter trays and demonstrated that the results obtained using this very efficient method were comparable to those obtained with the more laborious macrodilution method.

Recently, Hunfeld et al. (130) developed a new standardized colorimetric assay for the determination of susceptibility to antibiotics of several strains of *Borrelia*. This assay is based on color changes that result from actively metabolizing spirochetes after 72 hours of incubation. Briefly, *Borrelia* stock cultures were thawed, cultured in modified BSK medium at 33°C until the log phase of growth, and adjusted to 2.5×10^7 organisms/mL as determined by enumeration with a Kova counting chamber (Hycor, Garden Grove, CA) combined with dark-field microscopy. Final concentrations of the lyophilized antibiotics were reconstituted by adding of 200 µL of the final inoculum suspension (5×10^6 cells) in BSK containing phenol red (25 g/mL) as a growth indicator. Samples and growth controls were sealed with sterile adhesive plastic and cultured at 33°C with 5% CO_2. The presence or absence of growth was examined after 0, 24, 48, and 72 hours by kinetic measurement of indicator color shift at 562/630 nm applying a commercially available ELISA-reader (PowerWave 200, BioTek Instruments, Winooski, VT) in combination with a software-assisted calculation program (Microwin 3.0, Microtek, Overath, Germany). Colorimetric MICs of isolates were measured in triplicate by the quantification of growth achieved through the calculation of growth curves. Recently, two new techniques using fluorescent microscopy (BacLight viability staining) and dark-field microscopy have been successfully developed for antibiotic susceptibility testing of *B. burgdorferi* (131).

Results of Susceptibility Testing

The results of susceptibility testing for *B. burgdorferi* are presented in Table 7.6. *B. burgdorferi* strains of both European and North American origin have been tested against a variety of antimicrobials because of the increasing attention that this pathogen has recently attracted (125). It is evident that the macrolides, the tetracyclines, amoxicillin, and the third-generation cephalosporins all have good in vitro activity (127,132). Penicillin G activity is strain-dependent, with some strains being moderately resistant (133).

Treponema pallidum

Until recently, it was not possible to cultivate this organism. However, in 1981, Fieldsteel et al. (3) published a technique for the propagation of this treponeme in tissue culture. This cell culture was later confirmed (134) and has been used for drug susceptibility testing (126). Although there is no evidence of the emergence of resistance to benzylpenicillin (the treatment of choice for syphilis), clinically significant resistance to macrolides, an alternative to penicillin, has recently emerged in several developed countries due to point mutations

Table 7.6

Antimicrobial Susceptibility of *Borrelia burgdorferi*

Drug	MIC (μg/mL)	References
Aminoglycosides		
Amikacin	>32	(128,130)
Gentamicin	>32	(128)
Cephalosporins		
Cefixime	0.25–2	(130)
Cefoperazone	0.03–2	(130)
Cefotaxime	0.01–0.25	(130,194,195)
Ceftriaxone	0.01–0.25	(130,194–197)
Macrolides		
Azithromycin	≤0.015–0.06	(130,197)
Erythromycin	0.03–0.125	(195,196,198)
Roxithromycin	≤0.015–0.125	(130)
Penicillins		
Amoxicillin	0.06–2	(128,130,197)
Ampicillin	0.25–1	(128)
Penicillin	0.25–8	(128,195,196)
Piperacillin	≤0.06–0.125	(130)
Quinolones		
Ciprofloxacin	1–4	(195)
Tetracyclines		
Doxycycline	≤0.25–2	(133,197)
Minocycline	0.03–1	(130,133)
Tetracycline	0.06–2	(130,133,194,196)
Tigecycline	≤0.016	(194)
Miscellaneous		
Chloramphenicol	1–3	(128)
Imipenem	0.06–1	(195)
Sulfamethoxazole	>1,024	(128)

in 23S rRNA genes (135,136). However, no documented resistance to tetracyclines has been reported to date in *T. pallidum* (136). The failure of penicillin therapy for syphilis has been particularly noted in patients with AIDS. However, this is not because of any demonstrated resistance of the treponeme to penicillin, but rather because the therapy probably does not completely eliminate viable treponemes from the host and eradication of the infection depends on host defenses lacking in patients with AIDS.

Antimicrobial Susceptibility Testing

It has been shown that 24- to 100-fold multiplication of *T. pallidum* can be obtained in tissue culture using Sf1Ep cottontail rabbit epithelial cells (obtainable from the American Type Culture Collection, Rockville, MD) under 1.5% to 3.0% oxygen at 33°C to 34°C (134,137). However, continuous in vitro culture has not yet been achieved (126).

Results of Susceptibility Testing

The results of susceptibility testing of *T. pallidum* are presented in Table 7.7. Using this procedure, antimicrobial susceptibilities have been determined with penicillin, tetracycline, erythromycin, spectinomycin, oral cephalosporins, and quinolones. The MICs achieved with the tissue culture system correlate quite well with the clinical and experimental results obtained with these antimicrobials, with the exception of spectinomycin. The single clinical isolate that has been shown by the method of inhibition of protein synthesis to be resistant to erythromycin (135) had an A to G transition mutation at position 2058 of the 23S rRNA gene (138).

Table 7.7

Antimicrobial Susceptibility of *Treponema pallidum*		
Drug	**MIC (μg/mL)**	**References**
Amoxicillin	0.42	(199)
Ceftriaxone	0.01	(200)
Erythromycin	0.005	(126)
Penicillin G	0.0005	(126)
Spectinomycin	0.5	(126)
Tetracycline	0.2	(126)

Leptospira

Prior to 1989, the genus *Leptospira* was divided into two species, *Leptospira interrogans*, comprising all pathogenic strains, and *Leptospira biflexa*, comprising the strains from the environment. Within the species *L. interrogans*, there are approximately 200 serovars. The current classification of *Leptospira* is genotypic and now includes a number of genomospecies containing all serovars (139). A new species, *Leptospira fainei*, has been recently reported to cause infections in humans (140,141). Leptospirosis is a zoonosis acquired from a wide variety of domestic and wild animals. Although penicillin is considered the drug of choice because of its low MIC, there is concern that this antibiotic is not bactericidal for *Leptospira* species. Unfortunately, only limited in vitro studies with newer antimicrobials have been carried out.

Organism

Reference organisms obtained from the National Institute of Health (Tokyo, Japan) were used in a recent extensive study of antimicrobial susceptibility (142). These organisms are cultured in Korthof medium at 30°C, as described by Johnson and Harris (137).

Antimicrobial Susceptibility Testing

Tube dilution methodology may be used for determining the MIC and MBC (142). Inocula of 0.5 mL containing 0.5×10^8 to 1.5×10^8 organisms are put in each tube after the *Leptospira* species have been grown in Korthof medium for 5 days at 30°C. Inocula of 0.5 mL are added to tubes containing 4.5 mL of fresh Korthof medium with the desired concentration of antibiotics, and the tubes are incubated for 7 days at 30°C. The MIC is defined as the minimum concentration of antibiotic that inhibits all visible growth. The MBC was determined by taking 10 μL from each clear tube, subculturing this aliquot into 10 mL of fresh Korthof medium, and incubating these tubes for 3 weeks. The MBC is the minimum concentration of antibiotic that allows no growth in these subcultures, as determined by the absence of any visible growth.

Results of Susceptibility Testing

Oie et al. (142) studied the in vitro activity of 16 antibiotics against five serovar strains of the genus *Leptospira*. Five antibiotics (ampicillin, cefmetazole, moxalactam, ceftizoxime, and cefotaxime) yielded lower MICs than did penicillin G. Ceftizoxime and cefotaxime demonstrated the lowest MBCs and were more effective than penicillin G, streptomycin, tetracycline, ampicillin, and cefmetazole.

Because of the failure of penicillin to prevent a laboratory-acquired case of leptospirosis due to *L. interrogans* subgroup *icterohaemorrhagiae*, Broughton and Flack (143) determined MIC and MBC values for amoxicillin, erythromycin, lincomycin, tetracycline, oxytetracycline, and minocycline for the infecting strain. Amoxicillin and erythromycin were the most effective, with MBCs of 0.5 µg/mL and 0.1 µg/mL, respectively. Recently, the susceptibilities of 11 serovars (seven species) of *Leptospira* to 14 antibiotics have been reported (144). With the exception of chloramphenicol, all tested agents were at least as potent as penicillin and doxycyline, with the macrolide and ketolide drugs producing the lowest MICs (≤0.01 µg/mL).

CONCLUDING REMARKS

All of the organisms considered in this chapter, with the exception of the mycoplasmas, *B. burgdorferi*, and the *Leptospira* species, require either tissue culture or in vivo techniques for their propagation and susceptibility testing. Because of this, they frequently are not isolated from patients in whom they are causing disease.

If emerging resistance is to be detected, it is essential that recent clinical isolates are also tested, particularly those from patients who appear to be failing, or have failed, appropriate therapy. Our new real-time PCR assay could be useful in the future for the determination of the susceptibility to antibiotics of such fastidious bacteria (81). Moreover, recent development of new axenic culture media will also probably help to develop new, rapid, and simple antibiotic susceptibility assays in order to encourage laboratories to monitor the emergence of resistance for these intracellular bacteria in the future (8).

REFERENCES

1. Senterfit LB. Antibiotic sensitivity testing of mycoplasmas. In: Razin S, Tully JG, eds. *Methods in mycoplasmology.* New York: Academic Press, 1983:397–401.
2. Berger BW, Kaplan MH, Rothenberg IR, et al. Isolation and characterization of the Lyme disease spirochete from the skin of patients with erythema chronicum migrans. *J Am Acad Dermatol* 1985;13(3):444–449.
3. Fieldsteel AH, Cox DL, Moeckli RA. Cultivation of virulent *Treponema pallidum* in tissue culture. *Infect Immun* 1981;32(2):908–915.
4. Stapleton JT, Stamm LV, Bassford PJ Jr. Potential for development of antibiotic resistance in pathogenic treponemes. *Rev Infect Dis* 1985;7(Suppl 2):S314–S317.
5. Stamm WE. Potential for antimicrobial resistance in *Chlamydia pneumoniae*. *J Infect Dis* 2000;181(Suppl 3):S456–S459.
6. Ehret JM, Judson FN. Susceptibility testing of *Chlamydia trachomatis*: from eggs to monoclonal antibodies. *Antimicrob Agents Chemother* 1988;32:1295–1299.
7. Ridgway GL, Bebear C, Bebear CM, et al. Antimicrobial susceptibility testing of intracellular and cell-associated pathogens. *Clin Microbiol Infect* 2001;7(12):1–10.
8. Singh S, Eldin C, Kowalczewska M, et al. Axenic culture of fastidious and intracellular bacteria. *Trends Microbiol* 2012;21(2):92–99.
9. McCormack WM. Susceptibility of mycoplasmas to antimicrobial agents: clinical implications. *Clin Infect Dis* 1993;17(Suppl 1):S200–S201.
10. Jones RB, Van der Pol B, Martin DH, et al. Partial characterization of *Chlamydia trachomatis* isolates resistant to multiple antibiotics. *J Infect Dis* 1990;162(6):1309–1315.
11. Mourad A, Sweet RL, Sugg N, et al. Relative resistance to erythromycin in *Chlamydia trachomatis*. *Antimicrob Agents Chemother* 1980;18(5):696–698.
12. Johnson FW, Clarkson MJ, Spencer WN. Susceptibility of *Chlamydia psittaci* (ovis) to antimicrobial agents. *J Antimicrob Chemother* 1983;11(5):413–418.
13. Grayston JT, Kuo CC, Wang SP, et al. A new *Chlamydia psittaci* strain, TWAR, isolated in acute respiratory tract infections. *N Engl J Med* 1986;315(3):161–168.
14. Thompson SE, Washington AE. Epidemiology of sexually transmitted *Chlamydia trachomatis* infections. *Epidemiol Rev* 1983;5:96–123.
15. Crosse BA. Psittacosis: a clinical review. *J Infect* 1990;21(3):251–259.
16. Kuo CC, Grayston JT. In vitro drug susceptibility of *Chlamydia* sp. strain TWAR. *Antimicrob Agents Chemother* 1988;32:257–258.
17. Cross NA, Kellock DJ, Kinghorn GR, et al. Antimicrobial susceptibility testing of *Chlamydia trachomatis* using a reverse transcriptase PCR-based method. *Antimicrob Agents Chemother* 1999;43(9):2311–2313.
18. Dessus-Babus S, Belloc F, Bebear CM, et al. Antibiotic susceptibility testing for *Chlamydia trachomatis* using flow cytometry. *Cytometry* 1998;31(1):37–44.
19. Bailey JM, Heppleston C, Richmond SJ. Comparison of the in vitro activities of ofloxacin and tetracycline against *Chlamydia trachomatis* as assessed by indirect immunofluorescence. *Antimicrob Agents Chemother* 1984;26(1):13–16.
20. Wyrick PB, Davis CH, Raulston JE, et al. Effect of clinically relevant culture conditions on antimicrobial susceptibility of *Chlamydia trachomatis*. *Clin Infect Dis* 1994;19(5):931–936.

21. Paul TR, Knight ST, Raulston JE, et al. Delivery of azithromycin to *Chlamydia trachomatis*-infected polarized human endometrial epithelial cells by polymorphonuclear leucocytes. *J Antimicrob Chemother* 1997;39(5):623–630.

22. Kutlin A, Roblin PM, Hammerschlag MR. In vitro activities of azithromycin and ofloxacin against *Chlamydia pneumoniae* in a continuous-infection model. *Antimicrob Agents Chemother* 1999;43(9):2268–2272.

23. Roblin PM, Kutlin A, Reznik T, et al. Activity of grepafloxacin and other fluoroquinolones and newer macrolides against recent clinical isolates of *Chlamydia pneumoniae*. *Int J Antimicrob Agents* 1999;12(2):181–184.

24. Roblin PM, Reznik T, Kutlin A, et al. In vitro activities of gemifloxacin (SB 265805, LB20304) against recent clinical isolates of *Chlamydia pneumoniae*. *Antimicrob Agents Chemother* 1999;43(11):2806–2807.

25. Suchland RJ, Geisler WM, Stamm WE. Methodologies and cell lines used for antimicrobial susceptibility testing of *Chlamydia* spp. *Antimicrob Agents Chemother* 2003;47(2):636–642.

26 Hammerschlag MR. Activity of trimethoprim-sulfamethoxazole against *Chlamydia trachomatis* in vitro. *Rev Infect Dis* 1982;4(2):500–505.

27. Nagayama A, Nakao T, Taen H. In vitro activities of ofloxacin and four other new quinoline-carboxylic acids against *Chlamydia trachomatis*. *Antimicrob Agents Chemother* 1988;32(11):1735–1737.

28. Chirgwin K, Roblin PM, Hammerschlag MR. In vitro susceptibilities of *Chlamydia pneumoniae* (Chlamydia sp. strain TWAR). *Antimicrob Agents Chemother* 1989;33(9):1634–1635.

29. How SJ, Hobson D, Hart CA, et al. A comparison of the in-vitro activity of antimicrobials against *Chlamydia trachomatis* examined by Giemsa and a fluorescent antibody stain. *J Antimicrob Chemother* 1985;15(4):399–404.

30. Bowie WR. In vitro activity of clavulanic acid, amoxicillin, and ticarcillin against *Chlamydia trachomatis*. *Antimicrob Agents Chemother* 1986;29(4):713–715.

31. Chirgwin K, Roblin PM, Hammerschlag MR. In vitro susceptibilities of *Chlamydia pneumoniae* (Chlamydia sp. strain TWAR). *J Antimicrob Chemother* 1989;33:1634–1635.

32. Hammerschlag MR, Roblin PM, Bebear CM. Activity of telithromycin, a new ketolide antibacterial, against atypical and intracellular respiratory tract pathogens. *J Antimicrob Chemother* 2001;48(Suppl T1):25–31.

33. Roblin PM, Hammerschlag MR. In vitro activity of GAR-936 against *Chlamydia pneumoniae* and *Chlamydia trachomatis*. *Int J Antimicrob Agents* 2000;16(1):61–63.

34. Roblin PM, Hammerschlag MR. In vitro activity of a new antibiotic, NVP-PDF386 (VRC4887), against *Chlamydia pneumoniae*. *Antimicrob Agents Chemother* 2003;47(4):1447–1448.

35. Roblin PM, Reznik T, Kutlin A, et al. In vitro activities of rifamycin derivatives ABI-1648 (Rifalazil, KRM-1648), ABI-1657, and ABI-1131 against *Chlamydia trachomatis* and recent clinical isolates of *Chlamydia pneumoniae*. *Antimicrob Agents Chemother* 2003;47(3):1135–1136.

36. Segreti J, Kapell KS. In vitro activity of dirithromycin against *Chlamydia trachomatis*. *Antimicrob Agents Chemother* 1994;38(9):2213–2214.

37. Segreti J, Gvazdinskas L, Trenholme G. In vitro activity of minocycline and rifampin against staphylococci. *Diagn Microbiol Infect* 1989;12:253–255.

38. Cevenini R, Donati M, Sambri V, et al. Enzyme-linked immunosorbent assay for the in-vitro detection of sensitivity of *Chlamydia trachomatis* to antimicrobial drugs. *J Antimicrob Chemother* 1987;20(5):677–684.

39. Bianchi A, Scieux C, Salmeron CM, et al. Rapid determination of MICs of 15 antichlamydial agents by using an enzyme immunoassay (Chlamydiazyme). *Antimicrob Agents Chemother* 1988;32(9):1350–1353.

40. Khan MA, Potter CW, Sharrard RM. A reverse transcriptase-PCR based assay for in-vitro antibiotic susceptibility testing of *Chlamydia pneumoniae*. *J Antimicrob Chemother* 1996;37(4):677–685.

41. Schachter J. Rifampin in chlamydial infections. *Rev Infect Dis* 1983;5(Suppl 3): S562–S564.

42. Keshishyan H, Hanna L, Jawetz E. Emergence of rifampin-resistance in *Chlamydia trachomatis*. *Nature* 1973;244(5412):173–174.

43. Misyurina OY, Chipitsyna EV, Finashutina YP, et al. Mutations in a 23S rRNA gene of *Chlamydia trachomatis* associated with resistance to macrolides. *Antimicrob Agents Chemother* 2004;48(4):1347–1349.

44. Lenart J, Andersen AA, Rockey DD. Growth and development of tetracycline-resistant *Chlamydia suis*. *Antimicrob Agents Chemother* 2001;45(8):2198–2203.

45. Sandoz KM, Rockey DD. Antibiotic resistance in Chlamydiae. *Future Microbiol* 2010;5(9):1427–1442.

46. Dessus-Babus S, Bebear CM, Charron A, et al. Sequencing of gyrase and topoisomerase IV quinolone-resistance-determining regions of *Chlamydia trachomatis* and characterization of quinolone-resistant mutants obtained In vitro. *Antimicrob Agents Chemother* 1998;42(10):2474–2481.

47. Lo SC, Wear DJ, Green SL, et al. Adult respiratory distress syndrome with or without systemic disease associated with infections due to *Mycoplasma fermentans*. *Clin Infect Dis* 1993;17(Suppl 1):S259–S263.

48. Senterfit LB. Laboratory diagnosis of mycoplasma infections. *Isr J Med Sci* 1984;20(10):905–907.

49. Kenny GE, Cartwright FD, Roberts MC. Agar dilution method for determination of antibiotic susceptibility of *Ureaplasma urealyticum*. *Pediatr Infect Dis* 1986;5(Suppl 6):S332–S334.

50. Waites KB, Crabb DM, Bing X, et al. In vitro susceptibilities to and bactericidal activities of garenoxacin (BMS-284756) and other antimicrobial agents against human mycoplasmas and ureaplasmas. *Antimicrob Agents Chemother* 2003;47(1):161–165.

51. Waites KB, Figarola TA, Schmid T, et al. Comparison of agar versus broth dilution techniques for determining antibiotic susceptibilities of *Ureaplasma urealyticum*. *Diagn Microbiol Infect Dis* 1991;14(3):265–271.

52. Roberts MC, Koutsky LA, Holmes KK, et al. Tetracycline-resistant *Mycoplasma hominis* strains contain streptococcal *tetM* sequences. *Antimicrob Agents Chemother* 1985;28(1):141–143.

53. Tanner AC, Erickson BZ, Ross RF. Adaptation of the Sensititre broth microdilution technique to antimicrobial susceptibility testing of *Mycoplasma hyopneumoniae*. *Vet Microbiol* 1993;36(3–4):301–306.

54. Poulin SA, Perkins RE, Kundsin RB. Antibiotic susceptibilities of AIDS-associated mycoplasmas. *J Clin Microbiol* 1994;32(4):1101–1103.

55. Limb DI, Wheat PF, Hastings JG, et al. Antimicrobial susceptibility testing of mycoplasmas by ATP bioluminescence. *J Med Microbiol* 1991;35(2):89–92.

56. Tully JG, Whitcomb RF, Clark HF, et al. Pathogenic mycoplasmas: cultivation and vertebrate pathogenicity of a new spiroplasma. *Science* 1977;195(4281):892–894.

57. Waites KB, Cassell GH, Canupp KC, et al. In vitro susceptibilities of mycoplasmas and ureaplasmas to new macrolides and aryl-fluoroquinolones. *Antimicrob Agents Chemother* 1988;32(10):1500–1502.

58. Waites KB, Crouse DT, Nelson KG, et al. Chronic *Ureaplasma urealyticum* and *Mycoplasma hominis* infections of central nervous system in preterm infants. *Lancet* 1988;1(8575–8576):17–21.

59. Robertson JA, Coppola JE, Heisler OR. Standardized method for determining antimicrobial susceptibility of strains of *Ureaplasma urealyticum* and their response to tetracycline, erythromycin, and rosaramicin. *Antimicrob Agents Chemother* 1981;20(1):53–58.

60. Taylor-Robinson D, Furr PM. The static effect of rosaramicin on *Ureaplasma urealyticum* and the development of antibiotic resistance. *J Antimicrob Chemother* 1982;10(3):185–191.

61. Rylander M, Hallander HO. In vitro comparison of the activity of doxycycline, tetracycline, erythromycin and a new macrolide, CP 62993, against *Mycoplasma pneumoniae, Mycoplasma hominis* and *Ureaplasma urealyticum. Scand J Infect Dis Suppl* 1988;53:12–17.

62. Pereyre S, Guyot C, Renaudin H, et al. In vitro selection and characterization of resistance to macrolides and related antibiotics in *Mycoplasma pneumoniae. Antimicrob Agents Chemother* 2004;48(2):460–465.

63. Stopler T, Branski D. Resistance of Mycoplasma pneumoniae to macrolides, lincomycin and streptogramin B. *J Antimicrob Chemother* 1986;18(3):359–364.

64. Bebear C, Pereyre S, Peuchant O. *Mycoplasma pneumoniae*: susceptibility and resistance to antibiotics. *Future Microbiol* 2011;6(4):423–431.

65. Ishida K, Kaku M, Irifune K, et al. In vitro and in vivo activities of macrolides against *Mycoplasma pneumoniae. Antimicrob Agents Chemother* 1994;38(4):790–798.

66. Yamaguchi T, Hirakata Y, Izumikawa K, et al. In vitro activity of telithromycin (HMR3647), a new ketolide, against clinical isolates of *Mycoplasma pneumoniae* in Japan. *Antimicrob Agents Chemother* 2000;44(5):1381–1382.

67. Hammerschlag MR, Hyman CL, Roblin PM. In vitro activities of five quinolones against *Chlamydia pneumoniae. Antimicrob Agents Chemother* 1992;36:682–683.

68. Kaku M, Ishida K, Irifune K, et al. In vitro and in vivo activities of sparfloxacin against *Mycoplasma pneumoniae. Antimicrob Agents Chemother* 1994;38(4):738–741.

69. Kenny GE, Cartwright FD. Susceptibility of *Mycoplasma pneumoniae* to several new quinolones, tetracycline, and erythromycin. *Antimicrob Agents Chemother* 1991;35(3):587–589.

70. Krausse R, Schubert S. In-vitro activities of tetracyclines, macrolides, fluoroquinolones and clindamycin against *Mycoplasma hominis* and *Ureaplasma* ssp. isolated in Germany over 20 years. *Clin Microbiol Infect* 2010;16(11):1649–1655.

71. Taylor-Robinson D, Furr PM. Clinical antibiotic resistance of *Ureaplasma urealyticum. Pediatr Infect Dis* 1986;5(6)(Suppl):S335–S337.

72. Waites KB, Crouse DT, Cassell GH. Antibiotic susceptibilities and therapeutic options for *Ureaplasma urealyticum* infections in neonates. *Pediatr Infect Dis J* 1992;11(1):23–29.

73. Waites KB, Crouse DT, Cassell GH. Therapeutic considerations for *Ureaplasma urealyticum* infections in neonates. *Clin Infect Dis* 1993;17(Suppl 1):S208–S214.

74. Bebear CM, Bove JM, Bebear C, et al. Characterization of *Mycoplasma hominis* mutations involved in resistance to fluoroquinolones. *Antimicrob Agents Chemother* 1997;41(2):269–273.

75. MacKenzie CR, Nischik N, Kram R, et al. Fatal outcome of a disseminated dual infection with drug-resistant *Mycoplasma hominis* and *Ureaplasma parvum* originating from a septic arthritis in an immunocompromised patient. *Int J Infect Dis* 2010;14(Suppl 3):e307–e309.

76. Pereyre S, Gonzalez P, de Barbeyrac B, et al. Mutations in 23S rRNA account for intrinsic resistance to macrolides in *Mycoplasma hominis* and *Mycoplasma fermentans* and for acquired resistance to macrolides in *M. hominis. Antimicrob Agents Chemother* 2002;46(10):3142–3150.

77. Parola P, Paddock CD, Raoult D. Tick-borne rickettsioses around the world: emerging diseases challenging old concepts. *Clin Microbiol Rev* 2005;18(4):719–756.

78. Raoult D, Roussellier P, Vestris G, et al. In vitro antibiotic susceptibility of *Rickettsia rickettsii* and *Rickettsia conorii*: plaque assay and microplaque colorimetric assay. *J Infect Dis* 1987;155:1059–1062.

79. Raoult D, Roussellier P, Galicher V, et al. In vitro susceptibility of *Rickettsia conorii* to ciprofloxacin as determined by suppressing lethality in chicken embryos and by plaque assay. *Antimicrob Agents Chemother* 1986;29:424–425.

80. Rolain JM, Maurin M, Vestris G, et al. In vitro susceptibilities of 27 Rickettsiae to 13 antimicrobials. *Antimicrob Agents Chemother* 1998;42(7):1537–1541.

81. Rolain JM, Stuhl L, Maurin M, et al. Evaluation of antibiotic susceptibilities of three rickettsial species including *Rickettsia felis* by a quantitative PCR DNA assay. *Antimicrob Agents Chemother* 2002;46(9):2747–2751.

82. Ives TJ, Marston EL, Regnery RL, et al. In vitro susceptibilities of Bartonella and Rickettsia spp. to fluoroquinolone antibiotics as determined by immunofluorescent antibody analysis of infected Vero cell monolayers. *Int J Antimicrob Agents* 2001;18(3):217–222.

83. Ives TJ, Manzewitsch P, Regnery RL, et al. In vitro susceptibilities of *Bartonella henselae, B. quintana, B. elizabethae, Rickettsia rickettsii, R. conorii, R. akari,* and *R. prowazekii* to macrolide antibiotics as determined by immunofluorescent-antibody analysis of infected vero cell monolayers. *Antimicrob Agents Chemother* 1997;41:578–582.

84. Raoult D, Roussellier P, Tamalet J. In vitro evaluation of josamycin, spiramycin, and erythromycin against *Rickettsia rickettsii* and *R. conorii. Antimicrob Agents Chemother* 1988;32:255–256.

85. McLaren C, Ellis MN, Hunter GA. A colorimetric assay for the measurement of the sensitivity of herpes simplex viruses to antiviral agents. *Antiviral Res* 1983;3(4):223–234.

86. Wittwer CT, Ririe KM, Andrew RV, et al. The Light Cycler: a microvolume multisample fluorimeter with rapid temperature control. *Biotechniques* 1997;22(1):176–181.

87. Rolain JM, Raoult D. Prediction of resistance to erythromycin in the genus Rickettsia by mutations in L22 ribosomal protein. *J Antimicrob Chemother* 2005;56(2):396–398.

88. Drancourt M, Raoult D. Characterization of mutations in the rpoB gene in naturally rifampin-resistant *Rickettsia* species. *Antimicrob Agent Chemother* 1999;43(10):2400–2403.

89. Dumler JS, Barbet AF, Bekker CP, et al. Reorganization of genera in the families *Rickettsiaceae* and *Anaplasmataceae* in the order Rickettsiales: unification of some species of *Ehrlichia* with *Anaplasma, Cowdria* with *Ehrlichia* and *Ehrlichia* with *Neorickettsia*, descriptions of six new species combinations and designation of *Ehrlichia equi* and 'HGE agent' as subjective synonyms of *Ehrlichia phagocytophila. Int J Syst Evol Microbiol* 2001;51(Pt 6):2145–2165.

90. Dumler JS, Bakken JS. Ehrlichial diseases of humans: emerging tick-borne infections. *Clin Infect Dis* 1995;20:1102–1110.

91. Tachibana N, Kobayashi V. Effect of cyclophosphamide on the growth of *Rickettsia sennetsu* in experimentally infected mice. *Infect Immun* 1975;12:625–629.

92. Kobayashi Y, Ikeda O, Miaso T. Chemotherapy of sennetsu disease. *Progress in virology*. Tokyo, Japan: Bainukan, 1962:130–142.

93. Kelly DJ, LaBarre DD, Lewis GEJ. Effect of tetracycline therapy on host defense in mice infected with *Ehrlichia sennetsu*. In: Winkler HH, Ristic M, eds. *Microbiology*. Washington, DC: American Society for Microbiology, 1986:209–212.

94. Oyama T. Immunological studies of rickettsial infection—analysis of lymphoid cell subpopulations of the spleen of mice infected with *Rickettsia sennetsu* and *Rickettsia tsutsugamushi* [in Japanese]. *Kansenshogaku Zasshi* 1979;53:243–257.

95. Brouqui P, Raoult D. In vitro susceptibility of *Ehrlichia sennetsu* to antibiotics. *Antimicrob Agents Chemother* 1990;34:1593–1596.

96. Brouqui P, Raoult D. In vitro antibiotic susceptibility of the newly recognized agent of ehrhlichiosis in humans, *Ehrlichia chaffeensis*. *Antimicrob Agents Chemother* 1992;36:2799–2803.

97. Rolain JM, Maurin M, Bryskier A, et al. In vitro activities of telithromycin (HMR 3647) against *Rickettsia rickettsii*, *Rickettsia conorii*, *Rickettsia africae*, *Rickettsia typhi*, *Rickettsia prowasekii*, *Coxiella burnetii*, *Bartonella henselae*, *Bartonella quintana*, *Bartonella bacilliformis*, and *Ehrlichia chaffeensis*. *Antimicrob Agents Chemother* 2000;44(5):1391–1393.

98. Horowitz HW, Hsieh TC, Aguero-Rosenfeld ME, et al. Antimicrobial susceptibility of *Ehrlichia phagocytophila*. *Antimicrob Agents Chemother* 2001;45(3):786–788.

99. Klein MB, Nelson CM, Goodman JL. Antibiotic susceptibility of the newly cultivated agent of human granulocytic ehrlichiosis: promising activity of quinolones and rifamycins. *Antimicrob Agents Chemother* 1997;41:76–79.

100. Maurin M, Bakken JS, Dumler JS. Antibiotic susceptibilities of *Anaplasma* (Ehrlichia) *phagocytophilum* strains from various geographic areas in the United States. *Antimicrob Agents Chemother* 2003;47(1):413–415.

101. Maurin M, Abergel C, Raoult D. DNA Gyrase-mediated natural resistance to fluoroquinolones in Ehrlichia spp. *Antimicrob Agents Chemother* 2001;45(7):2098–2105.

102. Branger S, Rolain JM, Raoult D. Evaluation of antibiotic susceptibilities of *Ehrlichia canis*, *Ehrlichia chaffeensis*, and *Anaplasma phagocytophilum* by real-time PCR. *Antimicrob Agents Chemother* 2004;48(12):4822–4828.

103. Tantibhedhyangkul W, Angelakis E, Tongyoo N, et al. Intrinsic fluoroquinolone resistance in *Orientia tsutsugamushi*. *Int J Antimicrob Agents* 2010;35(4):338–341.

104. Maurin M, Benoliel AM, Bongrand P, et al. Phagolysosomes of *Coxiella burnetii*-infected cell lines maintain an acidic pH during persistent infection. *Infect Immun* 1992;60(12):5013–5016.

105. Maurin M, Raoult D. Q fever. *Clin Microbiol Rev* 1999;12(4):518–553.

106. Christopher GW, Cieslak TJ, Pavlin JA, et al. Biological warfare. A historical perspective. *JAMA* 1997;278(5):412–417.

107. Greenfield RA, Drevets DA, Machado LJ, et al. Bacterial pathogens as biological weapons and agents of bioterrorism. *Am J Med Sci* 2002;323(6):299–315.

108. Raoult D, Mege JL, Marrie T. Q fever: queries remaining after decades of research. In: Scheld WM, Craig WA, Hughes JM, eds. *Emerging infections*. Washington, DC: ASM Press, 2001:29–56.

109. Boulos A, Rolain JM, Maurin M, et al. Evaluation of antibiotic susceptibilities against *Coxiella burnetii* by real time PCR. *Int J Antimicrob Agents* 2004;23(2):169–174.

110. Brennan RE, Samuel JE. Evaluation of *Coxiella burnetii* antibiotic susceptibilities by real-time PCR assay. *J Clin Microbiol* 2003;41(5):1869–1874.

111. Rolain JM, Lambert F, Raoult D. Activity of telithromycin against thirteen new isolates of *C. burnetii* including three resistant to doxycycline. *Ann N Y Acad Sci* 2006;1063:252–256.

112. Beare PA, Sandoz KM, Omsland A, et al. Advances in genetic manipulation of obligate intracellular bacterial pathogens. *Front Microbiol* 2011;2:97.

113. Omsland A, Cockrell DC, Howe D, et al. Host cell-free growth of the Q fever bacterium *Coxiella burnetii*. *Proc Natl Acad Sci U S A* 2009;106(11):4430–4434.

114. Jabarit-Aldighieri N, Torres H, Raoult D. Susceptibility of *R. conorii*, *R.rickettsii* and *C.burnetii* to CI- 960 (PD 127,391), PD 131,628, pefloxacin, ofloxacin and ciprofloxacin. *Antimicrob Agents Chemother* 1992;36:2529–2532.

115. Maurin M, Raoult D. In vitro susceptibilities of spotted fever group rickettsiae and *Coxiella burnetii* to clarithromycin. *Antimicrob Agents Chemother* 1993;37:2633–2637.

116. Spyridaki I, Psaroulaki A, Vranakis I, et al. Bacteriostatic and bactericidal activities of tigecycline against *Coxiella burnetii* and comparison with those of six other antibiotics. *Antimicrob Agents Chemother* 2009;53(6):2690–2692.

117. Raoult D, Torres H, Drancourt M. Shell-vial assay: evaluation of a new technique for determining antibiotic susceptibility, tested in 13 isolates of *Coxiella burnetii*. *Antimicrob Agents Chemother* 1991;35(10):2070–2077.

118. Torres H, Raoult D. In vitro activities of ceftriaxone and fusidic acid against 13 isolates of *Coxiella burnetii*, determined using the shell vial assay. *Antimicrob Agents Chemother* 1993;37:491–494.

119. Baca OG, Akporiaye ET, Aragon AS, et al. Fate of phase I and phase II *Coxiella burnetii* in several macrophage-like tumor cell lines. *Infect Immun* 1981;33:258–266.

120. Roman MJ, Coriz PD, Baca OG. A proposed model to explain persistent infection of host cells with *Coxiella burnetii*. *J Gen Microbiol* 1986;132:1415–1422.

121. Raoult D, Drancourt M, Vestris G. Bactericidal effect of doxycycline associated with lysosomotropic agents on *Coxiella burnetii* in P388D1 cells. *Antimicrob Agents Chemother* 1990;34:1512–1514.

122. Rouli L, Rolain JM, El Filali A, et al. Genome sequence of *Coxiella burnetii* 109, a doxycycline-resistant clinical isolate. *J Bacteriol* 2012;194(24):6939.

123. Maurin M, Benoliel AM, Bongrand P, et al. Phagolysosomal alkalinization and the bactericidal effect of antibiotics: the *Coxiella burnetii* paradigm. *J Infect Dis* 1992;166:1097–1102.

124. Raoult D, Vestris G, Enea M. Isolation of 16 strains of *Coxiella burnetii* from patients by using a sensitive centrifugation cell culture system and establishment of strains in HEL cells. *J Clin Microbiol* 1990;28:2482–2484.

125. Agger WA, Callister SM, Jobe DA. In vitro susceptibilities of *Borrelia burgdorferi* to five oral cephalosporins and ceftriaxone. *Antimicrob Agents Chemother* 1992;36(8):1788–1790.

126. Norris SJ, Edmondson DG. In vitro culture system to determine MICs and MBCs of antimicrobial agents against *Treponema pallidum* subsp. *pallidum* (Nichols strain). *Antimicrob Agents Chemother* 1988;32(1):68–74.

127. Dever LL, Jorgensen JH, Barbour AG. In vitro antimicrobial susceptibility testing of *Borrelia burgdorferi*: a microdilution MIC method and time-kill studies. *J Clin Microbiol* 1992;30(10):2692–2697.

128. Preac-Mursic V, Wilske B, Schierz G. European *Borrelia burgdorferi* isolated from humans and ticks culture conditions and antibiotic susceptibility. *Zentralbl Bakteriol Mikrobiol Hyg A* 1986;263(1–2):112–118.

129. Donati M, Pollini GM, Sparacino M, et al. Comparative in vitro activity of garenoxacin against *Chlamydia* spp. *J Antimicrob Chemother* 2002;50(3):407–410.

130. Hunfeld KP, Kraiczy P, Wichelhaus TA, et al. Colorimetric in vitro susceptibility testing of penicillins, cephalosporins, macrolides, streptogramins, tetracyclines, and aminoglycosides against *Borrelia burgdorferi* isolates. *Int J Antimicrob Agents* 2000;15(1):11–17.

131. Sapi E, Kaur N, Anyanwu S, et al. Evaluation of in-vitro antibiotic susceptibility of different morphological forms of *Borrelia burgdorferi*. *Infect Drug Resist* 2011;4:97–113.

132. Levin JM, Nelson JA, Segreti J, et al. In vitro susceptibility of *Borrelia burgdorferi* to 11 antimicrobial agents. *Antimicrob Agents Chemother* 1993;37(7):1444–1446.

133. Johnson SE, Klein GC, Schmid GP, et al. Susceptibility of the Lyme disease spirochete to seven antimicrobial agents. *Yale J Biol Med* 1984;57(4):549–553.

134. Levy JA. Confirmation of the successful cultivation of *Treponema pallidum* in tissue culture. *Microbiologica* 1984;7:367–370.

135. Stamm LV, Stapleton JT, Bassford PJ Jr. In vitro assay to demonstrate high-level erythromycin resistance of a clinical isolate of *Treponema pallidum*. *Antimicrob Agents Chemother* 1988;32(2):164–169.

136. Stamm LV. Global challenge of antibiotic-resistant *Treponema pallidum*. *Antimicrob Agents Chemother* 2010;54(2):583–589.

137 Johnson RC, Harris VG. Differentiation of pathogenic and saprophytic letospires. I. Growth at low temperatures. *J Bacteriol* 1967;94(1):27–31.

138. Stamm LV, Bergen HL. A point mutation associated with bacterial macrolide resistance is present in both 23S rRNA genes of an erythromycin-resistant *Treponema pallidum* clinical isolate. *Antimicrob Agents Chemother* 2000;44(3):806–807.

139. Levett PN. Leptospirosis. *Clin Microbiol Rev* 2001;14(2):296–326.

140. Arzouni JP, Parola P, La Scola B, et al. Human infection caused by *Leptospira fainei*. *Emerg Infect Dis* 2002;8(8):865–868.

141. Petersen AM, Boye K, Blom J, et al. First isolation of *Leptospira fainei* serovar Hurstbridge from two human patients with Weil's syndrome. *J Med Microbiol* 2001;50(1):96–100.

142. Oie S, Hironaga K, Koshiro A, et al. In vitro susceptibilities of five *Leptospira* strains to 16 antimicrobial agents. *Antimicrob Agents Chemother* 1983;24(6):905–908.

143. Broughton ES, Flack LE. The susceptibility of a strain of *Leptospira interrogans* serogroup *icterohaemorrhagiae* to amoxycillin, erythromycin, lincomycin, tetracycline, oxytetracycline and minocycline. *Zentralbl Bakteriol Mikrobiol Hyg A* 1986;261(4):425–431.

144. Hospenthal DR, Murray CK. In vitro susceptibilities of seven *Leptospira* species to traditional and newer antibiotics. *Antimicrob Agents Chemother* 2003;47(8):2646–2648.

145. Bowie WR, Lee CK, Alexander ER. Prediction of efficacy of antimicrobial agents in treatment of infections due to *Chlamydia trachomatis*. *J Infect Dis* 1978;138(5):655–659.

146. Johannisson G, Sernryd A, Lycke E. Susceptibility of *Chlamydia trachomatis* to antibiotics in vitro and in vivo. *Sex Transm Dis* 1979;6(2):50–57.

147. Zurenko GE, Yagi BH, Vavra JJ, et al. In vitro antibacterial activity of trospectomycin (U-63366F), a novel spectinomycin analog. *Antimicrob Agents Chemother* 1988;32(2):216–223.

148. Bowie WR. Lack of in vitro activity of cefoxitin, cefamandole, cefuroxime, and piperacillin against *Chlamydia trachomatis*. *Antimicrob Agents Chemother* 1982;21(2):339–340.

149. Hammerschlag MR, Gleyzer A. In vitro activity of a group of broad spectrum cephalosporins and other beta-lactam antibodies against *Chlamydia trachomatis*. *Antimicrob Agents Chemother* 1983;23:493–494.

150. Martin DH, Pastorek JG, Faro S. In-vitro and in-vivo activity of parenterally administered beta-lactam antibiotics against *Chlamydia trachomatis*. *Sex Transm Dis* 1986;13(2):81–87.

151. Muytjens HL, Heessen FW. In vitro activities of thirteen beta-lactam antibiotics against *Chlamydia trachomatis*. *Antimicrob Agents Chemother* 1982;22(3):520–521.

152. Agacfidan A, Moncada J, Schachter J. In vitro activity of azithromycin (CP-62,993) against *Chlamydia trachomatis* and *Chlamydia pneumoniae*. *Antimicrob Agents Chemother* 1993;37(9):1746–1748.

153. Rumpianesi F, Morandotti G, Sperning R, et al. In vitro activity of azithromycin against *Chlamydia trachomatis*, *Ureaplasma urealyticum* and *Mycoplasma hominis* in comparison with erythromycin, roxithromycin and minocycline. *J Chemother* 1993;5(3):155–158.

154. Welsh LE, Gaydos CA, Quinn TC. In vitro evaluation of activities of azithromycin, erythromycin, and tetracycline against *Chlamydia trachomatis* and *Chlamydia pneumoniae*. *Antimicrob Agents Chemother* 1992;36:291–294.

155. Benson C, Segreti J, Kessler H, et al. Comparative in vitro activity of A-56268 (TE-031) against gram-positive and gram-negative bacteria and *Chlamydia trachomatis*. *Eur J Clin Microbiol* 1987;6(2):173–178.

156. Ridgway GL, Mumtaz G, Fenelon L. The in-vitro activity of clarithromycin and other macrolides against the type strain of *Chlamydia pneumoniae* (TWAR). *J Antimicrob Chemother* 1991;27(Suppl A):43–45.

157. Samra Z, Rosenberg S, Soffer Y, et al. In vitro susceptibility of recent clinical isolates of *Chlamydia trachomatis* to macrolides and tetracyclines. *Diagn Microbiol Infect Dis* 2001;39(3):177–179.

158. Stamm WE, Suchland R. Antimicrobial activity of U-70138F (paldimycin), roxithromycin (RU 965), and ofloxacin (ORF 18489) against *Chlamydia trachomatis* in cell culture. *Antimicrob Agents Chemother* 1986;30(5):806–807.

159. Miyashita N, Fukano H, Niki Y, et al. In vitro activity of telithromycin, a new ketolide, against *Chlamydia pneumoniae*. *J Antimicrob Chemother* 2001;48(3):403–405.

160. Miyashita N, Fukano H, Yoshida K, et al. In vitro activity of cethromycin, a novel antibacterial ketolide,

against *Chlamydia pneumoniae*. *J Antimicrob Chemother* 2003;52(3):497–499.

161. Kuo CC, Wang SP, Grayston JT. Antimicrobial activity of several antibiotics and a sulfonamide against *Chlamydia trachomatis* organisms in cell culture. *Antimicrob Agents Chemother* 1977;12(1):80–83.

162. Gieffers J, Solbach W, Maass M. In vitro susceptibilities of *Chlamydia pneumoniae* strains recovered from atherosclerotic coronary arteries. *Antimicrob Agents Chemother* 1998;42(10):2762–2764.

163. Miyashita N, Fukano H, Yoshida K, et al. In-vitro activity of moxifloxacin and other fluoroquinolones against *Chlamydia* species. *J Infect Chemother* 2002;8(1):115–117.

164. Maeda H, Fujii A, Nakata K, et al. In vitro activities of T-3262, NY-198, fleroxacin (AM-833; RO 23-6240), and other new quinolone agents against clinically isolated *Chlamydia trachomatis* strains. *Antimicrob Agents Chemother* 1988;32(7):1080–1081.

165. Roblin PM, Reznik T, Hammerschlag MR. In vitro activity of garenoxacin against recent clinical isolates of *Chlamydia pneumoniae*. *Int J Antimicrob Agents* 2003;21(6):578–580.

166. Roblin PM, Hammerschlag MR. In-vitro activity of gatifloxacin against *Chlamydia trachomatis* and *Chlamydia pneumoniae*. *J Antimicrob Chemother* 1999;44(4):549–551.

167. Hammerschlag MR. Activity of gemifloxacin and other new quinolones against *Chlamydia pneumoniae*: a review. *J Antimicrob Chemother* 2000;45(Suppl 1):35–39.

168. Heessen FW, Muytjens HL. In vitro activities of ciprofloxacin, norfloxacin, pipemidic acid, cinoxacin, and nalidixic acid against *Chlamydia trachomatis*. *Antimicrob Agents Chemother* 1984;25(1):123–124.

169. Segreti J, Kessler HA, Kapell KS, et al. In vitro activities of temafloxacin (A-62254) and four other antibiotics against *Chlamydia trachomatis*. *Antimicrob Agents Chemother* 1989;33(1):118–119.

170. Hardy DJ. Activity of temafloxacin and other fluoroquinolones against typical and atypical community-acquired respiratory tract pathogens. *Am J Med* 1991;91(6A):12S–14S.

171. Lefevre JC, Bauriaud R, Gaubert E, et al. In vitro activity of sparfloxacin and other antimicrobial agents against genital pathogens. *Chemotherapy* 1992;38(5):303–307.

172. Roblin PM, Kutlin A, Hammerschlag MR. In vitro activity of trovafloxacin against *Chlamydia pneumoniae*. *Antimicrob Agents Chemother* 1997;41(9):2033–2034.

173. Jones RB, Van der Pol B, Johnson RB. Susceptibility of *Chlamydia trachomatis* to trovafloxacin. *J Antimicrob Chemother* 1997;39(Suppl B):63–65.

174. Christensen JJ, Holten-Andersen W, Nielsen PB. *Chlamydia trachomatis*: in vitro susceptibility to antibiotics singly and in combination. *Acta Pathol Microbiol Immunol Scand B* 1986;94(5):329–332.

175. Gnarpe J, Eriksson K, Gnarpe H. In vitro activities of azithromycin and doxycycline against 15 isolates of *Chlamydia pneumoniae*. *Antimicrob Agents Chemother* 1996;40(8):1843–1845.

176. Kimura M, Kishimoto T, Niki Y, et al. In vitro and in vivo antichlamydial activities of newly developed quinolone antimicrobial agents. *Antimicrob Agents Chemother* 1993;37(4):801–803.

177. Harrison HR, Riggin RM, Alexander ER, et al. In vitro activity of clindamycin against strains of *Chlamydia trachomatis*, *Mycoplasma hominis*, and *Ureaplasma urealyticum* isolated from pregnant women. *Am J Obstet Gynecol* 1984;149(5):477–480.

178. Jones RB, Ridgway GL, Boulding S, et al. In vitro activity of rifamycins alone and in combination with other antibiotics against *Chlamydia trachomatis*. *Rev Infect Dis* 1983;5(Suppl 3):S556–S561.

179. Freidank HM, Losch P, Vogele H, et al. In vitro susceptibilities of *Chlamydia pneumoniae* isolates from German patients and synergistic activity of antibiotic combinations. *Antimicrob Agents Chemother* 1999;43(7):1808–1810.

180. Jenkin HM, Hung SC. Effect of vancomycin on the growth of psittacosis-trachoma agents cultivated in eggs and cell culture. *Appl Microbiol* 1967;15(1):10–12.

181. Jao RL. Susceptibility of *Mycoplasma pneumoniae* to 21 antibiotics in vitro. *Am J Med Sci* 1967;253(6):639–650.

182. Kenny GE, Cartwright FD. Susceptibilities of *Mycoplasma hominis*, *M. pneumoniae*, and *Ureaplasma urealyticum* to GAR-936, dalfopristin, dirithromycin, evernimicin, gatifloxacin, linezolid, moxifloxacin, quinupristin-dalfopristin, and telithromycin compared to their susceptibilities to reference macrolides, tetracyclines, and quinolones. *Antimicrob Agents Chemother* 2001;45(9):2604–2608.

183. Renaudin H, Bebear C. Comparative in vitro activity of azithromycin, clarithromycin, erythromycin and lomefloxacin against *Mycoplasma pneumoniae*, *Mycoplasma hominis* and *Ureaplasma urealyticum*. *Eur J Clin Microbiol Infect Dis* 1990;9(11):838–841.

184. Misu T, Arai S, Furukawa M, et al. Effects of rokitamycin and other macrolide antibiotics on *Mycoplasma pneumoniae* in L cells. *Antimicrob Agents Chemother* 1987;31:1843–1845.

185. Yu X, Fan M, Xu G, et al. Genotypic and antigenic identification of two new strains of spotted fever group rickettsiae isolated from China. *J Clin Microbiol* 1993;31:83–88.

186. Cassell GH, Waites KB, Pate MS, et al. Comparative susceptibility of *Mycoplasma pneumoniae* to erythromycin, ciprofloxacin, and lomefloxacin. *Diagn Microbiol Infect Dis* 1989;12(5):433–435.

187. Kenny GE, Hooton TM, Roberts MC, et al. Susceptibilities of genital mycoplasmas to the newer quinolones as determined by the agar dilution method. *Antimicrob Agents Chemother* 1989;33(1):103–107.

188. Osada Y, Ogawa H. Antimycoplasmal activity of ofloxacin (DL-8280). *Antimicrob Agents Chemother* 1983;23(3):509–511.

189. Waites KB, Crabb DM, Duffy LB. Inhibitory and bactericidal activities of gemifloxacin and other antimicrobials against *Mycoplasma pneumoniae*. *Int J Antimicrob Agents* 2003;21(6):574–577.

190. Kenny GE, Cartwright FD. Susceptibilities of *Mycoplasma pneumoniae*, *Mycoplasma hominis*, and *Ureaplasma urealyticum* to a new quinolone, trovafloxacin (CP-99,219). *Antimicrob Agents Chemother* 1996;40(4):1048–1049.

191. Bygdeman SM, Mardh PA. Antimicrobial susceptibility and susceptibility testing of *Mycoplasma hominis*: a review. *Sex Transm Dis* 1983;10(4)(Suppl):366–370.

192. Kenny GE, Cartwright FD. Susceptibilities of *Mycoplasma hominis*, *Mycoplasma pneumoniae*, and *Ureaplasma urealyticum* to new glycylcyclines in comparison with those to older tetracyclines. *Antimicrob Agents Chemother* 1994;38(11):2628–2632.

193. Brouqui P, Raoult D. Susceptibilities of Ehrlichia to antibiotics. In: Raoult D, ed. *Antimicrobial agents and intracellular pathogens.* 9th ed. Boca Raton, FL: CRC Press, 1993:179–199.

194. Ates L, Hanssen-Hubner C, Norris DE, et al. Comparison of in vitro activities of tigecycline, doxycycline, and tetracycline against the spirochete *Borrelia burgdorferi. Ticks Tick Borne Dis* 2010;1(1):30–34.

195. Mursic VP, Wilske B, Schierz G, et al. In vitro and in vivo susceptibility of *Borrelia burgdorferi. Eur J Clin Microbiol* 1987;6(4):424–426.

196. Johnson RC, Kodner C, Russell M. In vitro and in vivo susceptibility of the Lyme disease spirochete, *Borrelia burgdorferi*, to four antimicrobial agents. *Antimicrob Agents Chemother* 1987;31(2):164–167.

197. Sicklinger M, Wienecke R, Neubert U. In vitro susceptibility testing of four antibiotics against *Borrelia burgdorferi*: a comparison of results for the three genospecies *Borrelia afzelii, Borrelia garinii,* and *Borrelia burgdorferi* sensu stricto. *J Clin Microbiol* 2003;41(4):1791–1793.

198. Cinco M, Padovan D, Stinco G, et al. In vitro activity of rokitamycin, a new macrolide, against *Borrelia burgdorferi. Antimicrob Agents Chemother* 1995;39(5):1185–1186.

199. Goldmeier D, Hay P. A review and update on adult syphilis, with particular reference to its treatment. *Int J STD AIDS* 1993;4(2):70–82.

200. Korting HC, Walther D, Riethmuller U, et al. Comparative in vitro susceptibility of *Treponema pallidum* to ceftizoxime, ceftriaxone and penicillin G. *Chemotherapy* 1986;32(4):352–355.

Applications, Significance of, and Methods for the Measurement of Antimicrobial Concentrations in Human Body Fluids

Shelly Latte, Emilia Mia Sordillo, and Stephen C. Edberg

The proliferation of antimicrobial agents in recent years presents clinical laboratories with a potentially large number of antibiotics to assay. Many of the methods described in the previous edition of this book (367) remain the testing standard, whether for routine clinical therapeutic drug monitoring (e.g. automated immunoassay based methods) or for monitoring during the initial evaluation of a new antimicrobial agent (e.g. high pressure liquid chromatography/HPLC). Method modifications that have been introduced to increase assay sensitivity include improved sample preparation methods prior to HPLC and utilization of mass spectrometry for analyte detection following HPLC

Automated chemical methods for the determination of antibiotic concentrations in body fluids, most commonly serum or plasma, have become commonplace and can be performed with relative ease at reasonable costs. These automated methods have largely replaced bioassays, which are not routinely performed. Therapeutic drug monitoring of aminoglycosides is generally performed by enzyme immunoassay (EIA), particle-enhanced turbidimetric inhibition immunoassay (PETINIA), fluorescence polarization immunoassay (FPIA), cloned enzyme donor immunoassay (CEDIA), chemiluminescent microparticle immunoassay (CMIA), or similar labeled immunoassays because of their ease of performance, rapid turnaround times, and reasonable costs.

For example, Abbott Laboratories (Abbott Park, IL) produces CEDIAs, CMIAs, and PETINIAs for gentamicin, tobramycin, amikacin, and vancomycin which can be run on Abbott's Architect, an automated chemistry analyzer. Other immunoassay-based tests are available from numerous manufacturers including Beckman-Coulter (Jersey City, NJ), Roche Diagnostics (Indianapolis, IN), Siemens Diagnostics (Tarrytown, NY), and Vitros (Ortho Clinical Diagnostics Inc, Rochester, NY.)

The PETINIA assays previously produced by Dade Behring, Inc, for gentamicin, tobramycin, amikacin, and vancomycin were acquired by Siemens AG in 2007, and can be run on the company's Dimension and Dimension Vista instruments. These assays use latex particle antibiotic conjugates to compete for monoclonal antibody binding sites with the free, unconjugated antibiotic in the sample. The binding of unbound antibiotic to the antibody decreases the rate of aggregation of the particle-antibody complexes, which is inversely proportional to the concentration of antibiotic in the sample.

Roche Diagnostics' (Indianapolis, IN) CEDIA gentamicin II and tobramycin assays run on several of the company's automated chemistry analyzers. In the CEDIA assays, an inactive fragment of recombinant bacterial β-galactosidase that has been genetically engineered into two inactive fragments is conjugated to the study of antibiotic. Under assay conditions, the two enzyme fragments spontaneously reassociate to form a fully active enzyme that cleaves a chromogenic substrate. A color change is generated that is spectrophotometrically measured. Binding of a monoclonal antibody directed at the enzyme-drug conjugate interferes with enzyme reassociation. Free analyte in the sample competes with the conjugated drug for antibody sites. The quantity of enzyme that is formed and the resultant absorbance change are directly proportional to the amount of analyte that is present in the sample.

Vancomycin and chloramphenicol (CAM) levels are routinely obtained through the use of immunoassay or high-performance liquid chromatography (HPLC)–based methods. Determination of sulfonamide, trimethoprim, β-lactam, macrolide, quinolone, tetracycline, and other antimicrobial levels is largely confined to reference laboratories. Methods include HPLC, immunoassay, and bioassay, although this latter method has fallen into disfavor because of assay variability and potential interference when multiple drugs are administered. While radioimmunoassay (RIA) and gas chromatography techniques can also be used for antibiotic concentration analysis, these methods generally confer little advantage over existing immunoassays and are infrequently used.

Interestingly, despite the major advances in technology and the large increase in the number of antimicrobial drugs, the clinical indications for therapeutic monitoring of antibiotic concentrations are limited to a few select drugs and clinical settings. This is largely because of the improved toxicity profiles and large therapeutic windows of the majority of currently used antimicrobials. Most routine antimicrobial therapeutic drug monitoring involves aminoglycoside and glycopeptide (vancomycin) antibiotics and, to a lesser extent, CAM. Antituberculosis, antifungal, and antiretroviral therapies present additional applications in which therapeutic drug monitoring may prove to be of value.

Recently, concerns regarding increasing resistance among pathogenic organisms and the emergence of obesity as a major health issue have highlighted the importance of weight-based dosing paired with assessment of blood levels for many drugs. A notable example is the recommendation to maintain serum vancomycin through levels above 10 mg per L, and from 15 to 20 mg per L in serious infections, as outlined in the 2009 consensus guideline from the American Society of Health-System Pharmacists, the Infectious Diseases Society of America, and the Society of Infectious Diseases Pharmacists (373).

The assay of antibiotics or antibiotic material dates back to the demonstration of lysozyme in an agar diffusion assay system by Fleming (1) in 1922. Thus, the first use and many of the other initial uses of assay systems were for the detection of antibiotic activity that resulted from the in vivo production of antimicrobial substances. Assays of antibiotics in blood, urine, and other body fluids and tissues were primarily performed in conjunction with the determination of antibiotic pharmacology and pharmacokinetics.

In the late 1960s, accurate, rapid assays to measure blood levels of antimicrobial substances, particularly those with narrow toxic/therapeutic ratios, were sought (2–7). The value of such information for the optimal use of certain antibiotics eventually became apparent, but the popularization of rapid serum assays required most of the decade of the 1970s. Data from several laboratories demonstrated that the efficacy of some antibiotics correlated with their peak serum antibiotic levels (8,9; Williams DN et al., unpublished data, 1984). Primarily, as a consequence of this work, the measurement of aminoglycoside levels began to be performed in all seriously ill patients who received these drugs, irrespective of the patients' renal status (10).

Toxicity was also shown to be related to both peak and trough serum levels. Although the study by Line et al. (11) showed a correlation between streptomycin toxicity and trough levels, the concept that trough levels correlated better with toxicity than peak levels for aminoglycoside drugs remained in dispute for some time. Indeed, although it was quite clear from retrospective analyses that toxicity was associated with high serum levels of these antibiotics, it was difficult to prove that toxicity occurred at particular blood levels for a given drug. Table 8.1 demonstrates the toxic/therapeutic ratios of some commonly used aminoglycosides (12).

The measurement of antibiotic concentrations in various fluids has been a prominent aspect of the evaluation of new antibiotics and the quality control of their manufacture. With the availability of rapid, accurate assays, the measurement of antibiotic material in serum and other body fluids is feasible, desirable, and widely practiced for these purposes. Clinically, such assays have been used primarily for the determination of aminoglycoside levels in serum, for which peak levels primarily establish adequacy of therapy, while trough levels reflect potential drug accumulation and toxicity.

Although the most common reason for performing rapid serum antibiotic assays in hospitals is to regulate therapy with aminoglycoside antibiotics and vancomycin, there are other indications. For patients who have organ dysfunction, such as hepatic or renal failure, it is desirable to know whether or not antibiotics that are metabolized or

Table 8.1

Toxic/Therapeutic Ratios of Commonly Used Aminoglycoside Antibiotics				
Antibiotic	Average Daily Dose (mg/kg)	Therapeutic Concentration (μg/mL)	Toxic Concentrations (μg/mL)	
			Peak	Trough
Amikacin	15	8–16	>35	>10
Gentamicin	3–5	4–8	>12	>2
Kanamycin	15	8–16	>35	>10
Netilmicin	6.5	4–12	>16	>4
Tobramycin	3–5	4–8	>12	>2

eliminated (e.g., CAM) by damaged or imperfectly functioning organs accumulate. In some patients who are taking oral antibiotics, it may be important to know the extent to which they are absorbing the drugs from their gastrointestinal tracts (13–16). Therapeutic monitoring of β-lactam, macrolide, tetracycline, and other antibiotics with wide therapeutic windows occurs infrequently, but may be performed to assess compliance, and/or in patients with renal failure.

Aminoglycoside levels are usually ordered to establish the adequacy of therapy and to prevent toxicity. Retrospectively, there is a correlation between both peak and trough levels and toxicity. In one study, Black et al. (17) found a significant correlation between ototoxicity of amikacin and both peak and trough levels, with the *P* value being slightly lower for the peak than the trough value.

Another indication for the measurement of antibiotics from human body fluids has been the establishment of therapeutic levels of drugs in various body fluids. The field of the pharmacokinetics of antibiotics has developed rapidly, along with the number of drugs that are currently available to treat serious infections. The concept of the "class" or "type" antibiotic that is representative of all related members is no longer valid. For example, we can no longer predict the tissue distribution of all cephalosporins based on the activity of cephalothin. Many of the third-generation cephalosporins appear in extravascular body fluid compartments, while cephalothin does not. Therefore, the ability to assay each cephalosporin level in cerebrospinal fluid is desirable. As pharmaceutical chemists modify currently available antibiotics, additional generations and individual drugs will continue to be developed.

In the 1960s and 1970s, most work concentrated on microbiologic assay systems for the major classes of antibiotics. The 1970s witnessed the evolution of reference methods to rapid procedures that became available in clinical laboratories. By the late 1970s, approximately 75% to 85% of all assays in clinical laboratories were microbiologic in nature, with most of the remainder being RIAs (18). Subsequently, commercially available, nonisotopic immunoassays largely replaced microbiologic assays. Methods for the assay of virtually all classes of antibiotics by HPLC have become available and can be performed in a broad spectrum of laboratories. Immunoassays for aminoglycosides and vancomycin have become routine "black box" procedures because of the widespread availability of commercial kits. Assays for antituberculous, antifungal, and antiviral medications can be found in their respective chapters.

HOW TO CHOOSE AN ASSAY

The selection of an assay method depends on the clinical and research needs and on the capabilities and resources of the laboratory in which the assay is to be performed. For high-volume assays that require rapid turnaround, commercially sold immunoassays that use specific monoclonal antibodies and are performed on automated chemistry analyzers will be the methods of choice. Low-volume assays for which monoclonal antibodies, commercial kits, or automated chemistry analyzers are unavailable may be performed by HPLC or, in some instances, bioassay. As a rule of thumb, a laboratory that processes 10 or more specimens per day should select the most automated, least labor-intensive methods available, even if reagent and

Table 8.2

Antibiotic Assay Methods					
Factor	Microbiologic Assay	Radioenzymatic Assay	RIA	Nonradioactive Immunoassay	HPLC
Mean coefficient of variation (%)[a]	8.9	8.3	8.1	8.5	7.0
Variation range (%)[a]	3.3–17.0	6.0–10.4	4.3–17.3	5–10	5–9
Sensitivity (μg/mL)	0.5	0.5	0.1	0.25	0.1
Time required (h)	3–4	2–3	3–4	1	1
Technical time	10–20 min	1.5–2.5 h	1.5–2.5 h	30 min	30 min
Technical difficulty	Easy	Difficult	Difficult	Easy	Difficult
Availability	General	Specific	Specific	General	Specific
Cost	Inexpensive	Relatively inexpensive[b]	Expensive[b]	Moderate	Expensive

[a]From Stevens et al. (31), in part.
[b]Cost decreases as the number of specimens processed at one time increases.
RIA, radioimmunoassay; HPLC, high-performance liquid chromatography.

equipment costs are increased by doing so. Because the availability of assays to detect minimal deviations from the therapeutic range can be clinically important, sensitivity may take precedence over specificity (19). There remain circumstances in which microbiologic assays may still be useful with particular antibiotics. They have the advantage of being performed without costly or dedicated laboratory equipment. In addition, they determine the concentration of all active metabolites in one step.

There is an extremely broad array of microbiologic agar diffusion assays that are available for use. Each combination of agar, pH, and organism has been chosen to optimize the measurement of a given antibiotic, either alone or in combination with other antibiotics. For clinical purposes, however, the absolute sensitivity of the organism used is of less importance than such factors as the turnaround time of the test, the ability to store plates, and the resistance pattern of the organism. Rarely is it necessary for clinical assays to equal the sensitivity of research assays (20,21). When microbiologic assays in agar are well designed and measurements of zone sizes are made properly, these assays have shown excellent agreement with immunologic techniques (22–25).

A study was undertaken in Great Britain in the mid-1970s in which salted serum specimens of gentamicin were sent to numerous clinical laboratories that performed microbiologic assays for measurement of the drug in body fluids (26). This study classified the performance of fewer than 20% of laboratories, on average, as "good." Those laboratories with the least experience fared the worst.

Radioenzyme assays and RIAs were studied according to similar protocols. Repeated testing of the same laboratories demonstrated marked improvement because of either increased motivation or reexamination of and improvement in their techniques. Pocket calculators can be programmed to provide linear regression analysis with such factors as slope, intercept, and coefficient of variation, and it is recommended that such records be maintained as an internal quality control check of a bioassay (27). Deviations beyond 2 standard deviations (SDs), or 1 SD in the same direction, an inordinate number of times should prompt reexamination of the method.

Proficiency testing samples with serum samples spiked with antibiotics such as amikacin, gentamicin, tobramycin, and vancomycin are available from the College of American Pathologists and other authorized organizations. Participation in Centers for Medicare and Medicaid Services–approved proficiency testing programs for clinically tested antibiotic analytes for which such programs are available is required under the Clinical Laboratory Improvement Amendments of 1988 and for laboratory accreditation by certifying entities, irrespective of the testing method used. For antibiotics for which no Centers for Medicare and Medicaid Services–approved proficiency testing samples are available, laboratories must document biannual verification of the accuracy of their procedures.[a]

Table 8.2 summarizes the general advantages and disadvantages of the agar diffusion assay method.

---

[a]*12 CFR parts 493.803 and 493.1236 (2003).*

Almost all of the equipment necessary to perform the microbiologic assay successfully is familiar to microbiology technicians and is readily available in the microbiology laboratory. The only factor that needs to be rigidly controlled is the preparation of the antibiotic standards (28). For those laboratories without sensitive electrical balances or a person experienced in preparing such standards, the hospital pharmacy can be extremely helpful and is often willing to prepare standards. Skilled technical personnel are not required to perform the assay, and it generally takes less than 2 hours to train a technician to successfully complete it. Once the standards are made and familiarity with the calculation of results and preparation of media is attained, an antibiotic blood level can be set up within 10 to 20 minutes of receipt of the specimen. With most *Staphylococcus*, Enterobacteriaceae, and *Bacillus* assays, results are available within 2 to 4 hours (29–31). Finally, inexpensive equipment is used, limiting the cost of the assay and possible problems with instrument accessibility.

The major disadvantage of the microbiologic assay is the steep slope that is generated, especially for the assay of aminoglycoside antibiotics. As a consequence, a small difference in measurement can significantly alter the apparent concentration (32). Vernier calipers or automated instruments that are designed especially for this purpose, rather than millimeter rulers, should always be used to measure zone sizes. Rather than hand drawing a "best" straight line, x and y values should be interpolated from a regression curve. The regression curve can be generated with a pocket calculator. A second or third antibiotic that is present

in the specimen and unknown to the laboratory can, of course, lead to erroneously high results. Because a large percentage of hospitalized patients receive two or more antibiotics, it is incumbent on the assayist to contact the ward or the pharmacy to inquire as to what antibiotics the patient is receiving, irrespective of the information that is provided on the requisition form (33,34).

It is probably convenient when choosing a microbiologic assay to choose an organism, such as *Klebsiella*, that is inherently resistant to many antibiotics. The technician should be sure that likely combinations of antibiotics will not act synergistically on the organism that is selected. Inordinately high results should be confirmed by repeating the assay with the specimen diluted 1:5 and 1:10 in normal human serum and by determining whether an unknown second antibiotic is present (35).

Immunoassays are the method of choice for aminocyclitol/aminoglycoside antibiotics. The major advantages of these assays include specificity, automated analysis, microprocessor-controlled calculations, and versatility of analytes that can be measured with the required instrumentation. Immunoassays for aminoglycosides and other antibiotics are invariably competitive assays, in which bound or conjugated drug competes with free drug in the specimen for antibody binding sites. Some assay formats that are commonly used in clinical laboratories to measure aminoglycoside concentrations are listed in Table 8.3. For the measurement of gentamicin and tobramycin concentrations, the Abbott AXSYM FPIA (Abbott Laboratories, Abbott Park, IL), the Dade

Table 8.3

Assay Formats Commonly Used to Measure Aminoglycoside Concentrations	
ADVIA CENTAUR (Siemens)	Chemiluminescence enzyme immunoassay
Architect (Abbott)	Chemiluminescent Microparticle Immunoassay, turbidimetric inhibition immunoassay
CEDIA (Microgenics/Roche)	Homogeneous enzyme immunoassay (cloned donor immunoassay)
COBAS INTEGRA (Roche)	Fluorescence polarization immunoassay
DIMENSION (Siemens)	Turbidimetric inhibition immunoassay
DPC IMMULITE 2000 (Siemens)	Chemiluminescence enzyme immunoassay
Unicel DxC (Beckman)	Turbidimetric inhibition immunoassay
SYVA EMIT 2000 PLUS (Beckman)	Homogeneous enzyme immunoassay (enzyme multiplied immunoassay)
SYVA EMIT 2000 (Beckman, Siemens ADVIA)	Fluorescence polarization immunoassay

Dimension turbidimetric inhibition immunoassay (Siemens Diagnostics, Tarrytown, NY), and the Beckman Synchron (Beckman Coulter, Inc, Brea, CA) reagent are among the most commonly used assay systems in clinical laboratories. For the analysis of amikacin concentrations, the Abbott TDX/TDX FLEX (Abbott Laboratories, Abbott Park, IL) is a very popular assay format.

Although the material costs per test are higher for immunoassays than for microbiologic assays, the labor costs are significantly less. The necessary instrumentation costs significantly less than RIA or radioenzymatic assay equipment, and, in most cases, capital expenditures for instruments can be transferred to the costs of individual tests as disposable items. Because many reagents have refrigerated lifetimes of up to 12 weeks after they are constituted, these methods are applicable to laboratories of any size. Moreover, specialized technologists are not needed to perform immunoassays. In deciding between various assay methods and formats, one often must balance the costs of labor versus the costs of supplies. For clinical purposes, the sensitivity of nonisotopic immunoassays is no different from that of RIAs (36–43).

HPLC has become the method of choice for analysis of β-lactam concentrations in serum and other body fluids. Again, one must deal with the proviso that the equipment is expensive. However, one can process large numbers of specimens quite accurately in short periods of time (44,45). HPLC technology is the primary method of analysis of antibiotic concentrations in human body fluids in the research setting, especially when new drugs are being investigated. It is the method of choice when one wishes to analyze individual components of an antibiotic or its metabolites (46).

A particular advantage of HPLC is the ability to quantify closely related compounds in a mixture (47–53). HPLC procedures have been developed for the analysis of almost all antibiotics used for the treatment of human diseases (54–56). Unfortunately, the high cost of HPLC instruments makes it impractical for this technique to compete with immunoassays once a specific antibody has been produced for an antibiotic. In addition to the cost of the HPLC apparatus, the procedure generally requires a trained technologist and dedicated instrument to the analysis of particular antibiotics or classes of antibiotics for a defined period of time. Different antibiotic classes may require different columns and conditions. Unlike gas-liquid chromatography (GLC), however, the basic columns in HPLC technology (C_8 and C_{18}) may be used in the reverse-phase mode for all water-soluble antibiotics. The primary modifications that are required for the measurement of these drug concentrations are to the solvent systems. Because of the ability of HPLC to separate constituents in a mixture (e.g., the three gentamicin components), its analytical capabilities extend beyond those of RIAs (57–60).

SPECIMEN HANDLING

To achieve optimal results, specimens should be processed as soon as possible after they are obtained. Each antibiotic loses potency at its own rate. For example, aminoglycosides are much more stable than the penicillins.

Serum or ethylenediaminetetraacetic acid (EDTA)–treated plasma is the recommended specimen for measuring blood concentrations of aminoglycosides. Heparin in the concentrations present in heparin-containing blood collection tubes may inactivate aminoglycoside antibiotics through complex formation. This can cause underestimates of aminoglycoside concentrations. Heparin in therapeutic concentrations does not appear to have in vivo effects on aminoglycoside activity, but heparin-containing collection tubes should not be used unless their suitability has been verified by the manufacturer of an assay. Although sera of patients receiving gentamicin can be stored between 20°C and +25°C for up to 2 days without any significant effect, samples that are not tested within 2 hours should be stored at 0°C to 5°C to avoid possible inactivation by coadministered β-lactam antibiotics (61,62).

Acceptable samples for measurement of blood CAM concentrations include serum and EDTA or citrate anticoagulated plasma. These specimens should be kept protected from light and, if not analyzed immediately, stored frozen.

Serum or EDTA anticoagulated plasma are appropriate specimens for analysis of vancomycin concentrations. Heparin-containing samples are generally also considered acceptable. However, reports of vancomycin instability in the presence of heparin recommend exercising caution in testing such samples. Verification of specimen suitability is essential.

In general, if a specimen cannot be processed within 1 to 2 hours of its receipt, steps must be taken to ensure its potency. If it is to be processed the same day, it should be refrigerated at less than 4°C. If it cannot be processed the same day, it should be frozen. If the specimen can be processed within 3 to 4 days, freezing at −20°C should be sufficient. If storage is for a longer period, the specimen should be frozen at −70°C. If a tissue specimen cannot be processed within 2 to 3 hours, it should be frozen at −20°C for processing within 24 hours. If storage will be for more than 24 hours, the specimen should be frozen at −70°C (63).

FLUIDS OTHER THAN BLOOD

The clinical assay of antibiotics from sites other than serum or plasma has generally not been standardized (64). The determination of antibiotic concentrations in fluids other than blood involves all the variability that accompanies the measurement of antibiotic levels in serum and much more (65–68). These fluids can contain different types and amounts of proteins, chemical compounds, and cellular compounds and have different pH values as compared with serum. In order for an assay to be valid, standards must be prepared in the same milieu as the sample or in a matrix that has been demonstrated to be equivalent to it. In assaying a fluid, one must be sure that the specimen is not contaminated by blood. Although rather simplistic in practice, the avoidance of such contamination is difficult and sometimes not readily detectable (69).

No universal method is described that can be used for the assay of antibiotic concentrations in all fluids. The key to the assay of antibiotics in body fluids is that the standard antibiotic dilution curves should be prepared in the same media as the patient samples. For example, in assaying the level of an antibiotic in joint fluid, one should prepare standards in normal human joint fluid or in a solvent with a high protein content. In the determination of gentamicin concentrations in spinal fluid, it was found that if the standards were made in water, a 400% error could result. If the standards were made in 0.5% saline, the error was reduced to 50%. Finally, if the suspending medium was 150 mmol/L NaCl per 4.5 mmol/L CaCl$_2$, the results were not significantly different from those for cerebrospinal fluid (70).

One may determine the antibiotic concentration in fluids such as cerebrospinal fluid, joint fluid, or any other nonviscous fluid by diluting the antibiotic standards in normal fluid and performing the microbiologic assay, as described in the section "Elements Influencing Microbiologic Assays," for total biologic activity (71). When assaying an antibiotic that is not readily degraded

(e.g., aminoglycosides and CAM), an immunologic or chemical assay is best.

It is important to establish the concentration of antibiotic that was actually present in the fluid under study from that obtained in the presence of contaminating blood. One should analyze the fluid specimen for blood by weighing the fluid and measuring the amount of blood inside it (72). This may be done by spectrophotometric analysis. The fluid should be centrifuged at 3,000 rpm for 15 minutes and the supernatant placed in a 1-cm spectrophotometric cell. After brief aeration, the absorbance at 576 nm is recorded and corrected for turbidity produced by cellular debris by recording the absorbances at 600 and 624 nm. At these latter wavelengths, the hemoglobin absorption is less than 10% of the maximum.

To the absorbance at 600 nm is added the difference between the absorbances at 600 and 624 nm. The resulting absorbance represents the contributions made by the turbidity to the absorbance at 576 nm. This correction is then subtracted from total absorbance at 576 nm, with the remainder providing a measure of the tissue hemoglobin content. The absorbance value so obtained can be standardized in terms of hemoglobin concentration by making similar measurements with a sample of the patient's own blood, diluted 1:150.

Another potential problem in the assay of antibiotic concentrations in tissue is storage. When performing fluid assays, one tends to collect the fluid and freeze it until ready for use. In contrast, most clinical assays of antibiotic blood levels are performed soon after the specimen has been received.

The stability of an antibiotic depends on the medium in which it is suspended. An antibiotic that is stable in buffer for long periods of time at 20°C or at 4°C may be quite unstable at the same temperature in serum or tissue (73). One should store all body fluids at −70°C prior to assay. It is incumbent on the assayist, when storing antibiotics in a given tissue medium, to store a standard in parallel to assess any loss of activity (74). At this time, it is not possible to definitively predict how an antibiotic's stability will be affected by the particular fluid or tissue in which it is found (73,74). Antibiotics have been assayed successfully from many body sites by employing the principles described. Each fluid and antibiotic must be treated as a unique combination. Procedures that are satisfactory for one fluid and antibiotic pair will not necessarily prove satisfactory for another pair, even if the two are closely related.

Urine should be buffered to the optimum pH of the antibiotic in question, and its protein and sugar content should be recorded. Normal pooled urine from patients who are not receiving antibiotics, buffered in the same way, should be used as controls. The *Bacillus subtilis* technique has been used successfully for the determination of antibiotic concentrations in urine. As described in the section "Elements Influencing Microbiologic Assays," dilutions in a phosphate buffer provide good results. It has been reported that individuals may naturally excrete organic acids that can be antibacterial. Although this scenario is not common, the assayist should be on guard for spuriously high urine antibiotic levels due to the presence of such organic acids. One must filter-sterilize the urine if it contains microorganisms (75,76).

MICROBIOLOGIC ASSAYS

Microbiologic assays are relative rather than absolute (77). In one type of assay, an antibiotic concentration is determined from the microbiologic response of a strain of test organism to a series of standard antibiotic concentrations.

Agar Methods

Assays in agar fall into three broad categories: one-dimensional, two-dimensional, and three-dimensional. The one-dimensional assay employs a test tube or a capillary tube in which seeded agar has been poured and allowed to harden as the agar medium (Fig. 8.1). An antibiotic test suspension is pipetted onto the surface of the hardened agar, and zones of inhibition in one dimension are formed. The one-dimensional assay is especially appropriate for the assay of antibiotics under anaerobic conditions. This method never gained popularity in clinical laboratories in the United States, although it has been used frequently in Japan (78). The method does not lend itself to automation. Its major disadvantages are that it requires complex sample preparation and time-consuming dilution steps. The one-dimensional assay can be useful in determining the antibiotic fluid levels in a pediatric population or in other circumstances in which only a small amount of fluid is available for testing. A procedure for the one-dimensional tube assay is provided later in this chapter.

Clinical laboratories have most commonly used two-dimensional or three-dimensional assays. A two-dimensional assay is one in which the antibiotic diffuses directly against a wall of

seeded bacteria. This typically involves one of two designs. In the first technique, wells are cut in agar and seeded throughout with the test organism. In the second method, the test organism is swabbed onto the surface of the agar. Antibiotic disks are then placed on the agar surface. The assay is considered two-dimensional because the concentration of antibiotic as it diffuses radially is equal at any given distance from its source. In a three-dimensional assay, the antibiotic diffuses vertically to the bottom of the Petri plate, in addition to migrating along the surface of the agar. At a distance x from the disk, therefore, the concentration of antibiotic may not be identical in all dimensions. As the agar thickness in a three-dimensional system decreases, the likelihood that the antibiotic concentrations are equal at any given distance x from the source increases because the three-dimensional system is physically moving toward a two-dimensional system.

For clinical assays, the differences between the three- and two-dimensional systems are of little significance. In research settings, both systems should be compared to establish that they yield equal results before a three-dimensional system is used. The two-dimensional assay is theoretically somewhat sounder than the three-dimensional assay (79). The three-dimensional assay is one in which cylinders, fish spines, or disks are placed on the surfaces of seeded agar plates.

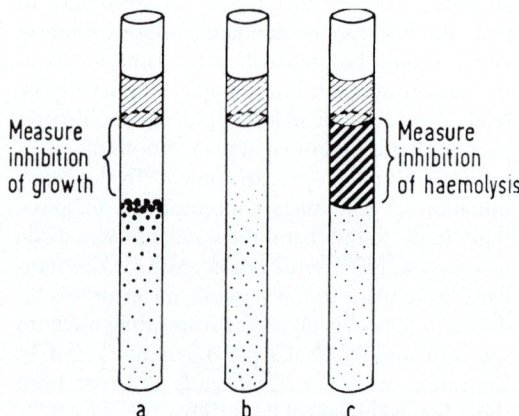

Figure 8.1 ■ Diagrammatic illustration of the one-dimensional assay. A: Assay of streptomycin with *Staphylococcus aureus* as test organism. **B:** Penicillin assay with *Staphylococcus aureus* as test organism. **C:** Penicillin assay with *Streptococcus pyogenes* in blood agar. (From Garrod LP, Lambert HP, O'Grady F. *Antibiotics and chemotherapy.* Edinburgh, United Kingdom: Churchill Livingstone, 1973, with permission.)

The well-type, two-dimensional assay and paper disk-type, three-dimensional assay have been extensively used clinically. One generally can determine the lower limits of antibiotic concentrations using well-type assays.

Elements Influencing Microbiologic Assays

In performing microbiologic assays, one must carefully account for the many conditions that affect the action of the antibiotic under study and the growth properties of the organism. Deviations from the use of rigid controls result in erroneous assay values (80). The most prominent factors that affect the performance of microbiologic assays follow.

Design

Basic to the assay of antibiotic concentrations is a system design that determines the levels accurately. One must be certain that the zone of inhibition around a source of antibiotic is produced in direct proportion to the amount of antibiotic that is contained within that source. One must also be certain that the response is linear within the range that is normally encountered in clinical specimens. Because dose-response curves are sigmoidal in shape, the assayist must test a sufficient number of specimens to be assured that they fall on the dose-response curve. Environmental factors such as temperature and pH must not affect the assay in either the high or low ranges.

Media

There are a wide variety of media from which to choose for the assay of antibiotic concentrations. Grove and Randall (81) in 1955 described 11 different media that were available for the assay of antibiotic concentrations in human specimens. Almost all subsequently published methods have used some variation of these 11 types of media. The choice of medium is related to the antibiotic under study, the assay design, and the test organism. Although a detailed discussion of the relative merits of each medium–antibiotic–organism combination is not within the scope of this chapter, the medium chosen should be optimized for the assayed antibiotic (79) (Table 8.4). A medium that is satisfactory for use with one antibiotic–organism combination may not be acceptable for the measurement of the same antibiotic concentration in an assay that uses a different organism (82).

The pH of the agar may vary with the mixture of ingredients and the method of preparation. Although the agars are made according to the same formulation, they may not be identical. This variability is the result of the undefined nature of many of the ingredients. For example, yeast extract and animal infusions are in no way standardized. Table 8.4 presents the effects that different agar preparations and pH values have on the results of an assay for the measurement of gentamicin concentrations. Although most researchers have not thought it necessary to use indicators in media, several have found it useful to add fermentable sugars that enable the determination of zones of inhibition by the accompanying pH changes (83). The spraying of plates with tetrazolium blue allows for the ascertainment of zone size more rapidly than by visible inspection alone (84). Agars differ in their susceptibilities to pH changes, crispness of zones, absolute sensitivities, and slopes of the standard curves that they produce (85). Because antibiotic standards and patients' specimens are included on the same plates in most clinical assays, such variations are internally controlled (Fig. 8.2).

Antibiotic Standards

The production of antibiotic standards is the most critical factor in these assays. Because microbiologic assays are relative assays, any inconsistency in the antibiotic standards results in erroneous concentration measurements. Each antibiotic is differentially active at different pH values (78,86). Because it is impractical to make antibiotic standards from powder each time an assay is to be performed, one may produce and store working concentrations of the antibiotic in small aliquots. Practically, the antibiotics are dissolved in appropriate buffers (Table 8.5) at high concentrations. These 1-mL aliquots can be stored at −20°C but should not be kept longer than 3 months. The aminoglycosides are extremely stable and probably can be held longer than the penicillins, which are more labile (79,87,88). Subsequent dilutions from these buffers are made in appropriate body fluids for assay use.

Antibiotics must be weighed using an analytical balance. The potency of the antibiotic should be calculated based on active micrograms per milligram of powder. In addition, the identical antibiotic must be present in the standard and the sample. For example, gentamicin is a compound composed of three molecular elements.

Table 8.4

Discriminatory Power, pH Susceptibility, and Reproducibility of Growth Inhibition Zones for Gentamicin on Five Media			
Medium and pH	**Discriminatory Power (ZDD, mm)[a]**	**Lateral Shift of Standard Curve by pH 7.0–8.5 Increase in Standard Solutions (mm)[b]**	**Reproducibility of Zone Diameters (SD of Mean, mm)[c]**
DST (Oxoid)			
6.5	2.9	±0.0	
7.5	3.6	±0.2($P >$.05)	0.21
8.5	(4.8)	± 0.0	
CAB (Oxoid)			
6.5	2.6	+0.6($P <$.05)	
7.5	2.8	+0.5($P <$.01)	0.24
8.5	(5.1)	+0.3($P >$.05)	
BAB (Oxoid)			
6.5	2.2	+0.6($P <$.001)	
7.5	3.0	+0.5($P <$.01)	0.24
8.5	(5.1)	+0.2($P >$.05)	
AM No. 2 (Oxoid)			
6.5	1.6	+0.9($P <$.001)	
7.5	1.9	+0.9($P <$.001)	0.22
8.5	(2.8)	+0.7($P <$.01)	
AM No. 2 (Difco)			
6.5	1.0	+1.1($P <$.001)	
7.5	1.6	+1.1($P <$.001)	0.20
8.5		+0.3($P >$.05)	

[a]Zone diameter difference (ZDD) between twofold dilutions of antibiotics. At agar pH 8.5, linearity in the semilogarithmic graph at concentrations below 2.0 mg/L was lost.
[b]A gentamicin standard series was divided and pH was adjusted to 7.0 or 8.5. Solutions were randomly distributed in wells 5 mm in diameter. Each value represents the mean of six determinations. Statistical analysis was by student's test for nonpaired observations.
[c]A solution of 4.0 mg/L gentamicin was applied to 50 wells (3 mm in diameter, filled to the brim) on five plates, and the standard deviation (SD) of mean zone diameters was calculated.

They should be present in the same proportion in the assay standards as they are in the pharmacy.

It is also important that there not be a second antibacterial substance present in the antibiotic standard. Because pharmacy materials may contain preservatives, they should not be used as standards except under emergency circumstances. It is necessary to make standards as close in composition to the patient's specimen as possible.

For the determination of antibiotic levels in blood, the specimen should be diluted in plasma or serum (89). As discussed subsequently, this principle also applies to the determination of

antibiotic levels from other tissue fluids. Considerable work has been performed to establish the types of sera that may be used for dilution. Horse serum, bovine serum, normal human serum, normal human serum inactivated at 56°C for 30 minutes, bovine serum albumin (BSA), and fetal calf serum have been the most extensively studied (61,90–92). It was found that, when antibiotics were suspended in different sera than that used in the test samples, errors of 80% to 367% in measured antibiotic concentrations resulted (6). In assaying antibiotics from cerebrospinal fluid, 150 mmol/L NaCl per 4.5 mmol/L CaCl$_2$

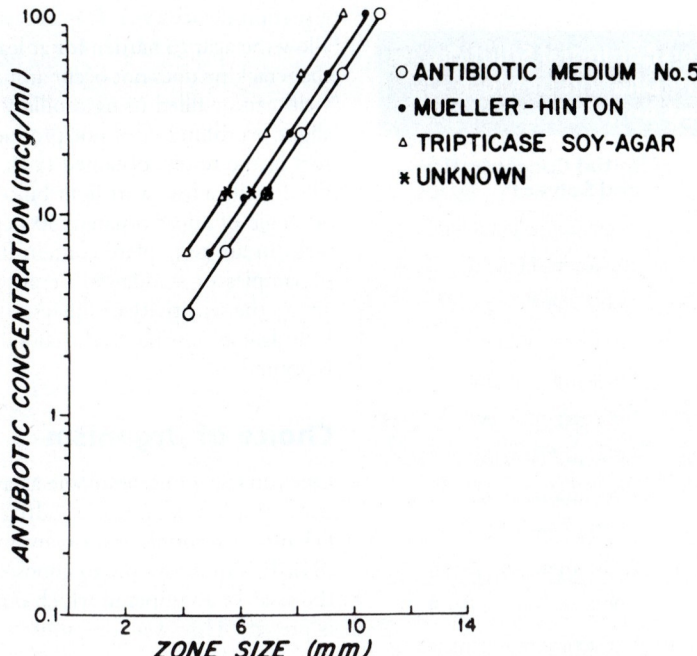

Figure 8.2 ■ **Determination of a CAM blood level using** *Escherichia coli* **ATCC strain 25922 as the test organism.** Although zone of inhibition diameters varied with each agar, all media yielded the same value, 10.4 μg/mL (±5%). (From Edberg SC, Chu A. Determining antibiotic levels in the blood. *Am J Med Technol* 1975;41:99–105, with permission.)

should be added to a phosphate buffer or inaccuracies occur (70). Apparently, it is not necessary to physically buffer the diluent serum (90). It also appears that cations present in sera at physiologic concentrations do not appreciably affect clinical assays (90).

Two factors that are present in sera may, however, exert some effect on microbiologic assays. The gentamicin recovery rate in normal serum has been reported to be between 80% and 90%. However, in uremic serum (blood urea nitrogen levels >50 mg/100 mL), the recovery rate of gentamicin has been shown to be only 50% to 69%. A more drastic decrease in the tobramycin level in the setting of uremia has been demonstrated. There has been some controversy about whether or not high levels of bilirubin in sera can interfere with the results of microbiologic assays of antibiotic concentrations. Blood bilirubin levels of greater than 23 mg/100 mL were shown to cause erroneous determinations of antibiotic concentrations (93). Bilirubin levels of 8 mg/100 mL did not affect the assay under study. Most workers have found that only assays in which bilirubin levels are above 20 mg/100 mL are adversely affected

(6,78). These levels are exceedingly rare in clinical samples. Suspending the antibiotic in a matrix equivalent medium that is similar to that from which it came corrects for several factors, the most important of which is protein binding.

Physical Factors

Disks must be known to be effective for assaying antibiotics. Schleicher & Schuell BioScience, Inc (Keene, NH) 740-E disks have been used extensively. Although individual investigators have used disks of different diameters, the smallest disk that produces good zone sizes in the range of the anticipated antibiotic levels should be used. If one is using the recommended 740-E disk, 20 μL of sample should be used in the assay. The maximum volume that this disk accurately holds is 25 μL. The filter paper must lie flat on the surface of the agar or irregular zone sizes will be produced. Supersaturation can lead to surface distortions.

The well technique is approximately five to six times more sensitive than techniques that use paper disks (93). Wells can be conveniently punched in agar with a metal cylinder that is attached to

Table 8.5

Standard Buffers for Initial Solution and Subsequent Dilution of Most Commonly Used Antibiotics

Antibiotic	Initial Concentration and Solvent[a]
Amikacin	1,000 μg/mL in buffer C
Ampicillin	100 μg/mL in dw
Azlocillin	1,000 μg/mL in dw
Bacitracin	100 μg/mL in buffer B
Cefamandole	1,000 μg/mL in dw
Cefoperazone	1,000 μg/mL in dw
Cefotaxime	1,000 μg/mL in dw
Cefoxitin	1,000 μg/mL in dw
Ceftriaxone	1,000 μg/mL in dw
Cephaloridine	1,000 μg/mL in buffer B
Cephalothin	1,000 μg/mL in buffer B
Chloramphenicol	10,000 μg/mL in ethanol
Clindamycin	1,000 μg/mL in dw
Cycloserine	1,000 μg/mL in dw
Dicloxacillin	1,000 μg/mL in buffer B
Erythromycin	10,000 μg/mL in methanol
Gentamicin	1,000 μg/mL in buffer C
Kanamycin	1,000 μg/mL in buffer C
Methicillin	1,000 μg/mL in buffer B
Mezlocillin	1,000 μg/mL in dw
Moxalactam	1,000 μg/mL in dw
Nafcillin	1,000 μg/mL in buffer B
Neomycin	1,000 μg/mL in buffer C
Netilmicin	1,000 μg/mL in buffer C
Oxacillin	1,000 μg/mL in buffer B
Penicillin G	1,000 units in buffer B
Piperacillin	1,000 μg/mL in dw
Streptomycin	1,000 μg/mL in buffer C
Tetracycline	1,000 μg/mL in 0.1 N HCl
Tobramycin	1,000 μg/mL in buffer C
Vancomycin	1,000 μg/mL in dw

[a]Buffer B, 1% phosphate buffer, pH 6.0 ± 0.05 (2 g of K_2HPO_4 plus 8 g of KH_2PO_4 in 1,000 mL of distilled water [dw]); buffer C, 0.1 mol/L phosphate buffer, pH 7.9 ± 0.1 (16.73 g of K_2HPO_4 plus 0.523 g of KH_2PO_4 in 1,000 mL of dw).
From Edberg SC, Chu A, Melnick G. Preparation of organisms for determining antibiotic concentrations from the blood. *Lab Med* 1973;4:36–37.

a suction device (94). It is necessary, however, to allow the agar to harden for at least 15 minutes so that cracking does not occur around the wells. The wells can be filled using capillary pipettes because slight overfilling does not produce significant errors in the results obtained (94). Wells should be filled while a low-watt light bulb is maintained at an angle of approximately 30 degrees so that the wells in an assay plate contain uniform amounts of samples or standards. Because the agar depth affects the sensitivity of the test, it is best to add as little agar as possible to the container when a plate is poured.

Choice of Organism

One can use a microbiologic assay to measure the concentration of almost any drug for which a sufficiently susceptible test organism can be isolated (84). It is quite simple to choose an organism for the assay of a sample in which only one antibiotic is present. However, one must exercise considerable caution in organism selection for an assay in which the specimen contains antibiotics in addition to the test drug.

The usual method is to use, as the test organism, a microorganism that is very sensitive to one of the antibiotics and insensitive to the other (81). This dictum appears simple but is often not reliable in practice (61). One must take into account synergy or antagonism, even though the test organism may appear to be resistant to one of the antibiotics. Thresholds at which one antibiotic interferes with another are published (95). The optimum way to assay antibiotics in a mixture is to chemically separate them by electrophoresis or chromatography prior to their measurement (96). This is probably not practical in clinical laboratories. Many test strains have been isolated that adequately take into account the physiologic levels of antibiotic combinations found in humans.

Organisms used for the clinical measurement of antibiotic blood levels most commonly include *Bacillus* (84,97–100), *Staphylococcus aureus* (82,93,101,102), *Sarcina lutea* (103,104), *Streptococcus* (102,105), *Clostridium* (99,106,107), *Klebsiella*, *Providencia* (108), and others (Fig. 8.3). Fungi and bacteria have been used for the assay of chemotherapeutic drugs (109,110). Assays that use bioluminescent bacteria (111,112) have also been employed. The actual choice of organism depends on the antibiotic to be measured, its susceptibility pattern, its ability to produce clear and

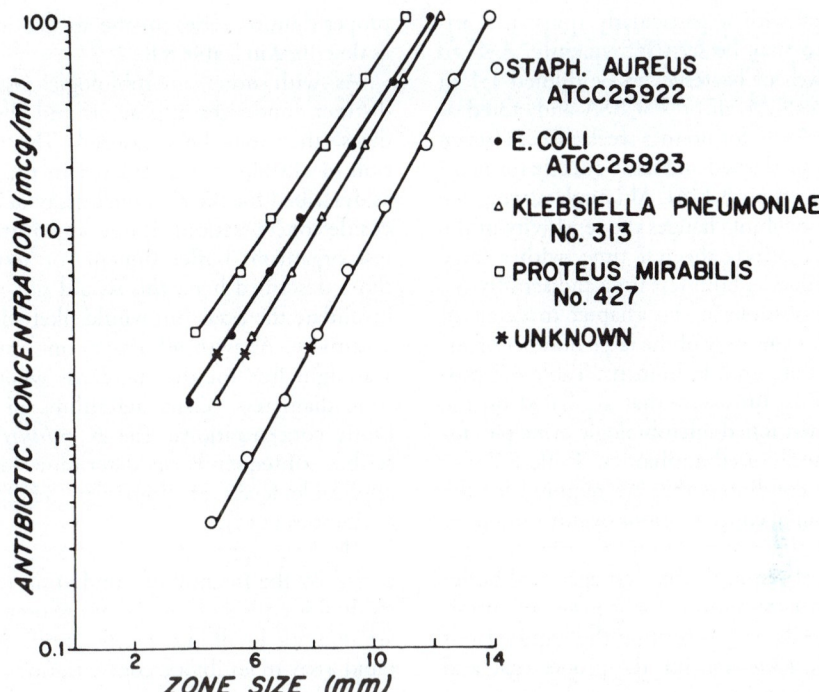

Figure 8.3 ■ **Determination of a gentamicin blood level using members of the family Enterobacteriaceae and *Staphylococcus aureus* as test organisms.** In each case, antibiotic medium 5 and an inoculum density of 0.5 McFarland standard was used. The *Proteus mirabilis* was not sensitive enough to yield a direct reading. All other test strains gave a gentamicin level of 2.4 μg/mL (±5%). (From Edberg SC, Chu A. Determining antibiotic levels in the blood. *Am J Med Technol* 1975;41:99–105, with permission.)

crisp zones on the given agar medium, and its ability to provide results within 4 hours. The organism that is selected impacts upon the minimum level of antibiotic that one can detect. Table 8.6 demonstrates the lower levels of detectability for some common antibiotics with assays that use Kirby-Bauer control strains *Staphylococcus aureus*, American Type Culture Collection (ATCC) strain

25923, and *Escherichia coli* ATCC strain 25922 as test organisms.

For the rapid determination of antibiotic levels, vegetative organisms must not be more than 24 hours old. The organism can be inoculated the night before the test is run or, more simply, swabbed off a plate, including a Kirby-Bauer sensitivity plate, that is no more than 1 day old (3).

Table 8.6

Approximate Lower Limits of Detectability Utilizing *Staphylococcus aureus* ATCC Strain 25923 and *Escherichia coli* ATCC Strain 25922 as Test Organisms

Limit of Detectability (μg/mL)

Organism	Ami	Amp	Carb	Meth	PenG	Ceph	Gm	Km	Col	Nal	Nit	Ery	Te	Tb	Chl	Cli
S. aureus	1	0.25	2	1	0.25	0.5	0.5	1.0	256	128	128	0.3	0.5	0.5	4.0	0.5
E. coli	2	8	8	256	128	8.0	1.5	3.0	1.0	4	4	64	1.0	1.0	8.0	128
B. subtilis	0.1	0.1	0.5	0.8	0.01	0.1	0.1	0.1	—	—	—	0.5	0.1	0.1	0.2	0.2

Ami, amikacin; Amp, ampicillin; Carb, carbenicillin; Meth, methicillin; PenG, penicillin G; Ceph, cephalothin; Gm, gentamicin; Km, kanamycin; Col, colistin; Nal, nalidixic acid; Nit, nitrofurantoin; Ery, erythromycin; Te, tetracycline; Tb, tobramycin; Chl, chloramphenicol; Cli, clindamycin. From Edberg SC, Chu A, Melnick G. Preparation of organisms for determining antibiotic concentrations from the blood. *Lab Med* 1973;4:36–37.

An organism with a particularly unusual sensitivity pattern may be seen infrequently. A 4- to 6-hour growth of bacteria can be diluted 1:1 in either fetal calf serum or 7% BSA and stored at $-20°C$ to $-70°C$ for up to 3 weeks. These frozen cultures can be thawed and used directly for rapid antibiotic assays (113,114). Although varying the size of the inoculum changes the sensitivity of the test, this also affects the test time, with a large inoculum reducing both test time and sensitivity.

It is not possible in this chapter to detail all conditions for the assay of the large number of antibiotics that are used in humans. Table 8.7 provides references for assays that are based on the previously mentioned microbiologic principles for some commonly used antibiotics. Table 8.7 also presents the conditions that are required for the determination of concentrations by diffusion assay for some of the major classes of antimicrobials. The choices of test organism, test agar, and buffer diluent shown are optimal for the class of antibiotic. One needs only substitute the required test organism for *Klebsiella*, use the proper agar and diluent described in Table 8.7, and choose the

proper dilution series for the antibiotic standard, as described in Table 8.8.

As with other microbiologic assays, when distinct zone sizes appear around the wells or disks, they may be measured. The concentration of antibiotic is calculated in the same way as described for the *B. subtilis* assay of aminoglycoside concentrations. If one substitutes another test organism, buffer diluent, or test agar for those described here, this would not necessarily invalidate the assay but would likely decrease its sensitivity. As with all assays, one must obtain a straight line for the standards when plotting zone diameters versus logarithms of the antibiotic concentrations. The *B. subtilis* assay described subsequently can determine the clinically applicable levels of almost all medically used antibiotics (115).

The basic approach used in bioassays is exemplified by the method of Lund et al. (116). This method is typical of those that use organisms that are resistant to all but specific antibiotics for the rapid assay of antibiotic concentrations in clinical material (4,114,117). Although any organism that

Table 8.7

Conditions for Assay of Major Classes of Antibiotics by Plate Diffusion Assay[a]

Antibiotic	Test Organism	Agar Type[b]	Dilution Buffer[c]
Penicillin G	*S. aureus* ATCC 6538P	AAM 1	B
Nafcillin	*S. aureus* ATCC 6538P	AAM 1	B
Oxacillin	*S. aureus* ATCC 6538P	AAM 1	B
Other semisynthetics (except ampicillin)	*S. aureus* ATCC 6538P	AAM 1	B
Cephalothins	*S. aureus* ATCC 6538P	AAM 1	B
Ampicillin	*S. lutea* ATCC 9341	AAM 11	C
Chloramphenicol	*S. lutea* ATCC 9341	AAM 1	B
Clindamycin	*S. lutea* ATCC 9341	AAM 11	C
Polymyxins	*Bordetella bronchiseptica* ATCC 4617	AAM 10	Same as B but 10 times as much salt
Erythromycin	*S. lutea* ATCC 9341	AAM 11	C
Rifampin	*B. subtilis* ATCC 6633	AAM 2	B
Tetracycline	*Bacillus cereus* var. *mycoides* ATCC 11778	AAM 8	A
Vancomycin	*B. cereus* var. *mycoides*	AAM 8	A

[a]For aminoglycosides, see the methods described in the text.
[b]Antibiotic media as described by Grove and Randall (81).
[c]Diluent buffers are those described in Table 8.5.

Table 8.8

Standard Curve Concentrations for Commonly Used Antibiotics

Antibiotic	Standard Curve Concentration (μg/mL)
Amikacin	5.0, 15.0, 25.0
Ampicillin	1.0, 5.0, 10.0
Aziocillin	2.0, 16.0, 64.0
Bacitracin	1.0, 1.25, 1.56
Cefamandole	2.0, 16.0, 64.0
Cefoperazone	2.0, 16.0, 64.0
Cefotaxime	2.0, 16.0, 64.0
Cefoxitin	2.0, 16.0, 64.0
Ceftriaxone	2.0, 16.0, 64.0
Cephaloridine	4.0, 8.0, 16.0
Cephalothin	2.0, 8.0, 32.0
Chloramphenicol	4.0, 8.0, 16.0
Clindamycin	1.0, 5.0, 10.0
Dicloxacillin	6.0, 12.0, 24.0
Erythromycin	2.0, 8.0, 32.0
Gentamicin	1.0, 5.0, 10.0
Kanamycin	5.0, 15.0, 25.0
Methicillin	1.0, 8.0, 16.0
Mezlocillin	2.0, 16.0, 64.0
Moxalactam	2.0, 16.0, 64.0
Nafcillin	0.5, 2.0, 8.0
Neomycin	2.0, 8.0, 32.0
Netilmicin	1.0, 5.0, 10.0
Oxacillin	1.0, 8.0, 16.0
Penicillin G	1.0, 4.0, 16.0
Piperacillin	2.0, 16.0, 64.0
Streptomycin	5.0, 15.0, 25.0
Tetracycline	1.0, 4.0, 25.0
Tobramycin	1.0, 5.0, 10.0
Vancomycin	5.0, 15.0, 25.0

From Edberg SC, Chu A, Melnick G. Preparation of organisms for determining antibiotic concentrations from the blood. *Lab Med* 1973;4:36–37.

possesses the appropriate sensitivity and meets the criteria described here can be used, the method of Lund et al. (116) provides a good model. The multiresistant *Klebsiella* strain they described is available from the ATCC. The method has been successfully field-tested. Prior to the substitution of another organism in this method, users should ensure that the new organism meets the criteria previously described. This strain of *Klebsiella* is resistant to most commonly used antibiotics, except gentamicin, tobramycin, and amikacin.

Presence of Aminoglycosides

Because the aminoglycoside antibiotics have broad activity, the assay of other classes of antibiotics that are present in combination with them has proved difficult. There are few bacteria that are resistant to aminoglycosides but sensitive to other classes of antibiotics. A group B *Streptococcus* has been used that allows the determination of clindamycin (CLD) concentrations in the presence of aminoglycosides (118). Care should be exerted when using any streptococcus if a patient is receiving penicillin-type antibiotics because of possible synergy between penicillin and aminoglycosides with this genus. Because aminoglycoside antibiotics are not active under anaerobic conditions, it is possible to determine the level of CLD in the presence of gentamicin using *Clostridium perfringens* (99). The addition of calcium and other divalent cations to the medium has proved effective (119). However, high levels of calcium may affect bacterial growth and render the medium somewhat turbid. Based on the same principle, cellulose phosphate powder can be incubated with the serum specimen to remove gentamicin (120).

Aminoglycoside antibiotics are inactivated by the polyanionic detergent sodium polyanetholesulfonate in a stoichiometric precipitation reaction (121). The addition of this material to media allows for the rapid determination of the levels of all other classes of antibiotics in the presence of all aminoglycosides (122). Using either nutrient agar or plate count agar, sterile 5% sodium polyanetholesulfonate solution (Grobax; Hoffmann-LaRoche, Nutley, NJ) is added to establish a final concentration of 0.8%. Using the Kirby-Bauer *S. aureus* ATCC strain 25923, or *E. coli* ATCC strain 25922, the standard well-type bioassay is run. For penicillin, cephalosporins, erythromycin, tetracycline, CAM, and vancomycin, *S. aureus* is the better choice. For antibiotics that are more active against gram-negative bacteria, such as ampicillin or the polymyxins, *E. coli* is preferred. The procedure described for the *Klebsiella* assay can be followed with either of these strains.

One-Dimensional Assays

As previously described, one-dimensional assays can be useful for the determination of antibiotic concentrations under anaerobic conditions and for assays for which only small amounts of specimen are available.

Medium

Nutrient agar is diluted with an equal amount of 1% peptone in water and brought to pH 7.8 (the pH varies depending on the type of antibiotic to be assayed). It is dispensed for storage in 19-mL amounts.

Procedure

The bacterial test strain (*S. aureus* 658P) is grown overnight in trypticase soy broth. It is diluted 1:100 and mixed well by shaking to break up clumps. Before use, the agar is melted and cooled to 48°C in a temperature-controlled water bath. Then 1 mL of the bacterial suspension is added to 19 mL of the test agar. The bacteria and the test agar are mixed well. The test agar is pipetted into conical test tubes that have an internal diameter of approximately 3 mm (K tubes used for determination of complement fixation in the Kolmer test in syphilis serology are satisfactory). The agar is added to a depth of 3 mm from the bottom of the tube. The agar is allowed to harden (at least 5 minutes). Standards for many commonly used antibiotics are described in Table 8.5. Each standard is pipetted into a different tube. Each standard should be repeated three times. The patient's serum is treated identically. The antibiotic standards and patient's serum should be added until they are 1.5 mm above the agar layers. Small deviations from this level do not affect the accuracy of the method. The tubes are incubated at 37°C overnight.

Interpretation

Typical assay results are presented in Figure 8.1. To determine inhibition of growth, each tube is laid on its side. Using an eyepiece with the ability to measure distances, the distance in millimeters from the point where the patient's specimen and the test agar meet (the meniscus of the test agar) to the point where growth of the test strain begins (often it is the place where large colonies are seen) is recorded. This measurement is repeated for each standard and the patient's specimen. The results are calculated as for any dose-response curve. On the ordinate (*y axis*), the logarithm of the antibiotic concentration is plotted. The depth of inhibition is plotted on the abscissa (*x axis*). The concentration of the patient's specimen is found by drawing a vertical line from the depth of inhibition on the *x axis* to the standard line and drawing a horizontal line from the point of intersection to the *y axis*, where the concentration of the antibiotic is read directly.

Amoxicillin and Clavulanic Acid

β-Lactamase inhibitors protect β-lactam antibiotics from destruction by these enzymes. Clavulanic acid, sulbactam, and tazobactam are those currently used. Because β-lactamase inhibitors are combined with β-lactam antibiotics in the same pharmaceutical preparations, a procedure for the assay of amoxicillin and clavulanic acids is presented (123).

Augmentin consists of amoxicillin trihydrate and the potassium salt of clavulanic acid as the anhydrous free acids in the ratio of two parts amoxicillin to one part clavulanic acid. Amoxicillin may be assayed in the presence of clavulanic acid. A conventional microbiologic assay technique with *S. lutea* as the assay organism can be used to measure amoxicillin concentrations in body fluids after the administration of Augmentin. This is not the case with clavulanic acid because its very low level of antibacterial activity precludes the use of a microbiologic assay technique that depends on measurement of antibacterial activity. Instead, clavulanic acid concentrations in body fluids can be assayed by a microbiologic agar diffusion method involving measurement of the inhibition of β-lactamase activity of a strain of *Enterobacter aerogenes*. In the method subsequently described, clavulanic acid does not interfere with the microbiologic assay of amoxicillin in clinical specimens, and amoxicillin does not influence the measurement of clavulanic acid.

This method uses a large-plate microbiologic assay technique in which samples are added to wells punched in agar. Modifications may be made as required; for example, Petri dishes may be used instead of large plates, and the specimens may be applied to the plates by assay cylinders, paper disks' fish spines, beads, and others. Moreover, the bacteriologic media used are not critical and individual laboratories may find their own modifications to be more suitable for their purposes than those described.

In principle, specimens should be assayed as soon as possible after collection and should not be stored for more than a few days before assays are performed. As a rule, β-lactam compounds are relatively unstable in aqueous solutions and in body fluids, and clavulanic acid is no exception. Consequently, care must be taken in the handling and storage of clinical specimens that contain amoxicillin and clavulanic acid. Serum specimens may be stored for up to 2 days in the refrigerator (4°C) or for up to 3 days in a freezer (−20°C). Clavulanic acid is relatively unstable in undiluted urine, particularly at alkaline pH, and is less stable (in urine) at −20°C than at 4°C. Accordingly, urine specimens for assay should be diluted 10-fold in citrate buffer, pH 6.5, as soon as possible after collection and stored at 4°C. Under these conditions, specimens of urine containing amoxicillin and clavulanic acid may be kept for up to 5 days at 4°C before assay.

The stability of clavulanic acid is influenced by the concentration, pH, and composition of the buffer solution that is used as a diluent. Solutions of clavulanic acid are most stable at pH 6.0 to 7.0, and preparations in citrate buffers or distilled water are more stable than those in phosphate buffers. Also, aqueous solutions that contain amoxicillin and clavulanic acid are more stable at 4°C than at −20°C. Consequently, aqueous solutions of Augmentin, clavulanic acid, or amoxicillin for microbiologic tests should be prepared in 0.1 mol/L of a citrate buffer, pH 6.5. Solutions that are prepared in this medium and contain up to 0.1 mol/L of amoxicillin or clavulanic acid may be stored at 4°C for up to 4 weeks.

Amoxicillin

Apparatus. The following equipment are required:

1. Large glass assay plates
2. Pasteur pipettes (nominally 30 drops/mL) or standard dropping pipettes (0.02 mL per drop)
3. Punches for cutting holes (7- to 8-mm diameter)
4. Lancets or broad needles
5. Test tubes, flasks, and pipettes as required
6. Leveling tripods or a level surface
7. Water bath at 50°C
8. Incubator at 30°C or 37°C
9. Needle-point calipers

Antibiotic medium 2 (81) is obtainable commercially in dehydrated form from Chesapeake Biological Laboratories (Baltimore, MD), Oxoid, Inc (Ogdensburg, NY), and Difco Laboratories (Sparks, MD). It is prepared by dissolving beef extract (1.5 g), yeast extract (3.0 g), peptone (6.0 g), and agar (15.0 g) in 1,000 mL of distilled water

and adjusting the pH to 6.5 or 6.6. Volumes of 300 mL are distributed in screw-capped bottles and sterilized at 15 psi for 15 minutes.

The required amount of medium is melted and maintained at 50°C in a water bath until the plates are ready to be poured. The assay plates are placed on a level surface or on leveling tripods and adjusted until they are level. The plates are sterilized by swabbing them with alcohol, followed by flaming. The swabbing and flaming procedure is performed twice. The inoculum is added to each bottle of agar and mixed thoroughly. The surface of the plate is flamed and the inoculated medium is poured evenly over the plate. The surface of the agar is again flamed to eliminate air bubbles, and the agar is allowed to solidify with the lid slightly open. The plates may be kept in a refrigerator at 4°C for up to 24 hours.

Buffer. Sorensen's buffer (0.1 mol/L citrate buffer, pH 6.5) is used. Solution A is 0.1 mol/L disodium citrate (21.0 g of citric acid in water, dissolved in 200 mL of 1 N NaOH [4.0 g/1,000 mL] and diluted to 1,000 mL). Solution B is 0.1 N NaOH (4.0 g/1,000 mL). Fifty-four milliliters of solution A is added to 46 mL of solution B. The pH of final solution is checked and, if necessary, adjusted by adding the required amounts of solution A or B.

Standard Solutions. Normal pooled human serum is sterilized by filtration and tested for the absence of antibacterial activity. The quantity of laboratory reference standard amoxicillin trihydrate that is equivalent to the required amount of amoxicillin pure, free acid is accurately weighed and dissolved in 0.1 mol/L citrate buffer, pH 6.5. Dilutions are made in pooled human serum for the assay of serum specimens or in 0.1 mol/L of a citrate buffer, pH 6.5, for the assay of other specimens or urine. Serial dilutions are prepared in the requisite diluent to give the necessary range of standard solutions. Each specimen is diluted to give a concentration that is estimated to fall within the range of the standard line.

Serum specimens are diluted in pooled human serum. Specimens of urine are diluted in 0.1 mol/L citrate buffer, pH 6.5. The required dilution depends on the dose of the drug that was administered and on the time at which the specimen was taken. The mean serum concentrations of amoxicillin and clavulanic acid in fasting volunteer subjects 1 hour after the administration of single oral 375 mg doses of Augmentin are 5.6 μg/mL for amoxicillin and 3.7 μg/mL for clavulanic acid. The mean urine concentration of clavulanic acid is 545 μg/mL.

Bacteria. A suspension of *S. lutea* (National Collection of Type Cultures strain 8340, ATCC strain 9341) is prepared by using a loop to inoculate 100 mL of nutrient broth in a 500 mL Erlenmeyer flask with organisms from a stock culture that has been grown on a nutrient agar slant and stored in the refrigerator at 4°C. The flask is incubated for 48 hours at 37°C and stored at 4°C. Stock cultures on agar slants may be kept for up to 4 months at 4°C. Broth suspensions may be held for 4 or 5 weeks at 4°C. An inoculum of 0.8 mL of the broth suspension into 100 mL of agar usually provides satisfactory growth on the large assay plates.

Procedure. Seeded plates are taken from the refrigerator and the agar surface is blotted dry with filter paper. Holes 8 mm in diameter are cut with a punch. The agar plugs are removed with a lancet or broad needle. The holes are filled with the specimens and standard solutions using a Pasteur or dropping pipette. The pipette is rinsed three times in buffer solution between each sample loading. The plates are incubated overnight at 30°C or 37°C.

Interpretation. The diameters of the inhibition zones are measured and the standard and sample responses are averaged. The mean inhibition zone diameters of the standard solutions are plotted against the logarithm of the antibiotic concentrations using semilogarithmic paper. The best fitting straight line connecting the points is constructed. The concentration of each dilution of specimen is determined by extrapolation from the straight line.

Clavulanic Acid

Clavulanic acid is a weak antibacterial agent. However, it is a potent inhibitor of certain β-lactamases. This latter property is the basis of a microbiologic assay for clavulanic acid in clinical specimens. In brief, a subinhibitory concentration (60 μg/mL) of benzylpenicillin is added to a nutrient agar that is inoculated with the β-lactamase–producing organism *E. aerogenes* BRL strain 1. Plates are poured and wells are cut in the agar in the usual fashion. At the concentrations tested, clavulanic acid has no inhibitory effect on the growth of the assay organism, but it does inhibit the β-lactamase

activity of the enterobacterium, thereby preventing destruction of the benzylpenicillin incorporated in the agar. As a consequence, inhibition zones are produced by the penicillin, the diameters of which are proportional to the concentration of clavulanic acid in the test sample.

The assay for the determination of clavulanic acid is identical to that for amoxicillin, with the following exceptions. The assay medium is adjusted to pH 7.4. The amount of laboratory standard material of potassium clavulanate that is equivalent to the required amount of the pure, free clavulanic acid is accurately weighed and dissolved in 0.1 mol/L of a citrate buffer, pH 6.5. Nutrient broth inoculated with a wire loop from a nutrient agar slant of *E. aerogenes* BRL strain 1 (or *Klebsiella pneumoniae* ATCC strain 29665) and incubated overnight at 37°C is used to inoculate the assay agar. A fresh culture should be used for each assay. An inoculum of 3.0 mL of overnight broth culture in 100 mL of agar produces satisfactory growth on large assay plates.

The inoculum is added to the agar and benzylpenicillin is added to the inoculated agar to give a final concentration of 6 μg of benzylpenicillin per milliliter of agar. The agar is poured into the plates, as described for the assay of amoxicillin. When the agar has set, the plates are stored in the refrigerator at 4°C and are used as soon as possible on the same day. This is essential because the assay organism is able to inactivate the penicillin incorporated in agar plates if they are allowed to stand at room temperature or overnight at 4°C. The results are interpreted as for the amoxicillin assay as previously described.

Three-Dimensional Assays

Antibiotic medium 11 (Difco Laboratories, Detroit, MI) is adjusted to pH 7.9. This agar may be stored in 25-mL aliquots in the refrigerator for up to 1 month. Prior to performing the assay, an appropriate number of tubes are melted and brought to 50°C; 0.4 mL of an overnight growth of *Klebsiella* in trypticase soy broth is added. The suspension is thoroughly mixed and 9 mL is poured into two 100 × 15-mm plastic Petri plates. Alternatively, 0.4 mL of a heavily inoculated 5-hour broth culture can be added to the agar.

Procedure

For each assay, 0.02 mL of the patient's serum is pipetted with sterile disposable capillary pipettes onto Schleicher & Schuell 740-E disks (Schleicher &

Schuell BioScience, Inc, Keene, NH). Alternatively, wells can be cut in the agar. The method described by Sabath et al. (6,93) is followed using the same number of standards and samples of the patient's serum.

Calculation of Results

Generally for a given antibiotic, results are obtained from a plot of the logarithm of the antibiotic concentration versus the zone diameter. This is quite adequate for calculations involving limited ranges of antibiotic concentrations. However, if the concentration range is greater than fourfold, it is better to plot the logarithm of the antibiotic concentration versus the square of the zone diameter. Lines that visually appear straight on plots of the logarithm of the antibiotic concentration versus zone diameter have frequently been shown by computer analysis to have low coefficients of variation (97). This caveat is particularly important if the slope of a line is steep. When using logarithmic paper to calculate antibiotic concentrations in this way, very small differences in values can produce large changes in the apparent concentrations, especially in the range of 10 to 100 μg/mL. It is best to use an assay system that provides the flattest possible line. Pocket calculators or handheld computers can provide "best fit" straight lines, coefficients of variation, SDs, and direct interpolations. Keeping permanent records of these calculations provides a strong internal quality control. One may, for example, detect the decay of antibiotic standards by changes in line slopes or differences in coefficients of variation.

When used to perform clinical assays, the microbiologic method produces results in 4 hours or less. Figures 8.4 and 8.5 illustrate that longer incubations affect the zone size only slightly. The size of the zone is, in effect, established approximately 2 or 3 hours after incubation. Small, uniform increases in zone size do not affect the slope of the line or the final calculation of antibiotic concentration.

Electrophoretic Separation of Antibiotics

Methods have been developed to separate antibiotics in a mixture by gel electrophoresis and to assay these separated compounds by covering the gel with an indicator bacterium in agar. After incubation, zones of inhibition are seen in the covering agar slab. These methods were especially useful before HPLC became available and may still have some applicability if one needs to assay for disparate classes of antibiotics in a mixture (124,125).

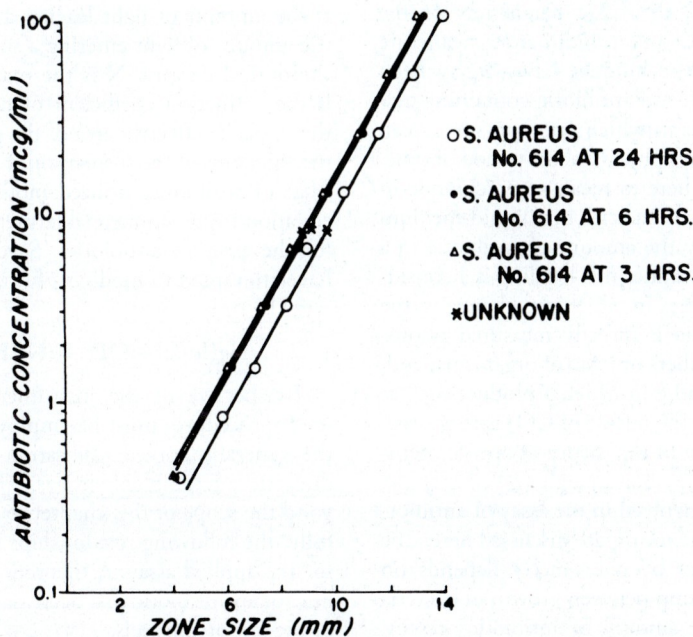

Figure 8.4 ■ **Determination of a gentamicin blood level with only the time of reading varied.** All levels were 8.2 μg/mL (±6%). The 2-hour reading was within 15% of the 24-hour reading by zone diameter measurement. (From Edberg SC, Chu A. Determining antibiotic levels in the blood. *Am J Med Technol* 1975;41:99–105, with permission.)

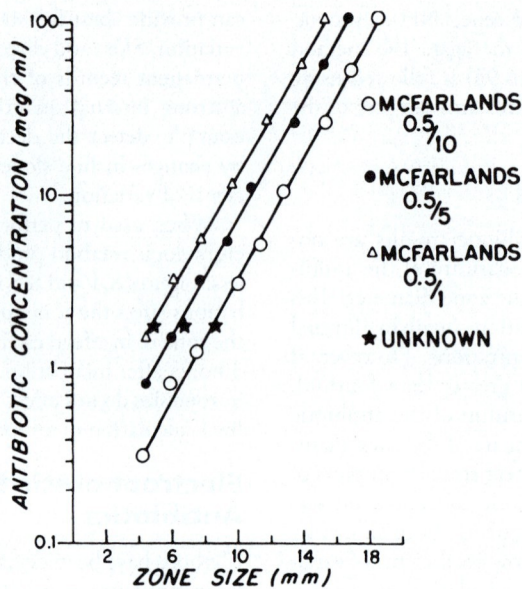

Figure 8.5 ■ Determination of a gentamicin level with only the inoculum density varied. Antibiotic medium 5 and *Staphylococcus aureus* were used in all tests. All inoculum densities yielded the same gentamicin level, 1.9 µg/mL (±5%). A large inoculum decreases the time the test requires but also decreases the sensitivity of the assay. (From Edberg SC, Chu A. Determining antibiotic levels in the blood. *Am J Med Technol* 1975;41:99–105, with permission.)

Broth Methods

Turbidimetric Assays

For completeness, the basic parameters of the assay of antibiotics by turbidimetric means are mentioned. These techniques have largely been relegated to the assay of antibiotic-containing materials in situations in which one wants to screen large numbers of samples in a short period of time. Turbidity is used here to mean any technique in which the growth of bacteria in a liquid medium is used to quantify the amount of antibiotic in a solution. Included under this heading is a consideration of techniques in which the change in the number of bacteria is directly measured photometrically (as numbers or mass of organisms) and, as an extension, those in which a product such as a change in pH or the release of CO_2 is measured.

An examination of the theory of optical methods was explored by Kavanaugh (79). Only the pertinent factors involved in the assay of antibiotics by turbidimetric means are discussed here. The assay of antibiotics by photometry depends on the direct relationship between growth of bacteria in culture and the amount of antibiotic present. Generally, this relationship is displayed in a plot of growth per unit time versus percent transmission or the optical density of the bacterial suspension. It should be noted that absorbance measures mass

or volume rather than the concentration of bacteria (79). This relationship can be stated as a form of Beer's Law or Beer-Lambert Law in which Io is the amount of light leaving a suspension, I is the amount of light entering a suspension, OD is the optical density, N is the mass of bacteria, E is the extinction coefficient of the particles, a is the optically effective area of the particle, and b is the thickness of the suspension. Early work on the assay of antibiotics utilized modifications of this equation from commercial fermentation processes for the assay of antibiotics. Several investigators have attempted to modify it for use in clinical assays (105).

$$\log(Io/I) = OD = (N)[Eab/2.3]$$

Irrespective of the instrument or technique used, procedures must be employed to straighten the generally curved calibration lines for turbidimetric microbiologic assays. Although it is beyond the scope of this chapter to treat the subject fully, the following relationships should be useful for the applied assay. A theoretical dose-response line for an antibiotic that decreases the growth rate of the test organism is

$$N_t = N_o \exp(k_o + f(v)k_M - k_aC)t,$$

where N_t is the concentration of the test inoculum after an incubation period of t, N_o is the concentration of the test inoculum at the beginning of the assay, k_o is the generation rate constant in the absence of antibiotic, C is the concentration of antibiotic with an inhibitory coefficient of k_a, k_M is the effect of the medium, and the function $f(v)$ is a function of the volume of the sample added to the assay. This is a theoretical expression because the major characteristics of the equation, although interrelated, are not absolutely known.

In an individual assay, N_o, k_o, $f(v)$, k_M, k_a, and t (time) are constant. Therefore, the variables of the equation may be related as follows:

$$\log N = G + BC,$$

where G and B are constants that are intrinsic to the assay. Because most spectrophotometers use absorbance (A), this equation may be translated into

$$\log A = E + FC.$$

To straighten the line, this equation may be modified as

$$\log (A + M) = O + PC.$$

The algebraic sign M is used to straighten the line over the particular concentration range in question. The constant M compensates for two sources of curvature: the nonlinear relationship between log N and C, and the inherent nonlinear responsiveness of photometers.

Because of this complexity, pure photometry has proven successful only in situations in which all conditions except the quantity of a single antibiotic in solution could be rigidly controlled. The Abbott Laboratories MS-2 instrument (Abbott Park, IL), a device that continually monitors bacterial growth in optical density units, has been used to determine antibiotic blood levels under clinical conditions using a growth curve analysis (126). The principle of this technique is that, for any dose-response curve, the response is the turbidity of bacteria in solution. The MS-2 instrument determines turbidity using red light–emitting diodes. The test culture is inoculated into the cuvette. After the culture reaches logarithmic growth phase, the culture is pulled down into compartments, each of which contains a disk. The disks can contain either a patient's serum or a standard. Generally, the patient's serum is tested in two compartments and each standard is repeated twice. After approximately 3 hours of incubation, the optical density (after minor corrections that are required because of the physical nature of the instrument) is plotted on the *y axis* and the logarithm of the antibiotic concentration

is plotted on the *x axis*. The instrument has a built-in computer that enables it to continuously monitor the growth of the test cultures. All calculations are automated. In the early 1980s, we used this instrument successfully with *S. aureus* as a test organism to determine the concentration of aminoglycosides in blood (126).

Broth Dilution Bioassay for Polymyxins

Broth dilution bioassay is rarely performed. However, this technique may prove useful for the measurement of polymyxin-class antibiotics. It was found that in normal agar, but not agarose, assays of colistin concentration yielded false-low blood and urine values (127). This was probably occurring because a highly diffusible precursor was being converted into a poorly diffusible active compound. The turbidimetric technique more accurately reflected what was actually occurring in the body than did agar techniques. Levels of the polymyxin group of antibiotics can be determined by a modification of the standard turbidimetric technique in which the number of viable organisms is counted.

Procedure. A strain of *Pseudomonas aeruginosa* that is sensitive to the polymyxins is employed as the test organism. The inoculum that is used for each antibiotic concentration determination is 0.05 mL of a 1- to 8-hour culture (grown in trypticase soy broth) that has been diluted at a 1:10,000 ratio in normal human serum. The patient's specimen is diluted in the same fluid that is to be assayed (serum specimens are diluted in serum, cerebrospinal fluid specimens are diluted in cerebrospinal fluid, and so on) to yield final percentage concentrations of 90%, 80%, 70%, 60%, 50%, 40%, 30%, 20%, 10%, and 0%. The final volume of each of these dilutions is 0.5 mL after the addition of 0.05 mL of the inoculum. Standards should be incubated with normal human serum for 18 hours at 37°C. This preincubation is necessary for activation of the polymyxin-type drugs.

Immediately after the addition of the inoculum, all tubes are incubated at 37°C for 30 minutes. After incubation, the tubes are plunged into an ice bath (0°C). The number of bacteria in each tube is determined by performing serial 10-fold dilutions with distilled water and plating 0.1 mL of each dilution on the surface of trypticase soy agar plates. The total number of viable bacteria per milliliter of inoculum is calculated from these colony counts after 18 hours of incubation at 37°C.

The end point for each titration of the poly-myxins in each patient's serum (or other fluid) is the smallest amount of patient's serum that results in a reduction of inoculum to 10% of the original viable count. To increase the precision of the end points, the concentration of the sub-ject's serum or the concentration of known anti-biotic that causes a reduction of 90% of the viable organisms is read from a curve that is drawn on semilogarithmic paper by plotting the number of organisms on the logarithmic axis versus the con-centration on the arithmetic axis. Performing the assay with normal human serum alone accounts for any reduction in bacteria that is caused by nonspecific factors.

Interpretation. The antibacterial activity of the polymyxin standards is compared with the antibacterial activity of the patient's specimen. The calculations are as set forth in the "Turbidimetric Assays" section. The titer of the patient's serum is multiplied by the minimum inhibitory concentration of the organism for the individual polymyxin to yield the amount of polymyxin-type antibiotic in the patient's serum.

pH Change Assays

Antibiotics act on bacteria by halting their growth and/or metabolism. Antibiotic-induced changes bacterial metabolic activity can be used to determine antibiotic concentrations in body fluids and tissues. The methods used are based on the principle that the larger the quantity of antibiotic that is in contact with a bacterial population, the greater will be the modifica-tion of the population's metabolic pathways. As with all dose-response assays, one must obtain a standard dose-response curve and calculate from only those points that fit the equation for a straight line.

The most popular method of this type employs a change in the pH of the growth medium as a measure of the amount of antibiotic that is pres-ent. If no antibiotic is present, the test strain grows and produces a change in the pH of the growth medium by metabolizing a constituent (e.g., a sugar, which would lower the pH, or urea, which would increase the pH). If an antibiotic is added to the system and the test organism is affected by it, the change in pH is lessened. The urease-based bioassay is representative of this group of assays and can be used by laboratories without special equipment.

Adenosine Triphosphate Measurement Assays

A potentially automatable assay that is a com-bination of a bioluminescence procedure and a chemical assay uses rates of endogenous adenos-ine triphosphate (ATP) production by *Klebsiella edwardsii* to determine antibiotic concentra-tions. The amount of ATP that is present in a broth reflects bacterial growth, which is inversely related to the amount of antibiotic present. Standards are inoculated with the test strain in parallel with the patient's serum. After 2 hours of incubation at 37°C, the tubes are extracted with an ethylenediaminetetraacetate/H_2SO_4 so-lution. The amount of bacterial ATP that is re-leased is determined by spectrophotometry (128). A plot of the antibiotic concentration versus the relative amount of ATP released is used to calcu-late the antibiotic blood level. One should heat the serum prior to performing the assay in order to destroy human adenosine triphosphatase. In-struments that enumerate bacteria in urine and other body sites based on this principle are avail-able from a number of vendors, including Cel-sis International (Newmarket, Suffolk, United Kingdom), Coral Biotechnology (San Diego, CA), and New Horizons Diagnostics Corpora-tion (Columbia, MD).

Bioluminescence

Methods that involve the use of luminescent bacteria have been proposed to determine the activity of antibiotics in serum (111,112). One type of assay called the *induced test* is based on the ability of some antibiotics to inhibit lucif-erase synthesis by luminescent bacteria (129). Ulitzur's (129) method, described in the follow-ing section, is sensitive, rapid, and potentially automatable.

Procedure. The serum is heated at 56°C for 30 minutes to eliminate bacterial activity. To 0.8 mL of serum, 0.2 mL of 10% NaCl containing 0.1 mol/L 3-(N-morpholino) propanesulfonic acid buffer and 1.5% glycerol is added. The final pH value of the mixture should be 7.9 for all antibiotics except CAM and tetracycline, which are tested at pH 6. A *Photobacterium leiognathi* 8SD18 cell suspension (200 μL, 3×10^8 cells/mL) is added to 0.8 mL of the serum, as well as to 1 mL of antibiotic-free pooled serum. After 10 minutes of preincubation at 30°C, proflavin is added to give a final concentration of 1.5 μg/mL for pH 7.9 or 25 μg/mL for pH 6.0. The vials are then incubated with gentle shaking at 30°C. Proflavin is a DNA-intercalating agent that induces the luminescence system of dark mutant luminescent bacteria. The results are recorded after 40 to 60 minutes of incubation. Luminescence is measured with a photometer/photomultiplier and is universely proportional to the concentration of the antibiotic in the specimen.

The bioluminescence test specifically determines the activity of the tested antibiotic as a de novo protein synthesis inhibitor. Antibiotics that act on DNA or cell wall synthesis are not detected by this test. The bioluminescence test is more sensitive than most available bioassays. This high sensitivity may be attributable to the greater susceptibility of newly synthesized proteins to the inhibitory actions of many antibiotics.

Serum Inhibitory Concentration and Serum Bactericidal Concentration

Broth dilution tests that employ patient serum as the antimicrobial milieu date to the work of Schlichter and McLean (130), who reported on the serum inhibitory concentrations (SIC) in 10 patients with streptococcal endocarditis. They obtained serum from these 10 patients, geometrically diluted each sample in broth, and inoculated each dilution with the patient's own organism (131). They obtained a titer of each patient's serum that reflected the serum's ability to inhibit macroscopic growth of the microbe. Fisher (132) subsequently extended this procedure by subculturing each tube that failed to exhibit macroscopic evidence of growth after overnight incubation. The highest dilution of a patient's serum, or titer, that was able to kill the microbial inoculum was called the *serum bactericidal concentration* (SBC). SIC/SBC tests have since been applied to specimens from patients receiving therapy for intravascular and other closed-space infections (133).

Procedure. The patient's infecting microbe is adjusted to yield between 10^5 and 10^6 colony-forming units (CFU)/mL in each tube (134). It is important that the actual CFU per milliliter value be determined. To do this, 0.1 mL each of a 1:100 and a 1:1,000 dilution of the inoculum is spread over the surface of the appropriate agar medium. After overnight incubation, the inoculum size is calculated from the number of colonies that are present on the plate that has between 20 and 200 colonies on it. For example, if there are 40 colonies on the plate that was inoculated with a 1:1,000 dilution, the original inoculum contained 4×10^5 CFU/mL.

The serum is diluted geometrically and the test is performed in a manner that is analogous to the minimum inhibitory concentration/minimum bactericidal concentration procedures. For most organisms, the broth can be Mueller-Hinton broth, with brain-heart or Levinthal medium used for fastidious microbes. To each of 12 tubes, 1 mL of broth is added. To the first tube is added 1 mL of serum, followed by thorough mixing. One milliliter from tube 1 is added to tube 2 and is thoroughly mixed. One milliliter from tube 2 is added to tube 3, and so forth. This process is continued through tube 12. However, 2 mL of broth is added to tube 12, rather than 1 mL as in the other tubes. One milliliter is removed from tube 12 and is transferred to a sterile test tube as a sterility control. A geometric dilution of the patient's serum has, therefore, been made from 2^1 to 2^{12}. One should also have a 14th tube that contains only the patient's undiluted serum. To each tube is added 1 mL of the patient's own microbe, diluted to yield a final concentration of 10^5 or 10^6 CFU/mL. All transfers should be made with sterile pipettes. All tubes are incubated in ambient air at 35°C for 18 to 24 hours. The lowest concentration (dilution) of the patient's serum that completely inhibits visible growth is the SIC. Concentration or dilution is converted to titer by the formula: titer = 1 per dilution. As the titer increases, the amount of serum in the tube decreases.

The SBC is determined by spreading 0.1 mL from each tube that does not show turbidity and the first tube that does show turbidity over the entire surface of a 100-mm diameter agar plate that contains the appropriate growth medium. A different pipette should be used for each transfer from a tube. The plates are incubated for 24 hours and preliminary colony counts are performed and recorded. The plates should be incubated for 48 hours when examining staphylococci and for up to 72 hours when examining other microbes. This extended incubation allows the organism to grow on the surface of agar and obviates any effects that transferred antibiotic may exert. The SBC is the lowest concentration (i.e., highest titer) of serum that produces 99.9% killing. For example, if the inoculum in each tube was 2.0×10^5 CFU/mL, killing would be defined as an agar plate that demonstrates no more than 20 colonies from a 0.1 mL subculture.

Interpretation. Much controversy surrounds the use of SIC/SBC tests (135,136). Importantly, few groups have performed the procedure in the same manner. Variations in protocols have involved inoculum size, type of broth, bactericidal end point, time of incubation, timing of the blood sample, volume of the broth sample, and the definition of the bactericidal end point. For these reasons, this test is no longer performed at Yale.

DIRECT CHEMICAL ASSAYS

Although considerable effort has gone into the determination of antibiotic concentrations in body fluids by direct chemical analysis, there are few instances in the clinical laboratory when one can use these methods. Because these assays are based on reactions that involve specific chemical groups on antibiotic molecules, the concentrations of antibiotics determined by many chemical assays include active drugs as well as metabolic breakdown products that retain the reacting moiety. Consequently, a chemical assay is most satisfactory in a pharmaceutical fermentation process in which one is dealing with a pure substance.

In vivo, from 0% to more than 95% of an administered drug may not exist in its native state. Because a clinical assay is intended to determine the amount of active material circulating, chemical assays may yield false-high values. In addition, for many antibiotics, all their breakdown products may not be known. When chemically assaying the amount of active drug from biologic sources for such antibiotics, it is dangerous to use estimates of average metabolically active fractions. In addition, secondary substances (either other chemotherapeutic agents or normal body constituents) may interfere with these assays. Because it is very difficult to exclude all possible agents in a given assay, falsely elevated values can unpredictably result.

Most chemical assays require extraction of the antibiotic prior to analysis. This extraction leads both to an inordinate number of technical procedures and to a greater possibility of error. Also, extracted material often requires specialized environmental safety conditions. Although these obstacles are not insurmountable in industry, they may be unwieldy for clinical laboratories.

The advantages of chemical assays for clinical laboratories are, at present, more theoretical than practical. Chemical assays can potentially be automated and should provide rapid turnaround times. Moreover, chemical analysis yields an absolute quantity, as opposed to a relative response, as in the microbiologic assay. This makes the standardization and implementation of controls easier. Only those assays that are useful in the routine and/or clinical research laboratory are discussed in the following paragraphs.

Colorimetric Assays

Aminoglycosides/Aminocyclitols

The thiobarbituric assay of streptomycin has been modified to allow it to determine clinically important levels of many deoxy sugars (137). Although the chromatogen that is produced when streptomycin and thiobarbituric acid react is quite stable, biologic homogenates that contain glycoproteins, sugars, and plasma proteins have been found to interfere with the assay. Changing the temperature of incubation from 100°C to 37°C eliminates all but plasma protein interference. Automated dialysis and computerized result analysis can potentially be used to design automated assays based on the method.

A crude solution of the enzyme is used in the reaction. The acetylated product, rather than being adsorbed to phosphocellulose paper, is not used at all. Thiol coenzyme A that is produced in the reaction is allowed to react with 5,5'-dithiobis(2-nitrobenzoic acid). The product of this reaction is thionitrobenzoic acid, a compound that has a maximum absorbance at 412 nm. The amount of thionitrobenzoic acid produced is a measure of the aminoglycoside concentration. For successful application of this assay, protein impurities must be removed. One should use a more pure enzyme suspension than that required for radioenzymatic assay procedures. With this assay system, gentamicin blood levels can be obtained within 15 minutes (138). Efforts to increase the sensitivity of the assay and to establish the optimal reaction conditions are underway. It should be noted that vancomycin, which is often used in conjunction with gentamicin and streptomycin, does not interfere in the chemical assays described in this chapter.

β-Lactam Antibiotics

Concentrations of the penicillins and related antibiotics in human specimens have been spectrophotometrically determined by a variety of methods. Most methods rely on a β-lactamase to hydrolyze the β-lactam ring of the drug and involve the measurement of the end products of the reaction (139,140). Historically, these methods have suffered from an inability to distinguish one form of penicillin from another. A relationship can be established between the consumption of iodine by a penicillin and the quantity of the penicillin in solution.

In one useful method, interfering protein is easily removed. Isopropyl alcohol is added to an aliquot of serum to remove the protein. The protein is precipitated by centrifugation (16,000 rpm in a Sorvall RC-2 centrifuge [Thermo Fischer Scientific, Inc., Waltham, MA, Norwalk, CT]). Two equal volume aliquots of the supernatant are taken. One aliquot is used as the sample, and the other is used as a blank. Iodine solution (0.01 N), buffered at pH 6.5, is added to each aliquot. A measured amount of aqueous penicillinase (Rikker penicillinase, 1,000 units/mL) is added to the sample while an equal amount of distilled water is added to the blank. After 25 minutes, the excess iodine in each tube is quantitated using a thiosulfate reagent and a starch indicator. The penicillin concentration can be calculated from the difference in iodine uptake between the specimen and the blank. The amounts of base and penicillinase that are required, as well as the incubation times, vary with the penicillins that are being measured. As a general formula, the amount of penicillin-type antibiotic (although susceptibility to penicillinase varies) can be calculated by the general formula:

$$\mu g/mL \text{ penicillin} = (V_2 - V_1)(MW/N)/\text{sample weight in mg}$$

where V_2 is the volume of 0.01 N iodine consumed after inactivation with alkali, V_1 is the iodine consumption before inactivation, MW is the molecular weight of the individual penicillin, and N is the number of iodine equivalents (141).

Another technique is to assay for a specific constituent of the penicillin molecule. This approach proved successful in the determination of 6-amino-penicillinoic acid with a glucosamine reagent (142). An additional method of analysis relies on the differential absorption of light in a given wavelength by different penicillin molecules to determine antibiotic levels when more than one drug is present. Ampicillin has a higher absorbance at 268 nm in a solution of pH 5 than in one at pH 9. This property has been used to measure concentrations of ampicillin in the presence of cloxacillin (143).

To avoid the difficulties inherent in the alkalized starch-iodine method, a procedure was developed that substituted chloroplatinic acid for base in the assay. Chloroplatinic acid degrades penicillin to penicillinoic acid, which can be measured colorimetrically. The color generated is more stable than that produced with the alkaline method. In the assay, 0.13 mL of 0.2% chloroplatinic acid is added to the penicillin-containing specimen and brought to a final volume of 4 mL with distilled water. The mixture is kept at room temperature for 30 minutes, after which time 1.5 mL of starch-iodine color reagent is added. The starch-iodine color reagent is prepared by adding equal volumes of water-soluble starch solution (0.8%) and 480 mol/L of a 4.8 mmol/L potassium iodine solution. After incubation for 5 minutes at room temperature, the amount of penicillin may be calculated from the absorbance measurement at 260 nm (101).

Active Sulfonamides

The body fluid is extracted into ethyl acetate from a nondeproteinized sample, yielding active unchanged sulfonamide and an acetylated inactive component. The acetylated component does not react in this assay.

Reagents. The following reagents are used:

1. McIlvain buffer, pH 5.5, which is made by mixing 8.6 volumes of a 0.2 mol/L aqueous solution of citric acid with 11.4 volumes of a 0.4 mol/L aqueous solution of disodium phosphate
2. Ethyl acetate
3. 2 N solution of HCl in acetone/water. The required quantity of this reagent must be freshly prepared immediately before each series of analyses by mixing one volume of 8 N HCl with three volumes of acetone. This product should not be kept for more than a few hours and should be discarded as soon as a brown color develops.
4. 0.1% sodium nitrate in a mixture of 3:1 acetone/distilled water
5. 5% solution of sulfaminic acid in 3:1 acetone/distilled water
6. 0.1% solution of α-naphthylethylenediamine dihydrochloride in a 3:1 mixture of acetone/distilled water
7. Methanol

Procedure. For plasma samples, 1 mL of McIlvain buffer is pipetted into a 10- to 15-mL shaking tube that is sealed by either an ether-tight glass or polyethylene stopper. Plasma (0.1 mL) and ethyl acetate (5 mL) are added. The tube is mixed by shaking for 10 minutes for extraction and simultaneous partial deproteinization and centrifuged 5 minutes at 3,000 rpm. The proteins settle between the two liquid phases as a fine precipitate.

Three milliliters of the supernatant is transferred to a test tube and 0.5 mL of HCl is added and mixed. Then 0.5 mL of 0.1% sodium nitrite solution is added, mixed, and allowed to stand for 6 minutes. One-half milliliter of sulfaminic acid solution is added and mixed well by shaking until there is no further liberation of gas bubbles. After 3 minutes, 0.5 mL of α-naphthylethylenediamine dihydrochloride solution is added and mixed. One-half milliliter of absolute methanol is then added. The tube is mixed until a homogeneous liquid phase is achieved. The tube is closed with a polyethylene stopper. In 20 minutes to 1 hour, one can determine the concentration of the product photometrically, as described in the following texts.

Total Sulfonamides

Reagents. The following reagents are used:

1. 20% trichloroacetic acid
2. 3 N aqueous HCl
3. 0.1% aqueous sodium nitrite
4. 0.5% aqueous sulfaminic acid
5. 0.1% aqueous solution of α-naphthylethylenediamine dihydrochloride (Note that all reagents can be stored at $-20°C$ for up to 1 year. Some reagents may freeze and should be well mixed after defrosting.)

Procedure. Four milliliters of distilled water is pipetted into a shaking tube that holds 10 to 15 mL and can be closed with either an ether-tight glass or polyethylene stopper. Then 0.2 mL of plasma is added and the tube is mixed well. The tube is placed in a boiling water bath for 4 minutes. One milliliter of 20% trichloroacetic acid is immediately added, followed by thorough mixing of the tube. The tube is centrifuged for 10 minutes at 3,000 rpm. Three milliliters of the supernatant is transferred to a test tube and 0.5 mL of 3 N HCl is added and mixed. The tubes are sealed and placed in a boiling water bath. After 1 hour, hydrolysis is complete. The tubes are allowed to cool and any condensation drops that may have formed along the walls are washed down. One-half milliliter of 0.1% sodium nitrite is added, mixed, and allowed to stand for 6 minutes. Sulfaminic acid (0.5%) is added to the tube, which is mixed by shaking until no gas bubbles are released. One-half milliliter of 0.1% aqueous α-naphthylethylenediamine

dihydrochloride is added and mixed. The solution can be measured spectrophotometrically, as described later, in approximately 20 to 60 minutes.

For urine samples, the procedure is the same as that described for plasma, except that in the assay for active sulfonamides, 0.15 mL of urine is mixed with 5 mL of McIlvain buffer, and 1 mL of this mixture is added to ethyl acetate. In the assay for total sulfonamides, 0.5 mL of urine is diluted with 20 to 50 mL of distilled water (depending on the amount of sulfonamide present). Standards in a similar solvent should be prepared to cover the range of sulfonamide concentrations that are expected in the sample and run in parallel with the patient samples. In addition, distilled water and a sample of the same type of specimen (e.g., plasma or urine) from a patient who has not received sulfonamides are also run as negative controls. All tubes are assayed at 554 nm. The value for each tube is determined by subtracting from the reading for each patient sample the reading obtained from the body fluid that does not contain sulfonamides. A standard Beer's Law or Beer-Lambert Law type of curve is constructed. One can interchange standard curves among the sulfonamides.

Occasionally, there may be so much sulfonamide present in a sample that it may not fall on the straight portion of the line. In these instances, samples should be diluted in the same body fluid from which they were collected and the assay should be repeated. If the identical body fluid is not available, distilled water can be used as a diluent with little error for all body fluids except bile. These methods are satisfactory for all sulfonamides.

Trimethoprim

Trimethoprim (TMP) can be extracted from body fluids with chloroform at a basic pH, extracted back into dilute H_2SO_4, and oxidized with $KMnO_4$ in an alkaline milieu to yield the fluorescent trimethoxybenzoic acid (TMBA) (144).

Reagents. The following reagents are used:

1. 0.1 N sodium carbonate solution
2. analytical-grade chloroform
3. 0.01 N H_2SO_4
4. 0.1 mol/L $KMnO_4$ in 0.1 N NaOH
5. 35% formaldehyde
6. 1 N H_2SO_4

Procedure. For the production of standard solutions of TMP, (a) 29.24 mg of TMBA is weighed in a 100-mL volumetric flask, which is then filled with chloroform; and (b) 5 mL of the solution from step (a) is added to a 100-mL volumetric flask, which is then filled with chloroform (this yields 20 μg/mL TMP). From this working standard solution, dilutions can be made in chloroform to cover the range of TMP that is encountered in biologic material.

To extract the antibiotic, 8 mL of Na_2CO_3, 10 mL of chloroform, and 1 or 2 mL of biologic fluid are added to a 25-mL shaking tube. The tube is stoppered and, to avoid emulsion, inverted gently head-over-tail for 4 minutes. The tube is centrifuged for 10 minutes at 3,000 rpm. As much of the aqueous phase as possible is aspirated into a new shaking tube and 4 mL of 0.01 N H_2SO_4 and 4 mL of the chloroform extract from the previous step are added. The tube is mixed by shaking for 10 minutes and centrifuged as described.

For oxidation of TMP to TMBA, 3 mL of the H_2SO_4 extract and 2 mL of the alkaline $KMnO_4$ solution are added to a shaking tube. The tube is mixed and placed in a 60°C water bath for 20 minutes. Then 0.3 mL of formaldehyde is added and the tube is mixed. One milliliter of 1 N H_2SO_4 is added, and the tube is placed in a 60°C water bath for 20 minutes. The tube is mixed and cooled to room temperature.

For extraction of TMBA, 2 mL of chloroform is added and the tube is mixed by vigorous shaking for 10 minutes, followed by centrifugation at 3,000 rpm. The clear chloroform phase is transferred into a quartz cuvette, and fluorescence is measured at an activation wavelength of 375 nm and a fluorescence wavelength of 360 nm. The amount of TMP is determined by

$$C = (Ma)(Cs)(F)/Ms,$$

where C is the concentration of TMP in the sample, Cs is the concentration of drug in the standard, Ma is the fluorescence of the TMP-containing sample after blank subtraction, Ms is the fluorescence reading of the standard after subtraction of the chloroform bank, and F is a constant that takes into account the conversion yield of TMP in TMBA (for 1 mL of body fluid, it is 5.442 and for 2 mL, it is 2.721).

Plotting the amount of TMBA and TMP (obtained through the conversion factor) versus fluorescent intensity should yield straight lines. The method is useful for the determination of TMP in samples from all body fluids. It has a sensitivity of 20 ng of TMP/mL of plasma. Other drugs, including the sulfonamides, do not react in this procedure. The method determines the concentration of unmetabolized, active TMP.

Chloramphenicol

CAM is used for the therapy of acute bacterial meningitis, rickettsial infections, typhoid fever, and brain abscesses. However, CAM may cause hematologic toxicity. Rarely, aplastic anemia with a high fatality rate occurs. In addition, CAM can cause bone marrow suppression, which is reversible and dose-related. Toxicity occurs in relation to dose when plasma levels exceed 80 mol/L (25 μg/mL). Therapeutic monitoring of serum CAM concentrations may be helpful in evaluating and maintaining effective levels of this potentially toxic antibiotic. This may be particularly important for patients with compromised liver status. In premature neonates, metabolism of the drug is unpredictable. High serum levels in these infants can produce the fatal gray baby syndrome.

In one useful chemical method for the determination of CAM concentrations, the drug is extracted from clinical specimens in isoamyl acetate. After extraction, the CAM concentration can be determined by analysis of the yellow color that develops when the extract reacts with isonicotinic acid hydrazine and sodium hydroxide (145). It appears that many of the biologic breakdown products of CAM are not extractable by this procedure.

Duplicate standards are prepared at 10, 20, and 30 μg/mL. Two milliliters of a phosphate buffer (0.1 mol/L; 2.21 μg of $NaH_2PO_4 \cdot H_2O$ and 7.61 g of $Na_2HPO_4 \cdot H_2O$ in 1 L of distilled water) is added to all tubes. Then 0.5 to 1.0 mL of serum or a standard solution is added. Distilled water is added to an additional tube as a negative control. Three milliliters of isoamyl acetate (Fisher Scientific Co, Hampton, NH) is pipetted into each tube. Each tube is tightly stoppered, mixed well by shaking for approximately 10 minutes, and centrifuged (16,000 rpm in a Sorvall RC-2 centrifuge [Thermo Fischer Scientific, Inc., Waltham, MA, Norwalk, CT] is optimal). To each tube that contains 2 mL of the supernatant solvent, 1.0 mL each of 1.5 N NaOH and 3% isonicotinic acid hydrazide (Eastman Kodak Co, Rochester, NY) are added. The tubes are then stoppered and incubated in a water bath at approximately 30°C for 45 minutes. The tubes are agitated periodically to ensure good mixing. After the incubation step has been completed, the yellow underlayer is aspirated with a Pasteur pipette and the absorbance is measured with a spectrophotometer at 430 nm. The blank is read as the negative control. The standard dose-response curve is then constructed by plotting the absorbance at 430 nm (the reading obtained from the test less the reading obtained with the blank) on the *x axis* versus the logarithm of antibiotic concentration on the *y axis*. Another colorimetric assay for CAM is described next.

Reagents. The enzyme reagent includes 200 mmol/L glycylglycine, pH 8, 1 mmol/L magnesium chloride, 7 mmol/L oxamic acid, 0.09 mmol/L acetyl coenzyme A, 60 U/L CAM acetyltransferase (CAT), 90.5 mmol/L nicotinamide adenine dinucleotide (NAD), 0.2 mmol/L thiamine pyrophosphate (TPP), 0.6 mmol/L 2-oxoglutarate, 20 U/L 2-oxoglutarate dehydrogenase (2-OGDH), and 0.01% GAFAC RE-610 (GAF Corp, Wayne, NJ). This reagent must be used within 2 hours of preparation. However, if the acetyl coenzyme A is omitted, the reagent can be stored at 4°C for 24 hours without a significant loss in activity of either enzyme. The color reagent, a solution of 0.2 mmol/L 2-(2-benzothiazolyl)-5-styryl-3-(4-phthalhydrazidyl) tetrazolium chloride in 12 mmol/L citric acid, that contains 0.02 mmol/L 1-methoxy-phenazine methosulfate, 0.04% Nonidet P-40, and 0.1% sodium azide, is stored in a dark bottle at 4°C. Citric acid provides maximum reagent stability.

Procedure. The enzymatic reactions are individually optimized with respect to buffer type, pH, and substrate and cofactor concentrations. To facilitate a rapid reaction, acetyl coenzyme A is required by CAT at a concentration that is in excess of the sample CAM concentration. The 2-OGDH reaction requires the substrate 2-oxoglutarate and the cofactors NAD, TPP, and magnesium ions. Oxamic acid is included as an inhibitor of endogenous serum lactate dehydrogenase activity. When the two enzymatic reactions are combined, glycylglycine buffer (200 mmol/L, pH 8) facilitates rapid reactions and gives maximum enzyme stability.

Dehydrogenase activity is detected by using reduction of the tetrazolium salt 2-(2-benzothiazolyl)-5-styryl-3-(4-phthalhydrazidyl) tetrazolium chloride (146) to a formazan dye, with the highest molar extinction coefficient under the prevailing assay conditions. CAT activity is determined by measuring the increase in absorbance at 412 nm of an assay mixture containing 100 mmol/L Tris-HCl, pH 8.0, 0.1 mmol/L acetyl coenzyme A, 0.1 mmol/L CAM, and 1 mmol/L

5,5-dithiobis (2-nitrobenzoic acid) (Ellman's reagent or DTNB). The reaction is initiated by adding 25 μL of CAT to 1 mL of assay mixture in a semimicrocuvette (path length of 1 cm).

2-OGDH (EC 1.2.4.2) activity is determined by measuring the increase in absorbance at 340 nm at 30°C of an assay mixture (1 mL) that contains 50 mmol/L of potassium phosphate buffer, pH 8.0, 1 mmol/L $MgCl_2$, 2.5 mmol/L NAD, 0.2 mmol/L TPP, 0.1 mmol/L coenzyme A, 2.5 mmol/L cysteine, and 2 mmol/L 2-oxoglutarate. The reaction is initiated with 25 μL of 2-OGDH.

The serum sample or CAM standard (0.1 mmol/L, 32 mg/L, 0.1 mL) is added to the enzyme reagent (0.5 mL) in a semimicrocuvette (path length of 1 cm), mixed well, and incubated at room temperature for 4 minutes. Color reagent (0.5 mL) is added and, after incubation at room temperature for exactly 2 minutes, the absorbance of the reaction mixture is measured at 575 nm. After 2 minutes, the reaction mixture exhibits a gradual increase in absorbance. A sample blank is prepared and its absorbance is measured by following the same procedure, except that glycylglycine buffer (200 mmol/L, pH 8) is substituted for the enzyme reagent.

The method is based on the reduction of a pale tetrazolium salt to a strongly colored formazan dye by NADH. The thiol groups of 2-OGDH also act as reducing agents, causing formazan production independent of the NADH reaction. Therefore, a reagent blank is required in addition to the sample blank, the absorbance of which is added to the sample blank value. The absorbance of the reagent blank is constant.

Performance. The assay is linear over the CAM range of 5 to 200 mol/L. The intra- and interbatch coefficients of variation (precision) are 1.4% to 4.9% and 4.3% to 6.3%, respectively. Mean recoveries (accuracy) from CAM-spiked (0.1 mmol/L and 0.025 mmol/L) serum samples from normal individuals and patients with renal failure were 98.4% and 105.6% for serum from normal individuals and 100.9% and 106.8% for serum from patients with renal failure. The method does not detect the inactive prodrug forms of CAM, that is, CAM succinate (intravenous preparations) and CAM palmitate (oral suspensions). Of the metabolites tested (CAM base, reduced base, and glycolic acid), only glycolic acid is recognized by CAT, with a cross-reactivity of 81%. However, this is a minor metabolite (<3%) and its detection is not considered important to the clinical utility of the assay.

Previous work indicates that CAT does not recognize CAM glucuronide (147). The method correlates well with reversed-phase high-performance liquid chromatography (RP-HPLC), which is specific for microbiologically active CAM. The assay also detects thiamphenicol, a CAM analog, with similar sensitivity and with a linear response up to a serum concentration of 100 μM. The endogenous colored compounds bilirubin and hemoglobin interfere with the color reaction when they are present in serum at concentrations above 200 μM and 0.2 mg/dL, respectively, because of a shift in the optimum wavelength of the final color. Thus, because of colorimetric interference, this assay is not recommended for use with grossly hemolyzed samples or when bilirubin concentrations exceed 200 μM.

A main advantage of this procedure is the speed with which an accurate CAM measurement can be obtained. The method requires no pretreatment of the sample such as heating or solvent extractions, as is required for HPLC, the more commonly employed assay for CAM. Moreover, a result is available within 6 minutes. The precision of the assay described here, when performed manually, is similar to that of the automated enzyme-multiplied immunoassay technique (EMIT) (148). However, it has the advantages of producing a linear response (allowing a single-point calibration) and requiring only a simple spectrophotometer to measure absorbance. Because it is a two-reagent system, the assay may also be adapted for a wide range of discrete analyzers. The method is specific and shows no significant interference by high concentrations of urea, creatinine, or phenolic compounds, which may be present in the serum of patients with renal failure (147).

RADIOENZYME ASSAYS

Bacteria are often resistant to antibiotics because they produce inactivating enzymes. Benveniste and Davies (149) and Davies et al. (150) provided the basis for radioenzymatic techniques in their description of a method by which they could determine the types of enzymes that inactivated certain antibiotics. Their basic method is used for the theoretical study of bacterial resistance.

Radioenzyme assays have been largely replaced. They were originally a by-product of the study of how enzymes destroy aminoglycosides and CAM. Table 8.2 presents the general advantages and disadvantages of radioenzymatic assays. Radioactive ATP in the presence of adenylating enzyme transfers radioactive ^{14}C to the aminoglycoside.

Aminoglycosides, which are positively charged, stick to negatively charged phosphocellulose papers. By enumerating the radioactive counts on these phosphocellulose papers, the extent to which adenylation occurred can be measured. Acetylating enzymes, which transfer acetyl groups from radioactive acetyl coenzyme A to aminoglycosides, can be similarly employed, with the measured counts on phosphocellulose paper reflecting the amount of acetylation that took place (149,150).

These adenylation and acetylation reactions provide the basis for radioenzymatic assays. It should be noted that the reactions are stoichiometric in that the amount of transfer in both adenylation and acetylation reactions is directly related to the quantity of antibiotic in the solution. The reaction takes place in several steps.

Many authors have used a method by which periplasmic enzymes are released from bacteria due to changes in osmotic pressure (151,152). By this method, less than 4% of the intracellular bacterial contents are released. However, the method is time-consuming and technically involved. Sonication has been investigated as a faster and easier method of obtaining the enzyme (153). The enzymes obtained by sonication appear to be as effective as those produced by osmotic shock. However, enzymes obtained by sonication may be somewhat more contaminated and unstable because of the release of proteolytic enzymes inside the bacteria (154). This could limit the length of time that the enzyme can be stored, a critical factor in the long-term usage of radioenzymatic techniques (155).

One may prepare the sonicate as follows. A 16-hour culture of *E. coli* RS/W677 is centrifuged at 14,000 × g for 5 minutes. The sediment is washed twice in 30 mmol/L NaCl plus 10 mmol/L Tris-HCl, pH 7.8. After the second wash, the pellet is suspended in 0.5 mmol/L MgCl$_2$ at 4°C (5 mL of 0.5 mmol/L MgCl$_2$ per 100 mL of original culture volume). The suspension is then sonicated for 20 seconds using a Dawe-type 3057A Soniprobe (Dawe Instruments Ltd, London, United Kingdom) set to give a 4 amp current. The cellular debris is removed by centrifugation at 25,000 × g for 20 minutes. The supernatant is divided into 0.1-mL aliquots and stored at 20°C (94).

Because it is undesirable to have to prepare the enzyme frequently, its stability has been studied under various conditions (154). Several methods have been developed to decrease enzyme lability. Keeping the enzyme frozen and in an ice bath are effective techniques (36,156). The enzyme has been shown to be stable for 24 hours at 4°C and 30 days at −20°C with BSA (157). Storing partially purified enzyme in reducing agents appears to increase its life span (158). Freezing the enzyme at low temperatures, such as −70°C, in quantities that will be used in a day's run, appears to be the most efficient and effective technique (159,160). It increases the storage life of the enzyme and significantly decreases the amount of technician time that is required to set up the assays.

DIRECT FLUORESCENT CHEMICAL ANALYSIS

A molecule is fluorescent when it can receive light at one wavelength and emit it at another wavelength. The wavelengths at which a given molecule receives and emits light are often specific to the molecule, a reactive group on a molecule, or a class of molecules. One major disadvantage of these assays is that other material present in the specimen, particularly radiologic fluorescein dyes and certain proteins, can fluoresce and interfere with the test. However, fluorescent assays typically are much more sensitive than chemical assays and can quantify compounds in the nanogram and often picogram per milliliter range.

Fluorescence can be determined in one of two ways. First, one may use the inherent fluorescent properties of the molecule. Second, for antibiotics that are either weakly fluorescent or nonfluorescent, one may covalently link a strongly fluorescent moiety to the drug in question. Because of the need for an extraction step, the possible need for coupling steps, the need for rather specialized equipment, the lack of standardized techniques, and the frequent inability to distinguish between active and inactive antibiotics, fluorescence methods have not been widely used in clinical laboratories, although they have been used in industry and U.S. Public Health Service laboratories. The reader is referred to the book by Undenfriend (161) for a general view of fluorescent analysis.

Although penicillins and cephalosporins are not generally inherently fluorescent, many produce fluorescent compounds under hydrolysis in the presence of acid (162). Attempts to simplify the extraction procedures and the number of technical manipulations that are required to generate such reactions have led to methods for measurement that can be clinically useful (141,163). For example, ampicillin concentrations can be determined in the absence of ampicillinoic acid by extraction. Standards should be prepared to cover the expected range of concentrations and serum blanks should be run to obtain measurements of background fluorescence.

Tetracyclines

Different tetracyclines require different fluorescent reagents to enhance their light-emitting properties (164). Each tetracycline should be tested individually to optimize these assays. Hall (165) has expanded the technique to measure the concentrations of tetracycline mixtures in plasma by using acid hydrolysis or alkaline degradation to convert the tetracycline into a fluorescent form. In these methods, aluminum salts are used to enhance the fluorescence of the end products. This fluorescence is measured with a spectrofluorometer. Each tetracycline exhibits a different structural arrangement of the chemical groups that surround the fluorescent nucleus of the anhydrous salts, creating individual fluorescent characteristics (165). A general method for the fluorometric determination of tetracyclines follows (166).

Apparatus

An Aminco-Bowman spectrophotofluorometer (American Instrument Company, Silver Spring, MD) fitted with a xenon arc lamp and an R 136 photomultiplier, or its equivalent, should be employed. Mirrors and 1-mm slits are placed in the cell housing.

Reagents

For most tetracyclines, one can use 0.5 mol/L magnesium acetate tetrahydrate plus 0.3 mol/L sodium barbitone in ethanedial. Minocycline, and other 7-aminotetracyclines, can be measured with a mixture of 0.2 mol/L magnesium acetate and 0.2 mol/L citric acid in ethanedial.

Procedure

A 0.2-mL aliquot of the sample (serum or other fluid) is mixed with 0.4 mL of a phosphate buffer (3 mol/L NaH_2PO_4 plus 1 mol/L Na_2SO_3) and thoroughly extracted with 2.5 mL of amyl acetate. The phases are separated by allowing them to settle or centrifuging the tube (approximately 500 × g). Two milliliters of the organic (top) phase are transferred to a Brown fluorometer cuvette. A suitable fluorescence reagent (0.6 mL) is added. (Fluorescence reagents are described later.) The tubes are mixed by shaking for 5 minutes. The turquoise fluorescence in the lower phase is read 20 minutes or more after shaking. If the lower phase is cloudy, the tubes are centrifuged ($500 \times g$ for 2 or 3 minutes) before reading. Standards (0.2 mL of a 10 mmol/L solution of the appropriate tetracycline) and blanks (0.2 mL of water) are also made.

For the determination of minocycline, a pH 6.5 buffer (0.5 mol/L NaH_2PO_4 plus 0.5 mol/L Na_2HPO_4) should be used instead of the phosphate sulfite buffer (137). Fluorescence is measured with excitation at 405 nm and emission at 490 nm. The fluorescence of 7-aminotetracyclines is read with excitation at 380 nm and emission at 480 nm (166).

IMMUNOLOGIC ASSAYS

Immunologic assays came into use in the mid-1970s. These assays were based largely on existing equipment and merely exploited procedures available for the assay of hormones. However, for the first time, the assay of antibiotics was removed from the realm of the specialist. These assays could be performed in a central location, with the instrument playing the primary role. The development of the means to elicit specific, high-titered antibodies to hapten antibiotics allowed RIA techniques to deliver a specificity that was impossible with biologic agents. As with any nonbiologic assay, however, one always had to be particularly careful not to measure a nonactive metabolite.

Because RIA equipment was expensive, the measurement of antibiotics was often mixed in with the assay of other drugs, resulting in significant delays in processing. The requirement to maintain a stock of highly active radioisotopes (often with short half-lives) gave impetus to the development of nonisotopic immunoassays. Unlike hormones, which are present in extremely small amounts and require highly sensitive methods of detection, antibiotics are generally present in levels above 0.5 µg/mL. Because other small molecules, such as antiepileptics and drugs of abuse, are also present in these levels, a technology was developed to measure small molecules by somewhat less sensitive, nonisotopic means. Unlike the stimulatory role played by existing RIA equipment in the development of RIA, the impetus for the development of the new nonisotopic immunoassays was largely the need to assay the aminoglycoside class of antibiotics.

Before the application of this technique to the measurement of antibiotic concentrations in 1975, RIA had been used for a number of years for the quantitation of hormonal substances

(167). All RIAs of antibiotics employ three broad reaction steps. The first step involves three components: radiolabeled antigen (antibiotic); high-titer, high-avidity antibody to that antigen; and unlabeled antigen (antibiotic obtained from the patient's serum). The reaction with either labeled or unlabeled antigen produces antibody combined with labeled antigen or antibody combined with unlabeled antigen. The more unlabeled antigen that is present in the reaction mixture, the less radiolabeled antigen combines with antibody.

After equilibrium is reached, one must quantify the amount of bound antibody in the mixture. This step involves either the removal of the bound antigen-antibody complex from solution by a precipitating agent or the removal of the unbound antigen from solution by chemical means. Because antigen/antibody reactions are stoichiometric in nature, the quantification of either the bound radiolabeled or the free radiolabeled antigen is directly proportional to the antibiotic level in a sample (168–170).

Although there are individual modifications, the test procedures follow a basic course (167). First, one incubates a known quantity of tritiated antibiotic with antibody (of known potency) to that antibiotic. A given amount of patient's serum is added and the mixture is allowed to come to equilibrium. These assays are heterogeneous and produce sigmoidal coprecipitation curves. Early investigators were hampered because only the relatively linear part of the sigmoidal curve could be used for the calculation of antibiotic concentrations. Robard et al. (171) devised a method in which the sigmoidal curve was converted to a straight line, thereby permitting the calculation of results over a much wider range of values. They found that the plot of $y = 100 \ (B/B^\circ)$ may be linearized by the equation representing a straight line in which logit $(y) = A + B \log x$, where x is the amount of unlabeled or patient drug, and y represents the percentage of antibiotic that is bound.

This logit conversion not only allowed a much wider range of antibiotic concentrations to be measured but also permitted the development of standard curves. As a result, one did not have to repeat all the controls each time a specimen was run. An advantage of immunologic assays is their within-class specificity. Although there may be cross-reactivity among members of the same drug class, there is no cross-reactivity among members of different classes (e.g., gentamicin and vancomycin).

Nonisotopic Immunoassays

The development of EIAs by Engvall and Perlmann (172,173) laid the foundation for design of nonradioisotopic immunoassays. In these immunoassays, an enzyme or fluorometric substance is coupled to the antigen or antibody in such a way that the activity of the parent compound is not appreciably affected. The significant difference between nonisotopic immunoassays and RIAs is the means of counting the label. In nonisotopic assays, the quantity label present is estimated from enzyme or fluorescence activity, which changes under the assay conditions.

Generally, when an enzyme–substrate reaction is used in an immunoassay, enzyme activity is measured as reaction velocity. In this situation, the reaction velocity must be proportional to the number of enzyme molecules that catalyze the reaction (174). In fluorescence immunoassays, a change in the nature of the interaction of light with the substrate is measured (175).

In many nonisotopic immunoassays, the label, whether fluorescent or nonfluorescent, is an enzyme. In order to distinguish RIAs from nonisotopic immunoassays, we must consider the characteristics of an enzyme label. First, it must be recognized easily as the label. The enzyme must be attached to the substrate in such a way that it maintains activity yet performs satisfactorily under the assay conditions. Second, the label must be stable. The label must not disintegrate when the assay is in process and it must be stable during storage. Invariably, the enzyme is covalently bound to the labeled molecule. Third, the enzyme must be quantitatively measurable. In nonisotopic immunoassays, one measures a secondary reaction product (i.e., produced by a substrate acting on the enzyme), rather than direct release of a radioisotope (176,177). Therefore, we do not measure the enzyme molecules themselves but instead measure the catalyzed reaction processes. With any enzymatic label, the product that is produced must be proportional to the amount of enzyme that catalyzes the reaction.

In considering the theory of enzyme activity and its relationship to the clinical assay, we must remember the Michaelis-Menten equation:

$$v = V\left[S/(S + K_m)\right],$$

where v is the measured reaction velocity, S is the concentration of substrate, and K_m is the calculated constant. In practice, one attempts to design the assay conditions so that S is much greater than K_m. In this case, we may assume that v is approximately equal to V and that

$$v = (k)E_2,$$

where E_2 is the total amount of enzyme that is present in the reaction mixture. It should be noted that this equation implies that the reaction velocity is independent of time.

The equations just described require that the reactions be followed continuously as they occur. One must measure the accumulation of product or the change in fluorescence as it occurs over time. There have been three primary means of quantitatively following enzyme reactions for the assay of haptens, including antibiotics, under these conditions. First is the spectrophotometric assay. The spectrophotometer is useful when the product of the reaction can be measured between 190 and 800 nm. Most workers have attempted to measure the release of the product directly. However, the product may first have to be transformed into a colored product. The advantage of using a spectrophotometer is that this instrument is readily available in clinical laboratories.

Much work has involved the study of fluorometric methods, which is the second approach. The outstanding feature of fluorometry is its high degree of sensitivity. Fluorometic methods are generally 100 to 1,000 times more sensitive than spectrophotometric methods. This sensitivity is especially manifested either when the initial substrate is nonfluorescent and becomes so during the reaction or when there is a change in fluorescence polarization as the reaction proceeds.

The third method, which employs electrodes, offers several advantages. Hydrogen ion concentrations and automatic titration apparatus may be employed to continuously measure a reaction as it proceeds. Considerable work has been performed on an oxygen electrode, which is a type of polarography (54).

Fundamental to nonisotopic immunoassays is the preparation of hapten–protein conjugates, in which haptens (antibiotic) and proteins (generally an enzyme) both function naturally. Most of the described methods have attached the hapten to the protein by free amino, hydroxyl, or carboxyl groups. Haptens with hydroxyl groups may be conjugated to a carrier protein by activation of the carboxyl group, followed by acylation of amino groups in the protein. The mixed-anhydride procedure has been commonly used for this purpose. Figure 8.6 demonstrates the principles of the reaction. The procedure is performed directly with the hapten and the conjugate.

Alternatively, one may use the carbodiimide procedure, in which uridine-5-carboxylic acid is coupled directly to poly-DL-alanyl-poly-L-lysine with dicyclohexylcarbodiimide in 95% dimethylformamide. The carrier or enzyme, excess hapten, and reagent are simply stirred together in water for 30 minutes each day for several days.

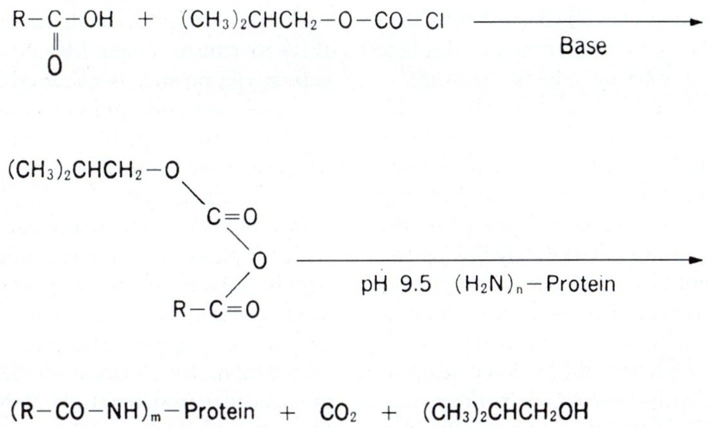

$$R-\underset{\underset{O}{\parallel}}{C}-OH \quad + \quad (CH_3)_2CHCH_2-O-CO-Cl \xrightarrow{\text{Base}}$$

$$(CH_3)_2CHCH_2-O \diagdown$$
$$C=O$$
$$\diagdown O \xrightarrow{\text{pH 9.5} \quad (H_2N)_n-\text{Protein}}$$
$$R-C \diagup O$$

$$(R-CO-NH)_m - \text{Protein} \quad + \quad CO_2 \quad + \quad (CH_3)_2CHCH_2OH$$

Figure 8.6 ■ **Mixed-anhydride reaction to label hapten antibiotics.** (From Kitagawa T, Kanamaru T, Wakamatsu H, et al. A new method for preparation of an antiserum to penicillin and its application for novel enzyme immunoassay of penicillin. *J Biochem* 1978;84:491–494, with permission.)

Haptens with amino groups, which include the aminocyclitol/aminoglycoside class of antibiotics, may be coupled to proteins. The reactions that are used to conjugate these haptens depend on whether the groups are aromatic or aliphatic amines. If the amino group is an aromatic amine, the hapten may be conjugated to proteins by the classic diazotization procedure. For example, CAM may be conjugated by this means (178). With this method, one must reduce the nitro group to an amino group before the conjugation reaction can occur. If the hapten contains an aliphatic amine, it can be reacted with carboxyl groups by the carbodiimide reagent. The conditions of this reaction are straightforward and similar to those employed for the conjugation of carboxyl groups. Optimally, amino groups of the hapten molecule can be acetylated by the hetero-bifunctional reagent *N*-(*m*-maleimidebenzoyloxy) succinimide to introduce a maleimide residue. As shown in Figure 8.7,

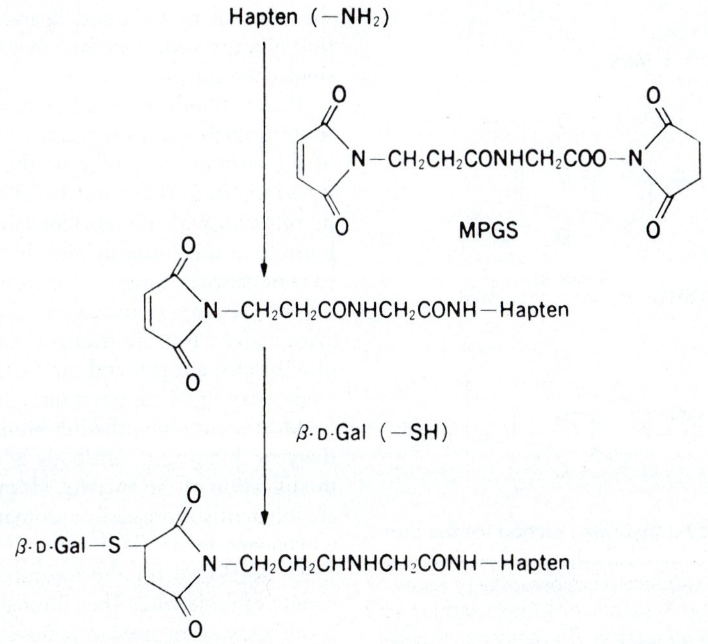

Hapten $(-NH_2)$

$$N-CH_2CH_2CONHCH_2COO-N$$
MPGS

$$N-CH_2CH_2CONHCH_2CONH-\text{Hapten}$$

β-D-Gal $(-SH)$

$$\beta\text{-D-Gal}-S \diagdown N-CH_2CH_2CHNHCH_2CONH-\text{Hapten}$$

Figure 8.7 ■ **Reaction with antibiotic and protein for the production of high-titered antibody.** β-D-*Gal*, β-D-*galactosidase*. (From Kitagawa T, Kanamaru T, Wakamatsu H, et al. A new method for preparation of an antiserum to penicillin and its application for novel enzyme immunoassay of penicillin. *J Biochem* 1978;84:491–494, with permission.)

the maleimide residue may be coupled with thiol groups, which are converted from the disulfide bonds of cystine residues by reductive cleavage.

Few enzymes have been used to label antibiotics. Peroxidase was coupled to gentamicin by a modified Nakne's method (8). One of the first enzymes used, which is still commonly employed in the EMIT system, is glucose-6-phosphate dehydrogenase. The means of covalently linking this enzyme to antibiotics is, however, a proprietary secret. β-D-Galactosidase has also been commonly employed. This reaction has been made possible through the use of hetero-bifunctional reagents such as N-(3-maleimidopropionylglycyloxy) succinimide (MPGS). A number of these reagents are equally useful. The general method is shown in Figure 8.8.

The bonding of ampicillin serves as a useful model of this type of antibiotic labeling. Fifty micromoles of ampicillin are dissolved in 0.05 mol/L of a phosphate buffer, pH 7.0. This is incubated with MPGS for 50 minutes at 30°C. After lyophilization, the powder is washed three times

Figure 8.8 ■ Mixed-anhydride reaction for the production of high-titered antibody to aminoglycoside antibiotics. *MBS*, *N*-(*m*-maleimidebenzoyloxy) succinimide. (From Kitagawa T, Kanamaru T, Wakamatsu H, et al. A new method for preparation of an antiserum to penicillin and its application for novel enzyme immunoassay of penicillin. *J Biochem* 1978;84:491–494, with permission.)

with 10 mL of ether/methylene chloride solution (2:1) to remove excess MPGS. Following desiccation, the powder is dissolved in 0.5 mol/L of a phosphate buffer, pH 6.0. Approximately 30% to 40% of the ampicillin is acetylated by MPGS. The acetylated ampicillin is coupled to the β-D-galactosidase enzyme by dissolving 1 mol in 1 mL of 0.05 mol/L phosphate buffer, pH 6.0, with 93 pmol of β-D-galactosidase and incubating the mixture overnight at room temperature. Thus, the conjugate is separated chromatographically using a Sepharose 6B column (1.8 × 30 cm) with 0.02 mol/L phosphate-buffered saline (PBS), pH 7.0, that contains 0.1% NaN_3, as the eluent. One unit of enzyme activity may be defined as the amount of enzyme that hydrolyzes 1 μmol of 7-β-D-galactopyanosyloxy-4-methylcoumarin per minute (178).

Nonisotopic immunoassays invariably use competition between labeled and unlabeled drug for antibody binding sites to derive the antimicrobial concentration in a specimen. These assays may be divided into two types: heterogeneous and homogeneous. The heterogeneous type was the first to be developed and is best exemplified by the enzyme-linked immunosorbent assay. Heterogeneous assays require wash steps to separate the bound and free ligands. Most commonly, these assays have been used to measure and detect large molecules. Homogeneous assays do not require the removal of unbound ligand from the reaction mixture and, therefore, may be performed as single-step assays.

If an antibody is bound to the antigen, the substrate is unable to gain access to the catalytic site of the enzyme. Accordingly, the enzyme's activity is inhibited. When unlabeled antigen is added, it competes with the enzyme-labeled antigen for binding to the antibody and the free form of the enzyme-labeled antigen is increased. As a result, enzyme activity is increased. Consequently, enzyme activity is proportional to the concentration of unlabeled antigen and can be used to quantitatively assay small hapten molecules.

Most commonly, the inhibition of enzyme activity on binding to antibody is caused by steric modification of the enzyme. Homogeneous assays are inherently more easily automated than are heterogeneous assays. These assays have been extensively developed for the measurement of a wide variety of molecules. The elimination in homogeneous assay of the need to remove unbound ligand from the reaction has made possible the generation of machinery that requires minimal technical input from the clinical laboratory. Automated instruments can measure enzyme activity through detection of reaction products and, with internally programmed computer analysis, derive the concentrations of the antibiotics in question.

Heterogeneous Nonisotopic Immunoassays

An assay for ampicillin is presented as a representative heterogeneous nonisotopic immunoassay. A mixture of 18 units of enzyme-labeled ampicillin (the production of which is described in the previous section) and 50 μL of 104-fold diluted rabbit ampicillin antiserum is incubated. A 0.1-mL sample or standard is added to 0.1 mL of the diluted ampicillin antiserum. To the sample or standard plus antiserum is added 0.5 mL of ampicillin–β-D-galactosidase conjugate and 0.05 mL of a 0.05 mol/L phosphate buffer, pH 6.0. This final volume of reactants is incubated for 6 to 8 hours at 4°C. Following incubation, 0.05 mL of normal rabbit serum, which has been

diluted 1:500, is added to 0.05 mL of goat antirabbit immunoglobulin G (IgG) serum, which has been diluted 1:5 and incubated with the reactant solution for 8 to 16 hours at 4°C. After this incubation period, 1 mL of 0.05 mol/L phosphate buffer, pH 6.0, is added and the entire mixture is centrifuged at 2,500 rpm for 20 minutes. The centrifugation step is repeated twice. To the reactant phase, 0.15 mL of substrate solution is added, with incubation at 30°C for 60 minutes. The amount of ampicillin present is calculated in a fluorometer, with excitation wavelength of 365 nm and emission wavelength of 448 nm (Fig. 8.9) (178–180).

To avoid the requirement for a centrifugation step, a method was developed that used antibody that was covalently linked to magnetizable particles (59). The sample is incubated with fluorescein-labeled gentamicin and antigentamicin serum to which has been attached magnetic particles. The magnetic particles are rapidly sedimented from the reaction mixture through contact with a polarized surface.

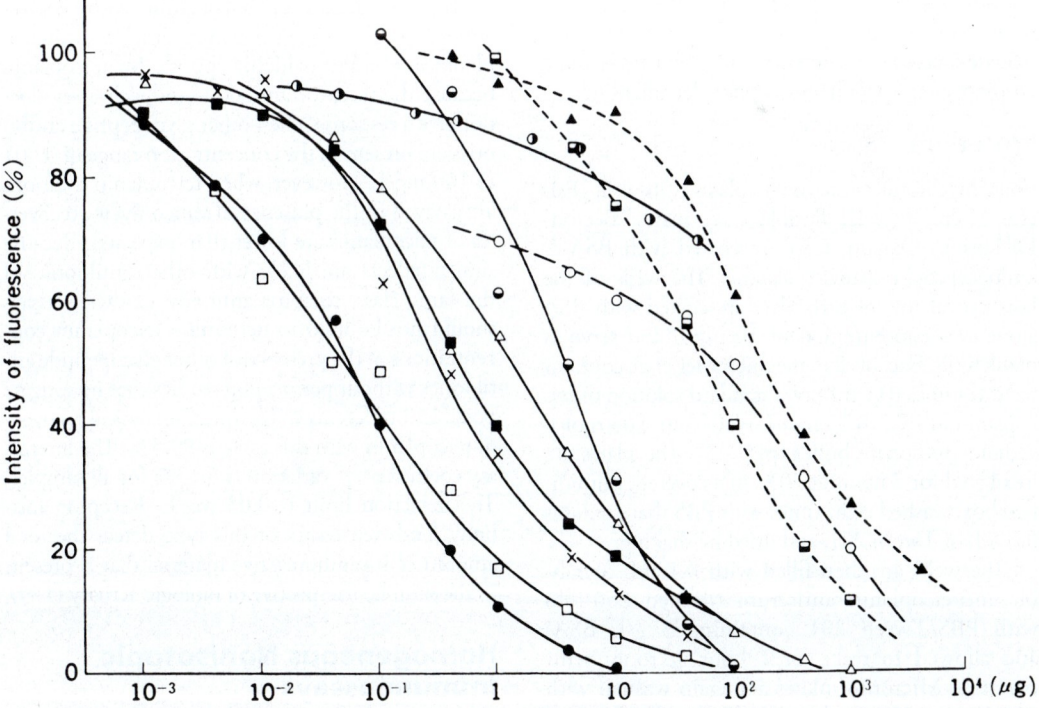

Figure 8.9 ■ **Heterologous nonisotopic immunoassay of ampicillin using an ampicillin-β-galactosidase conjugate.** ●, Ampicillin; ■, penicillin G; ✕, carbenicillin; □, sulbenicillin; ◔, flucloxacillin; ▣, cephalexin; ▲, cephaloglycin; ○, penicilloic acid. (From Kitagawa T, Kanamaru T, Wakamatsu H, et al. A new method for preparation of an antiserum to penicillin and its application for novel enzyme immunoassay of penicillin. *J Biochem* 1978;84: 491–494, with permission.)

Receptor Antibody Sandwich Assay for Teicoplanin

Teicoplanin, a glycopeptide antibiotic with activity similar to that of vancomycin, is currently used in Europe, Japan, and other countries to treat severe infections caused by gram-positive bacteria. Traditional methods for measuring concentrations of teicoplanin include microbiologic assays, HPLC, and solid-phase enzyme receptor assays (181). These methods have several limitations. First, the microbiologic assay is not specific for teicoplanin in the presence of other antibiotics and is of low accuracy when it is performed on biologic fluids. HPLC requires specialized equipment and laborious extraction procedures for sample preparation. Finally, the solid-phase enzyme receptor assay does not always yield accurate results in complex specimens such as bronchial expectorates or skin homogenates. The following method is a receptor antibody sandwich assay that is able to quantify teicoplanin in complex matrices. The method is based on bioselective adsorption of teicoplanin onto microtiter plates coated with BSA-ε-aminocaproyl-D-alanyl-D-alanine, a synthetic analog of the antibiotic's biologic target, followed by reaction with antiteicoplanin antibodies. The sandwich complexes are detected by incubation with peroxidase-labeled goat antibodies to rabbit IgGs and a chromogenic reaction with o-phenylenediamine.

Procedure

Polyvinylchloride microtiter plates (96-well, Falcon Micro Test III flexible assay plates; Becton-Dickinson, Oxnard, CA) are coated with BSA-ε-aminocaproyl-D-alanyl-D-alanine. The wells of the last vertical row of each plate are coated with BSA alone at a concentration of 10 mg/L and serve as blank wells. Each well in the microtiter plate contains fixed volumes (0.1 mL) of a standard solution of teicoplanin in PBS (0.15 mol/L NaCl and 0.05 mol/L sodium phosphate buffer, pH 7.3). The plates are incubated for 2 hours at 30°C in a covered, humidified box, washed eight times with PBS that contains 0.5 mL of Tween 201, and dried by shaking.

The wells are then filled with 0.1 mL of rabbit antiteicoplanin antiserum (diluted 250-fold with PBS/Tween 201 containing 3 g/L BSA) and allowed to react for 1 hour at room temperature. Microtiter plates are again washed with PBS/Tween 201. Each well is filled with 0.1 mL of peroxidase-conjugated goat antirabbit antibodies (diluted 1,500-fold with PBS/Tween 201/BSA). After reaction for 1 hour at room temperature and a wash step with PBS/Tween 201, 0.15 mL of chromogenic peroxidase substrate solution (1 g/L o-phenylenediamine and 3.5 mmol/L hydrogen peroxide in 0.1 mol/L sodium citrate buffer, pH 5) is added to each microtiter well. After 30 minutes of color development at 30°C, the reaction is stopped by adding 50 µL of 4.5 mol/L sulfuric acid to each well. Ten minutes later, the absorbance at 492 nm is measured in a Titertek Multiskan photometer (Titertek, Huntsville, AL). The binding curves are obtained by plotting, on semilogarithmic paper, the absorbances at 492 nm as a function of the teicoplanin concentration.

Performance

This assay has been used to detect teicoplanin in serum, ascitic fluid, skin homogenates, bronchial expectorates, pleural fluid, and prostate homogenates. Wells coated with only BSA, without BSA-ε-aminocaproyl-D-alanyl-D-alanine, have shown that nonspecific binding is negligible. A dose-response curve that is linear in the teicoplanin range of 0.004 to 0.15 mg/L indicates that the sandwich complex is formed despite the low molecular mass of the antibiotic.

The interaction of teicoplanin with BSA-ε-aminocaproyl-D-alanyl-D-alanine and the antiteicoplanin antibodies is highly specific for teicoplanin because the receptor antibody sandwich assay does not give a response when other glycopeptide antibiotics are present in the concentration range of 0.001 to 100 mg/L. However, when teicoplanin solutions are assayed in the presence of vancomycin, recoveries of teicoplanin are lower than expected. Because similar effects are likely with other antibiotics of the same class, receptor antibody sandwich assays should not be used to determine teicoplanin concentrations in the presence of other glycopeptide antibiotics without performing studies that investigate possible interferences. The mean analytical recovery of teicoplanin with this assay is 99.5%. The interassay coefficient of variation is 5.13% for all samples. The detection limit is 0.03 mg/L. Receptor antibody sandwich assays of this type detect the total amount of immunoreactive material that is present in the sample, irrespective of biologic activity (179).

Homogeneous Nonisotopic Immunoassays

Fluorescence Quenching

Fluorescence quenching was the first widely available, homogeneous, nonisotopic immunoassay procedure for the assay of antibiotic concentrations.

The method is based on the decrease in fluorescence that results from the combination of antibody with fluorescein-labeled antibiotic. This technique is rapid, sensitive, does not require an extraction step, and is automatable (182–184). The procedure is based on the same competitive binding principle that governs RIA.

Gentamicin

In a fluorescence quenching assay for gentamicin, a drug that has been made fluorescent through a reaction with fluorescein thiocarbamyl (FTC), is mixed with a serum specimen that contains both gentamicin and antigentamicin antiserum. Antigentamicin antiserum combines with FTC-gentamicin and stoichiometrically decreases the fluorescence of the conjugated antibiotic. As the amount of unconjugated gentamicin in the serum sample increases, the amount of antigentamicin antiserum available for binding to the FTC–gentamicin conjugate decreases, causing a proportional rise in the emitted fluorescence (183,185).

Apparatus

Fluorometric measurements are made with a xenon arc lamp in standard 1×1 cm glass cells.

Reagents

FTC-gentamicin is produced by the reaction of 0.425 g/L gentamicin free base with 0.50 g/L fluorescein isothiocyanate isomer (Sigma Biochemicals, Sigma-Aldrich, St. Louis, MO) in 50 nmol/L sodium carbonate–bicarbonate buffer, pH 9.0. The mixture is incubated for 2 hours at room temperature. Two milliliters of the reaction mixture is chromatographed on a 1×97-cm Sephadex G-15 column eluted at 1.8 mL/minute with a carbonate–bicarbonate buffer. The purity of the eluate can be determined by electrophoresing the products on Whatman no. 1 paper in 20 nmol/L of sodium carbonate–bicarbonate buffer, pH 9.0, at 10 V/cm for 2 hours. The band is visualized under shortwave ultraviolet (UV) light. Antigentamicin antiserum is prepared in rabbits, as for the RIA method (186).

Procedure

Excitation is at 495 nm and emission at 540 nm. In constructing a standard curve, the fluorescence value of a serum sample without gentamicin should be subtracted from both the patient serum and standard readings.

Antigentamicin antibody dilution curves are determined by making doubling dilutions in buffer of antigentamicin antiserum and pipetting 1-mL aliquots into two series of tubes. A 0.5-mL aliquot of a 1:200 dilution of stock FTC-gentamicin solution in buffer is added to each tube of one series and mixed. To each tube of the other series, 0.5 mL of the buffer is added. The tubes of the latter series serve as blanks that allow estimation of the fluorescence produced by the antiserum itself. Incubation is at room temperature for 5 minutes. The fluorescence of the test mixture and blanks is then measured. The corresponding blank signal is subtracted from the total signal of each test mixture. Figure 8.10 presents a typical antibody dilution curve.

The quenching fluorescence assay method is performed by diluting 50 μL of serum specimen 1:50 in buffer. To prepare standards, gentamicin concentrations are made in a geometric series from 0.25 to 32 μg/mL and diluted 1:50 in buffer. Aliquots of 0.5 mL of the diluted samples or standards are pipetted in duplicate into two series of small tubes. To each tube of one series, 0.5 mL of the 1:200 dilution in buffer of the stock FTC-gentamicin solution is added and mixed. Then 0.5-mL aliquots of a 1:80 dilution in buffer or antigentamicin serum are added to each tube and the contents are immediately mixed. To each tube of the other series, 1 mL of buffer is added and mixed. This latter

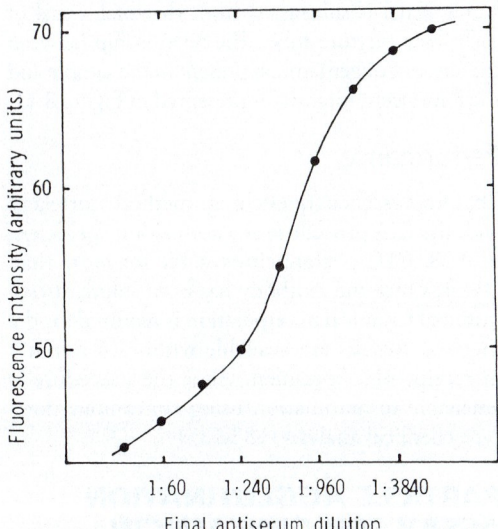

Figure 8.10 ■ Standard curve for antibody dilution in the fluorescent quenching assay. (From Shaw EJ. Immunoassays for antibiotics. *J Antimicrob Chemother* 1979;5:625–634, with permission.)

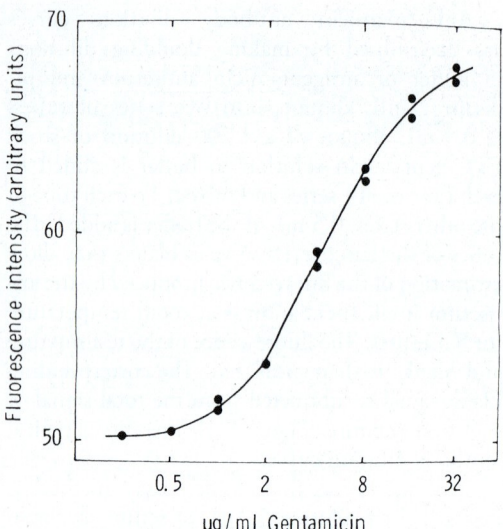

Figure 8.11 ■ **Quenching fluorescence immunoassay curve for the determination of a gentamicin blood level.** One must extrapolate on the straight portion of the curve. (From Shaw EJ. Immunoassays for antibiotics. *J Antimicrob Chemother* 1979;5:625–634, with permission.)

series serves for estimation of the fluorescence blank signals contributed by the intrinsic fluorescence of the serum samples or standards themselves.

The assay mixtures and blanks are incubated at room temperature for at least 5 minutes. All tubes are read in the fluorometer. The corresponding blank signal is subtracted from the total signal of each assay mixture tube. The relationship between the amount of gentamicin present in the sample and the fluorescent intensity is presented in Figure 8.11.

Performance

The fluorescence quenching method correlates with the RIA procedure at a correlation coefficient of 0.98. FTC-gentamicin is stable for more than 1 year. Once the antibody has been standardized, minimal technical manipulation is required for the method. Results are available within 15 minutes of receipt of a specimen. Also, the procedure is amenable to automation using continuous flow-type chemical analysis (183,185).

PARTICLE AGGLUTINATION ASSAY FOR GENTAMICIN

In an effort to develop a rapid and simple assay, the cost of which approaches that of the microbiologic assay, a hemagglutination inhibition assay for

gentamicin was developed (112). The technique applies to gentamicin that is covalently linked to BSA, which is covalently linked to sheep erythrocytes and fixed in formalin. This preparation is stable for up to 8 months in a refrigerator. The test is performed in Linbro microtiter plates (MP Biomedicals, Santa Ana, CA) with V wells. In principle, one drop of the patient's diluted serum is mixed with one drop of antiserum and, after 5 minutes at room temperature, one drop of gentamicin-bound sheep erythrocytes is added. The mixture is then incubated for 60 to 90 minutes at room temperature. Each of the reagents is standardized. If the patient's serum contains more gentamicin than is neutralized by the antiserum, agglutination of the gentamicin-coated sheep erythrocytes occurs. The lowest dilution of a patient's serum that causes agglutination is recorded.

A gentamicin standard containing 10 ng/mL is diluted to produce final concentrations of 0.31, 1.86, 2.97, 4.96, 6.51, 9.61, and 18.9 μg/mL in each microwell. Appropriate controls are added to adjacent wells. A given amount of reconstituted antiserum is added to all wells except the control well and the tray is mixed by gentle rotation. After 5 to 10 minutes, 50 μL of reconstituted cells is added to each well and the tray is mixed again by shaking. After 1 hour, the well number showing a pellet of cells equal to that of the control well is recorded. In effect, a titer, similar to cross-over broth dilution assays, is obtained. Although one can obtain only discontinuous values (values for which standard individual control wells are available), the method may prove effective if produced cheaply enough for clinical purposes. Based on the principle stated here, latex particles as carriers have also been marketed for the rapid semiquantitation of the major aminoglycoside/aminocyclitol antibiotics (187).

ENZYME-MULTIPLIED IMMUNOASSAY TECHNIQUE

The EMIT technique was developed from a free radical assay method that employed a spin label and detected drugs by electron spin resonance spectrometry. Electron spin resonance spectrometry requires expensive and very specialized equipment. EMIT was developed to bring the advantages of EIAs to clinical laboratories, without the requirement for large capital expenditures.

The heart of the EMIT is the attachment of an enzyme to the hapten. Commonly, lysozyme from egg whites, glucose-6-phosphate dehydrogenase from the bacterium *Leuconostoc mesenteroides,* malate dehydrogenase from pig heart mitochondria, and β-D-galactosidase from *E. coli* have been used as enzymes in EMIT assays. All these enzymes maintain significant activity after conjugation to the assayed drug.

Binding of antibody to the drug–enzyme conjugate inhibits the activity of the enzyme. The large protein antibody sterically hinders the association of the substrate with the active site of the enzyme, resulting in a reduction in the quantity of the product that is produced. The EMIT assay employs the stoichiometric competition between the antibiotic in the serum sample and the enzyme-conjugated drug for antibody binding sites to derive the serum antibiotic concentration. The activity of the conjugated enzyme is decreased on antibody binding and the amount of enzyme activity is directly proportional to the concentrations of free and bound enzymes present in the assay mixture. Therefore, one can derive the concentration of antibiotic in a sample from quantitative measurements of the reaction products by relating them to a standard curve. The major steps in immunoassay by EMIT are as follows:

1. Drug of unknown concentration + antibody → antibody–drug
2. Drug–enzyme conjugate + antibody → drug-enzyme-antibody
3. Substrate + antibiotic–enzyme → product

No separation step is required and the product is measured directly. Table 8.9 presents the major characteristics of the EMIT immunoassay. Table 8.10 lists the major advantages and disadvantages of the EMIT system.

Table 8.9

Major Characteristics of the Enzyme-Multiplied Immunoassay Technique Nonisotopic Immunoassay System

Parameter	Characteristic
Analysis time	>1 min
Technologist time	<1 min
Sample volume	<10 μL
Number of samples/time	30–40 samples/h
Reagent stability, lyophilized	1 y
Reagent stability, reconstituted	12 wk
Standard curve stability	8–72 h

Table 8.10

Advantages and Disadvantages of the Enzyme-Multiplied Immunoassay Technique System

Advantages
1. Small sample volume
2. Same technique for all antibiotics
3. Minimum technical skill and sample manipulation
4. Automatable
5. Results available quickly

Disadvantages
1. High cost of reagents
2. Analyzes drugs one at a time
3. May have interference from metabolites or similar compounds
4. May measure inactive metabolites

EMIT procedures have been modified for a wide variety of automated instruments. For example, Dade Behring's Syva EMIT Gentamicin 2000 (Siemens Diagnostics, Tarrytown, NY) homogeneous immunoassays are designed for used with most chemistry analyzers, including the company's Dimension (Siemens Diagnostics, Tarrytown, NY) combined chemistry/immunochemistry workstations. Many automated instruments automatically analyze the rate of change in absorbance of the sample or standard, correct for the absorbance from the drug-free control, and fit the data to a log-logit curve. In most cases, the coefficients of variation of the instruments range from 2% to 3%, but generally, 5% should be expected. It must be noted that, because the standard curves are not linear, small analytical errors may cause relatively large concentration errors at their limits. Thus, accurate timing and pipetting are crucial. For this reason, automated systems, even though they require larger capital investments and cost more per test, are less labor-intensive and require fewer repeat assays than manual procedures (188,189).

As with immunoassays in general, there are few limitations on the use of EMIT or interferences with its performance. The most common interference is the presence of the unconjugated enzyme in the specimen. For example, lysozyme and malate dehydrogenase may be endogenous in urine specimens. Lipemia, hemolysis, and hyperbilirubinemia do not interfere significantly with EMIT assays. When using EMIT to measure antibiotic concentrations in urine, changes in the pH or ionic strength may introduce errors into the system. This can be particularly pronounced when urease-splitting microbes in the urine increase its pH. It had been noted with the EMIT, as well as with other nonisotopic immunoassay systems, that the reproducibility of standard curves diminished when most of the reagent in a bottle had been used. Since this phenomenon appeared to have been caused by reagent evaporation, many manufacturers began packaging their reagents in smaller vessels (190).

The labor cost per test in the EMIT system is relatively small compared with the microbiologic assay. Approximately 20% of EMIT and 60% of biologic assay costs are for labor. In general, for the assay of antibiotics, the rapid availability of the assays overcomes the requirement for single-drug analysis (191,192).

The basic apparatus for EMIT includes a UV/visible light spectrophotometer with a temperature-controlled cuvette, a timer/printer, and a pipette/diluter. In general, serum or urine samples are diluted with buffer before the antibody–substrate and enzyme–antibiotic reagents are added. The mixture is aspirated into a spectrophotometer and absorbance is measured at two time points.

Amikacin

The assay of amikacin by EMIT is presented as a model for the assay of aminoglycoside/aminocyclitol antibiotics by this method. The principles, apparatus, and procedures are identical for other antibiotics. In the EMIT procedure, serum or plasma is mixed with reagent antibiotic that is coupled to glucose-6-phosphate dehydrogenase (reagent A). After incubation, antibodies to the particular drug are added. Glucose-6-phosphate serves as the substrate for the enzyme, and NAD is used as a cofactor.

The antidrug antibody competitively binds to both the free antibiotic and the enzyme-labeled drug. Antibody binding to the antibiotic–enzyme conjugate inactivates the enzyme. Consequently, as the antibiotic concentration in the specimen increases, the activity of glucose-6-phosphate dehydrogenase proportionally increases. Enzyme activity is reflected in the conversion of NAD to NADH. This reduction reaction produces a color change that is spectrophotometrically measured. Since NAD serves as a cofactor with bacterial, but not human glucose-6-phosphate dehydrogenase, interferences due to the presence of the human form of the enzyme are avoided by using bacterial glucose-6-phosphate dehydrogenase (from *L. mesenteroides*) in the assay.

Apparatus

A spectrophotometer that is capable of measurement at 340 nm at a constant temperature of 30°C must be used. A data-handling device must be attached to the spectrophotometer to analyze and print absorbance readings. In the past, recommended spectrophotometers have included the Syva S-111 (Dade Behring, Inc, Deerfield, IL) and Gilford Stasar 111 (Gilford Instrument Laboratories, Inc, Oberlin, OH). Each of these spectrophotometers should be set in the absorbance mode, with distilled water set to an optical density of 1.000. The switch mode control is set to concentration, and the set display is placed at 2.667 with the concentration calibrator knob. The display is zeroed with the zero control knob. Data handling has been performed with a Syva CP-5000 clinical processor (Siemens Diagnostics, Tarrytown, NY), Syva CP-1000 timer/printer (Siemens Diagnostics, Tarrytown, NY), or Syva timer/printer model 2400 (Siemens Diagnostics, Tarrytown, NY). Automatic sample handling has been accomplished with the Syva pipette/diluter model 1500 (Siemens Diagnostics, Tarrytown, NY). Any semiautomatic pipette/diluter that is capable of sampling 50 μL and delivering this sample along with 250 mL of assay buffer with sufficient force to ensure that there is adequate mixing of the reactants is satisfactory.

Reagents

Reagent A is amikacin to which has been covalently coupled glucose-6-phosphate dehydrogenase (the means of coupling is proprietary). This reagent, when reconstituted in buffer, is standardized to work with reagent B. Reagent A is reconstituted from the lyophilized form by adding 6.0 mL of distilled water. Following reconstitution, the reagent may be stored in the refrigerator overnight, but it must remain at room temperature for at least 2 hours before use. Reagent A should always be stored at 2°C to 8°C; it has a shelf life of 12 weeks.

Reagent B contains sheep antiamikacin antibody. This antibody–substrate reagent contains a standardized preparation of sheep γ-globulin, enzyme substrate glucose-6-phosphate, the coenzyme NAD, and preservatives in Tris buffer, pH 5.2. The lyophilized reagent is reconstituted with 6 mL of distilled water and must be allowed to remain at room temperature for at least 2 hours before use. Reagent B may be reconstituted and allowed to remain at 28°C overnight but must come to room temperature before use. It must be stored at 2°C to 8°C and is stable for 12 weeks.

The standard buffer solution used for dilution in the EMIT assay is 0.055 mol/L Tris-HCl buffer, pH 8.0, with a small amount of surfactant. The buffer solution is stable at room temperature for up to 12 weeks. Six amikacin calibrators and a control must be used. The calibrators are reconstituted with 1.0 mL of distilled water and the controls are reconstituted with 3.0 mL of distilled water. After reconstitution, the calibrators and controls must remain at room temperature for at least 2 hours before use. The calibrators and controls may be reconstituted and refrigerated overnight before use but must be at room temperature when the assays are run. The calibrators and controls must be stored at 2°C to 8°C and are stable for 12 weeks. The calibrators contain amikacin concentrations of 0, 2.5, 10, 20, and 50 μg/mL. The controls contain 15 μg/mL amikacin.

Procedure

Preparations for the test are made as follows: (a) All reagents are prepared as previously described; (b) all reagents must be well mixed and brought to room temperature; (c) all instruments must be properly calibrated; (d) the spectrophotometer must be zeroed with distilled water to 0.000; (e) the pipetter/diluter should be primed and flushed with buffer to ensure that there are no air bubbles in the lines; and (f) there must be a sufficient number of beakers present in the work rack. For calibrating, and for assaying unknowns, measurements should be made in duplicate and the results averaged. Duplicate readings that differ by more than six absorbance units should be repeated. The pipette tips must be carefully wiped with laboratory tissues both before and after the delivery of each solution. Solutions should not be held in the tubing for more than 5 seconds before delivery. The samples are analyzed as follows:

1. The calibrator, control, or specimen is diluted by delivering 50 μL of the appropriate solution and 250 μL of buffer to a 2.0-mL disposable beaker.
2. The sample is diluted again by adding 50 μL of the diluted sample from no. 1 to 250 μL of buffer solution and delivering this mixture to a second 2.0-mL disposable beaker.
3. Fifty microliters of reagent A is mixed with 250 μL of buffer solution, with delivery to the second beaker.
4. The spectrophotometer flow cell is purged.
5. Fifty microliters of reagent B plus 250 μL of buffer solution is added to the second beaker.

6. Immediately after the addition of reagent B, the contents of the second beaker are aspirated into the spectrophotometer flow cell. The printer/recorder should be automatically activated.
7. For the remaining samples, controls, and calibrators, steps 1 through 6 are repeated.
8. The spectrophotometer flow cell must be cleaned with the cleaning solution supplied with the instrument and the pipette/dilution lines must be stored in distilled water. After a 15-second delay, absorbance readings are made for each sample. The change in absorbance over a 30-second measurement period is used to calculate results.

The difference between the average calibrator zero reading (A_0) and the reading of each of the other calibrators (A), known as $A - A_0$, must be determined to plot a standard curve and to calculate the concentrations of the unknown samples. The Syva CP-5000 (Siemens Diagnostics, Tarrytown, NY) clinical processor automatically calculates the concentration of amikacin. The Syva CP-1000 timer/printer (Siemens Diagnostics, Tarrytown, NY) and Syva timer/printer model 2400 (Siemens Diagnostics, Tarrytown, NY) have built-in memory functions that store the A_0 reading so that the technologist may perform the necessary calculations on log-logit paper. The technologist derives the amikacin concentrations by preparing a standard curve and plotting $A - A_0$ for each calibrator against the calibrator concentrations on the lot-specific graph paper that is supplied with each reagent kit. A best fit line is constructed. Each time a new bottle of reagent A, reagent B, or buffer is used, a new standard line must be prepared. Furthermore, new standard lines must be drawn whenever duplicate controls vary by more than 10% or if any calibrator point lies more than six absorbance units off the line.

Performance

The EMIT amikacin assay is designed to measure the concentration of this antibiotic in serum or plasma. The major form of nontechnical error is generated by cross-reactivity with other compounds. Kanamycin significantly cross-reacts with the amikacin assay. Table 8.11 lists the concentration of a number of antibiotics that are required to produce a 30% measurement error in a sample that contains 10 μg/mL kanamycin. The assay range of quantitation is between 2.5 and 50 μg/mL. The coefficient of variation between runs is typically approximately 10%.

The EMIT has proven accuracy in clinical settings with the following limitations: (a) When β-lactam antibiotics are present in addition to

Table 8.11

Antibiotic Serum Concentrations Required to Produce 30% Error in a·Specimen Containing 10 μg/mL Kanamycin

Antibiotic	Concentration (μg/mL)
Carbenicillin	500
Cephalothin	500
Chloramphenicol	500
Clindamycin	500
Erythromycin	500
Gentamicin	100
Neomycin	500
Netilmicin	100
Penicillin	1,000
Tetracycline	1,000
Ticarcillin	500
Tobramycin	100
Sisomicin	100
Streptomycin	500
Sulfonamide	500

From Bastiani RJ. The EMIT system: a commercially successful innovation. *Antibiot Chemother* 1979;26:89–97.

amikacin, specimens must be assayed immediately or stored frozen; (b) severely hemolytic, lipemic, or icteric samples may interfere with the assay; and (c) kanamycin shows significant cross-reactivity with the amikacin assay. Table 8.9 describes the major performance characteristics of the EMIT immunoassay system (193,194).

Chloramphenicol

The recommended peak CAM concentration is from 10 to 20 mg/L (15 to 25 mg/L for meningitis). Because of CAM's potential toxicity, therapeutic monitoring of blood levels may be desirable with its use. Bioassays involve tedious preparation and lengthy incubation times. HPLC uses expensive equipment, and highly trained personnel are needed to perform HPLC assays. The following method describes a Syva EMIT assay (Dade Behring, Inc, Deerfield, IL) that was developed for measurement of CAM in human serum (58).

The Syva EMIT kit may be purchased from Dade Behring, Inc. Calibrators and buffers are reconstituted according to the manufacturer's

instructions. The assay has been performed with a Cobas-Bio centrifugal analyzer (Roche Analytical Instruments, Nutley, NJ) that was equipped with Data Reduction and Nonlinear Standard Curves (DENS) program version 8326. A standard curve for CAM is stored in the Cobas-Bio analyzer (Roche Analytical Instruments, Nutley, NJ) and the results from the individual serum samples are compared with the standard curve.

The sensitivity of the assay, defined as the smallest amount of CAM that can be accurately measured, is 2.5 mg/L (7.7 mol/L) for EMIT. Lower concentrations of CAM can be detected but not accurately quantified. The within-day precision coefficient of variation for EMIT is 4.0% at 5.0 mg/L, and the between-day coefficient of variation is less than 5.5%. When compared with HPLC and bioassay methods, the EMIT is specific for CAM and correlates well by regression analysis. The EMIT measures only the biologically active base form of the drug, uses a small sample size (0.2 mL), and provides rapid results. However, the reagents are expensive, and personnel need special training to perform the assay.

SUBSTRATE-LABELED IMMUNOFLUORESCENT ASSAY

The substrate-labeled immunofluorescent assay (SLIFA), like other immunoassays that are used to measure antibiotic concentrations, is based on competitive inhibition of the label of conjugated drug by drug that is present in the specimen. In the SLIFA procedure, the fluorescent moiety umbelliferone is generated from β-galactosylumbelliferone that is covalently bound to the antibiotic. In its usual state, the labeled antibiotic does not fluoresce. However, if the antibiotic–substrate reagent is cleaved by β-galactosidase, umbelliferone is released. When the β-galactosylumbelliferone–drug conjugate binds to the antidrug antibody, the conjugate is prevented from interacting with the enzyme. As in any competitive binding assay, the free antibiotic in serum sample competes with the conjugate for binding sites on the antibodies. The amount of conjugate available for the reaction is, therefore, directly related to the amount of free drug in the serum sample. In the SLIFA, the rate of increase in the intensity of fluorescence is proportional to the amount of antibiotic in the sample.

The reaction to label the aminoglycoside class of antibiotics with β-galactosylumbelliferone is a carbodiimide procedure. The reaction sequence proceeds in the same manner with all aminoglycoside/

aminocyclitol antibiotics. For the aminoglycoside amikacin, the β-galactosylumbelliferone reaction is performed by adding 50 mg of the potassium salt of β-[7-(3-carboxycoumarinoxyl)]-β-galactoside to 171 mg of amikacin sulfate in 2 mL of water. The pH is adjusted to 3.8 and the mixture is cooled to 0°C (in an ice bath). Thirty milligrams of 1-ethyl-[3-(3-dimethylaminopropyl)] carbodiimide hydrochloride are added.

After 2 hours, the mixture is chromatographed at 25°C on a 2.5 × 50-cm column of CM-Sephadex C-25 (Sigma-Aldrich, St. Louis, MO). The effluent is monitored at 345 nm. The column is washed with 200 mL of 50 mmol/L ammonium formate to elute the unreacted β-galactosylumbelliferone-amikacin. A linear gradient is formed with 400 mL of 50 mmol/L and 400 mL of 1.8 mol/L ammonium formate solution and applied to the column. A peak of material is eluted at a concentration of approximately 1.4 mol/L ammonium formate. The column is washed with 600 mL of 1.8 mol/L ammonium formate. The carbodiimide reaction appears to lead to the formation of amide bonds between the carboxylic acid of 1β-[7-(3-carboxycoumarinoxyl)] galactoside and the primary amino groups of the aminoglycoside antibiotic.

Amikacin

In the past, SLIFA kits have been commercially available for the assay of aminoglycoside/aminocyclitol antibiotics, including gentamicin, tobramycin, and amikacin (195,196). In addition, noncommercial antibiotic SLIFA kits have been produced for other aminoglycoside/aminocyclitol antibiotics. The procedure for the assay of amikacin in human serum or plasma is identical to other aminoglycoside/aminocyclitol assays. Only the absolute amounts of some of the reactants differ.

Apparatus

The SLIFA may be performed with any fluorescence spectrophotometer. Most commonly, either an Aminco-Bowman spectrophotofluorometer (American Instrument Company, Silver Spring, MD) or an Ames fluorocolorimeter (Miles Laboratories, Elkhart, IN) has been employed. The Aminco instrument is set for excitation at 400 nm and emission at 450 nm. The Ames instrument requires a 450 nm, narrow bandpass, interference filter for excitation, and a glass 5–56 (blue) filter on top of a glass 3–73 (yellow) filter for emission of light. The described SLIFA is not completely hands off in the sense that there are no microprocessors

and flow-through apparatus available to interpret the data. Accessory equipment includes (a) disposable fluorescence polystyrene cuvettes (Evergreen Scientific, Los Angeles, CA), (b) a pipetter/diluter equipped with a 250 μL reagent syringe and a 2.5 mL buffer syringe, (c) an accurate timer, and (d) 13 × 100-mm test tubes. It should be noted that aminoglycoside/aminocyclitol antibiotics may adsorb from dilute solutions onto glass. Therefore, plastic test tubes should always be used. (This physicochemical guideline applies to all assays, not just the SLIFA.)

Reagents

The antibody–enzyme reagent is composed of 1.5 units of β-galactosidase and antiserum-to-amikacin in 50 mmol/L bicine/0.1% sodium azide buffer (Worthington Biochemical, Inc, Freehold, NJ). Bicine buffer ([N, N-bis[2-hydroxyethyl] glysine) (grade A; Calbiochem, La Jolla, CA) is used at pH 8.5. The enzyme should be standardized at 25°C in 3-mL bicine buffer, pH 8.5, containing 3 mmol/L o-nitrophenyl-β-D-galactoside. The molar extinction coefficient for the product of this reaction, o-nitrophenyl, is 4.27 at 415 nm. One unit of enzyme activity hydrolyzes 1.0 mmol of substrate per minute. The antiserum has been commercially available (197). The antiserum must be of potency to inhibit the fluorescence to 10% to 20% of that in the absence of antiserum.

The antibiotic–drug conjugate consists of β-galacto-sylumbelliferyl-amikacin (0.007 absorbance units at 343 nm) in 5 mmol/L formate with 0.1% sodium azide buffer, pH 3.5. Each reaction mixture must contain 0.00035 absorbance units at 343 nm.

Standard amikacin concentrations should be made in normal human serum in the range of 0, 10, 20, 30, and 40 μg/mL amikacin. The range adjustment solution consists of a mixture of 7-hydroxycoumarin-3-(N-hydroxyethyl) carboxamide in 5 mmol/L formate, pH 3.5, with a final concentration of 0.1% sodium azide buffer. When 50 μL of the range adjustment solution is mixed with 1.5 mL of bicine buffer, the fluorescence intensity must be comparable to that absorbed with the high calibration samples at the end of a 20-minute incubation. The fluorescent antibiotic reagent must absorb maximally at 343 nm. However, on hydrolysis by β-galactosidase, the absorbance at 343 nm must decrease and a new maximum must appear at 405 nm. The absorbance of the enzyme–antibiotic conjugate at 405 nm after hydrolysis should be 1.6 times that at 343 nm before hydrolysis.

Procedure

After reconstitution, all components can be stored at 2°C to 3°C for up to 10 weeks. All components must be at room temperature before the assay is performed. The assay proceeds as follows.

1. Using a pipette/diluter, 1:50 dilutions of the calibrators and samples are made by diluting 50 μL of each specimen with 2.5 mL of diluted bicine buffer.
2. Fifty microliters of the antibody–enzyme reagent and 500 μL of buffer are dispensed, using the pipette/diluter, into the reaction cuvettes that are required for duplicate determinations of the calibrators and samples.
3. Fifty microliters of each of the diluted calibrators and samples is mixed with 500 μL of buffer and added to the reaction cuvettes.
4. Starting in the same calibrator sequence, the reactions are initiated at timed intervals by dispensing 50 μL of the amikacin fluorogenic reactant and 500 μL of buffer to each cuvette. The reactants must be thoroughly mixed.
5. After approximately 19 minutes, the reactions are read in sequence by zeroing the instrument with buffer and reading the first specimen in the fluorometer after adjusting the fluorescence reading to 90% of full scale.
6. At 20 minutes, the fluorescence intensity of the highest calibrator is read and recorded. Then the fluorescence intensity of the remaining cuvettes is read and recorded in the same sequence as that in which the reactions were initiated.
7. The concentration of amikacin in the assay is determined by constructing a standard line by plotting the average fluorescence readings for duplicate calibrators versus the amikacin concentrations.

The SLIFA performs comparably with other radiometric and nonisotopic immunoassays. Table 8.12 presents the salient performance characteristics of the assay for amikacin. As demonstrated in Figure 8.12, kanamycin and tobramycin cross-react at 2.4% and 0.2%, respectively, changing the response to the maximum dose by 50%. Other aminoglycoside/aminocyclitol antibiotics, including gentamicin, netilmicin, sisomicin, and streptomycin, do not significantly interfere with the assay. Additional antibiotics that have been tested, including carbenicillin, cephalothin, CAM, erythromycin, methicillin, and tetracycline, do not appear to affect the assay (198).

Table 8.12

Performance Characteristics for the Assay of Amikacin by the Substrate-Labeled Immunofluorescent Assay Technique

Characteristic	Parameter
Intraassay precision (15 μg/mL)	
Mean	15 μg/mL
Coefficient of variation	2.4%
Interassay precision (15 μg/mL control)	
Mean	15.5 μg/mL
Coefficient of variation	1.6%
Sensitivity	1.0 μg/mL
Correlation with RIA	
Correlation coefficient	0.99
Slope	0.95
Intercept	0.2 μg/mL
Standard error of estimate	1.6 μg/mL

RIA, radioimmunoassay.
From Provoost AP, Schalkwijk WP, Olusanya A, et al. Determination of aminoglycosides in rat renal tissue by enzyme immunoassay. *Antimicrob Agents Chemother* 1984;25:497–498.

The assay of amikacin by the SLIFA technique is accurate from 5 to 50 μg/mL. The accuracy of the SLIFA is affected by the same factors as other immunoassays of antibiotics (198).

Cycling Enzyme Assay

Cycling procedures are inherently appealing because they do not consume reagents during the course of reactions and can, therefore, use the same reagents for extended periods of time. Historically, the coenzymes NAD^+ and flavin adenine dinucleotide have been most frequently used as reaction cofactors. The assays have traditionally suffered from a lack of suitable detection systems for biologic samples. Cycling procedures have been described that use alcohol dehydrogenase and malate dehydrogenase as reagents. These assays are of limited use with biologic specimens because significant interference is generally present during the enzymatic cycling steps and in the final fluorometric measurements. An enzymatic cycling procedure with two irreversible reactions that are catalyzed by NAD^+ peroxidase and glucose-6-phosphate dehydrogenase has been devised. This cycling procedure is not adversely affected in an appreciable way by biologic fluids.

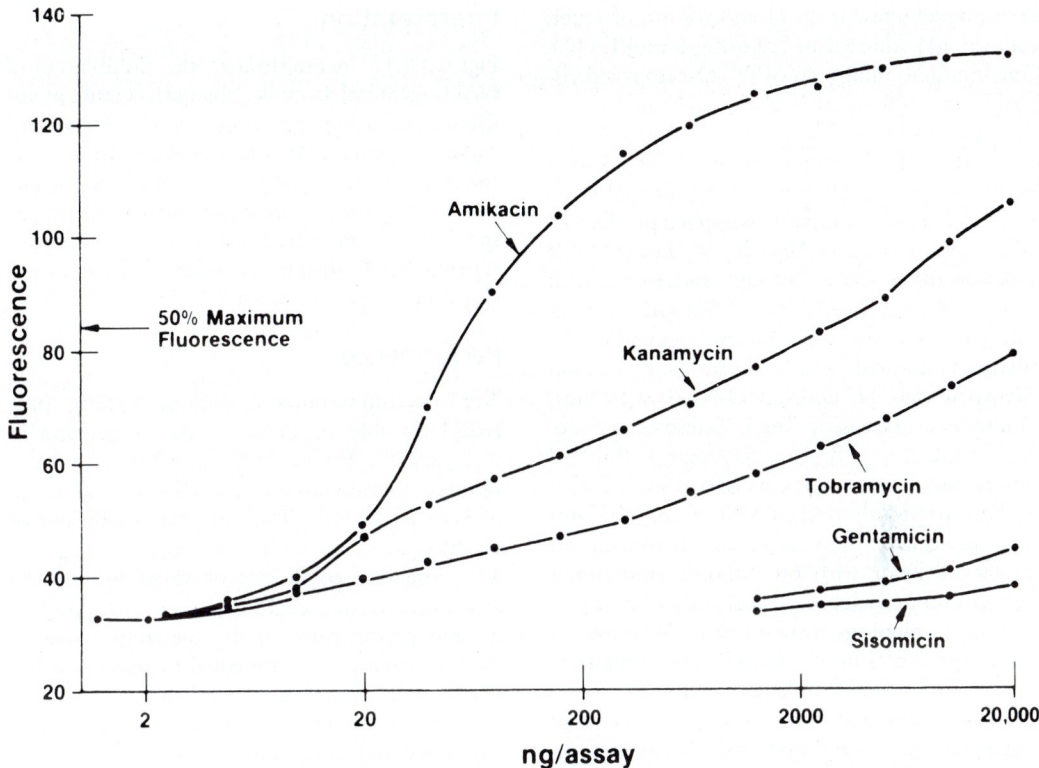

Figure 8.12 ■ **Cross-reactivity of aminoglycoside/aminocyclitol antibiotics in the SLIFA nonisotopic immunoassay.** (From Thompson SG, Burd JF. Substrate-labeled fluorescent immunoassay for amikacin in human serum. *Antimicrob Agents Chemother* 1980;18:264–268, with permission.)

The reaction has been designed to proceed as follows:

1. Gentamicin + (NAD^+-gentamicin) + antibody → gentamicin-antibody + (NAD^+-gentamicin)-antibody.
2. (NAD^+-gentamicin) + glucose-6-phosphate + glucose-6-phosphate dehydrogenase → (NADH-gentamicin) + H^+ + 6-phosphogluconate (cycling step).
3. 6-Phosphogluconate + NADP + glucose-6-phosphate dehydrogenase → NADPH + H^+ + ribulose-5-phosphate + CO_2 (indicator reaction).

Apparatus

A Perkin-Elmer model 555 UV/visible spectrophotometer (Perkin Elmer, Norwalk, CT) has been used for determining absorbance. This gentamicin assay has been performed with an Eppendorf model 1101M spectrophotometer (Eppendorf, Hamburg, Germany) that is equipped with a 334-nm filter.

Reagents

NAD^+ peroxidase (EC 1.11.1.1), glucose-6-phosphate dehydrogenase (EC 11.1.49), NAD phosphate ($NADP^+$) 1-oxoreductase from *L. mesenteroides*, 6-phosphogluconate dehydrogenase (EC 1.1.1.44), $NADP^+$ 2-oxoreductase, and β-D-glucose-6-phosphate crystallized monosodium salt were all obtained from Boehringer-Mannheim (Mannheim, Germany). Antigentamicin antibodies were obtained from Atlantic Antibodies (Scarborough, ME).

Procedure

For synthesis of NAD^+-labeled gentamicin, 5 g of gentamicin sulfate is dissolved in 15 mL of water. The pH of the solution is adjusted to 11.5 with 5 mol/L NaOH. The mixture is lyophilized and extracted in 2 L of boiling methanol. Free gentamicin base is dried in a vacuum. Gentamicin is conjugated to NAD^+ after the coenzyme has been converted to N^6-(2-carboxyethyl)-NAD^+. One gram of gentamicin base is dissolved in 5 mL of water, with the pH adjusted to 7.0 using 6 mol/L HCl. One hundred milligrams of N^6-(2-carboxyethyl)-NAD^+ and 500 mg of 1-ethyl-3-(3-dimethylaminopropyl) carbodiimide are dissolved in 2 mL of water. The pH is kept constant at 4.7 for a 3-hour incubation period. After incubation, the pH is adjusted to 7.0 and the mixture is applied to a Dowex 1-X2 column (Sigma-Aldrich, St. Louis, MO) (chloride form, 2.6 × 40 cm) and eluted with water (100 mL/hour). The UV-absorbing fraction is concentrated on a rotary evaporator. The mixture is desalted on a Sephadex G-15 column (Sigma-Aldrich, St. Louis, MO) (2.6 × 60 cm), with water as the eluent. The UV-absorbing material is applied to a BioRex 70 column (Bio-Rad Laboratories, Richmond, CA) (2.6 × 40 cm) that has been previously washed with 20 mmol/L ammonium acetate. The void volume is washed out at 100 mL/hour with 60 mmol/L ammonium acetate. Elution is accomplished with a linear gradient of ammonium acetate (20 to 50 mmol/L) over a period of 4 hours. The UV-absorbing fraction contains both NAD^+ and gentamicin.

The fraction that contains both NAD^+ and gentamicin is concentrated and fractionated on a Bio-Gel P4 column (Bio-Rad Laboratories, Richmond, CA) (2.6 × 60 cm) with water flowing at 40 mL/hour. After volume reduction to 10 mL, the two NADH and gentamicin peaks are stored at −30°C. These two peaks are analyzed for NAD^+ content using ethanol and alcohol dehydrogenase. Peak 1 has a molar absorptivity at 265 nm of 24.1×10^3/mol/L/cm in the oxidized form and 20.7×10^3/mol/L/cm in the reduced form. Peak 2 has absorptivity of 2.9×10^3/mol/L/cm in the oxidized form and 19.2×10^3/mol/L/cm in the reduced form. Peak 1 has a gentamicin content by RIA of 1.45 μg/mL and peak 2 has a gentamicin content of 0.99 μg/mL.

Fifty microliters of sample is added to 50 μL of the ice-cooled cycling reagent that contains 0.2 mol/L Tris, 0.28 mol/L potassium acetate, 12 mmol/L β-D-glucose-6-phosphate, 12 mmol/L hydrogen peroxide, 200 μg/mL NAD^+ peroxidase, and 200 μg/mL glucose-6-phosphate dehydrogenase, pH 8.5. The solution is mixed for 2 hours at 30°C. After cooling, 0.5 mL of 20 mmol/L Tris, 30 mmol/L ammonium acetate, 0.1 mmol/L ethylenediaminetetraacetate, 0.2 g/L BSA, 0.6 mmol/L $NADP^+$, and 10 μg/mL 6-phosphogluconate dehydrogenase, pH 7.7 (the spectrophotometric indicator reagent), is added. The absorbance at 334 nm is recorded after the mixture is incubated for 30 minutes at 25°C.

Interpretation

Figure 8.13 demonstrates the inhibition of NAD^+-gentamicin peak 2 by antigentamicin antiserum at various gentamicin levels. A standard curve for gentamicin was calculated from these values and is displayed in Figure 8.14. The absorbance values for gentamicin standards and patient specimens are measured at 334 nm, and after subtracting blank absorbance values, related to the gentamicin concentrations.

Performance

The spectrophotometric enzyme cycling procedure is able to detect 5 ng of gentamicin (0.1 μg/mL). The method is equal to other nonisotopic immunoassays and RIA in the range of 1 to 10 μg/mL. The intraassay coefficient of variation is 6.1% with a mean at 7.4 μg/mL. The intraassay coefficient of variation is 3.4% at a concentration of 13.1 μg/mL. The specificity and performance of the spectrophotometric cycling enzyme assay are equal to those of other nonisotopic immunoassays and the standard RIA method. In addition, reagents are not rapidly consumed and measurements may be made on a simple spectrophotometer (199).

FLUORESCENCE POLARIZATION IMMUNOASSAY

Like the other nonradioactive immunoassay techniques such as SLIFA and EMIT, the FPIA method was developed as a technology to assay small molecules. The theoretical basis for FPIA was described in the early 1970s by Dandliker et al. (200). Subsequently, Abbott Laboratories (Abbott Park, IL) accelerated the entry of this technology into clinical laboratories by developing an automated fluorescence polarization analyzer system (201).

A molecule naturally gravitates toward its lowest energy state but becomes excited after exposure to light. This excitation is the result of electrons moving from a lower energy shell to a higher energy shell. The leap to higher energy levels, governed by the laws of quantum mechanics, is temporary. The electron naturally returns to its original energy shell. The amount of energy gained during the first jump to a higher energy shell is greater than the amount of energy that the molecule loses when the electron returns to its normal orbit. The wavelength of light that is emitted during the return trip (emitted light) is longer than

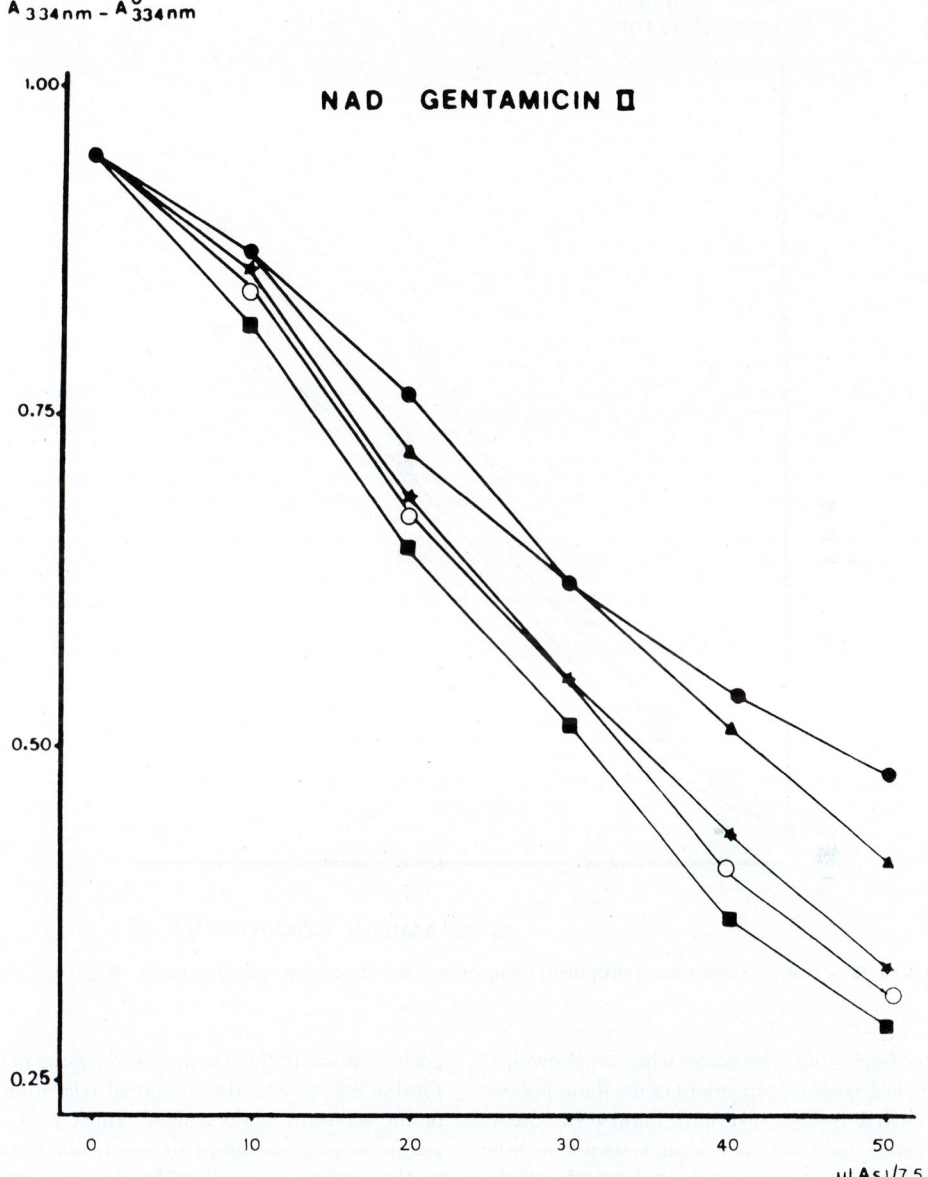

$A_{334nm} - A^0_{334nm}$

NAD   GENTAMICIN ▯

µl AS1/7 5

Figure 8.13 ■ Inhibition of NAD$^+$-gentamicin by antigentamicin antiserum for various levels of gentamicin (▶, 0 µg/mL; ▼, 0.3 µg/mL; ★, 0.5 µg/mL; ◀, 1 µg/mL; •, 1.5 µg/mL).

that which is absorbed during the primary jump (excitation light) and is measured as fluorescence. Ordinary (white) light contains a spectrum of wavelengths (white light). The electrical vectors of light waves that are produced by standard sources are randomly oriented. Excitation sources that are used in fluorometers can emit light at one, several, or a range of wavelengths of interest, depending on the applications for which the instrument is used. The intensity of the emitted fluorescent light is related to the excitation intensity of the initially absorbed light at the absorption wavelength.

Plane-polarized light is generated when light is passed through crystalline materials known as "polarizers." A polarizer orients the electrical vectors of incoming light waves in a single plane. Fluorescence polarization occurs when fluorophores that have been excited by polarized light also emit

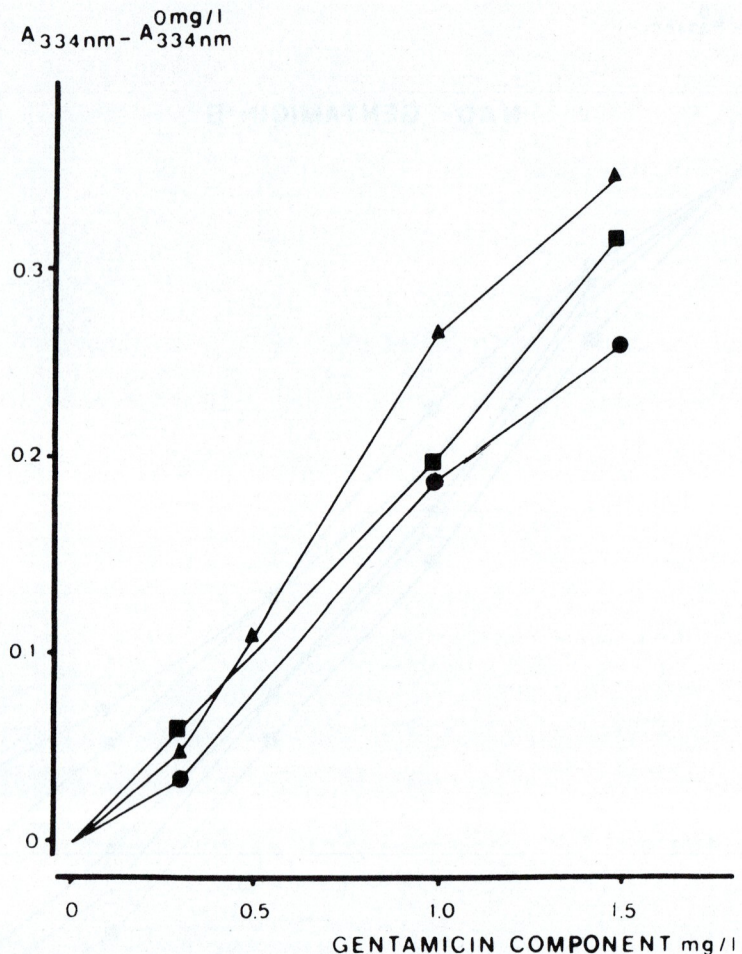

Figure 8.14 ■ **Standard curves for gentamicin components by the cycling immunoassay.** ◀, C_1; •, C_{1a}; ▶, C_2.

polarized light (366). This occurs when the Brownian movement (rotational relaxation) of the fluorophores under analysis is slower than their fluorescence decay times. Small molecules rotate rapidly, such that their rotational relaxation times are much shorter than their fluorescence decay times. Consequently, small fluorophores emit depolarized fluorescent light while large fluorophores emit polarized fluorescent light (202).

In developing the FPIA technique, the fluorescence decay times and rotational relaxation times of the molecules under study needed to be considered. The fluorescence decay time of the molecule is the time interval from the moment it is struck by polarized light until it releases its emitted light (203). The rotational relaxation time describes the molecule's Brownian motion and is the time an oriented molecule takes to leave alignment after an incoming burst of polarized light. To effectively determine

analyte concentrations with an FPIA assay that uses routine equipment, the rotational relaxation time of the molecule under analysis must be 1 nanosecond or less. This limits the use of the technique to the analysis of small molecules. For example, immunoglobulins have rotational relaxation times of approximately 100 nanoseconds.

The fluorescent light intensity that is produced by the sample is measured both parallel to and perpendicular to the plane of the polarized excitation light. The fluorescence polarization is measured by the following formula:

$$P = (I_{PAR} - I_{PERP})/(I_{PAR} + I_{PERP}),$$

where I_{PAR} (parallel) is the intensity of fluorescence parallel to the plane of the excitation light and I_{PERP} (perpendicular) is the intensity of fluorescence perpendicular to the plane of the excitation light.

In practice, the antibiotic is labeled with fluorescein. When the antibiotic binds to a specific antibody, the rotational relaxation time of the large antigen-antibody complex is increased so that it exceeds the fluorescence decay time of the label. The concentrations of antibody and fluorescent-labeled antigen are kept constant, with the only variable being the concentration of the antibiotic (unlabeled antigen) in the specimen. The higher the concentration of free antibiotic in the sample, the more this antigen limits binding of the labeled antibiotic to antibody, resulting in a proportional decrease in fluorescence polarization (204–208). Conversely, as the concentration of unlabeled antibiotic decreases, the amount of fluorescence polarization proportionately increases.

Fluorescence Immunoassay Method

Apparatus

A specially designed fluorometer with microprocessor controls is available from Abbott Laboratories (Abbott Park, IL). The instrument and specimen flow pathways are described in the following texts.

The filament of a General Electric EFM 50W tungsten/halogen lamp (Fairfield, CT) is focused through a 3-mm diameter entrance aperture. After passing through heat-absorbing glass (BD-38; Corion Corp, Holliston, MA), the light is collimated. All lenses in the system are Melles Griot plano-convex lenses (Albuquerque, NM) that have a focal length of 18 mm and a diameter of 15 mm. The collimated light is directed through a 10-nm bandwidth, 485-nm center wavelength, excitation filter (Corion Corp, Holliston, MA). Light reflected from the transparent glass beam splitter (Corning coverglass no. 1, Corning, NY) is focused onto a UV 215 B reference silicon detector (EG & G, Salem, MA). The reference detector signal is used to monitor the intensity of the lamp. The light transmitted through the beam splitter passes through an HN38S polarizer/crystalloid transmission–type liquid crystal combination (Polaroid, Cambridge, MA). This beam splitter also serves to rotate the plane of polarization. The excitation light is directed onto the sample, which is contained in a 12 × 75-mm glass tube. The emitted light is collimated through a lens, passed through a 10-nm band with a 525-nm interference filter, and then directed through a vertical HN38S polarizer. The emitted light is focused onto a 3 × 8-mm aperture and R928 photomultiplier tube (Hamamatsu Corp, Middlesex, NJ). The excitation optics and the emission optics are perpendicular. The polarizer/liquid crystal combination is rotated in an electric field applied to the liquid crystal. When voltage is directed through the liquid crystal, no rotation occurs and horizontal light passes through the sample. When there is no voltage, the liquid crystal rotates by 90% and the sample is excited by vertical light (209,210).

Measurements are made as directed by the microprocessor through emission fluorescence intensity measured by the photomultiplier tube. The gain of the photomultiplier tube is controlled by a model PMT-20 A/N high-voltage power supply (Bertran Associates, Syosset, NY). Both the excitation and fluorescent polarization intensities are captured in the vertical and horizontal modes and converted from voltages to frequencies, which are measured by a counter timer. Intensity values are presented as the ratio of the frequency channel counts to the reference clock channel counts (211).

Reagents

The fluorescein conjugate of amikacin is prepared by reacting the antibiotic with 5-[(4,6-dichlorotriazinyl) amino] fluorescein. The fluorescein compound is dissolved in methanol and added to amikacin in water at pH 9.0. The final concentration of the fluorescein reagent is 16 mol/L and that of amikacin is 160 mol/L. After 1 hour at room temperature, the mixture is applied to a diethylaminoethyl-cellulose chromatography column with 0.1 mol/L phosphate buffer, pH 8, as the eluent.

The amikacin–fluorescein conjugate is diluted in 0.1 mol/L Tris (hydroxymethyl) methylamine buffer, pH 7.5, that contains 1.212 g/L sodium dodecyl sulfate, 0.1 g/L bovine γ-globulin, and 0.1 g/L sodium azide. The concentration of the conjugate is approximately 100 nmol/L. Antiserum is diluted in a phosphate buffer, pH 7.5, that contains 0.1 g/L bovine γ-globulin, 0.1 g/L sodium azide, and 50 mg/L benzalkonium chloride. Standards and controls of amikacin are made as described for the SLIFA procedure.

Procedure

Amikacin is assayed by transferring 20 μL of sample or control into 1 mL of buffer. This step is repeated. After 20 μL of the diluted sample is dispensed into a 12 × 75-mm disposable culture tube, 200 μL of dilution buffer is added. To this solution, 40 μL of conjugate is added, followed by 700 μL of buffer. Finally, 40 μL of antiserum solution is added and dispensed into the reaction vessel, followed by 1.0 mL of buffer.

Table 8.13

Expected Performance of Assay of Amikacin by the Fluorescence Polarization Immunoassay Technique

Parameter	3 µg/mL	15 µg/mL	30 µg/mL
Mean (µg/mL)	2.8	15.14	30.68
Standard deviation within run (µg/mL)	0.17	0.30	0.65
Coefficient of variation within run (%)	6.11	2.01	2.12
Standard deviation between runs (µg/mL)	0.21	0.52	1.00
Coefficient of variation between runs (%)	7.50	3.51	3.26

From Jolley ME. Fluorescence polarization immunoassay for determination of therapeutic drug levels in human plasma. *J Anal Toxicol* 1981;5:236–240; Jolley ME, Stroupe SD, Schwenzer KS, et al. Fluorescence polarization immunoassay. III. An automated system for therapeutic drug determination. *Clin Chem* 1981;27:1575–1579.

Performance

Table 8.13 presents the salient characteristics of the FPIA for amikacin. The following antibiotics cross-react at a rate of less than 0.1% in the FPIA of amikacin: ampicillin, amphotericin, carbenicillin, cefamandole, cephalexin, cephaloglycin, cephaloridine, cephalothin, CAM, CLD, erythromycin, ethacrynic acid, 5-fluorocytosine, fortimicin A, fortimicin B, furosemide, fusidic acid, lincomycin, methicillin, methotrexate, oxytetracycline, penicillin, rifampin, sulfadiazine, sulfamethoxazole, tetracycline, ticarcillin, TMP, and vancomycin.

Table 8.14 presents the cross-reactivity of closely related compounds with the FPIAs of the aminoglycosides gentamicin, tobramycin, and amikacin. Figure 8.15 compares the FPIA results for

Table 8.14

Cross-reactivity of Aminoglycosides Gentamicin, Tobramycin, and Amikacin in the Fluorescence Polarization Immunoassay

Drug	Cross-reactivity (%)		
	Gentamicin	Tobramycin	Amikacin
Sagamicin sulfate	55.0	<0.1	<0.1
Sisomicin	30.0	<0.1	<0.1
Netilmicin	7.0	<0.1	<0.1
Gentamicin	100.0	<0.1	<0.1
Kanamycin A	<0.1	44.0	30.0
Kanamycin B	<0.1	43.0	3.0
3', 4'-Dideoxykanamycin B	<0.1	60.0	2.5
Tobramycin	<0.1	100.0	3.5
Amikacin	<0.1	1.5	100.0
Neomycin	<0.1	<0.1	<0.1
Spectinomycin	<0.1	<0.1	<0.1
Streptomycin	<0.1	<0.1	<0.1

From Jolley ME. Fluorescence polarization immunoassay for determination of therapeutic drug levels in human plasma. *J Anal Toxicol* 1981;5:236–240; Jolley ME, Stroupe SD, Schwenzer KS, et al. Fluorescence polarization immunoassay. III. An automated system for therapeutic drug determination. *Clin Chem* 1981;27:1575–1579.

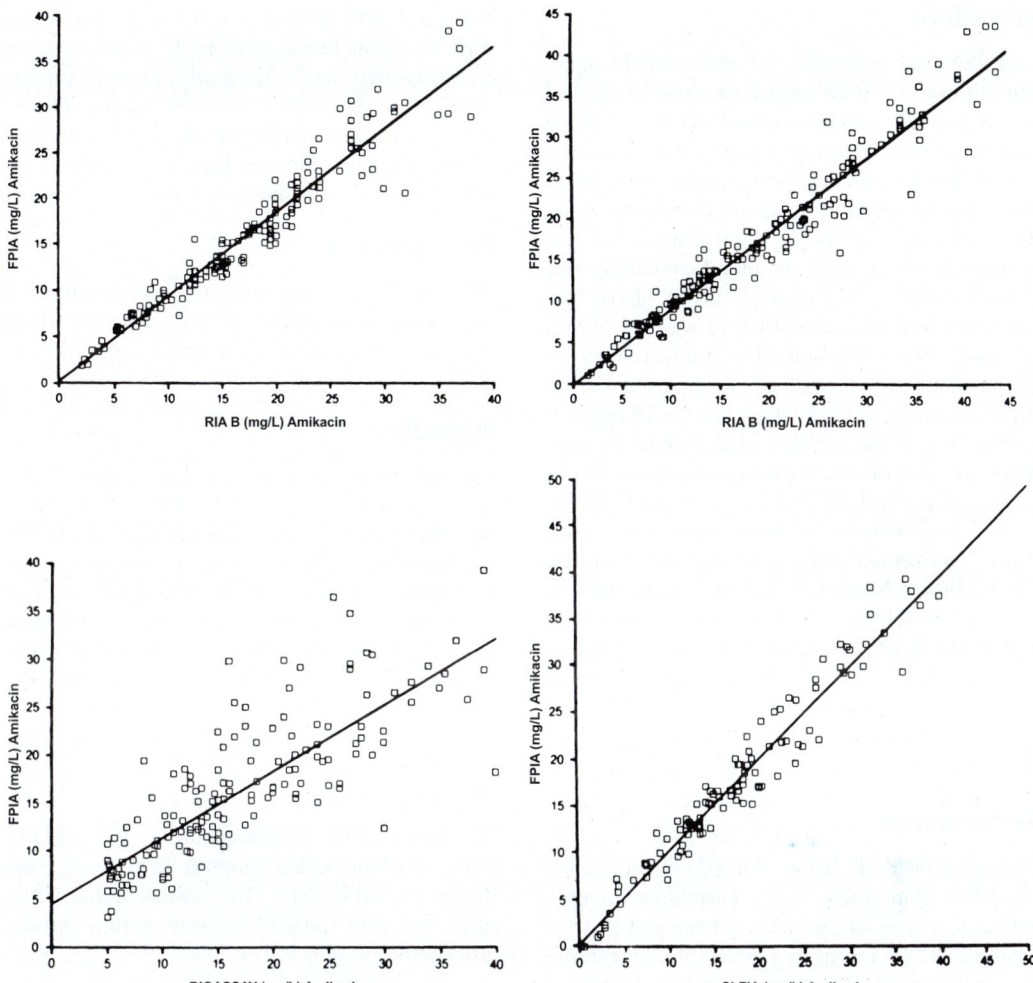

Figure 8.15 ■ Comparison of the analysis of amikacin by RIA, bioassay, and fluorescent nonisotopic immunoassay. (From Jolley ME. Fluorescence polarization immunoassay for determination of therapeutic drug levels in human plasma. *J Anal Toxicol* 1981;5:236–240, with permission.)

amikacin with those of RIA, bioassay, and SLIFA. Discrepancies between the slopes for the different assays are most likely attributable to the sources of the standards or their preparation and storage. Coefficients of variation between the immunoassays were 6.96% or greater. Results seen here with amikacin are also applicable to the aminoglycosides gentamicin and tobramycin (205,212).

Micromethod Fluorescence Polarization Immunoassay of Aminoglycosides

Gentamicin and netilmicin are aminoglycoside antibiotics that are used to treat gram-negative bacterial infections. Monitoring the concentrations of these drugs, usually in venous blood samples, helps optimize care by limiting the incidence of toxicity and therapeutic failure. However, venous samples are often difficult to obtain from infants and children. Capillary blood spotted on filter paper has been used successfully for detection of inborn errors of metabolism and for monitoring drug concentrations. For example, this technique has been used with an HPLC assay that has been previously described in this chapter to detect netilmicin and sisomicin. The following method is an FPIA that determines the gentamicin and netilmicin concentrations from blood samples spotted on filter paper.

Procedure

One hundred microliters of the standard aqueous solutions (0 to 20 μg/mL prepared in distilled water) and the gentamicin and netilmicin blood standards (0 to 20 μg/mL prepared with antibiotic-free pooled blood) are spotted onto filter paper. The spots are dried at 50°C for 10 minutes in an air-circulating oven or at room temperature for 5 hours. Using scissors, the blood-containing area is cut into five or six pieces and all are placed into one tube. Addition of 500 μL of warmed (35°C) 0.5 mol/L Na_2HPO_4 buffer to the tube is followed by incubation of the sample in an oven (35°C) for 60 minutes and centrifugation for 15 minutes (3,000 × g). The colorless clear filtrate is transferred to a well of a TDx cartridge (Abbott Laboratories, Abbott Park, IL) for measurement by FPIA.

The measurement of hemoglobin in extracts can be performed using a hemoglobin assay kit (Wako Pure Chemical Industries, Osaka, Japan). Twenty microliters of each extracted sample is mixed with 5 mL of cyanmethemoglobin reagent. After 5 minutes, the absorbance is measured at 540 nm and compared with that of the standard solution containing 3.58 of cyanmethemoglobin/5 mL.

Performance

Hemoglobin levels below 8.6 g/L do not affect the FPIA gentamicin assay. Ultrafiltration of a gentamicin-free sample with a hemoglobin level greater than 8.6 g/L gives a clear, colorless filtrate, demonstrating that the hemoglobin in the filtrate is almost completely removed by the ultrafiltration procedure. Maximum elution time from the spotted paper for both gentamicin and netilmicin is 60 to 90 minutes under the given extraction conditions. Recovery of gentamicin from dried blood-spotted samples in the concentration range of 1.5 to 20 μg/mL is from 92% to 115%. The lower limit of detection (LOD) of gentamicin or netilmicin with the FPIA reagent kits is 1 μg/mL each for samples spotted with 100 μL of whole blood.

The calibration curve for gentamicin or netilmicin in dried blood spots is linear over the concentration range of 1.0 to 20 μg/mL. The intraassay coefficients of variation are 5.6% and 6.3% for gentamicin concentrations of 5 and 10 μg/mL, and 4.6% and 1.6% for netilmicin concentrations of 10 and 20 μg/mL, respectively. The interassay coefficient of variation is 4.5% for a gentamicin concentration of 5 μg/mL and 9.7% for a netilmicin concentration of 10 μg/mL. Clinical samples from pediatric patients treated with netilmicin show excellent linear correlation when corrected for hematocrit levels. The applicability of the determination of gentamicin or netilmicin concentrations in dried blood spots by FPIA is limited because the quantification limit exceeds the effective range of the antibiotics (204).

Teicoplanin

Teicoplanin levels in serum can be determined by FPIA using fluorescein-labeled teicoplanin, which competes with unlabeled teicoplanin for antibody (213).

Procedure

For the generation of the calibration curve, standards containing 0, 5.0, 10.0, 25.0, 50.0, and 100.0 μg/mL teicoplanin are prepared. The International Bioclinical reagent system is used to prepare standards and serum samples for measurement by the American Bioclinical FP analyzer (Upland, CA). This instrument calculates the millipolarization values and extrapolates the teicoplanin concentration for each sample by comparing the values to those of the calibration curve.

Performance

The lower LOD of teicoplanin is 0.5 μg/mL. Other antibiotics that interfere in this assay are shown in Table 8.15. The results of the FPIA agree well with those of bioassay, with a correlation coefficient of 0.901.

Table 8.15

Specificity of Teicoplanin Fluorescence Polarization Immunoassay	
Drug	**Interference (%)**
Cefazolin	3.1
Ciprofloxacin	4.4
Daptomycin	3.0
Erythromycin	1.4
Gentamicin	0.2
Nafcillin	3.6
Piperacillin	2.8
Rifampin	6.3
Vancomycin	2.8

From Rybak MJ, Bailey EM, Reddy VN. Clinical evaluation of teicoplanin fluorescence polarization immunoassay. *Antimicrob Agents Chemother* 1991;35:1586–1590.

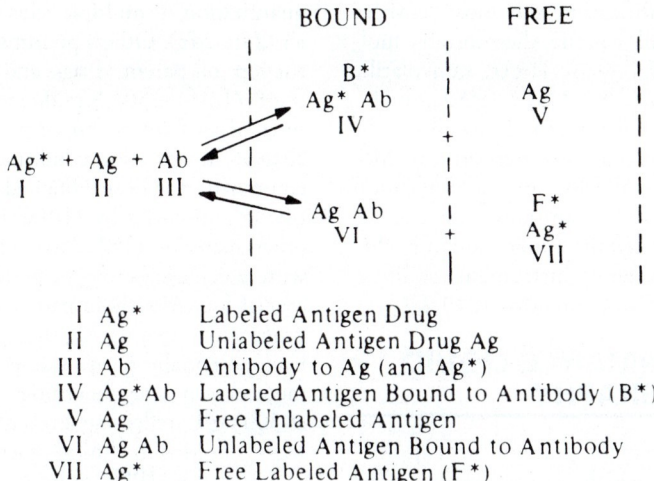

BOUND   FREE

$$B^*$$
$$Ag^* \; Ab$$
IV   Ag
                          V

Ag* + Ag + Ab
I   II   III   +

                        Ag Ab   F*
                        VI   Ag*
                                           VII
                                    +

I Ag*	Labeled Antigen Drug
II Ag	Unlabeled Antigen Drug Ag
III Ab	Antibody to Ag (and Ag*)
IV Ag*Ab	Labeled Antigen Bound to Antibody (B*)
V Ag	Free Unlabeled Antigen
VI Ag Ab	Unlabeled Antigen Bound to Antibody
VII Ag*	Free Labeled Antigen (F*)

Figure 8.16 ■ Reaction series of the RIA*, radiolabeled substances. (From Gentamicin radioimmunoassay. Newport Beach, CA: Monitor Science Corp, 1976, with permission.)

RADIOIMMUNOASSAYS

The general advantages and disadvantages of the RIA technique are shown in Table 8.2 (214,215) (Fig. 8.16). Because it is no longer in routine clinical use, it is not discussed further in this chapter.

CHROMATOGRAPHIC ASSAYS

Chromatography uses the ability of a compound in one type of medium to be selectively removed from that medium onto an adsorbent and to be quantitatively assayed. Most commonly, the compound is in a liquid and is adsorbed onto a solid (liquid chromatography) or is in the gas phase and is adsorbed onto a liquid (GLC). Inherent in any chromatographic method is the requirement for specialized adsorbent columns (which may be different for different antibiotics), the use of expensive equipment (especially in GLC), the use of various extraction procedures, and the requirement for a skilled technician to perform the assay.

The advantages of the procedure are that chromatography can separate even closely related compounds and analyze them separately. Generally, the method is quite sensitive, that is, able to quantitate between 1.0 and 0.5 μg/mL for most antibiotics and is quite rapid, requiring 30 to 60 minutes per specimen. The principles of chromatography have evolved from the early decades of the 20th century, with the most exciting applications occurring within the last 40 years.

Modern chromatography dates to 1941 when Martin and Synge (216) published their classic paper on liquid–liquid partition chromatography. They described individual rates of migration of substances that were a consequence of differing partition ratios between mobile and stationary liquid phases. Gas chromatography (GC) and thin-layer chromatography (TLC) appeared in the 1950s and were received enthusiastically. However, the time-consuming, crudely quantitative characteristics of TLC and the requirements of molecule volatility and thermostability for GC are disadvantages of these techniques. Building on chromatographic principles that evolved over five or more decades and experience gained from GC and TLC in particular, researchers developed HPLC in the late 1960s. The debut of HPLC was largely from the pioneering work of Horvath and Lipsky (217).

Although homogeneous and heterogeneous enzyme FPIA techniques may be viewed as competitive with HPLC, a more global view of the subject reminds us that each method has its own strengths and weaknesses and that the fields of therapeutic monitoring and pharmacokinetic assessment of antibiotics are strengthened by the appropriate application of each of these technologies. The advantages of HPLC are many. These will be amplified as improvements in instrumentation, packing materials, and methods are made. As with GC, mass spectroscopy (MS) is now being applied to HPLC (218). GC-MS will undoubtedly remain the method of choice for the most accurate identification and most sensitive quantitation of small, volatile, thermostable molecules. However, for many larger, nonvolatile, thermosensitive molecules, HPLC-MS has major potential as an analytic method. In this technique, HPLC is a preparatory step prior to MS, and allows the identification and quantification of molecules in the picogram range. Several papers have demonstrated the application of HPLC to MS and have presented instrument modifications to reduce MS contamination (219,220).

HIGH-PERFORMANCE LIQUID CHROMATOGRAPHY

HPLC is a reference method, if not the major reference method, by which all new antimicrobial agents are studied, from discovery to clinical application. It plays a major role in drug preparation, pharmacologic assessment, and clinical monitoring (50,64,91,216,221). Thus, an understanding of the analysis of antimicrobial agents by HPLC is essential in clinical laboratory practice.

HPLC as a technology has assumed a central role in the analysis of all water-soluble molecules in clinical laboratories. This technique is the method of choice for the analysis of penicillin and cephalosporin antibiotics. HPLC is especially useful clinically in the measurement of third-generation cephalosporins in the nonblood body compartments (222). It is also being used more frequently to measure parent antibiotics and their metabolites. This section discusses this powerful tool and provides specific examples of how it is used to determine concentrations of most of the major classes of antibiotics in use today.

Many antibiotics have been analyzed successfully by HPLC, including aminoglycosides (223–226), cephalosporins and penicillins (227–230), tetracyclines (231,232), trimethoprim-sulfamethoxazole (371), and others (44,233,234). The interested reader is referred to reviews by Nilsson-Ehle (235) and Jehl et al. (236) for discussions of the general method and its application to the analysis of drugs.

A number of factors stimulated the application of HPLC, a technique that was already in common use in science and industry, to the quantitation of antibiotics in biologic fluids (237–239). This technology was commonly used in modern laboratories to measure antiarrhythmic and anticonvulsant agents. The equipment and expertise were thus available. Several HPLC methods, using standard chromatographic equipment, have been developed that allow the simultaneous

quantitation of multiple, closely related antibiotics (240–243). Others permit simultaneous quantitation of parent drugs and some metabolites (9,48,71,244–250). Simultaneous analysis of mixtures of antibiotics can be performed with small changes in operating conditions (251). Once the equipment has been obtained, the cost of quantifying antibiotics by HPLC is competitive with other methods (252–256). Finally, the rapidity with which assays may be performed by HPLC is crucial for seriously ill patients who are receiving drugs with narrow toxic/therapeutic ratios or that have potentially severe side effects (257). HPLC methods can detect quantities of antibiotics as low as 500 ng/L, reflecting levels of sensitivity beyond what is needed in clinical practice (251).

Using the HPLC technique, highly reproducible, difficult separations are achieved rapidly and quantitatively (55,258–260). The majority of HPLC separations are accomplished in less than 1 hour, with many requiring only a few minutes. A wide variety of molecular species may be separated and quantitated by HPLC, including both large and small molecules, ions, isomers, polymers, polar molecules, and nonpolar molecules (261–263). Because HPLC is often performed at low or ambient temperatures, thermosensitive molecules are easily handled (264–266). After the analyte molecules pass the instrument detector, they may be collected quantitatively in unaltered form for further purification or investigation.

Prior to reviewing the practical application of the liquid–liquid partition principle in HPLC, let us first briefly consider its theoretical basis. All HPLC methods use the same basic steps:

1. Extraction of the drug with a specific solvent
2. Separation of the drug on the solid phase by HPLC
3. Detection of the effluent from the solid phase by spectrometry
4. Quantitation of the amount of antibiotic present by peak height analysis or peak area analysis

The aim of chromatography in general is the resolution or separation of different molecular species. To understand resolution in the context of HPLC, we must consider a few explanatory equations. These equations and a more in-depth discussion may be found in an excellent concise paper by Guiochon (267) or in the work of Giddings (268). First, let us assume that the groups of molecules eluting from the chromatographic column or peaks on the chromatogram are Gaussian in distribution (not entirely true but adequate for mathematical interpretation). The resolution (R) of two Gaussian peaks is defined by the equation

$$R = 2(t_{R2} - t_{R1})/(W_1 + W_2),$$

where t_{R1} and t_{R2} are the retention times of the first and second peaks, respectively, and W_1 and W_2 are the widths at the base of the chromatographic peaks. If the two peaks are close, the resolution is defined by the equation

$$R = (sq. rt. [N/4][(\alpha - 1)/\alpha] [k'_2/(1 + k'_2)].$$

To understand this equation, let us look at its component factors. First, remember that the width at the base of a Gaussian distribution is equal to 4 SD (σ). N, or the plate number of the column (a standard measure of its efficiency), is defined as

$$N = (16_{tR}/W)^2 = (t_R\sigma_t),$$

where σ_t is the SD of the peak in units of time and t_R and W are the retention time and base width of the peak, respectively. The relative retention of the two compounds being considered, σ, is described by the equation

$$\alpha = (t_{R2} - t_0)/(t_{R1} - t_0) = t'_{R2}/t'_{R1} = k'_2/k'_1,$$

where t_0 is the retention of an inert molecular species that theoretically is not retained by the column, t'_{R1} and t'_{R2} are the adjusted retention times, and k′ is the capacity factor of the column (how retentive it is in terms of these particular molecular species). The capacity factor, k, for each molecular species, may be redefined as

$$k = (t_R - t_0)/t_0 = r'_R/t_0$$

This factor, k, is important because it is proportional to the equilibrium constant that describes the distribution of molecules between the chromatographic phases.

Applying these formulas to HPLC, the mobile solvent phase passes over the stationary phase at a constant rate. The two phases possess different chemical polarities. As the analyte molecules in the mobile phase pass over the stationary phase, those with polarity closer to that of the stationary phase are retained selectively for a time on the column. Conversely, the analyte molecules with polarity closer to that of the mobile phase tend to remain in the mobile phase, passing through the column faster. Passing through the instrument monitor sequentially, these groups of molecules give rise to peaks on the chromatogram (Fig. 8.17).

The term *high-performance liquid chromatography* encompasses several different types of chromatography. Systems that have a polar stationary phase with a nonpolar mobile phase are termed *normal phase* or *straight phase*, while those having a nonpolar stationary phase with a polar mobile phase are termed *reverse phase*. A popular

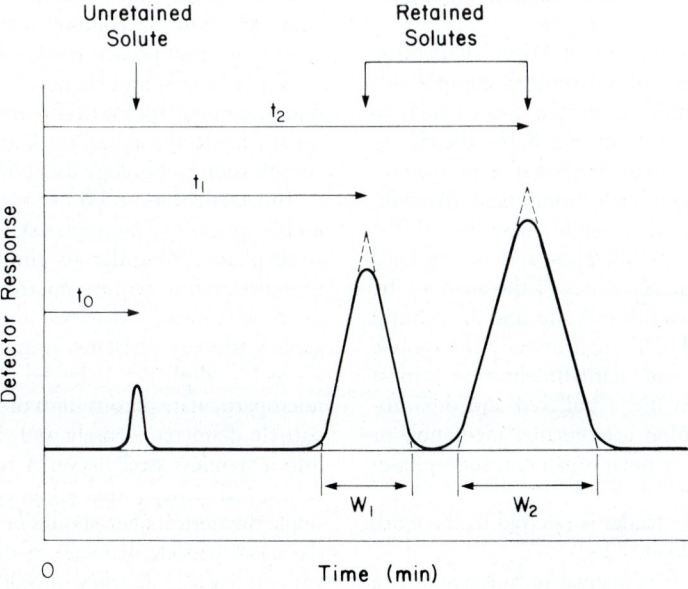

Figure 8.17 ■ **Theoretical chromatogram of unretained and retained solutes.**

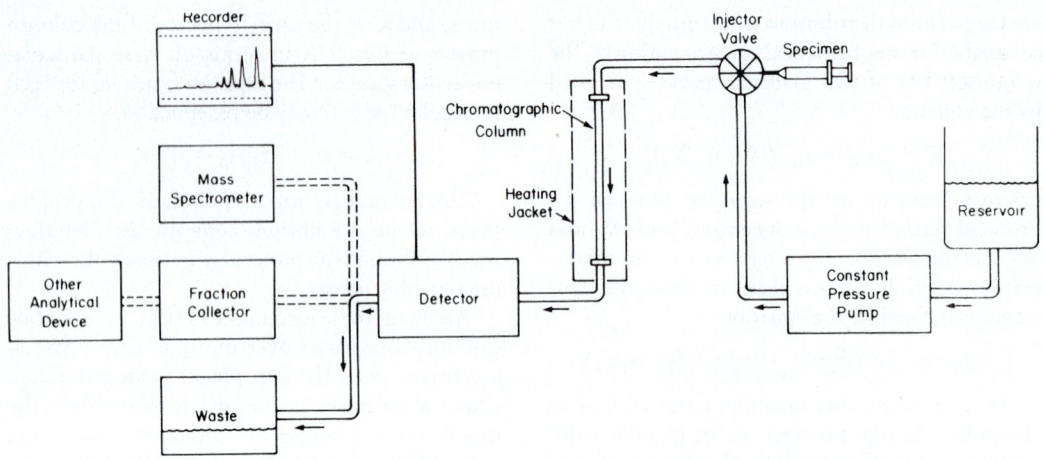

Figure 8.18 ■ Diagrammatic representation of HPLC.

variant of RP-HPLC is ion-pair chromatography, where the polarity (and thus the retention) of the analyte is changed by adding a second ion of opposite charge (counter-ion). Ion-exchange chromatography is based on competition between the analyte ion and a second, similarly charged molecule for oppositely charged sites on the exchange resin. An early form of HPLC using a solid stationary phase that separates molecules on the basis of differing size and weight is termed *size-exclusion* or *gel-permeation chromatography*. Gel-permeation chromatography has wide industrial and research applications but is rarely used for antimicrobial determinations in clinical laboratories.

Much of the versatility of HPLC is because of the wide variety of instrument components and chromatographic conditions from which to choose. In its simplest form (Fig. 8.18), the HPLC system is a closed system composed of an injector, pump, chromatographic column, and detector, with a reservoir for the mobile phase liquid. The composition of the mobile phase selected depends on the physical characteristics of the analyte, the complexity of the sample mixture, and the column packing employed. Although initially the mobile phase was usually nonpolar (straight phase), most recent applications use a buffered aqueous mobile phase containing acetonitrile, methanol, or some other relatively polar organic (reverse-phase) compound. For an extensive review of solvent phase selection, the reader is referred to the work of Snyder and Kirkland (269).

The injector, either manual or automatic, is a simple but very important component that allows the sample to be placed into the mobile phase

stream without disrupting the flow. The HPLC pump is critical in that it must present the mobile phase liquid to the chromatographic column at a constant pressure (usually <2,000 psi) to provide acceptable and reproducible analyte separations in a timely fashion. Pumps are available over a broad price range, with considerable variations in design that serve mainly to minimize pressure fluctuations.

Progress in the field of HPLC has been made through improvements in the chromatographic packing materials themselves and the consistency with which the columns are packed. High-quality, commercially prepared columns are available that offer improved batch-to-batch reliability and a wide selection of column lengths, efficiencies, types of support phases, particle sizes, shapes, pore sizes, pH ranges, and chemical specificities of the liquid stationary phase (270). The column sleeve is usually made of stainless steel, although the radial compression technology uses polyethylene (271).

In practice, most HPLC systems use a polar mobile phase and nonpolar stationary phase (reverse phase). In order to eliminate false peaks (bubbles) and to remove microparticulate matter, the mobile phase is degassed and filtered. The organic stationary phase is commonly composed of C_8 or C_{18} aliphatic chains bonded chemically to microparticulate porous silica of 5 to 10 μm mean particle diameter, densely and uniformly packed into a stainless steel sleeve. A rule of thumb for column efficiency is that for an efficient column, a single theoretical plate should be two to five times the mean particle diameter of the support phase, with an overall efficiency of 3,000 to 5,000 theoretical plates. The internal diameter of the sleeve is usually 2 to 5 mm, with the column length varying from 3 cm to several meters, although typically, it is less than 30 cm. The rate of flow of the mobile phase is usually 1 to 3 mL per minute, requiring a pressure of up to about 2,000 psi to maintain the flow and to attenuate chromatographic time.

Most current methods are performed at ambient temperature or at up to approximately 50°C. Above this, silica-based packing materials begin to deteriorate. The pH of the mobile phase is kept below 7 to 7.5 for the same reason, although non-siliceous packing materials are available that work well in the basic region.

The selection of the means by which the HPLC instrument "sees" the analyte molecules as they proceed in groups from the chromatographic column allows one to further tailor the instrument and the analysis for particular needs. Commonly used detectors include UV/visible, fluorescence, refractive index, electrochemical, infrared, and radiometric instruments, and mass spectrometry. UV detectors are most commonly used to monitor the effluent from the column, although fluorescence detectors, because of increased sensitivity and elimination of interfering peaks, are often preferred. State-of-the-art detectors tend to be microprocessor-controlled, with flow cell volumes down to 1 μL. However, less sophisticated detectors with flow cells of 10 μL are adequate for the majority of applications. Typically, 5 to 100 μL of the prepared sample is injected. The chromatographic time is usually less than 20 minutes. Current HPLC systems routinely work in the nanogram range. Between-day coefficients of variation are usually less than 5% to 7%. An internal standard is commonly used to minimize errors inherent in the system, particularly if some form of sample pretreatment is employed. For a concise review of the use of internal standards, the reader is referred to the work of Snyder and Kirkland (269).

Biologic fluids are typically complex mixtures that are composed of a wide variety of proteins, carbohydrates, lipids, and others. Beyond the deleterious effects these materials have on the injector, column packing material, and pump, their presence frequently interferes with the separation and quantitation of the analyte molecules under study. Consequently, some form of sample preparation is almost always required prior to the chromatography. Four major techniques are commonly employed to prepare samples for injection.

In most assays of biologic fluids, including antibiotic assays, it is essential to remove as much protein from the fluid under study as possible.

Most directly, one can precipitate the protein, for example, with trichloroacetic acid. However, acid precipitation leaves many interfering materials in the sample and the resultant pH change may be deleterious to the analyte molecules, metabolites, packing material, or other equipment components.

Alternatively, one may remove the protein with an ultrafilter such as those available from Millipore Corporation (Billerica, MA) (272), but not all low molecular weight proteinaceous material can be removed. Other interfering materials may pass through the filter as well. Additionally, analyte is lost if there is significant protein binding. In spite of its limitations, this method has been gaining popularity (273).

Solvent extraction has been the most common preparatory technique. Organic solvents extract specific organic molecules selectively from the specimen by solvent partitioning. In this process, protein in the sample is usually denatured and left at the liquid–liquid interface. By appropriate solvent selection and manipulation of the specimen pH, a satisfactory separation of the analyte from most of the other materials in the specimen can frequently be achieved. For example, piperacillin can be extracted into chloroform/1-pentanol at an acidic pH (274). The organic solvent containing the drug can be removed by evaporation, or the drug can be extracted back into an aqueous solution with a pH of 7, where the drug is ionized and water-soluble. This latter step further cleans the specimen and may be used to concentrate the analyte if a reduced quantity of the aqueous phase is used.

Many compounds may be isolated by first adsorbing them either onto an ion-exchange resin (275) if they are charged or onto a bonded reverse-phase packing material if they are not charged (276), followed by elution. For example, the aminoglycoside/aminocyclitol antibiotics are very polar and difficult to extract with an organic solvent. However, they may be easily adsorbed onto Amberlite resin (The Dow Chemical Company, Midland, MI) (275) or silicic acid (12), eluted, and analyzed.

The advantages of HPLC—rapid availability of results, sensitivity, specificity, and the ability to measure several drugs and their metabolites simultaneously—allow for easy therapeutic monitoring of antibiotics. At the same time, they enhance antibiotic development and pharmacokinetic evaluation. Nearly all of the antibiotics in use today have been assessed by HPLC. Concurrent with improvements in HPLC equipment and packing materials, methods have been developed for the quantitation of certain antibiotics by EMIT, RIA, fluorescence assays, FPIA, and other nonisotopic immunoassays. When a choice of technique is possible, some factors that should be considered before a selection is made include the equipment and expertise that is available within the laboratory, the positive and negative attributes of the specific methods under consideration, the laboratory's test volumes and costs, and the institution's clinical requirements (56,221,258,277–293).

Chloramphenicol

At present, CAM is probably the antibiotic most commonly quantified by HPLC in clinical laboratories. Several relatively simple methods are available that give sensitive and reproducible results rapidly and require only small quantities of specimen. Additionally, CAM and its succinate or palmitate prodrug esters may be measured simultaneously. HPLC conditions for their measurement are similar to those employed for quantitation of theophylline, acetaminophen, and some anticonvulsants, thus requiring minimal method modification for the many laboratories already measuring these drugs by HPLC (294). Radioenzymatic assays (158,295) are available to measure CAM, and a modification of these has been compared with HPLC (296). Table 8.16 presents a summary of the HPLC methods available for measuring CAM. The authors have preferred the method of Velagapudi et al. (297) because the procedure employs ethyl acetate extraction, is performed at ambient temperature, is monitored at the absorption maximum of CAM (278 nm), and uses a closely related compound (thiamphenicol) as the internal standard (298). Table 8.16 presents recent useful HPLC methods (299).

Cephalosporins

Factors to consider when deciding whether or not to monitor blood concentrations of cephalosporin drugs include the potential for toxicity and concerns about patient compliance (for the oral preparations), possible failure to reach or sustain therapeutic concentrations for other reasons, or inappropriate use of expensive medications. Blood concentrations of these drugs may also be monitored for the purposes of pharmacokinetic studies (256). Table 8.16 summarizes a number of available HPLC procedures for many of the cephalosporins (239,242,255,300–314). Several clinically important cephalosporin antibiotics are reviewed in this chapter.

Oral cephalosporins (cefaclor, cefadroxil, cephalexin, and cephradine) are widely used antibiotics. Cefixime, a newer member of this class of drugs, offers broader pharmacokinetic properties than older cephalosporin drugs, with enhanced gram-negative activity. Cefixime can be used for the treatment of otitis media, urinary tract infections, and respiratory tract infections (370). Initial HPLC methods were limited to the detection of one or two cephalosporins with the same assay system, and in their ability to measure drug concentrations in clinically significant ranges. Method enhancements including modifications of the mobile phase acqueous/organic ratio enabled multiple cephalosporins to be measured with a single assay system (369). The method outlined below uses a single HPLC system to measure five oral cephalosporins in a clinically significant drug concentration range (311).

Equipment

One Waters HPLC system (Millipore, Waters Division, Milford, MA) consists of a model 590 pump used to deliver the mobile phase and a model 481 variable wavelength detector set at 240 nm. Analysis may be performed using a 4.6-mm × 15-cm Altex Ultrasphere octyl C_8 column (5 μm particles; Beckman Instruments, Berkeley, CA) with a silica RCSS Guard Pak precolumn (Waters, Milford, MA). Linear least squares regression analysis is performed using a laboratory automation system (model 3357; Hewlett-Packard, Paramus, NJ).

Chromatographic Conditions

The mobile phase consists of methanol/12.5 mmol/L monobasic sodium phosphate buffer (20:80 by volume), adjusted to pH 2.6 with concentrated phosphoric acid. The mobile phase is filtered, degassed before use, and delivered at ambient temperature at a flow rate of 2 mL/minute. The order of elution for the five cephalosporins is cefadroxil, cefaclor, cefixime, cephalexin, and cephradine, between the times of 3 and 20 minutes.

Five milligrams of cefixime or 5 mg of cephalexin is dissolved in 10 mL of methanol to yield 500 mg/L stock solutions. Each standard is then serially diluted 10-fold. Working standards for the other drugs are prepared similarly, dissolving 5 mg of each compound (cefadroxil, cefaclor, and cephradine) in 10 mL of methanol to give 500 mg/L stock solutions, which are diluted by 10-fold serial dilutions to yield 50 mg/L and 5 mg/L working standards.

(continued on page 382)

Table 8.16

High-Performance Liquid Chromatography Methods

Author	Antimicrobial Compound Measured	Sample Preparation	Internal Standard	Mobile Phase	Stationary Phase (Reverse-Phase Unless Otherwise Indicated)	Temperature	Derivatization	Detection
Aravind et al. (125)	CAM, CAM-S	Ethyl acetate	5-Ethyl-5-p-toly-barbituric acid	ACN/H$_2$O (15:85)	C$_{18}$ (PE) ODS-HC-SIL-X-1	50°C	None	UV, 280 nm
Weber et al. (364)	CAM, CAM-S	ACN pptn	P-Nitropropionanilide	Methanol/H$_2$O (35:65)	C$_{18}$ μBondapak	RT	None	UV, 280/254 nm
Velagapudi et al. (297)	CAM, CAM-S	Ethyl acetate	Thiamphenicol	ACN/H$_2$O (20:80)	C$_{18}$ μBondapak	RT	None	UV, 278 nm
Brisson and Fourtillian (365)	Cefazolin, cephalothin, cefoxitin, cefotaxime, cefamandole, cefuroxime, cefoperazone	Chloroform/pentanol (3:1)	None	Methanol or ACN	C$_{18}$ μBondapak	RT	None	UV, 240/275 nm
Lecaillon et al. (250)	Cefsulodin, cefotiam, cephalexin, cefotaxime, deacetyl-cefotaxime, cefuroxime, cefroxadine	Methanol/TCA pptn	None, cephalexin or cefroxadine	Methanol/H$_2$O ± TBHS	LiChrosorb RP-8 or RP-18	RT	None	UV, 254 nm
Aravind et al. (359)	Moxalactam	Methanol pptn	8-Chlorotheophylline	Methanol/H$_2$O (4:96)	C$_{18}$(PE) HC-SIL-X	RT	None	UV, 230 nm

(Continued)

Table 8.16 (Continued)

High-Performance Liquid Chromatography Methods

Author	Antimicrobial Compound Measured[a]	Sample Preparation[b]	Internal Standard	Mobile Phase	Stationary Phase (Reverse-Phase Unless Otherwise Indicated)	Temperature[c]	Derivatization	Detection
Brisson and Fourtillan (274)	Piperacillin	Chloroform/pentanol	None	Methanol/H_2O (40:60)	C_{18} μBondapak	40°C	None	UV, 254 nm
Hildebrandt and Gundert-Remy (276)	Aziocillin, meziocillin	Sep-Pak C_{18}	None	ACN/H_2O (27:73)	C_{18} μBondapak	RT	None	UV, 220 nm
Maitra et al. (12)	Gentamicin	Silicic acid column	None	Methanol/H_2O (79:21)	C_{18} μBondapak	RT	Precolumn o-phthalaldehyde	Fluorescence, 36/430 nm
Bawdon and Madsen (319)	Sulbactam	Derivation: imidazole reagent + specimen; extraction: ACN/dichloromethaneprocedure	None	89% 0.1 mol/L phosphate buffer/11% ACN	Beckman ODS-5, stainless steel	RT	Imidazole	UV, 313 nm
LaFollette et al. (288)	Clindamycin	ACN	Triazolam	ACN/H_2O/phosphoric acid/76 mmol/L TMA (30:70:0.2:0.075), pH 6.7	Nova-Pak C_{18}	RT	None	UV, 198 nm
Jones and Chmel (329)	Meziocillin	TBAP	Piperacillin	Methanol/TBAP (25:75)	Econosphere C_{18}	RT	Precolumn	UV, 220 nm

Reference	Drug	Sample preparation	Internal standard	Mobile phase	Column	Temp		Detection
Godbillon et al. (324)	(5R,6S)2-Amino-6-[(1R)-hydroxyethyl]-2-penem-3-carboxylic acid	Serum: ammonium sulfate/phosphate buffer; urine: 25x dilution with phosphate buffer, pH 6.0	(5R,6S)2-Amino-6-[(1R)-hydroxyethyl]-2-penem-3-carboxylic acid	Phosphate buffer, pH 6.0	LiChrosorb RP-8	RT	None	UV, 320 nm
Pilkiewicz et al. (330)	Aztreonam	Serum: ACN; urine: 10x dilution with TBAHSO$_4$, pH 3.0	None	TBAHSO$_4$/ACN (80:20)	C$_{18}$ μBondapak on Corasll	RT	None	UV, 293 nm
Yamamoto et al. (344)	Pyrazinamide + metabolites (2,3-pyrazinedicarboxamide, 5-hydroxypyrazinoic acid, 5-hydroxypyrazinamide, pyrazinoic acid, pyrazinamide)	Perchloric acid	2,3-pyrazine dicarboxamide	KH$_2$PO$_4$	C$_{18}$ μBondapak	RT	None	Fluorescence, 410/365 nm
McAteer et al. (311)	Cefixime, cefaclor, cefadroxil, cephalexin, cephradine	ACN	Cefixime for other four cephalosporins; cephalexin for cefixime	Methanol/K$_2$HPO$_4$ (20:80)	C$_{18}$ Altex Ultrasphere	RT	None	UV, 240 nm
Leeder et al. (309)	Ceftazidime	Serum: methanol; urine: dilution with distilled H$_2$O within concentration range of standards	8-Chlorotheophyllin	Serum: KH$_2$PO$_4$/methanol (82:18); urine: KH$_2$PO$_4$/methanol (88:12)	C$_{18}$ μBondapak	RT	None	UV, 225 nm

(Continued)

Table 8.16 (Continued)

High-Performance Liquid Chromatography Methods

Author	Antimicrobial Compound Measured[a]	Sample Preparation[b]	Internal Standard	Mobile Phase	Stationary Phase (Reverse-Phase Unless Otherwise Indicated)	Temperature[c]	Derivatization	Detection
Barbhaiya et al. (301)	BMY-28142 (cephalosporin)	Plasma: ACN/TCA; urine: 3 × dilution with sodium buffer	Cefadroxil	ACN/octane sulfonic acid (12:88)	C18 Partisil 5 ODS-3RAC	RT	None	UV, 280 nm
			Ceftazidime	Methanol/sodium dodecyl sulfate/TCA/ phosphoric acid/ tetrahydrofuran (49.7:40.4:3.9: 0.7:5.3)				
Granich and Krogstad (308)	Ceftriaxone	Serum: ACN, CSF: ACN; urine; dilution 1:10 with normal saline	Moxalactam	ACN/H₂O (46:54) + ion-pairing agent (hexadecyltrimethyl- ammonium bromide dibasic potassium phosphate)	C18 μBondapak	RT	None	UV, 274 nm
Chan et al. (303)	Cephalothin, cefoxitin, cefaman- dole, cefuroxime, cefotaxime, moxa- lactam, ceftriaxone, ceftazidime	Plasma, serum, CSF, bile, perito- neal fluid, pleural fluid, ascitic fluid: ACN	Ceftazidime	N-Cetyl-N,N,N- trimethyl ammonium bromide, Titrisol/ phosphate buffer, glacial acetic acid/ ACN (350 mL)	LiChrosorb RP-18	RT	None	UV, 240 nm
		Urine, peritoneal dialysis fluid: diluted + ACN	Ceftazidime	As above with 600 mL ACN				

Reference	Drug	Sample preparation	Drug (IS)	Mobile phase	Column	Temperature		Detection
Demotes-Mainaird et al. (280)	Roxithromycin	Plasma, urine: dilution in phosphate buffer/dichloromethane	Erythromycin	ACN/ammonium acetate/methanol (55:23:22), pH 7.5	C$_{18}$ µBondapak	RT	None	Dual coulometric electrodes operated in oxidative screen mode (screen electrode = E1 + 0.7 V; sample electrode = E2 + 0.9 V)
Croteau et al. (279)	Erythromycin + esters (ethylsuccinate, estolate)	Plasma, saliva: diethylether, with residue reconstituted with ACN; urine: K$_2$HPO$_4$/diethylether, with residue reconstituted with ACN	Roxithromycin	Sodium acetate buffer/ACN/methanol (56:50:4), pH 7.0	C$_{18}$ µNovapak	RT	None	Single electrode cell in oxidative mode with amperometric cell potential at +0.9 V
Georgopoulos et al. (44)	Teicoplanin	SAX Bond Elut/Columns	Teicoplanin	Methanol/water (5:95)/n-heptanesulfonate, pH 4.0	LiChrosorb RP-8	30°C	None	UV, 240 nm

CAM-S, CAM succinate; ACN, acetonitrile; pptn, precipitation; TCA, trichloroacetic acid; TBAP, tetrabutylammonium phosphate; TBHS, tetrabutylammonium hydrogen sulfate; TMA, tetramethylammonium chloride; TBAHSO$_4$, tetrabutylammonium hydrogen sulfate; CSF, cerebrospinal fluid; cRT, room temperature; UV, ultraviolet.

Table 8.17

Performance Data for the Antibiotics Studied

Drug	Concentration Range (μg/mL)	Mean Coefficient of Variation (%)		Mean Net Recovery (%)
		Within-Day	Between-Day	
Cefixime	0.1–1	5.8	8.3	81.4
	1–10	4.7	4.2	
Cefaclor	1–20	5.7	6.0	72.6
	10–100	5.2	9.8	
Cefadroxil	1–20	8.8	7.1	90.1
	10–100	11.4	14.2	
Cephalexin	1–20	7.6	7.2	82.3
	10–100	4.0	5.6	
Cephradine	1–20	6.9	7.7	84.2
	10–100	7.3	8.6	

From McAteer JA, Hiltke MF, Silber BM, et al. Liquid-chromatographic determination of five orally active cephalosporins cefixime, cefaclor, cefadroxil, cephalexin, and cephradine in human serum. *Clin Chem* 1987;33:1788–1790.

Aliquots of the working standard solutions are added to polyethylene microcentrifuge tubes to give the desired drug concentrations. The solvent is then evaporated under a stream of nitrogen. The residue is reconstituted with 0.1 mL of serum, a known volume of internal standard (cefixime for the other four compounds, cephalexin for cefixime), and 0.1 mL of acetonitrile to precipitate serum proteins. Samples are vortex-mixed for 15 seconds and centrifuged at $14,000 \times g$ for 2 minutes. The clear supernatant is evaporated under a stream of nitrogen. The residue is reconstituted with 0.1 mL of the mobile phase, and 50 to 80 μL is delivered by a WISP autoinjector (Waters, Milford, MA) into the chromatograph.

Performance

The peak height ratio is linear over the concentration ranges studied (0.1 to 10 mg/L for cefixime and 1 to 100 mg/L for the others). The range for the coefficients of variation for intra- and interday measurements is less than 15%. With the exception of cefaclor, the recovery of each cephalosporin is greater than 81.4% over these concentration ranges. The lower recovery of cefaclor is probably because of its limited solubility in the mobile phase. This becomes a problem only at concentrations of more than 50 mg/L. These drug levels are not normally observed clinically. Other than salicylic acid, which absorbs UV light at 240 nm, commonly administered drugs do not generally interfere with the assay. Moreover, salicylic acid is eluted at 22.1 minutes, not in the same time

frame as any of the cephalosporins. The performance data for the cephalosporin assays are shown in Table 8.17.

By using a single system for all five cephalosporins, this HPLC method allows for monitoring without delays due to changes in equipment (311).

Measurement in Body Fluids Other Than Plasma

HPLC- based methods have also been used to determine achievable levels of a antibiotic in body fluids other than blood. For example, clinical trials of the oral cephalosporin cefditoren, which is currently approved in the United States for treatment of lower respiratory tract infections such as acute exacerbations of chronic bronchitis, community-acquired pneumonia, pharyngitis/tonsillitis, and uncomplicated skin-structure infections, included measurement of levels in urine (316) and lung epithelial lining fluid (315) in addition to plasma.

HPLC for Cefditoren Levels in Urine: Modifications to Equipment and Conditions

This HPLC method (316) specifies Nova-Pack C18, 15 cm × 0.39 mm (Waters Corporation, Milford, USA) as the stationary phase, a mobile phase of 75% 0.05 M disodium hydrogen phosphate dehydrated and 25% acetonitrile, adjusted to pH 7.0 by the addition of orthophosphoric acid, and a pump flow rate at 1.0 mL per minute. For cefditoren, the maximum ultraviolet (UV) absorbance is at a wavelength of 295 nm. The integrator was a Maxima 820 Waters data system.

Urine specimens are prepared by mixing 0.5 mL of each sample with 50 μL of an internal standard (aminopyrine, 0.1 mg per mL) plus 900 μL of water. A 25 μL aliquot of the prepared urine sample is injected onto HPLC for analysis. The retention times of ceftidoren and aminopyrine are 5.5 and 11.9 min, respectively. The reported intra- and interday variability (SD/mean × 100) is less than 9.15% for urine samples containing 10, 50 and 100 μg per mL cefditoren, with a limit of quantification of 10 mg per L for this assay method (316).

Liquid Chromatography-Tandem Mass Spectrometry LC-MS/MS for Cefditoren Levels in Lung Epithelial Lining Fluid (ELF)

This method (315) differs from the HPLC methods described above in that mass spectrometry rather than UV absorbance is used to detect the analyte after chromatographic separation, and in that all pipetting and centrifugation steps are carried out at 4°C.

As described earlier in this chapter, lung ELF samples collected by BAL must be centrifuged immediately after collection to remove cells, and the supernatants frozen and stored at −70°C until testing to maximize drug stability. The BAL samples must be concentrated, for example by freeze-drying, and reconstituted in a smaller volume of distilled water, before processing. For this method, the concentration of the internal marker urea is measured in the BAL sample [CBAL(urea)]and in a simultaneously collected serum or plasma sample [Cserum(urea)] to allow determination of a corrected cefditoren concentration in the lung ELF, according to the formula corrected cefditoren level = CBAL(cefditoren) X [Cserum(urea)/CBAL(urea)].

Procedure

To test for cefditoren, one mL of each reconstituted sample is mixed with 100 μL methanol. A 20 μL aliquot of each sample is chromatographed on a reversed-phase column, eluted with an isocratic (constant concentration rather than a gradient) solvent system, and monitored by liquid chromatography-tandem mass spectrometry (LC-MS/MS) with a selected reaction monitoring (SRM) method, in positive mode, with precursor → product ion for cefditoren, m/z 507 → m/z 241. The precursor → product ion for the internal standard

cefotaxime is m/z 456 → m/z 396. Under these conditions, cefditoren and the internal standard cefotaxime are eluted after approximately 1.2 min.

Calibration and inter-assay variation is assessed by testing samples in a range of concentrations (0.00200 mg per L, 0.0200 mg per L, 0.200 mg per L and 0.800 mg per L) prepared from a standard cefditoren solution in buffer in each run. An additional calibration standard such as cefotaxime prepared in a similar concentrations in buffer should be included. No interferences are noted between cefditoren and cefotaxime in this method. Calibration is performed by weighted (1/concentration) linear regression, and should show linearity between 0.00100 and 0.400 mg per L with quantification limits at the lowest calibration levels. The intra-day precision of the bronchoalveolar fluid assay is reported to ranges between 2.3 and 7.9%, and is 2.3% at 0.800 mg per L, 6.9% at 0.200 mg per L, 7.9% at 0.0200 mg per L, and 5.2% at 0.00200 mg per L. The analytical error of the bronchoalveolar fluid assay ranges from −5.0 to 4.7%, and is 4.7% at 0.800 mg per L, 1.0% at 0.200 mg per L, −3.4% at 0.0200 mg per L, and −5.0% at 0.00200 mg per L.

Calculation of the corrected cefditoren level in BAL requires that the urea concentration be determined. To determine the urea concentration in BAL samples by LC-MS/MS, 100 μl of an internal standard solution in Milli-Q-water and 1 ml gradient grade methanol are added to 1 ml of each human BAL sample, and a 10 μl aliquot of each sample is applied to a reversed-phase column, eluted with an isocratic solvent system, and monitored by LC-MS/MS with an SRM method in positive mode, with precursor to product ion for urea, m/z 157 3 m/z 114, and for the internal standard, m/z 160 3 m/z 115. Urea and the internal standard are eluted after approximately 2.3 min.

As for cefditoren, calibration and inter-assay variation is assessed by testing samples in a range of concentrations prepared from a standard urea solution in buffer and an additional calibration standard such as cefotaxime in each run. No interferences were observed for urea and the internal standard. Calibration by weighted (1/concentration) linear regression showed linearity of the urea calibration curves between 0.208 and 8.00 mg per L, and quantification limits at the lowest calibrator concentrations. The reported range for the inter-day precision and the analytical recovery of the spiked quality control standards is from 0.3 to 0.9%, and is 0.3% at 8.00 mg per L), 0.9% at 1.60 mg per L and 0.3% at 0.400 mg per L, with an analytical error of -1.4% at 8.00 mg per L), 4.2% at 1.60 mg per L, and 8.6% at 0.400 mg per L (315).

Penicillins and Aztreonam

Because new semisynthetic penicillins continue to be developed and require pharmaceutical, pharmacokinetic, and clinical assessment, HPLC has much to offer for this antibiotic group. Additionally, because of possible side effects, particularly those that are dose-related, selected therapeutic monitoring seems reasonable. Table 8.16 summarizes HPLC methods available for the penicillins. Note that some methods are designed for the assessment of pharmaceutical dosage forms but can probably be modified for use with biologic fluids (317–331). Assays for some major clinically useful penicillin and penicillin derivative antibiotics are presented in this chapter.

Aztreonam

Aztreonam is a totally synthetic, monocyclic, β-lactam antibiotic with low toxicity that exhibits specific activity against aerobic gram-negative bacteria and aminoglycoside and cephalosporin-resistant gram-negative organisms. Assays performed by microbiologic methods are lengthy and do not separate metabolites. The following assay describes an ion-pair HPLC method for the quantitative analysis of aztreonam and its metabolites in human and animal serum and urine.

Equipment

Two HPLC systems may be used interchangeably and yield equivalent results. One consists of the following components: two M-6000A solvent delivery pumps, a model 660 solvent gradient programmer and a model U6K injector (all from Waters Associates, Milford, MA), a model LC75 variable-wavelength UV detector set at 293 nm, an autocontroller (Perkin-Elmer, Inc., Welleshey, MA), and a model 3390A printer/plotter/integrator (Hewlett-Packard, Palo Alto, CA). The other HPLC system is a Hewlett-Packard model 1084B HPLC, which is equipped with a built-in variable-wavelength UV detector also set at 293 nm, an autosampler, and a printer/integrator. With both systems, the analysis is performed using the same column system, that is, a Bondapak C_{18} column (inside diameter, 3.9 mm; length, 3.0 cm) and a guard column (inside diameter, 3.9 mm; length, 3.0 cm). The guard column is packed with Bondapak C_{18} on Corasil (Waters, Milford, MA).

Chromatographic Conditions

The mobile phase consists of 0.005 mol/L tetra-butylammonium hydrogen sulfate/0.005 mol/L $(NH_4)_2SO_4$ and acetonitrile (80:20 by volume), adjusted to pH 3.0. The solution is filtered and degassed before HPLC use and is pumped at a flow rate of 2.0 mL/minute.

Procedure

Serum is diluted with an equal volume of acetonitrile and centrifuged for 2 minutes at ambient temperature at $15,000 \times g$. Supernatants are removed, and 50 μL is used for HPLC analysis. Urine samples are diluted 10-fold with 0.005 mol/L tetra-butylammonium hydrogen sulfate, pH 3.0. Fifty microliters of sample is used for analysis.

Standards of aztreonam for serum and urine are dissolved in the mobile phase and prepared at concentrations of 1,000, 500, 200, 100, 50, 20, 10, 5, 1, and 0.5 μg/mL. A standard curve is constructed using peak area versus concentration. Serum standards are prepared over the same concentration ranges as the mobile-phase standards but are diluted with an equal volume of acetonitrile and centrifuged. Supernatants are then used for HPLC analysis. Aztreonam urine standards are made in the same concentration ranges as described. Urine samples are diluted 10-fold with 0.005 mol/L tetrabutylammonium hydrogen sulfate and are analyzed by HPLC under the same conditions as the standards that are dissolved in the mobile phase. Peak areas for aztreonam obtained from the serum standards are plotted on the previously constructed standard curve of aztreonam standards dissolved in the HPLC mobile phase.

Performance

It is possible to analyze urine and serum from all species for aztreonam without encountering interfering peaks. The results are linear for serum and urine over the concentration range of 0.1 mg/mL to 0.5 μg/mL. Recovery of samples is between 96% and 102%, and total analysis time for either specimen type is less than 10 minutes per sample. Use of tetrabutylammonium hydrogen sulfate with acetonitrile and $(NH_4)_2SO_4$ to ion-pair the SO_3 group of aztreonam to the reverse-phase column gives a good retention time, a symmetrical peak shape for aztreonam, and also allows the drug to be separated from biologic fluid components. HPLC agrees well with a microbiologic assay for both sample types. The HPLC method offers the advantages of speed and the ability to separate chemical entities. Only a small sample is required for HPLC analysis (330).

Mezlocillin

Mezlocillin, an acylureidopenicillin, is a semisynthetic penicillin with a broad spectrum of antimicrobial activity against gram-positive and gram-negative organisms, including Enterobacteriaceae, *P. aeruginosa*, and *Bacteroides* spp. Previous assay methods, including HPLC, that have been developed to measure the drug's concentrations have not used internal standards. The following is a description of a reverse-phase, ion-pair, extraction HPLC assay that uses piperacillin as the internal standard.

Chromatographic Conditions

The mobile phase consists of 5 mmol/L of a phosphate buffer, pH 7.0, that contains 5 mmol/L tetrabutylammonium phosphate/acetonitrile (75:25). Fifteen microliters of the reconstituted eluate is injected onto a 250 × 4.5-mm Econosphere C_{18} column (5 μm particle size). Column effluent products are eluted at ambient temperature with the mobile phase at a flow rate of 1.0 mL/minute and are monitored at 220 nm.

Procedure

Solid-phase preparation is used for samples in the following manner: 0.5 mL of serum sample that contains 100 μL of tetrabutylammonium phosphate and 15 μL of piperacillin internal standard (1.0 g/L) are applied to solid-phase extraction columns that have been previously activated by washing with methanol and 5 mmol/L tetrabutylammonium phosphate. The column is then washed with water and dried by aspiration. The drug is eluted with 600 μL of an equivolume solution of chloroform/acetone. The eluate is then evaporated and reconstituted with 100 μL of the mobile phase. The assay is calibrated with drug-free serum spiked with mezlocillin (10 to 300 mg/L).

Performance

The peak area ratio of mezlocillin to the internal standard is linearly related to the mezlocillin concentration. The run-to-run coefficient of variation is less than 5%. Analytical recovery is 67%. There are no known interferences with other antibiotics that have been tested. The use of a solid-phase preparation and an internal standard had made this method unique compared with other HPLC assays for mezlocillin (329).

Carbapenems

Thienamycin, or (5*R*,6*S*)-2-aminomethyl-[(1*R*)-hydroxymethyl]-2-penem-3-carboxylic acid (Ciba-Geigy, Ardsley NY) belongs to a class of β-lactam antibiotics, the carbapenems, of which imipenem, meropenem, ertapenem, and doripenem are now used clinically in the United States. Carbapenems combine, in a single structure, the antimicrobial properties of penicillins and the cephalosporins, and are active against gram positive and gram negative organisms, although activity against *Pseudomonas aeruginosa* varies among member of the class. The following method is an HPLC assay for the determination of (5*R*,6*S*)-2-aminomethyl-6-[(1*R*)-hydroxyethyl]-2-penem-3-carboxylic acid in plasma and urine. It uses the closely related aminoethyl derivative of (5*R*,6*S*)-2-aminomethyl-6-[(1*R*)-hydroxyethyl]-2-penem-3-carboxylic acid as the internal standard.

Equipment

An RP-HPLC system consisting of a Hewlett-Packard (Palo Alto, CA) model 1084B instrument equipped with a variable-volume injector and a variable-wavelength detector that is set at 320 nm may be used. Analysis is performed using a prepacked column (20 cm × 4.6 mm, internal diameter) filled with LiChrosorb RP-8 (10 μM Hewlett-Packard) and a precolumn (1 cm × 4.6 mm, internal diameter) filled with Nucleosil C_{18} (30 μm). For the plasma assay, both columns must be replaced after 120 to 150 injections to prevent a decrease in separation efficiency. Peak areas are given by the integrator/recorder (79 850 A LC terminal), while peak heights are measured manually.

Chromatographic Conditions

The mobile phase consists of a phosphate buffer (8×10^{-3} mol/L Na_2HPO_4/5.9×10^{-3} mol/L KH_2PO_4), pH 6, and is degassed and filtered before use. The mobile phase is delivered at a flow rate of 1 mL/minute at room temperature.

Procedure

Plasma samples are prepared by adding 50 μL of internal standard solution (116.2 mol/L prepared in phosphate buffer, pH 6; 50 μL of phosphate buffer, pH 6; and 250 μL of a saturated solution of ammonium sulfate (53 μg of ammonium sulfate in 72 mL of water) to 250 μL of plasma in a glass tube. The solution is vortex-mixed for 30 seconds and centrifuged at 1,400 × g for 10 minutes. One hundred microliters of supernatant is used for analysis. For urine samples, a 1-mL volume of urine is diluted to 25 mL with phosphate buffer, pH 6. One milliliter of the diluted sample is added to 100 μL of the internal standard solution and 100 μL of phosphate buffer, pH 6, in a glass tube and vortex-mixed for 15 seconds. Thirty microliters of the mixture is used for analysis. For reasons of chemical stability, both samples needed to be injected as soon as possible after preparation.

Solutions of internal standards (116.2 μmol/L) as well as (5R,6S)-2-aminomethyl-6-[(1R)-hydroxyethyl]-2-penem-3-carboxylic acid stock solutions (2.05 mmol/L) are prepared in phosphate buffer, pH 6. Reference solutions are prepared by dilution with the same buffer. Plasma-calibrated samples are prepared by adding 50 μL of reference solution of (5R,6S)-2-aminomethyl-6-[(1R)-hydroxyethyl]-2-penem-3-carboxylic acid to 250 μL of drug-free plasma, and correspond to concentrations ranging from 1.64 to 410 μmol/L. Urine-calibrated samples are prepared by adding 100 μL of reference solutions of (5R,6S)-2-aminomethyl-6-[(1R)-hydroxyethyl]-2-penem-3-carboxylic acid to 1 mL of 25-fold diluted urine. Resulting concentrations range from 41 μmol/L to 1.025 mmol/L.

Performance

(5R,6S)-2-Aminomethyl-6-[(1R)-hydroxyethyl]-2-penem-3-carboxylic acid and the internal standard are well separated from plasma and urine components without any interferences. Calibration graphs for plasma and urine are obtained by plotting the (5R,6S)-2-aminomethyl-6-[(1R)-hydroxyethyl]-2-penem-3-carboxylic acid/internal standard peak area ratio against the concentration of (5R,6S)-2-aminomethyl-6-[(1R)-hydroxyethyl]-2-penem-3-carboxylic acid. Their equations are calculated using weighted linear regression. The coefficients of variation are 3% to 8.6% and recoveries are close to 100%. The method described is suitable for the determination of (5R,6S)-2-aminomethyl-6-[(1R)-hydroxyethyl]-2-penem-3-carboxylic acid in plasma and urine (324).

Measurement in Other Body Fluids, Urine, and Tissues

Reversed-phase HPLC with detection of separated drug by UV or by tandem mass spectrometry has also been used to evaluate the penetration of carbapenem antibiotics into body fluids other than plasma and into muscle and adipose tissue.

HPLC Measurement of Doripenem Penetration into Peritoneal Fluid

Doripenem is a parenteral carbapenem currently approved for treatment of intra-abdominal infections and complicated urinary tract infections including pyelonephritis. Ikawa et al. (333) used the HPLC method that follows to measure the total concentrations of doripenem in serum and peritoneal exudate to determine its peritoneal penetration. Samples were collected following intravenous administration of doripenem to uninfected patients who were undergoing abdominal surgery . To prepare serum or peritoneal exudate for HPLC, a sample (400 μL aliquot) was transferred to an ultrafiltration device (Nanosep 10K; Pall Corporation, Northborough, MA, USA) which was centrifuged at 12000 g for 10 min. A 20 μL aliquot of the filtrate was injected onto a chromatograph.

Chromatography was carried out using a reversed-phase column [XBridge C18 5μm (4.6 × 150 mm); Waters Corporation, Milford, MA, USA] and ultraviolet absorbance was detected at 300 nm. A mixture of 0.1 M sodium acetate buffer (pH 4.6) and acetonitrile (95:5, v/v) was used as a mobile phase at a flow rate of 1 mL per min. The column temperature was 40 C, and the retention time for doripenem was 5.9 min. The method was linear over a concentration range of 0.052100 mg per L and the lower limit of quantification was 0.05 mg per L in both serum and exudate. The precisions in intra- and inter-day assay (n = 6) were within 1.8% and 3.7%, respectively. The accuracies in the intra- and inter-day assay were 99.8% to 105.2% and 99.0% to 102.8%, respectively.

LC−MS/MS for Measurement of Carbapenems in Plasma, Urine and Tissue: Measurement of Doripenem and Its Metabolite, Doripenem-M-1, in Plasma and Urine

Cirillo et al. (332) described several methods based on reverse phase chromatography followed by tandem mass spectrometry (liquid chromatographic-triple quadrupole mass spectrometry [LC-MS/MS]) that were used in pharmacokinetic studies to detect doripenem and its inactive metabolite (doripenem-M-1) in human plasma and urine. Plasma and urine samples were processed at 4°C then stored frozen at −70°C until analyzed.

For the first method, plasma samples underwent solid phase extraction followed by separation with reverse phase chromatography. Chromatographic retention of doripenem was obtained on a Luna C18 column (150 × 4.6 mm; Phenomenex, Torrance, CA) with a mobile phase composed of 70:30 ammonium acetate:methanol. Column effluent was analyzed using the mass spectrometer (Sciex API 365, Concord, Ontario, Canada) equipped with Turbo ion spray in the positive ion mode. The lower limit of quantification for doripenem in plasma and urine was 0.200 μg per mL. For doripenem in plasma, mean accuracy for the quality control samples ranged from104% to 105%, and mean precision ranged from 5% to 6%. For doripenem in urine, mean accuracy for the quality control samples ranged from 103% to 107%, and mean precision ranged from 6% to 8%.

For the second method, 100 μL aliquots of the human plasma samples were prepared for HPLC by protein precipitation. Determination of levels of doripenem and its metabolite in plasma required the use of two different solid state and mobile phase systems. Chromatographic retention of doripenem and internal standards was obtained on an Atlantis HILIC Silica HPLC column (150 × 2.1 mm, 5-μm particle size; Waters, Milford, MA) under isocratic conditions with a mobile phase composed of acetonitrile and 20 mM ammonium formate containing 0.2% formic acid. Chromatographic retention of the metabolite doripenem-M-1 and internal standards was obtained on a Discovery HS F5, Supelco Analytical HPLC column (100 × 2.1 mm, 3-μm particle size; Sigma-Aldrich, St. Louis, MO) under isocratic conditions with a mobile phase composed of acetonitrile and water containing 0.05% formic acid.For both doripenem and doripenem-M-1, column effluent was analyzed by multiple reactions monitoring using the triple quadrupole mass spectrometer (Quattro Micro, Micromass, Waters, Milford, MA) equipped with electrospray in the positive ion mode. The validated linear range for doripenem was 0.100 to 20 μg per mL with the lower limit of quantitation at 0.100 μg per mL. The validated linear range for doripenem-M- 1 was 0.200 to 20 μg per mL with the lower limit of quantitation at 0.200 μg per mL.

For analysis in urine samples, chromatographic retention of doripenem, doripenem-M-1, and the internal standards was obtained on a Restek Allure PFP Propyl HPLC column (50 × 2.1 mm, 5-μm particle size; Bellefonte, Pennsylvania) under gradient conditions, with mobile phase A composed of 5:95 acetonitrile and water containing 0.1%

formic acid and mobile phase B composed of acetonitrile containing 0.1% formic acid. Column effluent was analyzed using the mass spectrometer (Sciex API 5000) equipped with Turbo ion spray in the positive ion mode. The lower limit of quantification for doripenem and doripenem-M-1 in urine was 0.200 μg per mL.

Measurement of Doripenem in Skeletal Muscle and Subcutaneous Tissues

Burian et al (334, with permission) used ultra-HPLC followed by tandem mass spectrometry (UHPLC-MS/MS) to determine doripenem levels in saliva, plasma, and extracellular space fluid of skeletal muscle and subcutaneous adipose tissue. Unbound drug concentrations were determined using The UHPLC-MS/MS system consisted of a Dionex UltiMate 3000 Rapid Separation (Germering, Germany) and an Applied Biosystems MDS Sciex API 4000 (MDS Sciex, Concord, Ontario, Canada) triple quadruple mass spectrometer fitted with an electrospray ionization source. Chromatographic separation was employed using a Waters Acquity CSH C18, 2.1 by 50 mm, 1.7 μm UHPLC column (Dublin, Ireland). The mobile phase consisted of aqueous formic acid (A) (pH 2.80) and acetonitrile (B). Three percent B was increased to 10% within 1.75 min, followed by 95% B for 2.25 min and re-equilibration for 3.70 min. The total run time for each sample was 7.70 min. The flow rate was kept at 0.500 mL per min at a temperature of 23°C. The autosampler was set at 10°C. The retention time of doripenem was 1.49 min +/−2.7%. The MS detection was performed with multiple reaction monitoring (MRM; positive ion mode) for quantification, and settings were optimized for doripenem analysis: nebulizer gas, heater gas, and curtain gas were set at 30, 30, and 40 L per min. Turbo IonSpray voltage was 5,500 V at 550°C. The collision activated dissociation (CAD) flow was used at 4 L per min, and the declustering and entrance potentials were 51 V and 10 V, respectively. The optimized collision energy (CE) for the analyte varied from 21 eV for the quantifier to 23 eV for the qualifier. The dwell time was adjusted to 120 ms per transition. Quantification of doripenem was employed using MRM of the transition m/z 420.9¡274.3 (quantifier), while the qualifier transition was m/z 420.9¡342.1. The Analyst 1.5 software (MDS Sciex,Concord, Ontario, Canada) was used to control the UHPLC-MS/MS system and to perform the measurement. The limit of detection (LOD, signal-to-noise ratio = 3) was

0.005 mg per L, and the limit of quantification (LOQ, signal-to-noise ratio = 10) was 0.025 mg per L.

Measurement of Ertapenem in Plasma and Tissue

A similar method using LC/MS has been developed by Koal et al. for the measurement of ertapenem in human plasma (369). This method also has been used to measure pharmacokinetics of ertapenem in colorectal tissue (340).

Column-Switching Approach for Pretreatment Before HPLC

Incorporation of column-switching before HPLC, which simplifies pretreatment of samples and has the potential for automation and analysis of multiple samples without loss of assay sensitivity or specificity, has been used in methods developed to assay levels of multiple beta-lactam antibiotics (337). The column switching approach is particularly useful for preparation of samples containing antibiotics such as ertapenem that are susceptible to hydrolysis during exposure to acids and solvents, and that can be altered or destroyed during harsh sample pretreatment procedures. During pretreatment, the antibiotic being assayed is concentrated on the head of the extraction column, while endogenous constituents that must be removed from the sample are passed through the column to waste; the exposure to acid is relatively short.

Assays for measurement of ertapenem in plasma and urine have been described that employ column-switching for on-line extraction at a neutral pH prior to reverse-phase HPLC.

The lower limits of quantization for the plasma and urine assays are 0.125 and 2.5, respectively (336,335).For this assay, a plasma sample is centrifuged and then injected onto an extraction column using 25 mM phosphate buffer, pH 6.5. After 3 min, using a column-switching valve, the analyte is back-flushed with 10.5% methanol-phosphate buffer for 3 min onto a Hypersil 5 mm C BDS 10034.6 mm analytical column and then detected by its absorbance at 300 nm. The sample preparation and HPLC conditions for the urine assay are similar, except for a longer analytical column 15034.6 mm. The plasma assay is specific and linear from 0.125 to 50 mg per mL; the urine assay is linear from 1.25 to 100 mg per mL. This assay has been used with minimal modification for detection of ertapenem in blister fluid, to determine its tissue penetration (338)

Further modification of the online extraction using an acidic mobile phase (0.1% formic acid,pH3) and a large injection volume (≥150 μL) has been reported to increase assay sensitivity to a LLOQ of 0.025 μg per mL, enabling its use for determination of ertapenem in cerebrospinal fluid. (339) This assay method is described in detail below (with permission).

Equipment

The HPLC autosampler (7l7plus) and loading pump for column-switching (pump 1, 600E) were from Waters (Milford, MA, USA). The elution pump (pump 2, Series 200 LC Micropump) and the UV-Vis detector (785A) were from Perkin-Elmer (Cupertino, CA, USA). Column-switching was performed by an Autochrom M10 column-switching valve (10-port) purchased from Valco Instruments Company (Houston, TX, USA). On-line extraction was performed using a Maxsil C18 (50 mm × 4.6 mm, 10m) column from Phenomenex (Torrance, CA, USA) and chromatography was performed using a BDS Hypersil C18 (100 mm × 4.6 mm, 5m) HPLC column from Keystone Scientific (Bellefonte, PA, USA). Data were collected, stored, and analyzed using Turbochrom Navigator Client/Server version 6.1 (Perkin-Elmer, Cupertino, CA, USA). An Eppendorf EDOS 5222 (Brinkmann Instruments, Westbury, NY, USA) pipettor was used for sample and standard aliquots.

Chromatorgraphic Conditions

Mobile phase 1 (MP1, 0.1% formic acid) and mobile phase 2 (MP2, ACN/0.1% formic acid, 15:85 (v/v)) were filtered and degassed through a 0.22m Magna R nylon filter (Whatman International, Maidstone, UK). The flow rates for pump 1 and pump 2 were 1.5 and 2.0 mL per min, respectively.

Procedure

CSF samples were thawed and then vortexed. Sample aliquots of 200 μL were mixed with 50 μL of buffer (0.1 M MES buffer, pH 6.5) and transferred to autosampler vials, which were capped, vortexed and stored in a 5°C autosampler until use. Each 150 μL sample was injected onto the extraction column for 3.5 min at a flow rate of 1.5 mL per min with MP 1.After 3.5 min, the analyte was back-flushed off of the extraction column and directed to the analytical column using MP 2, at a flow rate of 2.0 mL per min. At 5 min after injection, the switching valve returned MP 1 through the extraction column for equilibration prior to the next injection. Ertapenem eluted in 7 minutes. The total run time was 10 min.

Performance

The intraday precision and accuracy of this assay for calibration standards (0.025 − 10 μg per mL) and quality control samples (0.1, 0.5 and 2.5 μg per mL) were < 6.2% coefficient of variation and 96.8-104.0% of nominal concentration, respectively).

Sulbactam

Sulbactam, a penicillanic acid sulfone and a competitive and noncompetitive β-lactamase inhibitor, is administered with ampicillin and cefoperazone to expand the drug's antimicrobial spectrum to include β-lactam–resistant organisms. Assays that were described before the following method showed interference from metabolic products and lacked the sensitivity to determine sulbactam concentrations in tissue (368). The assay next presented is an HPLC method that is able to determine sulbactam and cefoperazone concentrations in plasma, urine, and prostate tissue.

Equipment

An RP-HPLC system that consists of a model 510B pump to deliver the mobile phase and a model 481 variable-wavelength detector (Waters Associates, Milford, MA) may be used. The detector settings include a wavelength of 313 nm, 0.05 absorbance units full-scale for plasma, and 0.01 absorbance units full-scale for tissues. The analysis is performed with a Beckman ODS-5 stainless steel column (Beckman Instruments, Fullerton, CA).

Chromatographic Conditions

The mobile phase consists of 89% of a 0.1 mol/L phosphate buffer, pH 6.1/11% acetonitrile. Tetra-butylammonium hydroxide (40%, 2 mL) is added to 1 L of buffer. The buffer is degassed and filtered before use. The mobile phase is delivered at a flow rate of 2.21 mL/minute. The retention time of the sulbactam imidazole derivative is 6.0 minutes.

Procedure

Sample preparation involves a two-step procedure: derivatization and extraction. The derivatization procedure for all three specimen types consists of adding 0.5 mL of an imidazole reagent to 1.0 mL of each specimen and standard. The specimens and standards are then vortex-mixed and stored at 4°C to allow the derivatization process to be completed. Imidazole reagent is prepared by dissolving 8.5 g of imidazole in water, adding 5 N HCl to bring the solution to pH 6.8, and adjusting the volume to 40 mL with water. Specimens are then extracted by using an acetonitrile/dichloromethane procedure. The procedure includes the addition of 2.0 mL of acetonitrile to the specimen test tube to precipitate the plasma proteins, centrifugation at 3,000 × g for 5 minutes, and the decanting of the supernatant into 3.0 mL of dichloromethane. The test tube is mixed and centrifuged. A WISP automated sample processor is used to deliver 15 μL of the upper aqueous layer that contains the sulbactam imidazole derivative.

Prostate tissue is blotted, weighed, diluted with phosphate buffer, pH 6.1, and homogenized. A standard curve for the determination of sulbactam concentrations in pooled plasma is prepared with concentrations ranging from 0 to 100 μg/mL. A standard curve for determination of sulbactam concentrations in prostate tissue is prepared by the addition of 2 to 25 μg of sulbactam per gram to a tissue supernatant. A standard curve for the determination of sulbactam concentrations in normal urine is prepared with concentrations of 0 to 100 μg/mL. No internal standard is added to any sample.

Chromatograms do not contain interfering peaks from body metabolites in plasma, urine, or prostate tissue, or show interference with cefoperazone or other antimicrobial agents (175). The two-step procedure is linear from 100 to 1.0 μg/mL. Extraction efficiency of the sulbactam imidazole derivative is more than 90% for all specimen types. The coefficient of variation for inter- and intrabatch studies for all specimens is generally less than 11.4%. The recovery of sulbactam from urine is more than 50%.

Aminoglycosides

A number of different methods are available for therapeutic monitoring of aminoglycoside levels. Most frequently, aminoglycoside levels in human specimens are obtained with nonisotopic immunoassays. Microbiologic assays, RIA, EMIT, HPLC, and several other assays have been compared for the monitoring of gentamicin concentrations (341,372). RIA, EMIT, FPIA, and HPLC are advantageous in that their results are available within a few hours, compared with 4 to 10 hours for microbiologic assays, depending on the method employed. However, interference from other aminoglycosides should be anticipated when using RIA or EMIT to quantify one of the members of this group. HPLC, although more complex and time-consuming than EMIT and, to a lesser extent, RIA, offers greater specificity than either method. Additionally, it is the only one of these methods that separates the components of gentamicin and other aminoglycosides. Table 8.16 provides information on several HPLC methods that are available to therapeutically monitor the aminoglycosides. If the decision is made to monitor an aminoglycoside by HPLC, the specific method selected will probably depend on the nature of the available equipment and the level of technical expertise within the laboratory (342,343). It has been the authors' opinion that the HPLC method of Marples and Oates (275) deserves initial consideration.

Examples of the major clinically useful aminoglycoside/aminocyclitol antibiotics are presented here. Gentamicin was the first major aminoglycoside to be analyzed by HPLC. Its assay serves as a model for the assay of the other aminoglycosides.

Reagents

A potassium borate buffer (0.4 mol/L) is prepared by the titration of 24.7 g of boric acid into 900 mL of distilled water. The pH is brought to 10.40 with concentrated potassium hydroxide solution. The solution is then diluted to 1 L.

o-Phthaldehyde (OPA) is prepared by dissolving 60 mg of OPA in 1 mL of methanol, followed by the addition of 2-mercaptoethanol (0.2 mL). The solution is gently stirred until complete decolorization occurs. Potassium borate buffer (100 mL) is added, and the mixture is vigorously stirred. The solution is placed in the supply vessel for OPA and flushed several times with nitrogen. It must be used within 2 days of preparation.

Stock gentamicin is prepared at a concentration of 1,000 μg/mL in 0.1 mol/L phosphate buffer, pH 8.0, and stored at −20°C until use. Appropriate dilutions of the stock solutions are made with water. A serum solution that contains 10 μg/mL gentamicin is prepared by the addition of gentamicin standard at 100 μg/mL to serum. Further dilutions from this serum standard are made in normal human serum.

Equipment

A Tracor model 990 pump (Tracor Instruments, Austin, TX) is used to deliver mobile phase. A Schoeffel model 970 fluorometer (Schoeffel Instrument Corp, Westwood, NJ) is used to detect the fluorescence product that is formed by continuous flow, postcolumn derivation with OPA. Fluorescence excitation is at 340 nm and a KV418 filter is used for emission. The photomultiplier voltage is varied between 1,000 and 1,100 V, depending on the sensitivity required. OPA is supplied to a mixing tee from a pressurized glass vessel. A Cheminer fitting (CJ-303 1; Laboratory Data Control, Riviera Beach, FL) is used for the mixing tee, and a delay coil consisting of a Teflon tube (2.0 × 0.6 mm i.d.) is used between the mixing tee and detector. Analysis is performed by using a Bondapak C_8 column (30 cm × 3.9 mm i.d.; Waters Associates, Milford, MA), with a precolumn (4.3 cm × 4.2 mm i.d.) packed with Micropart C_{18} phase-bonded silica gel (5 μm; Applied Science Laboratories, Deerfield, IL). The detector signal is processed and recorded by using a CDS 101 computing integrator (Varian) and a model 7123A recorder (Hewlett-Packard, Palo Alto, CA). Samples are injected using a Valco CV-6-VHPa-C20 injection valve with a 15-μL injection loop modified for variable-volume injection (Glenco Scientific, Houston, TX).

Chromatographic Conditions

Mobile phase compositions are expressed as the ratio of components, by volume, that are added to produce the final solution. No corrections need to be made for volume changes that occur as a result of mixing. Predominantly aqueous mobile phases are degassed before use by vacuum filtration through a Millipore type HA membrane filter (0.45 μm; Millipore Corp, Bedford, MA). Solutions that contain predominantly methanol are filtered through a solvent-resistant type of FH filter (0.5 μm). The mobile phase that is used for analysis contains 0.2 mol/L Na_2SO_4, 0.02 mol/L sodium pentasulfonate, and 0.1% (v/v) acetic acid in a water/methanol (97:3) mixture. The column flow rate is 2 mL/minute at 184 atm. The OPA flow rate is approximately 0.5 mL/minute.

Gentamicin is separated from interfering compounds in serum by ion-exchange gel chromatography. A 1.5-cm column with a bed volume of 1 mL is prepared with CM-Sephadex C-25 using 0.2 mol/L Na_2SO_4 as the initial buffer. Four hundred microliters of serum is applied to this column and eluted with 1 mL and 4 mL of the initial buffer in succession. The eluting buffer

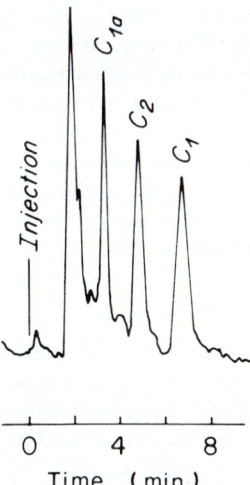

Figure 8.19 ■ HPLC assay of gentamicin compounds. The serum contained 1.0 μg/mL. Each gentamicin compound is distinctly separated and can be assayed. (From Anhalt JP. Assay of gentamicin in serum by high-pressure liquid chromatography. *Antimicrob Agents Chemother* 1977;11:651–655, with permission.)

is changed to 0.01 mol/L NaOH in 0.2 mol/L Na_2SO_4, and 600 μL of this buffer is added to the column. After the column has drained completely, a second volume of alkaline buffer (400 μL) is added and the eluate is collected. Fifteen microliters of this fraction are injected for chromatographic analysis. Figure 8.19 presents the results of a typical assay. The chromatogram of a mixture of C_{1a}, C_2, and C_1 gentamicin, all at 2.5 μg/mL, is pictured.

Teicoplanin

Equipment

The liquid chromatography system is from Kontron with a Uvikon photometric detector (Kontron AG, Eching). The LiChrosorb columns (Sigma-Aldrich, St. Louis, MO) are connected by an eco-tube cartridge system.

Chromatographic Conditions

The mobile phase is methanol/water (5:95, v/v) containing 0.01 mol/L disodium *n*-heptanesulfonate adjusted to pH 14.0 with sodium acetate and acetic acid. The HPLC system is operated at a flow rate of 0.8 mL/minute, a pressure of 59 bar, and a temperature of 30°C.

Procedure

A 1.0-mL plasma sample is extracted by dilution with *n*-heptanesulfonic acid and forced through a SAX Bond-Elut (Agilent Technologies, Inc, Santa Clara, CA) sample cleanup cartridge by vacuum. Plasma constituents are eluted from the cartridge with *n*-heptanesulfonic acid and teicoplanin is eluted with methanol. Detection is performed by measurement of the absorbance at 240 nm.

Performance

The calibration graph is linear in the range of 3 to 50 μg/mL. The detection limit is 0.2 to 0.4 μg/mL (44).

Clindamycin

CLD, synthesized from microbially fermented lincomycin, is an antibiotic that is often used to treat infections with gram-positive and gram-negative anaerobes, as well as gram-positive aerobes. Other analytical procedures, including GC and microbiologic assays, exist for the detection of CLD in biologic fluids. However, the GC assay requires lengthy extraction and derivatization procedures, while the microbiologic assay lacks specificity and is less accurate than HPLC. Both of these assays are time-consuming and labor-intensive. Previously used HPLC assays have been applied only to the analysis of CLD concentrations in sterile fluids or water and have not been used with biologic fluids. The following assay is an excellent HPLC assay for the quantification of CLD in biologic fluids, serum, and plasma.

Equipment

An RP-HPLC system is used that includes a model 510 pump (Waters Associates, Milford, MA) to deliver the mobile phase. A model 783 variable-wavelength UV detector (Spectros, Ramsey, NJ) with a detector wavelength of 198 nm and a filter response time of 0.1 second provides a reproducible, quantifiable peak that corresponds to 0.17 μg/mL. The monochromator of the detector is continuously purged with purified nitrogen to help decrease oxygen quenching and temperature-drift instability. Analysis is performed by using a Nova-Pak C_{18} octadecylsilane column (5 μm, 15 cm × 3.8 mm; Waters, Milford, MA) that has been wrapped in styrofoam to help stabilize the temperature. The detector signal is processed and recorded by using a Pro-840 computer printer (Waters, Milford, MA) for data collection, system operation, and data storage/retrieval.

Chromatographic Conditions

The mobile phase consists of acetonitrile/water/phosphoric acid/7.6 mmol/L trimethylammonium chloride (30:70:0.2:0.75), with a final pH of 6.7. The mobile phase is prepared in 2-L quantities in the following manner. A 600-mL volume of acetonitrile is transferred to a 2-L graduated cylinder. Nanopure (Millipore, Milford, MA) water is then poured into the cylinder until the fluid level reaches the 1,900-mL mark. Four milliliters of phosphoric acid is added along with 15 mL of a previously prepared 10% trimethylammonium chloride solution. Water is added to the 2-L mark and the contents are filtered under vacuum with a 0.45-μm membrane filter. The pH is adjusted to 6.7 with 1 mol/L sodium hydroxide and pumped through the column at a flow rate of 1.0 mL/minute and a pressure of 130 bar. A constant slow bubbling of helium through the mobile phase during operation is required to minimize the amount of oxygen in the system. Retention times for CLD and triazolam average 8 and 11.8 minutes, respectively.

Procedure

Heparinized plasma and serum samples (200 μL) are prepared by protein precipitation with 0.5 mL of acetonitrile that contains the internal standard triazolam (44 ng/100 mL). Samples are vortex-mixed for 20 seconds and centrifuged at 3,000 × g for 10 minutes. The resulting supernatant is poured off the protein pellet and evaporated under nitrogen to a volume of 250 μL. A WISP autoinjector is used to deliver 15 to 30 μL of the concentrated supernatant into the HPLC system. Standards are human plasma samples with the addition of the internal standard triazolam and CLD at 1.5 and 12 μg/mL, respectively.

Performance

Standard curves are constructed using an unweighted least squares ($y = mx + b$) method with the origin as a data point and a floating intercept. All chromatograms must be recalculated with forced baselines, as provided in a special chromatographic software package (Waters Associates, Milford, MA). The use of peak height provides better linearity than peak area when applied over the entire standard curve. Replicate standard curves run over a 36-hour period show no loss of integrity. The ranges for the coefficients of variation for intraday and interday measurement are 2.4% to 5.7%. The recovery range is 96% to 118%, and

there is no degradation of CLD in human plasma stored at −20°C for up to 56 days.

The use of a low-wavelength setting combined with the simple removal of oxygen from critical areas of the system allows for precise measurement of CLD concentrations in human plasma. This HPLC method also has the ability to measure CLD in other biologic fluids. It is fast, simple, and requires no extraction (288).

Roxithromycin

Roxithromycin is a macrolide antibiotic with an antibacterial spectrum of activity similar to that of erythromycin that exhibits enhanced, clinically desirable pharmacokinetic properties. Specifically, plasma levels are more sustained and are higher than for erythromycin, allowing for lower doses and less frequent administration. Previous assays for the macrolides have included microbiologic assays and HPLC using UV absorption fluorescence and electrochemical detection methods. Bioassays are lengthy and are not selective in the presence of active metabolites. HPLC that uses UV detection is limited because of weak macrolide absorbance in the low–UV wavelength range (<235 nm). Thus, large volumes of patient specimens (2 to 3 mL) are required to attain sufficient sensitivity and the weak macrolide absorbance results in increased background noise and large interferences from coextracted samples. The following HPLC assay uses electrochemical detection of roxithromycin in plasma and urine.

Equipment

An RP-HPLC system is used and consists of a solvent delivery pump (type 364.000; Knauer, Berlin, Germany), a manual injector (model U6K; Waters Associates, Milford, MA), and a dual-electrode electrochemical detector (ESA model 5100A; Coulochem Environmental Sciences, Bedford, MA). The electrochemical detector is equipped with a guard cell that has been placed in-line before the injector to electrolyze components of the mobile phase. The model 5010 dual-electrode cell is operated in the oxidative screen mode. The applied cell potential of the screen electrode E1 is set at + 0.7 V and the sample electrode E2 at + 0.9 V. This allows irreversible oxidation of many compounds in plasma and urine at the first electrode (E1) without a decrease in the response for roxithromycin and the internal standard. Analysis is performed using a Bondapak C_{18} reverse-phase column (30 cm × 3.9 mm, internal diameter; 10-μm particle size; Waters Associates, Milford, MA). The detector signal is recorded by an Omniscribe recorder (Houston Instruments, Houston, TX).

Chromatographic Conditions

The mobile phase consists of acetonitrile/83 mmol/L ammonium acetate/methanol (55:23:22 by volume), with the pH adjusted to 7.5 with acetic acid. The pH affects the retention times and oxidation of the macrolides. A pH of 7.5 is optimal. The low ionic strength of the buffer also helps provide adequate conductivity and minimizes background current. Before use, the mobile phase is filtered and pumped at ambient temperature through the column at a flow rate of 1.0 mL/minute. The retention times of roxithromycin and erythromycin base are 9.8 and 7.0 minutes, respectively.

Procedure

Two hundred–microliter aliquots of plasma or diluted urine (diluted 1:2 with isotonic NaCl solution), 100 μL of internal standard (10 μg/mL erythromycin), 600 μL of phosphate buffer, pH 9, and 3 mL of dichloromethane are pipetted into 10-mL glass extraction tubes, which are stoppered and mixed by shaking for 10 minutes. Following centrifugation at 2,000 × g for 5 minutes, the upper layer is discarded and the organic phase (2.5 mL) is evaporated at ambient temperature under a stream of nitrogen. The residue is reconstituted with 50 μL of methanol and vortex-mixed for 10 seconds. A 15-mL aliquot is injected into the HPLC system. Standards are human plasma and urine samples with roxithromycin at concentrations of 1 to 20 μg/mL. The internal standard erythromycin concentration is 10 μg/mL in doubly distilled water.

Chromatograms are recorded at a chart speed of 0.25 cm/minute and peaks are well resolved from endogenous plasma or urine compounds. Peak height ratios of roxithromycin to erythromycin are measured.

Performance

There is a linear relationship between concentration and response up to 25 μg/mL in plasma samples and diluted urine samples. Instrument precision as determined by repeated injection of 500 mg of roxithromycin is 2.3%. The ranges for the coefficients of variation for intraday and interday variation are 1.6% to 5.5% and 2.2% to 7.0%, respectively. The recovery ranges for roxithromycin and erythromycin are $6.82 \pm 1.0\%$ and $78.8 \pm 2.4\%$, respectively,

with no interfering peaks. Roxithromycin does not degrade upon storage at 37°C, 4°C, or −20°C. The use of dual coulometric electrodes that are operated in the oxidative screen mode allow for the rapid and sensitive detection of roxithromycin in small patient samples (280).

Pyrazinamide

Pyrazinamide, an analog of nicotinamide, exhibits antimycobacterial activity when it is administered with other drugs. The drug is well absorbed after oral administration and hydrolyzed and hydroxylated to the following metabolites: 5-hydroxypyrazinamide, pyrazinoic acid, and 5-hydroxypyrazinoic acid. All of these may be important in drug level monitoring to avoid the dose-related adverse effects of hyperuricemia and hepatotoxicity. Earlier assays, including an HPLC method that measures pyrazinamide and its three major metabolites, are time-consuming, tedious, and involve difficult extractions. The following method is rapid and allows simultaneous determination of pyrazinamide and its metabolites.

Equipment

The chromatographic system consists of an LC-6A chromatograph (Shimadzu, Kyoto, Japan) with an RF 530 HPLC fluorescence monitor (Shimadzu, Kyoto, Japan) set at 410/365 nm. Analysis is performed using a 10-μm Bondapak C_{18} column (30 cm × 3.9 mm, internal diameter; Waters Associates, Milford, MA) at a column temperature of 25°C. The signal is recorded using a C-R3A Chromatopac recorder (Shimadzu, Kyoto, Japan).

Chromatographic Conditions

The mobile phase consists of 0.02 mol/L KH_2PO_4, pH 2.56, and is delivered at a flow rate of 2.0 mL/minute. Peaks elute between 2 and 8 minutes in the following order: 2,3-pyrazinedicarboxamide, pyrazinoic acid, and pyrazinamide.

Procedure

A 100-μL aliquot of 2 mol/L perchloric acid is placed in a 5-mL glass tube that contains 0.5 mL of plasma, 0.3 mL of distilled water, and 100 μL of 10 mmol/L 2,3-pyrazinedicarboxamide (as the internal standard) and is thoroughly mixed for 10 seconds. After centrifugation at 1,500 × g for 10 minutes, a 200-μL aliquot of supernatant is neutralized with 48 μL of 1 mol/L sodium hydroxide solution. Sixty microliters of the supernatant is loaded onto the column.

The calibration graph is constructed by using 0.5 mL of drug-free plasma and adding 0.1 mL of a standard solution that contains pyrazinamide, its metabolites, and the internal standard plus 0.3 mL of distilled water to obtain a calibration between 5 and 80 μg/mL for pyrazinamide, between 2.5 and 50 μg/mL for pyrazinoic acid, between 1 and 10 μg/mL for 5-hydroxypyrazinamide, and between 2.5 and 0.25 μg/mL for 5-hydroxypyrazinoic acid. This allows creation of a calibration graph because a small peak of an endogenous compound in plasma overlaps the peak of 5-hydroxypyrazinamide under these chromatographic conditions.

Performance

Peak area versus concentration is linear with standards in aqueous solutions up to 100, 50, 10, 2.5, and 150 μg/mL for pyrazinamide, pyrazinoic acid, 5-hydroxypyrazinamide, 5-hydroxypyrazinoic acid, and 2,3-pyrazine-dicarboxamide, respectively. Detection limits for 5-hydroxypyrazinoic acid, 5-hydroxypyrazinamide, pyrazinoic acid, and pyrazinamide are 3, 3, 30, and 30 ng, respectively, with an apparatus detection limit of 0.45 ng/12 μL cell (344).

Linezolid

Linezolid, a new oxazolidinone antibiotic has broad activity against gram-positive organisms, including MRSA, vancomycin-resistant enterococci, and penicillin-resistant pneumococci. HPLC protocols for the measurement of linezolid levels in serum and other body fluids have been published (345–350). The following is a representative example of an HPLC assay for the measurement of linezolid concentrations in human serum. (345)

Equipment

The stationary phase consists of Hypersil 5ODS, 10 cm × 4.6 mm (Waters Corporation, Milford, MA). A Gina 50 autosampler (Dionex, Macclesfield, United Kingdom) for UV absorbance detection (λ_{max} 254), and the integrator is a Trilab 2000 (Trivector, Sandy, United Kingdom).

Chromatographic Conditions

The mobile phase consists of 1% *ortho*-phosphoric acid (BDH, Analar grade, Poole, United Kingdom), 30% methanol (Prolabs, Fontenay, France), and 2 g/L heptane sulfonic acid (Sigma-Aldrich, St. Louis, MO) adjusted to pH 5 by the addition of

10 M sodium hydroxide. The flow rate is 1.0 mL/min. Retention time for linezolid is 384 seconds.

Procedure

Samples are prepared by mixing aliquots (50:50) of the specimen with acetonitrile (Prolabs Fontenay, France). After mixing, the samples are incubated at room temperate for 10 minutes then centrifuged at 5,000 g for 5 minutes. Twenty microliters of the supernatant is injected.

Performance

The assay has been demonstrated to be reproducible, accurate, and linear at a concentration range from 0.0 to 30 mg/L. Intraday and interday reproducibility were less than 6% and 12.5%, with good correlation between drug concentration and peak for both aqueous and serum samples (r = 0.9999 for both). Linezolid recovery from serum approached 100% for concentrations tested. Accuracy of the assay expressed as percentage error was 4.0 for a 2.5 mg/L sample, 1.3 for an 8 mg/L sample, and 0.0 for an 18 mg/L sample. The lowest LOQ was 0.1 mg/L. No interference from 23 commonly used antimicrobial agents or unknown compounds in linezolid-free patient sera was found. Linezolid was shown to be stable in serum after sample preparation with acetonitrile for 24 hours at room temperature and was stable in serum alone for at least 7 days at room temperature and at 4°C.

GAS-LIQUID CHROMATOGRAPHY

GLC has been used successfully in the past to assay for antibiotics that could be volatilized. With the application of HPLC to virtually all antibiotic classes, the need for GLC analyses has become significantly reduced. The general principle of GLC analysis of antibiotics and an abbreviated assay of one drug, CAM, are presented. The method often includes a step that involves the conversion material to be assayed into a compound of high volatility so that it may be passed through a column in the gaseous phase. The general steps involved in GLC are the following:

1. Extraction of the drug from the serum sample
2. Conversion of the drug to a highly volatile form
3. Separation by GLC
4. Detection by flame ionization electron capture and so on
5. Quantitation of the drug by peak height or peak area

The finding that compounds can be rapidly converted to trimethylsilyl derivatives caused the gas chromatograph to become a tool for clinical laboratories. However, HPLC is the chromatographic technology of choice for the analysis of most antibiotics. The measurement of the concentrations of cephalosporin and (351) spectinomycin (352) antibiotics, CAM (353,354) and its chemically modified analogs (249,355), and the aminoglycosides have been determined using GLC.

Chloramphenicol

Equipment

A model 571 OA gas chromatograph equipped with dual flame ionization detector and a 1 mV model 7123A recorder (Hewlett-Packard, Palo Alto, CA), or the equivalent, is used. Glass columns are 122 cm $\times$ 2 mm (i.d.) (configuration 5) for on-column injection (Hewlett-Packard, Palo Alto, CA), packed with 3% OV-I on 100/120 Gas Chrom Q (Applied Science Laboratory Alltech Associates, Inc, Deerfield, IL). Septa are type HT-9 (high temperature, low speed; Applied Science Laboratory, Deerfield, IL).

The instrument conditions are as follows: injector temperature, 250°C; detector temperature, 300°C; oven temperature, programmed from 190°C to 270°C at 16°C per minute; gas flow rate, 40 mL/minute nitrogen, 250 mL/minute air, and 40 mL/minute hydrogen; and recorder chart speed, 13 mm/minute (Fig. 8.18).

Procedure

Serum (500 µL) is combined in 16 $\times$ 125-mm test tubes (Teflon-lined, screw cap) with 500 µL of a phosphate buffer (1 mol/L, pH 6.8) and 7 mL of ethyl acetate (Nanograde; Mallinckrodt Baker, Phillipsburg, NJ) that contains 21 µg of the internal standard. The tubes are mixed by shaking for 10 minutes in an Eberbach shaker at 350 oscillations/minute and centrifuged at 2,000 rpm in a desktop centrifuge for 10 minutes. The upper (organic) phase is transferred to fresh 16 $\times$ 125-mm tubes and is evaporated under a stream of nitrogen in a water bath at 40°C. Four milliliters of HCl (0.5 mol/L) is added and the tubes are held in an ultrasonic bath for 10 seconds to ensure that the residue completely dissolves. Seven milliliters of hexane is added and the tubes are mixed by shaking for 10 minutes in the Eberbach shaker (Eberbach Corporation, Ann Arbor, MI) and centrifuged for 3 minutes at 2,000 rpm. The upper (organic) phase is transferred into 7-mL screw-capped septum vials and evaporated under a stream of nitrogen in a 40°C water bath. Fifty microliters of Trisil (Pierce Chemical Co, Rockford, IL) is added to the residue and each vial is immediately capped. The vial contents are mixed on a vortex-type mixer and are allowed to stand for 8 minutes at room temperature. Two microliters of sample is injected into the gas chromatograph. One may sialylate the next sample immediately after injection to save time. The results are calculated by the peak height ratio method, using CAM and the acetyl analog of CAM as internal standards.

Standard curves are prepared by analyzing samples of normal serum containing known amounts of CAM. It is convenient to run 10, 20, 40, 60, and 80 µg/mL in normal serum as standards.

THIN-LAYER CHROMATOGRAPHY

TLC has been used in the clinical laboratory for many years to separate high molecular weight, biologically active compounds. Like all forms of chromatography, the unknown may be identified based on a comparison of the mobility of the unknown compound in a defined matrix with the mobility of standards. A TLC method has been developed that first separates antibiotics from a mixture based on their mobilities in the chromatograph and then, using a test strain of indicator organism, quantitates them by their biologic activities.

Tobramycin (Nebramycin Complex)

Apparatus

Thin-layer plates (20 $\times$ 20 cm) are prepared from silica gel G. Glass plates of sizes 20 $\times$ 2 $\times$ 0.03 cm and 16 $\times$ 2 $\times$ 0.3 cm are used for framing the chromatograms.

Reagents

All standard antibiotic solutions are dissolved in distilled water. Two developing solvents are employed: methylethyl ketone (96%)/ethanol (25%)/ammonium hydroxide (1:1:1) and chloroform/methanol (25%)/ammonium hydroxide (1:7:4). Solvent systems are made fresh before use (Table 8.18). Bioautograms are stained with 1% tetrazolium blue and 0.02% tetrazolium violet.

Table 8.18

R_F Values of Closely Related Antibiotics in a Chloroform/Methanol/Ammonium Hydroxide Solvent System

Antibiotic	$R_F \times 100$
Amikacin	6
Gentamicin (C_{1a}, C_1, C_2)	63
Kanamycin A	30
Neamine	37
Neomycin	12
Paromomycin	23
Sisomicin	60
Tobramycin (nebramycin) (2,5; 4,5; 5′)	32, 42, 51

From Pauncz JK, Harsanyi I. Aminoglycoside antibiotics: thin-layer chromatography, bioautographic detection and quantitative assay. *J Chromatogr* 1980;195:251–256.

Bacteria

The test organism used is *B. subtilis* ATCC strain 6633.

Procedure

Silica plates with a Camag or Desaga coater are made 0.25-mm thick, dried at room temperature for 2 days, and used without further pretreatment. Lines are drawn before use to ensure separate, 1.5-cm wide tracks. Tobramycin standard solutions are each diluted to a final content of 0.1 to 0.5 μg of the analyte. Patient specimens are dissolved in distilled water to also cover this range. Chromatography is allowed to proceed for a distance of 15 cm at room temperature. The plate is subsequently air-dried.

For the detection of microbiologic activity, nutrient agar is melted and the *B. subtilis* test organism is added to a final organism concentration of 1×10^8/mL. A 25-mL volume of this medium is poured onto the glass frame in order to cover the silica gel surface uniformly. The agar is covered with a 20×20-cm glass chromatographic plate and incubated for 10 to 16 hours at 37°C.

Interpretation

Quantitative determinations are performed using a calibration graph. The zones of inhibition of the *B. subtilis* test organism are measured with the standards and unknowns, and the concentration

of tobramycin is calculated in the same manner as for the analogous electrophoresis/bioautography procedure.

Performance

The TLC/bioautography method is able to measure as little as 0.1 to 0.3 μg of tobramycin (nebramycin complex). It is able to separate tobramycin into nebramycin 2, 4, 5′, 5, and 6. Furthermore, the TLC/bioautography method is able to differentiate between closely related aminoglycoside antibiotics by their gel mobilities.

The tetrazolium blue solution gives a colorless spot on a deep red background in order to measure the zones of inhibition more efficiently. In addition to tobramycin, the method is able to detect 0.2 μg of gentamicin and 0.1 μg of neomycin, paromomycin, and kanamycin (356). TLC is a useful method for the detection of tetracyclines (357,358).

ION-EXCHANGE CHROMATOGRAPHY OF AMINOGLYCOSIDES

A procedure based on the ion-exchange chromatographic separation of aminoglycosides from human body specimens has been developed for the spectrofluorometric assay of aminoglycosides/aminocyclitol antibiotics. The aminoglycosides are separated by elution from the column with sulfuric acid, followed by fluorometric analysis after derivatization.

Ion-Exchange Assay

Reagents

Reagents for ion-exchange chromatography include 0.1 mol/L sulfuric acid and 0.5 mol/L sulfuric acid. Reagents for the analysis of aminoglycoside concentrations include acetylacetone, formaldehyde (30%), and Britton-Robinson buffer, made by mixing 100 mL of solution 1 (0.2 mol/L phosphoric acid, 0.2 mol/L acetic acid, and 0.2 mol/L boric acid) with 15 mL of 1.0 mol/L sodium hydroxide (359). To 10 mL of the final buffer, which is at pH 2.6, 0.8 mL of acetylacetone and 2.0 mL of formaldehyde are added.

Procedure

The aminoglycosides are analyzed spectrophotometrically with a fluorescent dihydrolutidine derivative that is developed by the condensation of the primary amino group with acetylacetone and formaldehyde under acidic conditions. A 13.9 × 290-mm glass column is packed with 3 mL of Amberlite IRC 50 resin (sodium form). Either human urine (2 mL) or human serum (5 mL) is diluted to 10 mL with distilled water and applied to the column. Twenty milliliters of distilled water are applied to the column and impurities are diluted with 20 mL of 0.1 mol/L sulfuric acid. The aminoglycoside antibiotics are eluted from the column with 20 mL of 0.5 mol/L sulfuric acid. Two milliliters of this eluent is analyzed for the aminoglycoside concentration. The elution rate is approximately 0.5 mL/minute.

Two milliliters of the eluent is added to 2 mL of the analysis reagent and heated at 100°C for 10 minutes. After heating, the aminoglycoside is quantitated by determining its absorbance at an excitation wavelength of 421 nm and an emission wavelength of 488 nm in a 1-cm light path.

Performance

The method should be able to analyze any of the aminoglycoside antibiotics. Tobramycin, neomycin, sisomicin, kanamycin, and amikacin have been quantitated. The method is sensitive to 0.5 μg/mL.

MICELLAR ELECTROKINETIC CHROMATOGRAPHY OF ASPOXICILLIN

Micellar electrokinetic chromatography is a type of capillary zone electrophoresis in which a detergent forms micelles with electrically neutral substances, allowing their separation and detection by UV absorption (360). This method permits the quantitation of penicillin in plasma. Plasma proteins are solubilized by the detergent and thus do not interfere with the assay.

Micellar Method
Reagents

Sodium dodecyl sulfate is dissolved in a buffer of 0.02 mol/L sodium dihydrogen phosphate with 0.02 mol/L sodium tetraborate, passed through a 0.45-μm membrane filter, and degassed by sonication. Standards are dissolved in water to a concentration of 1 mg/mL.

Apparatus

A fused silica capillary tube with dimensions of 650 mm × 50 μm is used as a separation tube. Detection of antibiotic is achieved by on-column UV absorption measurement at 210 nm, using a Uvidec 100-V1 detector (Jasco, Tokyo, Japan) with a time constant of 0.05 second.

Performance

The calibration graph for aspoxicillin is linear in the range of 25 to 300 μg/mL. The detection limit is 1.3 μg/mL. The average recovery is 94% to 104%.

NUCLEAR MAGNETIC RESONANCE SPECTROSCOPY

Nuclear magnetic resonance techniques, while not widely available in the clinical setting, have been investigated for the measurement of antibiotic concentrations. When spinning nuclei in a magnetic field are irradiated by a second perpendicular field, they change their alignment to the new field. The amount of energy required for the transformation is characteristic of the molecule and depends on factors such as electronic configuration and intermolecular interactions. Nuclear magnetic resonance spectroscopy can provide information about the kinetic and structural aspects of the interactions between ligands and macromolecules, such as drugs and receptors. It offers both sensitivity and specific simultaneous identification and quantification of drugs and their metabolites in plasma, serum, and urine. Antibiotics that have been assayed include tetracyclines, penicillins, cephalosporins, and erythromycin (361).

POLAROGRAPHY OF CLAVULANIC ACID

Gonzalez Perez et al. (362) have described a method for the determination of levels of clavulanic acid in the presence of amoxicillin by differential pulse polarography. Clavulanic acid is hydrolyzed in a sulfuric medium to obtain an electroactive product with a reduction peak at 0.75 V. The procedure can detect clavulanic acid in the range of 8 to 2 mol/L.

REFERENCES

1. Fleming A. On a remarkable bacteriolytic element found in tissues and secretions. *Proc R Soc Lond [Biol]* 1922;93: 306–317.

2. Bartlett JG, Chang TW, Gurwith M, et al. Antibiotic-associated pseudomembranous colitis due to toxin-producing clostridia. *N Engl J Med* 1978;298:534.

3. Edberg SC, Chu A. Determining antibiotic levels in the blood. *Am J Med Technol* 1975;41:99–105.

4. Edberg SC, Young LS, Barry AL. Therapeutic drug monitoring: antimicrobial agents. In: *Cumitech 20.* Washington, DC: American Society for Microbiology, 1984:120.

5. Faine S, Knight DC. Rapid microbiological assay of antibiotic in blood and other body fluids. *Lancet* 1968;2: 375–378.

6. Sabath LD, Casey JI, Ruch PA, et al. Rapid microassay of gentamicin, kanamycin, neomycin, streptomycin, and vancomycin in serum or plasma. *J Lab Clin Med* 1971; 78:457–463.

7. Smith DH, Van Otto B, Smith AL. A rapid chemical assay for gentamicin. *N Engl J Med* 1972;286:583–586.

8. Kaye D, Levinson ME, Lebovitz ED. The unpredictability of serum concentrations of gentamicin: pharmacokinetics of gentamicin in patients with normal and abnormal renal function. *J Infect Dis* 1974;130:150–154.

9. Noone P, Parson TMC, Pattison JR, et al. Experience in monitoring gentamicin therapy during treatment of serious gram-negative sepsis. *Br Med J* 1974;1:477–481.

10. Edberg SC. Pharmacokinetics. In: Edberg SC, Berger SA, eds. *Antibiotics and infection.* New York: Churchill Livingstone, 1983:1–15.

11. Line DH, Poole GW, Waterworth PM. Serum streptomycin levels and dizziness. *Tubercle* 1970;51:7681.

12. Maitra SK, Yoshikawa TT, Hansen JL, et al. Serum gentamicin assay by high-performance liquid chromatography. *Clin Chem* 1977;23:2273–2278.

13. Chow AW, Montgomerie JZ, Guze LB. Parenteral clindamycin therapy for severe anaerobic infections. *Arch Intern Med* 1974;134:7882.

14. Fekety R. Vancomycin (symposium on antimicrobial therapy). *Med Clin North Am* 1982;66:175–181.

15. Issell BF, Bodey GP. Mezlocillin for treatment of infections in cancer patients. *Antimicrob Agents Chemother* 1980; 17:1008–1013.

16. Johnson GJ, Rao GHR, White JG. Platelet dysfunction induced by parenteral carbenicillin and ticarcillin. *Am J Pathol* 1978;91:85–106.

17. Black RE, Lau WK, Weinstein RJ, et al. Ototoxicity of amikacin. *Antimicrob Agents Chemother* 1976;9:956–961.

18. Thadepalli H, Rao B. Clinical evaluation of mezlocillin. *Antimicrob Agents Chemother* 1979;16:605–610.

19. Kallner A, Tryding N. Laboratory tests to evaluate drug administration. *Scand J Clin Lab Invest Suppl* 1989; 195:19–21.

20. LeFrock JL, Molavi A, Prince RA. Clindamycin (symposium on antimicrobial therapy). *Med Clin North Am* 1982;66:103–120.

21. Waterworth PM. Which gentamicin assay method is the most practicable? *J Antimicrob Chemother* 1977;3:18.

22. Dahlgren JC, Anderson ET, Hewitt WL. Gentamicin blood levels: a guide to nephrotoxicity. *Antimicrob Agents Chemother* 1975;8:58–62.

23. Daigneault R, Gagne M, Brazeau M. A comparison of two methods of gentamicin assay: an enzymatic procedure and an agar diffusion technique. *J Infect Dis* 1974;130:642–645.

24. Giamerellou H, Zimelis VM, Matulionis DO, et al. Assay of aminoglycoside antibiotics in clinical specimens. *J Infect Dis* 1975;132:399–406.

25. Smith AL, Waitz JA, Smith DH, et al. Comparison of enzymatic microbiological gentamicin assays. *Antimicrob Agents Chemother* 1974;6:316–319.

26. Reeves DS, Bywater MJ. Quality control of serum gentamicin assays: experience of national surveys. *J Antimicrob Chemother* 1975;1:103–116.

27. Melikian V, Wise R, Allum WH. Mezlocillin and gentamicin in the treatment of infections in seriously ill and immunosuppressed patients. *J Antimicrob Chemother* 1981; 7:657–663.

28. Sanders S, Bergan T, Fossberg E. Piperacillin in the treatment of urinary tract infections. *Chemotherapy* 1980;26: 141–144.

29. Phillips I, Warren C, Smith SE. Serum gentamicin assay: a comparison and assessment of different methods. *J Clin Pathol* 1974;27:447–451.

30. Shanson DC, Hince CD. Serum gentamicin assays of 100 clinical serum samples by a rapid 40°C Klebsiella method compared with overnight plate diffusion and acetyltransferase assays. *J Clin Pathol* 1977;30:521–525.

31. Stevens P, Young LS, Hewitt WL. Radioimmunoassay, acetylating radioenzymatic assay, and microbiological assay of gentamicin: a comparative study. *J Lab Clin Med* 1975;86:349–359.

32. Noone P, Pattison JR, Slack RCB. Rapid antibiotic assay. *Lancet* 1973;2:315–316.

33. Carling DC, Idelson BA, Casano AA, et al. Nephrotoxicity associated with cephalothin administration. *Arch Intern Med* 1975;135:797–801.

34. Rouan MC. Antibiotic monitoring in body fluids [review]. *J Chromatogr* 1985;340:361–400.

35. Broughall JM, Pugsley DJ, Reeves DS. Potential pitfall in bioassay of serum-gentamicin. *Lancet* 1975;2:1095.

36. Anders RJ, Lau A, Sharifi R, et al. Comparison of EMIT versus bioassay to evaluate inactivation of tobramycin by piperacillin. *Ther Drug Monit* 1987;9:472–477.

37. Andrews JM, Wise R. A comparison of the homogeneous enzyme immunoassay and polarization fluoroimmunoassay of gentamicin. *J Antimicrob Chemother* 1984;14:509–520.

38. Araj GF, Khattar MA, Thulesius O, et al. Measurements of serum gentamicin concentrations by a biological method, fluorescence polarization immunoassay and enzyme multiplied immunoassay. *Int J Clin Pharmacol Ther Toxicol* 1986;24:542–555.

39. Boyce EG, Lawson LA, Gibson GA, et al. Comparison of gentamicin immunoassays using univariate and multivariate analyses. *Ther Drug Monit* 1989;11:97–104.

40. Cavenaghi L, Corti A, Cassani G. Comparison of the solid phase enzyme receptor assay (SPERA) and the microbiological assay for teicoplanin. *J Hosp Infect* 1986;7(Suppl A): 85–89.

41. Cheng AF, Lam AW, French GL. Comparative evaluation of the Abbott TDX, the Abbott ABA200, and the Syva LAB5000 for assay of serum gentamicin. *J Antimicrob Chemother* 1987;19:127–133.

42. Ehret W, Probst H, Ruckdeschel G. Determination of aztreonam in faeces of human volunteers: comparison of reversed-phase high pressure liquid chromatography and bioassay. *J Antimicrob Chemother* 1987;19:541–549.

43. Lewis AS, Taylor G, Rowe HN, et al. Modified enzyme immunoassays for tobramycin using reduced sample and reagent volumes. *Am J Hosp Pharm* 1987;44:568–571.

44. Georgopoulos A, Czejka MJ, Starzengruber N, et al. High-performance liquid chromatographic determination of teicoplanin in plasma: comparison with a microbiological assay. *J Chromatogr* 1989;494:340–346.

45. Stobberingh EE, Hourben AW, Van Boven CP. Comparison of different tobramycin assays. *Clin Microbiol* 1982; 15:797–801.

46. Toothaker RD, Wright DS, Pachla LA. Recent analytical methods for cephalosporins in biological fluids [review]. *Antimicrob Agents Chemother* 1987;31:1157–1163.

47. Irwin WJ, Hempenstall JM, Li Wan Po A. Controlled-release penicillin complexes: high-performance liquid chromatography and assay. *J Chromatogr* 1984;278:85–96.

48. Kim H, Lin C. High-pressure liquid chromatographic method for determination of SCH 28191 in biological fluids. *Antimicrob Agents Chemother* 1984;25:45–48.

49. Kramer WG, Pickering LK, Culbert S, et al. Mezlocillin pharmacokinetics in pediatric oncology patients. *Antimicrob Agents Chemother* 1984;25:62–64.

50. Mattila J, Mannisto PT, Mantyla R, et al. Comparative pharmacokinetics of metronidazole and tinidazole as influenced by administration route. *Antimicrob Agents Chemother* 1983;23:721–725.

51. Mayhew JW, Fiore C, Murray T, et al. An internally-standardized assay for amphotericin B in tissues and plasma. *J Chromatogr* 1983;274:271–279.

52. McCormick EM, Echols RM, Rosano TG. Liquid chromatographic assay of ceftizoxime in sera of normal and uremic patients. *Antimicrob Agents Chemother* 1984;25: 336–338.

53. Ueda Y, Saita A, Fukuoka Y, et al. Interactions of β-lactam antibiotics and antineoplastic agents. *Antimicrob Agents Chemother* 1983;23:374–378.

54. Forchetti C. High-performance liquid chromatographic procedure for the quantitation of norfloxacin in urine, serum and tissues. *J Chromatogr* 1984;309:177–182.

55. Giese RW. Technical considerations in the use of high-performance liquid chromatography in therapeutic drug monitoring. *Clin Chem* 1983;29:1331–1343.

56. Knoller J, Konig W, Schonfeld W, et al. Application of high-performance liquid chromatography of some antibiotics in clinical microbiology. *J Chromatogr* 1988;427: 257–267.

57. Gravallese DA, Musson DG, Pauliukonis LT, et al. Determination of imipenem (N-formimidoyl thienamycin) in human plasma and urine by high-performance liquid chromatography: comparison with microbiological methodology and stability. *J Chromatogr* 1984;310:71–84.

58. Schwartz JG, Casto DT, Ayo S, et al. A commercial enzyme immunoassay method (EMIT) compared with liquid chromatography and bioassay methods for measurement of chloramphenicol. *Clin Chem* 1988;34:1872–1875.

59. Spencer RD, Toledo FB, William BT, et al. Design, construction, and two applications for an automated flow-cell polarization fluorometer with digital readout. *Clin Chem* 1973;19:838–844.

60. Svinarov DA, Dotchev DC. Simultaneous liquid-chromatographic determination of some bronchodilators, anticonvulsants, chloramphenicol, and hypnotic agents, with Chromosorb P columns used for sample preparation. *Clin Chem* 1989;35:1615–1618.

61. Jones SM, Blazevic DJ, Balfour HH. Stability of gentamicin in serum. *Antimicrob Agents Chemother* 1976;10:866–867.

62. Ulitzur S, Goldberg I. Sensitive, rapid and specific bioassay for the determination of antilipogenic compounds. *Antimicrob Agents Chemother* 1977;12:308–313.

63. Raahave D. Paper disc-agar diffusion assay of penicillin in the presence of streptomycin. *Antimicrob Agents Chemother* 1974;6:603–635.

64. Wagner JG. *Fundamentals of clinical pharmacokinetics.* Hamilton, IL: Drug Intelligence Publications, 1975.

65. Baer DM, Paulson RA. The effect of hyperlipidemia on therapeutic drug assays. *Ther Drug Monit* 1987;9:72–77.

66. Heimdahl A, Cars O, Hedberg M, et al. A micromethod for determination of antimicrobial agents in bone. *Drugs Exp Clin Res* 1988;14:649–654.

67. Raeburn JA. A method for studying antibiotic concentration in inflammatory exudate. *J Clin Pathol* 1972;24: 633–635.

68. Wade JD, Schimpff SC, Newman KA, et al. Potential of mezlocillin as empiric single-agent therapy in febrile granulocytopenic cancer patients. *Antimicrob Agents Chemother* 1980;18:299–306.

69. Barza M, Brusch J, Bergeron MG, et al. Penetration of antibiotics into fibrin loci in vivo. *J Infect Dis* 1974;129:73–78.

70. Deacon S. Assay of gentamicin in cerebrospinal fluid. *J Clin Pathol* 1976;29:749–751.

71. Harrison LI, Schuppan D, Rohlfing SR, et al. Determination of flumequine and a hydroxy metabolite in biological fluids by high-pressure liquid chromatographic, fluorometric, and microbiologial methods. *Antimicrob Agents Chemother* 1984;25:301–305.

72. Williamson J, Russel F, Doig WM, et al. Estimation of sodium fusidate levels in human serum, aqueous humor, and vitreous body. *Br J Ophthalmol* 1970;54:126–130.

73. Boylon JC, Simmons JL, Winchly GL. Stability of frozen solutions of sodium cephalothin and cephaloridine. *Am J Hosp Pharm* 1972;29:687–689.

74. Berti MA, Maccari M. Stability of frozen plasma containing different antibiotics. *Antimicrob Agents Chemother* 1975; 8:633–637.

75. Wells P, Robbins E, Cowley R, et al. Comparative analysis of two rapid automated methods and a semi-automated version of the urease method for determining aminoglycoside concentrations in serum. *J Clin Microbiol* 1987;25:1583–1586.

76. White LO, Edwards R, Holt HA, et al. The in vitro degradation at 37°C of vancomycin in serum, CAPD fluid and phosphate-buffered saline. *J Antimicrob Chemother* 1988;22:739–745.

77. Rake G, McKree CM, Jones H. A rapid test for the activity of certain antibiotic substances. *Proc Soc Exp Biol Med* 1942;51:273–274.

78. Garrod LP, Lambert HP, O'Grady F. *Antibiotics and chemotherapy.* Edinburgh, United Kingdom: Churchill Livingstone, 1973.

79. Kavanaugh F. *Analytical microbiology.* New York: Academic Press, 1972:11.

80. Foglesong A, Kavanagh F, Dietz JV. Possibility for error in FDA diffusion assays. *J Pharm Sci* 1978;68:797–798.

81. Grove DC, Randall WA. *Assay methods of antibiotics: a laboratory manual.* New York: Medical Encyclopedia, 1955.

82. Warren E, Snyder RJ, Washington JA. Four-hour microbiological assay of gentamicin in serum. *Antimicrob Agents Chemother* 1972;1:46–48.

83. Noone P, Pattison JR, Slack RB. Assay of gentamicin. *Lancet* 1973;1:49–50.

84. Liberman DF, Fitzgerald J, Robertson RG. Rapid disk test for determining clindamycin serum levels. *Antimicrob Agents Chemother* 1974;5:458–461.

85. Yamada Y, Sasaki J, Matsuzaki T, et al. Influence of medium and diluent pH and diffusion time on antibiotic bioassay. *Exp Clin Med* 1981;6:23–33.

86. Kohlstaedt KG. Propionyl erythromycin ester lauryl sulfate and jaundice. *JAMA* 1961;178:89–90.

87. Wilson C, Greenhood G, Remmington JS, et al. Neutropenia after consecutive treatment courses with nafcillin and piperacillin. *Lancet* 1979;1:1150.

88. Winston DJ, Murphy W, Young LW. Pipercillin therapy for serious bacterial infections. *Am J Med* 1980;69:225–261.

89. Arret B, Johnson DP, Kirshbarum A. Outline of details for microbiological assays of antibiotics: second revision. *J Pharm Sci* 1971;60:1689–1694.

90. Jarvis JD, Leung TWC. Some factors influencing the assay of gentamicin. In: Williams JD, Geddes AM, eds. *Chemotherapy*. Vol 2. New York: Plenum Press, 1975:143–146.

91. Shanson DC, Hince CJ, Daniels JV. Rapid microbiological assay of tobramycin. *J Infect Dis* 1976;134(Suppl):104–109.

92. Shanson DC, Hince C, Daniels JV. Assay of gentamicin and tobramycin by a reliable 2 1/2-hour Klebsiella plate method. In: Williams JD, Geddes AM, eds. *Chemotherapy*. Vol 2. New York: Plenum Press, 1975:147–153.

93. Sabath LD, Casey JI, Ruch PA, et al. Rapid microassay for circulating nephrotoxic antibiotics. *Antimicrob Agents Chemother* 1970;1969:83–89.

94. Bennett JV, Brodie JL, Benner EJ, et al. Simplified, accurate method for antibiotic assay of clinical specimens. *Appl Microbiol* 1966;14:170–177.

95. Arret B, Eckert J. New developments in antibiotic interference. *J Pharm Sci* 1968;57:871–878.

96. Lightbrown JW. Assay of individual antibiotics in drug combinations. In: PJ Watt, ed. *The control of chemotherapy*. London: E & S Livingstone, 1970:19.

97. Kabay A. Rapid quantitative microbiological assay of antibiotics and chemical preservatives of nonantibiotic nature. *Appl Microbiol* 1971;22:752–755.

98. Kondo S. Punch hole method, a new technique of antibiotic concentration bio-assay: a preliminary report. *Bull Osaka Med Sch* 1973;19:132–135.

99. Sabath LD, Toftegaard I. Rapid microassays for clindamycin and gentamicin when present together and the effect of pH and of each on the antibacterial activity of the other. *Antimicrob Agents Chemother* 1974;6:54–59.

100. Winters RE, Litwack KD, Hewitt WL. Relation between dose and levels of gentamicin in blood. *J Infect Dis* 1971;124:S90–S95.

101. Oden EM, Stander H, Weinstein MJ. Microbiological assay of gentamicin. *Antimicrob Agents Chemother* 1963;8:13–19.

102. Stroy SA. Modified microbiological assay for rapid estimation of antibiotic concentration in human sera. *Appl Microbiol* 1969;18:31–34.

103. Peromet M, Schoutens E, Vanderlinden MP, et al. Specific assay of gentamicin in the presence of penicillins and cephalosporins. *Chemotherapy* 1974;20:15.

104. Wagner JC, Novak E, Patel NC, et al. Absorption, excretion and half-life of clindamycin in normal adult males. *Am J Med Sci* 1968;256:25–37.

105. Joslyn DA, Galbraith M. A turbidimetric method for the assay of antibiotics. *J Bacteriol* 1950;59:711–716.

106. Levison ME. Microbiological agar diffusion assay for metronidazole concentrations in serum. *Antimicrob Agents Chemother* 1974;5:466–468.

107. Ralph ED, Clarke JT, Libke RD, et al. Pharmacokinetics of metronidazole as determined by bioassay. *Antimicrob Agents Chemother* 1974;6:691–696.

108. Marengo PB, Wilkins J, Overturf GD. Rapid specific microbiological assay for amikacin (BB-KB). *Antimicrob Agents Chemother* 1974;6:498–500.

109. Hanka LJ, Barnett MS. Microbiological assays and bioautography of maytansine and its homologues. *Antimicrob Agents Chemother* 1974;6:651–652.

110. Hanka LJ, Gerpheide SA, Spieles PR, et al. Improved methods for production, isolation, and assay of two new chloroisoxazoline amino acid antitumor antimetabolites: U-42,126 and U-43,795. *Antimicrob Agents Chemother* 1975;7:807–810.

111. Holmes RK, Sanford JP. Enzymatic assay for gentamicin and related aminoglycoside antibiotics. *J Infect Dis* 1974;129:519–527.

112. Mahon WA, Feldman RI, Scherr GH. Hemagglutination inhibition assay of gentamicin. *Antimicrob Agents Chemother* 1977;11:359–361.

113. Cosgrove RF. Rapid microbiological assay for chlorhydroxyquinoline that uses a cryogenically stored inoculum. *Antimicrob Agents Chemother* 1977;11:848–851.

114. Edberg SC, Chu A, Melnick G. Preparation of organisms for determining antibiotic concentrations from the blood. *Lab Med* 1973;4:36–37.

115. Fernandes PB, Ramer N, Rode RA, et al. Bioassay for A-56268 (TE-031) and identification of its major metabolite, 14-hydroxy-6-O-methyl erythromycin. *Eur J Clin Microbiol Infect Dis* 1988;7:73–76.

116. Lund ME, Blazevic DJ, Matsen JM. Rapid gentamicin bioassay using a multiple-antibiotic resistant strain of *Klebsiella pneumoniae*. *Antimicrob Agents Chemother* 1973;4:569–573.

117. Gentry LO, Jemsek JG, Natelson EA. Effects of sodium piperacillin on platelet function in normal volunteers. *Antimicrob Agents Chemother* 1981;19:532–533.

118. Jorgensen JH, Lee JC. Rapid bioassay for clindamycin alone in the presence of aminoglycoside antibiotics. *J Infect Dis* 1977;136:422–427.

119. Evrin FR, Bullock WE. Simple assay for clindamycin in the presence of aminoglycosides. *Antimicrob Agents Chemother* 1974;6:831–835.

120. Stevens P, Young LS. Simple method for elimination of aminoglycosides from serum to permit bioassay of other antimicrobial agents. *Antimicrob Agents Chemother* 1977;12:286–287.

121. Edberg SC, Bottenbley CJ, Singer JM. The mechanism of inhibition of aminoglycoside and polymyxin class antibiotics by polyanionic detergents. *Proc Soc Exp Biol Med* 1976;153:49–51.

122. Edberg SC, Bottenbley CJ, Gam K. Use of sodium polyanethol sulfonate to selectively inhibit aminoglycoside and polymyxin antibiotics in a rapid blood level antibiotic assay. *Antimicrob Agents Chemother* 1976;9:414–417.

123. Davidson AG, Stenlake JB. The spectrophotometric determination of ampicillin and cloxacillin in combined injections. *Analyst* 1974;99:476–481.

124. Alture-Werber E, Lowe L. A method for the routine determination of streptomycin levels in body fluids. *Proc Soc Exp Biol Med* 1946;63:277–280.

125. Aravind MD, Miceli JN, Kauffman RE, et al. Simultaneous measurement of chloramphenicol and chloramphenicol succinate by high-performance liquid chromatography. *J Chromatogr* 1980;221:176–181.

126. Edberg SC, Mishkin A. Turbidimetric determination of blood aminoglycoside levels by growth curve analysis. *J Pharm Sci* 1981;69:1442–1443.

127. Sande MA, Kaye D. Evaluation of methods for determining antibacterial activity of serum and urine after colistimethate injection. *Clin Pharmacol Ther* 1970;11:873–882.

128. Duda E, Marton L, Kiss G. Modification of the thiobarbituric acid assay of streptomycin. *Biochem Med* 1976; 15:330–332.

129. Ulitzur S. Determination of antibiotic activities with the aid of luminous bacteria. *Methods Enzymol* 1986;133: 275–284.

130. Schlichter JG, McLean H. Method of determining effective therapeutic level in treatment of subacute bacterial endocarditis with penicillin: preliminary report. *Am Heart J* 1947;34:209–211.

131. Schlichter JG, MacLean H, Milzer A. Effective penicillin therapy in subacute bacterial endocarditis and other chronic infections. *Am J Med Sci* 1949;217:600–608.

132. Fisher AM. A method for the determination of antibacterial potency of serum during therapy of acute infections: a preliminary report. *Bull Johns Hopkins Hosp* 1952;90:313–320.

133. Stratton CW, Reller LB. Serum dilution test for bactericidal activity: selection of a physiologic diluent. *J Infect Dis* 1977;136:187–195.

134. Barry AL, Sabath LD. Special tests: bactericidal activity and activity of antimicrobics in combination. In: Lenette EH, Spaulding EH, Truant JP, eds. *Manual of clinical microbiology*. 2nd ed. Washington, DC: American Society for Microbiology, 1974:431–435.

135. Rahal JJ Jr, Chan YK, Johnson G. Relationship of staphylococcal tolerance, teichoic acid antibody, and serum bactericidal activity to therapeutic outcome in *Staphylococcus aureus* bacteremia. *Am J Med* 1986;81:43–52.

136. Standiford HC, Tatem BA. Technical aspects and clinical correlations of the serum bactericidal test [review]. *Eur J Clin Microbiol* 1986;5:79–87.

137. Ace LN, Jaffe JM. Modified fluorometric assay for minocycline. *Biochem Med* 1975;12:401–402.

138. Williams JW, Langer JS, Northrop DB. A spectrophotometric assay for gentamicin. *J Antibiot* 1975;27: 982–987.

139. Durr A, Schatzmann HJ. A simple fluorometric assay for ampicillin in serum. *Experientia* 1975;31:503–504.

140. Fowler W, Khan MH. Mezlocillin in gonorrhea: a pilot study. *Curr Med Res Opin* 1979;5:790–792.

141. Davidson DF. A simple chemical method for the assay of amoxicillin in serum and urine. *Clin Chim Acta* 1976;69:67–71.

142. Shaikah K, Talati PG, Gang DM. Spectrophotometric method for the estimation of 6-aminopenicillinic acid. *Antimicrob Agents Chemother* 1973;3:194–197.

143. Harber MJ, Asscher AW. A new assay technique for antibiotics. In: Williams JD, Geddes AM, eds. *Chemotherapy*. Vol 2. New York: Plenum Press, 1975:125–131.

144. Schwartz DW, Koechlin BA, Weinfeld RE. Spectrofluorimetric method for the determination of trimethoprim in body fluids. *Chemotherapy* 1969;14(Suppl):22–29.

145. O'Gorman Hughes DW, Diamond LK. Chloramphenicol: simple chemical estimations in patients receiving multiple antibiotics. *Science* 1964;144:296–297.

146. Kalina M, Plapinger RE, Hoshino Y, et al. Nonosmiophilic tetrazolium salts that yield osmiophilic, lipophobic formazans for ultrastructural localization of dehydrogenase activity. *J Histochem Cytochem* 1972;20:685–695.

147. Morris HC, Miller J, Campbell RS, et al. A rapid enzymatic method for the determination of chloramphenicol in serum. *J Antimicrob Chemother* 1988;22: 935–944.

148. Dalbey M, Gano C, Izutsu A, et al. Quantitative chloramphenicol determination by homogeneous enzymeimmunoassay. *Clin Chem* 1985;31:933.

149. Benveniste R, Davies J. R-factor mediated gentamicin resistance: a new enzyme which modifies aminoglycoside antibiotics. *FEBS Lett* 1971;14:293–296.

150. Davies J, Brzezinska M, Benveniste R. R factors: biochemical mechanisms of resistance to aminoglycoside antibiotics. *Ann NY Acad Sci* 1971;182:226–233.

151. Heppel LA. Selective release of enzymes from bacteria. *Science* 1967;156:1541–1555.

152. Nossel NG, Heppel LA. The release of enzymes by osmotic shock from *Escherichia coli* in exponential phase. *J Biol Chem* 1966;241:3055–3062.

153. Broughall JM, Reeves DS. The acetyltransferase enzyme method for the assay of serum gentamicin concentrations and a comparison with other methods. *J Clin Pathol* 1975;28:140–145.

154. Forrey AW, Blair A, O'Neill M, et al. Enzymatic assay for gentamicin. *N Engl J Med* 1973;288:108.

155. Shaw WV. Comparative enzymology of chloramphenicol resistance. *Ann NY Acad Sci* 1971;182:234–242.

156. Shannon KP, Philips I. The use of aminoglycoside 2-N-acetyltransferase for the assay of gentamicin in serum, plasma and urine. *J Antimicrob Chemother* 1977;3: 25–33.

157. Smith AL, Smith DH. Gentamicin:adenine mononucleotide transferase: partial purification, characterization and use in the clinical quantitation of gentamicin. *J Infect Dis* 1974;129:391–401.

158. Smith AL, Smith DH. Improved enzymatic assay of chloramphenicol. *Clin Chem* 1978;24:1452–1457.

159. Butcher RH. Rapid serum gentamicin assay by enzymatic adenylation. *Am J Clin Pathol* 1977;68:566–569.

160. Tilton RC, Murphy JR, Mallet E. Assay for gentamicin. *N Engl J Med* 1972;287:1100.

161. Undenfriend S. *Fluorescence assay in biology and medicine*. New York: Academic Press, 1962.

162. Jusko WJ. Fluorometric analysis of ampicillin in biological fluids. *J Pharm Sci* 1971;60:728–732.

163. Barbhaiya RH, Turner P, Shaw E. A simple rapid fluorimetric assay of amoxicillin in plasma. *Clin Chim Acta* 1977;77:373–377.

164. Murthy VV, Goswami SL. A modified fluorimetric procedure for the rapid estimation of oxytetracycline in blood. *J Clin Pathol* 1973;22:548–550.

165. Hall D. Fluorimetric assay of tetracycline mixtures in plasma. In: Williams JD, Geddes AM, eds. *Chemotherapy*. Vol 2. New York: Plenum Press, 1975:111–114.

166. Lever M. Improved fluorometric determination of tetracyclines. *Biochem Med* 1972;6:216–222.

167. Jonsson S. Immunochemical study of the structural specificity of an antigentamicin antiserum, useful also for radioimmunoassay of sisomycin. In: Williams JD, Geddes AM, eds. *Chemotherapy*. Vol 2. New York: Plenum Press, 1975:165–168.

168. Broughton A. Monitoring antibiotic levels in body fluids. *Lab Manage* 1977;12:10–12.

169. Broughton A, Strong JE. Radioimmunoassay of antibiotics and chemotherapeutic agents. *Clin Chem* 1976; 22:726–732.

170. Broughton A, Strong JE, Pickering LK, et al. Radioimmunoassay of iodinated tobramycin. *Antimicrob Agents Chemother* 1976;10:652–656.

171. Robard D, Bridson W, Rayford PL. Rapid calculation of radioimmunoassay results. *J Lab Clin Med* 1969;74: 770–781.

172. Engvall E, Perlman P. Enzyme-linked immunosorbent assay, ELISA. *J Immunol* 1972;109:129–135.

173. Engvall E, Perlmann P. Enzyme-linked immunosorbent assay (ELISA): quantitative assay of immunoglobulin G. *Immunochemistry* 1971;8:871–874.

174. Murachi T. Knowledge reactions. In: Ishikawa E, Kawai T, Miyai K, eds. *Enzyme immunology*. New York: Igaku-Shoin, 1981:513.

175. Beezer AE, Miles RJ, Shaw EJ, et al. Antibiotic bioassay by flow microcalorimetry. *Experientia* 1980;36: 1051–1052.

176. Lu-Steffes M, Pittluck GW, Jolley ME, et al. Fluorescence polarization immunoassay. IV. Determination of phenytoin and phenobarbital in human serum and plasma. *Clin Chem* 1982;28:2278–2282.

177. Mattiasson B, Svensson K, Borrebaeck C, et al. Nonequilibrium enzyme immunoassay of gentamicin. *Clin Chem* 1978;24:1770–1773.

178. Kitagawa T, Kanamaru T, Wakamatsu H, et al. A new method for preparation of an antiserum to penicillin and its application for novel enzyme immunoassay of penicillin. *J Biochem* 1978;84:491–494.

179. Corti A, Cavenaghi L, Giani E, et al. A receptor-antibody sandwich assay for teicoplanin. *Clin Chem* 1987;33:1615–1618.

180. Corti A, Rurali C, Borghi A, et al. Solid-phase enzyme-receptor assay (SPERA): a competitive-binding assay for glycopeptide antibiotics of the vancomycin class. *Clin Chem* 1985;31:1606–1610.

181. Patton KR, Beg A, Felmingham D, et al. Determination of teicoplanin concentration in serum using a bioassay technique. *Drugs Exp Clin Res* 1987;13:547–550.

182. Shaw EJ. Immunoassays for antibiotics. *J Antimicrob Chemother* 1979;5:625–634.

183. Shaw EJ, Amina-Watson RA, Landon J, et al. Estimation of serum gentamicin by quenching fluoroimmunoassay. *J Clin Pathol* 1977;30:526–531.

184. Shaw EJ, Watson RAA, Smith DS. Continuous flow fluoroimmunoassay of serum gentamicin, with automatic sample blank correction. *Clin Chem* 1979;75:322–324.

185. Amina Watson RA, Landon J, Shaw EJ, et al. Polarization fluoroimmunoassay of gentamicin. *Clin Chim Acta* 1976;73:51–55.

186. Mahon WA, Ezer J, Wilson TW. Radioimmunoassay for measurement of gentamicin in blood. *Antimicrob Agents Chemother* 1973;3:585–589.

187. Khabbaz RF, Standiford HC, Bernstein D, et al. Measurement of amikacin in serum by a latex agglutination inhibition test. *J Clin Microbiol* 1985;22:669–701.

188. Bastiani RJ. The EMIT system: a commercially successful innovation. *Antibiot Chemother* 1979;26:89–97.

189. Voller A, Bidwell DE, Bartlett A. Enzyme immunoassays in diagnostic medicine. *Bull WHO* 1976;53:55–65.

190. Munro AJ, Landon J, Shaw EJ. The basis of immunoassays for antibiotics. *J Antimicrob Chemother* 1982;9:423–432.

191. Berry DJ. Chloramphenicol assay by EMIT [letter]. *J Antimicrob Chemother* 1988;21:684–685.

192. Warren C, Phillips I. A comparison of the homogeneous enzyme immunoassay (EMIT) autocarousel and quantitative single test (QST) systems with the radioenzymatic assay. *J Antimicrob Chemother* 1986;17:255–262.

193. Bolton AE, Hunter WM. The labelling of proteins to high specific radioactivities by conjugation to a 125I-containing acylating agent. *Biochem J* 1973;133:529–539.

194. Yeo KT, Traverse W, Horowitz GL. Clinical performance of the EMIT vancomycin assay. *Clin Chem* 1989;35: 1504–1507.

195. De Louvois J. A rapid method of assaying gentamicin and kanamycin concentrations in serum. *J Med Microbiol* 1974;7:11–16.

196. Kurta MJ, Billings M, Koh T, et al. Inexpensive double-antibody fluoroimmunoassay for aminoglycoside antibiotics, phenytoin, and theophylline in serum. *Clin Chem* 1983;29:1015–1019.

197. Thompson SG, Burd JF. Substrate-labeled fluorescent immunoassay for amikacin in human serum. *Antimicrob Agents Chemother* 1980;18:264–268.

198. Place JD, Thompson SG, Clements HM, et al. Gentamicin substrate-labeled fluorescent immunoassay containing monoclonal antibody. *Antimicrob Agents Chemother* 1983;24:246–251.

199. Filburn BH, Shull VH, Tempera YM, et al. Evaluation of an automated fluorescence polarization immunoassay for vancomycin. *Antimicrob Agents Chemother* 1983;24:216–220.

200. Dandliker WB, Kelly RJ, Dandliker J. Fluorescence polarization immunoassay: theory and experimental method. *Immunochemistry* 1973;10:219–227.

201. Blecka LJ. Fluorescence polarization immunoassay: a review of methodology and applications. *Ther Drug Monit* 1983;March:16.

202. Evenson M. Spectrophotmetric techniques. In: Burtis C, Ashwood E, eds. *Teitz textbook of clinical chemistry*. 3rd ed. Philadelphia: WB Saunders, 1999:96–98.

203. Watson RA, Landon J, Shaw EJ, et al. Polarisation fluoroimmunoassay of gentamicin. *Clin Chim Acta* 1976; 73:51–55.

204. Fujimoto T, Tsuda Y, Tawa R, et al. Fluorescence polarization immunoassay of gentamicin or netilmicin in blood spotted on filter paper. *Clin Chem* 1989;35:867–869.

205. Jolley ME. Fluorescence polarization immunoassay for determination of therapeutic drug levels in human plasma. *J Anal Toxicol* 1981;5:236–240.

206. Morse GC, Nairn DK, Bertino JS Jr, et al. Overestimation of vancomycin concentrations utilizing fluorescence polarization immunoassay in patients on peritoneal dialysis. *Ther Drug Monit* 1987;9:212–215.

207. Uematsu T, Mizuno A, Suzuki Y, et al. Evaluation of a fluorescence polarization immunoassay procedure for quantitation of isepamicin, a new aminoglycoside antibiotic. *Ther Drug Monit* 1988;10:459–462.

208. Uematsu T, Sato R, Mizuno A, et al. A fluorescence polarization immunoassay evaluated for quantifying astromicin, a new aminoglycoside antibiotic. *Clin Chem* 1988;34:1880–1882.

209. Perrin F. Polarization de la lumiere de fluorescence: vie moyenne des molecules dans l'etat excite. *J Phys Radium* 1926;7:390–401.

210. Weber G. Rotational Brownian motion and polarization of the fluorescence of solutions. *Adv Protein Chem* 1953;8:415–459.

211. Popelko SR, Miller DM, Holen JT, et al. Fluorescence polarization immunoassay. II. Analyzer for rapid, precise

measurement of fluorescence polarization with use of disposable cuvettes. *Clin Chem* 1981;27:1198–1201.

212. Jolley ME, Stroupe SD, Schwenzer KS, et al. Fluorescence polarization immunoassay. III. An automated system for therapeutic drug determination. *Clin Chem* 1981;27:1575–1579.

213. Rybak MJ, Bailey EM, Reddy VN. Clinical evaluation of teicoplanin fluorescence polarization immunoassay. *Antimicrob Agents Chemother* 1991;35:1586–1590.

214. Ackerman BH, Berg HG, Strate RG, et al. Comparison of radioimmunoassay and fluorescent polarization immunoassay for quantitative determination of vancomycin concentrations in serum. *J Clin Microbiol* 1983;18:994–995.

215. Sears SD, Standiford HC, Bernstein D, et al. Comparison of the latex agglutination inhibition assay for tobramycin with radioimmunoassay. *Eur J Clin Microbiol* 1986;5:347–350.

216. Martin AJP, Synge RLM. A new form of chromatogram employing two liquid phases. *Biochem J* 1941;35:1358–1368.

217. Horvath CS, Lipsky S. Use of liquid ion exchange chromatography for the separation of organic compounds. *Nature* 1966;211:748–749.

218. Dipiro JT, Taylor AT, Steele JCH Jr. Lack of influence of commonly used drugs on bioassay indicator organisms. *Antimicrob Agents Chemother* 1983;23:703–705.

219. Erni F. Liquid chromatography-mass spectrometry in the pharmaceutical industry: objectives and needs. *J Chromatogr* 1982;251:141–151.

220. Henlon JD, Thomson BA, Dawson PH. Determination of sulfa drugs in biological fluids by liquid chromatography/mass spectrometry/mass spectrometry. *Anal Chem* 1982;54:451–456.

221. Marunaka T, Maniwa M, Matsushima E, et al. High-performance liquid chromatographic determination of a new β-lactamase inhibitor and its metabolite in combination therapy with piperacillin in biological materials. *J Chromatogr* 1988;431:87–101.

222. Snyder LR, Kirkland JJ. *Introduction to modern liquid chromatography*. New York: John Wiley & Sons, 1979:552–556.

223. Anhalt JP. Assay of gentamicin in serum by high-pressure liquid chromatography. *Antimicrob Agents Chemother* 1977;11:651–655.

224. McClain JBL. Vancomycin quantitation by high-performance liquid chromatography in human serum. *J Chromatogr* 1982;231:463–466.

225. Peng GW, Gadella MAF, Peng A, et al. High-pressure liquid-chromatographic method for determination of gentamicin in plasma. *Clin Chem* 1977;23:1838–1844.

226. Peng GW, Jackson GG, Chiou WL. High-pressure liquid chromatographic assay of netilmicin in plasma. *Antimicrob Agents Chemother* 1977;12:707–709.

227. Buchs RP, Maxim TE, Allen N, et al. Analysis of cefoxitin, cephalothin and their deacylated metabolites in human urine by high-performance liquid chromatography. *J Chromatogr* 1974;99:609–618.

228. Carroll MA, White ER, Jancsik Z, et al. The determination of cephradine and cephalexin by reverse phase high-performance liquid chromatography. *J Antibiot* 1977;30:397–403.

229. Cooper MJ, Anders MW, Mirkin BL. Ion-pair extraction and high-speed liquid chromatography of cephalothin and diacetylcephalothin in human serum and urine. *Drug Metab Dispos* 1973;1:659–662.

230. Lauriault A, Awang DVX, Kindack D. High-performance liquid chromatographic determination of dicloxacillin in the presence of its degradation products. *J Chromatogr* 1984;283:449–452.

231. Butterfield AG, Hughes DW, Pound NJ, et al. Separation and detection of tetracycline by high-speed liquid chromatography. *Antimicrob Agents Chemother* 1973;4:11–15.

232. Nilsson-Ehle I, Yoshikawa TI, Schotz MC, et al. Quantitation of antibiotics using high-pressure liquid chromatography: tetracycline. *Antimicrob Agents Chemother* 1976;9:754–760.

233. Shaw FN, Sivner AL, Aarons L, et al. A rapid method for the simultaneous determination of the major metabolites of sulphasalazine in plasma. *J Chromatogr* 1983;274:393–397.

234. Wheals BB, Jane I. Analysis of drugs and their metabolites by high-performance liquid chromatography. *Analyst* 1977;102:625–644.

235. Nilsson-Ehle I. High-pressure liquid chromatography as a tool for the determination of antibiotics in biological fluids. *Acta Pathol Microbiol Scand Suppl* 1977;259:61–66.

236. Jehl F, Gallion C, Monteil H. High-performance chromatography of antibiotics. *J Chromatogr* 1990;531:509–548.

237. Adamovics J. Rapid determination of metronidazole in human serum and urine using a normal-phase high-performance liquid chromatographic column with aqueous solvents. *J Chromatogr* 1984;309:436–440.

238. Annesley T, Wilkerson K, Matz K, et al. Simultaneous determination of penicillin and cephalosporin antibiotics in serum by gradient liquid chromatography. *Clin Chem* 1984;30:908–910.

239. Ascalone V, Dal-Bo L. Determination of ceftriaxone, a novel cephalosporin, in plasma, urine and saliva by high-performance liquid chromatography on an NH2 bonded-phase column. *J Chromatogr* 1983;273:357–366.

240. Bowman DB, Aravind MK, Miceli JN, et al. Reversed-phase high-performance liquid chromatographic method to determine ceftriaxone in biological fluids. *J Chromatogr* 1984;309:209–213.

241. Brajtburg J, Elberg S, Bolard J, et al. Interaction of plasma proteins and lipoproteins with amphotericin B. *J Infect Dis* 1984;149:986–989.

242. Brendel E, Zschunke M, Meineke I. High-performance liquid chromatographic determination of cefonicid in human plasma and urine. *J Chromatogr* 1985;339:359–365.

243. Sharma JP, Berill RF. Improved high-performance liquid chromatographic procedure for the determination of tetracyclines in plasma, urine and tissues. *J Chromatogr* 1978;166:213–220.

244. Asukabe H, Sasaki T, Harada KI, et al. Improvement of chemical analysis of antibiotics. IV. Fluorodensitometric determination of polyether antibiotics. *J Chromatogr* 1984;295:453–461.

245. Campbell GW, Mageau RP, Schwab B, et al. Detection and quantitation of chloramphenicol by competitive enzyme-linked immunoassay. *Antimicrob Agents Chemother* 1984;25:205–211.

246. Fasching CE, Hughes CE, Hector RF, et al. High-pressure liquid chromatographic assay of Bay N 7133 in human serum. *Antimicrob Agents Chemother* 1984;25:596–598.

247. Gochin R, Kanfer I, Haigh JM. Simultaneous determination of trimethoprim, sulphamethoxazole and N4-acetylsulphamethoxazole in serum and urine by high-performance liquid chromatography. *J Chromatogr* 1981;223:139–145.

248. Golas CL, Prober CG, MacLeod SM, et al. Measurement of amphotericin B in serum or plasma by high-performance liquid chromatography. *J Chromatogr* 1983; 278:387–395.

249. Least CJ Jr, Wiegand NJ, Johnson GF, et al. Quantitative gas-chromatographic flame-ionization method for chloramphenicol in human serum. *Clin Chem* 1977;23:220–222.

250. Lecaillon JB, Rouan MC, Souppart C, et al. Determination of cefsulodin, cefotiam, cefalexin, cefotaxime, desacetyl-cefotaxime, cefuroxime and cefroxadin in plasma and urine by high-performance liquid chromatography. *J Chromatogr* 1982;228:257–267.

251. Holt DE, de Louvois J, Hurley R, et al. A high performance liquid chromatography system for the simultaneous assay of some antibiotics commonly found in combination in clinical samples. *J Antimicrob Chemother* 1990;26:107–115.

252. Lindberg RLP, Huupponene RK, Huovinen P. Rapid high-pressure chromatographic method for analysis of phenoxymethylpenicillin in human serum. *Antimicrob Agents Chemother* 1984;26:300–302.

253. Little JR, Little KD, Plut E, et al. Induction of amphotericin B-specific antibodies for use in immunoassays. *Antimicrob Agents Chemother* 1984;26:824–828.

254. Norrby SR, Alestig K, Ferber F, et al. Pharmacokinetics and tolerance of N-formimidoyl-thienamycin (MK0787) in humans. *Antimicrob Agents Chemother* 1983;23:293–299.

255. Oldfield N, Chang D, Garland W, et al. Quantitation of ceftetrame in human plasma and urine by high-performance liquid chromatography. *J Chromatogr* 1987;422:135–143.

256. Wold JS. Rapid analysis of cefazolin in serum by high-pressure liquid chromatography. *Antimicrob Agents Chemother* 1977;11:105–109.

257. Cummings KC, Torres AR, Edberg SC. The analysis of antimicrobial agents in biological fluids by high-performance liquid chromatography. II. Applications. *J Clin Lab Autom* 1984;4:244–255.

258. Chen ML, Chiou WL. Analysis of erythromycin in biological fluids by high-performance liquid chromatography with electrochemical detection. *J Chromatogr* 1983;278:91–100.

259. Falkowski AJ, Greger RJ. Hydroxylamine technique for in vitro prevention of penicillin inactivation of tobramycin. *Antimicrob Agents Chemother* 1984;26:643–646.

260. Hendrickx L, Roets E, Hoogmartens J, et al. Identification of penicillins by thin-layer chromatography. *J Chromatogr* 1984;291:211–218.

261. Fiore D, Auger FA, Drusano GL, et al. Improved micromethod for mezlocillin quantitation in serum and urine by high-pressure liquid chromatography. *Antimicrob Agents Chemother* 1984;26:775–777.

262. Schwertschlag U, Nakata LM, Gal J. Improved procedure for determination of flucytosine in human blood plasma by high-pressure liquid chromatography. *Antimicrob Agents Chemother* 1984;26:303–305.

263. Ueno H, Nishikawa M. Chromatographic separation and chemical analysis of polymers formed by penicillin G. *J Chromatogr* 1984;288:117–126.

264. Lovering AM, White LO, Reeves DS. Identification of aminoglycoside-acetylating enzymes by high-pressure liquid chromatographic determination of their reaction products. *Antimicrob Agents Chemother* 1984;26:10–12.

265. Myers CM, Blumer JL. Determination of imipenem and cilastin in serum by high-pressure liquid chromatography. *Antimicrob Agents Chemother* 1984;26:78–81.

266. Provoost AP, Schalkwijk WP, Olusanya A, et al. Determination of aminoglycosides in rat renal tissue by enzyme immunoassay. *Antimicrob Agents Chemother* 1984;25:497–498.

267. Guiochon G. Optimization in liquid chromatography. In: Horvath C, ed. *High-performance liquid chromatography: advances and perspectives.* New York: Academic Press, 1980;2:1–56.

268. Giddings JC. Theory of chromatography. In: Heftman E, ed. *Chromatography.* New York: Reinhold, 1967.

269. Snyder LR, Kirkland JJ. *Introduction to modern liquid chromatography.* New York: John Wiley & Sons, 1979: 246–268.

270. Kirkland KM, McCombs DA, Kirkland JJ. Rapid high-resolution high performance liquid chromatographic analysis of antibiotics. *J Chromatogr* 1994;A660:327–337.

271. Assenza SP, Brown PR. Evaluation of reversed-phase, radially-compressed, flexible-walled columns for the separation of low molecular weight, UV-absorbing compounds in serum. *J Liquid Chromatogr* 1980;3:41–59.

272. Amicon Corp. *Amicon micropartition system.* Lexington, MA: Amicon Corp, 1977.

273. Cummings KC, Jatlow PI. Sample preparation by ultra-filtration for direct gas chromatographic analysis of ethylene glycol in plasma. *J Anal Toxicol* 1982;6:324–326.

274. Brisson AM, Fourtillan JB. High-performance liquid chromatographic determination of piperacillin in plasma. *Antimicrob Agents Chemother* 1982;21:664–665.

275. Marples J, Oates MDG. Serum gentamicin, netilmicin and tobramycin assays by high-performance liquid chromatography. *J Antimicrob Chemother* 1982;10:311–318.

276. Hildebrandt R, Gundert-Remy U. Improved procedures for the determination of the ureidopenicillins azlocillin and mezlocillin in plasma by high-performance liquid chromatography. *J Chromatogr* 1982;228:409–412.

277. Barry AL, Packer RR. Roxithromycin bioassay procedures for human plasma, urine and milk specimens [corrected and issued with original pagination in Eur J Clin Microbiol 1986;5(6)]. *Eur J Clin Microbiol* 1986;5:536–540.

278. Bauchet J, Pussard E, Garaud JJ. Determination of vancomycin in serum and tissues by column liquid chromatography using solid-phase extraction. *J Chromatogr* 1987;414:472–476.

279. Croteau D, Vallee F, Bergeron MG, et al. High-performance liquid chromatographic assay of erythromycin and its esters using electrochemical detection. *J Chromatogr* 1987;419:205–212.

280. Demotes-Mainaird FM, Vincon GA, Jarry CH, et al. Micro-method for the determination of roxithromycin in human plasma and urine by high-performance liquid chromatography using electrochemical detection. *J Chromatogr* 1989;490:115–123.

281. Dow J, Lemar M, Frydman A, et al. Automated high-performance liquid chromatographic determination of spiramycin by direct injection of plasma, using column-switching for sample clean-up. *J Chromatogr* 1985;344: 275–283.

282. Haataja H, Kokkonen P. Determination of 2-acetyl erythromycin and erythromycin in human tonsil tissue by HPLC with coulometric detection. *J Antimicrob Chemother* 1988;21(Suppl D):67–72.

283. Holdiness MR. Chromatographic analysis of antituberculosis drugs in biological samples [review]. *J Chromatogr* 1985;340:321–359.

284. Hosotsubo H, Takezawa J, Taenaka N, et al. Rapid determination of amphotericin B levels in serum by

high-performance liquid chromatography without interference by bilirubin. *Antimicrob Agents Chemother* 1988;32:1103–1105.

285. Jehl F, Gallion C, Thierry RC, et al. Determination of vancomycin in human serum by high-pressure liquid chromatography. *Antimicrob Agents Chemother* 1985;27:503–507.

286. Jehl F, Monteil H, Tarral A. HPLC quantitation of the six main components of teicoplanin in biological fluids. *J Antimicrob Chemother* 1988;21(Suppl A):53–59.

287. Joos B, Luthy R. Determination of teicoplanin concentrations in serum by high-pressure liquid chromatography. *Antimicrob Agents Chemother* 1987;31:1222–1224.

288. LaFollette G, Gambertoglio J, White JA, et al. Determination of clindamycin in plasma or serum by high-performance liquid chromatography with ultraviolet detection. *J Chromatogr* 1988;431:379–388.

289. Levy J, Truong BL, Goignau H, et al. High-pressure liquid chromatographic quantitation of teicoplanin in human serum. *J Antimicrob Chemother* 1987;19:533–539.

290. Musson DG, Maglietto SM, Hwang SS, et al. Simultaneous quantification of cycloserine and its prodrug acetylacetonylcycloserine in plasma and urine by high-performance liquid chromatography using ultraviolet absorbance and fluorescence after post-column derivatization. *J Chromatogr* 1987;414:121–129.

291. Riva E, Ferry N, Cometti A, et al. Determination of teicoplanin in human plasma and urine by affinity and reversed-phase high-performance liquid chromatography. *J Chromatogr* 1987;421:99–110.

292. Skinner M, Kanfer I. High-performance liquid chromatographic analysis of josamycin in serum and urine. *J Chromatogr* 1988;459:261–267.

293. Woo J, Wong CL, Teoh R, et al. Liquid chromatographic assay for the simultaneous determination of pyrazinamide and rifampicin in serum samples from patients with tuberculous meningitis. *J Chromatogr* 1987;420:73–80.

294. Sood SP, Green VI, Bailey CL. Routine methods in toxicology and therapeutic drug monitoring by high performance liquid chromatography. II. A rapid microscale method for determination of chloramphenicol in blood and cerebrospinal fluid. *Ther Drug Monit* 1987;9:347–352.

295. Robison LR, Seligsohn R, Lerner SA. Simplified radioenzymatic assay for chloramphenicol. *Antimicrob Agents Chemother* 1978;13:25–29.

296. Weber AF, Opheim KE, Koup JR, et al. Comparison of enzymatic and liquid chromatographic chloramphenicol assays. *Antimicrob Agents Chemother* 1981;19:323–325.

297. Velagapudi R, Smith RV, Ludden TM, et al. Simultaneous determination of chloramphenicol and chloramphenicol succinate in plasma using high-performance liquid chromatography. *J Chromatogr* 1982;228:423–428.

298. Black SB, Levine P, Shinefield HR. The necessity for monitoring chloramphenicol levels when treating neonatal meningitis. *J Pediatr* 1978;92:235–236.

299. el-Yazigi A, Yusuf A, Al-Humaidan A. Direct, simultaneous measurement of chloramphenicol and its monosuccinate ester in micro-samples of plasma by radial-compression liquid chromatography. *Clin Chem* 1987;33:1814–1816.

300. Ackers IM, Myers CM, Blumer JL. Determination of cefsulodin in biological fluids by high-pressure liquid chromatography. *Ther Drug Monit* 1984;6:91–95.

301. Barbhaiya RH, Forgue ST, Shyu WC, et al. High-pressure liquid chromatographic analysis of BMY-28142 in plasma and urine. *Antimicrob Agents Chemother* 1987;31:55–59.

302. Bliss M, Mayersohn M. Liquid-chromatographic assay of cefamandole in serum, urine, and dialysis fluid. *Clin Chem* 1986;32:197–200.

303. Chan CY, Chan K, French GL. Rapid high performance liquid chromatographic assay of cephalosporins in biological fluids. *J Antimicrob Chemother* 1986;18:537–545.

304. Cowlishaw MG, Sharman JR. Liquid-chromatographic assay of cefoperazone from plasma and bile. *Clin Chem* 1986;32:894.

305. Emm TA, Leslie J, Chai M, et al. High-performance liquid chromatographic assay of cephalexin in serum and urine. *J Chromatogr* 1988;427:162–165.

306. Falkowski AJ, Look ZM, Noguchi H, et al. Determination of cefixime in biological samples by reversed-phase high-performance liquid chromatography. *J Chromatogr* 1987;422:145–152.

307. Friis JM, Lakings DB. High-performance liquid chromatographic method for the determination of cefpimizole in tissue. *J Chromatogr* 1986;382:399–404.

308. Granich GG, Krogstad DJ. Ion pair high-performance liquid chromatographic assay for ceftriaxone. *Antimicrob Agents Chemother* 1987;31:385–388.

309. Leeder JS, Spino M, Tesoro AM, et al. High-pressure liquid chromatographic analysis of ceftazidime in serum and urine. *Antimicrob Agents Chemother* 1983;24:720–724.

310. Marunaka T, Matsushima E, Maniwa M. Determination of cefodizime in biological materials by high-performance liquid chromatography. *J Chromatogr* 1987;420:329–339.

311. McAteer JA, Hiltke MF, Silber BM, et al. Liquid-chromatographic determination of five orally active cephalosporins cefixime, cefaclor, cefadroxil, cephalexin, and cephradine in human serum. *Clin Chem* 1987;33:1788–1790.

312. Najib NM, Suleiman MS, el-Sayed YM, et al. High-performance liquid chromatographic analysis of cephalexin in serum and urine. *J Clin Pharmacol Ther* 1987;12:419–426.

313. Turley CP, Kearns GL, Jacobs RF. Microanalytical high-performance liquid chromatography assay for cefpirome (HR 810) in serum. *Antimicrob Agents Chemother* 1988;32:1481–1483.

314. Wyss R, Bucheli F. Determination of cefetamet and its orally active ester, cefetamet pivoxyl, in biological fluids by high-performance liquid chromatography. *J Chromatogr* 1988;430:81–92.

315. Lodise TP, Kinziq-Schippers M, Drusano GL, et al. Use of population pharmacokinetic modeling and Monte Carlo simulation to describe the pharmacodynamic profile of cefditoren in plasma and epithelial lining fluid. *Antimicrob Agents Chemother* 2008;52(6):1945–1951.

316. Sádaba B, Azanza JR, Quetglas EG, et al. Pharmacokinetic/pharmacodynamic serum and urine profile of cefditoren following single-dose and multiple twice- and thrice-daily regimens in healthy volunteers: a phase I study. *Rev Esp Quimioter* 2007;20:51–60.

317. Abuirejeie MA, Abdel-Hamid ME. Simultaneous high-pressure liquid chromatographic analysis of ampicillin and cloxacillin in serum and urine. *J Clin Pharmacol* 1988;13:101–108.

318. Baskerville AJ, Flemingham D, Gruneberg RN. A high performance liquid chromatography method for the determination of FCE 22101, a novel penem antimicrobial, in serum. *Drugs Exp Clin Res* 1988;14:645–648.

319. Bawdon RE, Madsen PO. High-pressure liquid chromatographic assay of sulbactam in plasma, urine, and tissue. *Antimicrob Agents Chemother* 1986;30:231–233.

320. Carlqvist J, Westerlund D. Automated determination of amoxycillin in biological fluids by column switching in ion-pair reversed-phase liquid chromatographic systems with post-column derivatization. *J Chromatogr* 1985;344:285–296.

321. Egger HJ, Fischer G. Determination of the monocyclic-lactam antibiotic carumonam in plasma and urine by ion-pair and ion-suppression reversed-phase high-performance liquid chromatography. *J Chromatogr* 1987;420:357–372.

322. Fan-Havard P, Nahata MC. A rapid analysis of nafcillin using high-performance liquid chromatography. *Ther Drug Monit* 1989;11:105–108.

323. Forgue ST, Pittman KA, Barbhaiya RH. High-performance liquid chromatographic analysis of a novel carbapenem antibiotic in human plasma and urine. *J Chromatogr* 1987;414:343–353.

324. Godbillon J, Duval M, Gauron S, et al. High-performance liquid chromatographic determination of the penem antibiotic (5R,6S)-2-aminomethyl-6-[(1R)-hydroxyethyl]-2-penem-3-carboxylic acid in human plasma and urine. *J Chromatogr* 1988;427:269–276.

325. Haginaka J, Wakai J. Liquid chromatographic determination of penicillins by postcolumn alkaline degradation using a hollow-fiber membrane reactor. *Anal Biochem* 1988;168:132–140.

326. Haginaka J, Yasuda H, Uno T, et al. High-performance liquid chromatographic assay of clavulanate in human plasma and urine by fluorimetric detection. *J Chromatogr* 1986;377:269–277.

327. Hung CT, Lim JK, Zoest AR, et al. Optimization of high-performance liquid chromatographic analysis for isoxazolyl penicillins using factorial design. *J Chromatogr* 1988;425:331–341.

328. Jamaluddin AB, Sarwar G, Rahim MA, et al. Assay for cloxacillin in human serum utilising high-performance liquid chromatography with ultraviolet detection. *J Chromatogr* 1989;490:243–246.

329. Jones CW, Chmel H. Solid-phase ion-pair extraction and liquid chromatography of mezlocillin in serum. *Clin Chem* 1988;34:2155–2156.

330. Pilkiewicz FG, Remsburg BJ, Fisher SM, et al. High-pressure liquid chromatographic analysis of aztreonam in sera and urine. *Antimicrob Agents Chemother* 1983;23:852–856.

331. Watson ID. Clavulanate-potentiated ticarcillin: high-performance liquid chromatographic assays for clavulanic acid and ticarcillin isomers in serum and urine. *J Chromatogr* 1985;337:301–309.

332. Cirillo I, Vaccaro N, Turner K, et al. Pharmacokinetics, safety, and tolerability of doripenem after 0.5-, 1-, and 4-hour infusions in healthy volunteers. *J Clin Pharmacol* 2009;49:798.

333. Ikawa K, Morikawa N, Urakawa N, et al. Peritoneal penetration of doripenem after intravenous administration in abdominal-surgery patients. *J Antimicrob Chemother* 2007;60(6):1395–1397.

334. Burian B, Zeitlinger M, Donath O, et al. Penetration of doripenem into skeletal muscle and subcutaneous adipose tissue in healthy volunteers. *Antimicrob Agents Chemother* 2012;56(1):532–535.

335. Zhang J, Musson DG, Birk KL, et al. Direct-injection HPLC assay for the determination of a new carbapenem antibiotic in human plasma and urine. *J Pharm Biomed Anal* 2002;27:755–770.

336. Musson DG, Birk KL, Cairns AM, et al. High-performance liquid chromatographic methods for the determination of a new carbapenem antibiotic, L-749,345, in human plasma and urine. *J Chromatogr B Biomed Sci Appl* 1998; 720:99–106.

337. Gill CJ, Jackson JJ, Gerckens LS, et al. In vivo activity and pharmacokinetic evaluation of a novel long-acting carbapenem antibiotic, MK-826 (L-749,345). *Antimicrob Agents Chemother* 1998;42(8):1996–2001.

338. Laethem T, De Lepeleire I, McCrea J, et al. Tissue penetration by ertapenem, a parenteral carbapenem administered once daily, in suction-induced skin blister fluid in healthy young volunteers. *Antimicrob Agents Chemother* 2003;47(4):1439–1442.

339. Kitchen CJ, Musson DG, Fisher AL, et al. Column-switching technique for the sensitive determination of ertapenem in human cerebrospinal fluid using liquid chromatography and ultraviolet absorbance detection. *J Chromatogr B Analyt Technol Biomed Life Sci* 2004; 799(1):9–14.

340. Wittau M, Scheele J, Bulitta JB, et al. Pharmacokinetics of ertapenem in colorectal tissue. *Chemotherapy* 2011; 57:437–448.

341. Delaney CJ, Opheim KE, Smith AL, et al. Performance characteristics of bioassay, radioenzymatic assay, homogeneous enzyme immunoassay, and high-performance liquid chromatographic determination of serum gentamicin. *Antimicrob Agents Chemother* 1982;21:19–25.

342. Barends DM, Blauw JS, Smits MH, et al. Determination of amikacin in serum by high-performance liquid chromatography with ultraviolet detection. *J Chromatogr* 1983;276:385–394.

343. Rumble RH, Roberts MS. High-performance liquid chromatographic assay of the major components of gentamicin in serum. *J Chromatogr* 1987;419:408–413.

344. Yamamoto T, Moriwaki Y, Takahashi S, et al. Rapid and simultaneous determination of pyrazinamide and its major metabolites in human plasma by high-performance liquid chromatography. *J Chromatogr* 1987;413:342–346.

345. Tobin CM, Sunderland J, White LO, et al. A simple isocratic high-performance liquid chromatography assay for linezolid in human serum. *J Antimicrob Chemother* 2001;48:605–608.

346. Rana B, Butcher I, Grigoris P, et al. Linezolid penetration into osteo-articular tissues. *J Antimicrob Chemother* 2002;50:747–750.

347. Conte JE, Golden JA, Kipps J, et al. Intrapulmonary pharmacokinetics of linezolid. *Antimicrob Agents Chemother* 2002;46:1475–1480.

348. Tobin CM, Sunderland J, Lovering AM, et al. A high performance liquid chromatography (HPLC) assay for linezolid in continuous ambulatory peritoneal dialysis fluid (CAPDF). *J Antimicrob Chemother* 2003;51: 1041–1042.

349. Saralaya D, Peckham DG, Hulme G, et al. Serum and sputum concentrations following the oral administration of linezolid in adult patients with cystic fibrosis. *J Antimicrob Chemother* 2004;53:325–328.

350. Fiscella RG, Lai WW, Buerk B, et al. Aqueous and vitreous penetration of linezolid (Zyvox) after oral administration. *Ophthalmology* 2004;111:1191–1195.

351. Mullen PW, Mawer GE, Tooth JA. An indirect method for the determination of cephaloridine in serum by gas chromatography. *Res Commun Chem Pathol Pharmacol* 1974;7:85–94.

352. Bronson LW, Bowman PB. Gas chromatographic assay for the antibiotic spectinomycin. *J Chromatogr Sci* 1974;12: 373–376.

353. Resnick GL, Corbin D, Sandberg DH. Determination of serum chloramphenicol utilizing gas-liquid chromatography and electron capture spectrometry. *Anal Chem* 1966;38:582–585.

354. Shaw PD. Gas chromatography of trimethylsilyl derivatives of compounds related to chloramphenicol. *Anal Chem* 1963;35:1580–1582.

355. Nakagawa T, Masada M, Uno T. Gas chromatographic mass spectrometric analysis of chloramphenicol, thiamphenicol and their metabolites. *J Chromatogr* 1975;111:355–364.

356. Pauncz JK, Harsanyi I. Aminoglycoside antibiotics: thin-layer chromatography, bioautographic detection and quantitative assay. *J Chromatogr* 1980;195:251–256.

357. Oka H, Uno K. Improvement of chemical analysis of antibiotics. VI. Detection reagents for tetracyclines in thin-layer chromatography. *J Chromatogr* 1984;295:129–139.

358. Oka H, Uno K. Improvement of chemical analysis of antibiotics. VII. Simple method for the analysis of tetracyclines on reversed-phase thin-layer plates. *J Chromatogr* 1984;284:227–234.

359. Aravind MK, Miceli JN, Kauffman RE. Determination of moxalactam by high-performance liquid chromatography. *J Chromatogr* 1982;228:418–422.

360. Nishi H, Fukuyama T, Matsuo M. Separation and determination of aspoxicillin in human plasma by micellar electrokinetic chromatography with direct sample injection. *J Chromatogr* 1990;515:245–255.

361. Branch SK, Casy AF. Applications of modern high-field NMR spectroscopy in medicinal chemistry. *Prog Med Chem* 1989;26:355–436.

362. Gonzalez Perez C, Gonzalez Martin I, et al. Polarographic determination of clavulanic acid. *J Pharm Biomed Anal* 1991;9:383–386.

363. Gentamicin radioimmunoassay. Newport Beach, CA: Monitor Science Corp, 1976.

364. Weber A, Opheim KE, Wong K, et al. High-pressure liquid chromatographic quantitation of azlocillin. *Antimicrob Agents Chemother* 1983;24:750–753.

365. Brisson AM, Fourtillan JB. Determination of cephalosporins in biological material by reversed-phase liquid column chromatography. *J Chromatogr* 1981;223:393–399.

366. Bakerman S. Fluorescence polarization immunoassay. *Lab Manage* 1983;July:16–18.

367. Klein RD, Edberg SC. Applications, Significance of, and Methods for the Measurement of Antimicrobial Concentrations in Human Body Fluids. In: Lorian V, ed. *Antibiotics in Laboratory Medicine.* 5th edition. Lippincott Williams & Wilkins, 2005;290–364.

368. Foulds G, Gans DJ, Girard D, et al. Assays of sulbactam in the presence of ampicillin. *Ther Drug Monit* 1986;8:223–227.

369. Koal T, Deters M, Resch K, et al. Quantification of the carbapenem antibiotic ertapenem in human plasma by a validated liquid chromatography—mass spectrometry method. *Clin Chim Acta* 2006;364(1–2):239–245.

370. Signs SA, File TM, Tan JS. High-pressure liquid chromatographic method for analysis of cephalosporins. *Antimicrob Agents Chemother* 1984;26:652–655.

371. Spreaux-Varoquaux O, Chapalain JP, Cordonnier P, et al. Determination of trimethoprim, sulphamethoxazole and its N4-acetyl metabolite in biological fluids by high-performance liquid chromatography. *J Chromatogr* 1983;274:187–199.

372. Witebsky FG, Selepak ST. Feasibility of gentamicin measurement in icteric sera by the Syva EMIT system. *Antimicrob Agents Chemother* 1983;23:172–174.

373. Rybak M, Lomaestro B, Rotschafer JC, et al. Therapeutic monitoring of vancomycin in adult patients: a consensus review of the American Society of Health-System Pharmacists, the Infectious Diseases Society of America, and the Society of Infectious Diseases Pharmacists. *Am J Health Syst Pharm* 2009;66:82–98.

Chapter 9

Molecular Methods for Detection of Antibacterial Resistance Genes: Rationale and Applications

Kristin Hegstad, Ørjan Samuelsen, Joachim Hegstad, and Arnfinn Sundsfjord

THE CHALLENGE

The emergence and spread of antibiotic resistance in clinically important bacteria represent a multi-faceted challenge in clinical microbiology. Rapid identification of pathogens and prediction of their antimicrobial susceptibility has important thera-peutic and prognostic implications for individual patients (1). Detection of patients colonized by clinically important resistant bacteria is instru-mental for efficient infection control measures (2–4). Moreover, elucidation of antimicrobial resistance mechanisms at a molecular level is fun-damental in diagnostic interpretation of resistance phenotypes, understanding of the origins of resis-tance mechanisms, identification of transmission routes and vehicles for dissemination, and devel-opment of new antimicrobials (5,6).

Thus, we need specific and rapid diagnostic methods to guide antimicrobial therapy and infec-tion control interventions as well as accurate and efficient techniques for detection of genetic and biochemical mechanisms involved in the develop-ment and spread of antibiotic resistance. In this review, we describe the rationale for molecular detection of antimicrobial resistance genes, advan-tages, and limitations; address relevant technical aspects; and discuss the application of these meth-ods for specific clinical or epidemiologic purposes.

ANTIMICROBIAL RESISTANCE AT A MOLECULAR LEVEL

Enormous progress has been made in our un-derstanding of the genetics and biochemistry of antimicrobial resistance (5,7). This knowledge has important conceptual implications in a discussion of the use of molecular methods in detection of antimicrobial resistance. Most antimicrobials are nature's own products or derivatives developed by microorganisms in their competition for life and space. Thus, bacteria have evolved protective mechanisms that predate the antimicrobial era to avoid their own or others' inhibitory actions. Characterization of the antimicrobial resistome has revealed the presence of protoresistance genes with a phylogenetic relationship and potential to evolve into a resistance gene (5).

The genetic information encoding protective measures may be passed on to daughter cells (verti-cal transmission) or to other bacteria through trans-formation, transduction, or conjugation (horizontal gene transfer). The genetic basis for antimicrobial resistance includes (a) the acquisition, stabilization, and expression of new DNA by horizontal gene transfer or (b) mutations in cellular genes or acquired genes that alter antimicrobial target sites or affect gene expression. Recently, the concept of adaptive resistance has been introduced. Adaptive resistance involves transient alterations in gene and/or protein expression, including porins and efflux pumps, due to environmental stress that reverts after removal of the trigger (8). The genetic alterations or adaptations mediate a diversity of biochemical mechanisms of antimicrobial resistance: (a) enzymatic modification of antimicrobial agents; (b) target substitutions, am-plification, or modifications bypassing the binding or reducing the affinity for the antimicrobial agent; (c) barriers or efflux pumps reducing the access to the target.

Mutational resistance within a bacterial popula-tion and horizontal gene transfer events may not be frequent and the acquisition of modified or new genetic information mediates a biologic cost to the host that hamper expansion of the recipient. However, antimicrobial selection creates opportunities and ecologic niches for biologic amplification of antimicrobial resistance determinants and their hosts (9). Moreover, bacteria have developed compensatory mechanisms of fitness costs and host elements for capturing, stabilization, and mobilization of new genetic information, systems that favor long-term persistence of antimicrobial resistance genes without the exposure to selection (10,11).

Genetic and biochemical research in antimicrobial resistance have also provided insight into the molecular basis for cross- and coresistance (7). The concept of cross-resistance is based on mutations in overlapping antimicrobial targets, enzymatic modification, and drug efflux mechanisms affecting the susceptibility of antimicrobials across classes. The increased occurrence of genetically linked and coexpressed resistance determinants in R plasmids, integrons, and transposons illustrates the concept of coresistance and the selection of multiple resistance mechanism by the use of a single antimicrobial.

In clinical terms, the characterization of biochemical mechanisms for antimicrobial resistance and their genetic support has been important in the improvement of antimicrobial susceptibility testing and therapeutic interpretation of resistance phenotypes (12). Interpretive reading of antibiogram data involves the deduction of resistance mechanisms from susceptibility test results and interpretation of clinical susceptibility based on resistance mechanisms (13).

DETECTION OF ANTIMICROBIAL RESISTANCE GENES: ADVANTAGES AND LIMITATIONS

Phenotypic antimicrobial susceptibility testing requires growth of bacteria in pure culture and may routinely take at least 24 to 48 hours to obtain a valid result. Antimicrobial susceptibility testing of slow-growing organisms such as *Mycobacterium tuberculosis* may take even weeks or months (14). Thus, the development of rapid molecular assays may provide an attractive diagnostic approach as a guide to treatment options (15,16).

The advantages of genetic detection of antimicrobial resistance include the following: (a) A YES or NO answer if the presence of a defined resistance determinant is provided. (b) Not dependent on clinical categorization of susceptibility breakpoints, which may vary between countries and authoritative institutions. (c) Ability to detect resistance mechanisms involved in low-level resistance that could be difficult to detect by phenotypic methods. (d) Genetic assays can be performed directly with clinical specimens and bypass phenotypic expression reducing the time for detection. This is particularly important for difficult-to-culture organisms. (e) Easy and early interpretation allows early therapeutic predictions. (f) Genetic assays may reduce the biohazard risk associated with handling of culture-based techniques.

However, there are also drawbacks and pitfalls in the molecular approach: (a) Genetic predictions are based on screening for resistance determinants, whereas the preferred antimicrobial therapy is based on the detection of susceptibility. (b) You can, in principle, only detect what you already know and genetic methods do not take into account new resistance mechanisms. Thus, validated genetic methods generally have a high specificity but a lower sensitivity due to unknown resistance mechanisms not covered by current molecular assays. (c) There are silent genes, pseudogenes, or protoresistance genes that may cause false-positive results. (d) Mutations in primer binding sites may preclude PCR amplification generating false-negative results. (e) Low clinical sensitivity when performed directly on clinical samples due to inhibition of nucleic acid amplification or a limited number of targets. (f) Finally, regulatory environmental adaptations that only affect gene expression (adaptive resistance) are not detected unless a quantitative assessment of the specific mRNA is performed (8).

Hence, the genetic approach based on today's concepts cannot displace phenotypic methods in routine antimicrobial susceptibility testing of rapid-growing clinical relevant bacteria. Novel resistance mechanisms will arise continuously by mutations and regulatory adaptations, mobilization of unknown preexisting resistance genes from environmental reservoirs, and evolving protoresistance genes to resistance genes. However, genotypic methods should be endorsed for clinically important slow-growing organisms with increasing resistance problems based on chromosomal mutations such as *M. tuberculosis*. Moreover, the success of genetic assays in detection of antimicrobial resistance is also dependent on technical improvements; speed, accuracy, and user-friendliness may provide cost-saving formats of molecular assays. Apparently, the recent advances in whole genome sequencing (WGS) and bioinformatics workflows are of interest and, in particular, with regard to in silico antimicrobial susceptibility testing in surveillance and infection control (17–22).

MOLECULAR METHODS IN THE DETECTION OF ANTIMICROBIAL RESISTANCE: TECHNICAL ASPECTS AND APPLICATION STRATEGIES

New molecular diagnostics tools and new combinations of existing technology are continuously developed. Thus, the technology presented herein represents a snapshot as of early 2013 focusing mainly on nucleic acid amplification techniques (NAATs) and microarrays as well as giving a glimpse into the rapidly evolving technologies matrix-assisted laser desorption-ionization time-of-flight mass spectrometry (MALDI-TOF MS) and next generation sequencing for use in the molecular diagnostics of antimicrobial resistance.

Nucleic Acid Amplification Techniques

Many different NAATs have been developed. Some test principles and their relevant characteristics in the detection of antimicrobial resistance mechanisms are listed in Table 9.1. NAATs amplify restricted parts of DNA/RNA for the sample in question in a logarithmic manner, ending up with billions of copies per reaction tube. All these copies of DNA/RNA makes amplification techniques well suited for sensitive assays.

Table 9.1 descriptions include commonly used NAATs such as traditional polymerase chain reaction (PCR), multiplex PCR, real-time PCR, nucleic acid sequence-based amplification (NASBA), loop-mediated isothermal amplification (LAMP), and helicase-dependent amplification (HDA). Several detection systems used by real-time PCR are not mentioned, that is, Scorpions primers (Biosearch Technologies, Petaluma, CA), MGB Eclipse probes (EliTechGroup, Paris, France and Life Technologies, Grand Island, NY), Light-up probes (LightUp Technologies AB, Huddinge, Sweden), HyBeacon probes (Hain Lifescience GmbH, Nehren, Germany), Yin-yang probes (QuanDx, Menlo Park, CA), or Amplifluor (EMD Millipore, Billerica, MA). Examples of a real-time PCR melt curve and an amplification plot from real-time PCR probe detection are displayed in Figures 9.1 and 9.2, respectively.

Microarrays

The traditional Southern or Northern blot hybridization principles were used to develop microarrays for fast parallel, high-throughput detection and quantitation of nucleic acids (23). In nucleic acid arrays, hundreds or thousands of sequence-specific probes such as oligonucleotides or PCR products are deposited in fixed regions on a solid support or chip. Labelled targets applied to the solid support then hybridize to sequence-specific regions. The purposes for application of microarrays include large-scale genotyping (including single nucleotide polymorphism [SNP] analyses), gene expression profiling, and comparative genomic hybridizations (including copy number variation analysis). For a thorough introduction to microarray technology, including its applications, fabrication, target preparation, hybridization, detection, and data analysis, see Dufva (24). Both in-house and commercial microbial diagnostic microarrays have been developed to detect microbes as well as genes involved in antimicrobial resistance and virulence (25). The easy-to-use commercial microarray technology multiplexing power is attractive for antimicrobial resistance screening in central high-throughput facilities or hospital labs. A limitation of microarrays is that the signal does not provide any other information than the presence of the target. The size or complete sequence of the captured target molecule is not revealed.

The Application of Matrix-Assisted Laser Desorption-Ionization Time-of-Flight Mass Spectrometry Opens New Perspectives in the Detection of Antimicrobial Resistance

Bacterial identification based on mass spectral fingerprints obtained by MALDI-TOF MS is now routinely used in many clinical laboratories. The use of this technology in identification of antimicrobial resistance is rapidly increasing. For a detailed presentation of the use of MALDI-TOF MS in detection of antimicrobial resistance mechanisms, see Hrabak et al. (26). Briefly, antimicrobial resistance can either be revealed by changes in whole cell protein mass spectra when comparing susceptible and resistant isolates; by changes in mass spectra representing antimicrobials and their enzymatic degradation products or wild type and modified proteins/RNA; or by peptide, RNA, and DNA mini-sequencing (26–29).

The potential use of MALDI-TOF MS in detection of vancomycin-resistant enterococci (VRE) (30) and methicillin-resistant *Staphylococcus aureus* (MRSA) have been described but needs further refinements and validation (31). MALDI-TOF assays have also been developed to identify the enzymatic degradation of β-lactams by β-lactamases (32,33)

Table 9.1

Nucleic Acid Amplification Techniques and Their Relevant Characteristics in the Detection of Antimicrobial Resistance

Techniques	Detection	Test Principle, Advantages, and Limitations	Application	Clinical Examples
PCR	AGE[a], include restriction digestion or sequencing to detect SNPs	A segment of DNA between two known sequence regions is amplified in a thermocycler using oligonucleotide primers complementary to the target and a thermostable DNA polymerase. For detailed description, see Sambrook et al. (307). **Advantages:** may target long sequences, may discover insertions/deletions and information about the sequence size **Disadvantages:** time-consuming, not suitable for quantitative assay	Detection of acquired genes and SNPs	Glycopeptide resistance genes: *vanA, vanB1/B2/B3, vanC1/C2/C3* (16) Linezolid resistance gene: *cfr* (259)
Multiplex PCR	Multiple-sized fragments discriminated by AGE or multiple probes with different fluorophores measured in real-time	Multiplex PCR detects multiple targets in the same PCR reaction tube. **Advantages:** save runtime and reagents **Disadvantages:** more complex to optimize, not suitable for quantitative assay	Detection of acquired genes and SNPs	Extended-spectrum β-lactamase genes: *bla*CTX-M gr. 1, *bla*CTX-M gr. 2, *bla*CTX-M gr. 9, *bla*CTX-M gr. 8, *bla*CTX-M gr. 25 (176) Glycopeptide resistance genes: *vanA, vanB1/B2/B3, vanC1/C2/C3* (308)
Real-time PCR	Hybridization probes (fluorescence resonance energy transfer [FRET] probes), include locked nucleic acids (LNAs) to detect SNPs	Hybridization probes consisting of a donor and acceptor probe that binds the amplicon after one another. The light source of PCR instrument transfer energy to the donor probe which allows energy transfer to the acceptor probe, resulting in a detectable fluorescent signal. For detailed description, see Parks et al. (309). **Advantages:** faster than traditional PCR, high specificity **Disadvantages:** designed to work essentially on Roche LightCycler platforms	Detection of acquired genes and SNPs, quantification of target DNA/RNA	*Helicobacter pylori* clarithromycin resistance SNPs in 23S rRNA gene (310)
	Double-dye (dual-labelled, TaqMan) oligonucleotides/probes, include locked nucleic acids (LNAs) to detect SNPs	Double-dye probes labelled with a fluorophore at 5' and a quencher at 3'. Fluorescence is emitted due to cleavage of annealed probe during primer extension. For detailed description of the principle, see Holland et al. (311). **Advantages:** easy assay design, adaptable to many different real-time platforms **Disadvantages:** not suitable for AT-rich sequences without including expensive LNAs in the probe	Detection of acquired genes and SNPs, quantification of target DNA/RNA	MRSA *mecA, mecC, nuc,* PVL genes (63) *M. tuberculosis* resistance SNPs in *rpoB, katG, inhA* promoter (312)

(Continued)

Table 9.1 (Continued)

Nucleic Acid Amplification Techniques and Their Relevant Characteristics in the Detection of Antimicrobial Resistance

Techniques	Detection	Test Principle, Advantages, and Limitations	Application	Clinical Examples
	TaqMan minor groove binder (MGB) probes	TaqMan MGB probes binds to the minor groove of the DNA helix and produces fluorescence in the same fashion as ordinary double-dye probes. For detailed description, see Kutayavin et al. (313). **Advantages:** stronger and higher affinity than ordinary TaqMan probes; MGB increases the Tm of the probe resulting in shorter probe sequence, which fit tricky AT-rich target sequences; can discriminate on one base mismatch **Disadvantages:** higher cost than other double-dye probes	Detection of acquired genes and SNPs, quantification of target DNA/RNA	*M. tuberculosis* resistance SNPs in *rpoB, katG, embB* (314) Glycopeptide resistance genes: *vanA, vanB1/B2* (315)
	Molecular beacon (MB) probes, include melting-curve analysis for SNP detection	MB probes have a fluorophore at 5' and a quencher at 3'. When MB probes are in a hairpin stem structure, light is quenched. Light is not quenched when MB probes are in a stretched out structure hybridized to a complementary target. For detailed description, see Tyagi and Kramer (316) or Drake and Tan (317). **Advantages:** high specificity; the stem loop structure keeps a close proximity of the fluorophore and quencher moieties, which gives a good quenching and a high S/N **Disadvantages:** more complex probe design then, e.g., double-dye probes	Detection of acquired genes and SNPs, quantification of target DNA/RNA	MRSA/VRSA *vanA, mecA*, PVL genes (318)
				M. tuberculosis rifampin resistance SNPs in *rpoB* (319)
	SYBR Green I melt-curve analysis	SYBR Green I is used as a nonsaturated intercalating dye binding all double-stranded DNA (dsDNA). Different amplicons have specific Tm values. **Advantages:** low cost compared to probe detection, easy to use, sensitive **Disadvantages:** nonspecific SYBR green binds to all dsDNA; thus, primer dimers can be misinterpreted as a specific product; time-consuming compared to probe detections; not optimal for multiplex assays	Detection of acquired genes	Quinolone resistance genes: *qnrA, qnrB, qnrS, qnrC, qnrD, qepA* (297)

Method	Detection	Description	Capabilities	Examples
	High-resolution melting dyes (HRM dyes)	HRM dyes can, in contrast to SYBR Green I, saturate dsDNA without inhibiting the PCR reaction. Thus, changes in the Tm of the amplicons can be seen even for single base changes. For detailed description, see Taylor (320). **Advantages:** ease of use, high sensitivity and specificity, low cost, SNP detection **Disadvantages:** cannot get the actual sequence, so it cannot substitute sequencing	Detection of SNPs, DNA methylation analysis	*M. tuberculosis* resistance SNPs in *rpoB, katG, inhA* promoter (321) Linezolid resistant SNP in 23S rRNA gene (322)
Nucleic acid sequence–based amplification (NASBA)	Molecular beacon probes, include meting-curve analysis to detect SNP	Isothermal RNA amplification method. DNA detection requires denaturation. For detailed description, see Compton (323). **Advantages:** no requirement for thermal cycler; rapid kinetics; single-stranded RNA product does not require denaturation prior to detection **Disadvantages:** reagent not as robust as PCR reagents, laborious reagent preparation.	Detection of acquired genes and SNPs, quantification of target DNA/RNA	MRSA (324)
Loop-mediated isothermal amplification (LAMP)	Turbidity or SYBR Green I	One-step amplification reaction at isothermal conditions. For detailed description, see Notomi et al. (325). **Advantages:** no requirement for thermal cycler; rapid kinetics, cost-effective **Disadvantages:** complex assay design	Detection of acquired genes	Linezolid resistance gene *cfr* (268) MRSA *spa* and *mecA* genes (326) Carbapenemase resistance gene *bla*$_{NDM}$ (204)
Helicase-dependent amplification (HDA)	AGE, include LUX primers to quantify fluorescence in real-time	Isothermal amplification using DNA helicase to separate dsDNA and DNA polymerase for extension. For detailed description, see Vincent et al. (327). **Advantages:** no requirement for thermal cycler; rapid kinetics **Disadvantages:** higher reagent cost than PCR reagents	Detection of acquired genes, quantification of target DNA	*M. tuberculosis* rifampin resistance SNPs in *rpoB* (328) MRSA *nuc* and *mecA* genes (329)

aAGE, agarose gel electrophoresis.
MRSA, methicillin-resistant *Staphylococcus aureus*; PCR, polymerase chain reaction; SNP, single nucleotide polymorphism; S/N, signal/noise.

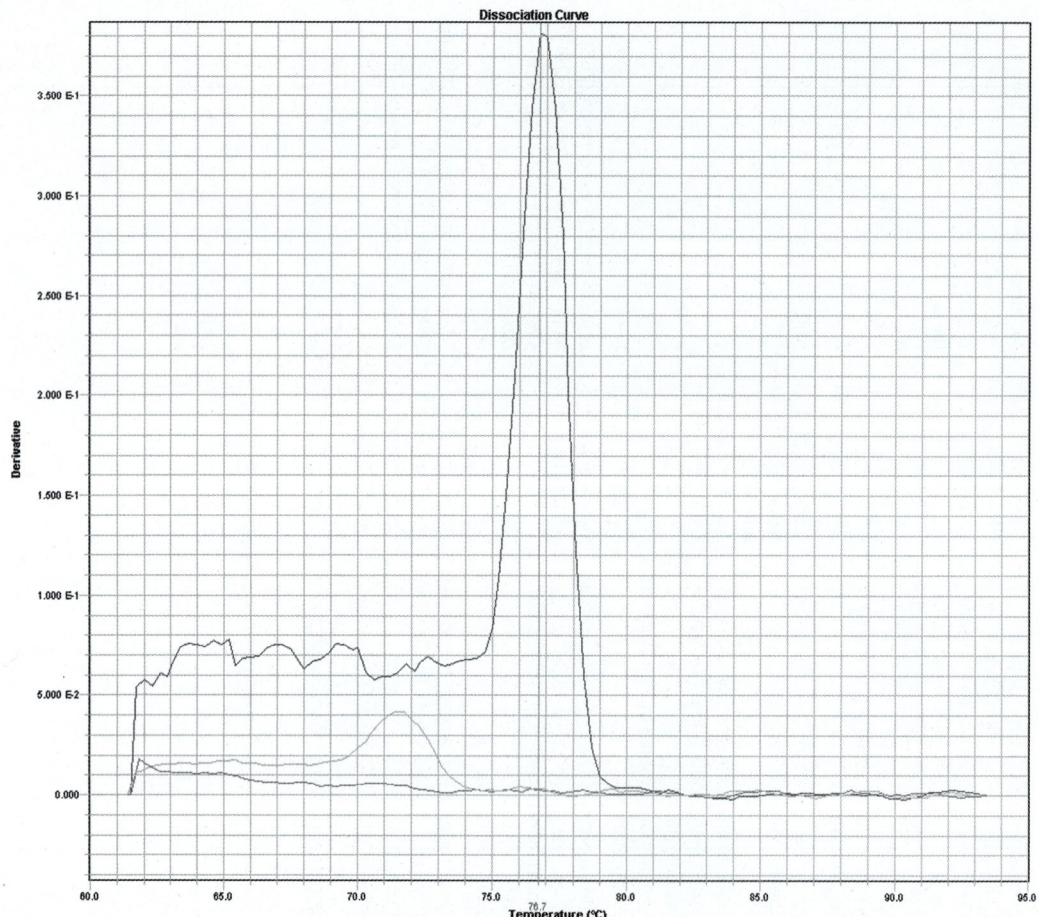

Figure 9.1 ■ SYBR Green I melting-curve analysis illustrating a positive *nuc* gene amplification with a Tm 76,7°C (*blue*), and two negative samples (*red* and *orange*). The *orange* melt-curve has an unspesific amplification most likely a primer dimer. (See Color Plate in the front of the book.)

or to reveal methylation of 23S rRNA by the *cfr* (chloramphenicol–florfenicol resistance) gene (34). Furthermore, MALDI-TOF MS–based mini-sequencing can reveal nucleotide polymorphisms responsible for antimicrobial resistance, that is, TEM-type extended-spectrum β-lactamase polymorphisms (35) and drug-resistant *M. tuberculosis* (36). Proteomic analyses using MALDI-TOF MS to identify proteins associated with resistance by peptide mass fingerprinting following sodium dodecyl sulfate polyacrylamide gel electrophoresis or 2D electrophoresis has been used to identify outer membrane or periplasmic proteins with different expression levels in resistant compared to susceptible isolates (37–41). Application of MALDI-TOF MS in proteomic analyses can complement molecular genetic techniques in reference or research laboratories. However, some

of their applications will be challenged by the use of WGS in the near future (26).

Nucleotide Sequencing Techniques and Their Application in Detection of Antimicrobial Resistance

Traditional Sanger dideoxy terminator sequencing, the gold standard for 30 years, has mainly been used to identify SNPs resulting in antimicrobial resistance rather than determining the presence of acquired resistance genes. Once the acquired genetic trait has been explored, the presence or absence of this is sufficient to reveal resistance mechanisms. The expanding need for whole genome sequence information has fuelled

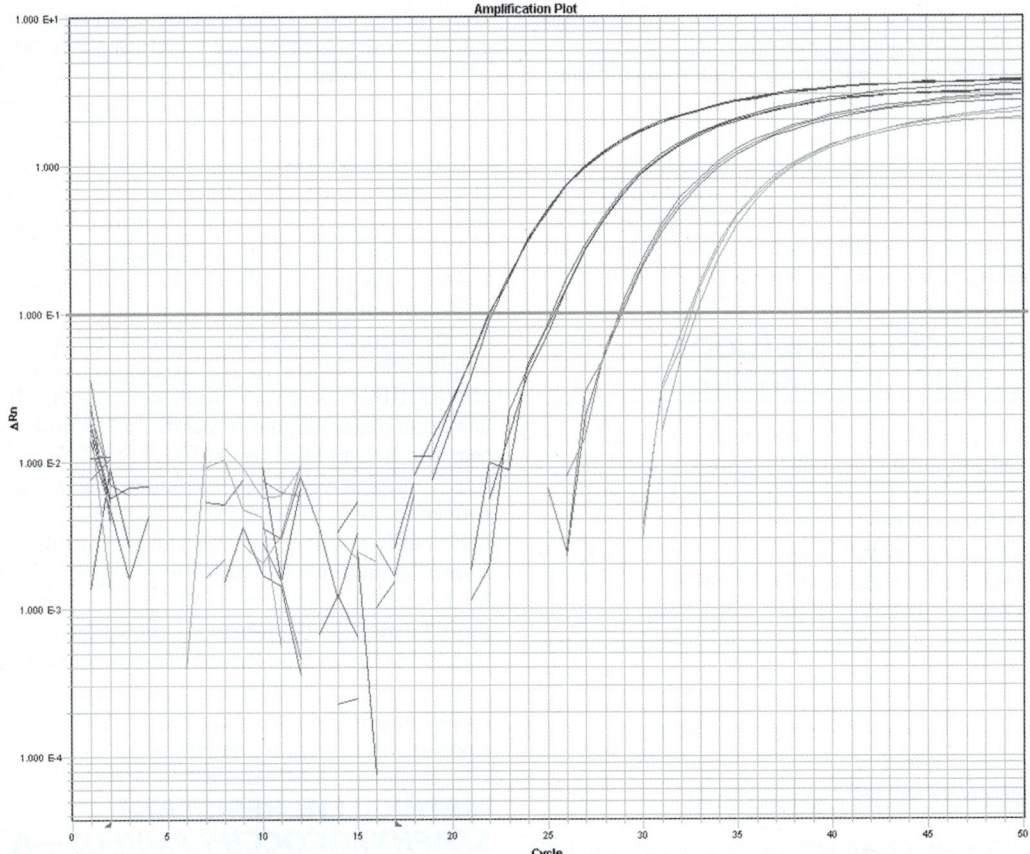

Figure 9.2 ■ Amplification plot showing four 10-fold dilutions of MRSA samples in triplicates, targeting SCC *mec* I gene. Detecion by molecular beacon probe, labeled with Fam in 5′and Dabcyl in 3′end. The *x axis* shows the number of PCR cycles, and the *y axis* shows fluorescent units in a logarithmic scale. The *green horizontal line* defines the cycle threshold value (CT-value) of each positive sample that crosses this line and is read at the *x axis*. A sample with a low CT-value has a higher starting concentration of the target compared to a sample with a higher CT-value. (See Color Plate in the front of the book.)

a technical revolution. Today's sequencers provided large volumes of genetic information in high resolution at dramatically decreased cost. Recent reviews have in detail described available first- to fourth-generation sequencing methods and their relevant characteristics and applications (42,43).

The turnaround time, cost, and user-friendliness of WGS have improved tremendously. Thus, whole bacterial genome sequencing is predicted to be a future routine method for species identification, the examination of antimicrobial resistance and virulence determinants as well as monitoring the evolution and clonal spread of bacterial pathogens (18).

Rapid WGS has already been used to investigate outbreaks of MRSA (44) and carbapenem-resistant

Klebsiella pneumoniae (45) and to unravel the molecular mechanisms in development of antimicrobial resistance during antimicrobial treatment of infections with multidrug-resistant *Acinetobacter baumannii* (46) and *K. pneumoniae* (45). Zankari et al. (47) have developed a continuously updated Web-based program (ResFinder at http://www .genomicepidemiology.org) presenting an easy way to identify acquired antimicrobial resistance genes in whole genome data. However, it is important when using this database to adjust the software ID threshold to less than 100% to find resistance genes that have mutations not recorded in the database. Furthermore, the results are categorized into different antimicrobial groups, but it is still important to understand the resulting genetic information in the context of the antimicrobial susceptibility profile.

The use of sequencing in clinical microbiology also call for a quality standard for sequence-based assays defining DNA sequence quality as well as quality of reference sequences from external databases. Extended comments on automated sequence quality assessments and the quality control of currently available databases have been pertinently outlined by Underwood and Green (48).

MOLECULAR METHODS: QUALITY ASSURANCE

It is critical that the molecular assays are sufficiently validated and quality assured for diagnostic purposes. This is not obvious even for methods published in peer review journals (authors own experiences). The validation of an assay has some key parameters to test such as sensitivity, specificity, accuracy, precision, limit of detection, detection range, repeatability and reproducibility, and external quality assessment (EQA)/proficiency testing, for example, Quality Control for Molecular Diagnostics (http://www.qcmd.org) (49,50).

Nucleic Acid Extraction

High-quality RNA/DNA provided by nucleic acid extraction is a prerequisite for the performance of NAAT. Both in-house and commercial as well as manual, semi-automated, and fully automated extraction systems are used for nucleic acid extraction. Silica solid-phase extraction by centrifugation or vacuum, coated and uncoated magnetic beads extraction, and magnetic silica beads extraction are commonly used in automated systems. The four main steps in nucleic acid extraction are cell disruption, lysis, wash and removal of cell debris and inhibitor buffer, and, finally, recovery of pure nucleic acid without inhibitors.

Inhibitors and enhancers can influence the sensitivity of a NAAT-based method at all stages. Inhibitors can originate from the clinical sample or extraction buffers, typically the lysis buffer or ethanol. The inhibitors can be the result of suboptimal extraction protocols not suitable for the test material or difficult-to-treat clinical samples such as sputum or whole blood.

The credibility of the sample result of a NAAT depends on the validation process of the assay and on types and number of controls that runs every time the assay is performed. The controls are meant to assure you that the process has been optimally performed. During nucleic acid extraction, positive and negative process controls (PPC and NPC) are needed. The PPC is a known positive reference strain that is diluted to 1 log above the limit of detection. Transport medium or ddH$_2$O is typically used as NPC. The purpose of the PPC is to confirm that the extraction process is performed optimally. If the PPC is negative after the NAAT, you need to rerun all samples from extraction. The purpose of the NPC is to check for cross-contamination during extraction.

An internal control (IC), also called internal amplification control (IAC) or internal positive control (IPC), is an inhibition control. The IC can be an oligo, plasmid or purified PCR product that will be amplified during the NAAT. Inhibition control is preferably introduced before the extraction step, for example, spiked in the magnetic beads solution, but can also be introduced from the amplification step, for example, spiked in the NAAT master mix. All negative samples should detect the IC; otherwise, the sample result should be discharged. The sample or nucleic acid elute should then be diluted 1:1 and rerun. When performing NAAT, it is recommended to include a positive and a negative amplification control.

METHICILLIN-RESISTANT *STAPHYLOCOCCUS AUREUS*—A TARGET FOR MOLECULAR DETECTION WITH INCREASING COMPLEXITY

Characteristics of Methicillin-Resistant *Staphylococcus aureus*

S. aureus is a major human pathogen within health care institutions and in the community. Thus, the overall resistance profile in clinical strains of *S. aureus* has an important impact on guidelines for empirical treatment of bacterial infections in general and bloodstream infection in particular. Wild-type *S. aureus* is naturally susceptible to β-lactam antimicrobials with the exception of monobactams. The high prevalence of penicillinase production in *S. aureus* has rendered the penicillinase-stable penicillins (oxacillin, cloxacillin, nafcillin, methicillin) the most active β-lactams.

Resistance toward penicillinase-stable penicillins in *S. aureus* is named methicillin resistance although this antimicrobial is not in clinical use. Methicillin resistance in *S. aureus* (MRSA) is caused by the acquisition of a *mecA* gene encoding a β-lactam low-affinity penicillin-binding protein

(PBP), termed PBP2a or PBP2'. PBP2a substitute the essential functions of the high-affinity PBPs in the presence of β-lactam antimicrobials, rendering the bacteria resistant to this important class of antimicrobials (51). The regulation of *mecA* expression is complex. Expression of *mecA* in a minor fraction of the bacterial population (heterogeneous expression) challenge phenotypic detection and requires molecular confirmation (52).

The new cephalosporins (ceftobiprole and ceftaroline) have a strong affinity for PBP2a and are active against MRSA (53). However, penicillinase-stable penicillins remain the reference β-lactams in the treatment of *S. aureus* infections in the absence of methicillin resistance. Infections with MRSA are associated with higher morbidity and mortality and increased hospital costs (54). Thus, rapid and accurate detection of MRSA from pure culture or directly in clinical samples are important for tailoring individual antimicrobial treatment as well as the implementation of appropriate infection control measurements to prevent the spread in health care institutions. Molecular techniques are used to confirm phenotypically suspected MRSA and to reduce the detection time in clinical samples.

Molecular Methods for Detection of Methicillin-Resistant *Staphylococcus aureus*

The development of molecular methods for detection of MRSA has been based on our current understanding of the genetic support of the *mecA* gene and its wide distribution in *S. aureus* and several coagulase-negative staphylococci (CoNS). The conserved 2.1 kb *mecA* gene is carried by a mobile genetic element in staphylococci, designated the *staphylococcal cassette chromosome mec* (SCC*mec*) (55). The SSC*mec* varies in size and content. A number of SCC*mec* types have been characterized (http://www.sccmec.org/Pages/SCC_HomeEN.html) and more diversity is to be expected. SSC*mec* encode recombinases (cassette chromosome recombinases [*ccr*]) that mediate excision and site-specific integration at the chromosomal *att*B site near the 3' end of *orfX*.

An array of different molecular strategies has been developed for the detection of MRSA, and selected publications are presented in Table 9.2. Some methods have targeted *mecA* itself and linked *S. aureus*–specific chromosomal genes (*nuc, femA*) in multiplex formats to differentiate between MRSA and other methicillin-resistant staphylococci (56–58). New insights into the detailed organization of SCC*mec* provided new concepts for MRSA-specific PCRs bridging the SSC*mec*-chromosomal *orfX* junction site (59). Developments of these strategies into real-time PCR assays have significantly improved their application in clinical microbiology. These methods are, together with the immunologic detection of PBP2', used as standard tests for MRSA detection and confirmation.

Challenges and Possibilities for Molecular Diagnostics of Methicillin-Resistant *Staphylococcus aureus*

The recent detection of a novel *mecA* homologue in human and bovine *S. aureus* populations has challenged our current molecular methods for

Table 9.2

Molecular Methods for Detection of Methicillin-Resistant *Staphylococcus aureus*			
Method	**Target**	**Substrate**	**Reference**
Multiplex PCR	*nuc, mecA*	Pure culture	Brakstad et al. (56)
Multiplex PCR	*nuc, mecA*	Pure culture	Vannuffel et al. (57)
Real-time multiplex PCR	SCC*mec, orfX*	Pure culture Clinical samples	Huletsky et al. (59)
Real-time multiplex PCR	*mecA, S. aureus* specific *femA*	Blood culture	Paule et al. (58)
Real-time multiplex PCR (BD gene Ohm/IDI-MRSA)	SCC*mec, orfX*	Clinical samples	Evaluated by Paule et al. (330) and Malhotra-Kumar et al. (66)
Real-time PCR	*mecC*	Pure culture	Stegger et al. (62)
Real-time multiplex PCR	*mecA, mecC, nuc*, PVL	Pure culture	Pichon et al. (63)

PCR, polymerase chain reaction.

detection of MRSA (60). The new *mecA* homologue is now classified as *mecC* in line with phylogenetic principles. *mecC* shows only 70% nucleotide sequence homology to *mecA*. Consequently, *mecC* and its corresponding PBP is not detected by conventional *mecA*-based PCRs or commercial immunologic PBP2' assays, respectively (61). Recent progress in molecular detection of MRSA has taken our extended knowledge on *mec*-alleles into consideration, both in the design of new PCR formats (62,63) and in a rapid micro-array-based detection (64).

The increasing repertoire of clinically relevant *mec*-homologues will also challenge the prospects for a rapid proteomic-based approach in the detection of MRSA. Both MALDI-TOF MS methods as well as surface-enhanced laser desorption-ionization time-of-flight (SELDI-TOF) MS has been described for the discrimination between methicillin-susceptible *S. aureus* (MSSA) and MRSA (31,65). A recent review on the application of MALDI-TOF MS in the detection of antimicrobial resistance concluded that the previously mentioned test needed further validation, although reproducible MRSA-specific profiles were obtained (26).

In conclusion, genetic detection of MRSA from pure cultures and complex clinical samples can be approached by a diversity of amplification-based techniques including in-house and commercial methods (66). Proteomic-based assays, except immunologic PBP2'-detection, need further refinements to be used in routine diagnostics. Methods based on the detection of *SCCmec* integration sites should take into account the increasing modular and sequence diversity in *SCCmec* types that may provide both false-positive and false-negative results. Moreover, antimicrobial selection will continue to facilitate transfer and stabilization of new *mec* homologues from commensals to *S. aureus* and challenge our molecular diagnostic repertoire targeting only known *mec* types (61).

DETECTION OF ACQUIRED GLYCOPEPTIDE RESISTANCE GENES

VRE and vancomycin-resistant *Enterococcus faecium* (VREfm) in particular are common nosocomial pathogens worldwide (67). The rates of vancomycin resistance monitored in medical centers in Europe, North and Latin America, and the Asia-Pacific region in 2004 to 2006 were less than 5% for *Enterococcus faecalis* and varied from 12% in Europe to 66% in North America for *E. faecium*

(68). The implementation of measures to control health care–associated VREfm are by many considered unmanageable with those resistance rates. However, the burden of VRE infections should not be belittled (70). VRE bloodstream infections are associated with increased mortality. Increased density of *van*-determinants and associated resistances will raise the risk of transfer to other gram-positive pathogens.

The *van* Alphabet

The vancomycin resistance cluster (*van*) alphabet in enterococci currently consist of nine gene clusters, namely the acquired *vanA*, *vanB*, *vanD*, *vanE*, *vanG*, *vanL* (69), *vanM* (71), and *vanN* (72), and the intrinsic *vanC* genotype in *Enterococcus gallinarum* and *Enterococcus casseliflavus*. Resistance is due to synthesis of altered peptidoglycan precursors with peptide side chains that terminate in D-lactate (*vanA*, *vanB*, *vanD* and *vanM*) or D-serine (*vanC*, *vanE*, *vanG*, *vanL*, and *vanN*) for which vancomycin has lower affinity than the normal D-alanine side chain terminus (73–76). Their characteristics and species distribution are summarized in Table 9.3. Both *vanA*, *vanB*, *vanG*, *vanM*, and *vanN* have been shown to be transferable between enterococci as part of large conjugative chromosomal elements or plasmids (69,71,72). However, the vast majority of VRE is associated with *vanA* and *vanB* determinants hosted by *E. faecium* or *E. faecalis*. Importantly, several independent cases of *vanA* transfer to *S. aureus* and MRSA have been reported (77). *S. aureus* may coexist with VRE in the gastrointestinal tract or superficial wounds, providing a likely reservoir for development of vancomycin-resistant *S. aureus* (VRSA) (78).

The *vanA* genotype is currently the most prevalent VRE genotype worldwide, but rates of infections with *vanB*-type VRE (mainly VREfm) infections are increasing in several European countries and are predominant in Australia (79–85). In contrast to *vanA*, the *vanB* ligase gene has been divided into three subtypes, *vanB1–3*, based on phylogenetic diversity (86–88). The most prevalent *vanB2* subtype (89–100) has been identified in adapted bacterial genera of the normal intestinal flora such as *Atopobium*, *Clostridium*, *Ruminococcus*, *Eggerthella*, and *Streptococcus* (101–104). The *vanB2* subtype has also been observed in two clinical samples of *Atopobium* and *Clostridium* (104). Interestingly, the *vanB2* subtype has a high prevalence in community and hospital human fecal specimens in the absence of cultivable VRE

Table 9.3

Glycopeptide Resistance due to *van*-Type Gene Clusters and Relevant Characteristics

Resistance	Acquired								Intrinsic
Level	High	Variable	High	Moderate	Low				Low
Type	VanA	VanB	VanM	VanD	VanE	VanG	VanL	VanN	VanC
MIC in mg/L:									
Vancomycin	≥16	≥2[a]	>256	≥16	6–32	12–16	8	12–16	2–32
Teicoplanin	>8[b]	0.5–1[c]	>0.75	0.25–64	0.5	0.5		0.5	0.5–1
van ligase gene	*vanA*	*vanB1-B3*	*vanM*	*vanD1-5*	*vanE*	*vanG1-2*	*vanL*	*vanN*	*vanC1-C3*
Modified target	D-alanine-D-lactate	D-alanine-D-lactate	D-alanine-D-lactate	D-alanine-D-lactate	D-alanine-D-serine	D-alanine-D-serine	D-alanine-D-serine	D-alanine-D-serine	D-alanine-D-serine
Transferable	Yes	Yes	Yes	No	No	Yes	No	Yes	No
Distribution	E. faecium E. faecalis E. avium E. casseliflavus E. durans E. gallinarum E. hirae E. mundtii E. raffinosus S. aureus S. epidermidis S. succinus S. saprophyticus Bacillus circulans Oerskovia turbata Arcanobacterium haemolyticum Paenibacillus Rhodococcus	E. faecium E. faecalis E. casseliflavus E. durans E. gallinarum E. hirae S. epidermidis S. succinus Streptococcus Clostridium Ruminococcus Eggerthella Atopobium	E. faecium	E. faecium E. faecalis E. avium E. gallinarum E. raffinosus Ruminococcus Nonenterococcal fecal flora	E. faecalis	E. faecalis Clostridium difficile Ruminococcus Nonenterococcal fecal flora	E. faecalis	E. faecium	E. gallinarum – vanC1 E. casseliflavus – vanC2/3

[a]Low-level MIC may occur in some strains due to weak induction of resistance expression. However, these strains are still important to diagnose, as glycopeptide treatment lead to selection of constitutively expressed glycopeptide resistance (331–335) and treatment failure.

[b]Some strains with *vanA* genotype are susceptible to teicoplanin and, thus, show a VanB phenotype; others are low-level resistant to vancomycin and intermediate-resistant to teicoplanin and, thus, show a VanD phenotype.

[c]Development of teicoplanin resistance of *vanB*-containing isolates may happen, but the majority of isolates are susceptible to teicoplanin.

(105–107). The high rates of nonenterococcal *vanB* in fecal samples result in a low predictive positive value for VRE using PCR detection of *vanB* directly from fecal samples (107–111), whereas *vanA* detection is more specific (111–113).

Possible Methods for Molecular Detection of *van* Genes

MALDI-TOF MS technology has been used to identify and investigate the epidemiology of an outbreak with *vanB*-positive VREfm (30), and an array of Raman-enhancing nanoparticles coated with vancomycin has been employed to capture VRE from human blood (114). Thus, the future holds promise for use of novel techniques to detect VRE. However, today, most described techniques for molecular detection of glycopeptide resistance involves amplification of the *van* genes.

A number of amplification techniques to detect the glycopeptide resistance genes have been developed. Methods that detect at least the two most common *van* genotypes (*vanA* and *vanB*) and evaluated on well-characterized strain collections or clinical specimens in comparison with in vitro susceptibility tests are listed in Table 9.4.

Amplification techniques are easy and useful tools for reference laboratories and routine labs that wish to confirm the phenotypic detection or investigate the molecular epidemiology of VRE. However, there are some aspects that are important to consider when applying these techniques. The *vanB*, *vanD*, and *vanG* determinants have subtypes. Thus, primers and probes described in the literature to hybridize to these *van* genotypes have been checked in silico against all subtypes to reveal ambiguities and notes of which subtypes they are likely to cover have been made in Table 9.4. Importantly, although the *vanB2* subtype is the most widespread subtype of *vanB*, not all PCR-based methods detect this subtype.

Because the *van* genes can be found in other bacterial genera than enterococci, it is important to consider when performing screening on biologic samples that many molecular methods detect the *van* genes and not VRE per se. Methods that detect only the *van* genes are thus expected to have a higher rate of false-positive results. Some of the methods listed in Table 9.4 include species-specific (*E. faecalis* and *E. faecium ddl, E. faecium recG*) or genus-specific (*tuf*) genes for identification of enterococci or staphylococci (*S. aureus nuc, Staphylococcus epidermidis* species-specific gene) to overcome this problem.

An oligonucleotide DNA microarray with 105 probes that target 42 genes of the glycopeptide resistance gene clusters *vanA, vanB, vanC, vanD, vanE,* and *vanG* including the subtypes of *vanB, vanD,* and *vanG* as well as detection of *ermB* and the *E. faecalis* specific gene *lsa* correctly identified the different genotypes of reference and other VRE strains with various phenotypes (115). This microarray give additional and complementary information compared to phenotype alone and is suitable for reference laboratories that wish to reveal the genetic content of the *van* clusters explaining defective gene clusters and identifying additional resistance elements masked by a similar resistance phenotype. This array is not commercially available. Moreover, all presently known *van* clusters are not included in this array. Thus, WGS will be a better research approach to identify all present resistance elements contributing to a phenotype because this will also give the opportunity to explore the unknown.

RESISTANCE TO MACROLIDES, LINCOSAMIDES, AND STREPTOGRAMINS: RELEVANT RESISTANCE ELEMENTS, PHENOTYPIC EXPRESSION, AND THEIR DETECTION

Characteristics of Resistance to Macrolide, Lincosamide, and Streptogramin Antibiotics

A multiplicity of clinical relevant mechanisms of macrolide, lincosamide, and streptogramin (MLS antimicrobials) resistance is found (116–119). A recently updated database on MLS resistance genes is available at http://faculty.washington.edu/marilynr/. The nomenclature review of MLS resistance genes in 1999 defined that a new MLS gene must have a 79% or less amino acid identity with all previously characterized MLS determinants before receiving a unique name (116). The conservative criteria are controversial for some of the genes, as determinants with higher identity score may have different host range and genetic support (118,120). Herein, we focus on the most prevalent and clinical relevant determinants of resistance and their molecular detection. Phenotypic antimicrobial susceptibility testing distinguishes between the main groups of MLS resistance mechanism and guides antimicrobial therapy. Thus, the main purpose for genotypic identification is related to molecular epidemiology issues, understanding the

Table 9.4

Amplification Methods for Detection of Glycopeptide Resistance Genes

Amplification Reaction	Genes Detected	Substrate	Extraction Method	Detection	Reference
PCR	vanA, vanB1/B2/B3, vanC1/C2/C3	Enrichment broth		AGE	Sundsfjord et al. (16)
PCR	vanA, vanB2/B3, maybe vanB1 (single mismatch in forward primer), vanD1/D2/D3/D4, maybe vanD5 (single mismatch in forward primer), vanE, vanG1/G2	Rectal swab		AGE	Domingo et al. (105)
Single and multiplex PCR	vanA, vanB1, maybe vanB2 (single mismatch in forward primer), vanC1, vanC2/C3, ddl E. faecalis, ddl E. faecium	Enrichment broth	Alkaline lysis with lysozyme	AGE	Dutka-Malen et al. (336)
Multiplex PCR-RFLP	vanA, vanB1/B3, maybe vanB2 (single mismatch in reverse primer)	Agar-grown colony	95°C 10 min	MspI restriction and AGE	Patel et al. (337)
Multiplex PCR	vanA, vanB1, some vanB2, maybe all vanB2 and vanB3 (single mismatch in forward primer)	Enrichment broth	95°C 20 min	AGE	Bell et al. (338)
Multiplex PCR	vanA, vanB1, maybe vanB2 (single mismatch in forward primer), 16S rDNA internal PCR control	Rectal swab	Chelex	AGE	Jayaratne and Rutherford (339)
Multiplex PCR	vanA, vanB1, maybe vanB2/B3 (single mismatch in both primers)	Rectal swab or stool specimen	XTRAX	Enzyme immunoassay	Petrich et al. (340)
Multiplex PCR	vanA, vanB1, vanC1/C2/C3, ddl E. faecalis, recG E. faecium, 16S rDNA internal PCR control	Agar-grown colony	Chelex	AGE	Kariyama et al. (341)
Multiplex PCR	vanA, vanB1/B2, maybe vanB3 (single mismatch in reverse primer), vanC1/C2/C3	Enrichment broth Agar-grown colony	QIAamp tissue kit Triton X	AGE	Lu et al. (342)
Multiplex PCR	vanA, vanB1/B2/B3, vanC1, vanC2/C3, ddl E. faecalis, recG E. faecium, 16S rDNA internal PCR control	Agar-grown colony		AGE	Elsayed et al. (308)
Multiplex PCR	vanA, vanB1, maybe vanB2 (single mismatch in forward primer), vanC1, vanC2/C3, tuf	Agar-grown colony	100°C 10 min	AGE	Perez-Hernandez et al. (343)
Multiplex PCR	vanA, vanB1, vanC1/C2/C3, ddl E. faecalis, ddl and recG E. faecium	Agar-grown colony	Chelex	AGE	Mac et al. (344)
Multiplex PCR	vanA, vanB1/B2/B3, vanC1/C2/C3, vanD1/D2/D3/D4, maybe vanD5 (single mismatch in both primers), vanE, vanG1, vanG2 (two mismatches in forward primer), ddl E. faecalis, ddl E. faecium, nuc S. aureus, S. epidermidis specific sequence	Enrichment broth	Alkaline lysis with lysozyme	AGE	Depardieu et al. (345)

(Continued)

Table 9.4 (Continued)

Amplification Methods for Detection of Glycopeptide Resistance Genes

Amplification Reaction	Genes Detected	Substrate	Extraction Method	Detection	Reference
TAAG Diagnostics QuickTAAG VRE kit (multiplex PCR)	vanA, vanB (not specified if targets all different subtypes of vanB), vanC1/C2/C3, sequences of E. faecium and E. faecalis species	Rectal swabs	DNExtract Swab kit	PCR fragment sizes estimated by TAAG multidetection system	Evaluated by Benadof et al. (346)
Seeplex VRE detection (dual-priming–based multiplex PCR)	vanA, vanB (not specified if targets all different subtypes of vanB)	Enrichment broth	100°C 10 min	AEG Screen tape system (auto-capillary electrophoresis)	Evaluated by Lee et al. (347) and Seo et al. (113)
High-resolution melt multiplex PCRs	vanA, vanB1, some vanB2, maybe all vanB2 and vanB3 (single mismatch in forward primer), enterococcal 16S-23S rRNA intergenic spacer region	Agar-grown colonies	95°C 10 min	High-resolution melt analyses	Gurtler et al. (348)
Real-time multiplex PCR	vanA, vanB1, maybe vanB2 (single mismatch in forward primer and VanB-640 probe)	Agar-grown culture Rectal swab Enrichment broth	Chelex QIAamp DNA Stool kit	Fluorescent hybridization probes signals detected by LightCycler	Palladino et al. (349,350)
Roche LightCycler vanA/vanB detection assay (real-time multiplex PCR)	vanA, vanB1/B2/B3, internal PCR control	Agar-grown culture Perianal swab in S.T.A.R. buffer Fecal specimens	100°C 10 min Total Nucleic Acid Isolation kit (Roche), MagNA Pure automatic extraction QIAamp DNA stool kit	Fluorescent hybridization probes signals or melting-curve analyses in LightCycler	Evaluated by Sloan et al. (351) and Young et al. (107)
BD GeneOhm VanR assay (real-time multiplex PCR)	vanA, vanB1/B2/B3, internal PCR control	Rectal/perianal swabs in BD GeneOhm VanR sample buffer Stool samples	BD GeneOhm VanR lysis tube containing glass beads	Fluorescent hybridization probes (molecular beacons) signals detected by SmartCycler	Evaluated by Usacheva et al. (108) and Gazin et al. (109)
Cepheid Xpert vanA/vanB (real-time multiplex PCR)	vanA, vanB (not specified if targets all different subtypes of vanB)	Rectal/perianal swabs Stool samples	Xpert vanA/vanB cartridge	GeneXpert	Evaluated by Bourdon et al. (110), Marner et al. (352), and Gazin et al. (109)
Real-time multiplex PCR	vanA, vanB1/B2	Enrichment broth	NorDiag Bullet system	TaqMan MGB probe signals in Applied Biosystems or LightCycler real-time PCR system	Fang et al. (315)

PCR, polymerase chain reaction; AGE, agarose gel electrophoresis; PCR-RFLP, polymerase chain reaction–restriction fragment length polymorphism; VRE, vancomycin-resistant enterococci.

dissemination and origins of MLS-related resistance determinants and their dynamics.

MLS antimicrobials have different chemical structures, but they share similar mechanisms of action. They are all inhibitors of bacterial translation. The structural analysis of bacterial ribosomal subunits in complex with antimicrobial inhibitors at an anatomic level has revealed their overlapping target sites (the peptidyl transfer center and the peptide exit tunnel) in the 50S subunit complex (121). Thus, they share many of the same resistance mechanisms (122).

The most commonly used macrolide antimicrobials include the natural product drug erythromycin and the semisynthetic derivatives clarithromycin and azithromycin. Macrolides are classified according to the number of atoms in the macrolactone ring: 14-membered (erythromycin and clarithromycin), 15-membered (azithromycin), and 16-membered (spiramycin). Ketolides (telithromycin) are semisynthetic derivatives of macrolides. Lincosamides (clindamycin and lincomycin) lacks the lactone ring. Streptogramin antimicrobials consist of a mixture of type A peptide–polyketide hybrids and type B cyclic depsipeptides that act synergistically by binding to the peptidyl transfer center and the peptide exit tunnel, respectively (5).

The spectrum of antibacterial activity of MLS antimicrobials is mainly restricted to gram-positive cocci (staphylococci and streptococci) and bacilli and gram-negative cocci. Gram-negative bacteria are, in general, inherently resistant to macrolides due to efflux mechanisms and drug inactivation. Exceptions include important human pathogens such as *Bordetella pertussis*, *Campylobacter* spp, Chlamydiales, *Helicobacter pylori*, and *Legionella* spp.

Mechanisms of Macrolide, Lincosamide, and Streptogramin Resistance and Their Genetic Determinants

There are three major mechanisms of MLS resistance: (a) target site modification by methylation or mutation that prevents the binding of the antimicrobial to its 50S ribosomal complex, (b) active efflux, and (c) enzyme-catalyzed drug inactivation. These mechanisms have been found in the bacteria producing these antimicrobials (5). The impact of the three mechanisms is unequal in terms of distribution and therapeutic implications in pathogenic bacteria. In large, modification of the ribosomal target complex confers broad-spectrum MLS resistance, whereas efflux and enzymatic inactivation

affect only specific molecules. Resistance phenotypes affecting MLS antimicrobials and their genetic counterparts are presented in Table 9.5.

High-level resistance to macrolides is most often mediated by the enzyme-catalyzed methylation of the 23S rRNA by Erm (*e*rythromycin *r*ibosome *m*ethylase) methyltransferases encoded by *erm* genes that confer constitutive or inducible macrolide-lincosamide-streptogramin B (MLSB) resistance phenotypes (122). The number of described *erm* genes has already passed 40 (http://faculty.washington.edu/marilynr/). Four major *erm* classes are detected in pathogenic bacteria: *erm*(A), *erm*(B), *erm*(C), and *erm*(F) (118,122). Although *erm*(A) and *erm*(C) are typically detected in staphylococci, *erm*(B) class genes are mostly observed in streptococci and enterococci, whereas *erm*(F) are mostly described in *Bacteroides* and other anaerobes. In addition to the *erm*(B) genes, the *erm*TR genes (a subset of the *erm*[A] class) are widely distributed in β-hemolytic streptococci (118). The notion that each *erm* class may have a relatively specific distribution, but not strictly confined to a bacterial genus, reflects their association to mobile genetic elements and various mechanisms for horizontal gene transfer (118,123).

Low-level macrolide resistance is mainly associated with streptococci and linked to the production of an efflux pump (M phenotype) conferring resistance to erythromycin but not to clindamycin and/or streptogramins (122). A macrolide efflux system in streptococci was firmly established in 1996 (124). This system was phenotypically recognized and characterized to confer low-level resistance to 14- and 15-membered macrolides only. Several *mef* determinants have been described and the number varies dependent on criteria for definition of new elements (118,120).

A number of reports has shown marked differences between *mef*(A) and *mef*(E) (118). For instance, the different genetic elements carrying *mef*(A) or *mef*(E) and their contexts have been studied (125). Moreover, the two genes have disseminated markedly different in an ever growing number of species (120).

Molecular Detection Macrolide, Lincosamide, and Streptogramin Resistance Determinants

It is not much of a surprise to find that PCR is by far the most established method for the detection of MLS resistance genes and their genetic support. The high degree of similarity between major

Table 9.5

Main Macrolide, Lincosamide, and Streptogramin Resistance Phenotypes in Staphylococci, Streptococci, and Enterococci

Mechanism	Gene Class			Phenotype	Resistance Phenotype[a]			
	staphylococci	streptococci	enterococci		14- and 15-M	16-M	L	S
Ribosomal methylation	erm(A), erm(C)	erm(A) ermTR subclass[b]		Inducible MLS$_B$	R	S[c]	S[c]	S
	erm(B)	erm(B)	erm(B)	Constitutive MLS$_B$	R	R	R	S[d]
Efflux	msr(A), msr(C)		msr(A), msr(C)	MS$_B$	R	S	S	S[e]
Efflux		mef(A)/mef(E)	mef(A)	M	R	S	S	S
Enzymatic modification	lnu(A)	lnu(B)	lnu(B)	L	S	S	R[f]	S
Efflux?	vga(A), vga(Av), lsa(B), unknown determinants			LS$_A$	S	S	I	S/I
Enzymatic modification of factor A or B ± efflux of factor A	vat(A), vat(B), vat(C), vga(A), vga(Av), vga(B), vgb(A), vgb(B), mph(C) in various combinations		vat(D), vat(E), vgb(A) in various combinations	S or LS[g]	S	S	S or I[g]	R

[a]-M, membered macrolides; L, lincosamide; S, streptogramins.
[b]Constitutive resistance has been reported.
[c]Risk of selection of resistant mutants.
[d]Reduced bactericidal activity.
[e]Fourteen- and 15-membered macrolides induce resistance to streptogramin B.
[f]Resistance to lincomycin and susceptibility to clindamycin.
[g]Possibility of lincomycin and clindamycin resistance in the presence of vga(A) and vga(Av) genes.
Adapted from Leclercq R. Macrolides, lincosamides, and streptogramins. In: Courvalin P, Leclercq R, Rice LB, eds. *Antibiogram*. Portland, OR: Eska Publishing, 2010:305–326.

groups of resistance determinants does not allow a reliable discrimination to be made by using DNA hybridization experiments. Recommended primers for detection of MLS genes are available at http://faculty.washington.edu/marilynr/. Moreover, a diversity of different PCR primer combinations for amplification of the *mef* gene have been reported creating amplification products ranging from 202 to 1,759 bp (Table 3 in [120]). However, when using PCR to target resistance determinants with nucleotide diversity, one must take into account mismatches and in particular those located at the ultimate 3′-end of the primer sequence or multiple mismatches that may be present along the sequence of the primer(s). The use of such primers may result in an inefficient PCR or preferential amplification of *mef* gene subpopulations without the mismatch. A straightforward method for discrimination between *mef*(A)

and *mef*(E) is based on the differential presence of restriction enzyme recognition sites in the two genes. Restriction enzyme digest resolved by agarose gel electrophoresis is sufficient to establish the difference (120).

The complexity of MLS-related resistance phenotypes are increasing. Several additional phenotypes affecting L or S antibiotics only (L phenotype) or in combination (LS phenotype) and their respective resistance determinants have been described lately (126–128). Importantly, lincosamide nucleotidyltransferases encoded by plasmid-mediated *lnu* genotypes and affecting the bactericidal activity of clindamycin have been described in staphylococci (117,122,127). Moreover, clinically relevant macrolide resistance in gram-negative bacilli has recently been described. Emerging plasmid-mediated *mph*(A) determinants encoding macrolide kinases was associated with azithromycin treatment failure in pediatric shigellosis (129).

In conclusion, the identification of MLS resistance mechanisms is important to guide the clinical use of MLS antimicrobials. The presence of various resistance determinants is highly dynamic and varies considerably between countries, species, and infections. Thus, it is important for empiric therapy guidelines that the phenotypic surveillance data on MLS susceptibility data are complemented with genotypic data showing the resistance determinants involved (122,130).

MOLECULAR DETECTION OF DRUG RESISTANCE IN *MYCOBACTERIUM TUBERCULOSIS*

The Problem

Drug-resistant *M. tuberculosis* (tuberculosis [TB]) represents a global public health threat (131). Diagnostic delays lead to increased mortality, selection for secondary resistance, and further transmission. Consequently, it is important to deliver reliable drug susceptibility test (DST) results in a clinically useful time frame.

Conventional phenotypic drug susceptibility testing of *M. tuberculosis* takes weeks to complete, although more rapid, commercialized, broth-based methods have been developed (132). Moreover, culture-based DSTs are labor-intensive and time-consuming and handling of TB cultures represents a potential biologic hazard. Thus, WHO has endorsed the development of molecular approaches to provide a rapid, relevant DST result to time-appropriate treatment.

Initial TB treatment is empirical, based on clinical suspicion and positive direct smears. Isoniazid (INH), rifampin (RMP), pyrazinamide (PZA), and ethambutol (EMB) are considered to be used as standard first-line treatment. Other antimicrobials including fluoroquinolones (FQs) are considered second-line drugs prescribed in case of resistance or intolerance. Multidrug-resistant TB (MDR-TB) is defined as resistant to at least the two main first-line anti-TB drugs, RMP and INH. In contrast, extensively drug-resistant TB (XDR-TB) is an MDR isolate that, in addition, express resistance to an FQ and at least one of the following second-line injectable drugs: amikacin (AMK), kanamycin (KAN), and capreomycin (CAP). The evolution of drug resistance in *M. tuberculosis*, including mechanisms and genetic regions involved in resistance formation has recently been reviewed (133).

Drug Resistance Mechanisms in *Mycobacterium tuberculosis* and Their Molecular Detection

M. tuberculosis is intrinsically resistant to a number of antimicrobials. This is partially due to a thick, lipid-rich cell wall that prevents antimicrobials for reaching their target as well as drug-inactivating enzymes such as β-lactamases (133). Thus, only a limited number of antimicrobials are effective treatment options. Acquired clinically relevant drug resistance in *M. tuberculosis* is not due to horizontal gene transfer. *M. tuberculosis* has not been shown to harbor plasmids. Further, the clonal population structure of TB indicates a limited role of horizontal gene transfer in the evolution of the species.

Hence, the genetic basis for acquired clinically relevant drug resistance in *M. tuberculosis* is chromosomal mutations that occur spontaneously during error-prone polymerization of DNA (134). Favorable mutations are selected for during antimicrobial selection and passed further through vertical transmission. The mutations are localized in genes for the antimicrobial target and affects drug–target affinity (RMP, FQs, aminoglycosides [AGs], and EMB). Mutations may also involve genes encoding drug-activation enzymes affecting the transformation of inactive antimicrobials to an active metabolite (INH, PZA, and para-amino salicylic acid [PAS]). A diverse array of commercial and in-house genotypic DSTs has been developed based on direct or indirect detection of resistance-conferring mutations of which some of them are selectively presented in Table 9.6 (135). Sequence- or hybridization-based detection of mutations in amplified products has become the standard techniques. Their success and limitations are partially based on the current knowledge of the factual mutations that account for phenotypic resistance (14).

The mechanisms conferring resistance to the two main first-line drugs, RMP and INH, are the most relevant diagnostic targets in genotypic DSTs. RMP and/or INH resistance trigger therapeutic modifications, extended DST, and individual drug tailoring. Detection of MDR-TB requires the use of second-line drugs, and monoresistance leads to therapeutic adjustments in the consolidation phase to avoid unintended monotherapy and resistance development. RMP inhibits the early steps in transcription, binding the β-subunit

Table 9.6

Molecular Methods for Detection of Drug Resistance in *Mycobacterium tuberculosis*

Method	Target	Substrate	Reference
PCR + pyrosequencing	Multiple somatic mutations/ MDR-/XDR-TB	Pure culture	Engström et al. (14)
PCR (Xpert MTB/RIF)	*rpoB*/MDR-TB	Sputum	Scott et al. (354)
Hemi-nested PCR (Xpert MTB/RIF)	*rpoB*/MDR-TB	Sputum	Boehme et al. (142)
PCR + hybridization	16S rRNA	Culture	Marme et al. (355)
PCR + hybridization (INNO-LiPA Rif)	*rpoB*/MDR-TB	Culture and sputum	De Beenhouwer et al. (356)
PCR + hybridization (GenoType MTBDR plus)	*rpoB, katG, inhA*/MDR-TB	Culture and sputum	Crudu et al. (357)
PCR + hybridization (GenoType MTBDRsl)	*gyrA, embB, rrs*/XDR-TB	Culture and sputum	Hillemann et al. (141)
Real-time PCR	*rpoB, katG*/MDR-TB	Culture and sputum	Espasa et al. (358)
Real-time PCR	16S rRNA/XDR-TB	Culture	Blaschitz et al. (359)
Real-time PCR	*rpoB, katG, inhA*, IS6110	Culture	Ramirez et al. (312)

PCR, polymerase chain reaction; MDR-TB, multidrug-resistant tuberculosis.

encoded by *rpoB* (136). Phenotypic resistance is mostly confined to *rpoB* mutations in an 81-bp region named RMP resistance-determining region (RRDR). INH is a prodrug, activated by the catalase-peroxidase enzyme encoded by *katG* (137). Activated INH is believed to target a mycolic acid synthesis enzyme, enoyl-acyl carrier protein reductase InhA (138). Thus, phenotypic resistance to INH has been associated with mutations in *katG* affecting the activation of INH as well as *inhA* promoter mutations mediating InhA hyperexpression. Several in-house and commercial tests are available and proven effective in detection of both RMP and INH resistance including point-of-care diagnostics (139–141).

Although resistance mechanisms toward RMP, INH, and other anti-TB drugs are extensively investigated, they remain to be completely resolved. A recent comprehensive study of 290 clinical *M. tuberculosis* strains from four continents comparing phenotypic DST with pyrosequencing targeting mutations associated with resistance to RMP, INH, EMB, FQ, AG, and CAP showed a very high specificity in detection of MDR- and XDR-TB strains (14). However, the sensitivity of genotypic detection of phenotypic resistance to individual drugs varied considerably from 95% for RMP and 94% for INH to 61% for EMB, reflecting our incomplete understanding of clinically relevant resistance mechanisms.

In conclusion, specific and sensitive rapid commercial molecular tests for detection of both *M. tuberculosis* and RMP resistance directly from sputum samples have been validated and made available (142). The choice of molecular methods must take into consideration the local or national prevalence of *M. tuberculosis* and MDR-TB as well as available resources, technology, and competencies. Implementation of these technologies for routine point-of-care diagnosis of *M. tuberculosis* and MDR-TB at the primary care level is quite promising (143). Although feasible, high-burden countries are often associated with limitations in resources, personnel, and technology, restricting the use of these techniques to reference laboratories. Thus, to make a real impact in TB control, large scale implementation needs sustainable financial and operational support to meet the urgent need of cost-effective, simplistic methods for rapid, sensitive, and specific detection of *M. tuberculosis* and clinically relevant drug resistance outside reference centers. This is very important, as empiric treatment of TB without timely DST in regions with a burden of drug-resistant TB will continue to amplify drug-resistant TB at a high cost (144).

DETECTION AND IDENTIFICATION OF GENES CODING FOR EXTENDED-SPECTRUM β-LACTAMASES AND CARBAPENEMASES IN GRAM-NEGATIVE BACTERIA

The Growing Diversity of β-Lactamase

The first β-lactamase was identified as early as 1940 (145), before β-lactams were introduced into clinical use. Since then, the introduction of new β-lactam antibiotics in clinical practice and the corresponding emergence of new β-lactamases in human pathogens have evolved in parallel. Currently, the number of identified β-lactamases and variants has probably reached more than 1,000 (146) (http://www.lahey.org/Studies). In the last two decades, the dissemination and alarming prevalence of extended-spectrum β-lactamases (ESBLs) and carbapenemases have been the main concern. They are now threatening the use of β-lactams, which has been our largest and most valuable group of antimicrobials (147,148).

ESBLs are characterized by their hydrolytic activity against extended-spectrum cephalosporins (oxyimino-β-lactams) such as ceftazidime and cefotaxime, as well as being inhibited by the classical β-lactamase inhibitors (146). Carbapenems and cephamycins (e.g., cefoxitin) are generally not affected by ESBLs. The first ESBLs identified were variants of the TEM-1 and SHV-1 β-lactamases (149). The ESBL variants of TEM-1 and SHV-1 only differs from their progenitors by a few to a single amino acid change (149). The current number of TEM- and SHV-ESBL variants and the amino acid changes can be found on the β-lactamase Web site (http://www.lahey.org/Studies). In addition to TEM- and SHV-ESBL variants, the CTX-M ESBLs have emerged as the most prevalent ESBLs on a global scale (147,149–151). Currently, more than 130 CTX-M variants have been identified (http://www.lahey.org/Studies). Based on the amino acid sequence, the CTX-M ESBL can be grouped into five to seven subgroups/clusters: CTX-M-1/-3, CTX-M-2, CTX-M-8, CTX-M-9/-14, CTX-M-25, CTX-M-45, and CTX-M-64 (151–153). Other less prevalent ESBLs include GES, VEB, PER, BEL, BES, TLA, SFO, IBC, and OXA variants (149,154).

In contrast, carbapenemases are β-lactamases with the ability to hydrolyze carbapenems such as meropenem, imipenem, ertapenem, and doripenem (146). In addition, many of the carbapenemases have hydrolytic activity against all β-lactams. Consequently, the presence of one carbapenemase can give resistance to the whole β-lactam group of antimicrobials. Currently, the most significant problem is the global dissemination of mobile or acquired carbapenemases among various gram-negative bacteria (148,155).

Acquired carbapenemases have been identified in three Ambler classes of β-lactamases (A, B, and D). Acquired class A carbapenemases includes KPC, IMI, NMC-A, and SME where KPC is the most prevalent and 18 different variants (KPC-2 to KPC-19) have been identified so far (http://www.lahey.org/Studies) (148,155). The acquired class B carbapenemases includes the metallo-β-lactamases (MBLs) such as VIM, IMP, NDM, SPM, GIM, SIM, AIM, DIM, KHM, TMB, and SMB (148,155). The MBLs VIM, IMP, and NDM have shown a global dissemination and are the most prevalent MBLs (148,155). For these MBLs, several variants have also been identified to date with 41 VIM variants, 48 IMP variants, and 12 NDM variants identified to date (http://www.lahey.org/Studies). The acquired class D carbapenemases includes the OXA-carbapenemases, which can be grouped into two subgroups: (a) the OXA-carbapenemases, OXA-23–like, OXA-24/-40–like, OXA-58–like, and OXA-143, which are almost exclusively found among *Acinetobacter* spp and (b) the OXA-48–like carbapenemases found among Enterobacteriaceae (156,157). Although variable, all of these acquired carbapenemases have activity toward carbapenems. However, their activity toward other β-lactams varies. OXA-carbapenemases have limited or no activities toward extended-spectrum cephalosporins, and MBLs have no activities toward monobactams (aztreonam) (156,157).

Molecular Detection of β-Lactamases

Molecular methods for detection of ESBLs and carbapenemases are challenging for the clinical microbiology laboratory due to the large number of β-lactamase groups and diversity within groups. Further, the continuously changing epidemiologic landscape and emergence of new ESBLs or carbapenemases requires molecular methods to be adaptable to these changes. The presence of ESBLs and carbapenemases does not always result in clinical resistance according to the current breakpoints set by clinical breakpoints committees such as the European Committee for Antimicrobial Susceptibility Testing (EUCAST, http://www.eucast.org) or Clinical and Laboratory Standards Institute (CLSI, http://www.clsi.org). Further, it is advised that susceptibility results can be "reported as found" irrespective of the presence of an ESBL or carbapenemase. Consequently, molecular identification of ESBL or carbapenemase genes is not required for guidance of treatment. It should be noted that these guidelines are controversial and discussed (158).

Biochemical Methods for Detection of Extended-Spectrum β-Lactamases and Carbapenemases

The gold standard method for detection of β-lactamase activity is analysis of β-lactam hydrolysis by spectrophotometry. This method is mainly used in reference laboratories, as it requires specialized equipment and training in interpretation of the hydrolytic curves. Further, the method is relatively slow, as it requires overnight growth of liquid bacterial cultures and preparation of a protein extract (159,160). Recent evaluations of this method also indicate that detection of carbapenem hydrolysis by NDM and OXA-carbapenemases in *A. baumannii* is difficult (161).

Another, novel biochemical approach has been described for detection of ESBLs and carbapenemases where the hydrolysis of β-lactams is detected due to color changes of a pH indicator (phenol red) as the pH changes during hydrolysis (162–164). Inclusion of β-lactamase inhibitors to these assays also allows the discrimination between subclasses of carbapenemases (164). These novel assays can be implemented in clinical laboratories, as they are relatively easy to perform and bacterial colonies can be used, resulting in a total turnover time of less than 2 hours (162).

The availability of MALDI-TOF MS in microbiologic laboratories has led to the investigation into its possible application for detection of antimicrobial resistance (26). Several promising reports are now emerging where MALDI-TOF MS has been used for the identification of β-lactamase activity, particularly carbapenemase activity, by detecting degradation products of different β-lactams with good results (32,33,165,166). The use of MALDI-TOF MS for detection of carbapenemase activity has the potential to be implemented in a routine clinical microbiologic laboratory. However, as no specialized software or kits have been developed, expertise in manual interpretation of the spectra is required.

DNA-Based Molecular Methods for Detection of Extended-Spectrum β-Lactamases and Carbapenemases

Over the years, various molecular methods, including conventional PCRs, real-time PCRs, LAMP, and DNA microarrays, have been described for detection of ESBLs and carbapenemases. The majority of methods are developed by the scientific community and there are only a limited number of methods that are commercially available. The description of molecular assays in the following texts is an attempt to provide examples of methods that have been described and used and to provide a platform for selection of methods based on the possibilities in different laboratories.

An important aspect before selecting a molecular method for detection of ESBLs or carbapenemases is the purpose of the assay. The large number of genes/variants and the constant emergence of new ESBLs and carbapenemases make it difficult for clinical laboratories to be up-to-date. Specific assays are therefore limited to reference laboratories. In epidemiologic studies, it might be important to use assays that cover a broad range of genes while in outbreak settings, and for infection control purposes, more targeted specific molecular assays could be considered. From epidemiologic studies, it is known that the dissemination of ESBL and carbapenemase genes is often associated with specific bacterial clones such as *Escherichia coli* sequence type (ST) 131 and $bla_{\text{CTX-M}}$, *K. pneumoniae* ST258 and bla_{KPC}, and *A. baumannii* clones and bla_{OXA}-carbapenemases (151,167,168). Molecular assays for rapid detection of some specific clones and associated ESBL or carbapenemase are developed, such as the detection of ST131 and $bla_{\text{CTX-M}}$ and ST258 and bla_{KPC} (169,170).

Conventional and Real-Time Polymerase Chain Reactions for Detection of Extended-Spectrum β-Lactamases and Carbapenemases

Conventional PCR and real-time PCR are the most commonly used molecular methods for detection of ESBLs and carbapenemases. Numerous PCRs, including conventional single and multiplex PCRs as well as real-time PCRs, have been described (Tables 9.7 and 9.8). For the detection of TEM and SHV ESBLs and variants of GES with carbapenemase activity, the identification of mutations are required to distinguish from the progenitor variants that are not ESBLs or lack carbapenemase activity. In conventional PCRs, sequencing of the bla_{TEM} or bla_{SHV} PCR products and analysis for mutations in the sequence are required either through standard Sanger sequencing (171) or pyrosequencing (172). Real-time PCR methods for discrimination of SHV variants and non-ESBL variants have also been described using melting-curve analysis (173).

A commercially available ligation-mediated real-time PCR from Check-Points designed for the detection of specific common mutations of SHV and TEM ESBL variants as well as CTX-M have been evaluated (174). Although PCR detection of CTX-M do not require discrimination from a non-ESBL variant, it is often desirable to determine which subgroup the CTX-M variant belongs to. Multiple PCR assays including conventional PCRs (175–177), conventional PCR followed by denaturing high-performance liquid chromatography (178), real-time PCR followed by pyrosequencing (179), and real-time PCR using probe-based detection or melting-curve analysis (173,180–182) have been developed. Real-time PCR assays for direct detection of bla_{CTX-M} in urine (181) and blood cultures (182,183) have also been reported. For the detection of the less

Table 9.7

Conventional Polymerase Chain Reactions for Detection of Extended-Spectrum β-Lactamase and Carbapenemase Genes		
Method	**Target Genes**	**Reference**
PCR and Sanger sequencing of bla_{TEM} and bla_{SHV} PCR products	bla_{TEM}, bla_{SHV}, bla_{CTX-M}	Tofteland et al. (171)
PCR and pyrosequencing	bla_{TEM} and bla_{SHV}	Jones et al. (172)
Multiplex PCRs	bla_{TEM}, bla_{SHV}, $bla_{OXA-1-like}$, $bla_{CTX-M\ gr.\ 1}$, $bla_{CTX-M\ gr.\ 2}$, $bla_{CTX-M\ gr.\ 9}$, $bla_{CTX-M\ gr.\ 8/25}$, bla_{GES-1} to bla_{GES-9}, bla_{GES-11}, bla_{PER-1}, bla_{PER-3}, bla_{VEB-1} to bla_{VEB-6}, $bla_{OXA-48-like}$, bla_{IMP} variants except $bla_{IMP-9,\ -16,\ -18,\ -22}$, and $_{-25}$, bla_{VIM-1}, bla_{VIM-2}, bla_{KPC-1} to bla_{KPC-5}	Dallenne et al. (175)
Multiplex PCR	$bla_{CTX-M\ gr.\ 1}$, $bla_{CTX-M\ gr.\ 2}$, $bla_{CTX-M\ gr.\ 9}$, $bla_{CTX-M\ gr.\ 8}$, $bla_{CTX-M\ gr.\ 25}$	Woodford et al. (176)
Multiplex PCR	$bla_{CTX-M\ gr.\ 1}$, $bla_{CTX-M\ gr.\ 2}$, $bla_{CTX-M\ gr.\ 9}$, $bla_{CTX-M\ gr.\ 25/26}$	Xu et al. (177)
Multiplex PCR and denaturing high-performance liquid chromatography	$bla_{CTX-M\ gr.\ 1}$, $bla_{CTX-M\ gr.\ 2}$, $bla_{CTX-M\ gr.\ 9}$, $bla_{CTX-M\ gr.\ 25/26}$	Xu et al. (178)
PCR and microchip gel electrophoresis, direct detection from blood cultures	bla_{CTX-M}	Fujita et al. (183)
PCR	bla_{PER}	Poirel et al. (186)
PCR	bla_{VEB}	Naas et al. (185)
PCR	bla_{BEL}	Bogaerts et al. (188)
PCR	$bla_{OXA-23-like}$, $bla_{OXA-24/-40-like}$, $bla_{OXA-58-like}$	Woodford et al. (189)
PCR	$bla_{OXA-23-like}$, $bla_{OXA-24/-40-like}$, $bla_{OXA-58-like}$, $bla_{OXA-143}$	Higgins et al. (190)
Multiplex PCRs	bla_{SME-1} to bla_{SME-3}, bla_{IMI-1} to bla_{IMI-3}, bla_{NMC-A}, bla_{GIM}, bla_{SIM}, bla_{NDM}, bla_{SPM}, $bla_{OXA-23-like}$, $bla_{OXA-24/-40-like}$, $bla_{OXA-48-like}$, $bla_{OXA-1\ group}$, $bla_{OXA-2\ group}$, $bla_{OXA-10\ group}$, $bla_{OXA-51\ group}$, $bla_{OXA-58\ group}$	Voets et al. (191)
Multiplex PCR	bla_{IMP}, bla_{VIM}, bla_{SPM}, bla_{GIM}, bla_{SIM}	Ellington et al. (192)
Multiplex PCRs	bla_{IMP}, bla_{VIM}, bla_{NDM}, bla_{SPM}, bla_{AIM}, bla_{DIM}, bla_{GIM}, bla_{SIM}, bla_{KPC}, bla_{BIC}, bla_{OXA-48}	Poirel et al. (193)

PCR, polymerase chain reaction.

prevalent ESBLs such as VEB (175,184,185), PER (175,184,186), GES (175,184,187), and BEL (188), conventional PCRs either as single or multiplex are mainly used for detection.

Various conventional PCRs and real-time PCRs have also been described for the detection of carbapenemase genes either as single or multiplex PCRs (Tables 9.7 and 9.8). There are also PCRs described which includes both detection of ESBLs and carbapenemases (175). Further, the developed PCRs vary with respect to the number of targets included. Conventional PCRs for detection of carbapenemases include a multiplex PCR for detection of the class D OXA-carbapenemases, $bla_{OXA-23-like}$, $bla_{OXA-24/-40-like}$, and $bla_{OXA-58-like}$, mainly identified in *Acinetobacter* spp (189). This PCR has been updated with the addition of primers for $bla_{OXA-143}$ (190). Further, different multiplex PCRs have

Table 9.8

Real-Time Polymerase Chain Reactions for Detection of Extended-Spectrum β-Lactamase and Carbapenemase Genes		
Method	**Target Genes**	**Reference**
Real-time PCR, melting-curve analysis and pyrosequencing	bla_{CTX-M}	Naas et al. (179)
Real-time PCR, melting-curve analysis	bla_{SHV}	Randegger et al. (173)
Multiplex real-time PCR, probe-based detection	bla_{CTX-M}, $bla_{CTX-M\ gr.\ 1}$, $bla_{CTX-M\ gr.\ 2}$, $bla_{CTX-M\ gr.\ 9}$	Birkett et al. (180)
Multiplex real-time PCR, probe-based detection, direct detection in urine samples	bla_{CTX-M}, $bla_{CTX-M\ gr.\ 1}$, $bla_{CTX-M\ gr.\ 2}$, $bla_{CTX-M\ gr.\ 9}$, $bla_{CTX-M\ gr.\ 8/25}$	Oxacelay et al. (181)
Real-time PCR, probe-based detection, direct detection in blood cultures	bla_{CTX-M}, $bla_{CTX-M\ gr.\ 1}$, $bla_{CTX-M\ gr.\ 2}$, $bla_{CTX-M\ gr.\ 9}$	Vanstone et al. (182)
Real-time PCR, melting-curve analysis	$bla_{CTX-M-15}$ and *E. coli* ST131	Dhanji et al. (169)
Real-time multiplex PCR, melting-curve analysis	bla_{IMP}, bla_{VIM}, bla_{SPM}, bla_{GIM}, bla_{SIM}	Mendes et al. (195)
Real-time multiplex, probe-based detection	bla_{KPC}, bla_{SME}, bla_{OXA-48}, bla_{IMI}, bla_{GES}	Swayne et al. (197)
Real-time multiplex, high-resolution melting-curve analysis	bla_{KPC}, bla_{NDM}, bla_{GES}, bla_{OXA-48}, bla_{VIM}, bla_{IMP}	Monteiro et al. (194)
Real-time PCR, probe-based detection	$bla_{KPC-1/-2}$ to bla_{KPC-12}	Richter et al. (198)
Direct detection perirectal and nasal swabs		
Real-time PCR, high-resolution melting-curve analysis	bla_{KPC}	Roth and Hanson (196)
Real-time PCR, probe-based detection	bla_{KPC}	Cole et al. (199)
Real-time PCR, probe-based detection, direct detection perianal/rectal swabs	bla_{KPC}	Hindiyeh et al. (205)
Real-time PCR, probe-based detection	bla_{KPC} and *K. pneumoniae* ST258	Chen et al. (170)
Real-time PCR, probe-based detection	bla_{NDM}	Diene et al. (200)
Real-time PCR, probe-based detection, evaluated on spiked stools	bla_{NDM}	Naas et al. (201)
Real-time PCR, probe-based detection	bla_{NDM}	Ong et al. (202)
Real-time PCR, probe-based detection	bla_{NDM}	Kruttgen et al. (203)
Ligation-mediated real-time PCR (Check-Points)	$bla_{CTX-M\ gr.\ 1}$, $bla_{CTX-M\ gr.\ 2}$, $bla_{CTX-M\ gr.\ 9}$, $bla_{SHV-238S}$, $bla_{TEM104K}$, $bla_{TEM164S}$	Nijhuis et al. (174)
Real-time PCR (bioMérieux NucliSENS)	bla_{KPC}	Spanu et al. (206)
Loop-mediated isothermal amplification	bla_{NDM}	Liu et al. (204)

PCR, polymerase chain reaction.

been described for the detection of class A and class B carbapenemases (191–193).

With respect to real-time PCRs for carbapenemases, different detection methods such as melting-curve analysis (194–196) or fluorescent probes (170,197–203) have been developed (Table 9.8). For the detection of bla_{NDM}, an assay using LAMP has been described with the potential of being a rapid test with low cost (204). Detection of bla_{NDM} and bla_{KPC} using real-time PCRs has been examined for their ability to detect these genes directly from clinical specimens such as perianal or rectal swabs (198,201,205). This can be particularly useful in outbreak settings or for screening of large populations. One commercially available real-time PCR assay from bioMérieux for the detection bla_{KPC} has been evaluated by Spanu et al. (206).

Oligonucleotide Array–Based Technology for Detection of Extended-Spectrum β-Lactamases and Carbapenemases

DNA microarray or oligo-based technology has the potential for detection of a large number of resistance genes and discrimination of variants within each class or family in a single test. In-house microarray assays have been developed for the detection of various resistance genes that also includes β-lactamases (207,208). However, the number of specific ESBL and carbapenemase genes in these arrays is limited. For the specific detection of ESBLs and carbapenemases, different approaches to this technology has been developed (Table 9.9). Grimm et al. (209) developed a DNA microarray for the detection of TEM ESBLs using Cy-labelled PCR products followed by hybridization on glass slides containing oligonucleotide probes. A further development of this assay has been done to include detection of SHV ESBL and CTX-M genes (210). A specific microarray for the direct detection and genotyping of bla_{KPC} variants also using Cy labelling and glass slides has been reported (211). This assay has also been evaluated using spiked urine samples.

An alternative approach by incorporating biotin into the DNA in the PCR reaction followed by hybridization to oligonucleotides on nitrocellulose membranes and detection using horseradish peroxidase have also been described for the detection of TEM, SHV, and CTX-M ESBLs (212). Two commercially available systems from AmplexDiagnostics (Gars Bahnhof, Germany)

Table 9.9

Oligonucleotide Arrays for Detection of Extended-Spectrum β-Lactamase and Carbapenemase Genes

Method	Target Genes	Reference
DNA microarray, evaluated with spiked urine samples	bla_{KPC} (including genotype separation, except bla_{KPC-12})	Peter et al. (211)
DNA microarray	bla_{CTX-M}, $bla_{SHV-ESBL}$, $bla_{TEM-ESBL}$	Leinberger et al. (210)
DNA microarray	$bla_{TEM-ESBL}$	Grimm et al. (209)
DNA microarray (Check-Points)	bla_{TEM}, bla_{SHV}, bla_{CTX-M}	Cohen Stuart et al. (214)
DNA microarray (Check-Points)	bla_{TEM}, bla_{SHV}, bla_{CTX-M}, bla_{KPC}, bla_{OXA-48}, bla_{VIM}, bla_{IMP}, bla_{NDM}	Naas et al. (215)
DNA microarray (Check-Points)	bla_{TEM}, bla_{SHV}, bla_{CTX-M}, bla_{KPC}, bla_{OXA-48}, bla_{VIM}, bla_{IMP}, bla_{NDM}	Woodford et al. (216)
DNA microarray (Check-Points)	bla_{TEM}, bla_{SHV}, bla_{CTX-M}, bla_{KPC}, bla_{OXA-48}, bla_{VIM}, bla_{IMP}, bla_{NDM},	Cuzon et al. (217)
DNA microarray (Check-Points)	bla_{TEM}, bla_{SHV}, bla_{CTX-M}, bla_{KPC}, bla_{OXA-48}, bla_{VIM}, bla_{IMP}, bla_{NDM}	Stuart et al. (218)
Oligonucleotide microarray	bla_{TEM}, bla_{SHV}, bla_{CTX-M}	Rubtsova et al. (212)
Multiplex PCR amplicon detection with reverse hybridization (AmplexDiagnostics)	bla_{VIM}, bla_{IMP}, bla_{NDM}, bla_{KPC}, bla_{OXA-48} (IMP-13 and IMP-14 not detected)	Kaase et al. (213)

PCR, polymerase chain reaction.

and Check-Points (Wageningen, The Nether-lands) using different approaches are described. The hyplex SuperBug ID (AmplexDiagnostics, Gars Bahnhof, Germany) includes a multiplex PCR for detection of KPC, VIM, NDM, and OXA-48 carbapenemases followed by detection of PCR products by reverse hybridization in microtiter plates precoated with specific oligonucleotide probes similar to a traditional antigen ELISA (213). The Check-Points (Wageningen, The Netherlands) technology includes a ligation-mediated PCR step where specific probes with primer sequences and zip codes will be ligated together if they match to the template DNA. This is followed by amplification PCR, hybridization, and detection in a microarray tube. Different Check-Points (Wageningen, The Netherlands) assays for detection of ESBLs and carbapenemases have been developed and evaluated (214–218).

DETECTION OF GENES ENCODING AMINOGLYCOSIDE RESISTANCE: AMINOGLYCOSIDE-MODIFYING ENZYMES AND 16S rRNA METHYLASES

Aminoglycosides—Mechanisms of Action and Resistance

Aminoglycosides (AGs) are an important group of antimicrobials often used in combination with β-lactams or glycopeptides for the treatment of invasive infections caused by both gram-negative and gram-positive bacteria. AGs include 4,6-disubstituted 2-deoxystreptamines (gentamicin, tobramycin, AMK, arbekacin, and KAN), 4,5-disubstituted deoxystreptamines (neomycin), monosubstituted deoxystreptamine (apramycin), and streptomycin, which has no deoxystreptamine ring (219). The primary target for AGs is the 16S RNA A-site located on the 30S subunit of the bacterial ribosome (220). Target site binding of AGs results in conformational changes of the A-site, which promotes mistranslation and concentration-dependent bactericidal effects.

Acquired antimicrobial resistance to AGs follows the major biochemical mechanisms of resistance: (a) enzymatic modification/inactivation, (b) mutations or modification of target, and (c) reduced accumulation in the cytoplasm through efflux or reduced permeability. The most prevalent mechanisms are associated with mobile genetic elements such as plasmids and/or transposons. The mechanisms mainly include aminoglycoside-modifying enzymes (AMEs) and 16S rRNA methylases (221,222). AMEs can be divided into three different classes based on the molecular mechanism of inactivation of AGs (221). Aminoglycoside *N*-acetyltransferases (AACs) uses acetyl coenzyme A to catalyze the acetylation of $-NH_2$ groups on AGs. Aminoglycoside O-nucleotidyltransferases (ANTs) modify AGs using adenosine triphosphate (ATP) to transfer adenosine monophosphate (AMP) to $-OH$ groups, whereas aminoglycoside O-phosphotransferases (APHs) catalyze the transfer of a phosphate group to the AG molecule (221). The modification and substrate specificity of the different AMEs and within each AME class varies. To date, numerous AMEs have been identified and the nomenclature is complex. For recent reviews, see Ramirez and Tolmasky (221), Shaw et al. (223), and Tolmasky (224).

Aminoglycoside Resistance Genes and Their Detection

The large number of genes encoding AMEs makes molecular detection of AMEs a complex and difficult exercise. DNA microarrays or WGS followed by bioinformatics analysis is probably the only methods that can offer the possibility of complete coverage for detection of all known AMEs. Various DNA microarrays that include probes for AME genes have been developed and used to characterize both gram-negative and gram-positive bacteria (208,225–229). The number of AME genes included in the DNA microarrays varies.

Aminoglycoside-Modifying Enzyme Genes in Gram-Positive Bacteria

Streptococci are considered intrinsically resistant to AGs due to reduced permeability. For enterococci and staphylococci, the number of AME genes identified in clinical isolates is relatively limited and conserved (230). The most prevalent AME genes in clinical samples include *aac(6′)-Ie-aph(2″)-Ia* encoding a bifunctional enzyme [AAC(6′)-APH(2″)], *ant(4′)-Ia* encoding ANT(4′)-Ia, and *aph(3′)-IIIa* encoding APH(3′)-III. Consequently, conventional PCR assays either as single or multiplex can often be sufficient and usually provide a good correlation with the phenotypic profile. Several

Table 9.10

Epidemiologic Studies on Aminoglycoside-Modifying Enzyme Genes in Enterococci and Staphylococci Describing Primers and Polymerase Chain Reaction Conditions		
AME Genes	**Species**	**Reference**
aac(6')-Ie-aph(2")-Ia, aph(2")-Ib, aph(2")-Id, aph(3')-IIIa, ant(4')-Ia	*Enterococcus* spp	Vakulenko et al. (360)
aac(6')-Ie-aph(2")-Ia, aph(3')-IIIa, ant(4')-Ia	*S. aureus*, CoNS	Schmitz et al. (361)
aac(6')-Ie-aph(2")-Ia, aph(3')-IIIa, ant(4')-Ia	*S. aureus*, CoNS	Ardic et al. (362)
aac(6')-Ie-aph(2")-Ia, aph(3')-IIIa, ant(4')-Ia	*S. aureus*	Ida et al. (363)
aac(6')-Ie-aph(2")-Ia, aph(2")-Ib, aph(2")-Ic, aph(2")-Id	*Enterococcus* spp	Qu et al. (364)
aac(6')-Ii, aac(6')-Im, aac(6')-Ie-aph(2")-Ia, ant(3")-Ia, ant(4')-Ia, ant(6)-Ia, ant(9)-Ia, ant(9)-Ib, aph(2")-Ib, aph(2")-Ic, aph(2")-Id, aph(3')-IIIa	*Enterococcus* spp	Mahbub Alam et al. (365)
aac(6')-Ie-aph(2")-Ia, aph(3')-IIIa, ant(4')-Ia, ant(6)-Ia, str	*Staphylococcus sciuri* group	Hauschild et al. (366)
aac(6')-Ie-aph(2")-Ia, aph(2")-Id/aph(2")-Ie, aph(3')-Ia, ant(6)-Ia, aac(6')-Ii	*Enterococcus* spp	Watanabe et al. (367)
aac(6')-Ie-aph(2")-Ia (aacA-aphD), aph(2")-Ib, aph(2")-Ic, aph(2")-Id, ant(3")-Ia, ant(6)-Ia	*Enterococcus* spp	Leelaporn et al. (368)

AME, aminoglycoside-modifying enzyme; CoNS, coagulase-negative staphylococci.

epidemiologic studies have described primers and conditions for detection of various AMEs in enterococci and staphylococci (Table 9.10).

Aminoglycoside-Modifying Enzyme in Gram-Negative Bacteria

The number of AME genes identified in gram-negative bacteria is more extensive compared to gram-positive bacteria making molecular detection more complex. However, specific AME genes are more prevalent than others (230). These include genes encoding AMEs belonging to the subclasses ANT(2")-I, AAC(6')-I, AAC(3)-I, AAC(3)-II, AAC(3)-III, AAC(3)-IV, and AAC(3)-VI. The epidemiology of AME genes varies by geographical location and selective pressure influencing the selection of AME genes to be targeted (230). Conventional PCR is the most used molecular method for detection of AME genes in gram-negative bacteria. Real-time PCRs have been designed for some specific AME genes. Particular attention has been given to *aac(6')-Ib* and detection of the *aac(6')-Ib-cr* variant that encodes a variant of *aac(6')-Ib* that are able to modify the FQs, ciprofloxacin, and norfloxacin (231–233). Table 9.11 shows illustrative studies describing PCRs for detection of AME genes in gram-negative bacteria.

Making Aminoglycosides Useless—The Emergence of Transferable 16S rRNA Methylases

16S rRNA methylases have recently emerged as a major mobile AG resistance mechanism among gram-negative bacteria (222). The enzymes methylate specific nucleotide residues in the binding site of AGs in the 16S rRNA conferring high-level and broad-spectrum AG resistance. Two subclasses of 16S rRNA methylases have been described: N7-G1405 and N1-A1408. To date, seven N7-G1405 16S rRNA methylases (ArmA, RmtA, RmtB, RmtC, RmtD, RmtD2, and RmtE) and one N1-A1408 16S rRNA methylase (NpmA) have been identified among gram-negative bacteria. The hallmark of N7-G1405 16S rRNA methylases is high level of resistance (minimum inhibitory concentration [MIC] ≥128 mg/L) to 4,6-disubstituted 2-deoxytreptamines such as gentamicin, tobramycin, AMK, arbekacin, and KAN. The dissemination of genes encoding 16S rRNA methylases is often associated with the spread of ESBL and carbapenemases. Molecular detection methods of 16S rRNA methylases described so far includes conventional multiplex PCRs (234,235). Bercot et al. (235) describe two multiplex PCRs that covers all 16S rRNA methylases identified

Table 9.11

Epidemiologic Studies of Aminoglycoside-Modifying Enzyme Genes in Gram-Negative Bacteria Describing Primers and Polymerase Chain Reactions Conditions			
Method	**AME Genes**	**Species**	**Reference**
PCR	*aac(2')-Ia, aac(3)-Ia, aac(3)-Ib, aac(3)-IIa, aac(6')-Ia, aac(6')-Ib, aac(6')-Ic, ant(2")-Ia, ant(3")-Ia, ant(4")-IIa, aph(3')-Ia, aph(3")-Ia, aph(3")-Ib*	Enterobacteriaceae	Miro et al. (369)
PCR	*aac(3)-I, aac(3)-II/VI, aac(3)-III/IV, aac(6')-I, aac(6')-II, ant(2")-I, ant(4')-II, aph(3')-VI*	*Pseudomonas aeruginosa*	Kim et al. (370)
PCR	*aac(6')-Ih, aac(6')-Ib, aph(3)-VI, aph(3')-Ia, ant(2")-Ia, aac(3)-Ia, aac(3)-IIa*	*Acinetobacter* spp	Noppe-Leclercq et al. (371)
PCR	*aac(3)-Ia, aac(3)-IIa, aac(6')-Ih, aph(3')-IV, ant(2")-Ia, aph(3')-Ia, aac(6')-Ib*	*Acinetobacter* spp	Akers et al. (372)
Real-time PCR	*aac(6')-Ib/aac(6')-Ib-cr, aac(3)-IIa/c*	*E. coli, K. pneumoniae*	Lindemann et al. (233)
Real-time PCR	*aac(6')-Ib/aac(6')-Ib-cr*	Enterobacteriaceae	Hidalgo-Grass and Strahilevitz (231)
Real-time PCR	*aac(6')-Ib/aac(6')-Ib-cr*	Enterobacteriaceae	Bell et al. (232)

PCR, polymerase chain reaction.

to date. The increasing diversity of 16S rRNA methylases may soon undermine the practical use of PCR in the detection of encoding genes and support the use of alternative molecular detection techniques such as MALDI-TOF MS (236). A recent review stated, however, that the template preparation needed to be simplified to be used for routine and reference purposes (45).

DETECTION OF LINEZOLID RESISTANCE IN STAPHYLOCOCCI, ENTEROCOCCI, AND STREPTOCOCCI

Linezolid Resistance Mechanisms

The overall high linezolid susceptibility rates (>99 %) for staphylococci, enterococci, and streptococci monitored in medical centers in Europe, Canada, Latin America, the United States, and the Asia-Pacific region remains stable (237–239). Linezolid inhibits bacterial protein synthesis by binding to the A-site pocket at the ribosomal peptidyltransferase center in domain V of the 23S rRNA (240). Resistance to linezolid is caused by target site modification. Point mutations in 23S rRNA domain V, in particular a G2576U mutation, and the presence of a transferable ribosomal methyltransferase encoded by the *cfr* gene are most often associated with linezolid resistance in clinical strains of staphylococci and enterococci (237–239,241,242). Mutations in ribosomal proteins L3 and L4 have also been shown to mediate linezolid resistance in staphylococci (237–239). In streptococci mutations in ribosomal protein, L4 have been the main mechanism identified in linezolid nonsusceptible clinical strains but 23S rRNA and L22 mutations (239,243–245) have also been reported.

The development of mutational-based linezolid resistance in staphylococci and enterococci was initially considered unlikely due to the presence of multiple copies of the 23S rRNA gene. The rate-limiting step in the development of linezolid resistance in enterococci appears to be the initial mutation occurring under antimicrobial selective pressure, as subsequent replacement of wild-type genes with mutant copies occurs rapidly by homologous recombination (246). The level of linezolid resistance expressed correlates with the number of mutated 23S rRNA genes (247). Mutations in a single copy of the 23S rRNA gene can contribute to increased linezolid MIC (248).

Linezolid Resistance Determinants

The transferable linezolid multiresistance gene, *cfr* (chloramphenicol–florfenicol resistance) gene, encodes a methyltransferase-catalyzing methylation of A2503 in the 23S rRNA V domain. Methylation of A2503 affects the binding of at least five antimicrobial classes (phenicols, lincosamides, oxazolidinones, pleuromutilins, and streptogramin A), leading to a multidrug-resistant phenotype (249).

The *cfr* gene has been reported as the underlying resistance mechanism in outbreaks of linezolid resistance *S. aureus* (250–252) and *S. epidermidis* (253) and has been detected on transferable plasmids in clinical isolates of *S. aureus* (254), CoNS (255,256), and recently also in *E. faecalis* (241). Acquisition of *cfr* in *S. aureus* was associated with a generally low fitness cost (257). The *cfr* encoding plasmids have, since their first discovery in year 2000 (258), been found in domestic animal isolates of staphylococci (259), enterococci (260,261), *Bacillus* (262–264), *Macrococcus caseolyticus*, *Jeotgalicoccus pinnipedialis* (265), and *E. coli* (266). The *cfr* gene has also been found on the chromosome of a *Proteus vulgaris* isolated from a pig (267). The *cfr* gene is expressed in both gram-positive and gram-negative bacteria (249) and is often located on plasmids that carry additional resistance genes (254,261–265) to important antimicrobial agents used in both human and veterinary medicine; thus, selection pressure and risk of further spread of *cfr* plasmids are likely.

Molecular Methods in Detection of Linezolid Resistance

The *cfr* gene can be amplified using PCR primers (cfr-fw TGA AGT ATA AAG CAG GTT GGG AGT CAC and cfr-rv ACC ATA TAA TTG ACC ACA AGC AGC) (259), giving a 100% match to the *cfr* genes detected as of early 2013 in both staphylococci and enterococci. Confirmation of PCR products of the correct size can be achieved either by restriction digestion or direct sequencing. Alternatively, the *cfr* gene may be detected by Southern blot (259) or LAMP (268).

Several approaches have been described to detect the most common 23S rRNA single nucleotide mutation (G2576T) conferring linezolid resistance in enterococci and staphylococci. Traditional SNP analysis used to detect the G2576T comprises PCR amplification of the domain V region of the 23S rRNA gene using primers for enterococci (247,269), staphylococci (270), or both (256) and restriction digestion by enzymes such as *Mae*I (247) or *Nhe*I (G↓CTAGC) (256,269,270). Mutated nucleotide generating new restriction sites is underlined. Quick and easy to perform

separation and analyses of the resulting restriction fragments has been tested with LabChip kit, Bioanalyzer, and BioSizing software (Agilent Technologies, Santa Clara, CA), which calculates both size and quantities of fragments (271). Other SNP detection approaches tested in enterococci include fluorescence in situ hybridization (FISH) assay with probes containing locked nucleic acids (LNAs) at the site of point mutation (272) as well as real-time PCRs with hybridization probes discriminating between mutant and wild-type alleles using either Taqman probes (271) or a LightCycler (Roche Diagnostics GmbH, Mannheim, Germany) assay including a fluorescent dye–labelled detection probe (273).

Pyrosequencing is a rapid technology ideal for processing a larger number of isolates that is useful for sequence determination of short DNA regions as well as for providing quantification of the number of mutant versus wild-type alleles. For a thorough description of the pyrosequencing method and suitable primers to detect the main SNPs responsible for linezolid resistance in enterococci (G2576T) and staphylococci (G2576T, T2500A, A2503G, T2504C, G2505A, G2445T, G2447T), see Woodford et al. (274). A modified assay spanning a larger area of the 23S rRNA gene has been used to cover both the G2576T and the C2534T mutations of linezolid-resistant *S. epidermidis* (275).

To reveal both known and novel mutations involved in linezolid resistance, PCR amplification and subsequent sequencing of individual 23S rRNA alleles has been described for *S. aureus* (248,276,277), *E. faecalis* (278), and *Streptococcus pneumoniae* (279,280). Others perform amplification and direct sequencing on 23S rRNA PCR products containing a mixture of alleles using primers suitable for enterococci and streptococci (281), staphylococci (270), streptococci (280), enterococci and staphylococci (256,282), or all three (283). Furthermore, amplification and sequencing of the genes *rplC* and *rplD* encoding ribosomal proteins L3 (284, 285) and L4 (270,284,285) in staphylococci and *rplD* encoding L4 in *S. pneumoniae* (280) to reveal mutations involved in linezolid resistance has been reported.

DETECTION OF PLASMID-MEDIATED QUINOLONE RESISTANCE GENES IN GRAM-NEGATIVE BACTERIA

The main mechanisms of resistance to quinolones and FQs have been the accumulation of mutations in the target enzymes DNA gyrase and DNA topoisomerase IV (286). These mutations occur in specific regions termed *quinolone resistance-determining regions* (QRDR) resulting in mutations in the target enzymes and reduced affinity for FQs. Methods for detection of chromosomal mutations in QRDR is generally determined by PCR followed by sequencing and will not be covered in this section. The dissemination of FQ resistance caused by chromosomal mutations would therefore be associated with clonal spread. Considering the rate of mutations, chromosomal mutations have not been sufficient to explain the relatively rapid frequency and nonclonality of resistance to FQs.

Plasmid-Mediated Quinolone Resistance Mechanisms

In 1998, the first plasmid-mediated quinolone resistance (PMQR) mechanism was reported in a *K. pneumoniae* isolate (287). The responsible PMQR gene was termed *qnr* for "quinolone resistance" and later renamed *qnrA1*. Subsequently, several *qnr* genes and variants have been discovered including *qnrA*, *qnrB*, *qnrS*, *qnrC*, and *qnrD*; for reviews, see Rodríguez-Martínez et al. (288) and Strahilevitz et al. (289). A classification scheme and database repository (http://www.lahey.org/qnrStudies/) for *qnr* genes have been set up to control the nomenclature (290). In addition to the *qnr* genes, two additional PMQR mechanisms have been identified. Robicsek et al. (291) showed that two amino acid mutations in the AME *aac(6')-Ib* resulted in a variant, *aac(6')-Ib-cr*, able to acetylate ciprofloxacin and norfloxacin. Further, two plasmid-mediated quinolone efflux pumps, QepA and OqxAB, have been identified (292,293).

Molecular Detection of Plasmid-Mediated Quinolone Resistance

The most common molecular method for detection of PMQR used has been PCR assays (Table 9.12). For detection of *qnr* genes, conventional multiplex PCRs have been described for the detection of different sets of *qnr* genes (294–296). Recently, a real-time multiplex using high-resolution melting (HRM) and ResoLight dye have been described for the detection of five *qnr* genes: *qnrA*, *qnrB*, *qnrS*, *qnrC*, and *qnrD* (297). Due to the large number and variety of *qnrB* variants, primer design has been a challenge and primer sequences should be evaluated against currently known *qnrB*

sequences in the database (http://www.lahey.org/qnrStudies/). False-positive *qnr* PCR products have also been observed by multiplex PCR but not by monoplex PCRs (296). Sequencing of the PCR products should therefore be considered for confirmation. Assays for detection of the more recently discovered *qnrC* and *qnrD* has mainly been performed with singleplex conventional PCRs (298,299) except for the inclusions of these genes in some multiplex PCRs as described earlier.

With respect to the two PMQR efflux mechanisms, QepA and OqxAB, methods for the detection of *qepA* have mainly been described. In addition to conventional PCR assays (293,300–302), Guillard et al. (297) have described a real-time PCR using SYBR Green I for the detection of *qepA*.

Detection of the *aac(6')-Ib-cr* variant of *aac(6')-Ib* requires the identification of mutations resulting in amino acid changes at codon 102 (Trp → Arg) and 179 (Asp → Tyr) (291). Various molecular methods have been applied for detection of *aac(6')-Ib-cr*. Because *aac(6')-Ib-cr* in contrast to *aac(6')-Ib* lacks the cut site for the restriction enzymes *Bst*F5I and *Bst*CI, restriction enzyme digestion of purified PCR products have been applied to identify the *aac(6')-Ib-cr* variant (303). Alternatively, Sanger sequencing or pyrosequencing of the *aac(6')-Ib* PCR product have also been applied (303,304). Two real-time PCR assays using HRM analysis have also been developed to detect the SNPs (231,232). To solve the issue of subtle changes observed with a T → A mutation responsible for the Trp → Arg conversion, Bell et al. (232) included an unlabelled probe with perfect match to the *aac(6')-Ib* allele and asymmetric concentrations of primer concentrations. For specific detection of the G535T mutation, a gap ligase chain reaction method has also been used (305).

CONCLUDING REMARKS

The exponential increase of acquired genes and SNPs involved in antimicrobial resistance makes it increasingly difficult to test for all possible mechanisms using molecular methods. It is also important to underline that guidance in antimicrobial therapy and individual treatment is based on susceptibility. Thus, phenotypic antimicrobial susceptibility methods will continue to be crucial in routine diagnostics. However, rapid and accurate genotypic detection of particular important resistance mechanisms (i.e., MRSA and carbapenemases) is important for

Table 9.12

Studies Describing Molecular Methods for Detection of Plasmid-Mediated Quinolone Resistance Genes		
Method	**PMQR Genes**	**Reference**
Conventional multiplex PCR	*qnrA, qnrB, qnrS*	Robiscek et al. (294)
Conventional multiplex PCR	*qnrA, qnrB, qnrS*	Cattoir et al. (295)
Conventional multiplex PCRs	I: *qnrA, qnrB, qnrC, qnrS* II: *aac(6')-Ib, qepA*	Kim et al. (296)
Real-time multiplex and singleplex PCR	I: *qnrA, qnrB, qnrS, qnrC, qnrD* II: *qepA*	Guillard et al. (297)
Conventional PCR	*qnrC, qnrD*	Veldmann et al. (299)
Conventional PCR	*qnrC*	Wang et al. (298)
Conventional PCR	*qepA*	Minarini et al. (300)
Conventional PCR	*qepA*	Yamane et al. (301)
Conventional PCR	*oqxA, oqxB*	Kim et al. (293)
Conventional PCR	*oqxA, oqxB*	Liu et al. (302)
Conventional PCR and *Bst*F5I/*Bts*CI restriction enzyme digestion or DNA analysis	*aac(6')-Ib-cr*	Park et al. (303)
Conventional PCR and pyrosequencing	*aac(6')-Ib-cr*	Guillard et al. (304)
Real-time PCR high-resolution melting analysis	*aac(6')-Ib-cr*	Bell et al. (232)
Real-time PCR high-resolution melting analysis	*aac(6')-Ib-cr*	Hidalgo-Grass and Strahilevitz (231)
Gap ligase chain reaction	*aac(6')-Ib-cr*	Warburg et al. (305)

PMQR, plasmid-mediated quinolone resistance; PCR, polymerase chain reaction.

efficient infection control measures. The need for rapid molecular detection of MDR- and XDR-TB is evident in primary health care settings in countries with a high burden of disease (144). Molecular methods are also fundamental in reference academic laboratories for detection of novel mechanisms, confirmation of unusual phenotypes, and emerging mechanisms of potential health importance.

WGS is on the verge of becoming a reality for molecular diagnostics in routine clinical microbiology, as the technological revolution of sequencing has reduced the time, effort, and cost. The potential use of WGS in antimicrobial resistance surveillance programs and infection control is evident (18,21,22). Their promising possibilities in routine diagnostic microbiology have also recently been evaluated (20,306). However, the bioinformatics workflow including more user-friendly programs for data analyses and quality-assured databases for reference sequences is important

tools that need to be solved in order for this methodology to become accessible in routine diagnostics (19,42,48).

The increasingly demanding technologies used for molecular diagnostic require skilled, highly trained personnel than currently may be found in the routine laboratories. Other obstacles may be costs of technology and lack of stable electricity. Thus, the advanced technologies may not be available in locations where the resistance problems are of most concern as illustrated by the increase in MDR- and XDR-TB in low- and middle-income countries worldwide associated with a high burden of HIV.

ACKNOWLEDGMENT

We apologize to all the authors whose work is not referred to in this review. The enormous amount of relevant publications made it impossible to include all.

REFERENCES

1. Kumar A, Roberts D, Wood KE, et al. Duration of hypotension before initiation of effective antimicrobial therapy is the critical determinant of survival in human septic shock. *Crit Care Med* 2006;34:1589–1596.

2. Diekema DJ, Dodgson KJ, Sigurdardottir B, et al. Rapid detection of antimicrobial-resistant organism carriage: an unmet clinical need. *J Clin Microbiol* 2004;42: 2879–2883.

3. Derde LP, Dautzenberg MJ, Bonten MJ. Chlorhexidine body washing to control antimicrobial-resistant bacteria in intensive care units: a systematic review. *Intensive Care Med* 2012;38:931–939.

4. Savard P, Perl TM. A call for action: managing the emergence of multidrug-resistant *Enterobacteriaceae* in the acute care settings. *Curr Opin Infect Dis* 2012;25: 371–377.

5. Morar M, Wright GD. The genomic enzymology of antibiotic resistance. *Annu Rev Genet* 2010;44:25–51.

6. Livermore DM, Winstanley TG, Shannon KP. Interpretative reading: recognizing the unusual and inferring resistance mechanisms from resistance phenotypes. *J Antimicrob Chemother* 2001;48(Suppl 1):87–102.

7. Courvalin P, Trieu-Cuot P. Minimizing potential resistance: the molecular view. *Clin Infect Dis* 2001;33(Suppl 3): S138–S146.

8. Fernandez L, Hancock RE. Adaptive and mutational resistance: role of porins and efflux pumps in drug resistance. *Clin Microbiol Rev* 2012;25:661–681.

9. Canton R, Morosini MI. Emergence and spread of antibiotic resistance following exposure to antibiotics. *FEMS Microbiol Rev* 2011;35:977–991.

10. Andersson DI, Hughes D. Persistence of antibiotic resistance in bacterial populations. *FEMS Microbiol Rev* 2011;35:901–911.

11. Depardieu F, Podglajen I, Leclercq R, et al. Modes and modulations of antibiotic resistance gene expression. *Clin Microbiol Rev* 2007;20:79–114.

12. Winstanley T, Courvalin P. Expert systems in clinical microbiology. *Clin Microbiol Rev* 2011;24:515–556.

13. Courvalin P. Interpretive reading of antimicrobial susceptibility tests. *ASM news* 1992;58:368–375.

14. Engström A, Morcillo N, Imperiale B, et al. Detection of first- and second-line drug resistance in *Mycobacterium tuberculosis* clinical isolates by pyrosequencing. *J Clin Microbiol* 2012;50:2026–2033.

15. Courvalin P. Genotypic approach to the study of bacterial resistance to antibiotics. *Antimicrob Agents Chemother* 1991;35:1019–1023.

16. Sundsfjord A, Simonsen GS, Haldorsen BC, et al. Genetic methods for detection of antimicrobial resistance. *APMIS* 2004;112:815–837.

17. Bennedsen M, Stuer-Lauridsen B, Danielsen M, et al. Screening for antimicrobial resistance genes and virulence factors via genome sequencing. *Appl Environ Microbiol* 2011;77:2785–2787.

18. Didelot X, Bowden R, Wilson DJ, et al. Transforming clinical microbiology with bacterial genome sequencing. *Nat Rev Genet* 2012;13:601–612.

19. Fricke WF, Rasko DA. Bacterial genome sequencing in the clinic: bioinformatic challenges and solutions. *Nat Rev Genet* 2014;15:49–55.

20. Hasman H, Saputra D, Sicheritz-Ponten T, et al. Rapid whole-genome sequencing for detection and characterization of microorganisms directly from clinical samples. *J Clin Microbiol* 2014;52:139–146.

21. Köser CU, Ellington MJ, Cartwright EJ, et al. Routine use of microbial whole genome sequencing in diagnostic and public health microbiology. *PLoS Pathog* 2012;8:e1002824.

22. Reuter S, Ellington MJ, Cartwright EJ, et al. Rapid bacterial whole-genome sequencing to enhance diagnostic and public health microbiology. *JAMA Intern Med* 2013;173:1397–1404.

23. Schena M, Shalon D, Davis RW, et al. Quantitative monitoring of gene expression patterns with a complementary DNA microarray. *Science* 1995;270:467–470.

24. Dufva M. Introduction to microarray technology. *Methods Mol Biol* 2009;529:1–22.

25. Bodrossy L, Sessitsch A. Oligonucleotide microarrays in microbial diagnostics. *Curr Opin Microbiol* 2004;7: 245–254.

26. Hrabak J, Chudackova E, Walkova R. Matrix-assisted laser desorption ionization-time of flight (maldi-tof) mass spectrometry for detection of antibiotic resistance mechanisms: from research to routine diagnosis. *Clin Microbiol Rev* 2013;26:103–114.

27. Wieser A, Schneider L, Jung J, et al. MALDI-TOF MS in microbiological diagnostics-identification of microorganisms and beyond (mini review). *Appl Microbiol Biotechnol* 2012;93:965–974.

28. Douthwaite S, Kirpekar F. Identifying modifications in RNA by MALDI mass spectrometry. *Methods Enzymol* 2007;425:1–20.

29. Blondal T, Waage BG, Smarason SV, et al. A novel MALDI-TOF based methodology for genotyping single nucleotide polymorphisms. *Nucleic Acids Res* 2003;31:e155.

30. Griffin PM, Price GR, Schooneveldt JM, et al. Use of matrix-assisted laser desorption ionization-time of flight mass spectrometry to identify vancomycin-resistant enterococci and investigate the epidemiology of an outbreak. *J Clin Microbiol* 2012;50:2918–2931.

31. Edwards-Jones V, Claydon MA, Evason DJ, et al. Rapid discrimination between methicillin-sensitive and methicillin-resistant *Staphylococcus aureus* by intact cell mass spectrometry. *J Med Microbiol* 2000;49:295–300.

32. Hrabak J, Studentova V, Walkova R, et al. Detection of NDM-1, VIM-1, KPC, OXA-48, and OXA-162 carbapenemases by matrix-assisted laser desorption ionization-time of flight mass spectrometry. *J Clin Microbiol* 2012;50:2441–2443.

33. Sparbier K, Schubert S, Weller U, et al. Matrix-assisted laser desorption ionization-time of flight mass spectrometry-based functional assay for rapid detection of resistance against beta-lactam antibiotics. *J Clin Microbiol* 2012;50:927–937.

34. Kehrenberg C, Schwarz S, Jacobsen L, et al. A new mechanism for chloramphenicol, florfenicol and clindamycin resistance: methylation of 23S ribosomal RNA at A2503. *Mol Microbiol* 2005;57:1064–1073.

35. Ikryannikova LN, Shitikov EA, Zhivankova DG, et al. A MALDI TOF MS-based minisequencing method for rapid detection of TEM-type extended-spectrum beta-lactamases in clinical strains of *Enterobacteriaceae*. *J Microbiol Methods* 2008;75:385–391.

36. Ikryannikova LN, Afanas'ev MV, Akopian TA, et al. Mass-spectrometry based minisequencing method for the rapid detection of drug resistance in *Mycobacterium tuberculosis*. *J Microbiol Methods* 2007;70:395–405.

37. Xu C, Lin X, Ren H, et al. Analysis of outer membrane proteome of *Escherichia coli* related to resistance to ampicillin and tetracycline. *Proteomics* 2006;6:462–473.

38. Siroy A, Cosette P, Seyer D, et al. Global comparison of the membrane subproteomes between a multidrug-resistant *Acinetobacter baumannii* strain and a reference strain. *J Proteome Res* 2006;5:3385–3398.

39. Vashist J, Tiwari V, Kapil A, et al. Quantitative profiling and identification of outer membrane proteins of beta-lactam resistant strain of *Acinetobacter baumannii*. *J Proteome Res* 2010;9:1121–1128.

40. Grobner S, Linke D, Schutz W, et al. Emergence of carbapenem-non-susceptible extended-spectrum beta-lactamase-producing *Klebsiella pneumoniae* isolates at the university hospital of Tubingen, Germany. *J Med Microbiol* 2009;58:912–922.

41. Imperi F, Ciccosanti F, Perdomo AB, et al. Analysis of the periplasmic proteome of *Pseudomonas aeruginosa*, a metabolically versatile opportunistic pathogen. *Proteomics* 2009;9:1901–1915.

42. McGinn S, Gut IG. DNA sequencing—spanning the generations. *N Biotechnol* 2013;30:366–372.

43. Shendure JA, Porreca GJ, Church GM, et al. Overview of DNA sequencing strategies. *Curr Protoc Mol Biol* 2011; Chapter 7:Unit 7.1.

44. Köser CU, Holden MT, Ellington MJ, et al, Rapid whole-genome sequencing for investigation of a neonatal MRSA outbreak. *N Engl J Med* 2012;366:2267–2275.

45. Snitkin ES, Zelazny AM, Thomas PJ, et al. Tracking a hospital outbreak of carbapenem-resistant *Klebsiella pneumoniae* with whole-genome sequencing. *Sci Transl Med* 2012;4:148ra116.

46. Rolain JM, Diene SM, Kempf M, et al. Real-time sequencing to decipher the molecular mechanism of resistance of a clinical pan-drug-resistant *Acinetobacter baumannii* isolate from Marseille, France. *Antimicrob Agents Chemother* 2013;57:592–596.

47. Zankari E, Hasman H, Cosentino S, et al. Identification of acquired antimicrobial resistance genes. *J Antimicrob Chemother* 2012;67:2640–2644.

48. Underwood A, Green J. Call for a quality standard for sequence-based assays in clinical microbiology: necessity for quality assessment of sequences used in microbial identification and typing. *J Clin Microbiol* 2011;49:23–26.

49. te Witt R, van Belkum A, MacKay WG, et al. External quality assessment of the molecular diagnostics and genotyping of meticillin-resistant *Staphylococcus aureus*. *Eur J Clin Microbiol Infect Dis* 2010;29:295–300.

50. Mattarucchi E, Marsoni M, Binelli G, et al. Different real time PCR approaches for the fine quantification of SNP's alleles in DNA pools: assays development, characterization and pre-validation. *J Biochem Mol Biol* 2005;38:555–562.

51. Chambers HF. Methicillin resistance in staphylococci: molecular and biochemical basis and clinical implications. *Clin Microbiol Rev* 1997;10:781–791.

52. Tomasz A, Nachman S, Leaf H. Stable classes of phenotypic expression in methicillin-resistant clinical isolates of staphylococci. *Antimicrob Agents Chemother* 1991;35:124–129.

53. File TM Jr, Wilcox MH, Stein GE. Summary of ceftaroline fosamil clinical trial studies and clinical safety. *Clin Infect Dis* 2012;55(Suppl 3):S173–S180.

54. Cosgrove SE, Sakoulas G, Perencevich EN, et al. Comparison of mortality associated with methicillin-resistant and methicillin-susceptible *Staphylococcus aureus* bacteremia: a meta-analysis. *Clin Infect Dis* 2003;36:53–59.

55. International Working Group on the Classification of Staphylococcal Cassette Chromosome Elements. Classification of staphylococcal cassette chromosome *mec* (SCCmec): guidelines for reporting novel SCCmec elements. *Antimicrob Agents Chemother* 2009;53:4961–4967.

56. Brakstad OG, Maeland JA, Tveten Y. Multiplex polymerase chain reaction for detection of genes for *Staphylococcus aureus* thermonuclease and methicillin resistance and correlation with oxacillin resistance. *APMIS* 1993;101:681–688.

57. Vannuffel P, Gigi J, Ezzedine H, et al. Specific detection of methicillin-resistant *Staphylococcus* species by multiplex PCR. *J Clin Microbiol* 1995;33:2864–2867.

58. Paule SM, Pasquariello AC, Thomson RB Jr, et al. Real-time PCR can rapidly detect methicillin-susceptible and methicillin-resistant *Staphylococcus aureus* directly from positive blood culture bottles. *Am J Clin Pathol* 2005;124:404–407.

59. Huletsky A, Giroux R, Rossbach V, et al. New real-time PCR assay for rapid detection of methicillin-resistant *Staphylococcus aureus* directly from specimens containing a mixture of staphylococci. *J Clin Microbiol* 2004;42:1875–1884.

60. Garcia-Alvarez L, Holden MT, Lindsay H, et al. Methicillin-resistant *Staphylococcus aureus* with a novel *mecA* homologue in human and bovine populations in the UK and Denmark: a descriptive study. *Lancet Infect Dis* 2011;11:595–603.

61. Ito T, Hiramatsu K, Tomasz A, et al. Guidelines for reporting novel *mecA* gene homologues. *Antimicrob Agents Chemother* 2012;56:4997–4999.

62. Stegger M, Andersen PS, Kearns A, et al. Rapid detection, differentiation and typing of methicillin-resistant *Staphylococcus aureus* harbouring either *mecA* or the new *mecA* homologue *mecA*(LGA251). *Clin Microbiol Infect* 2012;18:395–400.

63. Pichon B, Hill R, Laurent F, et al. Development of a real-time quadruplex PCR assay for simultaneous detection of *nuc*, Panton-Valentine leucocidin (PVL), *mecA* and homologue *mecA*$_{LGA251}$. *J Antimicrob Chemother* 2012;67:2338–2341.

64. Monecke S, Muller E, Schwarz S, et al. Rapid microarray-based identification of different mecA alleles in Staphylococci. *Antimicrob Agents Chemother* 2012;56:5547–5554.

65. Shah HN, Rajakaruna L, Ball G, et al. Tracing the transition of methicillin resistance in sub-populations of *Staphylococcus aureus*, using SELDI-TOF Mass Spectrometry and Artificial Neural Network Analysis. *Syst Appl Microbiol* 2011;34:81–86.

66. Malhotra-Kumar S, Haccuria K, Michiels M, et al. Current trends in rapid diagnostics for methicillin-resistant *Staphylococcus aureus* and glycopeptide-resistant enterococcus species. *J Clin Microbiol* 2008;46:1577–1587.

67. Hidron AI, Edwards JR, Patel J, et al. NHSN annual update: antimicrobial-resistant pathogens associated with healthcare-associated infections: annual summary of data reported to the National Healthcare Safety Network at the Centers for Disease Control and Prevention, 2006–2007. *Infect Control Hosp Epidemiol* 2008;29:996–1011.

68. Reinert RR, Low DE, Rossi F, et al. Antimicrobial susceptibility among organisms from the Asia/Pacific Rim, Europe and Latin and North America collected as part of TEST and the in vitro activity of tigecycline. *J Antimicrob Chemother* 2007;60:1018–1029.

69. Hegstad K, Mikalsen T, Coque TM, et al. Mobile genetic elements and their contribution to the emergence of antimicrobial resistant *Enterococcus faecalis* and *E. faecium*. *Clin Microbiol Infect* 2010;16:541–554.

70. Cattoir V, Leclercq R. Twenty-five years of shared life with vancomycin-resistant enterococci: is it time to divorce? *J Antimicrob Chemother* 2013;68:731–742.

71. Xu X, Lin D, Yan G, et al. *vanM*, a new glycopeptide resistance gene cluster found in *Enterococcus faecium*. *Antimicrob Agents Chemother* 2010;54:4643–4647.

72. Lebreton F, Depardieu F, Bourdon N, et al. D-Ala-d-Ser VanN-type transferable vancomycin resistance in *Enterococcus faecium*. *Antimicrob Agents Chemother* 2011;55:4606–4612.

73. Arthur M, Molinas C, Bugg TD, et al. Evidence for *in vivo* incorporation of D-lactate into peptidoglycan precursors of vancomycin-resistant enterococci. *Antimicrob Agents Chemother* 1992;36:867–869.

74. Billot Klein D, Gutmann L, Sable S, et al. Modification of peptidoglycan precursors is a common feature of the low-level vancomycin-resistant VANB-type *Enterococcus* D366 and of the naturally glycopeptide-resistant species *Lactobacillus casei, Pediococcus pentosaceus, Leuconostoc mesenteroides*, and *Enterococcus gallinarum*. *J Bacteriol* 1994;176:2398–2405.

75. Evers S, Courvalin P. Regulation of VanB-type vancomycin resistance gene expression by the VanS(B)-VanR (B) two-component regulatory system in *Enterococcus faecalis* V583. *J Bacteriol* 1996;178:1302–1309.

76. Handwerger S, Pucci MJ, Volk KJ, et al. The cytoplasmic peptidoglycan precursor of vancomycin-resistant *Enterococcus faecalis* terminates in lactate. *J Bacteriol* 1992;174:5982–5984.

77. Perichon B, Courvalin P. VanA-type vancomycin-resistant *Staphylococcus aureus*. *Antimicrob Agents Chemother* 2009;53:4580–4587.

78. Ray AJ, Pultz NJ, Bhalla A, et al. Coexistence of vancomycin-resistant enterococci and *Staphylococcus aureus* in the intestinal tracts of hospitalized patients. *Clin Infect Dis* 2003;37:875–881.

79. Werner G, Coque TM, Hammerum AM, et al. Emergence and spread of vancomycin resistance among enterococci in Europe. *Euro Surveill* 2008;13:1–11.

80. Granlund M, Carlsson C, Edebro H, et al. Nosocomial outbreak of *vanB2* vancomycin-resistant *Enterococcus faecium* in Sweden. *J Hosp Infect* 2006;62:254–256.

81. Werner G, Klare I, Fleige C, et al. Vancomycin-resistant *vanB*-type *Enterococcus faecium* isolates expressing varying levels of vancomycin resistance and being highly prevalent among neonatal patients in a single ICU. *Antimicrob Resist Infect Control* 2012;1:21.

82. Bourdon N, Fines-Guyon M, Thiolet JM, et al. Changing trends in vancomycin-resistant enterococci in French hospitals, 2001–08. *J Antimicrob Chemother* 2011;66:713–721.

83. Söderblom T, Aspevall O, Erntell M, et al. Alarming spread of vancomycin resistant enterococci in Sweden since 2007. *Euro Surveill* 2010;15:19620.

84. Bjørkeng EK, Rasmussen G, Sundsfjord A, et al. Clustering of polyclonal VanB-type vancomycin-resistant *Enterococcus faecium* in a low-endemic area was associated with CC17-genogroup strains harbouring transferable *vanB2*-Tn*5382* and pRUM-like *repA* containing plasmids with axe-txe plasmid addiction systems. *APMIS* 2011;119:247–258.

85. Johnson PD, Ballard SA, Grabsch EA, et al. A sustained hospital outbreak of vancomycin-resistant *Enterococcus faecium* bacteremia due to emergence of *vanB E. faecium* sequence type 203. *J Infect Dis* 2010;202:1278–1286.

86. Dahl KH, Simonsen GS, Olsvik Ø, et al. Heterogeneity in the *vanB* gene cluster of genomically diverse clinical strains of vancomycin-resistant enterococci. *Antimicrob Agents Chemother* 1999;43:1105–1510.

87. Gold HS, Unal S, Cercenado E, et al. A gene conferring resistance to vancomycin but not teicoplanin in isolates of *Enterococcus faecalis* and *Enterococcus faecium* demonstrates homology with *vanB, vanA*, and *vanC* genes of enterococci. *Antimicrob Agents Chemother* 1993;37:1604–1609.

88. Patel R, Uhl JR, Kohner P, et al. DNA sequence variation within *vanA, vanB, vanC-1*, and *vanC-2/3* genes of clinical *Enterococcus* isolates. *Antimicrob Agents Chemother* 1998;42:202–205.

89. Dahl KH, Lundblad EW, Røkenes TP, et al. Genetic linkage of the *vanB2* gene cluster to Tn*5382* in vancomycin-resistant enterococci and characterization of two novel insertion sequences. *Microbiology* 2000;146:1469–1479.

90. McGregor KF, Nolan C, Young HK, et al. Prevalence of the *vanB2* gene cluster in *vanB* glycopeptide-resistant enterococci in the United Kingdom and the Republic of Ireland and its association with a Tn*5382*-like element. *Antimicrob Agents Chemother* 2001;45:367–368.

91. Dahl KH, Røkenes TP, Lundblad EW, et al. Nonconjugative transposition of the *vanB*-containing Tn*5382*-like element in *Enterococcus faecium*. *Antimicrob Agents Chemother* 2003;47:786–789.

92. Zheng B, Tomita H, Inoue T, et al. Isolation of VanB-type *Enterococcus faecalis* strains from nosocomial infections: first report of the isolation and identification of the pheromone-responsive plasmids pMG2200, encoding VanB-type vancomycin resistance and a Bac41-type bacteriocin, and pMG2201, encoding erythromycin resistance and cytolysin (Hly/Bac). *Antimicrob Agents Chemother* 2009;53:735–747.

93. Demertzi E, Palepou MF, Kaufmann ME, et al. Characterisation of VanA and VanB elements from glycopeptide-resistant *Enterococcus faecium* from Greece. *J Med Microbiol* 2001;50:682–687.

94. Hanrahan J, Hoyen C, Rice LB. Geographic distribution of a large mobile element that transfers ampicillin and vancomycin resistance between *Enterococcus faecium* strains. *Antimicrob Agents Chemother* 2000;44:1349–1351.

95. Lee WG, Kim W. Identification of a novel insertion sequence in *vanB2*-containing *Enterococcus faecium*. *Lett Appl Microbiol* 2003;36:186–190.

96. Lopez M, Hormazabal JC, Maldonado A, et al. Clonal dissemination of *Enterococcus faecalis* ST201 and *Enterococcus faecium* CC17-ST64 containing Tn*5382-vanB2* among 16 hospitals in Chile. *Clin Microbiol Infect* 2009;15:586–588.

97. Lorenzo-Diaz F, Delgado T, Reyes-Darias JA, et al. Characterization of the first VanB vancomycin-resistant *Enterococcus faecium* isolated in a Spanish hospital. *Curr Microbiol* 2004;48:199–203.

98. Lu JJ, Chang TY, Perng CL, et al. The *vanB2* gene cluster of the majority of vancomycin-resistant *Enterococcus faecium* isolates from Taiwan is associated with the *pbp5* gene and is carried by Tn*5382* containing a novel insertion sequence. *Antimicrob Agents Chemother* 2005;49:3937–3939.

99. Torres C, Escobar S, Portillo A, et al. Detection of clonally related *vanB2*-containing *Enterococcus faecium* strains in two Spanish hospitals. *J Med Microbiol* 2006;55:1237–1243.

100. Valdezate S, Labayru C, Navarro A, et al. Large clonal outbreak of multidrug-resistant CC17 ST17 *Enterococcus faecium* containing Tn*5382* in a Spanish hospital. *J Antimicrob Chemother* 2009;63:17–20.

101. Ballard SA, Pertile KK, Lim M, et al. Molecular characterization of *vanB* elements in naturally occurring gut anaerobes. *Antimicrob Agents Chemother* 2005;49:1688–1694.

102. Dahl KH, Sundsfjord A. Transferable *vanB2* Tn*5382*-containing elements in fecal streptococcal strains from veal calves. *Antimicrob Agents Chemother* 2003;47:2579–2583.

103. Domingo MC, Huletsky A, Bernal A, et al. Characterization of a Tn*5382*-like transposon containing the *vanB2* gene cluster in a *Clostridium* strain isolated from human faeces. *J Antimicrob Chemother* 2005;55:466–474.

104. Marvaud JC, Mory F, Lambert T. *Clostridium clostridioforme* and *Atopobium minutum* clinical isolates with *vanB*-type resistance in France. *J Clin Microbiol* 2011;49:3436–3438.

105. Domingo MC, Huletsky A, Giroux R, et al. High prevalence of glycopeptide resistance genes *vanB*, *vanD*, and *vanG* not associated with enterococci in human fecal flora. *Antimicrob Agents Chemother* 2005;49:4784–4786.

106. Graham M, Ballard SA, Grabsch EA, et al. High rates of fecal carriage of nonenterococcal *vanB* in both children and adults. *Antimicrob Agents Chemother* 2008;52:1195–1197.

107. Young HL, Ballard SA, Roffey P, et al. Direct detection of *vanB2* using the Roche LightCycler *vanA/B* detection assay to indicate vancomycin-resistant enterococcal carriage—sensitive but not specific. *J Antimicrob Chemother* 2007;59:809–810.

108. Usacheva EA, Ginocchio CC, Morgan M, et al. Prospective, multicenter evaluation of the BD GeneOhm VanR assay for direct, rapid detection of vancomycin-resistant *Enterococcus* species in perianal and rectal specimens. *Am J Clin Pathol* 2010;134:219–226.

109. Gazin M, Lammens C, Goossens H, et al. Evaluation of GeneOhm VanR and Xpert *vanA/vanB* molecular assays for the rapid detection of vancomycin-resistant enterococci. *Eur J Clin Microbiol Infect Dis* 2012;31:273–276.

110. Bourdon N, Berenger R, Lepoultier R, et al. Rapid detection of vancomycin-resistant enterococci from rectal swabs by the Cepheid Xpert *vanA/vanB* assay. *Diagn Microbiol Infect Dis* 2010;67:291–293.

111. Mak A, Miller MA, Chong G, et al. Comparison of PCR and culture for screening of vancomycin-resistant enterococci: highly disparate results for *vanA* and *vanB*. *J Clin Microbiol* 2009;47:4136–4137.

112. Stamper PD, Cai M, Lema C, et al. Comparison of the BD GeneOhm VanR assay to culture for identification of vancomycin-resistant enterococci in rectal and stool specimens. *J Clin Microbiol* 2007;45:3360–3365.

113. Seo JY, Kim PW, Lee JH, et al. Evaluation of PCR-based screening for vancomycin-resistant enterococci compared with a chromogenic agar-based culture method. *J Med Microbiol* 2011;60:945–949.

114. Liu TY, Tsai KT, Wang HH, et al. Functionalized arrays of Raman-enhancing nanoparticles for capture and culture-free analysis of bacteria in human blood. *Nat Commun* 2011;2:538.

115. Cassone M, Del Grosso M, Pantosti A, et al. Detection of genetic elements carrying glycopeptide resistance clusters in *Enterococcus* by DNA microarrays. *Mol Cell Probes* 2008;22:162–167.

116. Roberts MC, Sutcliffe J, Courvalin P, et al. Nomenclature for macrolide and macrolide-lincosamide-streptogramin B resistance determinants. *Antimicrob Agents Chemother* 1999;43:2823–2830.

117. Luthje P, Schwarz S. Molecular basis of resistance to macrolides and lincosamides among staphylococci and streptococci from various animal sources collected in the resistance monitoring program BfT-GermVet. *Int J Antimicrob Agents* 2007;29:528–535.

118. Varaldo PE, Montanari MP, Giovanetti E. Genetic elements responsible for erythromycin resistance in streptococci. *Antimicrob Agents Chemother* 2009;53:343–353.

119. Le Bouter A, Leclercq R, Cattoir V. Molecular basis of resistance to macrolides, lincosamides and streptogramins in *Staphylococcus saprophyticus* clinical isolates. *Int J Antimicrob Agents* 2011;37:118–123.

120. Klaassen CH, Mouton JW. Molecular detection of the macrolide efflux gene: to discriminate or not to discriminate between *mef*(A) and *mef*(E). *Antimicrob Agents Chemother* 2005;49:1271–1278.

121. Tu D, Blaha G, Moore PB, et al. Structures of MLSBK antibiotics bound to mutated large ribosomal subunits provide a structural explanation for resistance. *Cell* 2005;121:257–270.

122. Leclercq R. Mechanisms of resistance to macrolides and lincosamides: nature of the resistance elements and their clinical implications. *Clin Infect Dis* 2002;34:482–492.

123. de Vries LE, Christensen H, Agersø Y. The diversity of inducible and constitutively expressed *erm*(C) genes and association to different replicon types in staphylococci plasmids. *Mob Genet Elements* 2012;2:72–80.

124. Sutcliffe J, Tait-Kamradt A, Wondrack L. *Streptococcus pneumoniae* and *Streptococcus pyogenes* resistant to macrolides but sensitive to clindamycin: a common resistance pattern mediated by an efflux system. *Antimicrob Agents Chemother* 1996;40:1817–1824.

125. Santagati M, Iannelli F, Oggioni MR, et al. Characterization of a genetic element carrying the macrolide efflux gene *mef*(A) in *Streptococcus pneumoniae*. *Antimicrob Agents Chemother* 2000;44:2585–2587.

126. Malbruny B, Werno AM, Murdoch DR, et al. Cross-resistance to lincosamides, streptogramins A, and pleuromutilins due to the *lsa*(C) gene in *Streptococcus agalactiae* UCN70. *Antimicrob Agents Chemother* 2011;55:1470–1474.

127. Luthje P, von Kockritz-Blickwede M, Schwarz S. Identification and characterization of nine novel types of small staphylococcal plasmids carrying the lincosamide nucleotidyltransferase gene *lnu*(A). *J Antimicrob Chemother* 2007;59:600–606.

128. Petinaki E, Guerin-Faublee V, Pichereau V, et al. Lincomycin resistance gene *lnu*(D) in *Streptococcus uberis*. *Antimicrob Agents Chemother* 2008;52:626–630.

129. Phuc Nguyen MC, Woerther PL, Bouvet M, et al. *Escherichia coli* as reservoir for macrolide resistance genes. *Emerg Infect Dis* 2009;15:1648–1650.

130. Seo YS, Srinivasan U, Oh KY, et al. Changing molecular epidemiology of group B streptococcus in Korea. *J Korean Med Sci* 2010;25:817–823.

131. World Health Organization. *Multidrug and extensively drug-resistant TB (M/XDR-TB): 2010 global report on surveillance and response*. Geneva: World Health Organization, 2010.

132. Van Deun A, Martin A, Palomino JC. Diagnosis of drug-resistant tuberculosis: reliability and rapidity of detection. *Int J Tuberc Lung Dis* 2010;14:131–140.

133. Müller B, Borrell S, Rose G, et al. The heterogeneous evolution of multidrug-resistant *Mycobacterium tuberculosis*. *Trends Genet* 2013;29:160–169.

134. Zhang Y, Yew WW. Mechanisms of drug resistance in *Mycobacterium tuberculosis*. *Int J Tuberc Lung Dis* 2009; 13:1320–1330.

135. Palomino JC. Molecular detection, identification and drug resistance detection in *Mycobacterium tuberculosis*. *FEMS Immunol Med Microbiol* 2009;56:103–111.

136. Campbell EA, Korzheva N, Mustaev A, et al. Structural mechanism for rifampicin inhibition of bacterial RNA polymerase. *Cell* 2001;104:901–912.

137. Johnsson K, Schultz PG. Mechanistic studies of the oxidation of isoniazid by the catalase peroxidase from *Mycobacterium tuberculosis*. *J Am Chem Soc* 1994;116:7425–7426.

138. Banerjee A, Dubnau E, Quemard A, et al. *inhA*, a gene encoding a target for isoniazid and ethionamide in *Mycobacterium tuberculosis*. *Science* 1994;263:227–230.

139. Helb D, Jones M, Story E, et al. Rapid detection of *Mycobacterium tuberculosis* and rifampin resistance by use of on-demand, near-patient technology. *J Clin Microbiol* 2010;48:229–237.

140. Hillemann D, Rusch-Gerdes S, Richter E. Evaluation of the GenoType MTBDRplus assay for rifampin and isoniazid susceptibility testing of *Mycobacterium tuberculosis* strains and clinical specimens. *J Clin Microbiol* 2007;45:2635–2640.

141. Hillemann D, Rusch-Gerdes S, Richter E. Feasibility of the GenoType MTBDRsl assay for fluoroquinolone, amikacin-capreomycin, and ethambutol resistance testing of *Mycobacterium tuberculosis* strains and clinical specimens. *J Clin Microbiol* 2009;47:1767–1772.

142. Boehme CC, Nabeta P, Hillemann D, et al. Rapid molecular detection of tuberculosis and rifampin resistance. *N Engl J Med* 2010;363:1005–1015.

143. Clouse K, Page-Shipp L, Dansey H, et al. Implementation of Xpert MTB/RIF for routine point-of-care diagnosis of tuberculosis at the primary care level. *S Afr Med J* 2012;102:805–807.

144. Moore DA, Shah NS. Alternative methods of diagnosing drug resistance—what can they do for me? *J Infect Dis* 2011;204(Suppl 4):S1110–S1119.

145. Abraham EP, Chain E. An enzyme from bacteria able to destroy penicillin. *Nature* 1940;146:837.

146. Bush K, Jacoby GA. Updated functional classification of beta-lactamases. *Antimicrob Agents Chemother* 2010;54: 969–976.

147. Pitout JD. Infections with extended-spectrum beta-lactamase-producing enterobacteriaceae: changing epidemiology and drug treatment choices. *Drugs* 2010;70: 313–333.

148. Tzouvelekis LS, Markogiannakis A, Psichogiou M, et al. Carbapenemases in *Klebsiella pneumoniae* and other *Enterobacteriaceae*: an evolving crisis of global dimensions. *Clin Microbiol Rev* 2012;25:682–707.

149. Paterson DL, Bonomo RA. Extended-spectrum beta-lactamases: a clinical update. *Clin Microbiol Rev* 2005;18: 657–686.

150. Canton R, Coque TM. The CTX-M beta-lactamase pandemic. *Curr Opin Microbiol* 2006;9:466–475.

151. Naseer U, Sundsfjord A. The CTX-M conundrum: dissemination of plasmids and *Escherichia coli* clones. *Microb Drug Resist* 2011;17:83–97.

152. Zhao WH, Hu ZQ. Epidemiology and genetics of CTX-M extended-spectrum beta-lactamases in Gram-negative bacteria. *Crit Rev Microbiol* 2013;39:79–101.

153. Bonnet R. Growing group of extended-spectrum beta-lactamases: the CTX-M enzymes. *Antimicrob Agents Chemother* 2004;48:1–14.

154. Naas T, Poirel L, Nordmann P. Minor extended-spectrum beta-lactamases. *Clin Microbiol Infect* 2008;14(Suppl 1): 42–52.

155. Walsh TR. Emerging carbapenemases: a global perspective. *Int J Antimicrob Agents* 2010;36(Suppl 3):S8–S14.

156. Poirel L, Naas T, Nordmann P. Diversity, epidemiology, and genetics of class D beta-lactamases. *Antimicrob Agents Chemother* 2010;54:24–38.

157. Poirel L, Potron A, Nordmann P. OXA-48-like carbapenemases: the phantom menace. *J Antimicrob Chemother* 2012;67:1597–1606.

158. Livermore DM, Mushtaq S, Barker K, et al. Characterization of beta-lactamase and porin mutants of *Enterobacteriaceae* selected with ceftaroline + avibactam (NXL104). *J Antimicrob Chemother* 2012;67:1354–1358.

159. Nordmann P, Gniadkowski M, Giske CG, et al. Identification and screening of carbapenemase-producing *Enterobacteriaceae*. *Clin Microbiol Infect* 2012;18:432–438.

160. Bernabeu S, Poirel L, Nordmann P. Spectrophotometry-based detection of carbapenemase producers among *Enterobacteriaceae*. *Diagn Microbiol Infect Dis* 2012;74: 88–90.

161. Bonnin RA, Naas T, Poirel L, et al. Phenotypic, biochemical, and molecular techniques for detection of metallo-beta-lactamase NDM in *Acinetobacter baumannii*. *J Clin Microbiol* 2012;50:1419–1421.

162. Nordmann P, Poirel L, Dortet L. Rapid detection of carbapenemase-producing *Enterobacteriaceae*. *Emerg Infect Dis* 2012;18:1503–1507.

163. Nordmann P, Dortet L, Poirel L. Rapid detection of extended-spectrum-beta-lactamase-producing *Enterobacteriaceae*. *J Clin Microbiol* 2012;50:3016–3022.

164. Dortet L, Poirel L, Nordmann P. Rapid identification of carbapenemase types in *Enterobacteriaceae* and *Pseudomonas* spp. by using a biochemical test. *Antimicrob Agents Chemother* 2012;56:6437–6440.

165. Burckhardt I, Zimmermann S. Using matrix-assisted laser desorption ionization-time of flight mass spectrometry to detect carbapenem resistance within 1 to 2.5 hours. *J Clin Microbiol* 2011;49:3321–3324.

166. Hrabak J, Walkova R, Studentova V, et al. Carbapenemase activity detection by matrix-assisted laser desorption ionization-time of flight mass spectrometry. *J Clin Microbiol* 2011;49:3222–3227.

167. Woodford N, Turton JF, Livermore DM. Multiresistant Gram-negative bacteria: the role of high-risk clones in the dissemination of antibiotic resistance. *FEMS Microbiol Rev* 2011;35:736–755.

168. Karah N, Sundsfjord A, Towner K, et al. Insights into the global molecular epidemiology of carbapenem non-susceptible clones of *Acinetobacter baumannii*. *Drug Resist Updat* 2012;15:237–247.

169. Dhanji H, Doumith M, Clermont O, et al. Real-time PCR for detection of the O25b-ST131 clone of *Escherichia coli* and its CTX-M-15-like extended-spectrum beta-lactamases. *Int J Antimicrob Agents* 2010;36:355–358.

170. Chen L, Chavda KD, Mediavilla JR, et al. Multiplex real-time PCR for detection of an epidemic KPC-producing *Klebsiella pneumoniae* ST258 clone. *Antimicrob Agents Chemother* 2012;56:3444–3447.

171. Tofteland S, Haldorsen B, Dahl KH, et al. Effects of phenotype and genotype on methods for detection of extended-spectrum-beta-lactamase-producing clinical isolates of *Escherichia coli* and *Klebsiella pneumoniae* in Norway. *J Clin Microbiol* 2007;45:199–205.

172. Jones CH, Ruzin A, Tuckman M, et al. Pyrosequencing using the single-nucleotide polymorphism protocol for rapid determination of TEM- and SHV-type extended-spectrum beta-lactamases in clinical isolates and identification of the novel beta-lactamase genes *bla*SHV-48, *bla*SHV-105, and *bla*TEM-155. *Antimicrob Agents Chemother* 2009;53:977–986.

173. Randegger CC, Hachler H. Real-time PCR and melting curve analysis for reliable and rapid detection of SHV extended-spectrum beta-lactamases. *Antimicrob Agents Chemother* 2001;45:1730–1736.

174. Nijhuis R, van Zwet A, Stuart JC, et al. Rapid molecular detection of extended-spectrum beta-lactamase gene variants with a novel ligation-mediated real-time PCR. *J Med Microbiol* 2012;61:1563–1567.

175. Dallenne C, Da Costa A, Decre D, et al. Development of a set of multiplex PCR assays for the detection of genes encoding important beta-lactamases in *Enterobacteriaceae*. *J Antimicrob Chemother* 2010;65:490–495.

176. Woodford N, Fagan EJ, Ellington MJ. Multiplex PCR for rapid detection of genes encoding CTX-M extended-spectrum (beta)-lactamases. *J Antimicrob Chemother* 2006;57:154–155.

177. Xu L, Ensor V, Gossain S, et al. Rapid and simple detection of *bla*CTX-M genes by multiplex PCR assay. *J Med Microbiol* 2005;54:1183–1187.

178. Xu L, Evans J, Ling T, et al. Rapid genotyping of CTX-M extended-spectrum beta-lactamases by denaturing high-performance liquid chromatography. *Antimicrob Agents Chemother* 2007;51:1446–1454.

179. Naas T, Oxacelay C, Nordmann P. Identification of CTX-M-type extended-spectrum-beta-lactamase genes using real-time PCR and pyrosequencing. *Antimicrob Agents Chemother* 2007;51:223–230.

180. Birkett CI, Ludlam HA, Woodford N, et al. Real-time TaqMan PCR for rapid detection and typing of genes encoding CTX-M extended-spectrum beta-lactamases. *J Med Microbiol* 2007;56:52–55.

181. Oxacelay C, Ergani A, Naas T, et al. Rapid detection of CTX-M-producing *Enterobacteriaceae* in urine samples. *J Antimicrob Chemother* 2009;64:986–989.

182. Vanstone GL, Yorgancioglu A, Wilkie L, et al. A real-time multiplex PCR assay for the rapid detection of CTX-M-type extended spectrum beta-lactamases directly from blood cultures. *J Med Microbiol* 2012;61:1631–1632.

183. Fujita S, Yosizaki K, Ogushi T, et al. Rapid identification of Gram-negative bacteria with and without CTX-M extended-spectrum beta-lactamase from positive blood culture bottles by PCR followed by microchip gel electrophoresis. *J Clin Microbiol* 2011;49:1483–1488.

184. Lee S, Park YJ, Kim M, et al. Prevalence of Ambler class A and D beta-lactamases among clinical isolates of *Pseudomonas aeruginosa* in Korea. *J Antimicrob Chemother* 2005;56:122–127.

185. Naas T, Poirel L, Karim A, et al. Molecular characterization of In*50*, a class 1 integron encoding the gene for the extended-spectrum beta-lactamase VEB-1 in *Pseudomonas aeruginosa*. *FEMS Microbiol Lett* 1999;176:411–419.

186. Poirel L, Cabanne L, Vahaboglu H, et al. Genetic environment and expression of the extended-spectrum beta-lactamase *bla*PER-1 gene in Gram-negative bacteria. *Antimicrob Agents Chemother* 2005;49:1708–1713.

187. Poirel L, Le Thomas I, Naas T, et al. Biochemical sequence analyses of GES-1, a novel class A extended-spectrum beta-lactamase, and the class 1 integron In*52* from *Klebsiella pneumoniae*. *Antimicrob Agents Chemother* 2000;44:622–632.

188. Bogaerts P, Bauraing C, Deplano A, et al. Emergence and dissemination of BEL-1-producing *Pseudomonas aeruginosa* isolates in Belgium. *Antimicrob Agents Chemother* 2007;51:1584–1585.

189. Woodford N, Ellington MJ, Coelho JM, et al. Multiplex PCR for genes encoding prevalent OXA carbapenemases in Acinetobacter spp. *Int J Antimicrob Agents* 2006;27:351–353.

190. Higgins PG, Lehmann M, Seifert H. Inclusion of OXA-143 primers in a multiplex polymerase chain reaction (PCR) for genes encoding prevalent OXA carbapenemases in *Acinetobacter* spp. *Int J Antimicrob Agents* 2010;35:305.

191. Voets GM, Fluit AC, Scharringa J, et al. A set of multiplex PCRs for genotypic detection of extended-spectrum beta-lactamases, carbapenemases, plasmid-mediated AmpC beta-lactamases and OXA beta-lactamases. *Int J Antimicrob Agents* 2011;37:356–359.

192. Ellington MJ, Kistler J, Livermore DM, et al. Multiplex PCR for rapid detection of genes encoding acquired metallo-beta-lactamases. *J Antimicrob Chemother* 2007;59:321–322.

193. Poirel L, Walsh TR, Cuvillier V, et al. Multiplex PCR for detection of acquired carbapenemase genes. *Diagn Microbiol Infect Dis* 2011;70:119–123.

194. Monteiro J, Widen RH, Pignatari AC, et al. Rapid detection of carbapenemase genes by multiplex real-time PCR. *J Antimicrob Chemother* 2012;67:906–909.

195. Mendes RE, Kiyota KA, Monteiro J, et al. Rapid detection and identification of metallo-beta-lactamase-encoding genes by multiplex real-time PCR assay and melt curve analysis. *J Clin Microbiol* 2007;45:544–547.

196. Roth AL, Hanson ND. Rapid detection and statistical differentiation of KPC gene variants in Gram-negative pathogens by use of high-resolution melting and ScreenClust analyses. *J Clin Microbiol* 2013;51:61–65.

197. Swayne RL, Ludlam HA, Shet VG, et al. Real-time TaqMan PCR for rapid detection of genes encoding five types of non-metallo- (class A and D) carbapenemases in *Enterobacteriaceae*. *Int J Antimicrob Agents* 2011;38:35–38.

198. Richter SN, Frasson I, Biasolo MA, et al. Ultrarapid detection of blaKPC(1)/(2)-(1)(2) from perirectal and nasal swabs by use of real-time PCR. *J Clin Microbiol* 2012;50:1718–1720.

199. Cole JM, Schuetz AN, Hill CE, et al. Development and evaluation of a real-time PCR assay for detection of *Klebsiella pneumoniae* carbapenemase genes. *J Clin Microbiol* 2009;47:322–326.

200. Diene SM, Bruder N, Raoult D, et al. Real-time PCR assay allows detection of the New Delhi metallo-beta-lactamase (NDM-1)-encoding gene in France. *Int J Antimicrob Agents* 2011;37:544–546.

201. Naas T, Ergani A, Carrer A, et al. Real-time PCR for detection of NDM-1 carbapenemase genes from spiked stool samples. *Antimicrob Agents Chemother* 2011;55:4038–4043.

202. Ong DC, Koh TH, Syahidah N, et al. Rapid detection of the *bla*NDM-1 gene by real-time PCR. *J Antimicrob Chemother* 2011;66:1647–1649.
203. Kruttgen A, Razavi S, Imohl M, et al. Real-time PCR assay and a synthetic positive control for the rapid and sensitive detection of the emerging resistance gene New Delhi Metallo-beta-lactamase-1 (*bla*(NDM-1)). *Med Microbiol Immunol* 2011;200:137–141.
204. Liu W, Zou D, Li Y, et al. Sensitive and rapid detection of the new Delhi metallo-beta-lactamase gene by loop-mediated isothermal amplification. *J Clin Microbiol* 2012; 50:1580–1585.
205. Hindiyeh M, Smollen G, Grossman Z, et al. Rapid detection of *bla*KPC carbapenemase genes by real-time PCR. *J Clin Microbiol* 2008;46:2879–2883.
206. Spanu T, Fiori B, D'inzeo T, et al. Evaluation of the New NucliSENS EasyQ KPC test for rapid detection of *Klebsiella pneumoniae* carbapenemase genes (*bla*KPC). *J Clin Microbiol* 2012;50:2783–2785.
207. Batchelor M, Hopkins KL, Liebana E, et al. Development of a miniaturised microarray-based assay for the rapid identification of antimicrobial resistance genes in Gram-negative bacteria. *Int J Antimicrob Agents* 2008;31:440–451.
208. Frye JG, Lindsey RL, Rondeau G, et al. Development of a DNA microarray to detect antimicrobial resistance genes identified in the National Center for Biotechnology Information database. *Microb Drug Resist* 2010;16:9–19.
209. Grimm V, Ezaki S, Susa M, et al. Use of DNA microarrays for rapid genotyping of TEM beta-lactamases that confer resistance. *J Clin Microbiol* 2004;42:3766–3774.
210. Leinberger DM, Grimm V, Rubtsova M, et al. Integrated detection of extended-spectrum-beta-lactam resistance by DNA microarray-based genotyping of TEM, SHV, and CTX-M genes. *J Clin Microbiol* 2010;48: 460–471.
211. Peter H, Berggrav K, Thomas P, et al. Direct detection and genotyping of *Klebsiella pneumoniae* carbapenemases from urine by use of a new DNA microarray test. *J Clin Microbiol* 2012;50:3990–3998.
212. Rubtsova MY, Ulyashova MM, Edelstein MV, et al. Oligonucleotide microarrays with horseradish peroxidase-based detection for the identification of extended-spectrum beta-lactamases. *Biosens Bioelectron* 2010;26:1252–1260.
213. Kaase M, Szabados F, Wassill L, et al. Detection of carbapenemases in *Enterobacteriaceae* by a commercial multiplex PCR. *J Clin Microbiol* 2012;50:3115–3118.
214. Cohen Stuart J, Dierikx C, Al Naiemi N, et al. Rapid detection of TEM, SHV and CTX-M extended-spectrum beta-lactamases in *Enterobacteriaceae* using ligation-mediated amplification with microarray analysis. *J Antimicrob Chemother* 2010;65:1377–1381.
215. Naas T, Cuzon G, Bogaerts P, et al. Evaluation of a DNA microarray (Check-MDR CT102) for rapid detection of TEM, SHV, and CTX-M extended-spectrum beta-lactamases and of KPC, OXA-48, VIM, IMP, and NDM-1 carbapenemases. *J Clin Microbiol* 2011;49:1608–1613.
216. Woodford N, Warner M, Pike R, et al. Evaluation of a commercial microarray to detect carbapenemase-producing *Enterobacteriaceae*. *J Antimicrob Chemother* 2011;66:2887–2888.
217. Cuzon G, Naas T, Bogaerts P, et al. Evaluation of a DNA microarray for the rapid detection of extended-spectrum beta-lactamases (TEM, SHV and CTX-M), plasmid-mediated cephalosporinases (CMY-2-like, DHA, FOX, ACC-1, ACT/MIR and CMY-1-like/MOX) and carbapenemases (KPC, OXA-48, VIM, IMP and NDM). *J Antimicrob Chemother* 2012;67:1865–1869.
218. Stuart JC, Voets G, Scharringa J, et al. Detection of carbapenemase-producing *Enterobacteriaceae* with a commercial DNA microarray. *J Med Microbiol* 2012;61: 809–812.
219. Veyssier P, Bryskier A. Aminocyclitol aminoglycosides. In: Bryskier A, ed. *Antimicrobial agents: antibacterials and antifungals*. Washington, DC: ASM Press, 2005: 453–469.
220. Majumder K, Wei L, Annedi SC, et al. Aminoglycoside antibiotics. In: Bonomo RA, Tolmasky M, eds. *Enzyme-mediated resistance to antibiotics: mechanisms, dissemination, and prospects for inhibition*. Washington, DC: ASM Press, 2007:7–20.
221. Ramirez MS, Tolmasky ME. Aminoglycoside modifying enzymes. *Drug Resist Updat* 2010;13:151–171.
222. Wachino J, Arakawa Y. Exogenously acquired 16S rRNA methyltransferases found in aminoglycoside-resistant pathogenic Gram-negative bacteria: an update. *Drug Resist Updat* 2012;15:133–148.
223. Shaw KJ, Rather PN, Hare RS, et al. Molecular genetics of aminoglycoside resistance genes and familial relationships of the aminoglycoside-modifying enzymes. *Microbiol Rev* 1993;57:138–163.
224. Tolmasky ME. Aminoglycoside-modifying enzymes: characteristics, localization, and dissemination. In: Bonomo RA, Tolmasky M, eds. *Enzyme-mediated resistance to antibiotics: mechanisms, dissemination, and prospects for inhibition*. Washington, DC: ASM Press, 2007: 35–52.
225. Perreten V, Vorlet-Fawer L, Slickers P, et al. Microarray-based detection of 90 antibiotic resistance genes of gram-positive bacteria. *J Clin Microbiol* 2005;43: 2291–2302.
226. Diarra MS, Rempel H, Champagne J, et al. Distribution of antimicrobial resistance and virulence genes in *Enterococcus* spp. and characterization of isolates from broiler chickens. *Appl Environ Microbiol* 2010;76: 8033–8043.
227. Champagne J, Diarra MS, Rempel H, et al. Development of a DNA microarray for enterococcal species, virulence, and antibiotic resistance gene determinations among isolates from poultry. *Appl Environ Microbiol* 2011;77: 2625–2633.
228. Garneau P, Labrecque O, Maynard C, et al. Use of a bacterial antimicrobial resistance gene microarray for the identification of resistant *Staphylococcus aureus*. *Zoonoses Public Health* 2010;57(Suppl 1):94–99.
229. Frye JG, Jesse T, Long F, et al. DNA microarray detection of antimicrobial resistance genes in diverse bacteria. *Int J Antimicrob Agents* 2006;27:138–151.
230. Vakulenko SB, Mobashery S. Versatility of aminoglycosides and prospects for their future. *Clin Microbiol Rev* 2003;16:430–450.
231. Hidalgo-Grass C, Strahilevitz J. High-resolution melt curve analysis for identification of single nucleotide mutations in the quinolone resistance gene *aac(6')-Ib-cr*. *Antimicrob Agents Chemother* 2010;54:3509–3511.
232. Bell JM, Turnidge JD, Andersson P. *aac(6')-Ib-cr* genotyping by simultaneous high-resolution melting analyses of an unlabeled probe and full-length amplicon. *Antimicrob Agents Chemother* 2010;54:1378–1380.

233. Lindemann PC, Risberg K, Wiker HG, et al. Aminoglycoside resistance in clinical *Escherichia coli* and *Klebsiella pneumoniae* isolates from Western Norway. *APMIS* 2012;120:495–502.

234. Doi Y, Arakawa Y. 16S ribosomal RNA methylation: emerging resistance mechanism against aminoglycosides. *Clin Infect Dis* 2007;45:88–94.

235. Bercot B, Poirel L, Nordmann P. Updated multiplex polymerase chain reaction for detection of 16S rRNA methylases: high prevalence among NDM-1 producers. *Diagn Microbiol Infect Dis* 2011;71:442–445.

236. Savic M, Lovric J, Tomic TI, et al. Determination of the target nucleosides for members of two families of 16S rRNA methyltransferases that confer resistance to partially overlapping groups of aminoglycoside antibiotics. *Nucleic Acids Res* 2009;37:5420–5431.

237. Flamm RK, Farrell DJ, Mendes RE, et al. ZAAPS Program results for 2010: an activity and spectrum analysis of linezolid using clinical isolates from 75 medical centres in 24 countries. *J Chemother* 2012;24:328–337.

238. Ross JE, Farrell DJ, Mendes RE, et al. Eight-year (2002–2009) summary of the linezolid (Zyvox) Annual Appraisal of Potency and Spectrum; ZAAPS) program in European countries. *J Chemother* 2011;23:71–76.

239. Flamm RK, Mendes RE, Ross JE, et al. Linezolid surveillance results for the United States: LEADER surveillance program 2011. *Antimicrob Agents Chemother* 2013; 57:1077–1081.

240. Wilson DN, Schluenzen F, Harms JM, et al. The oxazolidinone antibiotics perturb the ribosomal peptidyltransferase center and effect tRNA positioning. *Proc Natl Acad Sci U S A* 2008;105:13339–13344.

241. Diaz L, Kiratisin P, Mendes RE, et al. Transferable plasmid-mediated resistance to linezolid due to *cfr* in a human clinical isolate of *Enterococcus faecalis*. *Antimicrob Agents Chemother* 2012;56:3917–3922.

242. Gu B, Kelesidis T, Tsiodras S, et al. The emerging problem of linezolid-resistant *Staphylococcus*. *J Antimicrob Chemother* 2013;68:4–11.

243. Farrell DJ, Morrissey I, Bakker S, et al. In vitro activities of telithromycin, linezolid, and quinupristin-dalfopristin against *Streptococcus pneumoniae* with macrolide resistance due to ribosomal mutations. *Antimicrob Agents Chemother* 2004;48:3169–3171.

244. Wolter N, Smith AM, Farrell DJ, et al. Novel mechanism of resistance to oxazolidinones, macrolides, and chloramphenicol in ribosomal protein L4 of the pneumococcus. *Antimicrob Agents Chemother* 2005;49:3554–3557.

245. Ross JE, Anderegg TR, Sader HS, et al. Trends in linezolid susceptibility patterns in 2002: report from the worldwide Zyvox Annual Appraisal of Potency and Spectrum Program. *Diagn Microbiol Infect Dis* 2005; 52:53–58.

246. Lobritz M, Hutton-Thomas R, Marshall S, et al. Recombination proficiency influences frequency and locus of mutational resistance to linezolid in *Enterococcus faecalis*. *Antimicrob Agents Chemother* 2003;47:3318–3320.

247. Marshall SH, Donskey CJ, Hutton-Thomas R, et al. Gene dosage and linezolid resistance in *Enterococcus faecium* and *Enterococcus faecalis*. *Antimicrob Agents Chemother* 2002;46:3334–3336.

248. Meka VG, Pillai SK, Sakoulas G, et al. Linezolid resistance in sequential *Staphylococcus aureus* isolates associated with a T2500A mutation in the 23S rRNA gene and loss of a single copy of rRNA. *J Infect Dis* 2004;190:311–317.

249. Long KS, Poehlsgaard J, Kehrenberg C, et al. The Cfr rRNA methyltransferase confers resistance to phenicols, lincosamides, oxazolidinones, pleuromutilins, and streptogramin A antibiotics. *Antimicrob Agents Chemother* 2006;50:2500–2505.

250. Morales G, Picazo JJ, Baos E, et al. Resistance to linezolid is mediated by the *cfr* gene in the first report of an outbreak of linezolid-resistant *Staphylococcus aureus*. *Clin Infect Dis* 2010;50:821–825.

251. Sanchez Garcia M, De la Torre MA, Morales G, et al. Clinical outbreak of linezolid-resistant *Staphylococcus aureus* in an intensive care unit. *JAMA* 2010;303:2260–2264.

252. Locke JB, Morales G, Hilgers M, et al. Elevated linezolid resistance in clinical *cfr*-positive *Staphylococcus aureus* isolates is associated with co-occurring mutations in ribosomal protein L3. *Antimicrob Agents Chemother* 2010;54:5352–5355.

253. Bonilla H, Huband MD, Seidel J, et al. Multicity outbreak of linezolid-resistant *Staphylococcus epidermidis* associated with clonal spread of a *cfr*-containing strain. *Clin Infect Dis* 2010;51:796–800.

254. Gopegui ER, Juan C, Zamorano L, et al. Transferable multidrug resistance plasmid carrying *cfr* associated with *tet(L)*, *ant(4')-Ia*, and *dfrK* genes from a clinical methicillin-resistant *Staphylococcus aureus* ST125 strain. *Antimicrob Agents Chemother* 2012;56: 2139–2142.

255. Cai JC, Hu YY, Zhang R, et al. Linezolid-resistant clinical isolates of meticillin-resistant coagulase-negative staphylococci and *Enterococcus faecium* from China. *J Med Microbiol* 2012;61:1568–1573.

256. Bongiorno D, Campanile F, Mongelli G, et al. DNA methylase modifications and other linezolid resistance mutations in coagulase-negative staphylococci in Italy. *J Antimicrob Chemother* 2010;65:2336–2340.

257. LaMarre JM, Locke JB, Shaw KJ, et al. Low fitness cost of the multidrug resistance gene *cfr*. *Antimicrob Agents Chemother* 2011;55:3714–3719.

258. Schwarz S, Werckenthin C, Kehrenberg C. Identification of a plasmid-borne chloramphenicol-florfenicol resistance gene in *Staphylococcus sciuri*. *Antimicrob Agents Chemother* 2000;44:2530–2533.

259. Kehrenberg C, Schwarz S. Distribution of florfenicol resistance genes *fexA* and *cfr* among chloramphenicol-resistant *Staphylococcus* isolates. *Antimicrob Agents Chemother* 2006;50:1156–1163.

260. Liu Y, Wang Y, Wu C, et al. First report of the multidrug resistance gene *cfr* in *Enterococcus faecalis* of animal origin. *Antimicrob Agents Chemother* 2012;56: 1650–1654.

261. Liu Y, Wang Y, Schwarz S, et al. Transferable multiresistance plasmids carrying *cfr* in *Enterococcus* spp from swine and farm environment. *Antimicrob Agents Chemother* 2013;57:42–48.

262. Dai L, Wu CM, Wang MG, et al. First report of the multidrug resistance gene *cfr* and the phenicol resistance gene *fexA* in a *Bacillus* strain from swine feces. *Antimicrob Agents Chemother* 2010;54:3953–3955.

263. Wang Y, Schwarz S, Shen Z, et al. Co-location of the multiresistance gene *cfr* and the novel streptomycin resistance gene *aadY* on a small plasmid in a porcine *Bacillus* strain. *J Antimicrob Chemother* 2012;67:1547–1549.

264. Zhang WJ, Wu CM, Wang Y, et al. The new genetic environment of *cfr* on plasmid pBS-02 in a *Bacillus* strain. *J Antimicrob Chemother* 2011;66:1174–1175.

265. Wang Y, Wang Y, Schwarz S, et al. Detection of the staphylococcal multiresistance gene *cfr* in *Macrococcus caseolyticus* and *Jeotgalicoccus pinnipedialis*. *J Antimicrob Chemother* 2012;67:1824–1827.

266. Wang Y, He T, Schwarz S, et al. Detection of the staphylococcal multiresistance gene *cfr* in *Escherichia coli* of domestic-animal origin. *J Antimicrob Chemother* 2012;67:1094–1098.

267. Wang Y, Wang Y, Wu CM, et al. Detection of the staphylococcal multiresistance gene *cfr* in *Proteus vulgaris* of food animal origin. *J Antimicrob Chemother* 2011;66:2521–2526.

268. Qi J, Du Y, Zhu R, et al. A loop-mediated isothermal amplification method for rapid detection of the multidrug-resistance gene *cfr*. *Gene* 2012;504:140–143.

269. Bonora MG, Solbiati M, Stepan E, et al. Emergence of linezolid resistance in the vancomycin-resistant *Enterococcus faecium* multilocus sequence typing C1 epidemic lineage. *J Clin Microbiol* 2006;44:1153–1155.

270. Toh SM, Xiong L, Arias CA, et al. Acquisition of a natural resistance gene renders a clinical strain of methicillin-resistant *Staphylococcus aureus* resistant to the synthetic antibiotic linezolid. *Mol Microbiol* 2007;64:1506–1514.

271. Werner G, Strommenger B, Klare I, et al. Molecular detection of linezolid resistance in *Enterococcus faecium* and *Enterococcus faecalis* by use of 5' nuclease real-time PCR compared to a modified classical approach. *J Clin Microbiol* 2004;42:5327–5331.

272. Werner G, Bartel M, Wellinghausen N, et al. Detection of mutations conferring resistance to linezolid in *Enterococcus* spp. by fluorescence in situ hybridization. *J Clin Microbiol* 2007;45:3421–3423.

273. Woodford N, Tysall L, Auckland C, et al. Detection of oxazolidinone-resistant *Enterococcus faecalis* and *Enterococcus faecium* strains by real-time PCR and PCR-restriction fragment length polymorphism analysis. *J Clin Microbiol* 2002;40:4298–4300.

274. Woodford N, North SE, Ellington MJ. Detecting mutations that confer oxazolidinone resistance in Gram-positive bacteria. *Methods Mol Biol* 2007;373:103–114.

275. Zhu W, Tenover FC, Limor J, et al. Use of pyrosequencing to identify point mutations in domain V of 23S rRNA genes of linezolid-resistant *Staphylococcus aureus* and *Staphylococcus epidermidis*. *Eur J Clin Microbiol Infect Dis* 2007;26:161–165.

276. Locke JB, Rahawi S, Lamarre J, et al. Genetic environment and stability of *cfr* in methicillin-resistant *Staphylococcus aureus* CM05. *Antimicrob Agents Chemother* 2012;56:332–340.

277. Pillai SK, Sakoulas G, Wennersten C, et al. Linezolid resistance in *Staphylococcus aureus*: characterization and stability of resistant phenotype. *J Infect Dis* 2002;186:1603–1607.

278. Bourgeois-Nicolaos N, Massias L, Couson B, et al. Dose dependence of emergence of resistance to linezolid in *Enterococcus faecalis* in vivo. *J Infect Dis* 2007;195:1480–1488.

279. Farrell DJ, Douthwaite S, Morrissey I, et al. Macrolide resistance by ribosomal mutation in clinical isolates of *Streptococcus pneumoniae* from the PROTEKT 1999–2000 study. *Antimicrob Agents Chemother* 2003;47:1777–1783.

280. Tait-Kamradt A, Davies T, Cronan M, et al. Mutations in 23S rRNA and ribosomal protein L4 account for resistance in pneumococcal strains selected *in vitro* by macrolide passage. *Antimicrob Agents Chemother* 2000;44:2118–2125.

281. Prystowsky J, Siddiqui F, Chosay J, et al. Resistance to linezolid: characterization of mutations in rRNA and comparison of their occurrences in vancomycin-resistant enterococci. *Antimicrob Agents Chemother* 2001;45:2154–2156.

282. Sorlozano A, Gutierrez J, Martinez T, et al. Detection of new mutations conferring resistance to linezolid in glycopeptide-intermediate susceptibility *Staphylococcus hominis* subspecies hominis circulating in an intensive care unit. *Eur J Clin Microbiol Infect Dis* 2010;29:73–80.

283. Tsiodras S, Gold HS, Sakoulas G, et al. Linezolid resistance in a clinical isolate of *Staphylococcus aureus*. *Lancet* 2001;358:207–208.

284. Locke JB, Hilgers M, Shaw KJ. Mutations in ribosomal protein L3 are associated with oxazolidinone resistance in staphylococci of clinical origin. *Antimicrob Agents Chemother* 2009;53:5275–5278.

285. Miller K, Dunsmore CJ, Fishwick CW, et al. Linezolid and tiamulin cross-resistance in Staphylococcus aureus mediated by point mutations in the peptidyl transferase center. *Antimicrob Agents Chemother* 2008;52:1737–1742.

286. Hooper DC. Emerging mechanisms of fluoroquinolone resistance. *Emerg Infect Dis* 2001;7:337–341.

287. Martinez-Martinez L, Pascual A, Jacoby GA. Quinolone resistance from a transferable plasmid. *Lancet* 1998;351:797–799.

288. Rodriguez-Martinez JM, Cano ME, Velasco C, et al. Plasmid-mediated quinolone resistance: an update. *J Infect Chemother* 2011;17:149–182.

289. Strahilevitz J, Jacoby GA, Hooper DC, et al. Plasmid-mediated quinolone resistance: a multifaceted threat. *Clin Microbiol Rev* 2009;22:664–689.

290. Jacoby G, Cattoir V, Hooper D, et al. *qnr* Gene nomenclature. *Antimicrob Agents Chemother* 2008;52:2297–2299.

291. Robicsek A, Strahilevitz J, Jacoby GA, et al. Fluoroquinolone-modifying enzyme: a new adaptation of a common aminoglycoside acetyltransferase. *Nat Med* 2006;12:83–88.

292. Yamane K, Wachino J, Suzuki S, et al. New plasmid-mediated fluoroquinolone efflux pump, QepA, found in an *Escherichia coli* clinical isolate. *Antimicrob Agents Chemother* 2007;51:3354–3360.

293. Kim HB, Wang M, Park CH, et al. *oqxAB* encoding a multidrug efflux pump in human clinical isolates of *Enterobacteriaceae*. *Antimicrob Agents Chemother* 2009;53:3582–3584.

294. Robicsek A, Strahilevitz J, Sahm DF, et al. *qnr* prevalence in ceftazidime-resistant *Enterobacteriaceae* isolates from the United States. *Antimicrob Agents Chemother* 2006;50:2872–2874.

295. Cattoir V, Poirel L, Rotimi V, et al. Multiplex PCR for detection of plasmid-mediated quinolone resistance *qnr* genes in ESBL-producing enterobacterial isolates. *J Antimicrob Chemother* 2007;60:394–397.

296. Kim HB, Park CH, Kim CJ, et al. Prevalence of plasmid-mediated quinolone resistance determinants over a 9-year period. *Antimicrob Agents Chemother* 2009;53:639–645.

297. Guillard T, Moret H, Brasme L, et al. Rapid detection of *qnr* and *qepA* plasmid-mediated quinolone resistance genes using real-time PCR. *Diagn Microbiol Infect Dis* 2011;70:253–259.

298. Wang M, Guo Q, Xu X, et al. New plasmid-mediated quinolone resistance gene, *qnrC*, found in a clinical isolate of *Proteus mirabilis*. *Antimicrob Agents Chemother* 2009;53:1892–1897.

299. Veldman K, Cavaco LM, Mevius D, et al. International collaborative study on the occurrence of plasmid-mediated quinolone resistance in *Salmonella enterica* and *Escherichia coli* isolated from animals, humans, food and the environment in 13 European countries. *J Antimicrob Chemother* 2011;66:1278–1286.

300. Minarini LA, Poirel L, Cattoir V, et al. Plasmid-mediated quinolone resistance determinants among enterobacterial isolates from outpatients in Brazil. *J Antimicrob Chemother* 2008;62:474–478.

301. Yamane K, Wachino J, Suzuki S, et al. Plasmid-mediated *qepA* gene among *Escherichia coli* clinical isolates from Japan. *Antimicrob Agents Chemother* 2008; 52:1564–1566.

302. Liu BT, Wang XM, Liao XP, et al. Plasmid-mediated quinolone resistance determinants *oqxAB* and *aac(6')-Ib-cr* and extended-spectrum beta-lactamase gene *bla*CTX-M-24 co-located on the same plasmid in one *Escherichia coli* strain from China. *J Antimicrob Chemother* 2011;66:1638–1639.

303. Park CH, Robicsek A, Jacoby GA, et al. Prevalence in the United States of *aac(6')-Ib-cr* encoding a ciprofloxacin-modifying enzyme. *Antimicrob Agents Chemother* 2006;50:3953–3955.

304. Guillard T, Duval V, Moret H, et al. Rapid detection of *aac(6')-Ib-cr* quinolone resistance gene by pyrosequencing. *J Clin Microbiol* 2010;48:286–289.

305. Warburg G, Korem M, Robicsek A, et al. Changes in *aac(6')-Ib-cr* prevalence and fluoroquinolone resistance in nosocomial isolates of *Escherichia coli* collected from 1991 through 2005. *Antimicrob Agents Chemother* 2009;53:1268–1270.

306. Zankari E, Hasman H, Kaas RS, et al. Genotyping using whole-genome sequencing is a realistic alternative to surveillance based on phenotypic antimicrobial susceptibility testing. *J Antimicrob Chemother* 2013;68: 771–777.

307. Sambrook J, Fritsch EF, Maniatis T. *Molecular cloning: a laboratory manual.* New York: Cold Spring Harbor Laboratory Press, 1989.

308. Elsayed S, Hamilton N, Boyd D, et al. Improved primer design for multiplex PCR analysis of vancomycin-resistant *Enterococcus* spp. *J Clin Microbiol* 2001;39: 2367–2368.

309. Parks SB, Popovich BW, Press RD. Real-time polymerase chain reaction with fluorescent hybridization probes for the detection of prevalent mutations causing common thrombophilic and iron overload phenotypes. *Am J Clin Pathol* 2001;115:439–447.

310. Oleastro M, Menard A, Santos A, et al. Real-time PCR assay for rapid and accurate detection of point mutations conferring resistance to clarithromycin in *Helicobacter pylori*. *J Clin Microbiol* 2003;41:397–402.

311. Holland PM, Abramson RD, Watson R, et al. Detection of specific polymerase chain reaction product by utilizing the 5'—3' exonuclease activity of *Thermus aquaticus* DNA polymerase. *Proc Natl Acad Sci U S A* 1991;88:7276–7280.

312. Ramirez MV, Cowart KC, Campbell PJ, et al. Rapid detection of multidrug-resistant *Mycobacterium tuberculosis* by use of real-time PCR and high-resolution melt analysis. *J Clin Microbiol* 2010;48:4003–4009.

313. Kutyavin IV, Afonina IA, Mills A, et al. 3'-minor groove binder-DNA probes increase sequence specificity at PCR extension temperatures. *Nucleic Acids Res* 2000;28:655–661.

314. Wada T, Maeda S, Tamaru A, et al. Dual-probe assay for rapid detection of drug-resistant *Mycobacterium tuberculosis* by real-time PCR. *J Clin Microbiol* 2004;42:5277–5285.

315. Fang H, Ohlsson AK, Jiang GX, et al. Screening for vancomycin-resistant enterococci: an efficient and economical laboratory-developed test. *Eur J Clin Microbiol Infect Dis* 2012;31:261–265.

316. Tyagi S, Kramer FR. Molecular beacons: probes that fluoresce upon hybridization. *Nat Biotechnol* 1996;14: 303–308.

317. Drake TJ, Tan W. Molecular beacon DNA probes and their bioanalytical applications. *Appl Spectrosc* 2004;58: 269A–280A.

318. Sinsimer D, Leekha S, Park S, et al. Use of a multiplex molecular beacon platform for rapid detection of methicillin and vancomycin resistance in *Staphylococcus aureus*. *J Clin Microbiol* 2005;43:4585–4591.

319. Chakravorty S, Kothari H, Aladegbami B, et al. Rapid, high-throughput detection of rifampin resistance and heteroresistance in *Mycobacterium tuberculosis* by use of sloppy molecular beacon melting temperature coding. *J Clin Microbiol* 2012;50:2194–2202.

320. Taylor CF. Mutation scanning using high-resolution melting. *Biochem Soc Trans* 2009;37:433–437.

321. Choi GE, Lee SM, Yi J, et al. High-resolution melting curve analysis for rapid detection of rifampin and isoniazid resistance in *Mycobacterium tuberculosis* clinical isolates. *J Clin Microbiol* 2010;48:3893–3898.

322. Gabriel EM, Douarre PE, Fitzgibbon S, et al. High-resolution melting analysis for rapid detection of linezolid resistance (mediated by G2576T mutation) in *Staphylococcus epidermidis*. *J Microbiol Methods* 2012;90: 134–136.

323. Compton J. Nucleic acid sequence-based amplification. *Nature* 1991;350:91–92.

324. Deiman B, Jay C, Zintilini C, et al. Efficient amplification with NASBA of hepatitis B virus, herpes simplex virus and methicillin resistant *Staphylococcus aureus* DNA. *J Virol Methods* 2008;151:283–293.

325. Notomi T, Okayama H, Masubuchi H, et al. Loop-mediated isothermal amplification of DNA. *Nucleic Acids Res* 2000;28:E63.

326. Misawa Y, Yoshida A, Saito R, et al. Application of loop-mediated isothermal amplification technique to rapid and direct detection of methicillin-resistant *Staphylococcus aureus* (MRSA) in blood cultures. *J Infect Chemother* 2007;13:134–140.

327. Vincent M, Xu Y, Kong H. Helicase-dependent isothermal DNA amplification. *EMBO Rep* 2004;5:795–800.

328. Ao W, Aldous S, Woodruff E, et al. Rapid detection of *rpoB* gene mutations conferring rifampin resistance in *Mycobacterium tuberculosis*. *J Clin Microbiol* 2012;50:2433–2440.

329. Goldmeyer J, Li H, McCormac M, et al. Identification of *Staphylococcus aureus* and determination of methicillin resistance directly from positive blood cultures by isothermal amplification and a disposable detection device. *J Clin Microbiol* 2008;46:1534–1536.

330. Paule SM, Hacek DM, Kufner B, et al. Performance of the BD GeneOhm methicillin-resistant *Staphylococcus aureus* test before and during high-volume clinical use. *J Clin Microbiol* 2007;45:2993–2998.

331. Depardieu F, Courvalin P, Msadek T. A six amino acid deletion, partially overlapping the VanSB G2 ATP-binding motif, leads to constitutive glycopeptide resistance in VanB-type *Enterococcus faecium*. *Mol Microbiol* 2003;50:1069–1083.

332. Hayden MK, Trenholme GM, Schultz JE, et al. *In vivo* development of teicoplanin resistance in a VanB *Enterococcus faecium* isolate. *J Infect Dis* 1993;167:1224–1227.
333. Kawalec M, Gniadkowski M, Kedzierska J, et al. Selection of a teicoplanin-resistant *Enterococcus faecium* mutant during an outbreak caused by vancomycin-resistant enterococci with the *vanB* phenotype. *J Clin Microbiol* 2001;39:4274–4282.
334. Lefort A, Arthur M, Depardieu F, et al. Expression of glycopeptide-resistance gene in response to vancomycin and teicoplanin in the cardiac vegetations of rabbits infected with VanB-type Enterococcus faecalis. *J Infect Dis* 2004;189:90–97.
335. San Millan A, Depardieu F, Godreuil S, et al. VanB-type *Enterococcus faecium* clinical isolate successively inducibly resistant to, dependent on, and constitutively resistant to vancomycin. *Antimicrob Agents Chemother* 2009;53:1974–1982.
336. Dutka-Malen S, Evers S, Courvalin P. Detection of glycopeptide resistance genotypes and identification to the species level of clinically relevant enterococci by PCR. *J Clin Microbiol* 1995;33:24–27.
337. Patel R, Uhl JR, Kohner P, et al. Multiplex PCR detection of *vanA*, *vanB*, *vanC-1*, and *vanC-2/3* genes in enterococci. *J Clin Microbiol* 1997;35:703–707.
338. Bell JM, Paton JC, Turnidge J. Emergence of vancomycin-resistant enterococci in Australia: phenotypic and genotypic characteristics of isolates. *J Clin Microbiol* 1998;36:2187–2190.
339. Jayaratne P, Rutherford C. Detection of clinically relevant genotypes of vancomycin-resistant enterococci in nosocomial surveillance specimens by PCR. *J Clin Microbiol* 1999;37:2090–2092.
340. Petrich AK, Luinstra KE, Groves D, et al. Direct detection of *vanA* and *vanB* genes in clinical specimens for rapid identification of vancomycin resistant enterococci (VRE) using multiplex PCR. *Mol Cell Probes* 1999;13:275–281.
341. Kariyama R, Mitsuhata R, Chow JW, et al. Simple and reliable multiplex PCR assay for surveillance isolates of vancomycin-resistant enterococci. *J Clin Microbiol* 2000;38:3092–3095.
342. Lu JJ, Perng CL, Chiueh TS, et al. Detection and typing of vancomycin-resistance genes of enterococci from clinical and nosocomial surveillance specimens by multiplex PCR. *Epidemiol Infect* 2001;126:357–363.
343. Perez-Hernandez X, Mendez-Alvarez S, Claverie-Martin F. A PCR assay for rapid detection of vancomycin-resistant enterococci. *Diagn Microbiol Infect Dis* 2002;42:273–277.
344. Mac K, Wichmann-Schauer H, Peters J, et al. Species identification and detection of vancomycin resistance genes in enterococci of animal origin by multiplex PCR. *Int J Food Microbiol* 2003;88:305–309.
345. Depardieu F, Perichon B, Courvalin P. Detection of the *van* alphabet and identification of enterococci and staphylococci at the species level by multiplex PCR. *J Clin Microbiol* 2004;42:5857–5860.
346. Benadof D, San Martin M, Aguirre J, et al. A new multiplex PCR assay for the simultaneous detection of vancomycin-resistant enterococci from rectal swabs. *J Infect* 2010;60:354–359.
347. Lee SY, Park KG, Lee GD, et al. Comparison of Seeplex VRE detection kit with ChromID VRE agar for detection of vancomycin-resistant enterococci in rectal swab specimens. *Ann Clin Lab Sci* 2010;40:163–166.
348. Gurtler V, Grando D, Mayall BC, et al. A novel method for simultaneous *Enterococcus* species identification/typing and van genotyping by high resolution melt analysis. *J Microbiol Methods* 2012;90:167–181.
349. Palladino S, Kay ID, Flexman JP, et al. Rapid detection of *vanA* and *vanB* genes directly from clinical specimens and enrichment broths by real-time multiplex PCR assay. *J Clin Microbiol* 2003;41:2483–2486.
350. Palladino S, Kay ID, Costa AM, et al. Real-time PCR for the rapid detection of *vanA* and *vanB* genes. *Diagn Microbiol Infect Dis* 2003;45:81–84.
351. Sloan LM, Uhl JR, Vetter EA, et al. Comparison of the Roche LightCycler *vanA/vanB* detection assay and culture for detection of vancomycin-resistant enterococci from perianal swabs. *J Clin Microbiol* 2004;42:2636–2643.
352. Marner ES, Wolk DM, Carr J, et al. Diagnostic accuracy of the Cepheid GeneXpert *vanA/vanB* assay ver. 1.0 to detect the *vanA* and *vanB* vancomycin resistance genes in *Enterococcus* from perianal specimens. *Diagn Microbiol Infect Dis* 2011;69:382–389.
353. Leclercq R. Macrolides, lincosamides, and streptogramins. In: Courvalin P, Leclercq R, Rice LB, eds. *Antibiogram*. Portland, OR: Eska Publishing, 2010:305–326.
354. Scott LE, McCarthy K, Gous N, et al. Comparison of Xpert MTB/RIF with other nucleic acid technologies for diagnosing pulmonary tuberculosis in a high HIV prevalence setting: a prospective study. *PLoS Med* 2011;8:e1001061.
355. Marme N, Friedrich A, Müller M, et al. Identification of single-point mutations in mycobacterial 16S rRNA sequences by confocal single-molecule fluorescence spectroscopy. *Nucleic Acids Res* 2006;34:e90.
356. De Beenhouwer H, Lhiang Z, Jannes G, et al. Rapid detection of rifampicin resistance in sputum and biopsy specimens from tuberculosis patients by PCR and line probe assay. *Tuber Lung Dis* 1995;76:425–430.
357. Crudu V, Stratan E, Romancenco E, et al. First evaluation of an improved assay for molecular genetic detection of tuberculosis as well as rifampin and isoniazid resistances. *J Clin Microbiol* 2012;50:1264–1269.
358. Espasa M, Gonzalez-Martin J, Alcaide F, et al. Direct detection in clinical samples of multiple gene mutations causing resistance of *Mycobacterium tuberculosis* to isoniazid and rifampicin using fluorogenic probes. *J Antimicrob Chemother* 2005;55:860–865.
359. Blaschitz M, Hasanacevic D, Hufnagl P, et al. Real-time PCR for single-nucleotide polymorphism detection in the 16S rRNA gene as an indicator for extensive drug resistance in *Mycobacterium tuberculosis*. *J Antimicrob Chemother* 2011;66:1243–1246.
360. Vakulenko SB, Donabedian SM, Voskresenskiy AM, et al. Multiplex PCR for detection of aminoglycoside resistance genes in enterococci. *Antimicrob Agents Chemother* 2003;47:1423–1426.
361. Schmitz FJ, Fluit AC, Gondolf M, et al. The prevalence of aminoglycoside resistance and corresponding resistance genes in clinical isolates of staphylococci from 19 European hospitals. *J Antimicrob Chemother* 1999;43:253–259.
362. Ardic N, Sareyyupoglu B, Ozyurt M, et al. Investigation of aminoglycoside modifying enzyme genes in methicillin-resistant staphylococci. *Microbiol Res* 2006;161:49–54.
363. Ida T, Okamoto R, Shimauchi C, et al. Identification of aminoglycoside-modifying enzymes by susceptibility testing: epidemiology of methicillin-resistant *Staphylococcus aureus* in Japan. *J Clin Microbiol* 2001;39:3115–3121.

364. Qu TT, Chen YG, Yu YS, et al. Genotypic diversity and epidemiology of high-level gentamicin resistant *Enterococcus* in a Chinese hospital. *J Infect* 2006;52:124–130.

365. Mahbub Alam M, Kobayashi N, Ishino M, et al. Detection of a novel *aph(2")* allele (*aph[2"]-Ie*) conferring high-level gentamicin resistance and a spectinomycin resistance gene *ant(9)-Ia* (*aad 9*) in clinical isolates of enterococci. *Microb Drug Resist* 2005;11:239–247.

366. Hauschild T, Vukovic D, Dakic I, et al. Aminoglycoside resistance in members of the *Staphylococcus sciuri* group. *Microb Drug Resist* 2007;13:77–84.

367. Watanabe S, Kobayashi N, Quinones D, et al. Genetic diversity of enterococci harboring the high-level gentamicin resistance gene *aac(6')-Ie-aph(2")-Ia* or *aph(2")-Ie* in a Japanese hospital. *Microb Drug Resist* 2009;15:185–194.

368. Leelaporn A, Yodkamol K, Waywa D, et al. A novel structure of Tn*4001*-truncated element, type V, in clinical enterococcal isolates and multiplex PCR for detecting

aminoglycoside resistance genes. *Int J Antimicrob Agents* 2008;31:250–254.

369. Miro E, Grunbaum F, Gomez L, et al. Characterization of aminoglycoside-modifying enzymes in *Enterobacteriaceae* clinical strains and characterization of the plasmids implicated in their diffusion. *Microb Drug Resist* 2013;19:94–99.

370. Kim JY, Park YJ, Kwon HJ, et al. Occurrence and mechanisms of amikacin resistance and its association with beta-lactamases in *Pseudomonas aeruginosa*: a Korean nationwide study. *J Antimicrob Chemother* 2008;62:479–483.

371. Noppe-Leclercq I, Wallet F, Haentjens S, et al. PCR detection of aminoglycoside resistance genes: a rapid molecular typing method for *Acinetobacter baumannii*. *Res Microbiol* 1999;150:317–322.

372. Akers KS, Chaney C, Barsoumian A, et al. Aminoglycoside resistance and susceptibility testing errors in *Acinetobacter baumannii*-calcoaceticus complex. *J Clin Microbiol* 2010;48:1132–1138.

Chapter 10

Molecular Mechanisms of Action for Antimicrobial Agents: General Principles and Mechanisms for Selected Classes of Antibiotics

Charles William Stratton

INTRODUCTION

Importance of Understanding the Molecular Basis of Antimicrobial Action

Antimicrobial action can be defined as the interaction of the drug with the microorganism; this interaction is widely described as antimicrobial pharmacodynamics (1). The result of this interaction of the drug with the microorganism may be inhibition or death of the microbe or may instead be the emergence of a resistant subpopulation of microorganisms that can negate the effect of the antibiotic (2–5). Pharmacokinetics, on the other hand, is the interaction of the drug with the patient (6). The integration of pharmacodynamics with pharmacokinetics in the first decade of the 21st century has greatly improved optimal antimicrobial therapy (6–13). Integral to the application of pharmacodynamic and pharmacokinetic principles to antimicrobial therapy is an understanding of the molecular basis of antimicrobial action. Such an understanding begins with an understanding of the molecular targets for antimicrobial agents. These molecular targets include microbial RNA and DNA; microbial biosynthesis of proteins, folic acid, and cell wall (peptidoglycan); microbial membrane function; and microbial energy metabolism. The specific interaction of antimicrobial agents with each of these

molecular targets must be understood in order to optimally use pharmacodynamic and pharmacokinetic principles (14).

Although the global emergence of resistance may well be an inevitable and unavoidable result of the use of antimicrobial agents (3,15,16), the understanding and application of the molecular basis of antimicrobial action can minimize the degree of resistance that occurs (15–18). Moreover, understanding the molecular basis of antimicrobial action allows better appreciation of resistance mechanisms, which, in turn, allows these resistance mechanisms themselves to be targeted by antimicrobial agents (19). Moreover, understanding of the molecular targets provides a more rational approach for the use of combination antimicrobial therapy (20–23). The therapy of tuberculosis (TB) serves as an example of such a rational approach. Here, the use of combination therapy with new and/or different classes of antimycobacterial agents (24,25) that specifically target the dormant phase of mycobacteria has resulted in improved efficacy, whereas the use of specific therapeutic approaches such as directly observed therapy (26) has resulted in lower rates of resistance. It is therefore the purpose of this chapter to first review general principles that are useful for understanding the molecular basis of antimicrobial action and then to review mechanisms of action for selected classes of antimicrobial agents in current use or under investigation.

GENERAL PRINCIPLES OF ANTIMICROBIAL ACTION

Antimicrobial Mechanisms of Action in Relationship to the Cellular Structure and Physiology of Microbes

Importance of Microbial Physiology in Antimicrobial Action

The importance of the microbial growth phase for the in vitro effects of antimicrobial action has long been appreciated in clinical microbiology (27–31). However, this is only a small part of the microbial physiology that must be understood in order to optimally use antimicrobial agents. Microbial physiology is a complex subject with important implications for the effectiveness of antimicrobial agents, implications that have only recently become understood. Fortunately, there has been a great deal of progress made in understanding this microbial physiology and its influence on antimicrobial action. It is important to appreciate that microorganisms have mechanisms for replication, including synthesis of the cell wall (32–35), an important target of antimicrobial therapy (36,37). In addition to synthesis of the cell wall, a microorganism must also be able to focally lyse its cell wall so that replication can occur (33,36,38–40). The enzymes that mediate lysis of the cell wall must be tightly controlled; otherwise, they could cause destruction of the cell. These enzymes are preformed and are diffusely present in the cell wall until focally activated (39,40). Moreover, these enzymes can be globally activated as part of programmed cell death (i.e., apoptosis) or can be triggered by antimicrobial agents (41–45). Furthermore, microorganisms have evolved compensatory mechanisms to deal with times of starvation; these mechanisms ensure that the genome of some microorganisms survive until better times (46–48). Such mechanisms include quorum sensing, which may activate programmed cell death as the microbial population increases and nutrients become sparse (42,49,50). For example, programmed cell death in bacteria is a major factor in the development of biofilm (49,51,52). Microorganisms also have repair mechanisms when subjected to DNA damage, a reaction known as the "SOS" response; failing repair, programmed cell death is likely to occur (53–55). Finally, microorganisms often live in microcolonies in biofilm, and the behavior of a cell is greatly influenced by the location of the cell within the microcolony (52,56–58). Into this complex physiologic environment, antimicrobial agents are introduced. Attempting to understand the mechanism of action of these agents without understanding microbial physiology is futile. Accordingly, microbial physiology will be discussed in some detail.

Role of the Physiologic State of the Microbe in Antimicrobial Activity

The specific physiologic state of the microorganism, particularly its surface properties and rate of cell replication, markedly influences the activity of antimicrobial agents and partially determines whether they are bactericidal or bacteriostatic as well as their rate of killing (28–31,59–62). It has become clear that the pure in vitro broth culture, albeit the mainstay of antimicrobial susceptibility testing, is an artifact emphasizing free-floating mobile (planktonic) cells, which exist primarily in the laboratory setting and not in nature (i.e., infections) (29,62). This discriminates against the adherent (sessile) cells present in biofilm, which has now been acknowledged as the predominant growth form in natural ecosystems, including most infections (49,52,56–58,63). Moreover, microbial growth forms in biofilm have been associated with persistent infections and microbial resistance (49,60,63–65). Although noted long ago, it is no less true today: a solid support surface for the growth of bacteria provides a better approximation of the in vivo state than does broth medium (29).

Cellular Physiology of Microbial Life and Death

The growth of microorganisms in natural environments is characterized by periods of nutrient starvation, which results in growth rates that approximate zero (46–48,66). Nonetheless, bacteria are able to survive for prolonged periods of time despite the relative absence of nutrients. The survival of bacteria under these starvation conditions involves induction of a number of genes or proteins that mediate physiologic changes that enable the survival of some of the cells (46–48,66,67). These physiologic changes also can be seen as a microorganism transitions from the logarithmic phase of growth to the stationary phase, during which time the expression levels of a number of gene products produce marked phenotypic changes (31,66–69). Finally, these changes are seen after exposure of the microorganism to antimicrobial agents (70–72). The following examples are illustrative. Nutrient limitation in isolates of *Pseudomonas aeruginosa* has been shown to result in increased synthesis of exopolysaccharides (66,73,74). This phenotypic change, in turn, results in increased biofilm that appears to decrease the antimicrobial activity of a number of agents (75,76), including β-lactam agents such as piperacillin (77). Clinically, emergence of *P. aeruginosa* strains producing high levels of persister cells has been noted in patients with cystic fibrosis (65). Microbial stress can result in alteration of penicillin-binding proteins (PBPs) and cell walls. For example, heat shock protein ClpL in *Streptococcus pneumoniae* has been shown to induce a ClpL-dependent increase in the messenger RNA (mRNA) levels and protein synthesized by the cell wall synthesis gene pbp2x, which results in a thicker cell wall and higher resistance to penicillin (78). In response to a broad range of environmental stresses, wild-type strains of *Escherichia coli* become short coccobacillary forms that exhibit increased levels of resistance (79). These morphologic changes in *E. coli* are associated with alterations in the expression of PBPs, with an increase seen in the amount of PBP6 and a decrease in PBP3 (80–82). Similar changes in the PBPs of *Streptococcus pyogenes* (31) and *Haemophilus influenzae* (68) during the stationary phase have been reported. This suggests some common effects for PBPs during the stationary phase on microorganisms. Lack of certain nutrients also may play a role (47,83,84). For example, limitation of choline in the teichoic acids of *S. pneumoniae* results in replacement by ethanolamine, which subsequently inhibits the growing cells from splitting into diplococci (85). All of these changes and more appear to be triggered by stress, stationary phase, and/or limitation of nutrients and to be essential for continued cell survival during prolonged periods in the stationary phase (47,48,66,67,69,81,86).

Among other important changes that occur under starvation conditions are those associated with the stringent response (30,87). The stringent response is an adaptation to conditions of amino acid starvation. This response includes induction of specific enzymes such as guanosine tetraphosphate (ppGpp) in the initial stage, which then increases the transcription of both inducible and repressible enzyme operons involved in the stringent response (30,84,87–89). Examples of the stringent response include phenotypic changes seen in marine bacterial cells (83) as well as the latent infection caused by *Mycobacterium tuberculosis* (89). These changes in some microorganisms are characterized by rapid multiple divisions of starved cells, leading to the formation of ultramicrobacteria (<0.3 μm in diameter), which are also called dwarf forms (90). Rapid formation of multiple copies is presumed to improve the chances of individual genomes surviving. These cells are dormant forms and are quite resistant to many antimicrobial agents as well as to osmotic stress.

Starvation conditions are not the only conditions that may induce the stringent response. Other conditions that appear to induce the stringent response are exposure to certain antibiotics, including β-lactam agents. Lorian (91–93) demonstrated that staphylococci, when exposed to subinhibitory concentrations of penicillin, produced abnormally large cells that were actually clusters of smaller dwarf staphylococci crowded together within a single surrounding thickened cell wall and prevented from separating by the presence of many wide cross-walls. Comparison of the ultrastructure of staphylococci following penicillin exposure with that of staphylococci isolated from osteomyelitis in animal models revealed morphologies that were virtually indistinguishable (94). When incubated on drug-free media, these clusters of staphylococci separated into smaller clusters and eventually become normal-sized individual cells. This morphogenesis and fatal variations in the presence of penicillin of the staphylococcal cell wall are reviewed in more detail by Giesbrecht et al. (95).

These dwarf forms of staphylococci crowded together within a single thickened surrounding cell wall are likely to be dormant forms produced by the stringent response due to limited cell wall damage caused by subinhibitory concentrations of β-lactam agents. In contrast, higher levels of β-lactam agents cause enough cell wall damage to activate autolytic mechanisms (44,45,96). These differences, thus, may simply reflect a difference in the physiologic response to cell wall damage: limited cell wall damage triggers a stringent response, whereas extensive damage triggers apoptosis.

Multicellular forms of staphylococci also are seen in mutant staphylococci that have had their *scdA* gene inactivated (97). This aberrant cellular morphology is similar to those of staphylococci carrying *femA* and *femB* mutations (98). This suggests that the transient changes described by Lorian and colleagues (91,92,93) may become permanent after mutation of specific genes involved in this cellular morphology. Multiple dwarf copies of a microorganism within one thickened cell wall would presumably be more resistant to antimicrobial agents or other noxious substances and also would increase the chance of the genome surviving.

Similar effects have been described for other microorganisms. *Helicobacter pylori*, for example, has been shown to produce coccoid forms, which have been attributed to environmental stress such as starvation (69,99). These coccoid forms have also been found to emerge after exposure to antibiotics such as amoxicillin (100). They are not culturable in vitro but revert to culturable forms in mice (101). In *Bilophila wadsworthia*, scanning and transmission electron microscopy have demonstrated that subinhibitory concentrations of imipenem result in large multilobate cells, suggesting that new growth of cells was initiated while cell division or separation was inhibited (102). A similar effect of imipenem has been reported for *P. aeruginosa* isolates, where exposure to concentrations of imipenem greater than the relevant minimal inhibitory concentrations (MICs) results in large spheroplasts with evidence of cross-wall formation just before lysis (103). This effect presumably extends to the newer carbapenems such as meropenem. Dwarf forms of *P. aeruginosa* have been observed in microcolonies within the lung tissue of patients with cystic fibrosis (90,104,105). Each of these aberrant forms described most likely represents the entry of the microorganism into the stringent response phase.

It is of interest that, while long-starved cells are resistant to cell wall–active agents as well as agents that inhibit DNA synthesis, they remain somewhat susceptible to certain agents that inhibit protein synthesis (106) or interfere with bacterial membrane function (107). *Staphylococcus aureus* exposed to subinhibitory concentrations of antimicrobial agents that interfere with protein synthesis develop a thick cell wall (94) with one or two thick cross-walls, except in the case of tetracycline, where no cross-wall formation has been observed (108). This older observation has greater significance with the more recent demonstration of successful in vivo therapy of methicillin-resistant *Staphylococcus aureus* (MRSA) endocarditis with minocycline in the clinical setting (109) as well as in an experimental endocarditis model (110). In this experimental endocarditis model, minocycline was as effective as vancomycin. Recognition of the bactericidal effects of minocycline on microorganisms in a dormant phase may ultimately result in an additional antimicrobial agent for the therapy of methicillin-resistant staphylococci (111). This observation is likely to become more important as the incidence of community-acquired MRSA increases (112,113).

Cellular Physiology of Microbial Apoptosis and Repair

There are a number of physical or chemical agents in the natural environment of microbes that can cause damage to cells (114). The most vulnerable portions of microbial cells are the cell wall/membrane (36,37,107) and the cell genome (115–121). Therefore, it is not surprising that microbial cells have evolved repair systems for these vulnerable targets. If the damage to the microbial cell is severe and cannot be repaired, an apoptosis (programmed cell death) mechanism is activated (41,42,53–55,122,123). Programmed cell death may, for example, play a role in the elimination of bacterial cells that are damaged by cell wall–active agents such as penicillins (42–45,95–97,124). The balance between repair and programmed cell death may well be an unappreciated target of antimicrobial therapy; it is likely that rapid killing of microbes involves activation of such apoptotic mechanisms (44,45). Indeed, a number of major classes of bactericidal antimicrobial agents have been shown to induce hydroxyl radical formation that is an end product of an oxidative damage cellular death pathway that, in turn, leads to microbial cell death (44,45,125). For example, amoxicillin therapy in a rabbit endocarditis model has been shown to kill *Enterococcus faecalis* by two mechanisms (126). The first is autolysin independent and likely corresponds to the production of reactive oxygen species (44,45). The second is autolysin dependent and involves the loss of the osmoprotective function of the peptidoglycan at a high cell density. A similar dual mechanism of killing for penicillin against *S. pneumoniae* has been described (127). Apoptotic mechanisms may also explain species-specific bactericidal activity. An example is seen with chloramphenicol, which kills certain species such as *S. pneumoniae* and *H. influenzae* but not *Escherichia coli*. This may simply reflect differences in the activation of apoptotic mechanisms.

Prevention of damage to vital portions of the microbial cell is clearly an important prelude to cellular repair. Accordingly, microbial cells have developed an effective protective barrier for their cell wall/membrane called *biofilm* (52,56,57). Biofilm is discussed in detail due to its importance in infections and as a future target for antimicrobial therapy (49,52,57,63,64,128). Repair of this biofilm and of the underlying cell wall/membrane structure when damage occurs is an important microbial function. Biofilm repair involves synthesis of the precursors within the cytoplasm, translocation of these precursors to the outer portions of the cell wall/membrane, and final assembly of the biofilm matrix. Studies have shown that biofilm repair is dependent on a carbohydrate source, an energy source, certain enzymes, and functioning efflux pumps. With these components available, repair occurs very quickly (129). There is now intriguing evidence that macrolides can interfere with the synthesis and repair of biofilm; this process seems to involve inhibition of quorum-sensing as well as the elaboration of exotoxins by means of codon–anticodon interactions that inhibit the translation of mRNA for inducible enzymes (130–138). This important topic is also discussed in detail.

Repair of any damage to the cell wall/membrane of microbes appears to be most easily accomplished by replication, provided the damage is not extensive. This may be an important factor in combination antimicrobial therapy specifically directed at creating functional synergy of two antimicrobial agents against an infectious microbe. Such an approach, for example, might involve the use of cell wall disrupters combined with agents active against replicating microorganisms.

The repair of structural damage to DNA is also of considerable importance to the microbe, because this damage (and the repair) might result in mutations that could be lethal. Accordingly, the response to DNA damage by the microorganism is complex (53–55). There are three important mechanisms of DNA repair in microorganisms: (a) direct repair, which restores the original structure; (b) indirect repair, in which one DNA strand is bypassed during replication or is excised and then rebuilt by copying the intact strand; and (c) postreplication repair, in which the damage is eliminated by recombination between the sister strands after replication.

A major mechanism for indirect repair of damage that blocks chain elongation during replication is that provided by the SOS system (53–55,139). The SOS system is a set of approximately 20 damage-inducible (din) genes. The SOS response is controlled by two regulatory proteins, which are the products of the lexA and recA genes. The first protein product of the gene lexA normally represses the SOS response. Upon SOS induction, the recA gene produces RecA protein. Damaged DNA, in the presence of the single-strand–binding protein, binds RecA protein in a way that changes its configuration so that it becomes a protease that cleaves lexA. This results in derepression of the other genes. The induction of RecA protein can be inhibited by antimicrobial agents such as chloramphenicol, erythromycin, and tetracycline, which have codon–anticodon interactions that

inhibit the translation of mRNA needed for the synthesis of inducible enzymes.

Once activated, the SOS response has several effects. One of these is induction of DNA polymerases, which will be needed when cell division resumes (140). Another is cell division inhibition mediated by sfiA and sfiC, which target the ftsZ gene and protein, important factors in cell separation (141). Overproduction of the ftsZ protein has been shown to produce ultramicrobacteria. The SOS response is primarily involved in DNA repair (54,55). The major mechanism of repair of the activated SOS system is bypass repair. This particular mechanism of DNA repair tends to be error-prone and often results in mutants (54,55,140,142).

Cell Wall/Biofilm Structures of Gram-Positive and Gram-Negative Microorganisms

The cell walls of both gram-positive (Fig. 10.1) and gram-negative (Fig. 10.2) bacteria are similar, in that both possess inner cytoplasmic membranes as well as outer peptidoglycan (murein) layers (33,35,143–145). Gram-negative bacteria also have an additional outer cell membrane, which covers the peptidoglycan layer (82,143,145–147). Finally, the cell walls of both gram-positive and gram-negative bacteria interface with the external milieu via biofilm, which is a matrix-supported gel (52,56). Each of these structures plays a critical role in the interaction of antimicrobial agents with the microorganism (36,37,107,128).

The cytoplasmic membrane in each group of bacteria is a semipermeable membrane that regulates molecular flow, in turn determining pH (143,148,149), osmotic pressures (150), and availability of essential substances. The peptidoglycan layer in each group is a continuous cross-linked mesh that forms a polyionic and amphoteric network (33,34,143). The peptidoglycan mesh is composed of linear glycan chains that are interlinked by short peptides (33,34,82,143,144,151). This shell surrounds the entire microorganism, is known as a sacculus, and is found exclusively in eubacteria. The peptidoglycan sacculus is not a rigid shell but instead is elastic and flexible. This relatively porous peptidoglycan sacculus (exclusion limits of 100,000 Da) serves as a mechanical "exoskeleton" that helps to maintain the microorganism's shape, rigidity, and osmotic stability. The exoskeleton of gram-positive bacteria is thicker than that of gram-negatives, thus providing more rigidity. Although this polyanionic sacculus might appear to be an exclusion barrier, the exclusion

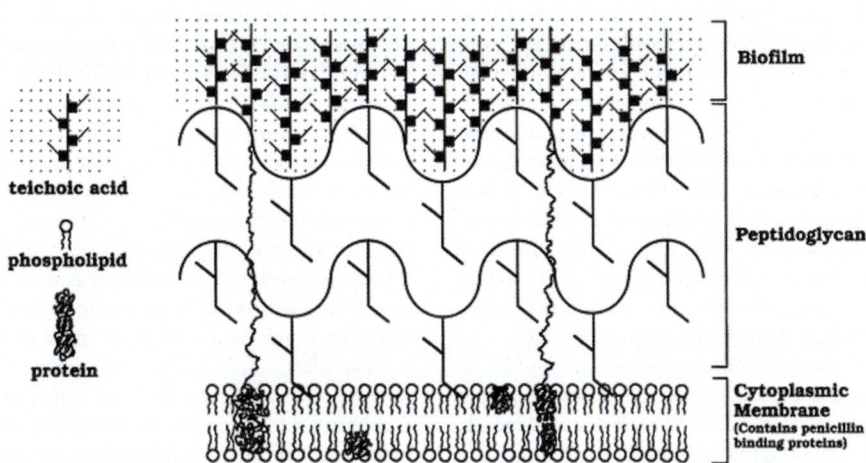

Figure 10.1 ■ Schematic representation of the cell wall of gram-positive microorganisms.

limits of 100,000 Da make this meshwork very coarse and thus allow molecules of lesser size, such as antimicrobial agents, which have sizes of 300 to 700 Da, to readily diffuse through the layer. Finally, the peptidoglycan structure is involved in the cell division process (32,34,152).

The molecular structures of the cytoplasmic membranes of gram-positive and gram-negative bacteria are essentially the same, consisting of lipid bilayers containing phospholipids and membrane proteins (143–145). There are, however, important differences in the peptidoglycan wall and the biofilm for these two groups of bacteria. Gram-positive bacteria have a relatively simple but thick cell wall constructed of peptidoglycan and teichoic acids, which are long-chain polymers consisting of glycerol or ribitol residues with phos-

phodiester links and various substituents such as uronic acids (85,144,153). Teichoic acids are found as either cell-bound or free soluble acids. The cell wall of gram-positive bacteria contains two forms of the cell-bound teichoic acid. In one form, lipoteichoic acid, one end of the chain is anchored to phospholipids in the cytoplasmic membrane while the other end transverses the peptidoglycan layer in such a way that it protrudes at the cell surface (153). In the second, a cell wall teichoic acid, one end is attached to *N*-acetylmuramyl residues in the peptidoglycan layer and the free end protrudes at the cell surface. Finally, free, soluble teichoic acid is present in large amounts in the outer portion of the cell wall.

At the surface of the gram-positive cell wall, the protruding teichoic acids can be linked with one

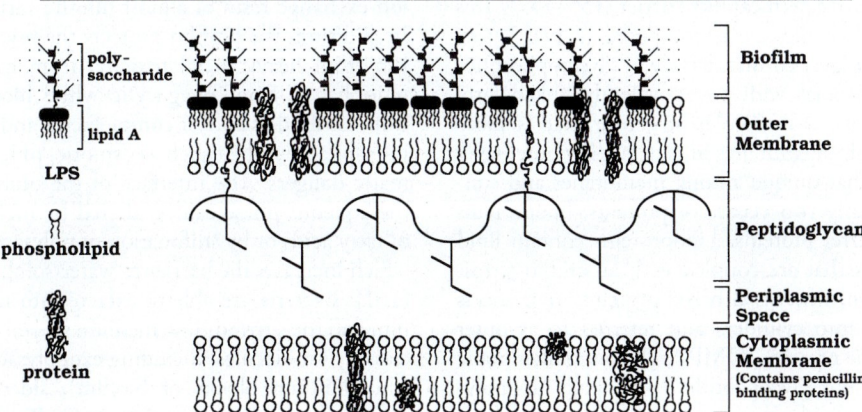

Figure 10.2 ■ Schematic representation of the cell wall of gram-negative microorganisms. LPS, lipopolysaccharide.

another via branching polysaccharides to form a matrix. The cross-linking of the biofilm matrix is accomplished using polysaccharides with repeating units of two or three sugars. The variety of possible hexose stereoisomers and of linkages, as well as the potential incorporation of unusual sugar residues, results in thousands of different trisaccharides in the matrix. Because the polysaccharide chains in the matrix are hydrophilic, water is absorbed into the matrix and transforms this outer layer into a gel. This matrix-supported gel (99% water) is known by a variety of names, including *biofilm*, *glycocalyx*, *slime*, *alginate*, and *capsule* (52,56).

One of the key components of the biofilm is phospholipids because of the covalent bonding they provide. In addition, this hydrated matrix depends on calcium and magnesium cations to maintain the negatively charged ends of the polysaccharides in close approximation. The availability of phospholipids and divalent cations in the medium greatly influences the final composition of the cell wall. This can be appreciated by considering the gram-positive cell wall. Under conditions of magnesium limitation, gram-positive bacteria increase the amount of teichoic acid produced while decreasing the amount of alanyl ester substitutions, which results in fewer polysaccharides present in the matrix and hence less biofilm. Phosphate limitation results in the replacement of teichoic acids by teichuronic acids, which have less covalent bonding. Starvation conditions, then, would be predicted to result in cell walls with minimal biofilm.

The cell walls of gram-negative bacteria differ from those of gram-positive bacteria in a number of ways (82,147,154). First, they have a relatively thin peptidoglycan layer, which provides less rigidity. Gram-negative cell walls also have an additional outer cell membrane (145–147) that serves as an effective permeability barrier (155–157). This outer cell membrane is composed of two layers. The inner layer consists largely of glycerophospholipid molecules with two covalently linked fatty acid chains, a molecular structure that is fairly common in membranes in general. The outer layer is somewhat unique among membranes and contains mainly two classes of proteins, lipoproteins and β-barrel proteins. Lipoproteins contain lipid molecules that are coupled with an amino-terminal cystein, whereas β-barrel proteins are β sheets wrapped into cylinders and referred to as outer membrane proteins (OMPs). The outer membrane also contains glycopeptides, principally lipopolysaccharides with six or seven covalently linked fatty acid chains. The fatty acids present in the lipopolysaccharides are saturated. This results in the interior of the lipid bilayer being less fluid, because there is no packing of carbons, as seen when the fatty acids are unsaturated (156). This serves to make this barrier more restrictive to hydrophilic agents.

Areas of adhesion between the outer cell membrane and the inner cytoplasmic membrane, called Bayer's junctions, have been described by a number of investigators. These adhesions of the inner cytoplasmic membrane to the cell peptidoglycan/outer membrane are probable sites of synthesis of the outer membrane and biofilm as well as synthesis of other substrates to be pumped from the cell cytoplasm into the periplasmic space or from the cell cytoplasm directly into the biofilm.

The periplasmic space is an aqueous cellular compartment delineated by the outer cell membrane and the inner cytoplasmic membrane (158). The periplasmic space contains various proteins that are densely packed, making this aqueous milieu more viscous than the cytoplasm. These proteins include potentially harmful proteins such as RNAse or alkaline phosphatase, thus making the periplasmic space an evolutionary precursor of the lysosomes of eukaryotic cells (159).

Gram-negative bacteria, like gram-positive bacteria, are surrounded by a polyanionic polysaccharide matrix, which differs mainly by being anchored by the lipooligosaccharides rather than by lipoteichoic acids. In some instances, the attachment is to the peptidoglycan layer, whereas in others the lipid A is anchored to the inner cytoplasmic membrane. This lipopolysaccharide matrix of gram-negative bacteria is also thought to provide some selectivity/hindrance via negative ionic charges and/or steric hindrance (160).

Biofilms of both gram-positive and gram-negative bacteria are essentially anionic polymeric diffusion barriers and can be thought of as an ion-exchange resin of almost infinite surface area. In addition, the biofilm protects the microorganism from heavy metal toxicity, from most bacteriophages, from phagocytic white blood cells, from antibodies and/or complement, and from an inhospitable milieu such as osmotic, pH, or enzymatic dangers. The interface of the biofilm with the aqueous phase can be altered by methylation of fatty acids or by sulfonation of polysaccharides, which increases the barrier to water-soluble agents (161). Bacteria are able to excrete into their biofilm and the surrounding medium several different classes of molecules, including exopolysaccharides (the building blocks of biofilm), siderophores, protein enzymes, and toxins (146). Biofilms also appear to serve as a repository for defensive substances such as β-lactamase (162).

In human infections, microbial cells are most often found with biofilm (52,57,58,63), even though microscopic examination may not readily reveal this. In clinical microbiology laboratories, the optimal growth conditions sought by microbiologists are far from the near-starvation circumstances the bacteria encounter in their natural environments. This is particularly true for broth media (29). However, the growth of gram-positive and gram-negative bacteria on agar plates in the laboratory may reflect, in part, the presence or absence of biofilm. Smooth colonies have more biofilm than do rough colonies, while mucoid or slimy colonies have the most. Deep rough colonies, on the other hand, have the smallest amount of biofilm, if any at all. These deep rough mutants have most of the core lipid A eliminated. Such strains are more susceptible to lysozyme and more permeable to hydrophobic antibiotics. Finally, in clinical microbiology laboratories, biofilm may be recognized and described microscopically as capsule.

Consequences of Biofilm Disruption

The disruption of the bacterial cell wall often results in the death of the microorganism (114). This is well appreciated by clinicians. Less well appreciated is that the disruption of biofilm surrounding an individual microbial cell is not without consequences (163–165). These may be related to osmotic pressure and the shifting of cell peptidoglycan by that pressure. There is a higher hydrostatic pressure within the cytoplasmic space of a microbe than that which is exerted on the cell by the external milieu. The presence of the biofilm matrix seems to assist in keeping this internal pressure in check (172). When a portion of the gel is removed, however, the internal pressure shifts the cell wall/membrane so that it protrudes through this disrupted area, resulting in a fingerlike projection containing cytoplasmic contents (164,166–168). Extrusion of this portion of the cell wall/membrane through the hole in the biofilm is a result of the cell wall/membrane shifting to adjust to the focused pressure directed at the area of disrupted biofilm. This shift in turn activates autolytic enzymes to dissolve the peptidoglycan component of the cell wall as the wall shifts during replication (169). This causes dissolution of cell wall peptidoglycan in this area, which, in conjunction with the high, focused internal pressure, effectively severs this protruding bleb (170), leaving a transient hole. If enough holes are formed, leakage of cytoplasmic contents results

in cellular death (171). The results of this process can be demonstrated by electron microscopy, which makes visible a range of ultrastructural changes, including narrow fingerlike projections, blebs, and extracellular cytoplasmic-filled vesicles. Disruption of the entire biofilm matrix, in contrast, tends to equalize the pressure over the entire cell wall/membrane. Consequently, when the autolytic enzymes dissolve the peptidoglycan of the entire cell, the result may be lysis of the entire cell or the creation of a spheroplast if the osmolarity of the external milieu is sufficiently high. When lysis is seen, it occurs rapidly, in contrast to the lysis seen after exposure to penicillin, where cells continue to grow for approximately half a generation before lysis (27,170). Finally, it appears that gram-negative bacteria are more susceptible to the effects of biofilm disrupters, perhaps because of their less rigid cell walls.

Disruption of biofilm can be accomplished by a number of physicochemical mechanisms (161). This disruption can be best appreciated by electron microscopy. The ultrastructure of normal cells of gram-negative or gram-positive bacteria has a slightly undulating smooth surface, which is transformed to a surface with blebs and tubular projections after displacement of Ca^{2+} and Mg^{2+} from the biofilm. Displacement of these cations from the biofilm by chelating agents such as ethylenediaminetetraacetic acid (EDTA) (155,170) or by polycationic agents (164,172) such as polymyxin B (166,167) and aminoglycosides (173,174) has been shown to be an effective way to disrupt biofilm, although this mechanism can be countered by the presence of excessive amounts of calcium and magnesium cations in the milieu (175–177). However, adding these cations after the damage has been done has no effect. The ultrastructural changes seen by electron microscopy are accompanied by a functional change, namely, increased permeability to hydrophobic agents such as antibiotics (146,163,178).

If the changes induced by the disruption of biofilm are not rapidly fatal and the cells are allowed to grow, the permeability barrier is repaired in about two-thirds of a generation (129). The addition of chloramphenicol or tetracycline or the omission of required amino acids does not affect the repair rate. A proton pump inhibitor such as 2,4-dinitrophenol, however, prevents repair. The activity of omeprazole and lansoprazole against *H. pylori* (179) may be related to their inhibitory effect on certain cellular membrane pumps. Omitting glucose also prevents biofilm repair. Interestingly, the addition of macrolides decreases the repair rate, possibly because of its inhibition of mRNA translation (180) as well as by the elaboration of exotoxins by means of codon–anticodon interactions that inhibit the translation of mRNA for inducible enzymes (130–138).

Effects of Antimicrobial Agents on the Production of Biofilm

Antimicrobial agents, not unexpectedly, can either increase or decrease the production of biofilm. This effect, in part, appears species-specific. For example, fluoroquinolones at concentrations of one-half the MIC of *Staphylococcus epidermidis* decrease the production of slime (i.e., biofilm) (181). On the other hand, exposure of *Klebsiella pneumoniae* to a fluoroquinolone such as ciprofloxacin (182) has been shown to increase the amount of biofilm by more than 100-fold. Similarly, exposure of *K. pneumoniae* as well as many other microorganisms to β-lactam agents results in increased production of biofilm (182). Reduction of biofilm can be seen with other agents such as salicylates (183). The reduction of biofilm appears to occur concomitantly with a decrease in porin proteins (184–186). If these porins are being utilized to pump the biofilm precursors to the cell wall outer surface for final assembly, the two events are probably cause and effect. The decrease in biofilm and porin protein has been shown to result in resistance (185,187,188). This phenomenon has been shown to inhibit the activity of cephalosporins (188), aminoglycosides (183), and carbapenems (186). If biofilm is increased by exposure to β-lactam agents, then antimicrobial agents that have an effect on biofilm should be enhanced by preexposure of the bacteria to β-lactam agents. Indeed, this has been noted in both in vitro (189) and in vivo (190) studies.

Effects of Biofilm on Antimicrobial Action

The establishment of biofilm is an important aspect of cell wall physiology for individual cells and is equally important for microorganisms collectively. Bacteria that live and metabolize in these dense biofilm-encased microcolonies gain a number of the advantages enjoyed by multicellular life forms (52,56,57,191). One such advantage is a circulatory system (although primitive) with which to receive nutrients and into which to discharge metabolic wastes. This circulatory system consists of permeable channels that pass through less dense areas of biofilm interspersed within the dense microcolonies (56,191). Along these channels live river populations of microorganisms. These channels have convective flow patterns that permit the penetration and distribution into the biofilm matrix of large (2,000 Da) molecules. Dissolved oxygen is another critical commodity that is distributed within the biofilm through these channels. Microelectrodes have determined that the concentrations of dissolved oxygen in dense microcolonies approach zero at the center, owing to diffusion limitations and oxygen utilization (192). Such direct observations explain the need for anaerobic pathways for microorganisms such as *P. aeruginosa* (90) and *M. tuberculosis* (193) that are considered to be strict aerobes. Similar redox-sensitive chemical probes and autoradiography (194) have been used to detect metabolic activity and have demonstrated that, within a microcolony, the majority of cells are metabolically active. Although metabolically active, bacteria within biofilm colonies grow very slowly and are considered to resemble stationary-phase cultures (19,60). Moreover, those microorganisms downriver receive fewer substrates and may therefore become nutritionally starved, setting into motion the complex set of events (59,61) previously described.

Changes in microbial growth rate and nutrient limitation have long been recognized to cause changes in cell envelope components, which, in turn, influence the susceptibility of the microbes to antimicrobial agents (27,59,61,195). Establishment of biofilm is a growth-related factor that influences the susceptibility of the microbes to antimicrobial agents (196). For example, exposure of planktonic cells of *P. aeruginosa* to a biofilm surface produced by cells of the same species triggers the expression of at least two genes, *algC* and *algG* (74). This influences the susceptibility of these cells to antimicrobial agents, because sessile cells encased in biofilm are phenotypically different from planktonic cells of the same species (57,58,197).

The presence of biofilm at the individual cellular level contributes to changes in the overall susceptibility patterns of microorganisms involved in chronic infections, because the encasement by biofilm allows aggregates of cells to exist together in microcolonies. In mature biofilms, bacterial cells occupy only 5% to 35% of the biofilm mass (49,58,63,64,197). There are currently two leading hypotheses for the persistence of chronic biofilm-associated infections: (a) decreased concentrations of antibiotics caused by impaired transport to some regions of the biofilm

(49,191,198,199) or by a dilutional effect (49) and (b) physiologic differences of sessile cells (197). A biofilm accumulation model has predicted that both mechanisms would result in reduced antimicrobial susceptibilities of 7-day-old biofilms compared with those of 2-day-old films (49). Growth rate–dependent killing was predicted to be decreased in thicker biofilms because of oxygen depletion, leading to reduced growth rates. The model also predicted resistance to the antibiotic due to depletion caused by increased biomass. The explanation was not that the antibiotic would fail to penetrate the biofilm but instead that the drug would be diluted in the bulk fluid. The binding of agents to biofilm is related to two factors: the relative availability of drug and the relative proximity. Relative availability is proportional to the amount of drug, whereas relative proximity is proportional to the concentration of the drug. The total amount of drug may remain the same as the biomass of polysaccharide increases, but the relative proximity decreases. Finally, many of the factors affecting antimicrobial susceptibility may change over time as the biofilm colony matures, because maturation alters the milieu for many microorganisms within the microcolony. For example, colonies deep within thick, mature biofilm may have reached the starvation stage.

Mechanisms of Antimicrobial Uptake

A factor that is clearly of great importance for effective antimicrobial action against bacteria is the penetration of the antimicrobial agent into both the human cell (200) and the microbial cell (201). Entry of the antimicrobial agents into human cells is considered a part of the pharmacokinetics of these agents (6). In this section, the entry of the antimicrobial agent into the microbial cell will be reviewed. In order to understand antimicrobial uptake, it is useful to understand the physiology of transport mechanisms located on microbial cell membranes.

In all microorganisms, the cytoplasmic membrane provides an osmotic barrier that is permeable to very few substances. It is porous to water and to uncharged organic molecules up to the size of glycerol. Gram-negative bacteria have an additional cell membrane, the outer membrane, which also acts as an effective barrier against antibiotics (155–157). In particular, hydrophobic antibiotics diffuse relatively poorly through the outer cell membrane in gram-negative bacteria

in comparison with diffusion through the cytoplasmic membrane. This is due to the lack of glycerophospholipid in the outer portion of the cell bilayer, which instead consists largely of lipopolysaccharides.

Antimicrobial agents derived from microorganisms bear little resemblance to natural substrates brought into the bacterial cell but instead are more akin to metabolites excreted by cells (202). Therefore, with few exceptions (e.g., fosfomycin, which uses a stereospecific nutrient transport system) (203), antibiotics do not utilize active transport mechanisms for substrate uptake into bacteria.

There are three general mechanisms for substrate uptake into the bacterial cell: simple diffusion, facilitated diffusion, and active transport (158,204). There is a fourth mechanism known as the self-promoted uptake pathway, which is used by certain bacteria for the uptake of polycationic antibiotics (205). Each is discussed.

Simple or passive diffusion is defined as movement of molecules across a permeable membrane in which the flux in either direction is proportional to the concentration on the entering side and the rate of net transfer is proportional to the concentration differences between the two sides. An important factor in this type of diffusion is the partitioning coefficient, which essentially indicates the ability of the substrate to dissolve into the membrane interior (i.e., permeability). Simple diffusion kinetics occurs with nonpolar organic molecules such as tetracycline, which penetrates by dissolving in the lipid of the membrane, as well as with antimicrobial agents that move across a membrane through water-filled membrane-protein channel (i.e., pore) that is known as a porin (201,205–208). Fluoroquinolones, for example, are taken into bacteria by passive diffusion through porins in a passive diffusion process that exhibits nonsaturable kinetics. Fluoroquinolones are amphoteric molecules and have both zwitterionic and uncharged forms at neutral pH. Generally, only uncharged molecules are involved in the passive diffusion process, with the amount of uncharged forms greatly influencing the penetrating ability of these agents. Charged molecules can also exhibit passive diffusion, provided there is an electrical gradient across the membrane (209).

Facilitated diffusion in theory involves a barrier-insoluble substance reacting with a carrier (i.e., transporter) within the barrier to form a complex that can shuttle across the membrane, where the substance is then released. This type of diffusion exhibits saturable Michaelis-Menten kinetics with a K_m and a V_{max}, but the K_m is the same on both sides of the membrane because this mechanism is not linked to an energy source. Another name for this type of uptake pathway is a passive carrier–mediated system. Facilitated diffusion is seen in yeasts (210) but has not yet been identified in bacteria.

Active transport means that the bacterial cell has the ability to concentrate molecules within the cell. This ability can be turned on or off (i.e., is inducible) and is linked to an energy source. Without this energy source, the molecules cannot pass across the membrane. The kinetics of active transport exhibits a K_m and a V_{max}, like the activity of an enzyme, and the carrier system can be saturated.

The self-promoted uptake pathway has been described for gram-negative bacteria and involves binding of the antibiotic to the lipopolysaccharide in the outer membrane (205,211,212). This is followed by outer displacement, by the antimicrobial agent, of magnesium and possibly calcium ions in the lipopolysaccharide matrix of the biofilm (213). This causes instability of the biofilm matrix, as described earlier, and leads to increased permeability (214). The presence of additional divalent cations prevents this by stabilizing the complex. The self-promoted pathway was first described as an uptake mechanism in *P. aeruginosa* for polycationic antibiotics such as polymyxin and the aminoglycosides (213). More recently, it has been noted for azithromycin in *E. coli* (215).

Cell membranes of microorganisms must be energized in order to concentrate nutrients needed for growth. The electrochemical gradient–induced proton motive force is a key factor in these energized cytoplasmic membranes. Microbial cell membranes are intrinsically impermeable to protons yet must move protons in or out of the cell. For example, any change in the intracellular pH of the microorganism would need to be absorbed by the buffering capacity of the cytoplasm (148) unless there was some method for expelling protons. Such a pH-homeostatic method exists and involves membrane-bound proton pumps (149). Proton-driven translocation of molecules is facilitated by reduced pH (216). These pumps may at times be responsible for the efflux of antibiotics by pumping out protons that are complexed with a negatively charged antibiotic.

The outer membrane in gram-negative bacteria, through changes in porin diffusion channels, can serve as a permeation barrier and thus greatly influences antimicrobial resistance (156,157,178,217,218). Moreover, the uptake of antimicrobial agents into bacterial cells also can be influenced by efflux mechanisms that may concomitantly act to remove the agent (150,156,219–222). In fact, the antimicrobial activity may be determined by the race between uptake and efflux. It is useful to appreciate the mechanisms of efflux, because these should themselves prove to be excellent targets for antimicrobial agents (222–225).

Membrane-bound proton pumps may be readily overcome by compounds with uncoupling activity (219). Classic uncouplers include carbonyl cyanide-*m*-chlorophenylhydrazine and 2,4-dinitrophenol (226). These uncouplers result in the abolition of respiratory control in the bacteria. This, in turn, results in stimulation of respiratory activity.

INHIBITORY OR LETHAL ANTIMICROBIAL ACTIVITY VERSUS FUNCTIONAL SYNERGY AGAINST MICROBES

Inhibitory and Lethal Effects

The goal of antimicrobial therapy, as appreciated by Lister and Ehrlich, is to destroy the invading microorganism without harming the host. The effectiveness of an antimicrobial agent has traditionally been measured by its ability to inhibit and kill bacteria. In theory, there are three basic ways to kill a bacterial cell: by causing irreparable damage to its genome, to its envelope, and to certain classes of its proteins (114–121). Antimicrobial agents have been developed that attempt to kill bacteria in each of these ways. Often, several antibiotics that use two of these three different ways are combined to enhance the lethal effect. Yet, as already noted, bacteria are not particularly easy to kill. This fact has not escaped microbiologists. It is well known that most antimicrobial agents exert their lethal effects on bacteria during the growth phase (2,27,195). Therefore, microbiologists have designed routine susceptibility tests to measure antimicrobial activity during the logarithmic growth phase in media that provide all of the ingredients for optimal growth (62). However, this is not the usual state of microorganisms in infected tissues. For example, *S. aureus* isolates from tissue-cage infections in rats have been shown to be in a state of dormancy and thus are relatively resistant to most antimicrobial agents (227). Perhaps the closest that broth susceptibility testing comes to mimicking a clinical infection is in the case of acute bacterial meningitis. Even then, there clearly is room for improvement (228). Susceptibility testing must be repositioned to provide test results that correlate with the clinical infection. Fortunately, clinical microbiologists have been working to accomplish this goal. An example is the integrated use of pharmacokinetic and pharmacodynamic models for the definition of breakpoints (9). As a result, the correlation of in vitro susceptibility testing with in vivo clinical effectiveness has markedly improved (14). Moreover, clinical microbiology laboratories are aware of emerging mechanisms of resistance and are particularly vigilant in detecting such resistance (229,230). Finally, antimicrobial susceptibility testing is frequently integrated with an antimicrobial stewardship program (231) that is aimed at controlling resistance.

Functional Synergy

Most clinical infections involve bacteria in a sessile state, as opposed to a planktonic state (63). However, antimicrobial agents that are able to kill bacteria in their sessile state are few in number (28,232,233). Of those agents currently available for clinical use, carbapenems and the fluoroquinolones have the greatest lethal effect against sessile bacteria—a lethal effect more readily obtained against gram-negative isolates than against gram-positive ones (233–235). Against gram-positive pathogens such as staphylococci, daptomycin has the greatest lethal effect against stationary-phase and nondividing organisms (236,237). This in vitro bactericidal activity, often defined as equal to or greater than a 3 $\log_{10}$ decrease in colony-forming units over a 24-hour period (62), may not be sufficient for total microbial killing against certain microorganisms (48) or with certain infections such as endocarditis (238). Total and rapid microbial killing is important in acute bacterial meningitis as well as in acute sepsis in immunodeficient hosts (2,7). Even the most rigorous in vitro susceptibility test methods, including time-kill kinetic methodology, may provide misinformation if the growth phase of the microorganism and the clinically desired end point are not correlated with the test method (14). This is shown by a report by investigators who found that clarithromycin, like other macrolides, demonstrated in vitro bactericidal activity against pneumococci by time-kill kinetic methodology (239). However, in a rabbit model for pneumococcal meningitis, clarithromycin was unable to cure pneumococcal meningitis despite susceptible isolates and cerebrospinal fluid levels of clarithromycin comparable

to those used to achieve in vitro killing (239). In chronic infections such as endocarditis and osteomyelitis, where involvement of biofilm is almost always present, rapid microbial killing is usually not achievable due to factors such as decreased biofilmpenetration/dilutional effects and dormant growth phase (240,241). Total microbial killing, on the other hand, is a well-recognized goal when treating these particular infections; antimicrobial therapy is usually given for 6 to 8 weeks in order to achieve total microbial killing (242,243).

The use of bactericidal drugs in order to achieve total microbial killing is not required for most infections (244,245). However, when bacterial eradication is deemed necessary, there are a number of ways that this may be predicted (246). Pharmacokinetic and pharmacodynamic parameters may be useful for predicting bacterial response (246,247). In addition, there are bactericidal tests including proposed reference methods available in most clinical microbiology laboratories (248).

The accumulated knowledge of antimicrobial mechanisms of action on different growth phases of bacteria has reached a point where it may encourage a multicomponent drug approach to antimicrobial therapy (21,249,250). This approach may involve using combination therapy that achieves functional synergy against the infecting microorganism. Functional synergy directed against the microorganism often can be achieved by using knowledge of the various physiologic states within which microorganisms exist combined with knowledge of specific antimicrobial agents that interfere with each of the physiologic states. When these agents are combined, their use may result in enhanced microbial killing that can be thought of as functional synergy. Although enhanced killing, as defined by a strict definition of synergy, may not be detected using in vitro methods, enhancement of total killing may be measured in other ways. For example, animal models have long been used to assess the ability of antimicrobial agents alone or in combination to eradicate microorganisms (251).

Functional synergy as a therapeutic approach is already in use but is not well appreciated. The therapy of TB is one of the oldest examples of this approach, for in such therapy, multiple antituberculous agents result in enhanced mycobacterial killing as well as minimizing the emergence of resistance. An example of this therapeutic approach is the recognition of the lethal effect of metronidazole on dormant forms of *M. tuberculosis* (252). This lethal activity appears to be related to the fact that the dormant state requires anaerobic pathways, which then provide the necessary electrons to activate metronidazole to its electrophilic degradation products (252). Metronidazole alone does not reduce the bacillary burden of *M. tuberculosis* in the guinea pig model (253). Exposing *M. tuberculosis* in its dormant state to metronidazole apparently kills the organism or triggers aerobic respiration. The return to aerobic pathways does not occur independently but instead occurs with resumption of mycobacterial replication. Thus, combining metronidazole or similar agents with agents that interfere with the replicating stage creates functional synergy that allows enhanced killing of the mycobacterium (24,254). Drug development strategies that target the different physiologic states of *M. tuberculosis* including the latent phase may allow improved treatment of TB (255). Indeed, the addition of metronidazole to isoniazid (INH) and rifampin in the macaque model has been shown to effectively treat animals with active TB within 2 months (256).

Another example of functional synergy is the use of an aminoglycoside with a β-lactam agent for the therapy of infections such as bacterial endocarditis caused by *P. aeruginosa*. The increased effectiveness of this combination is due to the disruption of the biofilm by the aminoglycoside (173,257), which enhances the β-lactam agent in two ways. The first is when disruption provides holes in the bacterial cell wall that allow increased penetration of the β-lactam agent. The second is when the dormant form is forced to replicate in an attempt to fix the damaged cell wall, thus providing a target for the β-lactam agent.

Other chronic infections that have benefited from a multidrug approach that provides functional synergy include pulmonary infections caused by *P. aeruginosa* in patients with cystic fibrosis. These infections involve the establishment in lung tissue of biofilm-encased microcolonies in which are found some dwarf forms, which may represent dormant forms that are utilizing anaerobic pathways (90,104,105). Clinical cure of these *Pseudomonas* pulmonary infections is rarely achieved (104). This is consistent with the in vitro observation that total microbial killing of sessile strains of *P. aeruginosa* is extremely difficult to achieve after the biofilm has matured for 5 to 7 days (196). Neither older synergistic combinations such as tobramycin and piperacillin (77) nor newer synergistic combinations such as fosfomycin and ofloxacin (258) are able to achieve total killing.

There are, however, some approaches that may allow functional synergy. The use of aerosolized tobramycin (259,260) or aerosolized colistin (261) is one of these; this approach provides greater concentrations of a biofilm disrupter (i.e., both tobramycin and colistin) as well as a bacterial cell membrane disrupter (i.e., colistin), which then can enhance the systemic use of other antipseudomonal agents. The prolonged use of aminoglycosides in chronic *Pseudomonas* infections is known to be followed by the emergence of aminoglycoside-resistant *Pseudomonas* strains characterized by a deep rough colony morphology on agar plates due to the lack of biofilm (257). The lack of a lipopolysaccharide/biofilm target for the primary action of the aminoglycoside is the mechanism of resistance, because these strains do not exhibit altered ribosomes or produce aminoglycoside-inactivating enzymes. The outer cell walls of these aminoglycoside-resistant strains are characterized by the lack of lipopolysaccharide and a marked increase in the amount of OprH OMP (257). Overproduction of this outer cell membrane protein decreases the accumulation of polymyxin and gentamicin by the self-promoted pathway (214). However, overproduction of OprH is associated with increased susceptibility to fluoroquinolone antibiotics (262). It appears that the overproduction of OprH is a mechanism that minimizes biofilm in order to counter the effects of biofilm disruption by polycationic agents, but in doing so, the altered cell wall seems to offer increased diffusion of lipophilic fluoroquinolones into the cytoplasm. The use of a fluoroquinolone and an antipseudomonal β-lactam agent along with the aerosolized aminoglycoside (264) thus allows functional synergy and provides an additional therapeutic option (265). Moreover, the addition of a macrolide such as azithromycin or clarithromycin to this regimen may prove useful. These macrolides have been shown to decrease the production of both biofilm (135,137,266) and exoenzymes (131,132) by *P. aeruginosa*, which creates yet another biofilm-related conflict while preventing further pulmonary damage by the exoenzymes (132,266–271). Macrolides and ketolides have been shown to have an effect on the outer membrane of *P. aeruginosa* (272,273) that appears to potentiate the activity of antipseudomonal agents and may allow functional synergy (274). Clinical experience with the use of aerosolized tobramycin (259,260), fluoroquinolones (264), and macrolides (275) for exacerbations of *Pseudomonas* infections in cystic fibrosis patients have shown that multidrug regimens that include one or more of these three agents result in reductions in *P. aeruginosa* sputum density and improvements in pulmonary function (265). Interestingly, a similar approach using a combination of clarithromycin and ceftazidime in a rat model for foreign body–related osteomyelitis caused by *P. aeruginosa* demonstrated that clarithromycin eradicated the biofilm and enhanced the bactericidal effect of ceftazidime (276).

There are other examples of functional synergy in microbes that can be purposely created by the selective use of antibiotics. Enhanced microbial killing is a frequent goal of combination antimicrobial therapy for infective endocarditis (20). Therefore, a number of examples of functional synergy demonstrated in experimental endocarditis are discussed. Temafloxacin has been shown to be effective in the therapy of experimental streptococcal endocarditis, and studies have found it to penetrate vegetations in a homogeneous manner (277). Dextranase is an enzyme capable of hydrolyzing 20% to 90% of streptococcal glycocalyx (biofilm). When used alone, dextranase has no in vitro antimicrobial effect on viridans streptococci nor does it have a beneficial effect on experimental streptococcal endocarditis (278). When dextranase is used in combination with temafloxacin, it significantly potentiates the effect of temafloxacin in vivo by reducing the amount of bacterial biofilm in infected vegetations and by altering the metabolic status of the microorganisms (279). The same effect has been seen when dextranase and penicillin have been combined in the treatment of experimental streptococcal endocarditis (278). Finally, an animal model for experimental *P. aeruginosa* endocarditis has shown an identical effect for alginase combined with amikacin (280). Of importance is the lack of beneficial effect demonstrated when the vegetation size is reduced by fibrinolytic therapy alone (281,282). The results of these studies are consistent with the theory that the bacteria in microcolonies embedded in biofilm have a lower metabolic rate (283). Reducing the amount of biofilm results in both an increased metabolic rate and increased replication, which each increases the antimicrobial activity of most antibiotics.

Another experimental approach to disrupting the biofilm as a method for creating functional synergy is to use the proteolytic enzyme serratiopeptidase (284). Serratiopeptidase is a metalloprotease produced by a strain of *Serratia* that is only partially inhibited by in vivo protease inhibitors and

has been used as an antiinflammatory drug because of its ability to increase the penetration of antibiotics into infected sites (285). This protease has been found to enhance the activity of ofloxacin on sessile cultures of *P. aeruginosa* and *S. aureus* (286). In addition, serratiopeptidase has been shown to reduce the ability of *Listeria monocytogenes* to form biofilm and to invade host cells (287).

Another commonly used drug with the potential for creating biofilm-related functional synergy in the therapy of microbial infections is aspirin (288). Aspirin has been noted to be a cell wall permeabilizer for *P. aeruginosa* (178). This role as a cell wall permeabilizer may be related to its effect on biofilm. Aspirin has been shown to cause a dose-dependent reduction in the weight of aortic vegetations in experimental endocarditis (289). In addition, when combined with vancomycin, aspirin improves the sterilization rate of aortic valve vegetations infected with *S. aureus*. These effects are similar to those of dextranase (279) and the protease of *Serratia* (286) and may be a result of functional synergy. Aspirin has been found to diminish the amount of microbial biofilm in a number of other studies (183,288). Salicylates also are known to depress the synthesis of porins in *E. coli*, *K. pneumoniae*, *Serratia marcescens*, *Burkholderia cepacia*, and *P. aeruginosa* (184–186,188). If these depressed porins are involved in the efflux of biofilm precursors as a part of biofilm maintenance, these two physiologic phenomena may be related. Finally, the combination of aspirin and amphotericin B has demonstrated functional synergy against biofilm cells of *Candida albicans* and *Candida parapsilosis* versus indifferent effects against planktonic cells of these microorganisms (290). Each of these antimicrobial strategies against infectious bacterial biofilm (291) is an example of the use of functional synergy.

Finally, rifampin combination therapy is a very controversial multidrug approach to a number of nonmycobacterial infections (292,293) that may owe its somewhat surprising albeit unpredictable efficacy to functional synergy. Rifampin combination therapy has been used clinically for various types of infections (293), but the predominant use seems to be for staphylococcal infections (292) that involve osteomyelitis and/or a prosthetic device–related infection. The controversy stems from a lack of convincing in vitro data that support the in vivo clinical findings. There are a number of clinical studies involving bone or joint infections that have demonstrated such in vivo efficacy, although these studies are generally underpowered

(294–301). Examples of a number of these clinical studies are provided. In one study (296), therapy with 900 mg/day rifampin plus 600 mg/day ofloxacin for 6 months was used for patients with prosthetic implants infected with *Staphylococcus* spp. The overall success rate was 74% among 47 patients, with 62% of patients being cured without removal of their orthopedic device (296). The success rate was 81% for the hip prosthesis group, 69% for the knee prosthesis group, and 69% for the osteosynthesis device group. A total of eight treatment failures were related to the isolation of a resistant microorganism. In another study (297), 33 patients with culture-proven staphylococcal infection associated with stable orthopedic implants and with a short duration of symptoms of infection were treated: 18 patients received ciprofloxacin and rifampin, whereas 15 patients received ciprofloxacin and a placebo. Twenty-four patients completed the trial; the cure rate was 12 of 12 (100%) for those who received ciprofloxacin plus rifampin versus 7 of 12 (58%) for those who received ciprofloxacin plus a placebo (297). In a third study (295), 10 patients with *Staphylococcus* spp–infected orthopedic implants were treated with various antibiotic regimens, all of which included rifampin. Of these patients, 8 were cured. Many of these studies (296–298,301) combined rifampin with a quinolone; indeed, early results with such oral therapy using rifampin combined with a quinolone have been encouraging (302).

Animal models of adjunctive rifampin for therapy of *Staphylococcus*-infected prosthetic devices/foreign bodies/osteomyelitis may offer some additional insight. A rat model of chronic staphylococcal foreign body infection (227) demonstrated that antimicrobial combinations of fleroxacin plus vancomycin and vancomycin plus fleroxacin and rifampin were highly effective and superior to single drugs. Further, the three-drug therapeutic regimen decreased bacterial counts more rapidly than the two-drug therapy and was curative in most cases (92% for three drugs versus 41% for two and less than 6% for monotherapy). No mutants resistant to these three agents were detected with combination therapy. A rabbit model of acute staphylococcal osteomyelitis caused by MRSA noted a 100% infection clearance with tigecycline and rifampin versus a 90% clearance with tigecycline alone, whereas vancomycin and rifampin showed a 90% infection clearance versus an 81.8% clearance with vancomycin alone (303). A guinea pig model assessing linezolid alone or combined with rifampin against a foreign body infection caused by MRSA demonstrated that the efficacy in the eradication of cage-associated MRSA infection was achieved only with the combination of rifampin and linezolid, with cure rates being between 50% and 60%; in this guinea pig model, a levofloxacin–rifampin combination achieved a 91% cure rate against a quinolone-susceptible MRSA strain (304). An MRSA knee prosthesis infection in rabbits was used to evaluate daptomycin or vancomycin alone and in combination with rifampin (305). This study demonstrated that daptomycin combined with rifampin sterilized 11 of 11 bones versus 2 of 12 for daptomycin alone, whereas vancomycin combined with rifampin sterilized 6 of 8 bones versus 0 of 12 for vancomycin alone (305). Moreover, rifampin prevented the emergence of daptomycin-resistant MRSA; the authors concluded that adjunctive rifampin is crucial to optimizing daptomycin efficacy against rabbit prosthetic joint infection due to MRSA (305). Additional studies in animal models have demonstrated similar efficacy of rifampin combinations (306–308).

The success of adjunctive rifampin for the therapy of *Staphylococcus*-infected prosthetic devices/foreign bodies/osteomyelitis may once again be due to functional synergy that targets biofilm (241,291). The efficacy of fluoroquinolones (302) is of interest because fluoroquinolones have been shown to decrease the production of slime (biofilm) by *S. epidermidis* (181), and it is likely that rifampin, through inhibition of protein synthesis, may decrease or prevent the availability of critical enzymes needed for ongoing maintenance of biofilm. As the biofilm microcolonies attached to the prosthetic device or glued into the bone begin to be slowly disrupted by the lack of ongoing maintenance, the staphylococci are forced to replicate, which further enhances the antimicrobial action of each antibiotic.

MECHANISMS OF ACTION FOR SELECTED CLASSES OF ANTIMICROBIAL AGENTS

Antimicrobial Classes in Current Clinical Use

β-Lactam Agents

As previously described, the main structural features of the peptidoglycan sacculus are linear glycan chains interlinked by short peptide bridges. A number of enzymatic activities are involved in the biosynthesis of the sacculus: catalyzation by glycosyltransferase enzymes of the formation of the linear glycan chains, cross-linking of the glycan chains by transglycosylase enzymes, and cross-linking via peptide bridges by transpeptidase enzymes (32,151). The latter peptide cross-links provide mechanical strength against osmotic pressure forces. Peptidoglycan structural modifications of completed cell wall are required in replicating cells as they grow, and each microorganism therefore possesses specific peptidoglycan hydrolases that are responsible for such structural adjustments (38–40,309). It is these transpeptidases/hydrolases (39,40,309), as well as other factors such as activation of newly recognized apoptotic death pathways (42–45), that appear to be important target(s) of β-lactam agents (36,40,96,310–314).

The mechanism of action of β-lactam agents is more complex than initially thought and likely involves three interrelated cellular processes (314). The first of these cellular processes is transpeptidation, which initially was thought to be the sole target of β-lactam agents (310). Penicillins, because of their structural similarity to the C-terminal D-alanyl-D-alanine end of the peptide stem, react chemically with the transpeptidases, also known as PBPs, to form stable acyl-enzymes, inactivating the PBPs and preventing further cross-linking. The inhibition of glycan cross-linking then leads to a weakened cell wall, which eventually ruptures due to osmotic pressure. However, it was noted that penicillins were able to cause inhibition of growth in certain bacteria without bacteriolysis. Therefore, triggering of autolytic cell wall enzymes was considered as a second and separate target of β-lactam agents (43,127,311). However, the mechanism for control of the autolytic system and how it was activated during treatment with β-lactam agents remained unknown until a number of observations suggested several possibilities. The electrophysiologic state of the cellular membrane is thought to be an important factor in the regulation of bacterial cell wall autolysis (107,315,316). There is increasing evidence that β-lactam agents may depolarize the membrane potential as a signal to induce autolysis (44,45,317). Moreover, there are a number of regulatory genes that are involved in bacterial autolysis (97,318,319). These genes may be activated after exposure to a sufficient concentration of β-lactam agent to cause irreparable damage (30,95,319). For example, a signal transduction pathway involved in regulating apoptotic death in pneumococci has been described (96). One of the death signals appears to be a peptide, which may function in a quorum-sensing manner. Finally, metabolism-related depletion of NADH, leaching of iron from iron-sulfur clusters, and stimulation of the Fenton reaction has been shown to lead to formation of harmful hydroxyl radicals that triggers an oxidative damage cellular death pathway (44,45). This pathway may be modulated by the stringent response in a manner yet to be detailed. Modulation of the stringent response under antimicrobial selection appears to create mutants that are virulent and not killed by a broad spectrum of antimicrobial agents (55). This resistance phenomenon has been described as physiologic tolerance (28,320).

Penicillins

Penicillins are characterized by a four-membered β-lactam ring fused to a five-membered thiazolidine ring containing a side chain (321). Manipulations of this side chain have been important in the pharmacokinetics and pharmacodynamics of penicillins. The ability to produce 6-aminopenicillanic acid (6-APA) by fermentation allowed chemists to replace the amino group of 6-APA with a large number of altered side chains, thus producing many different semisynthetic penicillins (322). The steric hindrance around the amide bond produced by bulky side chains such as carbocyclic or heterocyclic rings with substituents at the orthoposition of the 6-APA site produced the first semisynthetic penicillins with increased stability against staphylococcal β-lactamase. A number of such antistaphylococcal penicillins with bulky side chains have been synthesized, including methicillin; nafcillin; and the isoxazolyl penicillins, oxacillin, cloxacillin, dicloxacillin, and flucloxacillin.

Semisynthetic penicillins also include those created by a simple replacement of the α-carbon of the hydrophobic side chain at position 6 of benzylpenicillin by an amino (e.g., ampicillin), a carboxyl (e.g., carbenicillin), a ureido (e.g., mezlocillin), a piperazino (e.g., piperacillin) group, or a methoxy (e.g., temocillin). The result was the development of the extended-spectrum penicillins, which have been grouped as aminopenicillins, carboxypenicillins, ureidopenicillins, and methoxypenicillins (322–325). Such substitutions provided improved penetration through the outer cell membrane of gram-negative microorganisms as well as increased stability against β-lactamases produced by these pathogens. In particular, penetration through the restrictive pores of *P. aeruginosa* resulted in antipseudomonal activity for the carboxypenicillins (e.g., carbenicillin and ticarcillin) and the ureidopenicillins (e.g., mezlocillin, azlocillin, and piperacillin). The only methoxypen-icillin in clinical use is temocillin (324,325), which is not active against gram-positive organisms, an-aerobes, and *Pseudomonas* species; temocillin has not been approved for use in the United States. Temocillin is, however, resistant to most if not all classic and extended-spectrum β-lactamases as well as to AmpC β-lactamases (324). For this reason, it has been used in England as a carbapenem-sparing agent (324,325). Because the stability against β-lactamases did not include staphylococcal β-lactamase, a number of these extended-spectrum penicillins were combined with a β-lactamase inhibitor (e.g., clavulanate, sulbactam, or tazo-bactam) and are known as β-lactam–β-lactamase inhibitor combinations (323,326,327). To date, these combinations include amoxicillin/clavula-nate, ampicillin/sulbactam, ticarcillin/clavulanate, and piperacillin/tazobactam.

Cephalosporins

Cephalosporins are characterized by a four-membered β-lactam ring fused to a sulfur-con-taining ring-expanded system (328). One of the first cephalosporins, cephalosporin C, possessed an aminoadipic side chain, which could easily be chemically removed to give rise to 7-aminocepha-losporonic acid (7-ACA), which is analogous to 6-APA (329). From 7-ACA came the first-generation semisynthetic cephalosporins such as cefazolin. Substitutions at the C7 position as well as at the C3 position of the dihydrothiazine ring allow greater variation of semisynthetic cephalo-sporins than can be achieved with the penicillins (322,323). Consequently, more cephalosporins have been developed, and detailed reviews of these agents are available (322,323,328,330). Side chain substitution in the cephalosporins is built on the experience with penicillins and includes thiazolyl and phenylglycyl side chains. The substitutions at the C7 position are of particular importance in governing stability against β-lactamases. For ex-ample, substitution at the C7-α position of cepha-losporins with a methoxy group (e.g., cefoxitin and cefotetan, which are second-generation cephalo-sporins) resulted in the cephamycins, which have increased stability against β-lactamases, including those of the *Bacteroides fragilis* group. Substitution at the C7-β position with a methoxyimino group (e.g., cefotaxime, which is a third-generation cephalosporin) also increased the resistance of these agents to β-lactamases. Acyl side chains used with cephalosporins include aminothiazole

oximes, which may have charged carboxylates (e.g., ceftazidime, which is a third-generation cephalosporin) that improve penetration through gram-negative bacterial outer membranes. Cefepime, a fourth-generation cephalosporin, also has a positively charged quaternary ammonium in position C3, which creates a zwitterion that allows increased penetration of the gram-negative bacte-rial outer membrane. The 2-aminothiazolylaceta-mido group found in cefepime provides increased stability against β-lactamases. Ceftaroline is the first member of a new subclass of β-lactam agents, cephalosporins with activity against MRSA (331). A 1,3-thiazole ring attached to the 3-position of the cephalosporin nucleus and the oxime group in the C7 acyl moiety provide the basis for increased activity against MRSA with the 1,3-thiazole ring binding tightly to the MRSA PBP 2A following a conformational change in the protein allowing the active site to be exposed for binding (332). Cef-taroline is also active against multidrug-resistant *S. pneumoniae*.

Carbapenems

Carbapenems differ from conventional penicillins in having no sulfur atom in their five-membered ring and in having a double bond between car-bons 2 and 3 (332,333). This sterically alters the cis/trans configuration of the molecule in com-parison with other β-lactam agents and places the amide bond away from the water-containing groove of the serine-based β-lactamases. How-ever, carbapenems are susceptible to hydrolysis by metallo-β-lactamases. Four carbapenems (imi-penem, meropenem, ertapenem, and doripenem) are approved for clinical use in the United States.

Monobactams

There are two monocyclic β-lactams produced by microorganisms that possess antimicrobial activity, nocardicins and monobactams (334). The monobactam nucleus of these compounds exhibits only weak antimicrobial activity, and they, like the penicillins and cephalosporins, must have substitution around the central nucleus to achieve clinically useful antimicrobial activity. Side chain structure–activity relationships in monobactams parallel those of penicillins and cephalospor-ins. There is only one monobactam antibiotic, aztreonam, that has a 3-acyl aminothiazole-oxime side chain identical to that of ceftazidime, while the lactam ring has a *N*-sulfonate substituent on the other side (330,332,334). The *N*-sulfonate substituent is essential for β-lactamase stability. Like ceftazidime, aztreonam is useful only against gram-negative pathogens, with good activity against *P. aeruginosa*.

Aminoglycosides

All aminoglycoside antibiotics contain one or more amino sugar residues linked to a central, six-membered aminocyclitol ring by pseudoglycosidic bond(s). Spectinomycin is, strictly speaking, also an aminocyclitol with three fused rings but lacks amino sugars and pseudoglycosidic bonds. The primary mechanism of action of aminoglycosides is a decrease in protein synthesis after the drug has bound to the prokaryotic ribosome at the 16S ribosomal RNA (rRNA) site located in the small (30S) subunit of the ribosome (335–339). Aminoglycosides are hydrophilic sugars with multiple amino groups that function as polycations. Their polycationic nature allows binding to the polyanionic 16S rRNA on the 30S ribosome at the A site for aminoacyl–tRNA binding (338,339). The A site is composed of portions of the 530 loop, helix 34, and the base of helix 44; transfer RNA (tRNA) anticodons bind in a cleft formed between these individual domains of the A site. Binding of the aminoglycoside to the A site inhibits the translation process by causing misreading and/or hindering the translocation step. Analysis by X-ray crystallography suggests that the polycation binds to the RNA bases rather than to backbone atoms. Moreover, attachment at the A site suggests that aminoglycosides block a required transformational transition during the peptide bond–forming translocation process, bringing the translocation steps of protein synthesis in the ribosome to a halt. Aminoglycosides also bind to helix 69 of the large (50S) subunit of the ribosome (340,341). The result of this binding is reduction in the mobility of an adenine residue at position 1492 of the rRNA A-site; this reduction in mobility may be a key determinant in the antibacterial activity of aminoglycosides (342).

The polycationic nature of aminoglycosides also accounts for their recognized effect on biofilm and cell membranes (163,172). Aminoglycosides are bactericidal agents and often exhibit a rapid lethal effect on susceptible aerobic gram-negative bacilli. Such a rapid lethal effect has been noted to be contrary to the expected effect of agents acting on ribosomal targets (173). This lethal effect of aminoglycosides against aerobic gram-negative bacilli, moreover, is concentration-dependent, with

increasing concentrations achieving increased killing. Their effect against gram-positive cocci is, at best, inhibitory, unless a β-lactam agent is used in combination with the aminoglycoside.

Inhibition of protein synthesis, however, usually does not produce a bactericidal effect, let alone a rapid one. Therefore, binding to the 30S ribosome may not be the only mechanism of antimicrobial action for aminoglycosides; in fact, many susceptible gram-negative bacilli may be dead long before the drug arrives at the 30S ribosome (173,174,212). It is now recognized that aminoglycosides are polycations that competitively displace cell biofilm–associated Mg^{2+} and Ca^{2+} linking the polysaccharides of adjacent lipopolysaccharide molecules (174,211–213). The result is shedding of cell membrane blebs, with formation of transient holes in the cell wall and disruption of the normal permeability of the cell wall (163,170,173,174). This action alone may be sufficient to kill many susceptible gram-negative bacteria before the aminoglycoside has a chance to reach the 30S ribosome (Fig. 10.3). The surface effect of gentamicin has been investigated using bovine serum albumin–gentamicin complexes (174), which have been shown to be bactericidal against *P. aeruginosa*. These findings are in agreement with similar studies done with other immobilized surface agents (146,343–345).

Increased understanding of the mechanisms of action of aminoglycosides brought with it the realization that aminoglycosides have a concentration-dependent bactericidal effect (346) as well as a considerable postantibiotic effect (2). This allowed the dosing schedule to be modified to once per day (347). The modification integrated

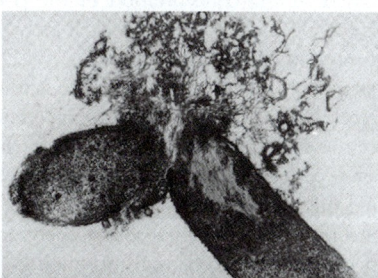

Figure 10.3 ■ *P. aeruginosa* **exposed to amikacin at 5 times the MIC for 5 hours.** Note the break in the cell wall, allowing the extrusion of the cell contents. (Reproduced with permission from Lorian V. Effects of low concentrations of antibiotics. In: Lorian V, ed. *Antibiotics in laboratory medicine*. 4th ed. Baltimore, MD: Williams & Wilkins, 1996:416.)

both pharmacokinetic and pharmacodynamic properties and offered the potential for greater efficacy and less toxicity (8,347–350). There has now been considerable experience with once-daily aminoglycoside regimens (347–350). Such regimens indeed appear to be clinically effective while reducing the incidence of nephrotoxicity. Moreover, they reduce the cost by decreasing ancillary service time and the need for serum aminoglycoside determinations.

Another question about the optimal utilization of aminoglycosides can be addressed. This concerns the timing of the doses when both an aminoglycoside and a β-lactam agent are administered. In vitro (189) and in vivo (190) studies have clearly demonstrated a remarkable advantage gained from nonsimultaneous administration of aminoglycosides and β-lactam agents when they are used in combination. The main benefit is a marked delay in bacterial regrowth regardless of the order in which the agents are given. However, the initial bactericidal effect is greater when the aminoglycoside is given first. The minimum time interval between doses of the aminoglycoside and the β-lactam agent for maximum delay of regrowth is 2 hours.

The reason for this phenomenon is clear if one accepts the premise that the aminoglycoside has its primary antimicrobial effect on biofilm. This effect would be greatest when there was no prior or concomitant use of cell wall–active agents, which have been shown to markedly affect the bacterial cell surfaces (103) and would thus lessen the opportunity for the aminoglycoside to have the optimal biofilm targets.

The bactericidal effects of aminoglycosides combined with β-lactam agents in vitro have been shown to be dependent on the concentrations of β-lactam agents used. If the concentration of the β-lactam agent is not optimized for bactericidal activity (i.e., four- to eightfold higher than the MIC), the effect of the β-lactam on the test microorganism is to stimulate increased production of biofilm (182) and thus enhance the effect of the aminoglycoside by providing a better target. Lorian and Ernst (351) have demonstrated this concept nicely. If, on the other hand, the concentration of the β-lactam agent is high enough to disrupt the cell wall morphology (103), then the biofilm target is lessened, which in turn lessens the lethal effect of the aminoglycoside (174,196). These two effects are exactly the opposite of what would be predicted to occur if the target of the aminoglycoside was the ribosome rather than biofilm. The overall lethal effect of aminoglycosides in vivo is enhanced by administering the aminoglycoside

before the β-lactam agent (190). Historically, aminoglycosides have been used in combination with other antimicrobial agents (most often a β-lactam agent) in order to enhance microbial killing and achieve increased efficacy (349). Most studies, however, fail to demonstrate improved outcomes (349); this may be due, in part, to not administering the aminoglycoside first.

Macrolides, Azolides, Lincosamides, Ketolides, and Streptogramins

The macrolides, azolides, lincosamides, ketolides, and streptogramins are grouped together despite structural differences because of similar biologic properties, including their mechanism of action against the 50S subunit of the bacterial ribosomes. Bacterial ribosomes are an important target for antimicrobial agents and have two specific subunits that are targeted, the 30S ribosomal subunit and the 50S ribosomal subunit (118). The specific target for the 50S ribosomal subunit for many of these agents appears to be domain V of the 23S rRNA, which is the peptidyltransferase center (352,353). Macrolides block the approach to the exit tunnel for elongating peptides and thus prevent polypeptide translation, causing premature release of peptidyl–tRNA intermediates. Lincosamides, however, inhibit the initiation of peptide chain formation (134,354), whereas the effect of the other macrolides is to prevent the extension of the growing peptide chain. Macrolides also block assembly of 50S subunits by their interaction with the 23S rRNA. There are interspecies variations in the ribosome structure that affect the binding of macrolides (355). These interspecies variations not only affect wild-type ribosomes but also affect ribosomes that have acquired resistance mutations. Thus, a mutation that results in high-level resistance to a specific macrolide in a particular species may only produce low-level resistance or none at all in a different species (355,356). Finally, it should be noted that the 23S rRNA of bacteria is the homolog of human mitochondrial 16S rRNA; antimicrobial agents that inhibit the bacterial 23S peptidyltransferase center may also impair human mitochondrial function (357).

Ketolides are the latest members of the macrolide group and are novel semisynthetic 14-membered–ring macrolides in which the main structural innovations are the lack of the neutral sugar cladinose in position C3 as well as a C11/C12 carbamate (358–360). When the C3 cladinose sugar moiety is removed, the resulting 3-hydroxy group is oxidized to a 3-keto group, hence the name *ketolide*. The macrolides, azolides, lincosamides, and ketolides all appear to bind to the same site or contiguous sites on the ribosome and so they may become competitive inhibitors if used together (359,361,362). This mechanism of action, inhibition of protein synthesis, results in bacteriostatic activity against most bacteria by all of these agents except ketolides, which have bactericidal activity (358–360). Inhibition of critical proteins in certain microbial species does, however, result in bactericidal activity of the macrolides. Such species-specific bactericidal activity is seen in vitro with the macrolide clarithromycin against *S. pneumoniae* but is less evident in vivo (239).

Macrolide antibiotics such as erythromycin, clarithromycin, and azithromycin appear to have the ability to decrease sputum production in patients with chronic respiratory infections (270,271,362–364). This has been attributed to a direct effect on the production of sputum (363) but may instead be due to inhibition of biofilm production by respiratory pathogens (266,270). Macrolides have been shown to markedly reduce the biofilm structure of microorganisms in their sessile phase (135) and to reduce the amount of virulent exotoxins (131,132). These microorganisms include *S. epidermidis* and *P. aeruginosa*. The mechanism seems to involve the suppression of a step or steps in the synthesis of monosaccharides, probably as a result of the suppression of mRNA (130,138). The use of macrolides such as erythromycin or azithromycin has been beneficial in chronic respiratory tract infections caused by *P. aeruginosa* (268–271).

Erythromycin. Erythromycin is a metabolic product of *Streptomyces erythreus* and consists of a 14-member lactone ring to which are attached two deoxy-sugars, desosamine and cladinose. The macrocyclic lactone ring is the source of the class name, *macrolide*. Erythromycin, like most macrolides, appears to act by binding in the ribosomal tunnel through which the nascent peptide moves and thus can be considered a peptidyltransferase inhibitor (130). Against some rapidly replicating bacteria, erythromycin exhibits in vitro bactericidal activity, but overall, it is considered to be bacteriostatic in clinical use.

Clarithromycin. Clarithromycin, like erythromycin, has a 14-member lactone ring structure that has been altered by the addition of a methoxy group at C6 of the lactone ring (133,361,362).

This substitution primarily results in better oral absorption, with little effect on the spectrum of activity. In fact, erythromycin, clarithromycin, and azithromycin appear to bind to the same receptor on the bacterial 50S ribosome subunit. Clarithromycin, like the other macrolides, has species-specific bactericidal activity (239), as defined by in vitro methods of assessment where a greater than or equal to 3 $\log_{10}$ decrease in colony-forming units over a 24-hour period is defined as bactericidal (62). The species usually considered to be killed by macrolides are *S. pneumoniae*, *S. pyogenes*, and *H. influenzae*. However, the bactericidal activity of clarithromycin against susceptible strains of *S. pneumoniae*, as demonstrated in vitro by time-kill kinetic curves, has been found to lack correlation with results from the rabbit model for pneumococcal meningitis (239). The use of an in vitro method to measure total microbial killing has been suggested as a way to better assess the bactericidal activity of antimicrobial agents used in bacterial meningitis (228).

Azithromycin. Azithromycin is derived from erythromycin and differs in having a methyl-substituted nitrogen in its 15-membered lactone ring (362,365). This class of drugs receives its name, *azolides*, from the presence of the nitrogen group. Azithromycin has the same mechanism of action as erythromycin, and these two drugs bind so close to each other on the ribosome that they are considered competitive inhibitors. Azithromycin, like erythromycin and other macrolides, is a bacteriostatic agent. Azithromycin, however, has a major advantage, namely, its absorption and prolonged intracellular/interstitial fluid levels. In particular, the intracellular levels should greatly enhance the therapy of infections caused by intracellular pathogens.

Dirithromycin. Dirithromycin is a semisynthetic derivative of erythromycin that is converted during absorption and distribution to an active metabolite 9-(*S*)-erythromyclamine, which is the predominant agent found in plasma and extravascular tissues (366,367). This macrolide demonstrates high and prolonged tissue concentrations, allowing once-daily dosing. The mechanism of action is identical to that of the other macrolides. The result is bacteriostatic activity against logarithmically growing microorganisms and may include bactericidal activity against bacteria in a static growth phase. Dirithromycin, like azithromycin, does not inhibit cytochrome P450 enzymes and thus does not cause clinically important drug–drug interactions, although its gastrointestinal side effects are similar to those of other macrolides (362,368). Macrolides appear to be able to suppress the initiation of mRNA synthesis (180) and thereby inhibit the production of biofilm (135,138), exoenzymes (131,132), and other such virulence factors by a diverse group of pathogens, including *P. aeruginosa* (131,269). If this proves to be clinically effective in chronic infections, a once-daily dosing that achieves high and prolonged tissue concentrations and has no significant drug–drug interactions will be extremely useful.

Telithromycin. Telithromycin is a ketolide (371) in which the C11/C12 carbamate residue includes a butyl chain linking an imidazole ring and a pyridine ring (358–360). The most important factors in terms of the structure and activity of telithromycin are the lack of the neutral sugar cladinose in position C3 as well as a C11/C12 carbamate group, which together markedly increase the affinity of telithromycin for its microbial target, the 23S ribosomal drug-binding pocket (352,353,369). Telithromycin interacts with the 23S rRNA portion of the 50S subunit in the upper portion of the peptide exit channel close to the peptidyl transferase center and prevents the peptide chain from passing through the peptide exit channel (352,353,369). The increased affinity of telithromycin for the 23S rRNA is seen even in macrolide-resistant strains (370) and also results in concentration-dependent bactericidal activity and a prolonged post–antimicrobial effect against important respiratory tract pathogens. The microbiologic spectrum of activity for telithromycin includes *S. pneumoniae*, *S. pyogenes*, *H. influenzae*, *Moraxella catarrhalis*, *Legionella* species, *Mycoplasma pneumoniae*, and *Chlamydia pneumoniae*, which suggest that telithromycin will play an important clinical role in the empirical treatment of community-acquired respiratory tract infections (371). The pharmacokinetic profile of telithromycin demonstrates that this drug can be administered once daily without regard for meals and requires no dose reduction in elderly patients or those having hepatic impairment (372). Telithromycin is well absorbed after oral administration, rapidly penetrates into respiratory tissues and fluids, and is highly concentrated within white blood cells. Integration of pharmacokinetic and pharmacodynamic properties reveals that telithromycin has a high AUC:MIC ratio compared with macrolide antimicrobial agents, which results in enhanced efficacy. Resistance, although rare to date, can occur (356). Finally, telithromycin is well tolerated and has a low propensity for drug interactions.

Clindamycin. Clindamycin is a member of the lincosamides, which are chemically unrelated to the macrolides (354). Lincosamides consist of an amino acid linked to an amino sugar. Clindamycin is a 7-deoxy-7-chloro derivative of lincomycin, the first member of the lincosamide class. These two agents, like the macrolides, act on the peptidyltransferase center of the 50S subunit of bacterial ribosomes (134). Clindamycin may exhibit in vitro bactericidal activity against susceptible microorganisms such as *S. aureus* and *B. fragilis*, but its in vivo activity is considered bacteriostatic. The reason for this species-specific bactericidal activity is unknown but may reflect differences in the apoptotic mechanisms of these microorganisms.

Streptogramins. The streptogramin group of antibiotics includes the mikamycins, the pristinamycins, the oestreomycins, and the virginiamycins. These compounds are classified into two main groups: polyunsaturated cyclic peptidolides and cyclic hexadepsipeptides. Both groups possess a wide variety of chemical functions. Quinupristin/dalfopristin (Synercid) is a semisynthetic antibiotic consisting of two water-soluble streptogramin components: pristinamycin IA, a peptidic macrolactone, and pristinamycin IIA, a polyunsaturated macrolactone (373–375). These two macrolactones are modified to be water-soluble and together demonstrate synergistic and concentration-independent lethal activity against gram-positive pathogens, including *S. aureus*, in contrast to the individual components, which are only inhibitory (376). This bactericidal effect is seen clinically as well, as evidenced by the successful treatment of bacterial endocarditis. It is thought that this activity is related to irreversible binding to ribosomes (377). The 70S ribosomal subunit appears to be the target, with binding, closing, or narrowing the extrusion channel. This combination also demonstrates a postantibiotic effect (378). Moreover, each component diffuses throughout cardiac vegetations and is more concentrated in these vegetations than in cardiac tissue. The peptide macrolactone is distributed homogeneously throughout each vegetation, while

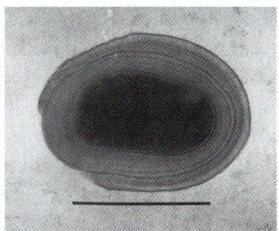

Figure 10.4 ■ *S. aureus* exposed to pristinamycin I and II in combination. Six layers of the cell wall are shown (original magnification ×100,000). (Reproduced with permission from Lorian V. Modes of action of antibiotics and bacterial structure: bacterial mass versus their numbers. In: Zak O, Sande MA, eds. *Handbook of animal models of infection.* London, United Kingdom: Academic Press, 1999;105–116.)

the polyunsaturated macrolactone reaches the core, with a gradient of decreasing concentrations from the periphery.

Exposure of *S. aureus* to quinupristin/dalfopristin results in two major cell alterations: an increase in cell size and an increase in the thickness of the cell wall. Some cells exhibit multilayered cell walls with as many as six layers (92) (Fig. 10.4), which is considerably thicker than the two- or three-layer cell wall that has been seen with exposure of *S. aureus* to chloramphenicol (94). This alteration is likely to be a stringent response.

Quinolones

The fluoroquinolones are synthetic antimicrobial agents that inhibit bacterial topoisomerases. Within several decades, these agents have proven their usefulness as a major class of broad-spectrum agents and have therapeutic potential yet to be realized (379). The first member of this group was nalidixic acid. The newer fluoroquinolones are all structurally similar to nalidixic acid and have a common skeleton, the four-quinolone planar heterocycle nucleus (380). Most also have a fluorine atom at position C6 of the structure (hence the name *fluoroquinolones*). Substitution on this skeleton is greatly aided by the vast knowledge accumulated regarding the structure–activity relationships, and the optimal groups for each position, in terms of size, shape, and electrical properties, have been well defined (380–384). Specific structural features that enhance the activity of fluoroquinolones are listed in Table 10.1.

These features can be used to predict the best configuration for a specific microorganism. For example, there are a number of new antibiotics that have demonstrated activity against *Mycobacterium* species (385). Among these are fluoroquinolones (386,387), despite the fact that *M. tuberculosis* does not possess homologs of the topoisomerase IV parC and parE genes (388). These fluoroquinolones can be evaluated by predicting their active structures (389). In addition, the most beneficial substituent of quinolones today holds not only for gram-positive and gram-negative bacteria but also for *Mycobacterium avium* (389); an N-substitution offers the greatest enhancement (390). This may be related to two factors: the amine groups may allow a greater concentration of the uncharged species to exist at neutral pH, and the N1-cyclopropylamine may also serve as a suicide inhibitor of redox enzymes, such as cytochrome P450 and methylamine dehydrogenase, which are present in bacteria. Alkylation of the N1-substituted moiety increased the activity of these agents against mycobacteria (390).

Table 10.1

Summary of Structure–Activity Relationships for Fluoroquinolone Antimicrobial Agents

Structure	Position	Activity
Halogen (F or Cl)	Position 6	Enhances overall effect
Pyrrolidine ring	Position 7	Enhances effect on gram-positive organisms
Piperazine ring	Position 7	Enhances effect on gram-positive organisms
Cyclopropyl ring	Position N1	Enhances overall effect
Amino group	Position 5	Enhances overall effect
Alkylation	Pyrrolidine or piperazine ring	Enhances effect on gram-positive organisms
Second halogen	Position 8	Enhances effect on anaerobic organisms

Fluoroquinolones interact with either or both of two topoisomerases, topoisomerase II and IV (115,117,325,391,392). Topoisomerase II (DNA gyrase) tends to be the primary target in gram-negative microorganisms; topoisomerase IV tends to be the primary target for gram-positive microorganisms. DNA gyrase is a vital bacterial enzyme that catalyzes the introduction of negative superhelical twists in circular DNA. Negative superhelical twists in circular DNA are needed for the following reasons. In order for DNA replication or transcription to take place, the two strands of double-helical DNA must first be separated. Separation, however, results in excessive positive supercoiling of the DNA in front of the point of separation. The bacterial enzyme DNA gyrase prevents this positive supercoiling by introducing negative supercoils into DNA. Gyrase consists of two functional subunits, the A subunit and the B subunit. The first catalyzes the step involving the passage of a segment of DNA through a double-stranded DNA break held open by the enzyme and then reseals the break. The second is responsible for adenosine triphosphate (ATP) hydrolysis, which is required for catalytic supercoiling by gyrase. Topoisomerase IV decatenates DNA and removes positive and negative supercoils: as in the case of topoisomerase II, there are two subunits involved. Quinolones rapidly bind to the topoisomerase-DNA complexes, and the resultant quinolone-topoisomerase-DNA complex is known as a cleaved complex (235). The cleaved complex essentially traps the topoisomerase and the single-stranded DNA and results in DNA double-stand breakage, resulting in chromosome fragmentation. The formation of these cleaved complexes also results in a variety of other quinolone-mediated phenomena. Binding of quinolones to GyrA (ParC helix-4 region) of DNA gyrase, which is located near the DNA gate region, results in rapid inhibition of nucleic acid biosynthesis. In contrast, binding of quinolones to GyrB (ParE) of topoisomerase IV results in a slower inhibition of nucleic acid biosynthesis. The inhibition of nucleic acid biosynthesis correlates with the bacteriostatic drug susceptibility (i.e., the MIC) but does not correlate with rapid cell death (235). Inhibition of nucleic acid biosynthesis combined with the double-stranded DNA breaks, in turn, induces the SOS response. Induction of the SOS response leads to production of a chromosomally encoded toxin, MazF, which alters protein carbonylation resulting in oxidative stress (393). Oxidative stress may then lead to an oxidative damage cellular death pathway resulting in rapid cell death (44,45,125). This oxidative damage cellular death pathway involves generation of highly destructive hydroxyl radicals through the Fenton reaction (44,45,394). Finally, induction of the SOS response also leads to filamentation of the bacteria although the role of filamentation in cell death, if any, is yet unclear (235).

In summary, fluoroquinolones are bactericidal agents that exhibit concentration-dependent killing with little postantibiotic effect at concentrations ranging from those equal to the MIC (1 times the MIC) up to approximately 10- to 20-fold higher (10 to 20 times the MIC). At higher concentrations (greater than 10 to 20 times the MIC), the SOS response appears to be evoked (44,45,235,395). This can result in a secondary bactericidal effect that is accompanied by a longer postantibiotic effect and a decrease in the emergence of resistant clones (234,396). This secondary bactericidal effect also may involve a signal to the apoptotic mechanism of the microbial cell, ultimately leading to rapid apoptosis (44,45,235). Cell death, therefore, may be relatively slow and related to a protein synthesis–dependent process or may be rapid and related to a protein synthesis–independent process.

DNA gyrase is the target of an increasing number of antibiotic classes. One of these classes consists of the synthetic quinolones, which act by interfering with the DNA-rejoining step involving the A subunit, while another class consists of the natural aminocoumarin-type compounds, which compete with ATP for binding to the B subunit of the enzyme. A related class, consisting of the 2-pyridones, is discussed later in "Antimicrobial Classes with Potential for Future Use."

Aminocoumarins

Aminocoumarin-type antimicrobial agents are characterized by their 3-amino-4,7-dihydroxycoumarin moiety and are produced by different strains of *Streptomyces* (397). Aminocoumarins include structurally similar agents, novobiocin, clorobiocin, and coumermycin as well more structurally complex agents, simocyclinone and rubradirin. Novobiocin, clorobiocin, and coumermycin share common structural features, which include the 3-amino-4,7-dihydroxycoumarin moiety as well as an L-noviosyl sugar and an aromatic acyl component attached to the amino group of the aminocoumarin moiety. Novobiocin and clorobiocin differ structurally only by substitution at two positions: CH3 versus Cl at position 8′ of the aminocoumarin ring and carbamoyl versus 5-methyl-pyrrol-2-carbonyl at the 3″-OH of novoise. Novobiocin, clorobiocin, and coumermycin interact with bacterial DNA gyrase with both the aminocoumarin moiety and the substituted deoxysugar moieties binding to the B subunit of DNA gyrase (398). The carbamoyl group of novobiocin and the 5-methyl-pyrrol-2-carbonyl group of clorobiocin are important for the binding of these agents to the GryB subunit. Moreover, the binding site of the aminocoumarin-type antimicrobial agents overlaps with the binding site of ATP; therefore, these agents competitively inhibit the ATP-dependent supercoiling of DNA. Topoisomerase IV is an additional target for clorobiocin but not novobiocin. Finally, the more structurally complex aminocoumarins simocyclinone and rubradirin do not have deoxysugar moieties at the 7-OH group of the aminocoumarin structure and thus do not bind with the GryB subunit of DNA gyrase. However, simocyclinone has been shown to bind to the N-terminal domain of the GryA subunit and thus also inhibits DNA gyrase (399,400). Although rubradirin does not inhibit DNA gyrase, it is structurally similar to the ansamycin/rifamycin family of antibiotics and is a potent inhibitor of RNA polymerase (401).

Novobiocin

Novobiocin is a glycosylated dihydroxycoumarin derivative of a natural aminocoumarin-type antibiotic produced by *Streptomyces niveus*. Novobiocin is the only member of the aminocoumarin-type agents that has been used clinically. Novobiocin acts on the B subunit of DNA gyrase and interferes with ATP hydrolysis (402). Novobiocin exhibits bactericidal activity in vitro and in vivo. Perhaps the greatest benefit would come from combining this agent with other DNA gyrase inhibitors (115) in order to decrease the selection of resistant mutants. However, other agents in the aminocoumarin family may be more useful in this regard.

Sulfonamides

The sulfonamides were the first effective chemotherapeutic agents to be used for the systemic therapy of bacterial infections in humans. Domagk (403) recognized this potential with Prontosil, which has sulfanilamide as its active metabolite, and later received the Nobel Prize in Medicine for this discovery. *Sulfonamide* is the generic name for

derivatives of *p*-aminobenzenesulfonamide. Sulfonamides inhibit the folate pathway in prokaryotic and primitive eukaryotic cells. These agents owe their activity to their being structural analogs and competitive antagonists of *p*-aminobenzoic acid (PABA); this antagonism is in part due to the attachment of the sulfa molecule directly to the benzene ring. Sulfa drugs exactly fit into the PABA-binding pocket, with the negatively charged oxygen atoms of the sulfonyl group and their common phenyl groups engaging the same hydrophobic site in the PABA-binding pocket (404). The result is competitive inhibition of dihydropteroate synthase, the bacterial enzyme that catalyzes the incorporation of PABA into dihydropteroic acid, the immediate precursor of folic acid (404–406). The in vitro and in vivo effects of this inhibition are bacteriostatic.

Trimethoprim

Trimethoprim chemically is 2,4-diaminopyrimidine and was specifically synthesized as a competitive inhibitor of dihydrofolate reductase (407,408). Trimethoprim selectively inhibits bacterial dihydrofolate reductase and does not interfere with mammalian dihydrofolate reductase due to the fact that trimethoprim does not fit into the nucleotide-binding site of the mammalian enzyme (409). This antibiotic inhibits folic acid synthesis, acting on the enzyme step that immediately follows that blocked by sulfonamides. The folic acid pathway is a small portion of a more complex pathway known as the aromatic biosynthetic pathway. The aromatic biosynthetic pathway is absent in mammals; the dietary requirements of mammals for phenylalanine, tryptophan, folic acid, and vitamin K reflect this absence. Bacteria, on the other hand, rely on this pathway, which makes it an attractive target for antimicrobial agents. Trimethoprim, like the sulfonamides, is bacteriostatic when used alone. The combination of these two inhibitors of folic acid synthesis, however, acts synergistically and produces a bactericidal effect (410–413).

Chloramphenicol

Chloramphenicol, also called Chloromycetin, is a broad-spectrum antibiotic produced by a variety of *Streptomyces* species, including *Streptomyces venezuelae* (414,415). This antimicrobial agent is unique among natural compounds in that it contains a nitrobenzene moiety that is connected to propanol as well as an amino group binding a derivative of dichloroacetic acid (414,416).

These latter moieties, propanol and dichloroacetic acid, must be intact for antimicrobial activity to occur, although substitution of the dichloroacetamide side chain is possible. A common mechanism of resistance is the acetylation of one or both hydroxyl groups on the propanediol moiety. These hydroxyl groups, however, cannot be substituted to prevent this type of resistance. The chloramphenicol molecule is one of the simplest antibiotic structures and was quickly and easily synthesized (414,417), becoming the first antibiotic whose chemical synthesis was feasible for large-scale commercial production.

Chloramphenicol is a small, uncharged, nonpolar molecule and readily diffuses through the cell wall/membrane. Although early work suggested that chloramphenicol is actively taken up by *E. coli*, later studies showed that there is actually an endogenous active efflux that depends on the proton motive force (418).

Chloramphenicol inhibits the peptidyltransferase reaction in bacterial protein synthesis by reversibly binding to a site in domain V of the 23S rRNA peptidyltransferase center of the 50S subunit of the 70S ribosome (417,419). This attachment prevents the attachment of the amino acid–containing end of the aminoacyl–tRNA complex to the ribosome, thereby inhibiting the formation of a peptide bond and causing translational inaccuracy (420). The site of action is near that of the macrolide antibiotics, clindamycin, and linezolid. Chloramphenicol thus may inhibit these agents competitively. This inhibition of protein synthesis in most susceptible microorganisms results in a bacteriostatic effect, although certain microbial pathogens, such as *H. influenzae*, *S. pneumoniae*, and *Neisseria meningitidis*, are readily killed in vivo by clinically achievable concentrations (421). This bactericidal activity may be due to the triggering of apoptotic mechanisms in these pathogens.

Chloramphenicol has other inhibitory effects in bacterial cells that are not related to inhibition of protein synthesis. Perhaps the most important effect is that on the bacterial translocase reaction in certain microorganisms. Chloramphenicol strongly inhibits the synthesis of teichoic acid in *Bacillus licheniformis* by inhibiting the function of undecaprenol-P (422).

Chloramphenicol is among the few agents that retain antimicrobial activity against bacteria in the stringent response phase (233). It therefore has potential for being combined with other agents that have similar effects, such as metronidazole and the

macrolides. Susceptibility testing methods, however, must reflect the nonreplicating growth phase when evaluating these combinations.

Ansamycins/Rifamycins

The rifamycins are a group of structurally similar macrocyclic antimicrobial agents produced by *Amycolatopsis mediterranei* (423,424). These agents belong to the family of ansamycin antibiotics, which are produced by various actinomycetes (423). The name ansamycin stems from the basket-like molecular architecture comprising an aromatic group bridged at nonadjacent positions by an aliphatic chain (423,424). The aromatic group for the rifamycins is a naphthalene ring system; thus, the basic structure of rifamycins is a naphthalene ring spanned by a long aliphatic loop. The target of rifamycins is bacterial RNA polymerase, which is a multi-subunit enzyme responsible for bacterial transcription (119–121,425–428). RNA polymerases are nucleotidyl transferase enzymes that are able to generate an RNA copy of a DNA or RNA template chain and thus control initiation and termination of transcription. RNA polymerases are found in nature in all eukaryotes, prokaryotes, and archaea as well as in many viruses; prokaryotic RNA polymerases differ from eukaryotic enzymes. Bacterial RNA polymerase is composed of four polypeptide subunits: α required for assembly of the enzyme, β involved in chain initiation and elongation, β' binds to the DNA template, and Ω constrains the β' subunit and aids its assembly into RNA polymerase. In the bacterial RNA polymerase, the large β and β' subunits form the pincers of a crab-claw molecule; a large channel between the pincers holds the following components: the RNA 3'-OH within the active site, an 8-9-base-pair RNA-DNA hybrid at the growing end of the transcript, at least 10 base pairs of duplex DNA downstream of the hybrid and approximately six nucleotides of single-stranded RNA upstream of the hybrid (119).

Rifampin

Rifampin is a semisynthetic derivative with modifications at the 4-position on the naphthalene ring of one of the natural rifamycins, rifamycin B. Other semisynthetic derivatives have been developed (429). Rifampin, like other rifamycins, acts by binding to the β subunit of the RNA polymerase and sterically blocks the extension of the nascent RNA chain after the first or second condensation step (119,425–428). The final result is inhibition of protein synthesis by prevention of chain initiation. Rifampin is a bactericidal agent in vivo as well as in vitro, but because of the high rate of resistant mutants, this antibiotic is always used in combination with another agent when treating serious infections.

Tetracyclines

The tetracyclines are broad-spectrum antibiotics discovered in the late 1940s following the isolation of chlortetracycline from *Streptomyces aureofaciens* (430–433). These agents were the first broad-spectrum antibiotics to be widely used in the therapy of bacterial infections in humans and are still in clinical use today (430,433).

Tetracycline antibiotics consist of a hydronaphthacene nucleus with four fused rings. Substitutions on this fused ring structure at carbons 4, 5, and 6 have resulted in semisynthetic agents; two of these are doxycycline and minocycline. These semisynthetic compounds are more lipophilic than their precursors and hence are more active.

At physiologic pH, many tetracyclines can exist in a mixture of two forms, a nonionized lipophilic form and a zwitterionic hydrophilic form (431). The lipophilic form assists passage through the cell membrane, while the hydrophilic form assists diffusion through the biofilm and the cytoplasm. Passage of tetracycline itself through gram-negative outer membranes involves the porins, with a preference for OmpF. OmpF porins are cation-selective, and tetracycline may pass through these channels as a cationic chelate of magnesium. The uptake of tetracycline across the cell membrane has been shown to involve an energy-dependent process that is now thought to be the result of a pH gradient. After tetracyclines enter bacteria via diffusion through the cell wall/membrane, these agents remain as a magnesium chelate or are complexed as such within the cytoplasm. These tetracycline/magnesium-chelated complexes, once inside the cytoplasm, appear to be membrane-impermeable.

Tetracycline derivatives can be classified into two categories based on their mechanism of action. The first category is known as the traditional tetracyclines and includes tetracycline, chlortetracycline, minocycline, and doxycycline (430–432). These traditional tetracyclines target the 16S ribosomal particle of the 30S ribosomal subunit (434) and inhibit protein synthesis at this ribosomal level due to disruption of codon–anticodon interactions between tRNA and mRNA in which

binding of aminoacyl–tRNA to the ribosomal acceptor site is prevented (118,431,432). This interaction appears to be reversible and is thought to account for the bacteriostatic nature of these agents.

The second category of tetracyclines is termed the atypical tetracyclines (435,436). In the atypical tetracyclines, substituents are introduced at carbon 9 without alteration of the basic structure of the classical tetracyclines, with the result that the primary target is not the ribosome but the cytoplasmic membrane (436). Examples of the atypical tetracyclines include chelocardin, anhydrotetracycline, and anhydrochlortetracycline; to date, none of the atypical tetracyclines are in clinical use (430,433,436). These modifications also allow the molecule to avoid recognition by a tetracycline efflux protein [TetA(B)]. The atypical lipophilic tetracyclines may exist primarily in the nonionized lipophilic form, which allows them to remain in the cell membranes. The interaction of these tetracycline analogs with the cell membrane is lethal, resulting in cellular lysis (435,436). This lethal effect may involve interruption of membrane-associated proton motive forces and energy metabolism (44,45,107).

Glycylcyclines

Glycylcyclines are a new class of semisynthetic tetracyclines (437–441) that contain the *N, N*-dimethylglycylamido substituent at the 9-position of minocycline and 6-demethyl-6-deoxytetracycline (437–444). The presence of this substituent overcomes the two major mechanisms responsible for tetracycline resistance in a wide variety of bacterial pathogens: active efflux of the drug out of the cell and protection of the ribosomes by the production of cytoplasmic proteins (432,437,439,445). Glycylcyclines have a higher binding affinity for ribosomes than earlier tetracyclines, which is thought to explain why cytoplasmic ribosomal protection proteins are unable to confer resistance to glycylcyclines (445). This accordingly extends the spectrum of these new agents to include multiresistant strains, including *Neisseria gonorrhoeae*, and in addition significantly improves their activity (at least fourfold), compared with the activity of minocycline and tetracycline (442,446).

Nitroimidazoles and Nitrofurans

Nitroimidazoles and nitrofurans are synthetic antimicrobial agents that are grouped together because both are nitro group ($-NO_2$)–containing ringed structures having similar antimicrobial effects (447). These antimicrobial effects require degradation of the agent within the microbial cell so that electrophilic radicals are formed. These reactive electrophilic intermediates then damage nucleophilic sites, including ribosomes, DNA, and RNA. The effect in vitro and in vivo against susceptible microorganisms is bactericidal.

Nitroimidazoles. The nitroimidazoles are organic nitroaromatic derivatives that are activated within the cytoplasm of microorganisms by electrons in order to exert their antimicrobial effect. The key to the antimicrobial activity of this class of drugs is the nitro group, which acts as a preferential electron acceptor (447,448). Electrons are needed to reduce the nitro group ($-NO_2$) to an amine or amino group ($-NH_2$). The reduction, however, does not proceed along the classical reduction pathway seen with nitrobenzene or its derivatives, such as chloramphenicol. Instead, the reduction leads to nitro radical anions, which undergo rapid decomposition to a nitrite ion and an imidazole radical. These short-lived electrophilic reduction products of the nitroimidazoles are produced within the microbial cell by enzymatic pathways utilized in anaerobic metabolism. Anaerobes depend on the ferredoxin-linked pyruvate oxidoreductase system as a major route of ATP generation. These pyruvate oxidoreductase pathways utilize ferredoxin, or similar electron transfer proteins, as electron acceptors from the oxidation of an enzyme-thiamine-pyrophosphate complex. The reduced ferredoxin normally transfers electrons to hydrogenase, but in the presence of nitroimidazoles, those electrons are transferred to the latter. Electrons from hydrogenase can also be transferred to nitroimidazoles. This transfer initiates the decomposition of the nitroimidazoles to radical electrophilic products. These products, most likely nitrite radicals, then react with nucleophilic protein sites and, among other effects, oxidize DNA, causing strand breaks and subsequent cell death.

Nitrofurans. Nitrofuran compounds consist of a primary nitro group ($-NO_2$) joined to a heterocycle ring; this group of nitroheterocyclic compounds includes various 5- and 2-nitroimidazoles and 5-nitrofurans (449). Susceptible microorganisms have been shown to possess reductases that reduce nitrofurans to reactive electrophilic metabolites, and an inverse correlation exists between reductase levels and MICs (450,451). These electrophilic metabolites produce a qualitatively nonspecific attack on nucleophilic sites, including ribosomal proteins and mRNA.

Metronidazole. Metronidazole is a nitroheterocyclic compound belonging to the nitroimidazole group of antimicrobial agents, and it was the first of this group of drugs to show useful clinical activity (448). This antibiotic has two metabolic derivatives, a hydroxy metabolite with significant antimicrobial activity and an acid metabolite with relatively little activity (452). The activity of metronidazole, like other members of the nitroimidazole group, is related to the production of nitrite radicals (450–454). Metronidazole is rapidly bactericidal, and its high killing rate of anaerobic bacteria is not affected by nutrients or growth rates.

Nitrofurantoin. Members of the nitrofuran class include nitrofurantoin and furazolidone, the latter being available only in Europe. Nitrofurantoin is metabolized by bacterial reductases, resulting in electrophilic radicals that nonspecifically attack nucleophilic sites and inhibit protein synthesis. In addition, nitrofurantoin appears to have another important mechanism of action. Nitrofurantoin has been found to increase the levels of Gp4, an enzyme implicated in the induction of the stringent response (451). At the same time, nitrofurans, including nitrofurantoin, have specific interactions with ribosome sites such as S18 in the platform region of the 30S subunit, which disrupts codon–anticodon interactions and thereby prevents mRNA translation (361,451). Therefore, it is possible that nitrofurantoin acts to induce Gp4 while preventing translation of the Gp4-stimulated mRNAs for inducible enzymes (361,451). This would effectively prevent bacterial entry into the stringent response and thus impair viability. In agreement with this possible mechanism is the fact that nitrofurantoin resistance has been shown to confer a reduction in fitness in *E. coli* in the absence of the antimicrobial agent (455).

Glycopeptides

Glycopeptide antimicrobial agents currently include vancomycin and teicoplanin (456–458). Vancomycin was originally isolated from the fermentation broths of *Amycolatopsis orientalis* (459), while teicoplanin was obtained from *Actinoplanes teichomyceticus* (460). Both agents possess a heptapeptide backbone but differ in substituents.

Both glycopeptides achieve their antimicrobial activity by binding to the terminal amino acyl-D-alanyl-D-alanine, which prevents the transfer of cell wall components from the lipid carrier to cell wall growth points (456,461). Therefore, they share similar antimicrobial spectra and potencies, which are essentially confined to gram-positive bacteria (462). Their activities are, however, not identical. There are several explanations for this fact. The two agents differentially bind to other peptide components of preformed peptidoglycan, which has no direct effect but reduces the available drug. In addition, structure–activity relationships for these two glycopeptide agents (vancomycin and teicoplanin) suggest dimerization of these antibiotics as a potentially important factor in their activity. Such dimerization has been shown to enhance the binding affinities of most glycopeptides for the peptidyl-D-alanyl-D-alanine sequence present in the growing cell wall, the notable exception being teicoplanin (463). Teicoplanin is unique among the glycopeptides in that it demonstrates no measurable propensity for dimerization (464). A dimerized agent has enhanced activity because the second binding event is essentially intramolecular, whereas the activity of an agent with a lipid anchor requires two steps for the same effect. Although perhaps subtle, this difference may account for some of the difference in the activities of these two agents against certain species of enterococci. The fatty acid chain that teicoplanin carries may diminish this difference by acting as a membrane anchor, thus increasing the affinity of the antimicrobial agent for the growing cell wall.

Vancomycin. Vancomycin is a narrow-spectrum antimicrobial agent that is mainly active against gram-positive cocci (465). It is a large, complex, tricyclic antibiotic with a molecular mass of 1,449 Da. Within the chlorine face of this large molecule, there is a pocket into which the D-alanyl-D-alanine precursor of the cell wall peptidoglycan is complexed, preventing polymerization of undecaprenyl pyrophosphoryl-*N*-acetylmuramyl-pentapeptide (UDP-MurNAc-pentapeptide) and *N*-acetylglucosamine into peptidoglycan (466). The in vitro and in vivo results of this inhibition of peptidoglycan synthesis, like that caused by a β-lactam agent, are bactericidal. However, it is important to appreciate that this bactericidal effect of vancomycin (and teicoplanin) is much slower than that of the β-lactam agents (467,468). Vancomycin, therefore, should be substituted for antistaphylococcal penicillins such as nafcillin only when absolutely

necessary, as in cases of penicillin allergy or methicillin resistance (465).

Teicoplanin. Teicoplanin differs chemically from vancomycin in a number of ways (469). First, teicoplanin has different carbohydrate substituents: D-glycosamine and D-mannose versus D-glucose and vancosamine in vancomycin. Next, teicoplanin has two dihydroxyphenylglycines rather than aspartic acid and *N*-methylleucine. Finally, teicoplanin is unique among the glycopeptides in having an acyl substituent, which is a fatty acid. This fatty acid makes teicoplanin much more lipophilic than vancomycin, accounting for its greater tissue and cellular penetration. This same property accounts for its activity against *M. tuberculosis*. The actual mechanism of action is identical to that of vancomycin, although the activity of these two agents is not always identical. Like vancomycin, teicoplanin is slowly bactericidal, in comparison with antistaphylococcal penicillins.

Lipoglycopeptides. Lipoglycopeptides are semisynthetic derivatives to the glycopeptides (vancomycin and teicoplanin) that contain the heptapeptide core that is common to all glycopeptides (470,471). This heptapeptide core allows members of the lipoglycopeptide family to inhibit transglycosylation by binding to D-alanyl-D-alanine stem termini in gram-positive bacteria in a manner identical to the glycopeptides. Lipoglycopeptides also possess hydrophobic and lipophilic substituents that help anchor the drug as well as target the bacterial cell membrane (107), resulting in membrane depolarization. It is the lipophilic side chains that distinguish these agents from glycopeptides such as vancomycin and also has resulted in these agents being categorized as lipoglycopeptides. The lipophilic side chains also prolong the half-life of these agents and help to anchor the drugs to the cell membrane. This dual mechanism of action results in more rapid bactericidal activity as well as activity against dormant bacteria (472). Members of the lipoglycopeptides include telavancin (approved for clinical use), oritavancin, and dalbavancin.

Telavancin and Oritavancin. Telavancin and oritavancin are members of the lipoglycopeptide class of antimicrobial agents; telavancin is in clinical use, whereas oritavancin is under development. Telavancin contains the heptapeptide core of vancomycin but possesses a hydrophobic (decylaminoethyl) side chain appended to the vancosamine sugar and a hydrophilic (phosphonomethyl aminomethyl) group on the 4 position of amino acid 7 (473). Oritavancin also contains the heptapeptide core of vancomycin but possesses a hydrophobic (N-r-[4-chlorophenyl]benzyl) group on the disaccharide sugar, the addition of a 4-epi-vancosamine monosaccharide to the amino acid residue in ring 6, and the replacement of the vancosamine moiety by 4-epi-vancosamine (474). These substitutions allow both agents to target both cell wall synthesis and cell membrane function. There are, however, some differences in the antimicrobial activity of these two lipoglycopeptides (472). Telavancin exhibits concentration-dependent bactericidal activity with the AUC/MIC being the pharmacodynamic parameter that best describes its activity. Oritavancin appears to exhibit concentration-dependent bactericidal activity in vitro and both concentration- and time-dependent bactericidal activity in vivo. Like telavancin, the AUC/MIC is the pharmacodynamic parameter that best describes the activity of oritavancin. Secondary binding of oritavancin to the pentaglycyl (Asp/Asn) bridging segment also occurs and contributes to oritavancin's activity against vancomycin-resistant organisms. Telavancin is active against vancomycin-intermediate *Staphylococcus aureus* (VISA) but has poor activity against vancomycin-resistant *Staphylococcus aureus* (VRSA). Oritavancin is active against both VISA and VRSA. Both telavancin and oritavancin are active against VanB vancomycin-resistant enterococci; enterococci exhibiting the VanA phenotype are resistant to telavancin while oritavancin retains activity. Of note is that these structural differences also result in differences in the pharmacokinetics of these two agents. Telavancin has a half-life of approximately 8 hours and requires daily dosing, whereas oritavancin has a half-life of almost 400 hours, which may allow for one dose per treatment course.

Phosphonomycin

Fosfomycin is a phosphoenolpyruvate analog that irreversibly inhibits phosphoenolpyruvate transferase. This agent is a unique antimicrobial agent unrelated to any other recognized class and is the only member, to date, of the phosphonomycin class (475). Fosfomycin is a broad-spectrum antibiotic produced by some strains of *Streptomyces* and by *Pseudomonas syringae*. The structure of fosfomycin is characterized by an epoxide ring and a carbon–phosphorus bond. This agent has an extremely low molecular mass of 138 Da and has been found to be nonreactive with negatively charged glycocalyx such as that produced by *P. aeruginosa*. Fosfomycin enters bacterial cells by active transport through the L-glycerophosphate and the hexose-6-phosphate uptake systems. Within the cell, fosfomycin blocks peptidoglycan synthesis through inhibition of the bacterial enzyme N-acetylglucosamine-3-O-enolpyruvyl transferase, which prevents the formation of N-acetylmuramic acid, an essential element of the peptidoglycan cell wall (203). The in vitro and in vivo results of this inhibition of polypeptide chain elongation are bactericidal in a time-dependent manner (475).

Fusidanes

Fusidanes are a family of naturally occurring tetracyclic triterpenoid antibiotics, of which fusidic acid is the only therapeutic representative. Fusidic acid is derived from the fungus *Fusidium coccineum*. This antibiotic exhibits a steroidlike structure but has no steroidlike activity due to the stereochemistry of the molecule. The mechanism of action for this antimicrobial agent appears to involve binding to elongation factor G, thus inhibiting polypeptide chain elongation (476). The in vitro and in vivo results of this inhibition of polypeptide chain elongation are slowly bactericidal (477). Fusidic acid is most active against *S. aureus*, including methicillin-resistant isolates (477,478). The MICs for methicillin-resistant isolates range from 0.03 to 1.0 g/mL. Fusidic acid was introduced into clinical practice in 1962, and despite more than three decades of limited use, the resistance rate is still low (479). However, *S. aureus* is able to develop resistance to fusidic acid when this agent is used alone; resistance is thought to be due to point mutations in the *fusA* gene (480). Fusidic acid is not available in the United States for general use, although efforts are being made to make this agent available (481,482).

Polymyxins and Colistin

The polymyxins are a group of polypeptide antibiotics that have molecular masses of approximately 1,000 Da and are isolated from different strains of *Bacillus* (483). These antimicrobial agents are characterized by a heptapeptide ring, a high content of diaminobutyric acid, and a side chain ending in fatty acid residues. Only polymyxin B and colistin (polymyxin E) are currently used clinically; colistin has found increasing use due to multidrug-resistant gram-negative bacterial infections (261,484). All of the polymyxins are cationic detergents that disrupt biofilm and interact with the phospholipids of the bacterial cell membrane resulting in altered bacterial cell membrane permeability, leakage of intracellular contents, and bacterial cell death. Colistin (polymyxin E) is a polymyxin B nonapeptide derivative that lacks the fatty acid tail. Polymyxin B covalently attached to agarose inhibits the respiration and growth of gram-negative bacteria but not gram-positive bacteria. Also, spheroplasts of *E. coli* are seen after exposure to immobilized polymyxin B (167,344,345,483). This is interpreted as indicating the activity is directed at the outer cell membrane. The effects of immobilized polymyxin B are identical to the effects of EDTA (129). The target, like that of EDTA, may involve biofilm via displacement of magnesium and calcium ions. This effect can be reversed by an excess of these divalent cations (166,175).

Cyclic Lipopeptides

Cyclic lipopeptides are a new class of potent antimicrobial agents with remarkable structural diversity (485). These agents are natural products produced by a variety of soil bacteria. Cyclic lipopeptides have nonribosomally synthesized peptide cores consisting of 11 to 13 amino acids that form a rigid 10-membered ring with an *N*-terminal fatty acid; this terminal fatty acid facilitates insertion into the lipid bilayer of bacterial membranes. Targeting the bacterial membrane of dormant bacteria is a relatively new approach to treating persistent infections (107). Structural diversity is a result of these agents containing multiple nonproteinogenic amino acids as well as different lipid tails. Among the members of this new class of antimicrobial agents are daptomycin, amphomycin, asparocin, friulimicin, glycinocin, laspartomycin, parvuline, and tsushimycin. Of these, only daptomycin is in clinical use (486).

Daptomycin

Daptomycin is a semisynthetic cyclic lipopeptide antibiotic that is the first of this class to enter clinical use (486,487). The A21978C lipopeptide complex to which daptomycin belongs is produced through the action of nonribosomal peptide synthetases in *Streptomyces roseosporus* (488). Daptomycin appears to dissipate membrane potential (487,489). The evidence for this is the activity of daptomycin on L forms of *Staphylococcus aureus*, which results in the leakage of intracellular potassium. In addition, scanning electron microscopy has shown gross morphologic alterations in the cytoplasmic membrane (490) that are consistent with disruption of the cell wall/membrane (166,167,174,345). Several reports have noted that daptomycin is capable of calcium-dependent interactions with bilayer membranes (191,192). Specifically, daptomycin in the presence of calcium ions oligomerizes to form a micelle-like amphipathic structure with the hydrophobic decanoyl side chain facing inward, which creates a pseudo–positively charged surface with increased affinity for the negatively charged microbial cell membrane (493). Daptomycin also has been shown to cause reorganization of the microbial cell membrane architecture and thus cause mislocalization of essential cell division proteins (494). These observations (493,494) suggest that daptomycin directly inserts into the bacterial cell membrane. Daptomycin demonstrates bactericidal action against both stationary-phase and nondividing *Staphylococcus aureus* cells, suggesting that it has a direct effect on the bacterial cell membrane (236). Daptomycin thus may exert its rapid bactericidal effect (468) by dissipating the transmembrane electrochemical potential of the cell membrane. This rapid killing may be due to activation of apoptotic mechanisms that are triggered following disruption of the bacterial cell membrane potential (44,45). A similar phenomenon of dissipation of membrane potential has been described for gentamicin and *Staphylococcus aureus* (209).

Oxazolidinones

Oxazolidinones are a new class of synthetic bacterial protein synthesis inhibitors (495,496). These agents are multicyclic compounds, some with fused rings, which represent a new series of antimicrobial agents unrelated by chemical structure to any other currently available antibiotics. Like the fluoroquinolones, another class of multicyclic compounds with fused rings, oxazolidinones are synthetic agents that offer many substitution sites for chemical modifications, as dictated by structure–activity relationships. Also, like the fluoroquinolones, some oxazolidinones have D- and L-isomers, only the latter of which is active against microorganisms (497). Salient structural features of representative agents in this class include tricyclic fused rings, which exhibit potent activity against MRSA and *S. epidermidis*; an appended thiomorpholine moiety, which confers potent in vitro activity against *M. tuberculosis*; fluorine substitution on the generic aromatic ring, which enhances activity against gram-positive cocci; and the addition of a piperazine ring, which also increases potency against gram-positive cocci (497,498). The spectrum of activity of oxazolidinones includes a diverse group of microorganisms such as *Enterococcus* spp, *M. tuberculosis*, and *Bacteroides* spp (495,498,499).

The mechanism of action is inhibition of protein synthesis because oxazolidinones inhibit ribosomal protein synthesis in a cell-free system (498,500). Like many antimicrobial agents that inhibit protein synthesis, oxazolidinones are bacteriostatic. However, their inhibition of protein synthesis is somewhat novel in that the oxazolidinones do not inhibit the peptide elongation step (498). Instead, the initial step of protein synthesis is inhibited, which in turn leads to codon–anticodon interactions where translation of mRNA for inducible enzymes is inhibited. In this respect, oxazolidinones are similar in action to lincosamides (134,354). This effect over time may result in cell death; both oxazolidinones and lincosamides are slowly bactericidal to certain microorganisms.

Resistance to oxazolidinones can occur by a single-step selection process, but this occurs at a frequency of less than 1 in 10^9. Resistance, when seen, is not associated with cross-resistance to other classes of antimicrobial agents.

Finally, oxazolidinones can be administered by both intravenous and oral routes. Peak levels in humans given 1 g orally reach 6 to 7 µg/mL, while the half-lives range from 2.4 to 12 hours (496). Oxazolidinones are metabolized by free radicals as well as excreted in the urine, with 40% to 60% of the drug intact.

Linezolid. Linezolid is the first member of the oxazolidinones in clinical use and is indicated in the therapy of nosocomial pneumonia and uncomplicated and complicated skin infections caused by select gram-positive bacteria (495,501,502). Linezolid is also active against *M. tuberculosis* (503), including multidrug-resistant strains (504) and has been used successfully for treatment of chronic, extensively drug-resistant TB (505). Linezolid is a morpholinyl analogue of the piperazinyl oxazolidinone and has a fluorine substitution at the phenyl

3-position (501). Although early studies suggested that linezolid inhibited protein synthesis (498), a more detailed explanation of this mechanism of action has only recently been described (506,507). The results of these studies suggest that linezolid binds in the A-site pocket at the peptidyltransferase center of the 50S ribosomal subunit. This A-site pocket is located within domain V of the 23S rRNA peptidyltransferase center near the interface with the 30S ribosomal subunit. Binding of linezolid to this A-site pocket thus interferes with the correct positioning of the aminoacyl–tRNA on the ribosome and blocks the initial step of protein synthesis. Lincosamides also inhibit the initiation of peptide chain formation (134,354), whereas the effect of the other macrolides is to prevent the extension of the growing peptide chain. It may be that blocking the initial step of protein synthesis accounts for the slowly bactericidal activity of both lincosamides such as clindamycin and linezolid.

Diarylquinolines

Diarylquinolines are a new class of antimicrobial agents that differ structurally and mechanistically from fluoroquinolones and other quinolone classes (508).

Antimicrobial Classes with Potential for Future Use

Diarylquinolines

Diarylquinolines are a new class of antimicrobial agents that differ structurally and mechanistically from fluoroquinolones and other quinolone classes (508). Although this class has a nitrogen-containing heterocycle nucleus that resembles the quinolone nucleus, it differs mainly in the specificity of the novel functionalized lateral 3' chains. Whereas fluoroquinolones target topoisomerases, diarylquinolines target microbial ATP synthase (508–511). Targeting respiratory ATP synthase, a component of the microbial energy metabolic pathway (107), is unique and interferes with the dormant phase of microbial pathogens as well as with the replicating phase (511). Diarylquinolines initially were developed for therapy against *M. tuberculosis* due to their activity against dormant strains (193,512). The first member of the diarylquinoline class, bedaquiline, has been successfully used for TB in clinical trials (25,513) and has been approved for use in the United States. Although bedaquiline does not have activity against bacteria other than mycobacteria, chemical derivatives with a core structure similar to bedaquiline have been developed and tested against gram-positive pathogens such as *Streptococcus pneumoniae* and *Staphylococcus aureus* with promising results (508).

2-Pyridones

The 2-pyridones are a new class of broad-spectrum antimicrobial agents that inhibit bacterial DNA gyrase (116,514,515). These compounds are similar to fluoroquinolones but differ by placement of the nitrogen atom in the ring juncture. Because the basic ring structure of the molecule is different from that of the quinolones or naphthyridines, 2-pyridones appear to bind differently at the DNA gyrase site. Accordingly, these agents have been found to be active against fluoroquinolone-resistant bacteria (116,516). The 2-pyridones exhibit in vitro bactericidal activity. Like fluoroquinolones, these agents are water-soluble and thus have excellent bioavailability when taken orally. Hundreds of 2-pyridones have been synthesized and evaluated in vitro and in vivo, with selected agents now moving toward human clinical trials (116,515). Moreover, triazoles have been introduced in position 8 and 2 of ring-fused bicyclic 2-pyridones (517). Several of these triazole functionalized ring-fused 2-pyridones are being evaluated for in vitro antibacterial properties.

Lantibiotics

Lantibiotics are a diverse group of ribosomally synthesized antimicrobial peptides produced by gram-positive bacteria (518). These small (19 to 38 amino acids) peptides are complex polycyclic molecules that contain the thioether amino acids lanthionine and/or 3-methyllanthionine (518–521). Moreover, such ribosomally synthesized polycyclic molecules are produced by macrocyclization, which is a common method used in nature to constrain the conformational flexibility of natural peptides of both ribosomal and nonribosomal origin (522,523). There are at least three genetic pathways to lanthionine-containing peptides, and these are widespread in nature (523). Lantibiotics are produced by a wide range of gram-positive bacteria, including a variety of lactic acid bacteria (518,524,525). Lantibiotics are primarily active against gram-positive bacteria (519,526) via a number of diverse mechanisms (518,527,528). Some of these peptides—class 1 lantibiotics such as nisin, subtilin, and Pep5—are positively charged, amphiphilic molecules that exert their primary bactericidal action on the cell membrane by causing pores (518,519,521,527). Nisin has a unique pore-

forming activity in that it uses the cell wall precursor lipid II as a docking molecule (524). Nisin also appears to have a dual mechanism of action due to binding to the cell wall precursor lipid II as this binding also inhibits cell wall biosynthesis (528). Class 2 lantibiotics such as cinnamycin and the related duramycins possess globular shapes and no net charge or a negative charge. These globular lantibiotics appear to inhibit phospholipases by binding phosphoethanolamine (518,520,521,527). Class 2 lantibiotics also include mersacidin; this lantibiotic does not form pores in plasma membranes but instead inhibits peptidoglycan synthesis, probably on the level of transglycosylation by complexing lipid II (518,520,521,527,529,530). Some class 2 lantibiotics appear to be bacteriostatic, whereas others appear to be bacteriocidal; this may be related to whether the lantibiotic possesses a dual mechanism of action or not. A third class of lantibiotics has been proposed (518); these lantionine-containing peptides lack significant antibiotic activity but instead have other functions for the producing cell. These lantibiotics include SapB, AmfS, and SapT (518).

Cationic Peptides

Cationic peptides, also called defensins, are short (20 to 50 amino acids) amphiphilic polycationic peptides that function as an important mechanism of innate immunity in plants and animals (531,532). These antimicrobial peptides are produced by phagocytic cells and lymphocytes as well as by the epithelial cell lining of the gastrointestinal and genitourinary tracts, the tracheobronchial tree, and keratinocytes (533). There are more than 800 sequences of antimicrobial peptides from the plant and animal kingdoms (534). Examples of these agents include cecropins (535), melittin (536), magainins (537), and epidermin (538). Defensins such as human α-defensin are known to have antimicrobial activity (532,539). In addition to direct antimicrobial activity, these "host-defense peptides" have important immune modulatory functions that include recruitment and activation of immune cells, neutralization of lipopolysaccharides, and enhancement of bacterial clearance (533,540,541). Some antimicrobial peptides are multifunctional and can enhance both cellular (Th1-dependent) and humoral (Th2-dependent) cytokine production and immune responses (533). The main targets of these antimicrobial cationic peptides are the bacterial cell membranes, with cell death resulting from interference of membrane-bound processes as well as from increased permeability. The antimicrobial activity of cationic peptides is due to physiochemical properties related to their amphiphilic nature, which allows these peptides to adopt conformations in which polar and positively charged amino acids orient to one side, whereas apolar structures orient to the other side. This arrangement enables these peptides to bind to negatively charged membrane surfaces and then integrate into the cytoplasmic membrane (532). Damage to the cytoplasmic membrane and/or pore formation may result in increased permeability (539,542). In addition, membrane-bound processes such as electron transport may be disrupted. Another effect of these cationic

peptides, like that of aminoglycosides, may be the disruption of the biofilm caused by these agents displacing Mg^{2+} and Ca^{2+}. Evidence for this is found in the fact that a number of these antimicrobial peptides have been noted to be active as insoluble complexes (343). This suggests that surface activity on the targeted microorganism is sufficient for lethal activity. Moreover, the interaction of antimicrobial peptides with biofilm is well served by the amphiphilic nature of these agents, which allows both amphipathic and hydrophobic portions and facilitates the passage of the molecule from the aqueous phase to the biofilm phase, where it displaces magnesium and calcium cations.

REFERENCES

1. Drusano GL. Antimicrobial pharmacodynamics: critical interactions of 'bug and drug.' *Rev Nat Microbiol* 2004;2:289–300.
2. Craig WA, Ebert SC. Killing and regrowth of bacteria *in vitro*: a review. *Scand J Infect Dis Suppl* 1991;74:63–70.
3. Davies J, Davies D. Origins and evolution of antibiotic resistance. *Microbiol Mol Biol Rev* 2010;74:417–433.
4. Paterson DL. "Collateral damage" from cephalosporin or quinolone antibiotic therapy. *Clin Infect Dis* 2004;38 (Suppl 4):S341–S345.
5. Stratton CW. Dead bugs don't mutate: susceptibility issues in the emergence of bacterial resistance. *Emerging Infect Dis* 2003;9:10–16.
6. Mouton JW, Dudley MN, Cars O, et al. Standardization of pharmacokinetic/pharmacodynamics (PK/PD) terminology for anti-infective drugs. *Int J Antimicrob Agents* 2002;19:355–358.
7. Craig WA, Leggett K, Totsuka K, et al. Key pharmacokinetic parameters of antibiotic efficacy in experimental animal infections. *J Drug Dev* 1988;1:7–15.
8. Ebert SC, Craig WA. Pharmacodynamic properties of antibiotics: application to drug monitoring and dosage regimen design. *Infect Control Hosp Epidemiol* 1990;11:319–326.
9. Stass H, Dalhoff A. The integrated use of pharmacokinetic and pharmacodynamic models for the definition of breakpoints. *Infection* 2005;33(Suppl 2):S29–S35.
10. Drusano GL. Pharmacokinetics and pharmacodynamics of antimicrobials. *Clin Infect Dis* 2007;45(Suppl 1): S89–S95.
11. MacGowan A. Revisiting beta-lactams—PK/PD improves dosing of old antibiotics. *Curr Opin Pharmacol* 2011;11:470–476.
12. Mouton JW, Ambrose PG, Canton R, et al. Conserving antibiotics for the future: new ways to use old and new drugs from a pharmacokinetic and pharmacodynamics perspective. *Drug Resist Updat* 2011;14:107–117.
13. Drusano GL, Lodise TP. Saving lives with optimal antimicrobial therapy. *Clin Infect Dis* 2013;56:245–247.
14. Stratton CW. In vitro susceptibility testing versus *in vivo* effectiveness. *Med Clin North Am* 2006;90:1077–1088.
15. Tenover FC. Development and spread of bacterial resistance to antimicrobial agents: an overview. *Clin Infect Dis* 2001;33(Suppl 3):S108–S115.
16. Canton R, Morosini MI. Emergence and spread of antibiotic resistance following exposure to antibiotics. *FEMS Microbiol Rev* 2011;35:977–991.
17. Russell AD, Chopra I. *Understanding antimicrobial action and resistance*. 2nd ed. New York: Ellis Horwood, 1996.
18. Drlica K. Antibiotic resistance: can we beat the bugs? *Drug Discov Today* 2001;6:714–715.
19. Poole K. Overcoming antimicrobial resistance by targeting resistance mechanisms. *J Pharm Pharmacol* 2001;53: 283–294.
20. Le T, Bayer AS. Combination antibiotic therapy for infective endocarditis. *Clin Infect Dis* 2003;36:615–621.
21. Yeh P, Tschumi AI, Kishony R. Functional classification of drugs by properties of their pairwise interactions. *Nat Genet* 2006;38:489–494.
22. Lim TP, Ledesma KR, Chang KT, et al. Quantitative assessment of combination antimicrobial therapy against multidrug-resistant *Acinetobacter baumannii*. *Antimicrob Agents Chemother* 2008;52:2898–2904.
23. Yuan Z, Ledesma KR, Singh R, et al. Quantitative assessment of combination antimicrobial therapy against multidrug-resistant bacteria in a murine pneumonia model. *J Infect Dis* 2010;201:889–897.
24. Filippini P, Iona E, Piccaro G, et al. Activity of drug combinations against dormant *Mycobacterium tuberculosis*. *Antimicrob Agents Chemother* 2010;54:2712–2715.
25. Diacon AH, Dawson R, von Groote-Bidlingmaier, et al. 14-day bactericidal activity of PA-824, bedaquiline, pyrazinamide, and moxifloxacin combinations: a randomized trial. *Lancet* 2012;380:986–993.
26. Weis SE, Slocum PC, Blais FX, et al. The effects of directly observed therapy of the rates of drug resistance and relapse in tuberculosis. *N Engl J Med* 1994;330:1247–1251.
27. Hobby GL, Dawson MH. Effect of growth rate of bacteria on action of penicillin. *Proc Soc Exp Biol* 1944;56:181–184.
28. Tuomanen E. Phenotypic tolerance: the search for beta-lactam antibiotics that kill nongrowing bacteria. *Rev Infect Dis* 1986;8(Suppl 3):S279–S291.

29. Lorian V. In vitro simulation of in vivo conditions: physical state of the culture medium. *J Clin Microbiol* 1989; 27:2403–2406.

30. Gilbert P, Collier PJ, Brown MRW. Influence of growth rate on susceptibility to antimicrobial agents: biofilms, cell cycle, dormancy and stringent response. *Antimicrob Agents Chemother* 1990;34:1865–1868.

31. Stevens DL, Sizhuang Y, Bryant AE. Penicillin-binding protein expression at different growth stages determines penicillin efficacy in vitro and in vivo: an explanation for the inoculum effect. *J Infect Dis* 1993;167:1401–1405.

32. Scheffers DJ, Pinho MG. Bacterial cell wall synthesis: new insights from localization studies. *Microbiol Mol Biol Rev* 2005;69:585–607.

33. Vollmer W. Peptidoglycan structure and architecture. *FEMS Microbiol Rev* 2008;32:149–167.

34. Mattei P-J, Neves D, Dessen A. Bridging cell wall biosynthesis and bacterial morphogenesis. *Curr Opin Struct Biol* 2010;20:749–755.

35. Silhavy TJ, Kahne D, Walker S. The bacterial cell envelope. *Cold Spring Harb Perspect Biol* 2010;2:a000414.

36. Vollmer W. The prokaryotic cytoskeleton: a putative target for inhibitors and antibiotics? *Appl Microbiol Bench Technol* 2006;73:37–47.

37. Schneider T, Sahl HG. An oldie but a goodie—cell wall biosynthesis as antibiotic target pathway. *Int J Med Microbiol* 2010;300:161–169.

38. Shockman GD, Daneo-Moore L, Higgins ML. Problems of cell wall and membrane growth, enlargement, and division. *Ann NY Acad Sci* 1974;235:161–197.

39. Shockman GD, Holtje J-V. Microbial peptidoglycan (murein) hydrolases. In: Ghuysen JM, Hakenbeck R, eds. *Bacterial cell wall*. Amsterdam: Elsevier, 1994:131–166.

40. Vollmer W, Joris B, Charlier P, et al. Bacterial peptidoglycan (murein) hydrolases. *FEMS Microbiol Rev* 2008;32:259–286.

41. Hochman A. Programmed cell death in prokaryotes. *Crit Rev Microbiol* 1997;23:207–214.

42. Lewis K. Programmed cell death in bacteria. *Microbiol Mol Biol Rev* 2000;64:503–514.

43. Kitano K, Tomasz A. Triggering of autolytic cell wall degradation in *Escherichia coli* by beta-lactam antibiotics. *Antimicrob Agents Chemother* 1979;16:838–848.

44. Kohanski MA, Dwyer DJ, Hayete B, et al. A common mechanism of cellular death induced by bactericidal antibiotics. *Cell* 2007;130:797–810.

45. Kohanski MA, Dwyer DJ, Collins JJ. How antibiotics kill bacteria: from targets to networks. *Nat Rev Microbiol* 2010;8:423–435.

46. Roszak DB, Colwell RR. Survival strategies of bacteria in the natural environment. *Microb Rev* 1987;51:365–379.

47. Kolter R. Life and death in stationary phase. *ASM News* 1992;58:75–79.

48. Lewis K. Persister cells. *Annu Rev Microbiol* 2010;64:357–372.

49. Stewart PS, Costerton JW. Antibiotic resistance of bacteria in biofilms. *Lancet* 2001;358:135–138.

50. Antunes LC, Ferreira RB, Buckner MM, et al. Quorum sensing in bacterial virulence. *Microbiology* 2010;156:227–282.

51. Bayles KW. The biological role of death and lysis in biofilm development. *Nat Rev Microbiol* 2007;5:721–726.

52. Lopez D, Vlamakis H, Kolter R. Biofilms. *Cold Spring Harb Perspect Biol* 2010;2:a000398.

53. Walker GC. Understanding the complexity of an organism's responses to DNA damage. *Cold Springs Harb Symp Quant Biol* 2000;65:1–10.

54. Foster PL. Stress response and genetic variation in bacteria. *Mutat Res* 2005;569:3–11.

55. Friedberg EC, Walker GC, Siede W, et al. *DNA repair and mutagenesis*. 2nd ed. Washington, DC: ASM Press, 2005.

56. Costerton JW, Lewandowski Z, Caldwell DE, et al. Microbial biofilms. *Annu Rev Microbiol* 1995;49:711–745.

57. Donlan RM, Costerton JW. Biofilms: survival mechanisms of clinically relevant microorganisms. *Clin Microbiol Rev* 2002;15:167–193.

58. Dunne WM Jr. Bacterial adhesion: seen and good biofilm lately? *Clin Microbiol Rev* 2002;15:155–166.

59. Brown MRW, Williams P. Influence of substrate limitation and growth phase on sensitivity to antimicrobial agents. *J Antimicrob Chemother* 1985;15(Suppl A):S7–S14.

60. Brown MRW, Allison DG, Gilbert P. Resistance of bacterial biofilms to antibiotic: a growth-rate related effect? *J Antimicrob Chemother* 1988;22:777–783.

61. Brown RW, Collier PJ, Gilbert P. Influence of growth rate on susceptibility to antimicrobial agents: modification of the cell envelope and batch and continuous culture studies. *Antimicrob Agents Chemother* 1990;34:1623–1628.

62. Stratton CW. Bactericidal testing. *Med Clin North Am* 1993;7:445–459.

63. Lynch AS, Robertson GT. Bacterial and fungal biofilm infections. *Ann Rev Med* 2008;59:415–428.

64. Costerton JW, Stewart PS, Greenberg EP. Bacterial biofilms: a common cause of persistent infections. *Science* 1999;284:1318–1322.

65. Mulcahy LR, Burns JL, Lory S, et al. Emergence of *Pseudomonas aeruginosa* strains producing high levels of persister cells in patients with cystic fibrosis. *J Bacteriol* 2010;192:6191–6196.

66. Nystrom T. Stationary-phase physiology. *Annu Rev Microbiol* 2004;58:161–181.

67. Colwell RR. Viable but nonculturable bacteria: a survival strategy. *J Infect Chemother* 2000;6:121–125.

68. Mendelman PM, Chaffin DO. Two penicillin-binding proteins of *Haemophilus influenzae* are lost after cells enter stationary phase. *FEMS Microbiol Lett* 1985;30:399–402.

69. Benaissa M, Babin P, Quellard N, et al. Changes in *Helicobacter pylori* ultrastructure and antigens during conversion from the bacillary to the coccoid form. *Infect Immun* 1996;64:2331–2335.

70. Singh VK, Jayaswal RK, Wilkinson BJ. Cell wall–active antibiotic-induced proteins of *Staphylococcus aureus* identified using a proteomic approach. *FEMS Microbiol Lett* 2001;199:79–84.

71. Shaw KJ, Miller N, Liu X, et al. Comparison of the changes in global gene expression of *Escherichia coli* induced by four bactericidal agents. *J Mol Microbiol Biotechnol* 2003;5:105–122.

72. Dorr T, Vulic M, Lewis K. Ciprofloxacin causes persister formation by inducing the TisB toxin in *Escherichia coli*. *PLoS Biol* 2010;8:e1000317.

73. Robertson JA, Trulear MG, Characklis WG. Cellular reproduction and extracellular polymer formation by *Pseudomonas aeruginosa* in continuous culture. *Biotechnol Bioeng* 1984;26:1409–1417.

74. Davies DG, Chakrabarty AM, Geesey GG. Exopolysaccharide production in biofilms: substratum activation of alginate gene expression by *Pseudomonas aeruginosa*. *Appl Environ Microbiol* 1993;59:1181–1186.

75. Stewart PS. Biofilm accumulation model that predicts antibiotic resistance of *Pseudomonas aeruginosa* biofilms. *Antimicrob Agents Chemother* 1994;38:1052–1058.

76. Drenkard E, Ausubel FM. *Pseudomonas* biofilm formation and antibiotic resistance are linked to phenotypic variation. *Nature* 2002;416:740–743.

77. Ahnwar H, Strap JL, Costerton JW. Dynamic interactions of biofilms of mucoid *Pseudomonas aeruginosa* with tobramycin and piperacillin. *Antimicrob Agents Chemother* 1992;36:1208–1214.

78. Tran TD, Kwon HY, Kim EH, et al. Decrease in penicillin susceptibility due to heat shock protein ClpL in *Streptococcus pneumoniae*. *Antimicrob Agents Chemother* 2011;55:2714–2728.

79. Henge-Aronis R. Survival of hunger and stress: the role of *rpoS* in early stationary phase gene regulation in *E. coli*. *Cell* 1993;72:165–168.

80. Dougherty T, Pucci MJ. Penicillin-binding proteins are regulated by *rpoS* during transitions in growth states of *Escherichia coli*. *Antimicrob Agents Chemother* 1994;38:205–210.

81. Denome SA, Elf PK, Henderson TA, et al. *Escherichia coli* mutants lacking all possible combinations of eight penicillin binding proteins: viability, characteristics, and implications for peptidoglycan synthesis. *J Bacteriol* 1999;181:3981–3993.

82. Vollmer W, Bertsche U. Murein (peptidoglycan) structure, architecture and biosynthesis in *Escherichia coli*. *Biochim Biophys Acta* 2008;1778:1714–1734.

83. Moyer CL, Morita RY. Effect of growth rate and starvation-survival on the viability and stability of a psychrophilic marine bacterium. *Appl Environ Microbiol* 1989;55:1122–1127.

84. Matin A. The molecular basis of carbon-starvation-induced general resistance in *Escherichia coli*. *Mol Microbiol* 1991;5:3–10.

85. Ward JB. Teichoic and teichuronic acids: biosynthesis, assembly, and location. *Microbiol Rev* 1981;45:211–243.

86. Wrangstadh M, Conway PL, Kjelleberg S. The role of an extracellular polysaccharide produced by the marine *Pseudomonas* sp. S9 in cellular detachment during starvation. *Can J Microbiol* 1989;35:309–312.

87. Chatterji D, Ojha AK. Revisiting the stringent response, ppGpp and starvation signaling. *Curr Opin Microbiol* 2001;4:160–165.

88. Magnusson LU, Farewell A, Nystrom T. ppGpp: a global regulator in *Escherichia coli*. *Trend Microbiol* 2005;13:236–242.

89. Primm TP, Anderson SJ, Mizrahi V, et al. The stringent response of *Mycobacterium tuberculosis* is required for long-term survival. *J Bacteriol* 2000;182:4889–4898.

90. Costerton JW, Lam K, Chan R. The role of the microcolony in the pathogenesis of *Pseudomonas aeruginosa*. *Rev Infect Dis* 1983;5(Suppl):S867–S873.

91. Lorian V. Some effects of subinhibitory concentrations of penicillin on the structure and division of staphylococci. *Antimicrob Agents Chemother* 1975;7:864–870.

92. Lorian V, Atkinson B. Effects of subinhibitory concentrations of antibiotics on cross walls of cocci. *Antimicrob Agents Chemother* 1976;9:1043–1055.

93. Lorian V, Atkinson B, Lim Y. Effect of rifampin and oxacillin on the ultrastructure and growth of staphylococci. *Rev Infect Dis* 1983;5(Suppl):S419–S427.

94. Gemmell CG, Lorian V. Effects of low concentrations of antibiotics on bacterial ultrastructure, virulence, and susceptibility of immunodefenses: clinical significance. In: Lorian V, ed. *Antibiotics in laboratory medicine*. 4th ed. Baltimore: Williams & Wilkins, 1996:397–452.

95. Giesbrecht P, Kersten T, Maidhof H, et al. Staphylococcal cell wall: morphogenesis and fatal variations in the presence of penicillin. *Microbiol Mol Biol Rev* 1998;62:1371–1414.

96. Novak R, Charpentier E, Braun JS, et al. Signal transduction by a death signal peptide: uncovering the mechanism of bacterial killing by penicillin. *Mol Cell* 2000;5:49–57.

97. Brunskill EW, Bayles KW. Identification and molecular characterization of a putative regulatory locus that affects autolysis in *Staphylococcus aureus*. *J Bacteriol* 1996;178:611–618.

98. Henze U, Sidow T, Wecke J, et al. Influence of *femB* on methicillin resistance and peptidoglycan metabolism in *Staphylococcus aureus*. *J Bacteriol* 1993;175:1612–1620.

99. Catrenich C, Makin K. Characterization of the morphological conversion of *Helicobacter pylori* from bacillary to coccoid form. *Scand J Gastroenterol* 1991;26(Suppl 181):S58–S64.

100. Berry V, Jennings K, Woodnutt G. Bactericidal and morphological effects of amoxicillin on *Helicobacter pylori*. *Antimicrob Agents Chemother* 1995;39:1859–1861.

101. Cellini L, Allocati N, Angelucci D, et al. Coccoid *Helicobacter pylori* not culturable in vitro reverts in mice. *Microbiol Immunol* 1994;38:843–850.

102. Summanen F, Wexler HM, Lee K, et al. Morphological response of *Bilophia wadsworthia* to imipenem: correlation with properties of penicillin-binding proteins. *Antimicrob Agents Chemother* 1993;37:2638–2644.

103. Elliot TS, Greenwood D. The morphological response of *Pseudomonas aeruginosa* to aztreonam, cefoperazone, ceftazidime, and formimidoyl thienamycin. *J Med Microbiol* 1984;17:159–169.

104. Koch C, Hiby N. Pathogenesis of cystic fibrosis. *Lancet* 1993;341:1065–1069.

105. Lam JS, Chan R, Lam K, et al. The production of mucoid microcolonies by *Pseudomonas aeruginosa* within infected lungs in cystic fibrosis. *Infect Immun* 1980;28:546–556.

106. Sterstrom T-A, Conway P, Kjelleberg S. Inhibition by antibiotics of the bacterial response to long-term starvation of *Salmonella typhimurium* and the colon microbiota of mice. *J Appl Bacteriol* 1989;67:53–59.

107. Hurdle JG, O'Neill AJ, Chopra I, et al. Targeting bacterial membrane function: an underexploited mechanism for treating persistent infections. *Nat Rev Microbiol* 2011;9:62–75.

108. Hash JH, Davis MC. Electron microscopy of *Staphylococcus aureus* treated with tetracycline. *Science* 1962;138:8–28.

109. Lawlor MT, Sullivan MC, Levitz RE, et al. Treatment of prosthetic valve endocarditis due to methicillin-resistant *Staphylococcus aureus* with minocycline. *J Infect Dis* 1990;161:812–814.

110. Nicolau DP, Freeman CD, Nightingale CH, et al. Minocycline versus vancomycin for treatment of experimental endocarditis caused by oxacillin-resistant *Staphylococcus aureus*. *Antimicrob Agents Chemother* 1994;38:1515–1518.

111. Yuk JH, Dignani MC, Harris RL, et al. Minocycline as an alternate antistaphylococcal agent. *Rev Infect Dis* 1991;13:1023–1024.

112. David MZ, Daum RS. Community-associated methicillin-resistant *Staphylococcus aureus*: epidemiology and clinical consequences of an emerging epidemic. *Clin Microbiol Rev* 2010;23:616–687.

113. Moellering RC. MRSA: the first half century. *J Antimicrob Chemother* 2012;67:4–11.

114. Hugo WB, ed. *Inhibition and destruction of the bacterial cell*. New York: Academic Press, 1971.

115. Couturier M, el Bahassi M, Van Melderen L. Bacterial death by DNA gyrase poisoning. *Trends Microbiol* 1998;6:269–275.

116. Mitscher LA. Bacterial topoisomerase inhibitors: quinolones and pyridone antibacterial agents. *Chem Rev* 2005;105:559–592.

117. Kathiravan MK, Khilare MM, Nikoomanesh K, et al. Topoisomerase as target for antibacterial and anticancer drug discovery. *J Enzyme Inhib Med Chem* 2013;28:419–435.

118. Poehlsgaard J, Douthwaite S. The bacterial ribosome as a target for antibiotics. *Nat Rev Microbiol* 2005;3:870–881.

119. Artsimovitch I, Vassylyeva DG. Is it easy to stop RNA polymerase? *Cell Cycle* 2006;5:399–404.

120. Chopra I. Bacterial RNA polymerase: a promising target for the discovery of new antimicrobial agents. *Curr Opin Invest Drugs* 2007;8:600–607.

121. Mariani R, Maffioli SI. Bacterial RNA polymerase inhibitors: an organized overview of their structure, derivatives, biological activity and current clinical development status. *Curr Med Chem* 2009;16:430–454.

122. Bayles KW. Are the molecular strategies that control apoptosis conserved in bacteria? *Trends Microbiol* 2003;11:306–311.

123. Rice KC, Bayles KW. Death's toolbox: examining the molecular components of bacterial programmed cell death. *Mol Microbiol* 2003;50:729–738.

124. Bayles KW. The bacterial action of penicillin: new clues to an unsolved mystery. *Trends Microbiol* 2000;8:274–278.

125. Wang X, Zhao X, Malik M, et al. Contribution of reactive oxygen species to pathways of quinolone-mediated bacterial cell death. *J Antimicrob Chemother* 2010;65:520–524.

126. Dubee B, Chau F, Arthur M, et al. The in vitro contribution of autolysins to bacterial killing elicited by amoxicillin increases with inoculum size in *Enterococcus faecalis*. *Antimicrob Agents Chemother* 2011;55:910–912.

127. Moreillon P, Markiewicz Z, Machman S, et al. Two bactericidal targets for penicillin in pneumococci: autolysis-dependent and autolysis-independent killing mechanisms. *Antimicrob Agents Chemother* 1990;34:33–39.

128. Sintim HO, Smith JA, Wang J, et al. Paradigm shift in discovering next-generation anti-infective agents: targeting quorum sensing, c-di-GMP signaling and biofilm formation in bacteria with small molecules. *Future Med Chem* 2010;2:1005–1035.

129. Leive L. Studies on the permeability change produced in coliform bacteria by ethylenediaminetetraacetate. *J Biol Chem* 1968;243:2373–2380.

130. Haight TH, Finland M. Observations on mode of action of erythromycin. *Proc Soc Exp Biol Med* 1952;81:188–193.

131. Kita E, Sawaki M, Nishikawa F, et al. Suppression of virulence factors of *Pseudomonas aeruginosa* by erythromycin. *J Antimicrob Chemother* 1991;27:273–284.

132. Mizukane R, Hirakata Y, Kaku M, et al. Comparative *in vitro* exoenzyme-suppressing activities of azithromycin and other macrolide antibiotics against *Pseudomonas aeruginosa*. *Antimicrob Agents Chemother* 1994;38:528–533.

133. Neu HC. The development of macrolides: clarithromycin in perspective. *J Antimicrob Chemother* 1991;27 (Suppl A):S1–S9.

134. Reusser F. Effect of lincomycin and clindamycin on peptide chain initiation. *Antimicrob Agents Chemother* 1975;7:32–37.

135. Yasuda H, Ajiki Y, Koga T, et al. Interaction between biofilms formed by *Pseudomonas aeruginosa* and

136. Naica Y, Jansch L, Bredenbruch F, et al. Quorum-sensing antagonistic activities of azithromycin in *Pseudomonas aeruginosa* PAO1: a global approach. *Antimicrob Agents Chemother* 2006;50:1680–1688.

137. Hoffmann N, Lee B, Hentzer M, et al. Azithromycin blocks quorum sensing and alginate polymer formation and increases the sensitivity to serum and stationary-growth-phase killing of *Pseudomonas aeruginosa* and attenuates chronic *P. aeruginosa* lung infection in Cftr(-/-) mice. *Antimicrob Agents Chemother* 2007;51:3677–3687.

138. Perez-Martinez I, Haas D. Azithromycin inhibits expression of the GacA-dependent small RNAs RsmY and RsmZ in *Pseudomonas aeruginosa*. *Antimicrob Agents Chemother* 2011;55:3399–3405.

139. Little JW, Mount DW. The SOS regulatory system of *Escherichia coli*. *Cell* 1982;29:11–22.

140. Yeiser B, Pepper ED, Goodman MF, et al. SOS-induced DNA polymerases enhance long-term survival and evolutionary fitness. *Proc Natl Acad Sci U S A* 2002;99:8737–8741.

141. Corton JC, Ward JE Jr, Lutherhaus J. Analysis of cell division gene *ftsZ* (*sulB*) from gram-negative and gram-positive bacteria. *J Bacteriol* 1987;169:1–7.

142. Walthers RN, Piddock LJV, Wise R. The effect of mutations in the SOS response on the kinetics of quinolone killing. *J Antimicrob Chemother* 1989;24:863–873.

143. Rogers HJ, Perkins HR, Ward JB. *Microbial cell walls and membranes*. London: Chapman & Hall, 1980.

144. Shockmann GD, Barrett JF. Structure, function, and assembly of cell walls of gram-positive bacteria. *Ann Rev Microbiol* 1983;37:501–527.

145. Beveridge TJ. Structures of gram-negative cell walls and their derived membrane vesicles. *J Bacteriol* 1999;181:4725–4733.

146. Hancock REW. Bacterial outer membranes: evolving concepts. *ASM News* 1991;57:175–182.

147. Lugtenberg B, Van Alphen L. Molecular architecture and functioning of the outer membrane of *Escherichia coli* and other gram-negative bacteria. *Biochim Biophys Acta* 1983;737:51–115.

148. Booth IR. Regulation of cytoplasmic pH in bacteria. *Microb Rev* 1985;49:359–378.

149. Padan E, Schuldiner S. Intracellular pH regulation in bacterial cells. *Methods Enzymol* 1986;25:337–352.

150. Borges-Walmsley MI, Walmsley AR. The structure and function of drug pumps. *Trends Microbiol* 2001;9:71–79.

151. van Heijenoort J. Formation of the glycan chains in the synthesis of bacterial peptidoglycan. *Glycobiology* 2001;11:25–36.

152. Nanninga N. Morphogenesis of *Escherichia coli*. *Microbiol Mol Biol Rev* 1998;62:110–129.

153. Morath S, Von Aulock S, Hartung T. Structure/function relationships of lipoteichoic acids. *J Endotoxin Res* 2005;11:348–356.

154. Gan L, Chen S, Jensen GJ. Molecular organization of Gram-negative peptidoglycan. *Proc Natl Acad Sci U S A* 2008;105:18953–18957.

155. Leive L. The barrier function of the gram-negative envelope. *Ann NY Acad Sci* 1974;235:109–129.

156. Nikaido H. Prevention of drug access to bacterial targets: role of permeability barriers and active efflux. *Science* 1994;264:382–388.

157. Delcour AH. Outer membrane permeability and antibiotic resistance. *Biochim Biophys Acta* 2009;1794:808–816.

158. Erhmann M. *The periplasm*. Washington, DC: ASM Press, 2007.
159. De Duve C, Wattiaux R. Functions of lysosomes. *Annu Rev Physiol* 1966;28:435–492.
160. Schearer BG, Legakis NJ. *Pseudomonas aeruginosa*: evidence for the involvement of lipopolysaccharide in determining outer membrane permeability to carbenicillin and gentamicin. *J Infect Dis* 1985;152:351–355.
161. Magnusson K-E. Physiochemical properties of bacterial surfaces. *Biochem Soc Trans* 1989;17:454–458.
162. Giwercman B, Jensen ET, Hiby N, et al. Induction of beta-lactamase production in *Pseudomonas aeruginosa* biofilm. *Antimicrob Agents Chemother* 1991;35:1008–1010.
163. Vaara M. Polycations sensitize enteric bacteria to antibiotics. *Antimicrob Agents Chemother* 1983;24:107–113.
164. Stratton CW, Warner RR, Coudron PE, et al. Bismuth-mediated disruption of the glycocalyx-cell wall of *Helicobacter pylori*: ultrastructure evidence for a mechanism of action for bismuth salts. *J Antimicrob Chemother* 1999;43:659–666.
165. Toney JH. Biofilms—a neglected antibacterial target? *Curr Opin Investig Drugs* 2007;8:598–599.
166. Kaye JJ, Chapman GB. Cytological aspects of antimicrobial antibiosis. III. Cytologically distinguishable stages in antibiotic action of colistin sulfate on *Escherichia coli*. *J Bacteriol* 1963;86:536–543.
167. Schindler PRG, Teuber M. Action of polymyxin B on bacterial membranes: morphological changes in the cytoplasm and in the outer membrane of *Salmonella typhimurium* and *Escherichia coli* B. *Antimicrob Agents Chemother* 1975;8:95–104.
168. Yoshida T, Hiramatsu K. Potent bactericidal activity of polymyxin B against methicillin-resistant *Staphylococcus aureus* (MRSA). *Microbiol Immunol* 1993;31:853–859.
169. Tetsuaki T, Svarachorn A, Soga H, et al. Lysis and aberrant morphology of *Bacillus subtilis* cells caused by surfactants and their relation to autolysin activity. *Antimicrob Agents Chemother* 1990;34:781–785.
170. Rogers SW, Gilleland HE, Eagon RG. Characterization of a protein-lipopolysaccharide complex released from cell walls of *Pseudomonas aeruginosa* by ethylenediaminetetraacetic acid. *Can J Microbiol* 1964;15:743–748.
171. Dixon RA, Chopra I. Leakage of periplasmic proteins from *Escherichia coli* mediated by polymyxin B nonapeptide. *Antimicrob Agents Chemother* 1986;29:781–788.
172. Vaara M, Vaara T. Polycations as outer membrane-disorganizing agents. *Antimicrob Agents Chemother* 1983; 24:114–122.
173. Martin NL, Beveridge TJ. Gentamicin interaction with *Pseudomonas aeruginosa*. *Antimicrob Agents Chemother* 1986;29:1079–1087.
174. Kadurugamuwa JL, Clarke AJ, Beveridge TJ. Surface action of gentamicin on *Pseudomonas aeruginosa*. *J Bacteriol* 1993;175:5798–5805.
175. Newton BA. Reversal of the antimicrobial activity of polymyxin by divalent cations. *Nature* 1953;172: 160–161.
176. Nicas TI, Hancock REW. Alteration of susceptibility to EDTA, polymyxin B and gentamicin in *Pseudomonas aeruginosa* by divalent cation regulation of outer membrane protein H1. *J Gen Microbiol* 1983;129: 509–517.
177. Turakhia MH, Characklis WG. Activity of *Pseudomonas aeruginosa* in biofilms: effect of calcium. *Biotechnol Bioeng* 1989;33:406–414.
178. Hancock REW. Alterations in outer membrane permeability. *Annu Rev Microbiol* 1984;38:237–264.
179. Rubinstein G, Dunkin K, Howard AJ. The susceptibility of *Helicobacter pylori* to 12 antimicrobial agents, omeprazole and bismuth salts. *J Antimicrob Chemother* 1994;34:409–413.
180. Menninger JR. Functional consequences of binding macrolides to ribosomes. *J Antimicrob Chemother* 1985;16(Suppl A):S23–S24.
181. Pérez-Giraldo C, Rodriguez-Benito A, Morán FJ, et al. In-vitro slime production of *Staphylococcus epidermidis* in the presence of subinhibitory concentrations of ciprofloxacin, ofloxacin, and sparfloxacin. *J Antimicrob Chemother* 1994;33:845–848.
182. Held TK, Adamczik C, Trautmann M, et al. Effects of MICs and sub-MICs of antibiotics on production of capsular polysaccharide of *Klebsiella pneumoniae*. *Antimicrob Agents Chemother* 1995;39:1093–1096.
183. Domenico P, Hopkins T, Schoch PE, et al. Potentiation of aminoglycoside inhibition and reduction of capsular polysaccharide production in *Klebsiella pneumoniae* by sodium salicylate. *J Antimicrob Chemother* 1990;25:205–214.
184. Sawal T, Hirano S, Yamaguchi A. Repression of porin synthesis by salicylate in *Escherichia coli*, *Klebsiella pneumoniae* and *Serratia marcesans*. *FEMS Microbiol Lett* 1987;40:233–237.
185. Burns JL, Clark DK. Salicylate-inducible antibiotic resistance in *Pseudomonas cepacia* associated with absence of a pore-forming outer membrane protein. *Antimicrob Agents Chemother* 1992;36:2280–2285.
186. Sumita Y, Fukasawa M. Transient carbapenem resistance induced by salicylate in *Pseudomonas aeruginosa* associated with suppression of outer membrane protein D2 synthesis. *Antimicrob Agents Chemother* 1993;37:2743–2746.
187. Rosner JL. Nonheritable resistance to chloramphenicol and other antibiotics induced by salicylates and other chemotactic repellents in *Escherichia coli* K-12. *Proc Natl Acad Sci U S A* 1985;82:8771–8774.
188. Foulds J, Murray DM, Chai T, et al. Decreased penetration of cephalosporins through the outer membrane of *Escherichia coli* grown in salicylate. *Antimicrob Agents Chemother* 1989;33:412–417.
189. Barclay ML, Begg EJ, Chambers ST, et al. Improved efficacy with nonsimultaneous administration of first doses of gentamicin and ceftazidime *in vitro*. *Antimicrob Agents Chemother* 1995;39:132–136.
190. Guggenbichler JP, Allerberger F, Dierich MP, et al. Spaced administration of antibiotic combinations to eliminate *Pseudomonas* from sputum in cystic fibrosis. *Lancet* 1988;2:749–750.
191. Gilbert P, Maira-Litran T, McBain AJ, et al. The physiology and collective recalcitrance of microbial biofilm communities. *Adv Microb Physiol* 2002;46:202–256.
192. Rodriguez GG, Phipps D, Ishiguro K, et al. Use of a fluorescent redox probe for direct visualization of actively respiring bacteria. *Appl Environ Microbiol* 1992;58:1801–1808.
193. Islam MS, Richards JP, Ojha AK. Targeting drug tolerance in mycobacteria: a perspective from mycobacterial biofilms. *Expert Rev Anti Infect Ther* 2010;10: 1056–1066.
194. Stewart PS, Karel SF, Robertson CR. Characterization of immobilized cell growth rates using autoradiography. *Biotechnol Bioeng* 1991;37:824–833.

195. Tuomanen E, Cozens R, Tosch W, et al. The rate of killing of *Escherichia coli* by beta-lactam antibiotics is strictly proportional to growth rate. *J Gen Microbiol* 1986;132:1297–1304.

196. Evans DJ, Brown MRW, Allison DG, et al. Susceptibility of bacterial biofilms to tobramycin: role of specific growth rate and phase in division cycle. *J Antimicrob Chemother* 1990;25:585–591.

197. Gristina AG, Hobgood CD, Webb LX, et al. Adhesive colonization of biomaterials and antibiotic resistance. *Biomaterials* 1987;8:423–426.

198. Kumon H, Tomochika K, Matunaga T, et al. A sandwich cup method for the penetration assay of antimicrobials through *Pseudomonas* exopolysaccharides. *Microbiol Immunol* 1994;38:615–619.

199. Westrin BA, Axelsson A. Diffusion in gels containing immobilized cells: a critical review. *Biotechnol Bioeng* 1991;38:439–446.

200. Mandell GL. Uptake, transport, delivery, and intracellular activity of antimicrobial agents. *Pharmcotherapy* 2005;25(Suppl):S130–S133.

201. Braun V, Bos C, Braun M, et al. Outer membrane channels and active transporters for the uptake of antibiotics. *J Infect Dis* 2001;183(Suppl 1): S12–S16.

202. Hancock REW, Bellido F. Antibiotic uptake: unusual results for unusual molecules. *J Antimicrob Chemother* 1992;29:235–243.

203. Kahan FM, Kahan JS, Cassidy PJ, et al. The mechanism of action of fosfomycin. *Ann NY Acad Sci* 1974;235:364–385.

204. Ames GF. Bacterial periplasmic transport systems: structure, mechanism, and evolution. *Annu Rev Biochem* 1986;55:397–425.

205. Hancock RE, Bell A. Antibiotic uptake into gram-negative bacteria. *Eur J Clin Microbiol Infect Dis* 1988;7:713–720.

206. Ceccarelli M, Danelon C, Laio A, et al. Microscopic mechanism of antibiotics translocation through a porin. *Biophys J* 2004;87:58–64.

207. Ceccarelli M, Ruggerone P. Physical insights into permeation of and resistance to antibiotics in bacteria. *Curr Drug Targets* 2008;9:779–788.

208. James CE, Mahendran KR, Molior A, et al. How beta-lactam antibiotics enter bacteria: a dialogue with the porins. *PLoS One* 2009;4:e5453.

209. Mates SM, Eisenberg ES, Mandel LJ, et al. Membrane potential and gentamicin uptake in *Staphylococcus aureus. Proc Natl Acad Sci U S A* 1982;79:6693–6697.

210. Mansfield BE, Oltean HN, Oliver BG, et al. Azole drugs are imported by facilitated diffusion in *Candida albicans* and other pathogenic fungi. *PLoS Pathog* 2010;6:e1001126.

211. Peterson AA, Hancock REW, McGroaty EJ. Binding of polycationic antibiotics and polyamines to lipopolysaccharide of *Pseudomonas aeruginosa. J Bacteriol* 1985;164:1256–1261.

212. Kadurugamuwa JL, Lam JS, Beveridge TJ. Interaction of gentamicin with the A band and B band lipopolysaccharides of *Pseudomonas aeruginosa* and its possible lethal effect. *Antimicrob Agents Chemother* 1993;37: 715–721.

213. Hancock REW, Raffle VJ, Nicas TI. Involvement of the outer membrane in gentamicin and streptomycin uptake and killing in *Pseudomonas aeruginosa. Antimicrob Agents Chemother* 1981;19:777–785.

214. Iida K, Koike M. Cell wall alterations in gram-negative bacteria by aminoglycoside antibiotics. *Antimicrob Agents Chemother* 1974;5:95–97.

215. Farmer S, Li Z, Hancock REW. Influence of outer membrane mutations on susceptibility of *Escherichia coli* to the dibasic macrolide azithromycin. *J Antimicrob Chemother* 1992;29:27–33.

216. McLaughlin SGA, Dilger JP. Transport of protons across membranes by weak acids. *Physiol Rev* 1980;60: 825–863.

217. Nikaido H. Bacterial resistance to antibiotics as a function of outer membrane permeability. *J Antimicrob Chemother* 1988;22(Suppl A):S17–S22.

218. Pages JM, James CE, Winterhalter M. The porin and the permeating antibiotic: a selective diffusion barrier in Gram-negative bacteria. *Nat Rev Microbiol* 2008;6:893–903.

219. Paulsen IT, Brown MH, Skurray RA. Proton-dependent multidrug efflux systems. *Microbiol Rev* 1996;60:575–608.

220. Nikaido H. Antibiotic resistance caused by gram-negative multidrug efflux pumps. *Clin Infect Dis* 1998;27(Suppl 1): S32–S41.

221. Putman MY, van Veen HW, Konings WN. Molecular properties of bacterial multidrug transporters. *Microbiol Mol Biol Rev* 2000;64:672–693.

222. Li XZ, Nikaido H. Efflux-mediated drug resistance in bacteria: an update. *Drugs* 2009;69:1555–1623.

223. Lomovskaya O, Warren MS, Lee A, et al. Identification and characterization of inhibitors of multidrug resistance efflux pumps in *Pseudomonas aeruginosa*: novel agents for combination therapy. *Antimicrob Agents Chemother* 2001;45:105–116.

224. Lomovskaya O, Watkins W. Inhibition of efflux pumps as a novel approach to combat drug resistance in bacteria. *J Mol Microbiol Biotechnol* 2001;3:225–236.

225. Bhardwaj AK, Mohanty P. Bacterial efflux pumps involved in multidrug resistance and their inhibitors: rejuvinating the antimicrobial therapy. *Recent Pat Antiinfect Drug Discov* 2012;7:73–89.

226. Russell JB. Another explanation for the toxicity of fermentation acids at low pH: anion accumulation versus uncoupling. *J Appl Bacteriol* 1992;73:363–370.

227. Chuard C, Herrmann M, Vaudaux P, et al. Successful treatment of experimental chronic foreign body infection due to methicillin-resistant *Staphylococcus aureus* by antimicrobial combinations. *Antimicrob Agents Chemother* 1991;35:2611–2616.

228. Stratton CW, Aldridge KE, Gelfand MS. *In vitro* killing of penicillin-susceptible, -intermediate, and -resistant strains of *Streptococcus pneumonia* by cefotaxime, ceftriaxone, and ceftizoxime: a comparison of bactericidal and inhibitory activity with CSF levels. *Diagn Microbiol Infect Dis* 1995;22:35–42.

229. Jorgensen JH, Ferraro MJ. Antimicrobial susceptibility testing: a review of principles and contemporary practices. *Clin Infect Dis* 2009;49:1749–1755.

230. Holland TL, Woods CW, Joyce M. Antimicrobial susceptibility testing in the clinical laboratory. *Infect Dis Clin N Am* 2009;23:757–790.

231. McGowan JE. Antimicrobial stewardship—the state of the art in 2011: focus on outcome and methods. *Infect Control Hosp Epidemiol* 2012;33:331–337.

232. Tuomanen E. Antibiotics which kill non-growing bacteria. *Trends Pharmacol Sci* 1987;8:121–122.

233. Eng RHK, Padberg FT, Smith SM, et al. Bactericidal effects of antibiotics on slowly growing and non-growing bacteria. *Antimicrob Agents Chemother* 1991;35:1824–1828.

234. Carrer G, Flandrois JP, Lobry JR. Biphasic kinetics of bacterial killing by quinolones. *J Antimicrob Chemother* 1991;27:319–327.

235. Drlica K, Malik M, Kerns RJ, et al. Quinolone-mediated bacterial death. *Antimicrob Agents Chemother* 2008;52: 385–392.

236. Mascio CT, Alder JD, Silverman JA. Bactericidal action of daptomycin against stationary-phase and nondividing *Staphylococcus aureus* cells. *Antimicrob Agents Chemother* 2007;51:4255–4260.

237. Dominguez-Herrera J, Docobo-Perez F, Lopez-Rojas R, et al. Efficacy of daptomycin versus vancomycin in an experimental model of foreign-body and systemic infection caused by biofilm producers and methicillin-resistant *Staphylococcus epidermidis*. *Antimicrob Agents Chemother* 2012;56:613–617.

238. Upton A, Drinkovic D, Pottumarthy S, et al. Culture results of heart valves resected because of streptococcal endocarditis: insights into duration of treatment to achieve valve sterilization. *J Antimicrob Chemother* 2005;55:234–239.

239. Schmidt T, Froula J, Tauber MG. Clarithromycin lacks bactericidal activity in cerebrospinal fluid in experimental pneumococcal meningitis. *J Antimicrob Chemother* 1993;32:627–632.

240. Jung CJ, Yeh CY, Shun CT, et al. Platelets enhance biofilm formation and resistance of endocarditis-inducing streptococci on the injured heart valve. *J Infect Dis* 2012;205:1066–1075.

241. Brady RA, Leid JF, Calhoun JH, et al. Osteomyelitis and the role of biofilms in chronic infection. *FEMS Immunol Med Microbiol* 2008;52:13–22.

242. Que Y-A, Moreillon P. Infective endocarditis. *Nat Rev Cardiol* 2011;8:322–336.

243. Lew DP, Waldvogel FA. Osteomyelitis. *N Engl J Med* 1997;336:999–1007.

244. Pankey GA, Sabath LD. Clinical relevance of bacteriostatic versus bactericidal mechanisms of action in the treatment of Gram-positive bacterial infections. *Clin Infect Dis* 2004;38:864–870.

245. Finberg RW, Moellering RC, Tally FP, et al. The importance of bactericidal drugs: future directions in infectious diseases. *Clin Infect Dis* 2004;39:1314–1320.

246. Jacobs MR. How can we predict bacterial eradication? *Int J Infect Dis* 2003;7(Suppl 1):S13–S20.

247. Nicolau DP. Predicting antibacterial response from pharmacodynamics and pharmacokinetic profiles. *Infection* 2001;29(Suppl 2):S11–S15.

248. Peterson LR, Shanholtzer CJ. Tests for bactericidal effects of antimicrobial agents: technical performance and clinical standards. *Clin Microbiol Rev* 1992;5:420–432.

249. Kalan L, Wright GD. Antibiotic adjuvants: multicomponent anti-infective strategies. *Expert Rev Mol Med* 2011;13:e5.

250. Wood K, Nishida S, Sontag ED, et al. Mechanism-independent method for predicting response to multidrug combinations in bacteria. *Proc Natl Acad Sci U S A* 2012;109:12254–12259.

251. Belmatoug N, Fantin B. Contribution of animal models of infection for the evaluation of the activity of antimicrobial agents. *Int J Antimicrob Agents* 1997;9:73–82.

252. Wayne LG, Sramek HA. Metronidazole is bactericidal to dormant cells of *Mycobacterium tuberculosis*. *Antimicrob Agents Chemother* 1994;38:2054–2058.

253. Hoff DR, Caraway ML, Brooks EJ, et al. Metronidazole lacks antibacterial activity in guinea pigs infected with *Mycobacterium tuberculosis*. *Antimicrob Agents Chemother* 2008;52:4137–4140.

254. Iona E, Giannoni F, Pardini M, et al. Metronidazole plus rifampin sterilizes long-term dormant *Mycobacterium tuberculosis*. *Antimicrob Agents Chemother* 2007;51:1537–1540.

255. Barry CE 3rd, Boshoff HI, Dartois V, et al. The spectrum of latent tuberculosis: rethinking the biology and intervention strategies. *Nat Rev Microbiol* 2009;7:845–855.

256. Lin PL, Dartois V, Johnston PJ, et al. Metronidazole prevents reactivation of latent *Mycobacterium tuberculosis* infection in macaques. *Proc Natl Acad Sci U S A* 2012;109:14188–14193.

257. Nicas TI, Hancock REW. Outer membrane protein H1 of *Pseudomonas aeruginosa*: involvement in adaptive and mutational resistance to ethylenediaminetetraacetate, polymyxin B, and gentamicin. *J Bacteriol* 1980;143:872–878.

258. Kumon H, Ono N, Iida M, et al. Combined effect of fosfomycin and ofloxacin against *Pseudomonas aeruginosa* growing in a biofilm. *Antimicrob Agents Chemother* 1995;39:1038–1044.

259. Ramsey BW, Dorkin HL, Eisenberg JD, et al. Efficacy of aerosolized tobramycin in patients with cystic fibrosis. *N Engl J Med* 1993;328:1740–1746.

260. Parkins MD, Elborn JS. Tobramycin Inhalation Powder™: a novel drug delivery system for treating chronic *Pseudomonas aeruginosa* infection in cystic fibrosis. *Expert Rev Respir Med* 2011;5:609–622.

261. Michalopoulos A, Papadakis E. Inhaled anti-infective agents: emphasis on colistin. *Infection* 2010;38:135–142.

262. Young M, Hancock REW. Fluoroquinolone supersusceptibility mediated by outer membrane protein OprH overexpression in *Pseudomonas aeruginosa*: evidence for involvement of a non-porin pathway. *Antimicrob Agents Chemother* 1992;36:2365–2369.

263. Young M, Hancock REW. Fluoroquinolone supersusceptibility mediated by outer membrane protein OprH overexpression in *Pseudomonas aeruginosa*: evidence for involvement of a non-porin pathway. *Antimicrob Agents Chemother* 1992;36:2365–2369.

264. Stockmann C, Sherwin CM, Zobell JT, et al. Optimization of anti-pseudomonal antibiotics for cystic fibrosis pulmonary exacerbations: III. Fluoroquinolones. *Pediatr Pulmonol* 2013;48:211–220.

265. Mesaros N, Nordmann P, Plesiat P, et al. *Pseudomonas aeruginosa*: resistance and therapeutic options at the turn of the new millennium. *Clin Microbiol Infect* 2007;13:560–578.

266. Ichimiya T, Takeoka K, Hiramatsu K, et al. The influence of azithromycin on the biofilm formation of *Pseudomonas aeruginosa in vitro*. *Chemotherapy* 1996;42:186–191.

267. Doring G, Goldstein A, Roll A. Role of *Pseudomonas aeruginosa* exoenzyme in lung infections of patients with cystic fibrosis. *Infect Immun* 1985;49:557–562.

268. Kudoh S, Azuma A, Yamamoto M, et al. Improvement of survival in patients with diffuse panbronchiolitis treated with low-dose erythromycin. *Am J Respir Crit Care Med* 1998;157:1829–1832.

269. Molinari G, Guzmán A, Pesce A, et al. Inhibition of *Pseudomonas aeruginosa* virulence factors by subinhibitory concentrations of azithromycin and other macrolide antibiotics. *J Antimicrob Chemother* 1992;31:681–688.

270. Saiman L, Marshall BC, Mayer-Hamblett N, et al. Azithromycin in patients with cystic fibrosis chronically

infected with *Pseudomonas aeruginosa. JAMA* 2003;290: 1749–1756.

271. Sawaki M, Mikami R, Mikasa K, et al. The long-term chemotherapy with erythromycin in chronic lower respiratory tract infections second report: including cases with *Pseudomonas* infections. *J Jpn Assoc Infect Dis* 1986; 60:45–50.

272. Imamura Y, Higashiyama Y, Tomono K, et al. Azithromycin exhibits bactericidal effects on *Pseudomonas aeruginosa* through interaction with the outer membrane. *Antimicrob Agents Chemother* 2005;49:1377–1380.

273. Buyck JM, Plesiat P, Traore H, et al. Increased susceptibility of *Pseudomonas aeruginosa* to macrolides and ketolides in eukaryotic cell culture media and biological fluids due to decreased expression of oprM and increased outer membrane permeability. *Clin Infect Dis* 2012;55:534–542.

274. Lutz L, Pereira DC, Paiva RM, et al. Macrolides decrease the minimal inhibitory concentrations of antipseudomonal agents against *Pseudomonas aeruginosa* from cystic fibrosis patients in biofilm. *BMC Microbiol* 2012;12:196.

275. Cai Y, Chai D, Wang R, et al. Effectiveness and safety of macrolides in cystic fibrosis patients: a meta-analysis and systematic review. *J Antimicrob Chemother* 2011;66: 968–978.

276. Kandemir O, Oztuna V, Milcan A, et al. Clarithromycin destroys biofilm and enhances bactericidal agents in the treatment of *Pseudomonas aeruginosa* osteomyelitis. *Clin Ortho Relat Res* 2005;430:171–175.

277. Cremieux AC, Saleh-Mghir A, Vallois JM, et al. Efficacy of temofloxacin in experimental *Streptococcus adjacens* endocarditis and autoradiographic diffusion pattern of [^{14}C] temofloxacin in cardiac vegetations. *Antimicrob Agents Chemother* 1992;36:2216–2221.

278. Dall L, Barnes WG, Lane JW, et al. Enzymatic modification of glycocalyx in the treatment of experimental streptococcal endocarditis due to viridans streptococci. *J Infect Dis* 1987;156:736–740.

279. Mghir AS, Cremieux AC, Jambou R, et al. Dextranase enhances antibiotic efficacy in experimental viridans streptococcal endocarditis. *Antimicrob Agents Chemother* 1994;38:953–958.

280. Bayer A, Susan P, Ramos MC, et al. Effects of alginase on the natural history and antibiotic therapy of experimental endocarditis caused by mucoid *Pseudomonas aeruginosa. Infect Immun* 1992;60:3979–3985.

281. Dewar HA, Jones MR, Barnes WS, et al. Fibrinolytic therapy in bacterial experimental studies in dogs. *Eur Heart J* 1986;7:520–527.

282. Buiting AGM, Thompson J, Emeis JJ, et al. Effects of tissue-type plasminogen activator (t-PA) on the treatment of experimental *Streptococcus sanguis* endocarditis. *J Infect Dis* 1989;159:780–784.

283. Sande MA, Courtney KB. Nafcillin-gentamicin synergism in experimental staphylococcal endocarditis. *J Lab Clin Med* 1976;88:118–124.

284. Miyata K, Maejima K, Tomada K, et al. *Serratia* protease. I. Purification and general properties of the enzyme. *Agric Biol Chem* 1970;34:310–318.

285. Yamazaki H, Tsjuji H. Anti-inflammatory activity of TSP, a protease produced by a strain of *Serratia. Folia Pharmacol Jpn* 1967;63:302–314.

286. Selan L, Berlutti F, Passariello C, et al. Proteolytic enzymes: a new treatment strategy for prosthetic infections? *Antimicrob Agents Chemother* 1993;37:2618–2621.

287. Longhi C, Scoarughi GL, Poggiali F, et al. Protease treatment affects both invasion ability and biofilm formation in *Listeria monocytogenes. Microb Pathog* 2008;45:45–52.

288. Al-Bakri AG, Othman G, Bustanji Y. The assessment of the antibacterial and antifungal activities of aspirin, EDTA and aspirin-EDTA combination and their effectiveness as antibiofilm agents. *J Appl Microbiol* 2009;107:280–286.

289. Nicolau DP, Marangos MN, Nightingale CH, et al. Influence of aspirin on development and treatment of experimental *Staphylococcus aureus* endocarditis. *Antimicrob Agents Chemother* 1995;39:1748–1751.

290. Zhou Y, Wang G, Li Y, et al. In vitro interactions between aspirin and amphotericin B against planktonic cells and biofilm cells of *Candida albicans* and *C. parapsilosis. Antimicrob Agents Chemother* 2012;56:3250–3260.

291. Simoes M. Antimicrobial strategies effective against infectious bacterial biofilms. *Curr Med Chem* 2011;18: 2129–2145.

292. Perlroth J, Kuo M, Tan J, et al. Adjunctive use of rifampin for the treatment of *Staphylococcus aureus* infections. A systematic review of the literature. *Arch Intern Med* 2008;168:805–819.

293. Forrest GN, Tamura K. Rifampin combination therapy for nonmycobacterial infections. *Clin Microbiol Rev* 2010;23:14–34.

294. Norden CW, Fierer J, Bryant RE. Chronic staphylococcal osteomyelitis: treatment with regimens containing rifampin. *Rev Infect Dis* 1983;5(Suppl 3):S495–S501.

295. Widmer AF, Gaechter A, Ochsner PE, et al. Antimicrobial treatment of orthopedic implant–related infections with rifampin combinations. *Clin Infect Dis* 1992;14:1251–1253.

296. Drancourt M, Stein A, Argenson JN, et al. Oral rifampin plus ofloxacin for the treatment of *Staphylococcus*-infected orthopedic implants. *Antimicrob Agents Chemother* 1993;37:1214–1218.

297. Zimmerli W, Widmer AF, Blatter M, et al. Role of rifampin for treatment of orthopedic implant-related staphylococcal infections: a randomized controlled trial. Foreign-Body Infection (FBI) Study Group. *JAMA* 1998;279:1537–1541.

298. Senneville E, Yazdanpanah Y, Cazaubiel M, et al. Rifampicin-ofloxacin oral regimen for the treatment of mild to moderate diabetic foot osteomyelitis. *J Antimicrob Chemother* 2001;48:927–930.

299. Antony SJ. Combination therapy with daptomycin, vancomycin, and rifampin for recurrent, severe bone and prosthesis joint infections involving methicillin-resistant *Staphylococcus aureus. Scand J Infect Dis* 2006;38:293–295.

300. Barberan J, Aguilar L, Carroquino G, et al. Conservative treatment of staphylococcal prosthetic joint infections in elderly patients. *Am J Med* 2006;119:993.e7–993.e10.

301. Barberan J, Aguilar L, Gimenez MJ, et al. Levofloxacin plus rifampin conservative treatment of 25 early staphylococcal infections of osteosynthetic devices for rigid internal fixation. *Int J Antimicrob Agents* 2008;32:154–157.

302. Rissing JP. Antimicrobial therapy for chronic osteomyelitis in adults: role of the quinolones. *Clin Infect Dis* 1997;25:1327–1333.

303. Yin LY, Lazzarini L, Li F, et al. Comparative evaluation of tigecycline and vancomycin, with and without rifampicin, in the treatment of methicillin-resistant *Staphylococcus aureus* experimental osteomyelitis in a rabbit model. *J Antimicrob Chemother* 2005;55:995–1002.

304. Baldoni D, Haschke M, Rajacic Z, et al. Linezolid alone or combined with rifampin against methicillin-resistant *Staphylococcus aureus* in experimental foreign-body infection. *Antimicrob Agents Chemother* 2009;53: 1142–1148.

305. Saleh-Mghir A, Muller-Serieys C, Dinh A, et al. Adjunctive rifampin is crucial to optimizing daptomycin efficacy against rabbit prosthetic joint infection due to methicillin-resistant *Staphylococcus aureus*. *Antimicrob Agents Chemother* 2011;55:4589–4593.

306. Garrigos C, Murillo O, Euba G, et al. Efficacy of usual and high doses of daptomycin in combination with rifampin versus alternative therapies in experimental foreign-body infection by methicillin-resistant *Staphylococcus aureus*. *Antimicrob Agents Chemother* 2010;54: 5251–5256.

307. Lefebvre M, Jacqueline C, Amador G, et al. Efficacy of daptomycin combined with rifampicin for the treatment of experimental methicillin-resistant *Staphylococcus aureus* (MRSA) acute osteomyelitis. *Int J Antimicrob Agents* 2010;36:542–544.

308. Vergidis P, Rouse MS, Euba G, et al. Treatment with linezolid or vancomycin in combination with rifampin is effective in an animal model of methicillin-resistant *Staphylococcus aureus* foreign body osteomyelitis. *Antimicrob Agents Chemother* 2011;55:1182–1186.

309. Sauvage E, Kerff F, Terrak M, et al. The penicillin-binding proteins: structure and role in peptidoglycan biosynthesis. *FEMS Microbiol Rev* 2008;32:234–258.

310. Tipper DJ, Strominger JL. Mechanism of action of penicillins: a proposal based on their structural similarities to acyl-D-alanyl-D-alanine. *Proc Natl Acad Sci U S A* 1965;54:1133–1141.

311. Tomasz A. The mechanism of the irreversible antimicrobial effects of penicillins: how the beta-lactam antibiotics kill and lyse bacteria. *Annu Rev Microbiol* 1979; 33:113–137.

312. Demain AL, Elander RP. The beta-lactam antibiotics: past, present, and future. *Antonie Van Leeuwenhoek* 1999;75:5–19.

313. Koch AL. Penicillin binding proteins, beta-lactams, and lactamases: offensives, attacks, and defensive countermeasures. *Crit Rev Microbiol* 2000;26:205–220.

314. Goo KS, Sim TS. Designing new β-lactams: implications from their targets, resistance factors and synthesizing enzymes. *Curr Comput Aided Drug Des* 2011;7:53–80.

315. Harold FM. Ion currents and physiological functions in microorganisms. *Ann Rev Microbiol* 1977;31:181–203.

316. Jolliffe LK, Doyle RJ, Steips UN. The energized membrane and cellular autolysis in *Bacillus subtillis*. *Cell* 1981;25:753–763.

317. Penyige A, Matko J, Deak E, et al. Depolarization of the membrane potential by beta-lactams as a signal to induce autolysis. *Biochem Biophys Res Comm* 2001;290:1169–1175.

318. Brunskill EW, de Jonge BLM, Bayles KW. The *Staphylococcus aureus scdA* gene: a novel locus that affects cell division and morphogenesis. *Microbiol* 1997;143:2877–2882.

319. Groicher KH, Friek BA, Fujimoto DF, et al. The *Staphylococcus aureus* irgAB operon modulates murein hydrolase activity and penicillin tolerance. *J Bacteriol* 2000;182:1794–1801.

320. Normark BH, Normark S. Antibiotic tolerance in pneumococci. *Clin Microbiol Infect* 2002;8:613–622.

321. Wright AJ. The penicillins. *Mayo Clin Proc* 1999;74: 290–307.

322. Hamilton-Miller JM. Development of the semi-synthetic penicillins and cephalosporins. *Int J Antimicrob Agents* 2008;31:189–192.

323. Martin SI, Kaye KM. Beta-lactam antibiotics: newer formulations and newer agents. *Infect Dis Clin North Am* 2004;18:603–619.

324. Livermore DM, Tulkens PM. Temocillin revived. *J Antimicrob Chemother* 2009;63:243–245.

325. Balakrishnan I, Awad-El-Kariem FM, Aali A, et al. Temocillin use in England: clinical and microbiological efficacies in infections caused by extended-spectrum and/or derepressed AmpC β-lactamase-producing *Enterobacteriaceae*. *J Antimicrob Chemother* 2011;66: 2628–2631.

326. Lee N, Yuen KY, Kumana CR. Clinical role of beta-lactam/beta-lactamase inhibitor combinations. *Drugs* 2003;63:1511–1524.

327. Drawz SM, Bonomo RA. Three decades of beta-lactamase inhibitors. *Clin Microbiol Rev* 2010;23:160–201.

328. Marshall WF, Blair JE. The cephalosporins. *Mayo Clin Proc* 1999;74:187–195.

329. Abraham EP, Newton GG. The structure of cephalosporin C. *Biochem J* 1961;79:377–393.

330. Asbel LE, Levison ME. Cephalosporins, carbapenems, and monobactams. *Infect Dis Clin North Am* 2000;14: 435–447.

331. Laudana JB. Ceftaroline fosamil: a new broad-spectrum cephalosporin. *J Antimicrob Chemother* 2011;66(Suppl 3):S11–S18.

332. Hellinger WC, Brewer NS. Carbapenems and monobactams: imipenem, meropenem, and aztreonam. *Mayo Clin Proc* 1999;74:420–434.

333. Nicolau DP. Carbapenems: a potent class of antibiotics. *Expert Opin Pharmacother* 2008;9:32–37.

334. Bonner DP, Sykes RB. Structure activity relationship among the monobactams. *J Antimicrob Chemother* 1984;14:313–327.

335. Carter AP, Clemons WM, Brodersen DE, et al. Functional insights from the structure of the 30S ribosomal subunit and its interactions with antibiotics. *Nature* 2000;407:340–348.

336. Kotra LP, Haddad J, Mobashery S. Aminoglycosides: perspectives on mechanisms of action and resistance and strategies to counter resistance. *Antimicrob Agents Chemother* 2000;44:3249–3256.

337. Vicens Q, Westhof E. RNA as a drug target: the case of aminoglycosides. *Chembiochem* 2003;4:1018–1023.

338. Magnet S, Blanchard JS. Molecular insights into aminoglycoside action and resistance. *Chem Rev* 2005;105: 477–497.

339. Silva JG, Carvalho I. New insights into aminoglycoside antibiotics and derivatives. *Curr Med Chem* 2007;14: 1101–1119.

340. Kaul M, Barbieri CM, Pilch DS. Defining the basis for the specificity of aminoglycoside-rRNA recognition: a comparative study of drug binding to the A sites of *Escherichia coli* and human rRNA. *J Mol Biol* 2005; 346:119–134.

341. Scheunemann AE, Graham WD, Vendeix FA, et al. Binding of aminoglycoside antibiotics to helix 69 of 23S rRNA. *Nucleic Acids Res* 2010;38:3094–3105.

342. Kaul M, Barbieri CM, Pilch DS. Aminoglycoside-induced reduction to nucleotide mobility at the ribosomal RNA A-site as a potentially key determinant of antibacterial activity. *J Am Chem Soc* 2006;128: 1261–1271.

343. Haynie SL, Crum GE, Doele BA. Antimicrobial activities of amphiphilic peptides covalently bonded to a water-insoluble resin. *Antimicrob Agents Chemother* 1995;39:301–307.

344. LaPorte DC, Rosenthal KD, Storm DR. Disruption of *Escherichia coli* growth and respiration by polymyxin B covalently attached to agarose beads. *Biochemistry* 1977;16:1642–1648.

345. Rosenthal KS, Storm DR. Disruption of the *Escherichia coli* outer membrane permeability barrier by immobilized polymyxin B. *J Antibiot* (Tokyo) 1977;30:1087–1092.

346. Moore RD, Lietman PS, Smith CR. Clinical response to aminoglycoside therapy: importance of the ratio of peak concentration to minimal inhibitory concentration. *J Infect Dis* 1987;155:93–99.

347. Gilbert DN. Once-daily aminoglycoside therapy. *Antimicrob Agents Chemother* 1991;35:399–405.

348. Nicolau DP, Freeman CD, Belliveau PP, et al. Experience with a once-daily aminoglycoside program administered to 2,184 adult patients. *Antimicrob Agents Chemother* 1995;39:650–655.

349. Craig WA. Optimizing aminoglycoside use. *Crit Care Clin* 2011;27:107–121.

350. Pagkalis S, Mantadakis E, Mavros MN, et al. Pharmacological considerations for the proper clinical use of aminoglycosides. *Drugs* 2011;71:2277–2294.

351. Lorian V, Ernst J. Activity of amikacin and ampicillin in succession and in combination. *Diagn Microbiol Infect Dis* 1988;11:163–169.

352. Douthwaite S, Champney WS. Structures of ketolides and macrolides determine their mode of interaction with the ribosomal target site. *J Antimicrob Chemother* 2001;48(Suppl T1):1–8.

353. Wilson DN. On the specificity of antibiotics targeting the large ribosomal subunit. *Ann N Y Acad Sci* 2011;1241:1–16.

354. Spizek J, Novotna J, Rezanka T. Lincosamides: chemical structure, biosynthesis, mechanisms of action, resistance, and applications. *Adv Appl Microbiol* 2004;56:121–154.

355. Kannan K, Mankin AS. Macrolide antibiotics in the ribosome exit tunnel: species-specific binding and action. *Ann N Y Acad Sci* 2011;1241:33–47.

356. Vester B, Douthwaite S. Macrolide resistance conferred by base substitutions in 23S rRNA. *Antimicrob Agents Chemother* 2001;45:1–12.

357. Cohen BH, Saneto RP. Mitochondrial translational inhibitors in the pharmacopeia. *Biochim Biophys Acta* 2012;1819:1067–1074.

358. Bryskier A. Ketolides-telithromycin, an example of a new class of antibacterial agents. *Clin Microbiol Infect* 2000;6:661–669.

359. Zhanel GG, Walters M, Noreddin A, et al. The ketolides: a critical review. *Drugs* 2002;62:1771–1804.

360. Ackermann G, Rodloff AC. Drugs of the 21st century: telithromycin (HNR 3647)—the first ketolide. *J Antimicrob Chemother* 2003;51:497–511.

361. Contreras A, Vasquez D. Cooperative and antagonistic interactions of peptidyl-tRNA and antibiotics with bacterial ribosomes. *Eur J Biochem* 1977;74:539–547.

362. Zuckerman JM, Kaye KM. The newer macrolides, azithromycin and clarithromycin. *Infect Dis Clin North Am* 1995;9:731–745.

363. Goswami SK, Kivity S, Marom Z. Erythromycin inhibits respiratory glycoconjugate secretion from human airways *in vitro*. *Am Rev Respir Dis* 1990;141:72–78.

364. Tamaoki J, Takeyama K, Tagaya E, et al. Effect of clarithromycin on sputum production and its rheological properties in chronic respiratory tract infections. *Antimicrob Agents Chemother* 1995;39:1688–1690.

365. Ballow CH, Amsden GW. Azithromycin: the first azalide antibiotic. *Ann Pharmacother* 1992;26:1253–1261.

366. Kirst HA, Creemer LC, Paschal JW, et al. Antimicrobial characterization and interrelationships of dirithromycin and epidirithromycin. *Antimicrob Agents Chemother* 1995;39:1436–1441.

367. Wintermeyer SM, Abdel-Rahman SM, Nahata MC. Dirithromycin: a new macrolide. *Ann Pharmacother* 1996;30:1141–1149.

368. Watkins VS, Polk RE, Stotka JL. Drug interactions of macrolides: emphasis on dirithromycin. *Ann Pharmacother* 1997;31:349–356.

369. Hansen LH, Mauvais P, Douthwaite S. The macrolide-ketolide antibiotic binding site is formed by structures in domains II and V of 23S ribosomal RNA. *Mol Microbiol* 1999;31:623–631.

370. Douthwaite S, Hansen LH, Mauvais P. Macrolide-ketolide inhibition of MLS-resistant ribosomes is improved by alternative drug interaction with domain II of 23S rRNA. *Mol Microbiol* 2000;36:183–193.

371. Nguyen M, Chung EP. Telithromycin: the first ketolide antimicrobial. *Clin Ther* 2005;27:1144–1163.

372. Zeitlinger M, Wagner CC, Heinisch B. Ketolides—the modern relatives of macrolides: the pharmacokinetic perspective. *Clin Pharmacokinet* 2009;48:23–38.

373. Allington DR, Rivey MP. Quinupristin/dalfopristin: a therapeutic review. *Clin Ther* 2001;23:24–44.

374. Delgado G Jr, Neuhauser MM, Bearden DT, et al. Quinpristin-dalfopristin: an overview. *Pharmacotherapy* 2000;20:1469–1485.

375. Manfredi R. A re-emerging class of antimicrobial agents: streptogramins (quinupristin/dalfopristin) in the management of multiresistant gram-positive nosocomial cocci in hospital setting. *Mini Rev Med Chem* 2005; 5:1075–1081.

376. Kang L, Rybak MJ. Pharmacodynamics of RP 595000 alone and in combination with vancomycin against *Staphylococcus aureus* in an *in vitro*–infected fibrin clot model. *Antimicrob Agents Chemother* 1995;39:1505–1511.

377. Aumercier M, Bouhallab S, Capmau ML, et al. RP 59500: a proposed mechanism for its bactericidal activity. *J Antimicrob Chemother* 1992;30(Suppl A):S9–S14.

378. Nougayrede A, Berthaud N, Bouanchaud DH. Post-antibiotic effects of RP 59500 with *Staphylococcus aureus*. *J Antimicrob Chemother* 1992;30(Suppl A):S101–S106.

379. Appelbaum PC, Hunter PA. The fluoroquinolone antibacterials: past, present and future perspectives. *Int J Antimicrob Agents* 2000;16:5–15.

380. Chu DTW, Fernandes PB. Structure-activity relationships of the fluoroquinolones. *Antimicrob Agents Chemother* 1989;33:131–135.

381. Maxwell A. The molecular basis of quinolone action. *J Antimicrob Chemother* 1992;30:409–416.

382. Domagala JM. Structure-activity and structure-side-effect relationships for the quinolone antibacterials. *J Antimicrob Chemother* 1994;33:685–706.

383. Fabrega A, Madurga S, Giralt E, et al. Mechanisms of action and resistance to quinolones. *Microb Biotechnol* 2009;2:40–61.

384. Hawkey PM. Mechanisms of quinolone action and microbial response. *J Antimicrob Chemother* 2003;51(Suppl 1):29–35.

385. Khardoli N, Nguyen H, Rosenbaum B, et al. *In vitro* susceptibilities of rapidly growing mycobacteria to newer antimicrobial agents. *Antimicrob Agents Chemother* 1994;38:134–137.

386. Pranger AD, Alffenaar JW, Aarnoutse RE. Fluoroquinolones, the cornerstone of treatment of drug-resistant tuberculosis: a pharmacokinetic and pharmacodynamic approach. *Curr Pharm Des* 2011;17:2900–2930.

387. Takiff H, Guerrero E. Current prospects for the fluoroquinolones as first-line tuberculosis therapy. *Antimicrob Agents Chemother* 2011;55:5421–5429.

388. Mdluli K, Ma Z. *Mycobacterium tuberculosis* DNA gyrase as a target for drug discovery. *Infect Discord Drug Targets* 2007;7:159–168.

389. Klopman G, Li J-Y, Wang S, et al. *In vitro* anti–*Mycobacterium avium* activities of quinolones: predicted active structures and mechanistic considerations. *Antimicrob Agents Chemother* 1994;38:1794–1802.

390. Haemers A, Leysen DC, Bollaert W, et al. Influence of N substitution on antimycobacterial activity of ciprofloxacin. *Antimicrob Agents Chemother* 1990;34:496–497.

391. Berger JM, Gamblin SJ, Haarrison SC, et al. Structure and mechanism of DNA topoisomerase II. *Nature* 1996;379:225–232.

392. Shen LL, Mitscher LA, Sharma PN, et al. Mechanism of inhibition of DNA gyrase by quinolone antibacterials: a cooperative drug-DNA binding model. *Biochemistry* 1989;28:3886–3894.

393. Kolodkin-Gal L, Engelverg-Kulka. Indiction of *Escherichia coli* chromosomal *mazEF* by stressful conditions causes and irreversible loss of viability. *J Bacterol* 2006; 188:3420–3423.

394. Imlay JA. Pathways of oxidative damage. *Annu Rev Microbiol* 2003;52:395–418.

395. Lewin CS, Howard BMA, Ratcliffe NT, et al. 4-Quinolones and the SOS response. *J Med Microbiol* 1989;29: 139–144.

396. Piddock LJV, Walters RN. Bactericidal activities of five quinolones for *Escherichia coli* strains with mutations in genes encoding the SOS response or cell division. *Antimicrob Agents Chemother* 1992;36:819–825.

397. Heide L. The aminocoumarins: biosynthesis and biology. *Nat Prod Rep* 2009;28:1241–1250.

398. Flatman RH, Eustaquio A, Li SM, et al. Structure-activity relationships of anminocoumarin-type gyrase and topoisomerase IV inhibitors obtained by combinatorial biosynthesis. *Antimicrob Agents Chemother* 2006; 50:1136–1142.

399. Flatman RH, Howells AJ, Heide L, et al. Simocyclinone D8, an inhibitor of dNA gyrase with a novel mode of action. *Antimicrob Agents Chemother* 2005;49: 1093–1100.

400. Edwards MJ, Flatman RH, Mitchenall LA, et al. A crystal structure of the bifunctional antibiotic simocyclinone D8, bound to DNA gyrase. *Science* 2009;326: 1415–1418.

401. Reusser F. Inhibition of ribosomal and RNA polymerase functions by rubradirin and its aglycone. *J Antibiot* 1979;32:1186–1192.

402. Contreras A, Maxwell A. *GyrB* mutations which confer resistance also affect DNA supercoiling and ATP hydrolysis by *Escherichia coli* DNA gyrase. *Mol Microbiol* 1992;6:1617–1624.

403. Domagk G. Ein Beitrag zur Chemotherapie der Bakteriellen Infektionen. *Dtsch Med Wochenschr* 1935;7: 250–253.

404. Yun MK, Wu Y, Li Z, et al. Catalysis and sulfa drug resistance in dihydropteroate synthase. *Science* 2012; 335:1110–1114.

405. Woods DD. Relation of *p*-aminobenzoic acid to mechanism of action of sulphanilamide. *Br J Exp Pathol* 1940;21:74–90.

406. Achari A, Somers DO, Champness JN, et al. Crystal structure of the anti-bacterial sulfonamide drug target dihydropteroate synthase. *Nat Struct Biol* 1997;4: 490–497.

407. Bushby SRM, Hitchings GH. Trimethoprim, a sulphonamide potentiator. *Br J Pharmacol* 1968;33:72–90.

408. Quinlivan EP, McPartin J, Weir DG, et al. Mechanism of the antimicrobial drug trimethoprim revisited. *FASEB J* 2000;14:19–24.

409. Matthews DA, Bolin JT, Burridge JM, et al. Dihydrofolate reductase. The stereochemistry of inhibitor selectivity. *J Biol Chem* 1985;260:392–399.

410. Hitchings GH. Mechanism of action of trimethoprim-sulfamethoxazole—I. *J Infect Dis* 1973;128(Suppl 3);S433–S436.

411. Masters PA, O'Bryan TA, Zurlo J, et al. Trimethoprim-sulfamethoxazole revisited. *Arch Intern Med* 2003;163: 402–410.

412. Richards RM, Taylor RB, Zhu ZY. Mechanism for synergism between sulphonamides and trimethoprim clarified. *J Pharm Pharmacol* 1996;48:981–984.

413. Sköld O. Sulfonamides and trimethoprim. *Expert Rev Anti-infect Ther* 2010:1–6.

414. Bartz QR. Isolation and characterization of chloromycetin. *J Biol Chem* 1948;172:445–450.

415. Powell DA, Nahata MC. Chloramphenicol: new perspectives on an old drug. *Drug Intell Clin Pharm* 1982;16:295–300.

416. Vining LC, Stuttard C. Chloramphenicol. *Biotechnology* 1995;28:505–530.

417. Johansson D, Jessen CH, Pohlsgaard J, et al. Design, synthesis and ribosome binding of chloramphenicol nucleotide and intercalator conjugates. *Bioorg Med Chem Lett* 2005;15:2079–2083.

418. Levy SB. Active efflux mechanisms for antimicrobial resistance. *Antimicrob Agents Chemother* 1992;36: 695–703.

419. Pongs O, Bald R, Erdmann VA. Identification of chloramphenicol-binding protein in *Escherichia coli* ribosomes by affinity labeling. *Proc Natl Acad Sci U S A* 1973; 70:2229–2233.

420. Thompson J, O'Connor M, Mills JA, et al. The protein synthesis inhibitors, oxazolidinones and chloramphenicol, cause extensive translational inaccuracy *in vivo*. *J Mol Biol* 2002;322:273–279.

421. Rahal JJ, Simberkoff MS. Bactericidal and bacteristatic action of chloramphenicol against meningeal pathogens. *Antimicrob Agents Chemother* 1979;16:13–18.

422. Stow M, Starkey BJ, Hancock IC, et al. Inhibition by chloramphenicol of glucose transfer in teichoic acid biosynthesis. *Nature* 1971;229:56–57.

423. Rinehart KL Jr, Shield LS. Chemistry of ansamycin antibiotics. *Fortschr Chem Org Naturst* 1976;33:231–307.

424. Sensi P. History of the development of rifampin. *Rev Infect Dis* 1983;5(Suppl):S402–S406.

425. McClure WR, Cech CL. On the mechanism of rifampicin inhibition of RNA synthesis. *J Biol Chem* 1978;253:8949–8956.

426. Wehrli W. Rifampin: mechanisms of action and resistance. *Rev Infect Dis* 1983;5(Suppl 3):S407–S411.

427. Campbell EA, Korazheva N, Mustaev A, et al. Structural mechanism for rifampin inhibition of bacterial RNA polymerase. *Cell* 2001;104:901–912.

428. Floss HG, Yu TW. Rifamycin—mode of action, resistance, and biosynthesis. *Chem Rev* 2005;105:621–632.

429. Aristoff PA, Garcia GA, Kirchhoff PD, et al. Rifamycins—obstacles and opportunities. *Tuberculosis (Edinb)* 2010;90:94–118.

430. Nelson ML, Levy SB. The history of the tetracyclines. *Ann N Y Acad Sci* 2011;1241:17–32.

431. Chopra I, Roberts M. Tetracycline antibiotics: mode of action, applications, molecular biology, and epidemiology of bacterial resistance. *Microbiol Mol Biol Rev* 2001;65:232–260.

432. Agwuh KN, MacGowan A. Pharmacokinetics and pharmacodynamics of the tetracyclines including glycocyclines. *Chemother* 2006;58:256–265.

433. Roberts MC. Tetracycline therapy: update. *Clin Infect Dis* 2003;36:462–467.

434. Moazed D, Noller HF. Interaction of antibiotics with functional sites in 16S ribosomal RNA. *Nature* 1987;327:389–394.

435. Rasmussen B, Noller HF, Doubresse G, et al. Molecular basis of tetracycline action: identification of analogs whose primary target is not the bacterial ribosome. *Antimicrob Agents Chemother* 1991;35:2306–2311.

436. Oliva B, Gordon G, McNicholas P, et al. Evidence that tetracycline analogs whose primary target is not the bacterial ribosome cause lysis of *Escherichia coli*. *Antimicrob Agents Chemother* 1992;36:913–919.

437. Sum PE, Lee VJ, Testa RT. Glycylcyclines. I. A new generation of potent antimicrobial agents through modification of 9-aminotetracyclines. *J Med Chem* 1994;37:184–188.

438. Tally FP, Ellestad GA, Testa RT. Glycylcyclines: a new generation of tetracyclines. *J Antimicrob Chemother* 1995;35:449–452.

439. Sum PE, Sum FW, Projan SJ. Recent developments in tetracycline antibiotics. *Curr Pharm Des* 1998;4:119–132.

440. Chopra I. Glycylcyclines: third generation tetracycline antibiotics. *Curr Opin Microbiol* 2001;1:464–469.

441. Chopra I. New developments in tetracycline antibiotics: glycylcyclines and tetracycline efflux pump inhibitors. *Drug Resist Updat* 2002;5:119–125.

442. Testa RT, Petersen PJ, Jacobus NV, et al. *In vitro* and *in vivo* antibacterial activities of the glycylcyclines, a new class of semisynthetic tetracyclines. *Antimicrob Agents Chemother* 1993;37:2270–2277.

443. da Silva LM, Nunes Salgado HR. Tigecycline: a review of properties, applications, and analytical methods. *Ther Drug Monit* 2010;32:282–288.

444. Yahav D, Lador A, Paul M, et al. Efficacy and safety of tigecycline: a systematic review and meta-analysis. *J Antimicrob Chemother* 2011;66:1963–1971.

445. Bergeron J, Ammirati M, Danley D, et al. Glycylcyclines bind to the high-affinity tetracycline ribosomal binding site and evade Tet(M) and Tet(O)-mediated ribosomal protection. *Antimicrob Agents Chemother* 1996;40:2226–2228.

446. Noskin GA. Tigecycline: a new glycylcycline for treatment of serious infections. *Clin Infect Dis* 2005;41(Suppl 5):S303–S314.

447. Chung MC, Bosquesi PL, dos Santos JL. A prodrug approach to improve the physicochemical properties and decrease the genotoxicity of nitro compounds. *Curr Pharm Des* 2011;17:3515–3526.

448. Ingham HR, Selkon JB, Hale JH. The antibacterial activity of metronidazole. *J Antimicrob Chemother* 1975;1:355–361.

449. Raether W, Hanel H. Nitroheterocyclic drugs with broad spectrum activity. *Parasit Res* 2003;90(Suppl 1):S19–S39.

450. Edwards DI. Nitroimidazole drugs—action and resistant mechanisms. I. Mechanisms of action. *J Antimicrob Chemother* 1993;31:9–20.

451. McOster CC, Fitzpatrick PM. Nitrofurantoin: mechanism of action and implications for resistance development in common uropathogens. *J Antimicrob Chemother* 1994;33:23–33.

452. Pendland SL, Piscitelli SC, Schreckenberger PC, et al. *In vitro* activities of metronidazole and its hydroxy metabolite against *Bacteroides* spp. *Antimicrob Agents Chemother* 1994;38:2106–2110.

453. Samuelson J. Why metronidazole is active against both bacteria and parasites. *Antimicrob Agents Chemother* 1999;43:1533–1541.

454. Lofmark S, Edlund C, Nord CE. Metronidazole is still the drug of choice for treatment of anaerobic infections. *Clin Infect Dis* 2010;50(Suppl):S16–S23.

455. Sandegren L, Lindqvist A, Kahimeter G, et al. Nitrofurantoin resistance mechanism and fitness cost in *Escherichia coli*. *J Antimicrob Chemother* 2008;62:495–503.

456. Van Bambeke F, Van Laethem Y, Courvalin P, et al. Glycopeptide antibiotics: from conventional molecules to new derivatives. *Drugs* 2004;64:913–936.

457. Finch RG, Eliopoulos GM. Safety and efficacy of glycopeptides antibiotics. *J Antimicrob Chermother* 2005;55(Suppl 2):S5–S13.

458. Jeya M, Moon HJ, Lee KM, et al. Glycopeptide antibiotics and the novel semi-synthetic derivatives. *Curr Pharm Biotechnol* 2011;12:1194–1204.

459. Griffith RS, Peek FB. Vancomycin, a new antibiotic: preliminary clinical and laboratory studies. In: Welch H, Martini-Ibanez F, eds. *Antibiotics annual 1955–1956*. New York: Medical Encyclopedia, 1956:619–622.

460. Williams AH, Gruneberg RN. Teicoplanin. *J Antimicrob Chemother* 1984;22:397–401.

461. Nagarajan R. Structure-activity relationships of vancomycin-type glycopeptide antibiotics. *J Antibiot* (Tokyo) 1993;46:1181–1195.

462. Svetitsky S, Leibovici L, Paul M. Comparative efficacy and safety of vancomycin versus teicoplanin: systematic review and meta-analysis. *Antimicrob Agents Chemother* 2009;53:4069–4079.

463. Beauregard DA, Williams DH, Gwynn MN, et al. Dimerization and membrane anchors in extracellular targeting of vancomycin group antibiotics. *Antimicrob Agents Chemother* 1995;39:781–785.

464. Gerhard U, Mackay JP, Maplestone RA, et al. The role of the sugar and chlorine substituents in the dimerization of vancomycin antibiotics. *J Am Chem Soc* 1993;115:232–237.

465. Rybak MJ. The pharmacokinetic and pharmacodynamic properties of vancomycin. *Clin Infect Dis* 2006;42(Suppl):S35–S39.

466. Nagarajan R. Antibacterial activities and modes of action of vancomycin and related glycopeptides. *Antimicrob Agents Chemother* 1991;35:605–609.

467. Nagarajan R. Antibacterial activities and modes of action of vancomycin and related glycopeptides. *Antimicrob Agents Chemother* 1991;35:605–609.

468. Stratton CW, Liu C, Weeks LS. Bactericidal activity of daptomycin compared with methicillin, cefazolin,

cefamandole, cefuroxime, ciprofloxacin, and vancomycin against staphylococci as determined by kill-kinetic studies. *Antimicrob Agents Chemother* 1987;31:1210–1215.

469. Jung HM, Jeya M, Kim SY, et al. Biosynthesis, biotechnical production, and application of teicoplanin: current state and perspectives. *Appl Microbiol Biotechnol* 2009;84:417–428.

470. Guskey MT, Tsuji BT. A comparative review of the lipoglycopeptides: oritavancin, dalbavancin, and telavancin. *Pharmacotherapy* 2010;30:80–94.

471. Zhanel GG, Calic D, Schweizer F, et al. New lipoglycopeptides: a comparative review of dalbavancin, oritavancin, and telavancin. *Drugs* 2010;70:859–886.

472. Arhin FF, Belley A, McKay GA, et al. Characterization of the *in vitro* activity of novel lipoglycopeptide antibiotics. *Curr Protoc Microbiol* 2010;Chapter 17:Unit 17.1.

473. Saravolatz LD, Stein GE, Johnson LB. Telavancin: a novel lipoglycopeptide. *Clin Infect Dis* 2009;49:1908–1914.

474. Zhanel GG, Schweizer F, Karlowsky JA. Oritavancin: mechanism of action. *Clin Infect Dis* 2012;54(Suppl 3):S214–S219.

475. Michalopoulos AS, Livaditis IG, Gougoutas V. The revival of fosfomycin. *Int J Infect Dis* 2011;15:e732–e739.

476. Von Daehne W, Godtfredsen WO, Rasmussen RR. Structure-activity relationships on fusidic acid–type antibiotics. *Adv Appl Microbiol* 1979;25:95–146.

477. Turnidge J. Fusidic acid pharmacology, pharmacokinetics and pharmacodynamics. *Int J Antimicrob Agents* 1999;12(Suppl 2):S23–S34.

478. Verbist L. The antimicrobial activity of fusidic acid. *J Antimicrob Chemother* 1990;25(Suppl B):S1–S15.

479. Shanson DC. Clinical relevance of resistance to fusidic acid. *J Antimicrob Chemother* 1990;25(Suppl B):S15–S21.

480. Farrell DJ, Castanheira M, Chopra I. Characterization of global patterns and the genetics of fusidic acid resistance. *Clin Infect Dis* 2011;52(Suppl 7):S487–S492.

481. Tsuji BT, Okusanya OO, Bulitta JB, et al. Application of pharmacokinetic-pharmacodynamic modeling and the justification of a novel fusidic acid dosing regimen: raising Lazarus from the dead. *Clin Infect Dis* 2011;52(Suppl 7):S513–S519.

482. Fernandes P, Pereira D. Efforts to support the development of fusidic acid in the United States. *Clin Infect Dis* 2011;52(Suppl 7):S542–S546.

483. Landman D, Georgescu C, Martin A, et al. Polymyxins revisited. *Clin Microbiol Rev* 2008;21:449–465.

484. Falagas ME, Kasiakou SK. Colistin: the revival of polymyxins for the management of multidrug-resistant gram-negative bacterial infections. *Clin Infect Dis* 2005;40:1333–1341.

485. Strieker M, Marahiel MA. The structural diversity of acidic lipopeptide antibiotics. *Chembiochem* 2009;10:607–616.

486. Eisenstein BI, Olesson FB Jr, Baltz RH. Daptomycin: from the mountain to the clinic, with essential help from Francis Tally, MD. *Clin Infect Dis* 2010;50(Suppl 1):S10–S15.

487. Tally FP, DeBruin MF. Development of daptomycin for gram-positive infections. *J Antimicrob Chemother* 2000;46:523–526.

488. Debono M, Barnhart M, Carrell CB, et al. A21978C, a complex of new acidic peptide antibiotics: isolation, chemistry, and mass spectral structure elucidation. *J Antibiot (Tokyo)* 1987;40:761–777.

489. Alborn WE Jr, Allen NE, Preston DA. Daptomycin disrupts membrane potential in growing *Staphylococcus aureus*. *Antimicrob Agents Chemother* 1991;35:2282–2287.

490. Wale LJ, Shelton AP, Greenwood D. Scanning electron microscopy of *Staphyococcus aureus* and *Enterococcus faecalis* exposed to daptomycin. *J Med Microbiol* 1989;30:45–49.

491. Lakey JH, Ptak M. Fluorescence indicates a calcium-dependent interaction between the lipopeptide antibiotic LY146032 and phospholipid membranes. *Biochemistry* 1988;27:4639–4645.

492. Allen NE, Alborn WE Jr, Hobbs JN Jr. Initiation of membrane potential–dependent amino acid transport by daptomycin. *Antimicrob Agents Chemother* 1991;35:2639–2642.

493. Straus SK, Hancock RE. Mode of action of the new antibiotic for Gram-positive pathogens daptomycin: comparison with cationic antimicrobial peptides and lipopeptides. *Biochim Biophys Acta* 2006;1758:1215–1223.

494. Pogliano J, Pogliano N, Silverman JA. Daptomycin-mediated reorganization of membrane architecture causes mislocalization of essential cell division proteins. *J Bacteriol* 2012;194:4494–4504.

495. Livermore DM. Linezolid *in vitro*: mechanism and antibacterial spectrum. *J Antimicrob Chemother* 2003;51 (Suppl 2):S9–S16.

496. Shaw KJ, Barbachyn MR. The oxazolidinones: past, present, and future. *Ann N Y Acad Sci* 2011;1241:48–70.

497. Eustice DC, Brittelli DR, Feldman PA, et al. An automated pulse labeling method for structure-activity relationship studies with antibacterial oxazolidinones. *Drugs Exp Clin Res* 1990;16:149–155.

498. Daley JS, Eliopoulos GP, Reiszner E, et al. Activity and mechanism of action of DuP 105 and DuP 721, new oxazolidone compounds. *J Antimicrob Chemother* 1988;21:721–730.

499. Slee AM, Wuonola MA, McRipley RJ, et al. Oxazolidines, a new class of synthetic antibiotic agents: *in vitro* and *in vivo* activities of DuP 105 and DuP 721. *Antimicrob Agents Chemother* 1987;31:1791–1797.

500. Patel U, Yan YP, Hobbs FW, et al. Oxazolidinones' mechanism of action: inhibition of the first peptide bond formation. *J Biol Chem* 2001;276:37199–37205.

501. Fung HB, Kirschenbaum HL, Ojofeitimi BO. Linezolid: an oxazolidinone antimicrobial agent. *Clin Ther* 2001;23:356–391.

502. Leach KL, Brickner SJ, Noe MC, et al. Linezolid, the first oxazolidinone antibacterial agent. *Ann N Y Acad Sci* 2011;1222:49–54.

503. Cremades R, Rodriguez JC, Garcia-Pachon E, et al. Interaction between linezolid and *Mycobacterium tuberculosis* in an experimental *in vitro* model. *APMIS* 2011;119:304–308.

504. Schecter GF, Scott C, True L, et al. Linezolid in the treatment of multidrug-resistant tuberculosis. *Clin Infect Dis* 2011;50:49–55.

505. Lee M, Lee J, Carroll MW, et al. Linezolid for treatment of chronic extensively drug-resistant tuberculosis. *N Eng J Med* 2012;367:1508–1518.

506. Ippolito JA, Kanyo ZF, Wang D, et al. Crystal structure of the oxazolidinone antibiotic linezolid bound to the 50S ribosomal subunit. *J Med Chem* 2008;51:3353–3356.

507. Wilson DN, Schluenzen F, Harms JM, et al. The oxazolidinone antibiotics perturb the ribosomal peptidyl-transferase center and effect tRNA positioning. *Proc Nat Acad Sci U S A* 2008;105:13339–13344.

508. Balemans W, Vranckx L, Lounis N, et al. Novel antibiotics targeting respiratory ATP synthesis in Gram-positive pathogenic bacteria. *Antimicrob Agents Chemother* 2012; 56:4131–4139.

509. Andries K, Verhasselt P, Guillemont J, et al. A diarylquinoline drug active on the ATP synthase of *Mycobacterium tuberculosis*. *Science* 2005;307:223–227.

510. Koul A, Dendouga N, Vergauwen K, et al. Diarylquinolines target subunit c of mycobacterial ATP synthase. *Nat Chem Biol* 2007;3:323–324.

511. Haagsma AC, Podasca I, Koul A, et al. Probing the interaction of the diarylquinoline TMC207 with its target mycobacterial ATP synthase. *PLoS One* 2011;6:e23575.

512. Koul A, Vranckx L, Dendouga N, et al. Darylquinolines are bactericidal for dormant mycobacteria as a result of disturbed ATP homeostasis. *J Biol Chem* 2008;283:25273–25280.

513. Diacon AH, Pym A, Grobusch M, et al. The diarylquinoline TMC207 for multidrug-resistant tuberculosis. *N Engl J Med* 2009;360:2397–2405.

514. Eliopoulos GM, Wennersten CB, Cole G, et al. In vitro activity of A-86719.1, a novel 2-pyridone antimicrobial agent. *Antimicrob Agents Chemother* 1995;35:850–853.

515. Li Q, Mitscher LA, Shen LL. The 2-pyridone antibacterial agents: bacterial topoisomerase inhibitors. *Med Res Rev* 2000;20:231–293.

516. Alder J, Clement J, Meulbroek J, et al. Efficacies of ABT-719 and related 2-pyridones, members of a new class of antibacterial agents, against experimental bacterial infections. *Antimicrob Agents Chemother* 1995;39:971–975.

517. Bengtsson C, Lindgren AE, Uvell H, et al. Design, synthesis and evaluation of triazole functionalized ring-fused 2-pyridones as antibacterial agents. *Eur J Med Chem* 2012;54:637–646.

518. Willey JM, van der Donk WA. Lantibiotics: peptides of diverse structure and function. *Annu Rev Microbiol* 2007;61:477–501.

519. McAuliffe O, Ross RP, Hill C. Lantibiotics: structure, biosynthesis and mode of action. *FEMS Microbiol Rev* 2001;25:285–308.

520. Pag U, Sahl HG. Multiple activities in lantibiotics: models for the design of novel antibiotics? *Curr Pharm Des* 2002;8:815–833.

521. Cotter PD, Hill C, Ross RP. Bacterial lantibiotics: strategies to improve therapeutic potential. *Curr Protein Pept Sci* 2005;6:61–75.

522. Walsh C. *Antibiotics: actions, origins, resistance.* Washington, DC: ASM Press, 2003.

523. Goto Y, Li B, Claesen J, et al. Discovery of unique lanthionine synthetases reveals new mechanistic and evolutionary insights. *PLoS Biol* 2010;8:e1000339.

524. Bierbaum G, Sahl HG. Lantibiotics: unusually modified bacteriocin-like peptides from gram-positive bacteria. *Zentralbl Bakteriol Paraitenkd Infektionskr Hyg Abt I Orig* 1993;278:1–22.

525. Twomey D, Ross RP, Ryan M, et al. Lantibiotics produced by lactic acid bacteria: structure, function

and applications. *Antonie Van Leeuwenhoek* 2002;82: 165–185.

526. Moll GN, Roberts GC, Konings WN, et al. Mechanism of lantibiotic-induced pore-formation. *Antonie Van Leeuwenhoek* 1996;69:185–191.

527. Chatterjee C, Paul M, Xie L, et al. Biosynthesis and mode of action of lantibiotics. *Chem Rev* 2005;105:633–684.

528. Bierbaum G, Sahl HG. Lantibiotics: mode of action, biosynthesis and bioengineering. *Curr Pharm Biotechnol* 2009;10:2–18.

529. Brotz H, Bierbaum G, Markus A, et al. Mode of action of the lantibiotic mersacidin: inhibition of peptidoglycan biosynthesis via a novel mechanism. *Antimicrob Agents Chemother* 1995;39:714–719.

530. Hasper HE, Kramer NE, Smith JL, et al. An alternative bacteriocidal mechanism of action for lantibiotic peptides that target lipid II. *Science* 2006;313: 1636–1637.

531. Ganz T. Defensins: antimicrobial peptides of innate immunity. *Nat Rev Immunol* 2003;3:710–720.

532. Findlay B, Zhanel GG, Schweizer F. Cationic amphiphiles, a new generation of antimicrobials inspired by the natural antimicrobial peptide scaffold. *Antimicrob Agents Chemother* 2010;54:4049–4058.

533. Oppenheim JJ, Biragyn A, Kwak LW, et al. Roles of antimicrobial peptides such as defensins in innate and adaptive immunity. *Ann Rheum Dis* 2003;62(Suppl 2):S17–S21.

534. Boman HG. Antibacterial peptides: basic facts and emerging concepts. *J Intern Med* 2003;254:197–215.

535. Boman HG, Faye I, Gudmundsson GH, et al. Cell-free immunity in *Cecropia*: a model system for antibacterial proteins. *Eur J Biochem* 1991;201:23–31.

536. Dempsey CE. The actions of melittin on membranes. *Biochim Biophys Acta* 1990;1031:143–161.

537. Zasloff M. Magainins, a class of antimicrobial peptides from *Xenopus* skin: isolation, characterization of two active forms and partial cDNA sequence of a precursor. *Proc Natl Acad Sci U S A* 1987;84:5449–5453.

538. Schnell N, Entian K-D, Schneider U, et al. Prepeptide sequence of epidermin, a ribosomally synthesized antibiotic with four sulphide-rings. *Nature* 1988;333: 276–278.

539. Zhang Y, Lu W, Hong M. The membrane-bound structure and topology of a human α-defensin indicate a dimer pore mechanism for membrane disruption. *Biochemistry* 2010;49:9770–9782.

540. Yeaman MR, Yount NY. Unifying themes in host defense effector polypeptides. *Nature Rev Microbiol* 2007;5:727–740.

541. Scott MG, Dullaghan E, Mookherjee N, et al. An anti-infective peptide that selectively modulates the innate immune response. *Nature Biotechnol* 2007;25:465–472.

542. Tang M, Waring AJ, Hong M. Phosphate-mediated arginine insertion into lipid membrane and pore formation by cationic membrane peptide from solid-state NMR. *J Am Chem Soc* 2007;129:11438–11446.

Chapter 11

Antiviral Agents for HIV, Hepatitis, Cytomegalovirus, and Influenza: Susceptibility Testing Methods, Modes of Action, and Resistance

Daniel Amsterdam

Antiviral compounds have now been available for several decades. However, more recently, there has been a surge in the development of antivirals sparked by the AIDS epidemic and influenza pandemics. As was the case for antimicrobial agents, the question of their evaluation in clinical practice is an ongoing challenge. The correlation of in vitro activity, determined either by phenotypic or genotypic assays with patient outcome required continued research and outcome determinations. Although the initial approach for determining in vitro activity was to identify a phenotype, antiviral evaluations were conducted using genotypic assays. This was made possible through sequencing techniques that were applied to portions of viral RNA and DNA related to the targets of available compounds. As will be seen, phenotypic testing is a more complex, time-consuming, and costly procedure.

The representative viruses reviewed in this chapter establish chronic infection in their hosts. They invade and, as such, behave as quasispecies—that is, complex mixtures of genetically related but distinct viral populations in equilibrium within a given replicative environment. For this reason, at any given time, patients harbor a large number of different viral genomes, which can lead to unreliable evaluations of susceptibility/resistance when using phenotypic methodologies.

Over the past decade, the field of molecular virology testing has evolved to provide broadened dynamic range and increased assay sensitivity, leading to more actionable decision points for clinicians. Viral load monitoring of HIV, the hepatitis viruses, and human cytomegalovirus, is a routine barometer of a patient's infected viral status and is typically used by physicians to gauge a patient's response to therapy.

GENERAL CONSIDERATIONS FOR ANTIVIRAL SUSCEPTIBILITY TESTING

Unlike the case for bacterial pathogens where antimicrobial susceptibility testing is typically routine, antiviral susceptibility testing, because of complexity and cost, has more limited applicability. Antiviral susceptibility testing is necessary for evaluating new antiviral agents, defining mechanisms of resistance, determining the frequency of emergence of drug-resistant viral mutants, and for testing cross-resistance to alternative agents.

Aside from spontaneous mutations, most of the available agents are able to induce mutations, at least at their active site, resulting in modified viral replication capacity. This varies according to mutations, some of which may be beneficial in reducing viral replication (i.e., viral fitness). However, reciprocal interaction between mutations can only be measured by phenotypic testing. For the viral infections presented in this chapter (i.e., HIV, hepatitis B and C, CMV, and influenza), phenotypic and genotypic approaches will be presented.

VARIABLES OF ANTIVIRAL SUSCEPTIBILITY TESTING

Currently, there are limited standards for performing antiviral susceptibility testing. The Clinical and Laboratory Standards Institute (CLSI) has published one approved standard applicable to herpes simplex virus (HSV) (1), which will not be addressed in this chapter.

Variables that influence the final results of these assays include cell culture line, viral inoculum titer, incubation temperature and interval, concentration range of the antiviral agent studied, reference strains, assay method, and end point determination and interpretation. The virus inoculum titer has been shown to affect the end point evaluation; a large inoculum can render a susceptible isolate appear resistant, whereas a reduced inoculum can make all isolates appear susceptible (2). The duration of incubation must be sufficient to permit detection of small plaques in the plaque reduction assay (PRA) or to allow growth of a potentially resistant subpopulation, which may replicate at reduced rates compared to the wild-type virus. The important consideration of the viral inoculum is the heterogeneity within the virus population. A single clinical isolate can represent a mixture of drug-susceptible and drug-resistant phenotypes (3–5).

ASSESSING ANTIVIRAL EFFICACY

Phenotypic versus Genotypic Assays

Phenotypic assays evaluate the inhibitory effect of antiviral agents on the virus population recovered from a patient. Various end point determinations have been measured and include plaque reduction as in the PRA; inhibition of viral nucleic acid synthesis; reduction in the yield of viral structural proteins such as the p29 antigen of HIV or the hemagglutinin (HA) of influenza; and the diminution in the enzymatic activity of a functional protein, for example, the reverse transcriptase (RT) of HIV-1 and the neuraminidase (NA) of influenza virus. Currently used phenotypic assays include PRA, dye uptake (DU), DNA hybridization, enzyme immunoassay (EIA), NA inhibition and yield reduction assays (YRAs), and peripheral blood mononuclear cell (PBMC)–based cocultivation and recombinant virus assay (RVA) for HIV-1. It should be noted that all assays have not been used for every viral group. Genotypic assays evaluate viral nucleic acid to detect the presence of specific sequence that causes antiviral drug resistance. Genotyping has been applied to all virus groups discussed in this chapter. The approach for genotypic assays encompass nucleic acid sequencing by automated sequencers, PCR amplification and restriction enzyme digestion of the products, and hybridization of microarrays of oligonucleotide probes. Phenotypic assays assess the combined effect of multiple resistant mutations (if present), whereas genotypic assays can only detect resistance mutation within the selected target.

Phenotypic Assays

The historical standard method of antiviral susceptibility testing has been the PRA. It is the method to which new methods are usually compared. Many variations of the PRA have been reported; a standard exists as developed by CLSI (1). The principle of the PRA is the inhibition of viral plaque formation in the presence of viral agent. The concentration at which the antiviral agent inhibits plaque formation by 50% is referred to as the IC_{50}. Although the PRA is labor-intensive and uses reagents to a greater extent than other methods, it is appropriate for small-scale testing of isolates. As discussed earlier, titers of the viral isolate need to be adjusted to ensure an inoculum appropriate for the surface area of the testing unit, wells, or plates.

The DU assay, based on preferential uptake of a vital dye (neutral red) by living but not by nonviable cells, has been used mainly for testing HSV and will not be discussed in detail here.

DNA hybridization assays are semiquantitative measures of the amount of viral DNA produced in the absence and presence of antiviral drugs. The IC_{50}s are calculated from these end points. This approach has been used to measure the effect of different antiviral compounds on DNA synthesis. The procedure has been detailed and good correlation between the PRA and a dot blot hybridization assay has been demonstrated (6,7).

EIA susceptibility testing methods for various viruses including influenza A have been developed (8). EIAs permit quantitative measurement of viral activity by spectrophotometric analysis. The IC_{50}s are calculated as the concentrations of antiviral agents that reduce absorbance to 50% of the virus control. Susceptibility testing of influenza A virus by PRA is tedious; the EIA methodology is technically easier and is more suitable for testing multiple isolates. For influenza, the EIA approach uses antibodies to influenza A virus HAs (H1 or H3). Viral growth correlates with expression of viral HA.

Another approach for assessing antiviral activity is the use of YRAs. These assays reflect the ability of an antiviral agent to inhibit the production of infectious virus instead of the formation of a plaque. For testing antiinfluenza A compounds, cell monolayers are infected with virus in the presence and absence of antiviral compound and virus replication is determined by measuring HA titers. The test virus isolate is considered drug susceptible if the HA titer is reduced at least fourfold compared to untreated virus (9,10).

Genotypic Assays

The investigation of antiviral susceptibility or the converse resistance has been studied extensively for viral agents discussed in this chapter; more recently, these studies have addressed influenza viruses. Although not all mutations that cause resistance are known, many have been defined, permitting the application of genotypic and/or sequence analysis. Genotypic assays may be more costly than phenotypic approaches but their relatively rapid turnaround time compared to phenotypic assays confers a distinct advantage. Applicable assays will be discussed for each of the viruses.

Currently, aside from spontaneous mutations, most of the available antiviral compounds are able to induce mutations, at least at their active site, resulting in a modified viral replication capacity. This varies according to the mutations, some of which may be beneficial in reducing viral replication (viral fitness). However, reciprocal interaction between mutations can only be measured by phenotypic testing. Resistance testing is currently used in clinical practice for HIV infection. These mutations in proviral DNA are being investigated. For the other viral infections presented in this chapter, that is, HBV and HCV, cytomegalovirus (CMV), and influenza, sequencing procedures for clinical practice are still at the early stage and are typically restricted to treatment failure, but rarely for treatment choice, for lack of a significant number of available compounds. However, their use for epidemiologic purposes has been amply demonstrated. This has provided data on viral variability among different countries.

ANTIVIRAL AGENTS FOR HIV: MODE OF ACTION AND ANTIVIRAL RESISTANCE

Considerable progress has been made in defining the indications for resistance testing and determining the cost-effectiveness of strategies that use testing in the management of HIV-infected individuals. Prospective, randomized trials have shown at least short-term virologic benefits for resistance testing (11). Moreover, emerging data indicate that viral drug resistance is a problem whenever treatment is used, and it may be increasing in importance. It has also become clear that knowledge concerning patterns of resistance and cross-resistance is critical to the development of successful sequential antiretroviral (ARV) regimens.

In developed countries, resistance testing has been adopted as the standard of care in case of failure to respond to ARV treatments for HIV infection (12,13). Drug resistance testing became an essential tool to assist clinicians in the selection of potent ARV drug regimens that will enhance the likelihood of favorable treatment responses. In the United States, more than 20 ARV drugs are approved for use; they belong to six classes of drugs based on their mechanism of action (Fig. 11.1). The ARV types are nucleoside/nucleotide reverse transcriptase inhibitors (NRTIs), nonnucleoside/nucleotide reverse transcriptase inhibitors (NNRTIs), protease inhibitors (PIs), chemokine receptor 5 (CCR5) antagonists, integrase strand transfer inhibitors (INSTIs), and fusion inhibitors.

To better understand the modes of action and antiviral resistance of HIV the basic structure of the virus should be appreciated. HIV is a member of the *Lentivirus* genus in the *Retroviridae* family. The retrovirus genome consists of two RNA molecules transmitted as a single stranded positive sense enveloped virus. Upon entry into the target cell, viral RNA is reverse transcribed into double-stranded DNA by virally encoded reverse transcriptase that is transported with the viral genome in the virus particle. Two different approaches are used to assess HIV drug resistance: genotyping and phenotyping. Understanding the characteristics, performances, and the interpretation of these assays is needed to use them optimally (14–16). Genotypic assays detect mutations expressed as nucleotide disarray resulting in amino acid changes that have been shown to correlate with in vitro and/or in vivo resistance to a particular drug or class of drugs. Phenotypic assays provide quantitative measure of drug susceptibility by

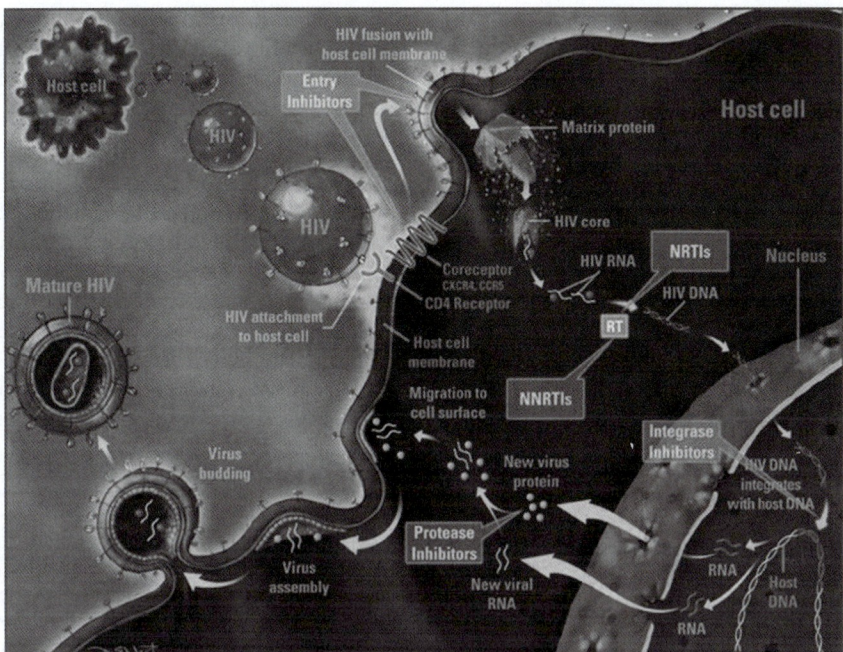

Figure 11.1 ■ Replication cycle of HIV: sites of antiviral action. (See Color Plate in the front of the book.)

determining the concentration of drug required to inhibit virus replication in cell culture.

ARV resistance due to viral gene mutations accounts for a large portion of treatment failures. The emergence of these genetic changes in HIV type 1 (HIV-1) is fostered by ongoing viral replication in the presence of subinhibitory concentrations of ARVs. Poor penetration of drugs into certain body compartments (sanctuary sites), inadequate adherence, and variable pharmacokinetic factors may contribute to subtherapeutic drug levels in vivo. This, in turn, may allow for selection of either preexisting (archived) or newly generated drug-resistant mutants. The critical problem in the clinical setting is that a mutant selected by a failing regimen may have some degree of cross-resistance to other drugs in the same class that have not yet been prescribed to that patient. The development of cross-resistance may lead to a reduced virologic or immunologic response to subsequent regimens. As scientists develop new agents active against resistant virus (see Fig. 11.1), clinical medicine is also implementing diagnostic strategies designed to detect ARV resistance and individualize subsequent regimens.

ARV resistance develops when viral replication continues in the presence of the selective pressure of drug exposure. As previously noted, the 20 approved ARV drugs belong to six classes based upon their mechanism of action (see Fig. 11.1).

For some drugs, such as the NRTI lamivudine and all available NNRTIs, a single mutation induces high-grade resistance in a predictable manner. For others such as zidovudine, abacavir, tenofovir, and most PIs, high-grade resistance requires the serial accumulation of multiple mutations and is thus slower to emerge.

Nucleoside and Nucleotide Reverse Transcriptase Inhibitors

Although most of the mutations associated with NRTI resistance are not at the active site of the enzyme, they do lead to conformational changes that affect the active site aspartate residues. Different mutations lead to two different mechanisms for resistance: decreased substrate binding and increased phosphorolysis (removal of the chain-terminating substrate that has already been incorporated into the growing proviral DNA chain). Both mechanisms lead to an overall net decrease in termination of the elongating chain of HIV DNA by the NRTI.

Nonnucleoside Reverse Transcriptase Inhibitors

Two patterns of multi-NNRTI resistance have been described. One is the K103N RT mutation. This single mutation confers resistance to all currently available NNRTIs, presumably by stabilizing the closed-pocket form of the enzyme, thus inhibiting the binding of the drug to its target. The fact that all available agents in this class bind to the same domain explains the broad pattern of cross-resistance and has prompted the development of new agents that interact with this domain more favorably. Indeed, another pattern of multi-NNRTI resistance is the accumulation of multiple mutations including L100I, V106A, Y181C, G190S/A, and M230L. Rarely, Y188L causes multi-NNRTI resistance.

Enhanced susceptibility to NNRTIs (i.e., hypersusceptibility) has been described in association with multiple mutations conferring broad cross-resistance to NRTIs and a lack of NNRTI resistance mutations. Longer duration of NRTI use, prior use of zidovudine, and abacavir or zidovudine resistance all have been associated with hypersusceptibility. This phenomenon appears to have biologic significance, with its presence enhancing the response to efavirenz-based regimens. A significantly greater short-term reduction in plasma HIV-1 RNA level, showing hypersusceptibility to efavirenz, was noted in patients who received that drug for salvage therapy.

Protease Inhibitors

The sequential use of certain PIs may be possible in some situations because several drugs in this class have distinctive major resistance mutations. This is particularly true for nelfinavir and has been suggested for atazanavir. All other PIs retain activity in vitro and in vivo against D30N isolates selected by nelfinavir. Less commonly, nelfinavir failure is associated with L90M, which is more likely to add to cross-resistance to other PIs. The I50V amprenavir resistance mutation alters the hydrophobic interaction with the target and had been thought to alter the binding of other drugs in this class only minimally. Clinical evidence to support particular PI sequencing, except that for nelfinavir, is lacking.

The presence of two key mutations (e.g., D30N, G48V, I50V, V82A/F/T/S, I84V, and L90M) generally confers broad cross-resistance to most currently available PIs. One strategy to avoid the accumulation of multiple mutations is to use low-dose ritonavir to increase the circulating levels (or "boost") of other PIs (e.g., lopinavir, indinavir, amprenavir, and saquinavir), which may result in higher and more prolonged drug concentrations and greater suppression of viral variants that contain a limited number of mutations. Thus, resistance depends not only on intrinsic properties of the virus but also on the achievable plasma levels of the drug.

Fusion Inhibitors

The fusion inhibitor operates by interfering with the fusion of viral and cellular membrane and thus entry into the CD4 cell. It binds to the initial heptad repeat (HR1) in the gp41 subunit of the viral envelope glycoprotein and prevents conformational changes required for fusion of the viral and cellular membranes. Enfuvirtide is the currently available fusion inhibitor delivered by subcutaneous injection. This agent is typically reserved for salvage therapy.

Integrase Strand Transfer Inhibitors

ARVs of this category obstruct integrase by binding in the catalytic core domain of the enzyme and competing for binding with host DNA. This action prevents integrase from inserting the viral genome into host DNA. Raltegravir is the currently available compound. Dolutegravir is a once-daily alternative to raltegravir.

When initiating therapy for HIV-infected patients that are considered naive, that is, never before been treated for infection, the U.S. Food and Drug Administration (FDA) panel recommends that therapy consist of two NRTIs and at least one ARV from another ARV class including a NNRTI, INSTI, or PI. The reference Web site provides up-to-date preferred regimens and weighs the strength of recommendations (Panel on Antiretroviral Guidelines for Adults and Adolescents. Guidelines for the Use of Antiretroviral Agents in HIV-1-Infected Adults and Adolescents. http://www.aidinfo.nih.gov).

Entry Inhibitors

Entry of HIV-1 into target cells is a multistep process involving attachment (mediated by gp120 binding to CD4), chemokine coreceptor binding, and association of two trimeric helical coils (HR-1 and HR-2) located in the ectodomain of gp41 into a six-helix bundle that brings the virus and cell membranes into close approximation, allowing membrane fusion to occur. A number of drugs currently in development block HIV-1 infection by interfering with one of these steps. The recently approved fusion inhibitor enfuvirtide (known as T-20) blocks the association of HR-1 with HR-2 by binding to the trimeric HR-1 complex, thereby inhibiting fusion and blocking virus entry (17). Mutations in HR-1 that reduce enfuvirtide susceptibility are selected by in vitro passage of HIV-1 in the presence of the drug and have been identified in isolates obtained from patients receiving enfuvirtide in clinical trials.

Identification of the presence of drug resistance by means of genotypic or phenotypic resistance assays can help a health care provider select a combination of ARVs that is likely to suppress HIV-1 replication (i.e., "active drugs" to which that patient's virus population is not cross-resistant). To maximize the therapeutic benefit and minimize toxicity, information collected from the viral genotype or phenotype must be used in conjunction with the patient's ARV treatment history, response to past regimens, immunologic status, pharmacologic data, and the clinician's own knowledge of ARV drugs. Knowing when and how to use resistance testing in a clinical practice will lead to better clinical management of HIV-1–infected patients.

METHODS

Resistance assays use different technologies that provide complementary information about ARV resistance. As noted earlier, the two different types of drug resistance tests available are genotypic and phenotypic assays. Genotype assays provide information about viral mutations that may result in changes in viral susceptibility to particular drugs or classes of drugs. Phenotype assays directly quantitate the level of susceptibility of a patient's virus sample to specific drugs in vitro. The values measured from the patient sample are compared with values measured from a standard wild-type reference strain. The degree of phenotypic resistance is the difference in susceptibility to a particular drug between the patient sample and the reference strain. In most cases, both genotype and phenotype testing methods require the use of polymerase chain reaction (PCR) technology to amplify the HIV-1 genes of interest (PR and RT) from patients' plasma samples. However, there are numerous differences between these two resistance testing methods.

Phenotypic Testing

Several phenotypic assays have been in use for testing HIV-1. A serious limitation of some of these procedures is that not all clinical isolates grow in the cell culture lines used in these assays.

In the late 1980s, the first developed phenotypic assays were PBMC assays that required isolation of the virus by cocultivating patient's PBMCs with mitogen-stimulated PBMCs obtained from HIV-seronegative donors, then titration of the virus stock. Subsequently, the inhibition of virus growth, in the presence of several concentrations of the drug, was evaluated by measurement of p24 Ag or RT activity in comparison with the replication in the absence of drug (18,19). These PBMC assay methods had several limitations regarding the difficulties in standardization, the interassay variability, and the burdensome workload for laboratory personnel. Overall, the PBMC compartment does not represent the actively replicating virus population present in the plasma compartment.

The development of RVA method, first described in 1994 (20), enabled the measurement of phenotypic resistance on a large scale. Since 1998, two companies have developed RVA assays: Antivirogram (Virco BVBA, Mechelen, Belgium) and PhenoSense (ViroLogic Inc, San Francisco, CA) (21). Antivirogram was the first RVA adapted to commercial development. The overall approach of the three commercial phenotypic assays is similar, but each assay is performed using different protocols (extraction, amplification) and reagents (viral vectors, cell lines, titration of the virus) (Table 11.1). Assays use PCR to amplify the entire protease, much of RT, and a part of the 3′ end of gag gene, including cleavage sites (p4/p2, p2/p7, p7/p1, p1/p6) from HIV-1 RNA extracted from patient plasma. Phenotypic PI resistance may be modulated by mutations at gag-pol cleavage sites, and four of the nine cleavage sites in the recombinant virus come from the patient virus and five from the laboratory virus construct. The amplified material is incorporated into vectors that derive from full-length molecular clones of HIV-1 but lack the protease and RT regions of the pol gene to create a recombinant HIV-1 isolate. After amplification, two strategies have been used to insert patient PR and RT sequences into vectors: The Antivirogram test (Virco BVBA, Mechelen, Belgium) uses homologous recombination following cotransfection of cell lines, whereas the PhenoSense assay (ViroLogic Inc, San Francisco, CA) uses site-specific endonuclease cleavage and direct ligation. Ligation products that are capable of propagating the vectors to high copy number are then introduced into bacterial cells. High virus stocks are generated by transfecting the recombinant viral vector DNA.

Table 11.1

	Antivirogram	PhenoSense
Characteristics of Commercial Phenotypic Resistance Assays		
Requirements:		
Viral load	• 1,000 copies/mL	• 500 copies/mL
Volume	• <500 μL (ideal, 3 mL)	• 1 mL
Amplification of PR and RT	• RT-PCR (two rounds, PCR) • PR/RT amplified together PR (10–99), RT (1–500)	• Purification of viral RNA • RT-PCR (one round, PCR) • PR/RT amplified together: 3'gag, PR (1–99), RT (1–305)
Assembly of recombinant virus	Transfected producer cells: MT4 and homologous recombination between: • PR/RT products (2.2 kB) • Infectious ΔPR/RT HIV vector	DNA ligation between: • PR/RT products (1.5 kB) • ΔPR/RT HIV vector with luciferase gene in envelope. Propagation of retroviral vector as bacterial plasmid
Preparation of virus stock	Multiple rounds of replication competent virus in MT4 after homologous recombination	Single burst of virus after transfection of HEK293 cells by: • Recombinant vector • Plasmid encoding the envelope of A-MLV • PI added to transfected cells • RT added at the infection step (fresh HEK293)
Drug susceptibility	• Titration of recombinant viruses using cells containing a fluorescent reporter gene	
Assay readout	Fluorescent readout of indicator cells	Luciferase indicator gene in virus vector; bioluminescence readout
Turnaround time	3–4 weeks	2 weeks

PR, protease; RT, reverse transcriptase; RT-PCR, reverse transcriptase polymerase chain reaction; PCR, polymerase chain reaction; kB, kilobase; HEK293, human embryonic kidney 293 cell line; A-MLV, amphotropic murine leukemia virus.

PhenoSense assay (ViroLogic Inc, San Francisco, CA) is a single-cycle assay using recombinant viruses that are limited to a single round of viral replication by a specific deletion in the HIV *env* gene of the vector. In this assay, evaluation of reverse transcriptase inhibitors (RTIs) involve serial dilutions of drugs added to the target cell line at the time of virus inoculation to block RT activity at the cell entry. PIs are evaluated by adding serial dilutions of drug to the transfected cells producing the virus stocks. In the Antivirogram (Virco BVBA, Mechelen, Belgium) assay, generation of high virus stocks is obtained by cultivating the recombinant viruses for several replication cycles (1 to 2 weeks). Then the virus stock is titrated before testing for drug susceptibility. Either PIs or RTIs can be evaluated using the same format by adding serial dilutions of drug to the cultures at the time of virus inoculation.

Commercially available RVA systems exploit the use of sensitive reporter genes that have been engineered into the target cells or the retroviral vector. Transcription of the reporter gene is placed under the regulatory control of the HIV-1 promoter/enhancer within the long terminal repeat (LTR). With infection with the recombinant virus, reporter gene expression is transactivated by the HIV-1 tat protein that is produced early in the HIV-1 replication cycle.

Drug susceptibility is assessed by comparing the IC_{50} of the patient virus to the IC_{50} of a drug-susceptible reference strain derived from the NL4–3 or HXB2 strain. Assay data are analyzed by plotting the percent inhibition of virus replication versus the log_{10} drug concentration. The final results are expressed as fold change or resistance indices, which are calculated as the IC_{50} of the patient virus divided by the IC_{50} of the reference virus. The Antivirogram (Virco BVBA, Mechelen,

Belgium) assay results report IC_{50} values with graphic- and numerical-fold change values.

These phenotypic methods have been adapted to measure drug susceptibility to the entry inhibitors (22). The first results showed a very large variability in the IC_{50} of isolates from drug-naive patients. Such variability of up to 3 logs difference in IC_{50} is not yet explained.

Studies evaluating the comparative performances of the different phenotyping assays are limited. Excellent concordance was observed between the Antivirogram (Virco BVBA, Mechelen, Belgium) and PhenoSense (ViroLogic Inc, San Francisco, CA) assays (23) but the majority of the viruses tested were of the wild type.

Phenotypic Assays

Several phenotypic assays are available for determining the susceptibility of an HIV-1 isolate to nucleoside analog RT inhibitors. As noted earlier, a serious limitation of some of these procedures is that the clinical isolate recovered may not grow in the designated cell culture lines used in these assays. In order to meet this challenge, the AIDS Clinical Trials Group developed an assay performed in PBMCs that allows for most clinical isolates at HIV-1 (24). Viral end point is measured by quantitating p-24 antigens. To circumvent the typical drawbacks of phenotypic assays, a new iteration was developed, the RVAs. The two RVAs commercially available were previously noted: the Antivirogram (Virco BVBA, Mechelen, Belgium) assay (25) and the PhenoSense (ViroLogic Inc, San Francisco, CA) assay (21). In addition to the lengthy turnaround time of these phenotypic assays (~10 days) is the requirement for a minimum of 500 to 1,000 copies of HIV-1 RNA/mL plasma.

An unusual phenotypic assay exploits the requirement for HIV-1 to bind to a coreceptor, in addition to CD-4 for the virus to gain entry into the host cell; CXC chemokine receptor type 4 (CXCR4) and CCR5 are two major coreceptors for HIV-1 expressed on T lymphocytes and macrophages, respectively. A recently introduced entry inhibitor, Maraviroc, exploits the necessity for HIV-1 to bind to CCR5, preventing fusion of HIV-1 and T-lymphocyte membrane, thus blocking entry into cells. However, some HIV-1 strains exhibit "dual-tropism," that is, they use both CXCR4 and CCR5 receptors; patient isolates must be characterized prior to initiation of Maraviroc therapy by means of a tropism assay to discern the required receptor(s). Commercially available tropism assay(s) are extant:

the Phenoscript assay and the Trofile (Laboratory Corporation of America Holdings, Burlington, NC) assay. For integrase inhibitors such as raltegravir, an alternative specific phenotypic assay, PhenoSense Integrase (ViroLogic Inc, San Francisco, CA), is available. Mutations that confer resistance to integrase inhibitors have been elucidated and encompass two different pathways with a major mutation of either Q148/K/R or N155H. Using this information, laboratories can develop genotypic assays to detect this resistance capability.

Phenotypic drug susceptibility assay results are interpreted by comparing the replication of patient-derived viruses to replication of well-characterized laboratory strains at equivalent drug concentrations. The phenotypic assay cutoffs (change in IC_{50}) defining whether the patient viral strain is susceptible or resistant are evolving. Former assays used "technical" cutoffs that refer to the interassay variability of the controls (one- to twofold for PhenoSense [ViroLogic Inc, San Francisco, CA] and two- to fourfold for Antivirogram [Virco BVBA, Mechelen, Belgium]). The "biologic" cutoff was obtained by testing a large number of viruses from treatment-naive individuals and defining the natural distribution of drug susceptibility in HIV-1 strains. The most relevant interpretation of phenotypic assay results is based on "clinical" cutoffs, which are distinct for each ARV drug and different for each assay system. Clinically relevant cutoffs available for a limited number of drugs are based on analysis of the relationship between baseline phenotype and reduction in viral load (Table 11.2).

In the Antivirogram (Virco BVBA, Mechelen, Belgium) assay, biologic cutoff values are the basis for reporting assay results for all drugs tested except tenofovir and lopinavir/ritonavir, which are based on clinical response data. In the PhenoSense (ViroLogic Inc, San Francisco, CA) assay, results for lopinavir/ritonavir (26), abacavir (27), tenofovir (28), stavudine, and didanosine (29,30) are reported using clinically derived cutoffs. The PhenoSense (ViroLogic Inc, San Francisco, CA) assay can also measure increased susceptibility, often referred to as *hypersusceptibility*. This phenomenon has been mainly described for NNRTI drugs and is associated with resistance to nucleoside analogs (31). In a retrospective analysis of virologic outcome in patients who were NNRTI naive and NRTI experienced, increased susceptibility to efavirenz (as defined as less than 0.4-fold in susceptibility) was independently predictive of reduction in virologic failure (32). Even partial activity may be clinically useful when treatment options are limited (26).

There are ongoing efforts to develop clinical cutoffs for all approved ARV drugs, but some clinical cutoffs are difficult to establish as they are too close to the technical cutoff or the variability of the assay (33). When interpreting the results of phenotypic assay, the clinician should consider how each cutoff was derived (Table 11.2).

Genotypic Testing

The presence of resistance mutations by genotypic assays is identified by DNA sequencing or point mutation assays such as hybridization assays. Most diagnostic laboratories developed their own assays, which are referred to as *home-brew* assays. All genotypic assays require extraction of the virus genome, usually from the plasma specimen, then retrotranscription of the viral RNA in cDNA. Subsequently, the DNA is amplified in a single or nested PCR. Dideoxynucleotide sequencing is the standard approach to HIV genotyping (34).

Mutations in the nucleic acid sequence cause amino acid substitutions when messenger RNA (mRNA) is translated into protein. Some mutations are "silent mutations"; that is, the nucleic acid changes do not alter the amino acid sequence. Mutations are designated in a short-hand format using single-letter abbreviations for the amino acids encoded by a particular triplet of nucleotides (a codon). The normal, or wild-type, amino acid present at a particular location in a protein is given, followed by the location (amino acid position, or codon number), followed by the new amino acid that has replaced the wild-type amino acid. The designation L90M, for example, indicates that the amino acid methionine (M) has been substituted for the wild-type amino acid leucine (L) at position 90, which is one of the codons in the region that codes for the protease enzyme, and is designated PR. The region that codes for the reverse transcriptase enzyme is designated RT.

In 2001, a commercial HIV-1 RT and protease genotyping kit was approved by the FDA and European Medical Evaluation Agency (EMEA) for use in clinical settings. A second kit was FDA- and EMEA-approved in 2002 (Table 11.3). The advantages of using approved kits include standardization and consistency of results across laboratories, making them preferable to laboratory-developed tests (LDTs), previously known as *home-brew tests* in local laboratories with low experience in molecular biology. However, the commercial kits are more expensive and may not provide the flexibility of home-brew methods.

Table 11.2

Commercial Phenotypic Assays: Biologic or Clinical Cutoffs

Drug	Antivirogram	PhenoSense
Zidovudine	4.0	2.2
Lamivudine	4.5	2.5
Didanosine	3.5	1.7[a]
Zalcitabine	3.5	1.7
Stavudine	3.0	1.7[a]
Abacavir	3.0	4.5–6.5[a,b]
Tenofovir	4.0[a]	1.4–4[a,b]
Nevirapine	8.0	2.5
Delavirdine	10.0	2.5
Efavirenz	6.0	2.5
Indinavir	3.0	2.5
Ritonavir	3.5	2.5
Nelfinavir	4.0	2.5
Saquinavir	2.5	2.5
Amprenavir	2.5	2.5
Lopinavir	10.0[a]	10.0[a]

[a]Clinical cutoff.
[b]The lowest cutoff corresponds to a possible virologic response and the highest to the absence of response.

Overview of a Laboratory-Developed Test Sequencing Method: HIV-1 RNA Extraction, cDNA Synthesis, Amplification, and Sequencing

Genotypic Assays

The interactions between different mutations complicate the interpretation of genotypic assays. Mutations are designated by the wild-type amino acid present at a particular position of the RT or protease gene, followed by the amino acid position, then by the new amino acid that has replaced the wild-type amino acid. For example, M184V indicates that the methionine (M) wild-type amino acid at position 184 of the RT gene is replaced by the valine (V) amino acid. A large number of genotypic-resistance interpretation tools have been developed in recent years. These include mutation lists, rule-based algorithms, and interpretations based on databases correlating genotypes with corresponding phenotypic

Table 11.3

Characteristics of Commercial HIV-1 Genotypic Assays		
	TruGene HIV-1 Genotyping Kit	**ViroSeq HIV-1 Genotyping System**
Requirements	1,000 copies/mL	1,000 copies/mL
Sequenced region	RT: codons 39–244 PR: codons 1–99	RT: codons 1–335 PR: codons 1–99
Contents of the kit	• RT-PCR • Clip sequencing • Electrophoresis • Software for interpretation	• RNA extraction • RT-PCR • Sequencing • Software for interpretation
Interpretation and reporting	• List of resistance mutations • Interpretation by rule-based algorithm available in the package	• List of resistance mutations • List of unknown mutations as compared with HXB2 • Interpretation by proprietary algorithm

RT, reverse transcriptase; PR, protease; RT-PCR, reverse transcriptase polymerase chain reaction.

susceptibilities. The listing of mutations associated with resistance is available through the expert panel of International AIDS Society (IAS)-USA (http://www.iasusa.org) or Los Alamos National Laboratory (http://hiv-web.lanl.gov).

The interpretation of genotypic assays is based on interpretation systems called algorithms. They have the objective, in treated patients, to predict the response to each ARV according to the combination of mutations present on the RT and protease genes. More than 20 algorithms are available from different sources. Some algorithms are public and available on Web sites, such as the algorithms from Stanford University (http//hivdb.stanford .edu), the Rega Institute (http://www.kuleuven .ac.be), and the Agence Nationale de Recherches sur le Sida et les hépatites virales (http://www .hivfrenchresistance.org).

The early approach to interpreting genotypes was based on the in vitro correlation studies relating genotype with phenotype. However, recent data showed difficulty in determining reliable phenotypic cutoffs for some drugs such as stavudine, didanosine, and amprenavir (33,35). Correlation studies analyzing the virologic response in treatment-experienced patients according to the genotypic profile at baseline should provide the most relevant information for establishing algorithms. Such algorithms are still limited and available for some ARV drugs such as abacavir (36), stavudine (37,38), amprenavir (39), lopinavir (26,40,41) and tenofovir (28). The method issues for correlating baseline phenotype with virologic response also apply to analyses of baseline genotype and

response. To build up such algorithms, a strict method is needed that is not standardized. Multivariate analyses must show the predictive value of the algorithm when there are confounding factors such as viral load at baseline, previous drug history, duration of past treatment, and new drugs in the regimen (42). Then the validation step must confirm that the algorithm is also predictive of the virological response in a different data set (37). These correlation studies are based on retrospective analyses of patients enrolled in therapeutic trials that are sometimes several years old. The accuracy of these algorithms depends on the prevalence of specific resistant mutations at baseline; some mutations, relevant to the resistance but underrepresented in the genotype profile, will be ignored by the algorithm.

No single study can be expected to provide a full picture of the relationship between genotype and response. The genotypic profile of patients is changing as new drugs become available that may select for previously unknown mutations. There is a need for wide-ranging databases containing appropriately quality-controlled data from genotypic resistance assays and international efforts to be developed to pool databases and to establish standardized analyses for constructing algorithms that need to be frequently refined.

Different reporting formats and interpretation systems are provided by the wide diversity of clinical virology laboratories providing HIV genotyping. Laboratories using home-brew assays have varied approaches to reporting the results. Some laboratories provide only a list of mutations, and understanding by clinicians is poor. In addition to listing each resistance mutation detected in RT and PR genes, the interpretation must be provided with the precise indication of the algorithm used.

Reports of genotypic resistance usually score virus isolates as "resistant," "possible resistant," or "no evidence of resistance." Some algorithms classify patient isolates in four or five categories. Possible resistance corresponds to different situations according to the algorithm and the drugs: The detected mutations may have been associated with diminished virologic response in some but not all patients. This classification may also refer to a limited knowledge on resistance to this particular drug.

The use of expert advice in interpreting a genotype result has been shown to lead to a better choice in the alternative regimen compared with a regimen chosen in the absence of expert advice (43). Unfortunately, such expert advice is not always available. The role of the expert is to know the bases of the algorithm and to modulate the interpretation according to the clinical and immunologic parameters of the patient.

The discordances in interpretations seem to be drug-related, low for NNRTI, and more important for some ARVs such as stavudine, didanosine, abacavir, and amprenavir (44,45). Several studies retrospectively analyzed the relationship between the different interpretations of resistance genotypes by several algorithms and the outcome of salvage treatment in cohorts of drug-experienced patients (45,46). These studies show generally significant discordances between available algorithms that are associated with different predictions of subsequent virologic outcomes.

Virtual Phenotype

Another approach to interpreting genotype is employed by Virco (47). This company maintained a large proprietary database of specimens for which both genotype and phenotype are known for each drug. From this database, viruses with the same genotype as that of the patient's virus are identified and the average IC_{50} of these matching viruses is calculated, estimating the likely phenotype of the patient's virus. Several reports support the validity of the virtual phenotype for interpreting genotypes (48). However, the accuracy of the predicted phenotype depends on the number of database matches with the patient's isolate. For the new or investigational agents, the system is

delayed by the need to accumulate genotype–phenotype data; with the availability of new drugs and the selection of new mutations, the number of matches may decrease.

INTERPRETATION OF DRUG RESISTANCE ASSAYS: DISCORDANCES BETWEEN GENOTYPE AND PHENOTYPE RESULTS

Appropriate interpretation of the results of drug resistance testing is a challenging problem for both phenotype and genotype assays (12). These interpretation tools show variability, which may modulate the choice of drugs to be used and therefore affect the therapeutic outcome. More attention is being focused on the importance of a standardized approach to interpret resistance results. Interpretation of resistance testing and choice of new therapy must be performed in light of all clinical information, including past therapies, previous viral load and immunologic responses, adherence, tolerance, and toxicities. Previous resistance test results must be considered when available.

Several studies comparing phenotype and genotype results on a large number of clinical samples showed that discordances between results are not uncommon (49,50). The clinical usefulness of genotypic testing has been demonstrated in most prospective, randomized studies; in contrast, phenotypic testing has been shown to be clinically useful in a few prospective studies. Genotypic testing is also used more commonly than phenotypic testing because of its lower cost, wider availability, and shorter turnaround time. Unlike genotyping assays, phenotyping assays involving sophisticated laboratory procedures are not available as test kits for widespread distribution.

Genotypic testing may detect a single drug resistance mutation within a virus population that will affect the virologic response but will not reduce phenotypic drug susceptibility. For example, the Y181C mutation confers in vitro susceptibility to efavirenz (51) but is associated with absence of clinical response to this drug (52). Genotypic assays detect mutations present as mixtures even if the mutation is present at a level that is too low to affect drug susceptibility in a phenotypic assay and identify reversal mutations that do not cause phenotypic drug resistance but indicate the presence of previous drug pressure. Decreased phenotypic susceptibility to some drugs may be suppressed (resensitization) by other mutations in the sequence. In the presence of thymidine mutations that decrease susceptibility to zidovudine, the presence of M184V or L74V or K65R may restore the in vitro susceptibility to this drug. Such in vitro–increased susceptibility has not been proved to be clinically relevant.

Phenotypic testing in research settings is essential for establishing genotype-phenotype correlations, which provide the first bases for interpreting genotype tests and for designing new antiviral drugs that are effective against existing drug resistance strains.

Relationship of Genotype and Phenotype Results to Drug Levels

Virus drug susceptibility is likely to be a continuous phenomenon because of partial remaining activity of the drugs against mutant viruses and variability of drug exposure.

Data correlating drug concentrations with virologic response have been generated for most PIs and NNRTIs. The concept of inhibitory quotients (IQs) characterizes the relationship between drug exposure and drug susceptibility of the virus and is defined as the C_{min} of drug divided by measure of resistance either by phenotype (IQ: C_{min}/IC_{50}), "virtual" phenotype (vIQ: C_{min}/value of IC_{50} according to the virtual phenotype), or genotype (GIQ: C_{min}/number of mutations). This concept has begun to be applied to prediction of response to PIs (53). The concept is particularly suitable for PIs that exhibit very large interindividual drug concentration variability. Although IQs have yet to be prospectively evaluated as a tool for managing HIV infection, they have been shown to be better predictors of virologic response in treatment-experienced patients receiving lopinavir boosted by ritonavir than plasma drug concentrations and/or resistance testing alone (53). The virtual IQ was the best predictor of viral load reduction in response to ritonavir boosting indinavir-based therapy in patients with ongoing viremia (54). The accurate adjustment of the in vitro–calculated IC_{50} to the in vivo protein binding remains to be determined. In PI-experienced patients receiving boosted amprenavir, the genotype IQ, using the C_{min} measured at week 8 and the number of PI resistance mutations evaluated at baseline, was the best predictor of the virologic response at week 12 (55). These approaches need to be validated in prospective clinical trials.

Practical Considerations

All genotypic and recombinant phenotypic assays use initial amplification through reverse transcriptase polymerase chain reaction (RT-PCR) as the first step in the process. Because these assays require amplification of a larger segment of the HIV-1 genome than assays designed only to detect the presence of HIV-1 RNA, they are generally less sensitive than viral load assays and require samples with at least 1,000 copies per milliliter of HIV-1 RNA to obtain amplification from plasma, although amplification is possible in some samples at lower viral load.

Plasma is the main source of virus used for testing HIV-1 drug resistance in the clinical setting. Because the half-life of HIV-1 in plasma is approximately 6 hours, only actively replicating virus can be isolated from this source; thus, the sequence of plasma virus represents the quasispecies most recently selected by ARV drugs (56). Specialized testing for research purposes can use a variety of other tissue compartments such as cerebrospinal fluid, genital secretions, PBMCs, or lymph nodes.

Blood samples may be drawn in either EDTA or acid citrate dextrose vacutainers. Heparin must be avoided as it inhibits PCR reactions. Plasma separation should be performed within a maximum of 6 hours after blood collection. Sample volume consists of 1 to 3 mL of plasma that can be stored at −80°C. Samples taken for viral load should be stored frozen within the laboratory in order that retrospective resistance testing can be undertaken.

These tests are technically demanding, and external quality control is essential. This is addressed by national and international pathology laboratory accreditation programs. Laboratories undertaking resistance testing should provide clinical support to HIV clinics and demonstrate participation in external quality control programs and accreditation by national and international agencies. In addition to quality assurance of the assay, quality assurance of the laboratory performing the assay is also required. Currently, all the laboratories in the United States that perform genotyping or phenotyping assays must have certification according to the Clinical Laboratory Improvement Act (CLIA) 1988 indicating some level of review of the laboratory's performance standard (CLIA Related Federal Register, FDA, 1995. Available at http//www.fda.gov/cdrh/clia/fr/hsq230n.html). In Europe, some hospital laboratories participate in proficiency testing programs for genotyping.

Drug costs are driving the overall total *cost* of HIV-1 care in developed countries. A National Institutes of Allergy and Infectious Diseases and Centers for Disease Control and Prevention (CDC)–funded study analyzed cost-effectiveness in genotypic resistance testing using an HIV-1 stimulation model of 1 million patients (57). The authors reported that the cost-effectiveness of genotypic resistance is similar or better than that of recommended interventions for HIV-1-infected patients, such as *Mycobacterium avium* complex prophylaxis.

There is large geographical variability in reimbursement of HIV drug resistance assays. Lack of or low levels of reimbursement may still limit access in some areas or countries. However, proper implementation of resistance assays may reduce the overall cost of patient management by prompting more appropriate choices in therapy and avoiding drugs that are likely to induce toxicities.

LIMITATIONS OF RESISTANCE TESTING

Quasispecies

Resistance testing has technical limitations. Both genotypic and phenotypic testing depends on PCR amplification of virus from plasma and therefore do not address the properties of different virus components (i.e., whole virus vs. viral genome alone). The likelihood of generating sufficient genome product to undertake further analysis depends on the starting concentration of virus. The nature of direct PCR sequencing techniques limits the detection of minority strains of virus within the plasma virus population to 20% (17,58–61). Smaller proportions of mutant virus may contribute to subsequent therapy failure and will not be detected. This component of the variable-limited portion of the virus population contributes to the concept of "quasispecies." This limitation is particularly troublesome in patients with complicated treatment histories or in those who have discontinued one or more ARV drugs. To maximize the likelihood of identifying drug resistance mutations present within the virus population of a patient, it is important to analyze plasma samples for resistance testing before changing or discontinuing ARV therapy and to consider the patient's treatment history when interpreting the results of resistance testing.

Direct PCR is done in clinical settings because it is quicker and more affordable than testing multiple clones individually. Clonal sequencing of individual strains is performed in research settings to answer questions about the pathways and evolution of HIV-1 drug resistance. Multiple quasispecies with distinct resistance genotypes coexist at any given time and some initially minority populations, with or without additional changes, can subsequently emerge as majority populations (62,63).

Cellular Reservoirs

The evolution of HIV-1 drug resistance mutations in proviral DNA in PMBCs lags behind that in plasma HIV-1 RNA. In patients with multiple virologic failures, proviral DNA may contain multiple archived mutations that are not present in plasma (64–67). Discrepancies in protease and RT resistance profiles have been described between plasma and other compartments such as cerebrospinal fluid or semen. The variable penetration of ARV drugs into sanctuary sites may contribute to the differential evolution of HIV and the emergence of drug resistance (68–70). However, the utility of sequencing virus from PBMC or from other sanctuary sites has not been evaluated in either prospective or retrospective clinical trials.

Non-B Subtypes

HIV-1 group M has evolved into multiple subtypes that differ from one another by 10% to 30% along their genomes. In North America and Europe, most HIV-1 isolates belong to subtype B. However, subtype B accounts for only a small proportion of HIV-1 isolates worldwide and non-B isolates are being identified with increasing frequency in Europe. Technically, primers used for RT, PCR, and sequencing may have a lower rate of annealing for non-B compared with subtype B templates. The performances of the different phenotypic and genotypic assays are currently being investigated. The ViroSeq HIV-1 genotyping system (Celera, Alameda, CA) was used to determine protease and RT sequences from a panel of 126 non-B subtypes isolates. Four specimens that could not be amplified included three subtype D isolates and one CRF02-AG isolate (71). The TruGene assay (Visible Genetics Inc, Toronto, Canada) using prototype 1.5 RT-PCR primers and the ViroSeq (Celera, Alameda, CA) assay were both successful for sequencing 34 non-B isolates, although five isolates (two belonging to subtype C, one to subtype B, one to subtype E, and one to subtype H) lacked double-strand sequence coverage in the ViroSeq assay (Celera, Alameda, CA) (72,73).

When mutation sequences were studied in subtype B and non–subtype B population, it was determined that all known subtype B resistance mutations were extant in the non-B subtypes and 80% were correlated with ARV treatment of patients with the non-B subtypes (74). Based on this conclusion, it appears reasonable to continue to focus on known subtype B resistance mutations for global monitoring of resistance.

It should be recognized that in general genotypic assays regardless of the methodologic approach can only detect known resistance-associated mutations. A concern with each genotypic methodology is that mutant variants may be present in the patient's infection at low frequencies and may not be detectable so that mixtures of HIV-1 strains with minor sequence variations may not be distinguishable.

OUTLOOK: HIV AND ANTIRETROVIRALS

As resistance to ARVs is anticipated to be ongoing, there will be pressure to develop new drugs and approaches to therapy for HIV infection. Clearly, the testing methodology will be genotypic, with whole genome sequencing of the virus and interpretation and resistance testing being a key component.

HEPATITIS B: STRUCTURE OF THE VIRUS AND DISCUSSION OF ANTIVIRAL AGENTS

Hepatitis B virus (HBV) was the first of the hepatitis viruses to be discovered. Whereas infection during adulthood is frequently cleared, vertical transmission from mother to child leads to persistent infection. More than *350* million people worldwide are currently persistently infected with HBV and are at risk of developing liver cirrhosis and hepatocellular carcinoma (75).

The HBV is a noncytopathic, parenteral DNA virus. The outcome of HBV infection depends on the kinetics of the virus–host interaction and particularly on the strength of the innate and adaptive, humoral, and cellular immune response. Whereas patients with acute hepatitis B have a vigorous and polyclonal immune response to HBV antigens, individuals with chronic hepatitis B have a weak and restricted immune response to HBV (76). Studies demonstrated that the latent, immune-mediated clearance mechanisms become activated spontaneously in chronically infected individuals undergoing hepatitis B e antigen (HBeAg)

clearance (77). In addition, it has been shown that immune clearance of HBV can occur via cytolytic as well as noncytolytic mechanisms (78).

The asymmetric replication of the HBV genome, via RT of an RNA intermediate, makes it prone to mutations. Although mutations can occur randomly along the HBV genome, the overlapping open reading frames (ORFs) limit the number and location of viable mutations. Viable variants are selected on the basis of replication competence of the virus, selection pressure from the host's immune system, and in some instances, exogenous factors such as antiviral therapy. The divergence of HBV sequences results in HBV quasispecies, variants, and genotypes with epidemiologic and clinical significance.

Structure of Hepatitis B

Virions

The HBV is an enveloped virus containing 3.2-kb, partially double-stranded DNA contained in a relaxed circular genome; it is the prototype member of the family Hepadnaviridae (79), which includes genetically similar viruses that infect primates and monkeys, woodchucks and ground squirrels, and herons and ducks. Electron microscopic examination of the serum of a highly viremic carrier reveals three types of virus-associated particles. The HBV virion, which is 42 nm in diameter, comprises an outer envelope formed by the hepatitis B surface antigen (HBsAg). This envelope surrounds an inner nucleocapsid made up of the hepatitis B core antigen (HBcAg) that packages the viral genome and associated polymerase. Abundant spherical particles 17 to 25 nm in diameter in numbers up to 10^{13} per milliliter and less numerous tubular structures or filaments approximately 20 to 22 nm in diameter and of variable length in numbers up to 10^{11} per milliliter do not contain HBV DNA and thus are not infectious.

Viral Genotypes

There are currently seven recognized genotypes of HBV, designated A to G, that vary by 8% at the nucleotide level over the entire genome (80). The HBV genotype designation is based on the entire genomic sequence and thus is more reliable than the serologic subtype nomenclature that was used previously, which was based on the immunoreactivity of particular antibodies to a limited number of amino acids in the envelope protein. The relationship between the four major subtypes (*adw, adr, ayw,* and *ayr*) and genotypes has been determined (Table 11.4) (81).

Table 11.4

Major Hepatitis B Virus Genotypes

Genotype	Subtype	Genome Length (nt)	Global Distribution
A	adw2, ayw1	3,221	USA, Western Europe, Central Africa, India
B	adw2, ayw1	3,215	Asia
C	adw2, adr, ayr	3,215	East Asia, Polynesia
D	ayw	3,182	Mediterranean area, India
E	ayw	3,212	West Africa
F	adw, ayw	3,215	Central and South America, Polynesia
G	adw	3,248	USA, Europe

Important pathogenic and therapeutic differences do exist among HBV genotypes (82). For example, genotype C is associated with more severe disease than genotype B, and genotype D is associated with more severe disease than genotype A (83). Genotypes C and D are associated with a lower response rate to interferon therapy than genotypes B and A (81,83). Recombination between two HBV genotypes has been reported for genotypes B and C (84) and genotypes A and D (85), generating more diversity.

Genome and Common Mutants of Hepatitis B Virus

The genome of HBV is a partially double-stranded, relaxed, circular DNA molecule about 3,200 nucleotides (nt) in length (Fig. 11.2) (79). The two linear DNA strands are held in a circular configuration by a 226-base pair (bp) cohesive overlap between the 5′ ends of the two DNA strands that contain 12-nt direct repeats called DR1 and DR2 (79). All known complete HBV genomes are gapped and circular, comprising between 3,181 and 3,221 bases, depending on the genotype (see Table 11.4). Within the virion, the minus strand has a fixed length with defined 5′ and 3′ ends and a terminal redundancy of 8 to 9 nt (86). The minus strand is not a closed circle and has a nick near the 5′ end of the plus strand. The viral polymerase is covalently bound to the 5′ end of the minus strand. The 5′ end of the plus strand contains an 18-base-long oligoribonucleotide, which is capped in the same manner as mRNA (86). The 3′ end of the plus strand is not at a fixed position,

so most viral genomes contain a single-stranded gap region of variable length ranging from 20% to 80% of genomic length that can be filled in by the endogenous viral DNA polymerase.

The minus strand contains four ORFs and carries all the protein-coding capacity of the virus (79). Importantly, these overlap in a frame-shifted manner with one another so that the minus strand is read one and a half times (79). The longest ORF encodes the viral polymerase (POL). The ORF for the envelope (PreS/S) genes is completely located within the POL ORF, and the ORF for the core (PreC/C) and X genes partially overlap with POL ORF. Thus, the HBV encodes more than one protein from one ORF by using multiple internal AUG codons within an ORF, creating additional start sites for protein biosynthesis. Nested sets of proteins with different N-termini are thus synthesized (80).

The HBV mutation frequency has been estimated to be approximately 1.4 to 3.2 × 10^{-5} nt substitutions per site per year, approximately 10-fold higher than for other DNA viruses (87). The HBV POL is an RT and lacks proofreading function. The mutation rate of HBV is also influenced by the clinical phase of the patients, such as immune tolerance versus immune elimination, and clinical settings such as immunosuppression and transplantation (88). The predominant HBV exists in an infected individual as the major population of the HBV quasispecies pool. The stability of the predominant HBV within this pool is maintained by particular selection pressures from the host's immune system and the constraints imposed by the overlap in reading frames, viability, and replication competence of the virus. Furthermore, the

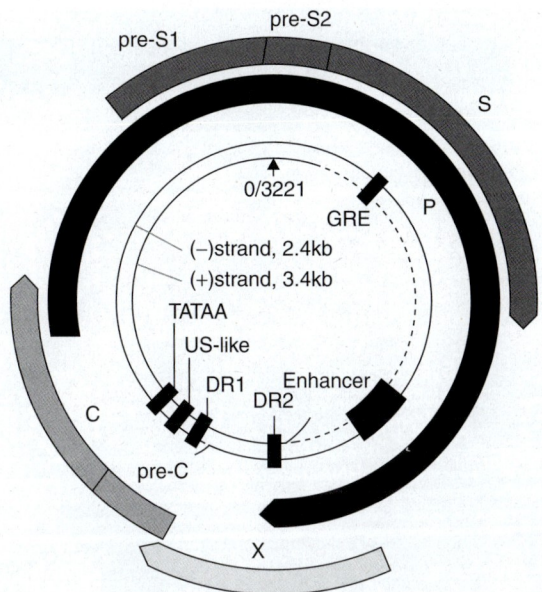

Figure 11.2 ■ Genome of hepatitis B virus (HBV). The genome of HBV, within virus particles or spherical virion, is composed of relaxed, circular, partially double-stranded DNA. The long, full-length, minus-strand is approximately 3,200 nt in length and has a protein (the viral polymerase) covalently bound to its 5′ terminus. The plus strand, which varies in length, depending on species and subtype, has a capped oligoribonucleotide at its 5′ end. The plus strand maintains genome circularity by a cohesive overlap across the 5′ and 3′ termini of the minus strand. The HBV genome includes four ORFs that encode at least seven translation products through the use of varying in-frame initiation codons. These translation products include three surface antigens (HBsAg): the envelope glycoproteins preS1, preS2, and S; core (C) and e antigens (HBcAg and HBeAg); viral polymerase (P); and the X protein (HBx). The genome is also replete with important cis-elements required for the regulation of HBV gene expression and replication. These include viral promoters, enhancers, and signal regions. The 5′ terminus of both strands contain regions of short (11-nucleotide) repeats, DR1 and DR2, which are essential for priming the synthesis of their respective DNA strands during replication.

magnitude and rate of virus replication are important, with the total viral load in serum frequently approaching 10^{11} virions per milliliter. Most estimates place the mean half-life of the serum HBV pool at about 1 to 2 days, so that the daily rate of the de novo HBV production may be as great as 10^{11} virions.

The high viral loads and turnover rates, coupled with poor replication fidelity, all influence mutation generation and the extent of the HBV quasispecies pool. Furthermore, the availability of "replication space" requires that the eventual takeover by a mutant virus depends on the loss of the original wild-type virus, which is itself governed by factors such as replication fitness and the turnover and proliferation of hepatocytes (89,90). Replication space can be understood in terms of the potential of the liver to accommodate new HBV covalently closed circular DNA molecules (cccDNA; Fig. 11.3). Synthesis of new cccDNA molecules can occur only if uninfected cells are generated by growth within

the liver, hepatocyte turnover, or loss of cccDNA from existing infected hepatocytes (91,92). Thus, the expansion of a (drug-) resistant mutant in the infected liver can be possible only with the creation of new replication space.

Mutations in the Precore/Core Promoter, Precore, and Core Genes

Two major groups of mutations have been identified that result in reduced or blocked HBeAg expression. The first group includes a translational stop codon mutation at nt 1896 of the precore gene (93). The second group of mutations affect the precore/core (pre-C/C) promoter, also called basic core promoter, at nt 1762 and nt 1764, resulting in a transcriptional reduction of the pre-C/C mRNA (Table 11.5).

The single-base substitution (G-to-A) at nt 1896 gives rise to a translational stop codon (TGG to TAG) in the second last codon (codon 28) of the

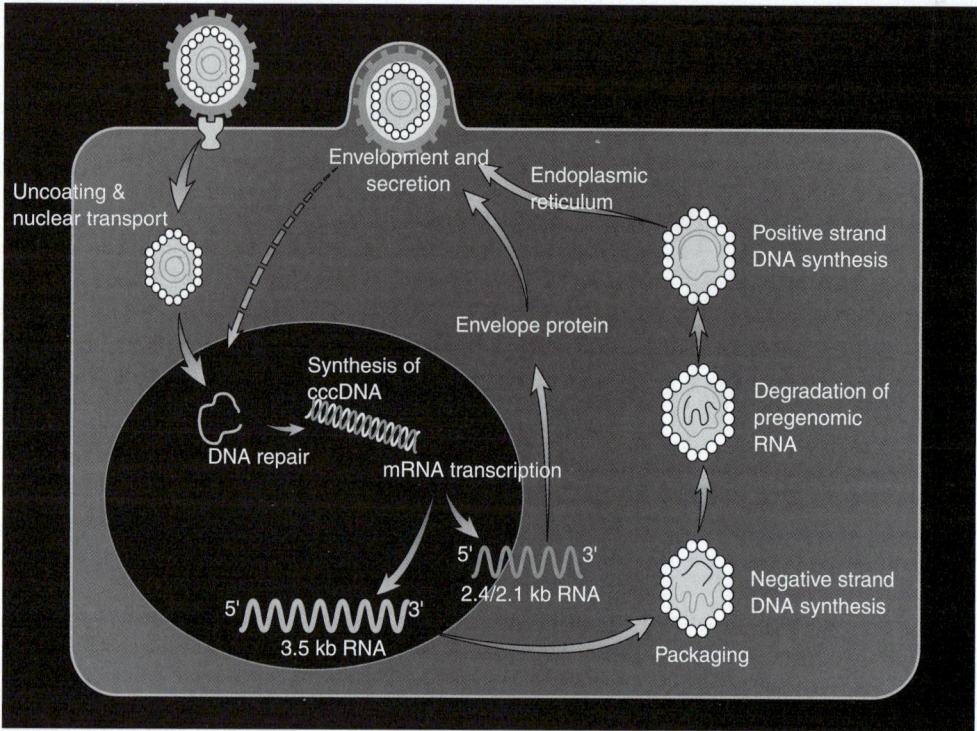

Figure 11.3 ■ Schematic illustration of the hepatitis B viral infection and replicative cycle within the hepatocyte. Infectious virions attach to a cellular receptor(s) and uncoat, releasing nucleocapsids that migrate to the cell nucleus. The partially double-stranded DNA genome is converted to cccDNA, which is the template for the transcription of four viral transcripts. Translation occurs following transcript export to the cytoplasm. The pgRNA interacts with two gene products, P and C, to form immature, RNA-packaged nucleocapsids. The pgRNA is reverse-transcribed into DNA by P. The DNA genome can be either redelivered to the nucleus, or nucleocapsids can be coated by surface glycoproteins (in the Golgi and endoplasmic reticulum) before being exported as enveloped virions.

Table 11.5

Main Forms of Hepatitis B Virus Variants/Mutants

Precore gene
 G-A at nt 1896, tryptophan-stop at codon 28 (G1896A)
 G-A at nt 1899, glycine-aspartate at codon 29 (G1889A)

Precore/core promoter gene

A-T at nt 1762 and G-A at nt 1764 (A1762T, G1764A)

Envelope gene
 Glycine-arginine at codon 145 (sG145R)
 Aspartate-alanine at codon 144 (sD144A)

Polymerase gene
 Lamivudine-resistant mutants
  Methionine-valine or isoleucine at codon 204 (rtM204V/I)
  Leucine-methionine at codon 180 (rtL180M)
 Adefovir dipivoxil–resistant mutants
  Asparagine-threonine at codon 236 (rtN236T)

precore gene located in the epsilon (ϵ) structure. The ϵ structure is a highly conserved stem loop structure, with the nt G1896 forming a base pair with nt 1858 at the base of the stem loop. In HBV genotypes B, D, E, G, and some strains of genotype C, the nt 1858 is a thymidine (T). Thus, the stop codon mutation created by G1896A (T-A) stabilizes the ϵ structure. In contrast, the precore stop codon mutation is rarely detected in HBV genotype A, F, and some strains of HBV genotype C, as the nt at position 1858 is a cytidine (C), maintaining the preferred Watson-Crick (G-C) base pairing.

Three other mutations (at nt positions 1817, 1874, and 1897) that cause truncations in HBeAg have been reported (88). In addition, changes that affect the initiation codon at nt 1814, 1815, and 1816 have been described. The mutation at G1899A is frequently detected in association with the precore stop mutation of G1896A. Early studies implicated the HBV precore stop codon mutant, leading to HBeAg negativity, as a possible virulence factor for severe liver disease and fulminant hepatitis B (94,95). However, this strain has also been found in asymptomatic carriers (96).

The pre-C/C promoter mutations, such as A1762T plus G1764A, may be found in isolation or conjunction with precore mutations, depending on the genotype (see Table 11.5). The double mutation of A1762T plus G1764A results in a decrease in HBeAg production of up to 70% (97). This mutant strain display reduced binding of liver-specific transcription factors, resulting in less pre-C/C mRNA transcripts and thus less precore protein. However, this mutation does not affect the transcription of pregenomic RNA (pgRNA) or the translation of the core or polymerase protein. Thus, by removing the inhibitory effect of the precore protein on HBV replication, the pre-C/C promoter mutations appear to enhance viral replication by suppressing pre-C/C mRNA relative to pgRNA (97). As with the precore mutations, the pre-C/C promoter mutations have not been conclusively identified as a potential virulence marker.

The core gene possesses both B cell and cytotoxic T-lymphocyte epitopes, and for the virus to persist in the infected host, during the elimination phase of hepatitis B, escape mutations within those epitopes are readily selected (88,97). Akarca and Lok (98) have demonstrated that the frequency of core gene mutations is associated with the presence of precore stop codon mutations, HBeAg negativity, and active liver disease.

Mutations in the X Gene

Mutations in the X region can involve the regulatory elements that control replication such as the pre-C/C promoter and the enhancer 1. Because the pre-C/C promoter encompasses nt 1742 to 1802 and overlaps with the X gene in the concomitant reading frame, the A1762T plus G1764A pre-C/C promoter mutations also change in the X gene at xK130M and xV131I. A novel class of HBx mutants has been found in patients with hepatocarcinoma exhibiting increased clonal outgrowth and decreased apoptosis, implying a possible role in hepatocarcinogenesis (99).

Mutations in the Envelope Gene

Most hepatitis B vaccines contain the major HBsAg, and an immune response to the major hydrophilic region induces protective immunity. Mutations in this epitope have appeared under pressure generated by vaccine-induced antibodies (100). In addition, mutations have been detected after treatment of liver-transplant patients with hepatitis B immunoglobulin (101). Most isolates have a mutation from glycine to arginine at residue 145 of HBsAg (sG145R) or aspartate to alanine at residue 144 (sD144A) (see Table 11.5). The former mutation has been shown to evade the known protective anti-HBs response.

Viral Life Cycle

An understanding of the HBV life cycle is crucial for the identification of potential antiviral targets (102,103). HBV replication begins when the virion attaches to an as yet unidentified receptor on the hepatocyte surface (see Fig. 11.3). Following viral entry, the virus uncoats and is transported to the nucleus where the relaxed circular genome is converted by the host cellular machinery to the cccDNA; the cccDNA is, in turn, organized into viral minichromosomes. This key replicative intermediate is the transcriptional template for production of the various HBV RNAs, including the pgRNA, that are necessary for viral replication and represents one of the major obstacles in the development of effective treatments for the control of HBV infection. Transcription of the 3.5-kb pgRNA serves three important roles. First, its translation leads to production of the core and POL proteins. Second, it participates in the nucleocapsid packaging reaction, the specificity of which is provided by a unique stem-bulge-stem structure known as epsilon (ϵ) on the 5′ and 3′ ends of the pgRNA (104). Following translation of the pgRNA, the POL protein binds to the 5′-end ϵ. Host proteins such as heat shock protein 90 (Hsp90) stabilize this POL–ϵ interaction (104). The *cis*-translated core proteins dimerize around the pgRNA-pol complex and self-assemble to form viral nucleocapsids (105).

Once packaged into a nucleocapsid, the pgRNA serves its third and most important role as the template for reverse transcription and DNA synthesis. The POL protein is bound to the 5′ ϵ structure and acts as its known primer for initiation and synthesis of the first three nucleotides of the negative-strand DNA (102,103). This nascent DNA is then translocated to the 3′ end of the pgRNA where it binds to the complementary sequence within a 12-nt region known as direct repeat 1 (DR1). From here, negative-strand DNA synthesis proceeds and the RNase H activity of the POL protein degrades all but the last few nucleotides of the template pgRNA. This RNA oligomer is translocated to the 3′ copy of the 12-nt repeat known as DR2, from which point positive-strand DNA synthesis begins. Elongation of the positive-strand DNA proceeds to the 5′ end of the negative strand where a third strand transfer occurs. This is facilitated by a short redundancy (r) in the negative-strand DNA template, which anneals to the r region on the 5′ end positive-strand DNA, thereby circularizing the genome (102,103). Premature termination of the positive-strand DNA synthesis by the POL protein results in the characteristic partially double-stranded genome. The HBV nucleocapsid containing the partial double-strand DNA is either recycled back to the nucleus to increase the supply of cccDNA, or undergoes further processing in the endoplasmic reticulum and Golgi for virion assembly. Mature virions are subsequently exported from the cell via the constitutive secretory pathway.

Antiviral Drugs

Success in HIV drug development in the 1990s revolutionized treatment of hepatitis B. Several antiviral agents that were developed for the treatment of HIV infection proved to be effective in inhibiting HBV replication. Several therapeutic interventions are now available encompassing five nucleoside analogs: 2′,3′-dideoxy-3′-thiacytidine (3TC), adefovir dipivoxil, telbivudine, tenofovir, and entecavir. All treatments have limited long-term efficacy. Although there have been few direct comparison trials, the short-term efficacy for both HBeAg-positive and HBeAg-negative hepatitis B appears comparable; factors predictive of response are similar. Thus, the advantages and disadvantages of each treatment, the durability of response, and the patient's preference must be carefully weighed before a decision is made (106).

The review of the HBV life cycle reveals that apart from reverse transcription, most viral processes depend on host cell machinery. The most important of these is the generation and persistence of cccDNA. Conventional antiviral inhibitors of viral DNA synthesis such as nucleoside/nucleotide analogs (Table 11.6) can prevent or reduce the development of new molecules of cccDNA. However, successful elimination of the existing pool of hepadnaviral cccDNA has only been achieved by either a noncytolytic T helper type 1 (Th1) immune response (107,108) or immune-mediated cell killing followed by hepatocyte division (109,110). In this context, it is important to note that treatment of hepatitis B with nucleoside analogs can result in the partial restoration of specific immunoresponsiveness, which appears necessary for durable host-mediated control of infection (111). Thus, the concept of successful therapy for hepatitis B is converging on the use of both antiviral and immunomodulating approaches. In this chapter, the focus is on antiviral drugs.

Evaluation of Drug Efficacy

The major role of serum HBV DNA assays in patients with hepatitis B is to assess HBV replication and candidacy for antiviral therapy. Quantitative HBV DNA testing in serum is also important in assessing the response to antiviral treatment. Historically, the molecular assays for HBV DNA detection and quantification were not well standardized. However, over the past several years

Table 11.6

Hepatitis B Antiviral Compounds		
Drug	**Class**	**Mechanism of Action**
IFN-α	Interferon	Immune-mediated clearance
IFN-α2b and pegylated lamivudine	NRTI	Cytidine analog
Adefovir dipivoxil	NRTI	dATP analog, chain terminator
Entecavir	2-Deoxyguanoside analog	Inhibits polymerase priming activity and chain elongation
Telbivudine	NRTI	dTTP analog
Tenofovir disoproxil fumarate	NRTI	dATP analog (chain terminator)
Emtricitabine	NRTI	Nucleoside analog of cytidine

IFN, interferon; NRTI, nucleoside reverse transcriptase inhibitor.

with the onset of real-time PCR, there have been significant advances. Several commercial "cleared" (approved) assays using real-time PCR or transcription-mediated amplification (TMA) from five different manufacturers have become available. The lower limit of detection (LLOD) ranges from 6 to 30 IU/mL of HBV with the upper end of the dynamic range at 8.0 $\log_{10}$ IU/mL. These assays have been reviewed by Valsamakis (112) and more recently by Chevaliez and colleagues (113) detailing LLODs and dynamic ranges.

A National Institutes of Health workshop on the management of hepatitis B proposed that the definitions and criteria of the response to antiviral therapy of hepatitis B be standardized. An arbitrary value of more than 10^5 viral copies per milliliter has been chosen as a diagnostic criterion for hepatitis B (106). However, this definition is not perfect. The proposal categorized responses as biochemical, virologic or histologic, and as on-therapy or sustained off-therapy (106) (Table 11.7).

As for HIV-1, both phenotypic and genotypic assays have been used to characterize HBV drug resistance mutations. Various phenotypic methods have been studied; several are reviewed by Shaw et al. (114). In methods involving the development of point mutations associated with drug resistance, the phenotype is deduced by

comparing replications of cell lines with or without mutations in the presence/absence of drugs. As with HIV-1, virtual phenotyping has been established that correlates patient clinical results with viral mutational data to assign a viral phenotype (114). Known mutations associated with resistance to HBV antiviral compounds are discussed by Chao and Hu (115).

Lamivudine and Virogram

Hepadnaviruses replicate through an RNA template that requires RT activity. HBV DNA polymerase was shown to share homologies with the RT from retroviruses. Inhibitors for RT of oncogenic RNA viruses may suppress HBV DNA replication. Lamivudine (Epivir) is the minus enantiomer of 3TC. It was developed as an RTI for use in HIV infection. Lamivudine has been shown to be a potent inhibitor of HBV replication in 2.2.15 cells (116). The 2.2.15 cells were clonal cells derived from Hep G2 cells that were transfected with a plasmid containing HBV DNA. These cells secreted hepatitis B virions. The 2.2.15 cells were maintained in minimal essential medium supplemented with 10% (vol/vol) fetal bovine serum (FBS). Cells were incubated at 37°C in a moist atmosphere containing 5% CO_2/95% air. The 2.2.15 cells were inoculated at a density of 3×10^5 cells per 5 mL in a 25-cm^2 flask.

The drugs studied were added to the medium 3 days after the inoculation. Cells were grown in the presence of drugs for 12 days with changes of medium every 3 days. After incubation, the medium was centrifuged (10 minutes at 2,000 $\times$ g) and polyethylene glycol (M_r, 8,000) was added to the supernatant to a final concentration of 10% (wt/vol). The virus was pelleted (10 minutes at 10,000 $\times$ g). The pellet was resuspended at 1% the original volume in TNE (10 mM Tris HCl, pH 7.5/100 mM NaCl/1 mM EDTA). The suspension was adjusted to 1% sodium dodecyl sulfate (SDS) and proteinase K at 0.5 mg/mL and incubated for 2 hours at 55°C. The digest was extracted with phenol/chloroform, 1:1 (vol/vol), and the DNA was precipitated with ethanol. The DNA pellet was dissolved in TE$_{80}$ (10 mM Tris-HCl, pH 8.0/1 mM EDTA) and then electrophoresed in a 0.8% agarose gel followed by blotting onto Hybond-N membrane. The blot was hybridized with a ^{32}P-labeled HBV DNA (*Bam* HI insert from plasmid pam6; American Type Culture Collection [ATCC]) probe, washed twice with standard saline citrate (SSC)/0.2% SDS at room temperature for 1 hour and 0.1 $\times$ SSC/0.2%

Table 11.7

Definition of Response to Antiviral Therapy of Chronic Hepatitis B

Category of Response	Criteria
Biochemical	Decrease in serum ALT to within the normal range
Virologic	Decrease in serum HBV DNA to undetectable levels (<105 copies/mL in unamplified assays) and loss of HBeAg in patients who were initially HbeAg
Histologic	Decrease in histology activity index by at least two points in comparison with pretreatment liver biopsy
Complete	Loss of HBsAg and fulfillment of criteria of biochemical and virologic response

ALT, alanine transferase; HBV, hepatitis B virus; HBeAg, hepatitis B e antigen; HBsAg, hepatitis B serum antigen.

SDS at 55°C for 30 minutes, and then autoradiographed. The intensity of the autoradiographic bands was quantified by a scanning densitometer. HBID$_{50}$ was defined as the drug concentration that inhibited HBV viral DNA yield in the medium by 50%. The values were obtained by plotting percentage inhibition compared with control versus the drug concentration.

No cell growth retardation or effects on mtDNA was observed after the administration of lamivudine at concentrations at least 100 times higher than concentrations that completely block HBV replication. Lamivudine did not affect the integrated HBV DNAs. Since the RNA replicative intermediates are transcribed from the integrated DNA, it is not surprising that HBV-specific transcripts were not affected by drug treatment. Thus, interruption of drug treatment resulted in a return of HBV virus to intra- and extracellular populations (116). Lamivudine is phosphorylated in vivo to the active triphosphate (3TC-TP) that competes with deoxycytidine triphosphate (dCTP) for DNA synthesis. It inhibits DNA synthesis by terminating the nascent proviral DNA chain.

Emergence of the YMDD mutation was associated with duration of therapy. Sixty-seven percent of patients who received lamivudine for 4 years showed evidence of the YMDD mutation, 40% of patients showing evidence after 104 weeks, 31% of patients showing evidence between weeks 52 and 104, and 14% showing evidence after 52 weeks (117,118). Drug resistance can be detected as early as 49 days after taking lamivudine (119), but clinical evidence (phenotypic expression) of drug resistance, which is indicated by a rise in serum alanine transferase (ALT), does not occur before 6 months. Mutations in the catalytic polymerase/RT domain of the gene for HBV polymerase have been associated with lamivudine resistance in patients receiving treatment for HBV infection (120). This is one of the four functional domains of HBV polymerase, which also possesses a priming region, a spacer domain, and a region with ribonuclease H activity (91). The identification of several regions of conserved sequences within the polymerase/ RT domain has led to its further subdivision into subdomains A to F. A sequence of four amino acids within the C subdomain consisting of tyrosine (Y) followed by methionine (M) and two aspartic acid (D) residues is highly conserved among viral polymerase/RTs. Termed the *YMDD motif*, it is essential for polymerase activity because of its involvement in binding nucleotide substrates in the catalytic site (120). Lamivudine resistance has

been associated with substitution of isoleucine (I) or valine (V) for methionine in the YMDD motif at position 552 (rtM204I/V) of HBV polymerase/ RT (see Table 11.5) (121). In vitro assays have confirmed that the YMDD motif mutations conferred reduced susceptibility of HBV to lamivudine (120,122). However, in vitro experiments also suggested that YMDD mutant HBV had reduced replicative efficiency in the absence of lamivudine, compared with wild-type HBV (120).

In most cases, YMDD mutations occur in combination with an additional mutation in the B subdomain rtL180M (L528M) that is located in the catalytic site near the YMDD motif in the three-dimensional model of HBV polymerase. The combined L528M/M552I or L528M/ M552V mutations have been shown to restore the in vitro viral replication capacity of HBV containing YMDD motif mutations (120). These data reaffirm the growing body of clinical data indicating that patients who develop lamivudine-resistant HBV undergo rebound in serum HBV DNA that returns to level similar to those seen prior to therapy with lamivudine (123). Modeling suggests that mutation of the YMDD motif methionine at position 552 to valine or isoleucine causes steric hindrance between the methyl group on the β-branched side chain of valine/isoleucine and the sulfur atom in the unnatural L-oxathiolane ring of lamivudine (91,121). Besides reducing the strength of binding of lamivudine to the polymerase, steric hindrance results in a different orientation of the inhibitor when bound to the mutant enzyme that reduces the efficiency of incorporation of lamivudine triphosphate into replicating viral DNA. Resistance because of steric hindrance may be a problem common to all L-nucleosides (91). These mutations do not affect binding of the natural substrate dCTP to the same degree because the deoxyribose ring is in the natural D-configuration. Thus, the effect on natural substrates is small compared with the effect on lamivudine, and the polymerase enzyme can preserve a significant, but decreased, level of activity (121).

Adefovir Dipivoxil

Adefovir dipivoxil is an oral prodrug of adefovir (9-[2-phosphonylmethoxyethyl] adenine, PMEA), a phosphonate nucleotide analog of adenosine monophosphate. It is an acyclic nucleoside phosphonate (ANP) compound (124). The antiviral effect of the ANP analogs is the result of a selective interaction of their diphosphate metabolite with the viral DNA polymerase. Based on the structural resemblance to natural deoxynucleoside triphosphates (i.e., dATP in this case), this diphosphate metabolite acts both as a competitive inhibitor and an alternative substrate during the DNA polymerase reaction. PMEA inhibited HBV release from human hepatoma cell lines Hep G2 2.2.15 and HB611 cells (transfected with human HBV) (125). The cells were seeded in 25 cm^2 tissue culture flasks (Costar, Sigma-Aldrich, St. Louis, MO) at a density of 4×10^4 cells/cm^2 in Dulbecco's modified Eagle minimum essential medium (EMEM) supplemented with 2 mmol/L L-glutamine (Flow Laboratories, Rockville, MD), garamycine (40 μg/mL), amphotericin B (2.5 μg/mL), the neomycin analog G418 (360 μg/mL for HepG2 cells; 200 μg/mL for HB611 cells), and 10% FBS. Medium was changed every 3 days. When cells reached confluency at day 6, FBS concentration was reduced to 2%. Cell cultures were maintained in 5% CO_2 atmosphere at 37°C. At day 3, the culture medium was supplemented with various concentrations of PMEA. Cell culture supernatants and cells were harvested at day 12 and subjected to HBV DNA and HBsAg analysis.

The 50% cytotoxic concentration of PMEA was determined in 24-well tissue plates (cell density: 4×10^4 cells/cm^2) by inhibition of [^{3}H] methyl-dThd incorporation during 24 hours starting at 3 days after seeding. HBsAg secretion was inhibited by PMEA in a concentration-dependent manner in HB611 cells. Moreover, in congenital duck hepatitis B virus (DHBV)–infected ducklings, PMEA at a dose of 30 mg/kg/day was found to affect a marked decrease in DHBV DNA (122). PMEA has been found to have immunostimulating effects in mice, reflected by the induction of interferon (mainly α/β) and a significant enhancement of natural killer cell activity (126,127). The interferon levels induced by PMEA, given for 5 consecutive days at a dose of 25 mg/kg^{-1}, were comparable with those achieved with the known interferon-inducer poly I:C. The natural killer enhancement by PMEA appeared to be coupled, at least in part, to interferon production. However, cytokines other than interferon may be involved, since prolonged administration of PMEA (5 mg/kg/day for 20 days) resulted in sustained natural killer enhancement in the absence of interferon production.

In two phase III clinical studies, although mutations in the polymerase sites of HBV had been described (rtS119A, rtH133L, rtV214A, rtH234Q) in 4 of 271 patients treated with adefovir dipivoxil

for 48 weeks, no adefovir resistance mutations were identified in this large group of hepatitis B patients (128). However, in 1 patient during the second year of treatment with adefovir dipivoxil, the rise of HBV DNA and the exacerbation of liver disease led to the identification of a novel asparagine-to-threonine mutation at residue rt236 in domain D of the HBV polymerase (see Table 11.5). In vitro testing of a laboratory strain encoding the rtN236T mutation and testing of patient-derived virus confirmed that the rtN236T substitution caused a marked reduction in susceptibility to adefovir dipivoxil (129).

Resistance to adefovir dipivoxil is significantly less common than for lamivudine. The emergence of resistance to adefovir dipivoxil appears to be delayed and infrequent. Adefovir is an acyclic nucleotide analog and is smaller than the bulkier oxathiolanes (121). Molecular modeling studies suggest that adefovir can be accommodated more effectively in the more constrained and "crowded" deoxynucleoside triphosphate-binding pocket that carries the rtM204V/I mutations (129). Finally, the adefovir-resistant HBV was sensitive to lamivudine (130).

Entecavir

Entecavir, a cyclopentyl guanosine analog, is a potent inhibitor of HBV DNA polymerase, inhibiting both the priming and elongation steps of viral DNA replication (106,131,132). Entecavir is phosphorylated to its triphosphate, the active compound, by cellular kinases. It is a selective inhibitor of HBV DNA. It has little or no inhibitory effect on the replication of other DNA viruses such as herpes simplex, CMV, and RNA viruses such as HIV. Entecavir is also effective against lamivudine-resistant mutants but less effective than against wild-type HBV (131,133,134). In an in vitro assay using Hep G2 2.2.15 human liver cells, the EC$_{50}$ for entecavir was 0.00375 μM compared with 0.116 μM for lamivudine. Therefore, entecavir is 30 times more potent than lamivudine in suppressing viral replication. In woodchucks with chronic woodchuck infection, doses of 0.1 mg/kg of entecavir reduced woodchuck hepatic virus (WHV) titers by 7 logs (135). In addition, after 14 months of entecavir therapy, viral core antigen, WHV, and cccDNA were undetectable in liver biopsy samples of nine WHV tested (136). There is also a decrease of the incidence of hepatocellular carcinoma and an increase of survival in treated WHVs as compared with untreated WHVs.

Entecavir has been evaluated in phase I/II clinical studies. The viral dynamics during and after entecavir therapy were studied in a small number of patients with hepatitis B receiving different doses of entecavir ranging from 0.05 to 1.0 mg/day of entecavir. The median effectiveness in blocking viral production was 96%. The median half-life of viral turnover was 16 hours and the median half-life of infected hepatocytes was 257 hours (10.7 days). Rebound of viral replication also followed a biphasic return to baseline levels (137). During short-term therapy, entecavir seems to show stronger antiviral activity than lamivudine, but this assumption should be validated by head-to-head studies. In addition, entecavir shows continuous activity in patients with detectable lamivudine-induced mutant virus (138).

Until now, no entecavir-resistant viral mutants have been described (132). Prolonged therapy as well as prophylactic therapy, for example, in liver-transplant recipients, is feasible and not limited by breakthrough infections. Different ongoing multi-center phase III studies are currently evaluating the efficacy and safety of entecavir in HBeAg-positive and HBeAg-negative patients and in patients resistant to lamivudine. These studies are comparing entecavir with lamivudine for 48 weeks with extended treatment (96 weeks).

Emtricitabine and Tenofovir

Emtricitabine (FTC) is a cytosine nucleoside analog with antiviral activity against both HBV and HIV. It differs from lamivudine in having a fluorine at the 5-position of the nucleic acid. In a pilot study, five different doses of FTC were evaluated (25, 50, 100, 200, and 300 mg daily for 8 weeks) in 49 patients with HBeAg-positive hepatitis B (106,139). At the end of treatment, serum HBV DNA decreased by 2 to 3 logs in patients receiving the higher doses.

Phase III clinical trials are underway to determine the long-term safety and efficacy of FTC. However, the role of FTC in the treatment of hepatitis B may be limited by its structural similarity to lamivudine and hence the potential for cross-resistance and the development of HBV drug-resistant mutants.

Tenofovir is a nucleotide analog approved for the treatment of HIV infection. It has in vitro activity against both wild-type and lamivudine-resistant HBV (140). A report of five patients with HBV and HIV coinfection demonstrated a $4 \log_{10}$ drop in HBV DNA levels during 24 weeks of treatment (141).

β-L-Nucleosides

The natural nucleosides in the β-L-configuration (β-L-thymidine (L-dT), β-L-2-deoxycytidine (L-dC), and β-L-2-deoxyadenosine [L-dA]) represent a newly discovered class of compounds with potent, selective, and specific activity against hepadnavirus. In vitro studies have shown that these compounds are not active against other viruses such as herpes viruses or HIV, but these compounds have marked effects on HBV replication. It is not yet clear if these compounds are active against lamivudine-resistant HBV mutants (106,142–145).

L-dT is at the most developed stage of clinical investigation and has a remarkably clean preclinical toxicology profile. So far, it does not have mitochondria toxicity and it appears not to be mutagenic. After 1 year of therapy, antiviral activity was significantly greater for L-dT compared with lamivudine, and ALT normalization was greatest for L-dT monotherapy (146). Combination therapy of L-dT and lamivudine was not more efficacious than L-dT alone.

Another promising β-L-nucleoside compound is Val-L-dC. Preliminary results in phase I/II testing indicate substantial antiviral activity with a good safety profile (106).

Combinations of β-L-nucleoside appear to have additive or synergistic effect against HBV. In vitro studies and animal testing showed that there is no evidence of cellular or mitochondrial toxicity. The combination of L-dT and Val-L-dC was analyzed in a woodchuck study. Over a 12-week treatment period, the combination of L-dT and Val-L-dC cleared WHV DNA in all of the five animals tested with no significant side effects noted.

Other Antiviral Drugs

Several compounds have been developed that have a mechanism of HBV inhibition that is unrelated to the viral polymerase. The first of these are the phenylpropenamide derivates, AT-61 and AT-130. King et al. (147) showed that AT-61 did not affect total HBV RNA production or HBV DNA polymerase activity but did significantly reduce the production of encapsidated RNA. Importantly, both AT-61 and AT-130 have identical antiviral activity against wild-type strains as well as a number of different lamivudine-resistant strains of HBV (148). In vitro studies using AT-130 showed significant inhibition of the production of encapsidated HBV RNA but had no effect on total HBV RNA and did not affect core protein or nucleocapsid production, indicating an interference with the encapsidation process itself (149). Steric inhibition or interaction with the host cell chaperone proteins such as Hsp90 may be a possible mechanism. Phenylpropenamides are not water soluble and have very low bioavailability. Their future successful development as antiviral agents will depend on overcoming potential toxicity and medicinal chemistry issues.

A second class of compounds, the heteroaryldihydropyrimidines, are also potent nonnucleoside inhibitors of HBV replication both in vitro and in vivo (150). The heteroaryldihydropyrimidine compounds include the candidate molecule Bay 41–4109 and congeners Bay 38–7690 and Bay 39–5493. Exposure of HBV-infected cells to Bay 41–4109 resulted in increased degradation of core protein through improper formation of viral nucleocapsids. These heteroaryldihydropyrimidine compounds were shown to have efficacy against HBV in the HBV-transgenic mouse model and to possess suitable preclinical pharmacokinetic and toxicologic profile (150). Their novel mechanism of action and highly specific antiviral activity indicates that future clinical studies may be warranted.

A third compound, LY582563, is a 2-amino-6-arylthio-9-phosphonomethoxyethylpurine bis (2,2,2,-trifluoro-ethyl) ester, a novel nucleotide analog derivative of phosphonomethoxyethyl purine. It belongs to a structural class that is similar to adefovir. This compound has excellent antiviral activity against HBV with a good preclinical toxicity profile (151). It is also effective against lamivudine-resistant HBV (152). Its mechanism of action and early clinical development are under investigation.

Outlook: Hepatitis B Therapies

The long-term success of therapy for hepatitis B depends on safe, effective suppression of HBV replication for a long period of time without giving rise to resistant viral strains. As the long-term efficacy of current therapy for hepatitis B is limited, the patient's age, severity of liver disease, and likely response must be weighed against the potential for adverse events and complications before treatment is initiated. Recommendations for the management of patients with hepatitis B have been recently published by an international panel (153).

In the past several years, the treatment of hepatitis B has been improved. It is now possible to contemplate combination therapy for hepatitis B. The future question is which agents to combine: two or more nucleoside/nucleotide analogs or antiviral agents plus immunomodulatory drugs. A recent report reviews several alternative rescue therapies for chronic hepatitis B (115).

Gene therapy is defined as the introduction of new genetic material into a target cell with a therapeutic benefit to the individual represents a novel approach (154). Several genetic antiviral strategies including ribozymes, antisense oligonucleotides, interfering peptides or proteins, and therapeutic DNA vaccine have been explored for the molecular therapy of hepatitis B (154,155). A novel molecular strategy that holds promise is the use of small interfering RNAs (siRNA). RNA interference is a cellular process of sequence-specific gene silencing in which small duplexes of RNA target a homologous sequence for cleavage by cellular ribonucleases (156). The introduction of approximately 22-nt siRNAs into mammalian cells can lead to specific silencing of cellular mRNAs without induction of the nonspecific interferon responses that are activated by longer RNA duplexes. Posttranscriptional gene silencing mediates resistance to both endogenous, parasitic, and exogenous pathogenic nucleic acids and can regulate the expression of protein-coding gene (156). This approach has been successfully applied to HBV (157). The siRNA molecules dramatically reduced virus-specific protein expression and RNA synthesis, and these antiviral effects were independent of interferon. Although this approach holds great promise, issues such as gene delivery, stability, toxicity, resistance, and safety need to be resolved.

HEPATITIS C VIRUS INFECTION: VIROLOGY AND CULTURE SYSTEMS FOR ANTIVIRAL DRUG STUDIES

Hepatitis C virus (HCV) is a major pathogen, harbored by over 250 million people worldwide, with a 70% risk of chronic infection for contaminated individuals (158). Chronic hepatitis may lead not only to limited histologic lesions in 20% of patients but also to severe fibrosis and cirrhosis. Complications arising from chronic HCV infection include the development of cirrhosis, end-stage liver disease, and hepatocellular carcinoma. Among the latter, at least 30% will develop hepatocellular carcinoma in the following 20 years (158,159). Accordingly, complications arising from chronic HCV are the leading cause of death from liver disease and the most common indication for liver transplantation throughout the world. Although recent progress has been made in the knowledge of the HCV life cycle, thanks to new experimental tools such as selectable subgenomic replicons, we are still limited in our understanding by the lack of an efficient cell culture system and of an easy-to-use animal model (160). Consequently, the identification of new therapeutic targets is particularly difficult. Interferon-α (IFN-α) and ribavirin have been the mainstay of available therapies for chronic HCV infection for years. Therapeutic results may appear disappointing as, at best, 50% of the treated patients will have undetectable HCV viremia when these drugs are used in combination therapy (161).

Therapeutic improvements resulted from the progression of using standard IFN-α monotherapy to pegylated interferons coupled with ribavirin when measured in the rates of sustained virologic response (SVR). Despite these improvements, the rates of cure in genotype 1 infection remained around 40% to 50% for treatment-naive individuals with poorer outcomes for African Americans, individuals with cirrhosis, prior treatment failure, and HIV coinfection (162–165).

Ongoing research in the elucidation of the HCV life cycle and crystal structures of several viral proteins has broadened the development of drug targeted at specific points in the HCV life cycle (166–169) (Table 11.8). Specifically, it has been the nonstructural (NS) protein required for ongoing viral replication and spread that have been the primary targets of drug development.

Direct-acting antiviral agents (DAAs), which include NS3/4A PIs, replication complex inhibitor (NS5A), and NS5B polymerase inhibitor, have been developed (see Table 11.8). Additionally, agents that target host protein involved in viral replication have been studied

Biology of Hepatitis C Virus

HCV is an enveloped virus containing a single-strand, positive-sense RNA (170). It belongs to the *Hepacivirus* genus of the Flaviviridae family, also containing two other genera: pestivirus and flavivirus. The most closely related virus is GBC-B, a hepatotropic virus infecting tamarins (171). The HCV genome contains approximately 9,600 nt with one ORF, encoding for a single polyprotein.

Genetic Variability of Hepatitis C Virus

Despite this apparently basic genetic structure, the polyprotein may vary, depending on the genotype. In fact, HCV RNA shows wide genetic variability as the estimated rate of nucleotide change is around 10^3 substitutions per site per year (172), although this rate of nucleotide change depends on the considered genomic region. For example, the polyprotein is flanked by two nontranslated regions that are highly conserved and in contrast, some hot spots of mutations have been recognized, particularly in the E2 envelope protein, which contains two hypervariable sequences (173). It is noteworthy that this genetic variability

Table 11.8

Antiviral Agents for Hepatitis C Virus		
Drug	**Class**	**Mechanism of Action/Features**
Boceprevir	NS3/4A serine PI	Inhibits cleavage of viral protein during and after translation by blocking viral protease/metabolized via P450 system; associated with drug–drug interactions
Danoprevir		
Telaprevir		Low genetic barrier to resistance
Vaniprevir		
Mericitabine	NS5B nucleoside polymerase inhibitor	Nucleoside analogue that binds active site of NS5B polymerase enzyme and terminates viral RNA generation; effective vs. all genotypes
Filibuvir		
Alisporvir	Cyclophilin inhibitor	Targets host cyclophilin enzyme which may modulate NS5A function; effective vs. all HIV genotypes

From Fox AN, Jacobsen IM. Recent successes and noteworthy future prospects in the treatment of chronic hepatitis C. *Clin Infect Dis* 2012;55(Suppl 1):S16–S24.

complicates study designs of HCV pathogenesis since a single viral protein may lead to different in vitro reactivity with host proteins, depending on the amino acid sequence. Thus, over 90 genotypes have been screened around the world, and six main HCV types are now distinguished, according to the proposed classification (174). Prevalence of genotypes may vary around the world; for example, genotype 1b represents more than 45% of the isolates in Europe and only 17% in the United States (175). This genetic variability is obvious within the host, representing quasispecies (176). These facts are, at least in part, related to the high viral turnover, since the estimated viral production is 10^{12} per day (174,177).

Since infectious virions are permanently selected through their interactions with the host, this may partly explain immune failure to eradicate HCV and resistance to antiviral drugs (160,178). However, the identification of some highly conserved amino acid sequences among both structural and nonstructural proteins suggest essential functions for viral life cycle and could constitute the target of new antiviral drugs.

Viral Life Cycle

The polyprotein is processed by viral and cellular proteases in 10 structural and nonstructural proteins. Structural proteins include the core (i.e., the viral nucleocapsid) and the envelope proteins El and E2. The NS proteins are NS2 to NS5B, required for viral replication. These two groups of proteins are separated by the short membrane peptide p7 (160,179). Recently, the p7 function appeared to act as an ion channel (180). This assemblage results in a complete virion exhibiting a diameter of 30 to 50 nm (181). However, particles isolated from plasma may vary as a result of complex formation with very-low-density lipoproteins or immunoglobulins (182).

The main cellular target for HCV is the hepatocyte (177). But extrahepatic sites allowing viral replication have been identified, such as PBMCs (essentially B cells and monocytes), lymph nodes, and possibly biliary cells (177,183,184). More than one cellular receptor should exist for HCV: CD81 was the first one to be discovered (185), but experimental animal models showed that it did not allow viral replication by itself (186). Accordingly, very-low-density lipoprotein receptors and glycosaminoglycans are potential coreceptors for HCV (187).

The life cycle of HCV is more hypothetical beyond the stage of target cell infection because our progress in this field is hampered by the absence of a relevant model for HCV entry, replication, and release. Clearly, El and E2 are involved in membrane fusion operating between the virus and the endoplasmic reticulum (188). For this purpose, these two viral products interact through heterodimerization, allowing endoplasmic reticulum retention (189). Thus, viral RNA translation may proceed, beginning by the internal ribosome entry site binding to ribosome (190,191). The positive-stranded viral RNA serves as a template for the production of RNA negative strands, which allow the synthesis of viral genome, and thus virions, by interactions with copies of the core protein (190). As an example, the core protein produced in bacteria allows the formation of nucleocapsids when incubated with RNA molecules (192). However, NS proteins such as NS3 helicase and NS5B RNA-dependent RNA-polymerase obviously play a major role in this viral life cycle, but our understanding of their molecular interactions needs to be improved (160).

Experimental Systems for Antiviral Drug Study

Attempts to explore and understand the antiviral activity of IFN-α and ribavirin have been studied (193–195). For an in-depth understanding of the mechanism of action, several investigators consider that an experimental system is necessary. Toward this end, HCV protein functions and their interaction with the crystal structure of the RNA-dependent RNA polymerase has been determined (196). Dellamonica et al. (196) described several culture model systems using cellular or animal models. These include fetal liver cells, hepatoma cell lines, immortalized T or B cell lines, and a simian model that mirrors the natural history of HCV infection (197–204).

All this information is required to fully understand the current procedure to study the antiviral effects of licensed drugs. However, the mechanisms accounting for the antiviral activity of both IFN-α and ribavirin are essentially unidentified (158,161,193,194). IFN-α is thought to induce an antiviral cellular state and may upregulate the destruction of infected cells. Ribavirin is a synthetic guanosine analog mostly used for the treatment of respiratory syncytial virus infection. The inhibition of HCV is hypothetical and it seems that most of its antiviral effect is indirect through synergic interaction with IFN-α, upregulating antiviral immune responses (195).

Evaluating Antiviral Therapy

For HCV infection, viral load monitoring to measure HCV RNA levels in serum or plasma has played a critical role in assessing the efficacy of antiviral therapy. Achievement of SVR, defined as undetectable HCV RNA in serum or plasma, 12 to 24 weeks after completion of therapy is a primary objective of anti-HCV treatment and has been interpreted as clinical "cure" (205–207). Undetectable levels are typically interpreted as 15 IU/mL of HCV RNA. A report of "undetectable" HCV RNA does not necessarily mean the absence of virus but rather that the assay may be unable to detect HCV RNA because the level is below the lower limit of quantitation (LLOQ) and outside of the linear range where the manufacturer (or laboratory) can attest to a highly reproducible and accurate measurement.

An additional use of viral load monitoring of HCV RNA levels during treatment is to guide duration of therapy, known as response-guided therapy (RGT). RGT has become a necessary and complementary component of patient management protocols because it represents a personalized approach that can optimize treatment, safety, and outcomes (208,209).

Outlook: Hepatitis C

Despite many unresolved aspects of HCV infection, considerable efforts have been made since the definitive identification of the virus. A better understanding of HCV epidemiology will allow improved prevention; meanwhile, detection of infected patients is easy to achieve early in the natural history of their disease. Therefore, treatment combinations may be prescribed in cases of mild liver disease, increasing chances of cure for patients. Moreover, current tools for the study of the HCV life cycle should provide the opportunity to develop new antiviral drugs.

There appears to be a dynamic drug pipeline for HCV treatment where the goal will be an HCV regimen free of interferon with orally administered treatment. The landmark introduction in 2011 of the initial two DAAs telaprevir and boceprevir for HCV genotype 1 infections may have been the prelude to this goal. However, it was disappointing that results from clinical trials preclude their administration as monotherapy. Both compounds have a low barrier to resistance and require concomitant administration of pegylated interferon and ribavirin to prevent the emergence of resistant mutants.

HUMAN CYTOMEGALOVIRUS: ANTIVIRAL DRUGS, RESISTANCE, AND SUSCEPTIBILITY TESTING METHODS

Human cytomegalovirus (HCMV), a member of the herpesvirus family, is a ubiquitous agent that commonly infects human beings. As with other herpesviruses, primary infection is followed by latent infection. Recurrent infections are most often caused by reactivation of latent virus but reinfection also occurs. HCMV infections are generally mild or asymptomatic in immunocompetent adults, but HCMV is a major cause of defects in neonates and is a major pathogen in immunosuppressed individuals, including recipients of bone marrow and solid-organ transplants and patients with AIDS. In particular, HCMV was the most common cause of sight- and life-threatening opportunistic infection in patients with AIDS prior to the availability of highly active ARV therapy.

The cornerstone of antiviral therapy is ganciclovir, which was the first compound licensed in the United States specifically for treatment of CMV infections. Ganciclovir is a synthetic acyclic nucleoside analog, structurally similar to guanine. Its structure is similar to acyclovir and, like acyclovir, requires phosphorylation to achieve antiviral activity. Following phosphorylation by the viral protein pUL97, cellular enzymes phosphorylate the monophosphate form to di- and triphosphate metabolites. Subsequently, the ganciclovir-triphosphate metabolite then exerts its antiviral effect on CMV-infected cells.

Other compounds currently approved for the treatment of severe HCMV infections include the deoxyguanosine analog ganciclovir and its prodrug valganciclovir, the ANP cidofovir, and the pyrophosphate analog foscarnet. All of these compounds are inhibitors of the viral DNA polymerase encoded by gene *UL54*.

As cidofovir already contains a phosphate-mimetic group, it needs only two phosphorylation steps to reach the active stage. These phosphorylations are performed by host cellular enzymes. Thus, cidofovir does not depend on the virus-induced kinase to exert its antiviral action. Cidofovir diphosphate interacts as competitive inhibitor with the normal substrate (deoxycytosine triphosphate) for the viral polymerase. Two consecutive incorporations at the 3' end of the DNA chain are required to efficiently shut off DNA elongation. Incorporation of one cidofovir diphosphate molecule causes a marked decrease in the rate of DNA elongation. Foscarnet does not require intracellular activation to exert its antiviral activity. It is not incorporated into the growing DNA and it reversibly blocks the pyrophosphate binding site of the viral DNA polymerase and inhibits the cleavage of pyrophosphate from deoxynucleoside triphosphates.

Patients receiving long-term suppressive anti-HCMV therapy may develop antiviral resistance. In AIDS patients before the era of highly active ARV therapy, epidemiologic studies have shown that the frequency of resistance increased with the duration of therapy and reached 27% of patients after 9 months of ganciclovir (210), 13% of patients after 1 year of valganciclovir (211), and 37% of patients after 1 year of foscarnet (212). In solid organ recipients, 7% of the HCMV infection were resistant to ganciclovir after a median delay of 10 months (213).

Methods used in the laboratory to determine the susceptibility of HCMV strains to antiviral drugs are classified as phenotypic or genotypic. Phenotypic methods aim to determine the concentration of an antiviral agent that inhibits the virus in culture. Genotypic assays are designed to detect mutations known to confer antiviral resistance in the genome of the viruses being studied.

Phenotypic Antiviral Assays

A variety of phenotypic assays have been used in different studies to determine the antiviral susceptibilities of HCMV strains. Each of these methods measures the inhibition of HCMV growth in tissue cultures in the presence of serial dilutions of antiviral drugs. The 50% inhibitory concentration (IC_{50}) is defined as the concentration of antiviral agent resulting in a 50% reduction in viral growth. The methods usually performed include the PRAs that measure the inhibition of replication of infectious virus, the assays based on DNA hybridization that measure the inhibition of viral DNA synthesis, and enzyme-linked immunosorbent and flow cytometry–based assays that measure production of one or more viral proteins. The IC_{50} values determined with these different phenotypic assays depend on the nature of the replication marker chosen.

Clinical Specimens to Study

HCMV can be recovered from various clinical specimens such as peripheral blood leukocytes, bronchoalveolar liquid, cerebrospinal fluid, organ biopsy, urine samples, and vitreous fluid. Strains recovered from blood are usually chosen to be tested because viremia reflects blood dissemination and active infection. However, resistance profiles of a blood strain may differ from those of strains recovered from other body compartments and directly responsible for the disease because antiviral drug selection pressure may differ from one compartment to another. In addition, patients may shed multiple strains of HCMV either concurrently or sequentially (214).

Constitution of Viral Stocks

All the assay methods require the constitution of viral stocks obtained after sequential passaging of the viral isolate. Viral stocks are constituted by either extracellular virus recovered from culture supernatants or intracellular virus present in infected cells. Constitution of extracellular virus stocks requires at least 8 to 10 passages and is therefore time-consuming. Moreover, some isolates remain cell associated and no extracellular virions are produced. On the contrary, constitution of a stock of infected cells may be achieved after only one to three passages; however, it may require more passages (215).

Tissue culture supernatants containing extracellular virus are clarified by centrifugation at 1,000 rpm for 10 minutes and divided into aliquots and kept frozen at $-80°C$ until use. Titers of extracellular virus stocks are determined from a thawed aliquot using a plaque assay or a rapid immunocytochemistry assay. Infected fibroblast monolayers are trypsinized; cells are then counted and used for the phenotypic assay.

Plaque Reduction Assay

PRA has been considered as the "gold standard" for antiviral phenotypic testing. A standardized assay has been proposed by Landry et al. (216).

Human fibroblasts grown as just confluent monolayers in 24-well plates are inoculated with a standardized inoculum of a stock virus (50 to 100 plaque-forming units per well). After adsorption for 90 minutes, the medium is aspirated and the wells are overlaid with a 0.4% agarose medium containing serial dilutions of the drug to be tested. Concentrations usually tested are between 1 and 50 µM for ganciclovir, 50 and 800 µM for foscarnet, and 0.1 and 20 µM for cidofovir. Each drug concentration is tested at least in triplicate, as well as controls without drug. The cultures are incubated for 7 days at 37°C. Monolayers are fixed in 10% formalin in phosphate-buffered saline (PBS) and stained with

0.8% crystal violet in 50% ethanol. The IC_{50} of the antiviral agent for the isolate is defined as the concentration causing a 50% reduction in the number of plaques produced as compared with controls. Alternatively, a medium without agarose can be used. The plates are then incubated for 4 days and the foci are revealed by immunoperoxidase staining using monoclonal antibody E-13 (214).

DNA Hybridization Assay

Cell cultures are inoculated with a standardized amount of virus and incubated in the presence of different concentrations of antiviral agent until control wells show 60% to 80% cytopathic effect. Then the cells are lysed and whole DNA is extracted and hybridized to a radiolabelled HCMV probe. Radioactivity is counted. The IC_{50}s of the antiviral agents are the concentrations that reduce by 50% the DNA hybridization values compared with the hybridization values of controls (217).

Detection of Human Cytomegalovirus Antigens

Viral production is measured by using immunofluorescence-, immunoperoxidase-, or flow cytometry–based methods for detection and quantification of cells expressing HCMV antigens or by using enzyme-linked immunosorbent assay–based methods for quantification of HCMV antigens produced in cells (218,219).

Limitations of Phenotypic Assays

Phenotypic assays are limited by the excessive time required to complete the assay (1 to 2 months). To reduce the turnaround time involved in PRAs, a modified assay has been performed directly in primary cultures of clinical specimens such as urine, amniotic fluid, and bronchoalveolar lavage samples (220). Blood leukocytes from patients with documented HCMV viremia were also used as inoculum in a PRA (221). These methods provided results within 4 to 6 days. Their major limitation is that the virus titers of the clinical specimens are often too low to allow them to be used.

Resistant strains in a mixture may not be detected because of strain selection that occurs during passaging. Therefore, the virus stock studied may be not representative of the original population of virus. If antiviral drug is added to the cell culture medium in order to favor growth of mutant virus, de novo resistant strains may be selected in cell culture (222).

Interpretation

Dose-inhibition curves are constructed to determine the IC_{50} values of the antiviral agents of the studied strains. The type of cell culture used, the size of the viral inoculum, the method used, and the laboratory performing the test are factors that affect the results. Therefore, there is a significant variability among methods and laboratories. When feasible, a baseline isolate from the same patient should be tested in parallel with the isolate of interest. However, baseline isolates are often missing. Reference susceptible and resistant strains must be included in each susceptibility assay. Antiviral drug IC_{50} values for the isolate to test are compared with the results obtained for the reference strains. A comparison with the results obtained for a panel of susceptible strains tested in the laboratory can assist in the interpretation.

The IC_{50} cutoff values proposed to define resistance to antiviral compounds are as follows: more than 12 μM for ganciclovir, more than 400 μM for foscarnet, and more than 2 or 4 μM for cidofovir. HCMV strains for which ganciclovir IC_{50} is more than 6 μM and less than 12 μM are considered to have decreased susceptibility to ganciclovir (215,216,223). However, cutoff values are to be determined in each laboratory.

Genotypic Antiviral Assays

Ganciclovir resistance results mostly from changes in the *UL97* phosphotransferase responsible for the primophosphorylation of ganciclovir (Table 11.9) (224,225). Mutations in the *UL54* DNA polymerase gene appear after prolonged ganciclovir therapy (226). They contribute to a high level of resistance to ganciclovir and induce cross-resistance to cidofovir. All foscarnet and cidofovir resistance mutations that are currently known map to the *UL54* gene (Table 11.10) (223,227–231).

Viral DNA Extraction

Viral DNA is extracted from cultures in 25-cm^2 flasks using the procedure described by Hirt (232). Briefly, infected cell monolayers exhibiting at least 50% cytopathic effect are washed twice in PBS and then 0.4 mL of Hirt solution (100 mM Tris-HCl, pH 7.5, 10 mM EDTA, 0.5% SDS) is added. After incubation at room temperature for 20 minutes, the lysate is transferred to a microtube and 0.1 mL of 5 M NaCl solution is added. The mixture is incubated for 12 hours at 4°C and centrifuged at 15,000 rpm

Table 11.9

UL97 Changes in Cytomegalovirus Strains Resistant to Ganciclovir

Role in Conferring Resistance to Ganciclovir	Residue	Amino Acid Change
Proven by marker transfer experiments	460	Methionine to isoleucine/valine
	520	Histidine to glutamine
	590–593	Deletion of alanine-alanine-cysteine-arginine
	591–594	Deletion of alanine-cysteine-arginine-alanine
	594	Alanine to valine/glycine
	595	Deletion of leucine, leucine to serine/phenylalanine
	603	Cysteine to tryptophane
	607	Cysteine to tyrosine
Suspected	590	Alanine to threonine
	591	Alanine to valine/aspartic acid
	592	Cysteine to glycine
	595	Leucine to tryptophane/threonine
	596	Glutamic acid to glycine/aspartic acid
	597	Asparagine to isoleucine
	598	Glycine to valine
	599	Lysine to methionine
	600	Deletion of leucine
	601	Deletion of threonine
	603	Cysteine to tyrosine
	606	Alanine to aspartic acid
	665	Valine to isoleucine

for 5 minutes. The resulting supernatant is digested with proteinase K (1 mg/mL) at 56°C for 1 hour and then extracted with phenol chloroform and precipitated with ethanol. By this procedure, a purified DNA preparation enriched in viral DNA is obtained. Alternatively, infected monolayers are trypsinized, washed twice in PBS, and centrifuged. The cell pellet is submitted to lysis in a buffer containing 10 mM Tris-HCl, pH 8.0, 50 mM KCl, 2 mM MgCl$_2$, 0.9% Nonidet P-40, and 100 μg/mL of proteinase K for 1 hour at 56°C (215). The mixture is centrifuged for 5 minutes at 15,000 rpm and the supernatant containing DNA is collected. DNA is extracted from clinical samples using commercially available purification columns according to the manufacturer's instructions.

Rapid Genotypic Methods

Detection of Ganciclovir Resistance-Related Mutations in Gene UL97. Rapid screening methods have been designed to detect the mutations at codons 460, 594, 591, 592, 594, 595 (the most frequently observed in clinical isolates), and at codon 520 (233–236). They are based on restriction enzyme analysis of three selected PCR products amplified from HCMV-infected cultures or from clinical samples (Tables 11.11 and 11.12). The PCR reaction mixtures include 5% dimethyl sulfoxide, deoxynucleosides triphosphate at 200 μM each, primers at 1μM each, 2.5 units of Taq polymerase (Roche Diagnostics, Basel, Switzerland), and 500 ng of DNA. The reactions are cycled 40 times as follows: 95°C for 1 minute, 55°C for 45 seconds, and 72°C for 45 seconds.

The restriction enzymes *Nla* III, *Alu* I, *Hha* I, *Mse* I, *Taq* I, and *Hae* III are used to digest the PCR products (Table 11.13) (233,235,236). The digests are analyzed on a 15% polyacrylamide gel and stained with ethidium bromide.

The diagnostic screening assays based on restriction enzyme analysis of selected PCR products allow the detection of the most frequent *UL97* mutations involved in resistance to ganciclovir and can identify minority mutants if they reach 10% of the viral population. The disadvantage of these rapid and simple tests is that they miss specific mutations that do not result in a change in the restriction enzyme pattern and previously unmapped mutations.

Table 11.10

UL54 Changes in HCMV Strains Resistant to Antiviral Compounds[a]

Region	Modification	Viral Phenotype		
		Ganciclovir	Cidofovir	Foscarnet
ExoI	D301N	R	R	S
IV	N408D	R	R	S
	F412C	R	R	S
	F412V	R	R	S
	D413E	R	R	S
δC	L501I	R	R	S
	K513E	R	R	S
	P522S	R	R	S
	L545S	R	R	S
	D588E	S	S	R
II	T700A	S	S	R
	V715M	S	S	R
	I722V	R	R	S
VI	V781I	S	S	R
III	L802M	R	S	R
	K805Q	S	R	S
	T821I	R	S	R
V	A987G	R	R	S
	Del 981–982	R	R	R
Other	E756D	S	S	R
	E756K	I	I	R

[a]Data derived from Chou E, Lurain NS, Thompson KD, et al. Viral DNA polymerase mutations associated with drug resistance in human cytomegalovirus. *J Infect Dis* 2003;188:32–39. Cihlar T, Fuller MD, Cherrington J. Characterization of drug resistance-associated mutations in the human cytomegalovirus DNA polymerase gene by using recombinant mutant viruses generated from overlapping DNA fragments. *J Virol* 1998;72:5927–5936. Erice A. Resistance of human cytomegalovirus to antiviral drugs. *Clin Microbiol Rev* 1992;12(Suppl 2): S286–S297.
R, resistant; S, sensitive; I, intermediate; del, deletion.

Table 11.11

Restriction Enzyme Digestion Screening for *UL97* Mutations Related to Ganciclovir Resistance

PCR Product			Enzyme	*UL97*	Fragment Size (Base Pair)	
Forward Primer	Reverse Primer	Size (Base Pair)		Codon	Wild-type Sequence	Mutant Sequence
CPT1088 M	CPT1619	532	*Nla* III	460	198, 168, 126, 9	324, 168, 9
CPT1088 M	CPT1587 M	501	*Alu* I	520	314, 187	297, 187, 17
CPT1713	CPT1830	118	*Hha* I	594	50, 38, 18, 12	62, 38, 18
			Mse I	595 = >F	76, 42	46, 42, 30
			Taq I	595 = >S	99, 19	71, 48, 19
			Hae III	591 + 592	59, 59	63, 55
			Hae III	591		118

PCR, polymerase chain reaction.

Table 11.12

Sequence of the Primers Used for Rapid Screening for *UL97* Mutations[a]	
Primer	**5'-3' Sequence**
CPT 1088	ACGGTGCTCACGGTCTGGAT
CPT 1619	AAACGCGCGTGCGGGTCGCAGA
CPT 1587 M	CTGCAGCGGCATGGGTCGGAAAGCAAG
CPT 1713	CGGTCTGGACGAGGTGCGCAT
CPT 1830 M	AATGAGCAGACAGGCGTCGAAGCA
	GTGCGTGAGCTTGCCGTTCTT

[a]Isolated base changes have been introduced in primer CPT 1830 to create recognition sites for *Taq* I (TCGA) in S595 mutants and a recognition site for *Mse* I (TTTA) in F595 mutants. Primer CPT 1587 creates an additional *Alu* I site in presence of Q520.

Detection of Resistance-Related Mutations in Gene UL54. Restriction enzyme analysis of PCR fragments have been used to detect the ganciclovir and cidofovir resistance change L501F and the ganciclovir and foscarnet resistance change A809V in the DNA polymerase (228,237).

Sequence Analysis Methods

Sequencing is the nucleotide sequence analysis that is proven to be the most accurate method for genotypic resistance determination of HCMV strains. However, no standardized assay is available to routinely achieve the analysis of the *UL97* and *UL54* genes. The complete genes or the gene regions involved in resistance are amplified by PCR and then PCR products are directly sequenced (Tables 11.14 to 11.16) (215,238,239). Amplification of *UL97*, either with the primer set CPL97-F and CPL97-R or the primer set HLF97-F and HLF97-R, is performed using the GeneAmp XL PCR kit (Applied Biosystems, Foster City, CA). The reactions are cycled 30 times as follows: 94°C for 1 minute and 60°C for 10 minutes. The entire gene *UL54* is amplified using the GeneAmp XL PCR kit (Applied Biosystems, Foster City, CA). The *UL54* region of interest is amplified using high-fidelity polymerase. PCR products are purified using QIAquick PCR (Qiagen, Valencia, CA) purification kits and are then submitted to sequence reaction. When analysis of sequences are to be performed on an ABI automated DNA sequencer, the purified templates (10 or 20 ng) are sequenced using ABI Prism BigDye Terminator

Table 11.13

Rapid Screening for *UL97* Mutations: Conditions of Polymerase Chain Reaction Product Digestion with Restriction Enzymes[a]			
	Enzyme Unity Number Per Reaction	**Incubation**	
Enzyme		**Length Time (Hours)**	**Temperature (°C)**
Nla III	3	2	37
Alu I	5	2	37
Hha I	3	2	37
Hae III	3	2	37
Taq I	3	2	65
Mse I	3	2	37

[a]A 10-µL sample of polymerase chain reaction product is digested in a final volume of 20 µL.

Table 11.14

Primer Sequences for Polymerase Chain Reaction Amplification of the *UL97* Gene[a]	
Fragment Amplified	**Sequence**
Entire gene (2,254 bp)	CPL97-F
	5′-GGAAGACTGTCGCCACTATGTCC-3′
	CPL97-R
	5′-CTCCTCATCGTCGTCGTAGTCC-3′
Codons 400 to 707 (1,038 bp)	HLF97-F
	5′-CTGCTGCACAACGTCACGGTACATC-3′
	HLF97-R
	5′-CTCCTCATCGTCGTCGTAGTCC-3′

bp, base pair.
Adapted from Lurain NS, Weinberg A, Crumpacker CS, et al. Sequencing of cytomegalo-virus UL97 gene for genotypic antiviral resistance testing. *Antimicrob Agents Chemother* 2001;45:2775–2780.

Table 11.15

Primer Sequences for Polymerase Chain Reaction Amplification of the *UL54* Gene		
Fragment Amplified[a]	**Primer Sequence**	**Reference**
Entire gene (3.7 kbp)	Forward: 5′-GTCAGCCTCTCACGGTCCGCTAT-3′ Reverse: 5′-CTCAGTCTCAGCAGCATCATCAC-3′	Chou et al. (238)
Codons 363 to 1,005 (1,926 bp)	Forward: 5′-ATC TCT TTA CGA TCG GCA CC-3′ Reverse: 5′-ATC CTC AAA GAG CAG GGA GAG-3′	Fillet et al. (239)

[a]bp, base pair.

Table 11.16

Primer Sequences for Sequencing of *UL97* and *UL54* Coding Strands[a]			
Gene	**Sequence**	**Nucleotide Position**	**Reference(s)**
UL97	5′-ATCGACAGCTACCGACGTGCC-3′ 5′-GTCGGAGCTGTCGGCGCTGGG-3′	1285–1305 1651–1671	Lurain et al. (215)
UL54	5′-CGCCTCTCACTCGATGAAGT-3′ 5′-TCAGGAAGACTATGTAGTGG-3′ 5′-GCCCACAACCTCTGCTACTC-3′ 5′-CAGCAGATCCGTATCT-3′ 5′-CGGCCGCCACCAAGGTGTAT-3′ 5′-AGATCTCGTGCGTGTGCTACG-3′	3708–3727 3260–3279 2840–2859 2391–2406 2071–2090 1627–1647	Sullivan et al. (231) Ducancelle et al. (214) Fillet et al. (239)

[a]*UL97* nucleotides are numbered from codon 1. Nucleotide positions in *UL54* gene are identified.

version 3.0 (Applied Biosystems, Foster City, CA) ready reaction cycle sequencing kit according to the manufacturer's instructions. Depending on the sequencing method chosen, minority mutants in a mixture can be detected if they reach 20% to 40% of the viral population. Sequences of *UL97* and *UL54* are aligned with the AD169 strain reference sequence (EMBL accession no. X17403) using Align Plus, version 4.0 (Scientific and Educational Software, Durham, NC).

The interpretation of genetic assays requires the distinction of resistance-associated mutations to natural interstrain variation. Some of the mutations observed in resistant strains have been validated as resistance markers by a process of marker transfer, but others have not. To date, resistance mutations in *UL97* have been found at one of three sites. At two of those, there are point mutations in a single codon (460 and 520), and at the third site, there are point mutations or deletions within the codon range 590 to 607. On the contrary, resistance-associated mutations in *UL54* are widely dispersed across the coding sequence. The interstrain sequence homology is above 98% and 99% for *UL54* and *UL97*, respectively (215,238,239). *UL54* sequences determined in HCMV isolates sensitive to antiviral drugs have been deposited in GenBank under accession numbers AF133589 through AF133628 and under accession numbers AY422355 through AY422377 (238,239). *UL97* sequences of ganciclovir-sensitive strains have been deposited under accession numbers AF34548 through AF345573 (215).

Outlook: Human Cytomegalovirus Assays

Phenotypic assays are still important to corroborate genotypic results. However, the time required to perform the assays is too long to provide useful therapeutic information. Results obtained by both types of susceptibility testing are usually concordant. However, it should be noted that viruses harboring mutations responsible for resistance can be classified as susceptible in phenotypic assays. Because some *UL97* or *UL54* mutations are associated with a slow growth of HCMV in culture, it has been proposed that the presence of these mutations could introduce bias in the interpretation of phenotypic assays. As patients can be infected by multiple HCMV strains, cell culture–based assays can select a different virus population from that selected by PCR-based assays.

In the specialized area of CMV viral load testing for organ transplant donors and recipients, a

notable development was recently unveiled, which is expected to transform clinical practice. WHO revised the solid organ transplant guidelines, which require reporting viral load results using an international standard (240). The revised guidelines clearly demonstrate that CMV monitoring has become part of the PCR era with quantitative PCR viral load testing as the standard of care for monitoring patients. Toward this end, FDA recently approved the first CMV viral load assay with traceability to the WHO international CMV standard. These developments have garnered significant optimism in this field because it will make possible universal clinical recommendations for CMV patient management and will positively impact outcomes.

ANTIVIRAL AGENTS FOR INFLUENZA VIRUSES: MODE OF ACTION AND ANTIVIRAL RESISTANCE

Influenza continues to be an important public health concern in the 21st century. This infection is responsible for annual epidemics with significant mortality and morbidity (241,242). During recent outbreaks, pandemic strain of influenza A emerged from the animal reservoir, leading to devastating influenza with high attack rates, as during the H1N1 "swine flu" pandemic in 2009 to 2010 (243,244). Pandemics were observed three times during the 20th century (245,246) and most recently in the 21st century during 2009 to 2010 (242,244). Influenza is highly contagious, with person-to-person contagion spread easily via aerosol droplets that infect epithelial cells of the respiratory tract (247–249).

Human and animal influenza viruses belong to the family Orthomyxoviridae. There are three genera corresponding to influenza virus types A, B, and C (250,251). Influenza viruses are divided into subtypes based on major antigenic specificities of their surface glycoproteins HA and NA. To date, 16 different HAs and 9 different NAs have been described. The name of the influenza virus each season reflects the HA and NA segments present in the strain following gene reassortment. In 2013, influenza A (H1N1) and A (H3N2) represented the typical seasonal influenza A virus subtypes. Influenza A (H1N1) is the same strain that caused the 2009 influenza pandemic and in 2013 is circulating as seasonal influenza (242). Two influenza B viruses also cause seasonal influenza. Influenza B strains are named after the communities in which they first appeared, Victoria and Yamagata strains (242). Type C influenza causes sporadic and only minor outbreaks, although occasionally may cause more severe illness in children (252). In recent years, sporadic transmission of influenza viruses from animals to humans has occurred. In 2011, swine influenza virus subtype A (H3N2) was detected in people; the label "variant" influenza (vH3N2) was used to distinguish these viruses from human viruses of the same strain (242,244).

Among influenza viruses, influenza A is most notable. In recent years, influenza B caused less than 20% of clinical cases of influenza. Once infection occurred, however, it was able to produce significant morbidity (244). Both viruses together cause annual outbreaks and epidemics during cold winter seasons in temperate climates. These organisms are also responsible for epidemic illness throughout the world (245). During some recent warmer winters attributed to climate change, fewer people became infected with influenza and hence had waning immunity. These seasons were followed by more severe epidemics during subsequent years (253).

Influenza is associated with nonspecific signs and symptoms (250). The definition for influenza-like illness is the triad linking fever plus one respiratory and one general sign. Briefly, following a short incubation period of 24 to 48 hours, the disease is usually characterized by the sudden onset of high fever with chills, headache, dry cough, myalgia, asthenia, diarrhea, and nasal congestion with or without mild rhinorrhea (249,250,254). This disease is observed in all age groups. In some cases, bacterial superinfection can be observed, leading to severe pulmonary infection and increased morbidity and mortality (255,256). In classic influenza illness, spontaneous recovery is observed after 5 to 7 days of infection, depending on the patient's age and the immune status. In the recent outbreaks, populations more susceptible to complications and mortality included the elderly, young children, pregnant women, those with chronic respiratory diseases, the morbidly obese, as well as immunocompromised individuals (249,257,258). People older than 65 years of age accounted for 90% of seasonal influenza–associated deaths, even though these individuals made up only about 15% of the population (259). In general, the disease lasts 7 to 8 days in young children and can last several months in immunocompromised patients.

Prevention strategies for high-risk populations have been implemented, given the seriousness of this disease. Since 2010, annual influenza vaccination has been recommended for everyone older than 6 months of age (249,260). Most hospitals and health care institutions mandate vaccination of all health care workers as well (260). Because influenza C has minimal population disease risk as compared to influenza A and B, only the A and B strains are included in seasonal influenza vaccines (242). Many institutions prohibit health care workers from coming to work when they have respiratory symptoms and fever during times of epidemic. Wearing of face masks, compliance with handwashing protocols, and respiratory droplet isolation are all important components of influenza prevention programs (244). Public health considerations include administration of antiviral agents to nonvaccinated patients within 48 hours of influenza exposure, especially to those who are at high risk of influenza complications due to premorbid conditions or who are severely immunosuppressed (244).

Influenza Virus Structure

Influenza A and B viruses share common features (250). They are pleomorphic, 80- to 120-nm virus particles. Influenza A, B, and C viruses can be differentiated by their viral-specific nucleoprotein and matrix proteins (252). The viral membrane is covered with a large quantity of evenly spaced glycoproteins: HA and NA, with four times more HA than NA molecules. Influenza A viral RNA has eight segments of single-stranded negative-sense RNA and many copies of nucleoprotein (NP), along with the polymerase complex. Six of the eight segments of RNA (see Table 11.17 for a list of names and functions) each produce a single viral protein, and two segments (7 and 8) produce two proteins each. The seventh segment encodes for the matrix 2 protein (M2) and the matrix 1 protein (M1). The ribonucleoprotein (RNP) and the lipid envelope are connected by the M1 protein. Influenza B and C also contain polymerase proteins and NP. However, influenza B has only four membrane proteins (HA, NA, influenza B matrix 2 protein, and NB, a membrane protein specific to influenza B); influenza C contains only two proteins, influenza C matrix 2 (CM2) and the HA-esterase-fusion (HEF) protein, which functions as HA and NA combined (251,261).

TABLE 11.17

List of Different Virus Proteins of Influenza A

Segment	Gene Size in Nucleotides	Protein(s)	Protein Size in Amino Acids	Protein Name and Function
1	2,341	PB2	759	Polymerase basic protein 2; Polymerase (subunit basic 2)
2	2,341	PB1 PB1-F2	757 87	Polymerase basic protein 1; Polymerase (subunit basic 1) Polymerase basic protein 1-F2; Proapoptotic mitochondrial protein
3	2,233	PA	716	Polymerase acidic protein ; Polymerase (subunit acidic)
4	1,778	HA	566	Hemagglutinin; receptor binding site and fusion, main target of neutralizing antibodies
5	1,565	NP	498	Nucleoprotein; role in virus entry into host nucleus
6	1,413	NA	454	Neuraminidase; sialidase enzymatic activity (virion release)
7	1,027	M1 M2	252 97	Matrix 1; matrix protein Matrix 2; proton channel activity
8	890	NS1 NS2/NEP	230 121	Nonstructural protein 1; interferon inhibitor, gene regulation Nonstructural protein 2 = nuclear export protein; nuclear export of viral proteins

From Samji T. Influenza A: understanding the viral life cycle. *Yale J of Biol and Med* 2009;82:153–159; Barik S. New treatment for influenza. *BMC Med* 2012;10:104.

These are all enveloped viruses. Influenza A viral envelope is made of a lipid bilayer containing three transmembrane proteins: HA (which makes up 80% of the membrane protein), NA (17% of the membrane protein), and M2 protein (making up a minor component of the membrane, with up to only 20 molecules per virus) (251). HA and NA are exclusively within the viral envelope membrane and M2 forms tetramers through the membrane. M1 protein is under the lipid bilayer (251).

Protein Function

Matrix 1 Protein

M1 protein is responsible for the stability of the membrane and interacts with the virus RNA segments. M1 lies just beneath the lipid membrane and attaches to the viral ribonucleoproteins (vRNPs). vRNPs are composed of single-stranded, negative-sense RNAs wrapped around nonstructural protein 1 (NSP1) and nonstructural protein 2 (NSP2; also called nuclear export protein or NEP).

Three viral polymerase proteins make up the rest of this complex (250,251,262).

Influenza RNA is surrounded by NP. The complexed RNP is transcribed by the viral RNA polymerases to make mRNAs leading to viral protein synthesis. The NP-RNA complex sits in the lipid bilayer membrane, together with the HA and NA glycoproteins and the proton channel M2 protein. NS1 is not packaged into new virus particles but has important interactions with the host innate immune system and plays a role in viral growth and pathogenicity. NS2/NEP controls interaction between viral RNA and vRNP complexes to assist in the export new viral particles from the host cell (259).

Matrix 2 Protein

Matrix 2 (M2) channel protein found within the viral envelope is identified in influenza A viruses only (250,262). To be active, M2 molecules are organized as disulfide-linked tetramers, located as integral membrane proteins, with their N terminus expressed at the virus surface. They are encoded by a spliced mRNA from genome RNA segment 7 of the virus (250). The active part of M2 in the ion channel is located in the 19 residue transmembrane domain (251). During acidification of the endosome, these tetramers form an important channel for hydrogen ions between the interior of the virus and its environment, providing a low pH within the virus, leading to uncoating. Acidification via the M2 channel also allows the M1 protein to dissociate from the RNP-NP complex, permitting viral RNP to enter the nucleus of the cell and begin viral replication.

Hemagglutinin

HA is one of two major virus surface proteins and is encoded from genome RNA segment 4 in influenza A and B viruses (250). HA is a complex protein with key functions in initiating the infection process through binding to sialic acid receptors (263,264). It is synthetized as a precursor protein, HA0, which has to undergo a proteolytic cleavage to become active. Cleavage generates two proteins (HA1 and HA2) bonded by two disulfide bonds (Fig. 11.4). HA1 is of globular form and contains

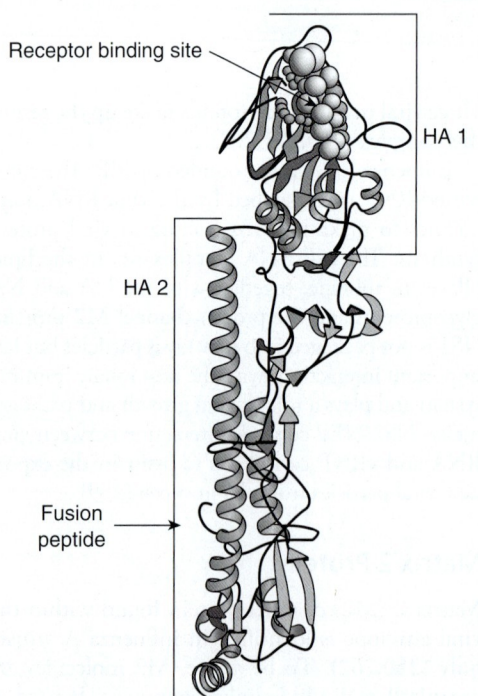

Receptor binding site

HA 1

HA 2

Fusion peptide

Figure 11.4 ■ Structure of the hemagglutinin (monomeric).

the major antigenic sites as well as the receptor binding site (RBS), which is highly conserved between types and subtypes (265,266). On host cells, specificity of viral binding to glycoproteins are determined by two species-restricted linkages: $\alpha(2,3)$ (avian recognition) and $\alpha(2,6)$ (human recognition). Viruses from swine recognize and bind to either. HA molecule attachment to cell surface sialic acid receptors are strongly dependent on these binding sites (251). HA2 is a long, fibrous stem that forms triple-stranded, coiled-coil protein that contains the transmembrane domain and the fusion peptide; this fusion peptide is available after HA0 cleavage (267). At the virus surface, the HA glycoproteins are trimeric and very abundant. When submitted to low pH, HA undergoes conformational changes that allow HA-mediated membrane fusion (263). Subsequently, endosomes form, allowing the M2 ion channel to open which acidifies the viral core, releasing vRNP to enter host cell cytoplasm (251). vRNP must then enter the host nucleus in order for viral transcription and replication to take place, culminating in development of host infection.

Neuraminidase

NA is the second major surface glycoprotein (250,268). It is encoded from genome RNA segment 6 in influenza A and B viruses. It is organized into two domains, the stalk and the head. The head of the NA contains the active site of the enzyme (Fig. 11.5). These proteins are organized as homotetramers at the virus surface (250). Among influenza viruses, the structure of the catalytic site of NA is highly conserved. This protein is a sialidase. The role of NA is to cleave sialic acids from adjacent glycoproteins, preventing HA from aggregating with the cell surface sialic acids. Effectively, NA facilitates release of newly produced viruses from the host cell surface after budding. Without this process, viral particles would not be released from the plasma membrane (251). Efficient interplay of HA and NA activities is necessary for optimal viral infection. After release, NA enables the virus to find target cells despite the large amount of protein covered with sialic acids in nasal mucus (268). Compared with influenza A, on the surface of influenza B, NA is present in very low quantity (252).

BM2 Protein

Influenza B matrix 2 protein (BM2) is found in influenza B only (250,252). It is a tetramer protein similar to the M2 influenza A matrix protein.

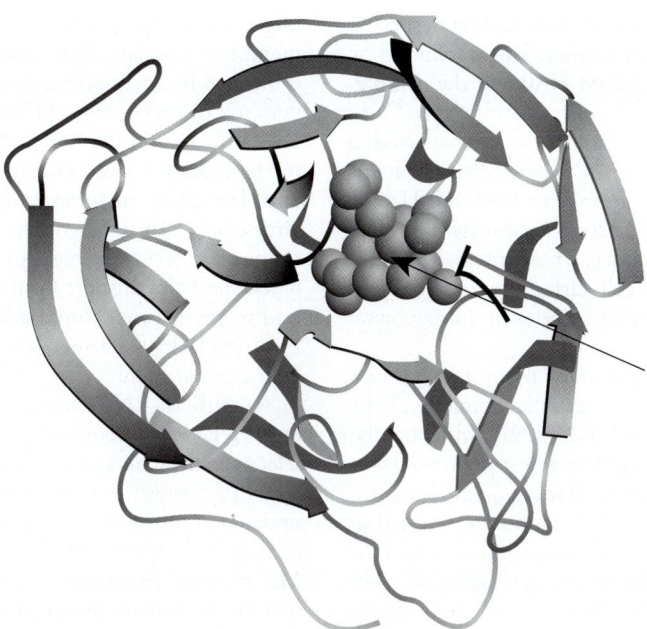

Figure 11.5 ■ **Structure of the neuraminidase (monomeric).** *Arrow* shows sialic acid in the catalytic site of the neuraminidase.

The RNA segment 7 of the influenza B virus codes for this protein, similar to the M2 protein of influenza A. BM2 protein produces a pH-sensitive proton channel that is mandatory for successful virus replication. These proteins appear to have dual functions of transmembrane proton conductance as well as recruitment of other proteins during virus replication (252).

Although M2 and BM2 are structurally and functionally similar, there is limited homology between their amino acid sequence and only in the transmembrane portion of the protein. These differences in function are highlighted by the observation that the M2 channel but not the BM2 channel is inhibited by the antiviral drug amantadine (261).

Viral Infection and Pathogenic Mechanisms

The first step in cellular infection by influenza viruses is the attachment of the virus to its cellular receptor (246,250,251,263). These receptors are identical for influenza A and B viruses. This attachment is performed by interaction between the RBS located at the end of the HA and the sialic acids of the target cell. Virus attachment depends on the recognition of the specific sialic acid by the RBS (251,263). There are sialic acids with different structures; the one recognized by human influenza viruses is linked to galactose by the $\alpha(2-3)$ linkage. This attachment mediates endocytosis. After endocytosis, the pH in the endosome is lowered, leading to HA conformational change and subsequent membrane fusion. The fusion peptide of several HA trimers intercalate into lipid bilayers to be efficient (251,252,263). Concomitantly, the M2 ion channel conducts H^+ ions inside the viral particle to allow uncoating and subsequent release of vRNPs in the cytoplasm of the infected cell and its transport to the nucleus. vRNAs are then transcribed into mRNAs and replicated.

Viral mRNA synthesis in the nucleus requires initiation by host cell primers. Replication of virion RNA occurs in two steps: the synthesis of the RNA template (full-length copies) and the copy of these templates into vRNAs. Viral mRNA is translated into viral proteins. HA, NA, and M2 are integral membrane proteins and are synthesized in the Golgi apparatus, while M1, NP, PA, PB1, PB2, NS1, and NEP are not. During synthesis in the Golgi apparatus, M2 protein acts as an ion channel to prevent HA molecules from undergoing early, irreversible, pH-induced conformational changes. Synthesis of HA in the endoplasmic reticulum is a stepwise conformational maturation of the protein with independent folding of specific domains in the HA monomer. This is followed by trimerization of uncleaved HA0 and the completion of folding to a pH-neutral form of HA. Once properly assembled and folded, it is transported to the Golgi apparatus where oligosaccharide chains are added and HA0 cleavage to HA1 and HA2 is performed. NA and M2 are eventually are transported to the cell surface. These integral proteins are expressed at the cell surface, preferentially in lipid raft microdomains, and can initiate viral budding (251).

The budding process starts by protein–protein interaction between intracellular domains of the NA, M2, and HA and M1 (269). Subsequently, vRNPs assemble themselves as a structure of eight RNPs with one of each viral segment; this complex interacts with the M1 monolayer located at the budding area in the envelope. This initiates the budding process with proper packaging of eight RNA segments (270). NA is needed to release fully formed virions from the cell surface because these virions are covered with sialic acids and, hence, aggregate, and/or adhere to the cell surface. NA removes HA-sialic acid links, releasing viral particles (251,271). Release of the newly formed viral particles yields between 5 log and 6 log viral particles per milliliter of nasal mucus.

Antiviral Agents for Influenza

Given the incidence of influenza causing significant global morbidity and mortality, approaches to manage seasonal outbreaks mandate both therapeutic and public health interventions. However, influenza virus is continually evolving; it may either be altered through small gradual changes (antigenic drift) or abrupt major changes (antigenic shift) due to genetic reassortments, leading to resistant strains. Influenza resistance increases the risk of recurrence of worldwide pandemics, as in 1918 and 2009 (272). Since the introduction of amantadine in 1962, it was realized that therapeutic interventions could control and prevent such devastation (Fig. 11.6).

Anti-M2 Products Adamantines: Amantadine and Rimantadine

The first description of antiinfluenza activity of the M2 channel blocker amantadine was reported in 1962. Both amantadine and its derivative, rimantadine, inhibit in vitro replication of influenza A viruses at concentrations achievable in vivo. The

target site is the M2 ion channel protein transmembrane domain (262). The ion channel activity is blocked by amantadine. As a result, M1 protein does not dissociate from the vRNPs blocking viral uncoating within the host cell, which is necessary for replication (246,250). Amantadine has a second, late effect on some subtypes of influenza A virus whose HA undergoes fusion-conformational changes at relatively high pH. Amantadine can block the H^+ transport from the Golgi. This can lead to premature conformational changes of the HA from lack of control of the pH in this intracellular compartment.

As with all RNA viruses, influenza virus mutates relatively frequently. Mutations provide selective advantages, including resistance to antiviral drugs as well as to vaccines, which need to be updated annually due to this fact (259). As demonstrated by analysis of resistant mutants, altered M2 proteins containing a change in the transmembrane domain display resistant phenotype to amantadine and rimantadine. Sequencing of RNA segment 7 from resistant isolates has demonstrated that nucleotide changes in the transmembrane domain, such as single nucleotide changes at residues 26, 27, 30, 31, and 34, can result in a resistant phenotype (246). Among clinical cases, the most frequent resistant mutation observed is in codon 31. All amino acid residues involved in resistance are located in the drug binding site. Influenza BM2 protein is intrinsically resistant to adamantine therapy (252,261).

The use of amantadine or rimantadine results in the frequent emergence of resistant strains (246,273,274). Current strains of influenza A H3N2 and H1N1 are already resistant to these agents (274). Resistance can be observed by day 2 of use, and in up to 45% of treated patients by day 7. These resistant isolates have been found to be as contagious and as pathogenic as the wild-type strain. By 2005 to 2006, more than 90% of seasonal influenza strains were resistant to the adamantines (275). Given the high frequency of resistance, there is rarely a role to use these agents to treat influenza nowadays. The CDC no longer recommends use of either of these drugs (244,249).

Neuraminidase Inhibitors: Zanamivir and Oseltamivir

The most commonly prescribed influenza treatment nowadays target NA since the decline in use of the M2 inhibitors due to high resistance. Influenza

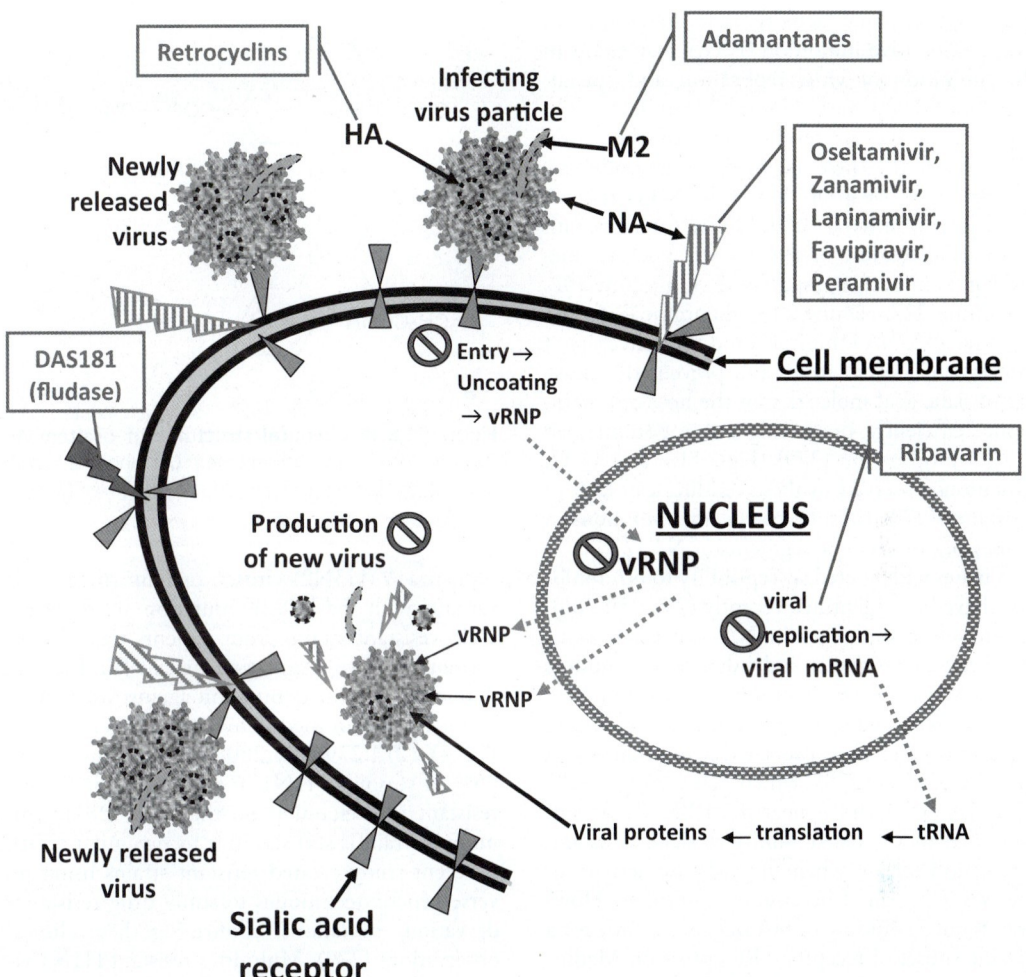

Figure 11.6 ■ Therapeutic targets for treatment of influenza A. Schematic of the life cycle of influenza A and its viral proteins. Old and new drugs targeting influenza pathways are identified in red boxes. Future targets for influenza viral/host immune response and cellular interactions are identified as red crossed circles ⊘. Influenza enters the host cell through the sialic acid receptor via neuraminidase alteration of the receptor. Then, viral RNA synthesis occurs in the infected host nucleus using RNP as a template. Viral translation occurs in host cytoplasm. New virus is produced then exported from host cells. Neuraminidase and the experimental agent DAS181 (Fludase) "cut" the sialic acid receptor at the cell membrane (sawtooth). NA, neuraminidase; HA, hemagglutinin; M2, matrix 2 protein ion channel; vRNP, viral ribonucleoproteins; viral mRNA, viral messenger RNA; tRNA, transfer RNA. (Adapted from Samji T. Influenza A: understanding the viral life cycle. *Yale J of Biol and Med* 2009;82:153–159; Centers for Disease Control and Prevention. Influenza antiviral medications: summary for clinicians. http://www.cdc.gov/flu/pdf/professionals/antiviral-summary-clinicians.pdf. Accessed December 15, 2013; Hayden FG. Newer influenza antivirals, biotherapeutics and combinations. *Influenza Other Respir Viruses* 2013;7[Suppl 1]:63–75.) (See Color Plate in the front of the book.)

NA functions as a sialidase and has a role in the release of the newly assembled virions from infected cells (246,268). This enzyme cleaves the linkage between a terminal sialic acid and the adjacent D-galactose or D-galactosamine. It is responsible for (a) the removal of sialic acids and (b) the release of budding virions. It also enables the transport of the virus through the mucin layer of the respiratory tract to bind to the target epithelial cell. The NA is a homotetramer, and each monomer harbors one catalytic site. This catalytic site is highly conserved among the different A subtypes and the B viruses.

It has long been postulated that sialic acid analogs may function as inhibitors to sialidases and may have antiviral activity (246,268,276,277). This competitive inhibition of NA may result in the inhibition of virus replication and spreading. Since 1999, new NA inhibitors have been licensed for use in several parts of the world (259,268,278). These licensed compounds display very effective inhibition of the NA enzymatic activity. The antiviral NA inhibitor interacts with amino acid residues of the catalytic pocket, especially glutamine 119, aspartate 151, arginine 152, glutamine 227, alanine 246, glutamine 276, and arginine 292. NA inhibitors bind the active site of influenza A and B viruses and prevent the cleavage of sialic acid molecules on the host cell membrane, efficiently preventing an important step in viral propagation (279) (Figs. 11.7 and 11.8). Mutations observed in these residues can lead to resistance (277) via subtype-specific mutations in framework or catalytic segments of NA (279).

Viruses with altered susceptibility to NA inhibitors have been identified recently (249,259,280). Given subtle variations in NA structures, resistance can be unique to individual NA inhibitors (274). Viruses with mutations in position 119, 152, 274, and 292 were resistant. In some viruses, mutations were also associated with changes in the HA protein (278), which acts synergistically with NA (259) and is near the RBS. These mutants lead to a reduced affinity to sialic acids and ease virion release when the sialidase activity of the NA is impaired because of mutations. However, reduced binding of HA may occur only for a specific subset of receptors. Receptors on Madin-Darby canine kidney (MDCK) cells, which are most often used for influenza virus growth inhibition assays, have both α-2,3– and α-2,6–linked terminal sialic acid residues, whereas human cells have only α-2,6–linked sialic acids (250). Hence, this system may not detect a virus with decreased binding capacities to α-2,6–linked sialic acids. In

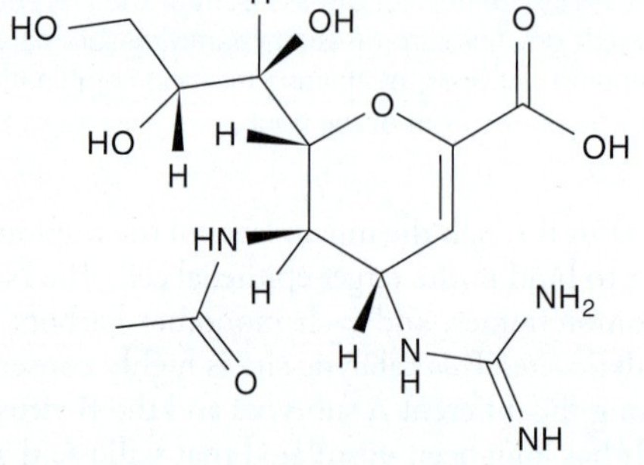

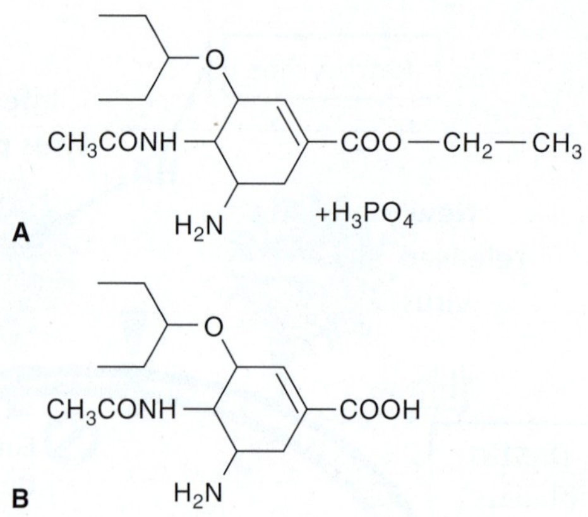

Figure 11.8 ■ Chemical structures of oseltamivir. Prodrug (oseltamivir [phosphate]) **(A)** and the active product (oseltamivir [carboxylate]) of oseltamivir **(B)**.

influenza A (H3N2) viruses, oseltamivir-resistant variants with the R292K mutation are reported. Drug-resistant strains from patients treated with oseltamivir have a mutation in E119V. The predominant resistance mutation against oseltamivir and peramivir in the influenza A (H1N1) virus is H274Y (274,279). By 2008 to 2009, more than 95% of seasonal H1N1 in the United States was resistant to oseltamivir on this basis (281). This mutant strain is still sensitive to zanamivir (274). A recent study created resistant strains using reverse genetic techniques to study drug resistance of various mutations, confirming these clinical observations (279). Multidrug-resistant H1N1 viruses may be due to certain NA mutations such as E119G and E119V. This severe form of resistance may produce increased risk for immunocompromised patients. It is thought that the potential for viral transmission is low, however (279). The I222V mutation increases resistance to oseltamivir as well as peramivir and raises concern about the potential public health implications of this double mutant strain of influenza (279).

A recent review found that oral oseltamivir reduces mortality in high-risk populations. Both oseltamivir and inhaled zanamivir also appear to reduce hospitalizations and decrease the duration of influenza symptoms (282). Oseltamivir-resistant strains predispose patients to develop pneumonia more often, particularly in immunocompromised individuals (272), increasing their morbidity and mortality.

The therapeutic regimen of neuraminidase inhibitors (NAIs) is shown in Table 11.18. Zanamivir is administered by oral or nasal aerosol. It

Figure 11.7 ■ Chemical structure of zanamivir.

Table 11.18

Zanamivir and Oseltamivir Treatment[a] and Chemoprophylaxis[b] Regimens for Influenza A and B

Drug		Age (Years)		
	1–4 or 6	**7–9**	**10–12**	**13–64 and ≥65**
Zanamivir[c,f]				
Treatment	NA[d] ages 1–6	10 mg BID by inhalation	10 mg BID by inhalation	10 mg BID by inhalation
Prophylaxis	NA ages 1–4	10 mg daily by inhalation ages 5–9	10 mg daily by inhalation	10 mg daily by inhalation
Oseltamivir[e,f]				
Treatment	NA	<15 kg 30 mg × 2/d		
		16–23 kg 45 mg × 2/d		75 mg twice daily
		23–40 kg 60 mg × 2/d		
		>40 kg adult dose		
Prophylaxis	NA	<15 kg 30 mg		75 mg daily
		16–23 kg 45 mg		
		23–40 kg 60 mg		
		>40 kg adult dose		

[a]Treatment regimens are generally administered for 5 days but can be extended for patients who remain severely ill.
[b]Chemoprophylaxis regimens are generally administered for 7 to 10 days but can be extended to 2 weeks for control of outbreaks in hospitals and chronic care facilities.
[c]Reduce dosage if creatinine clearance is less than 30 mL/min. Do not administer for persons with asthma and/or reactive airway disease.
[d]Not applicable/not approved.
[e]Reduce dose to 75 mg per day in case creatinine clearance is less than 30 mL/min; NA if creatinine clearance is less than 10 mL/min.
[f]Possible seasonal prevention in unvaccinated at-risk patient groups.
Adapted from Fiore AE, Fry A, Shay D, et al. Antiviral agents for the treatment and chemoprophylaxis of influenza—recommendation for the Advisory Committee on Immunization Practices (ACIP). *MMWR Recomm Rep* 2011;60:1–24.

is poorly absorbed (4% to 17%). It has a half-life of 3.4 hours and it has a bioavailability of 10% to 20% (283). After administration of a single 10-mg dose by using an inhaling device to administer the micronized formulation, the peak is observed at 2.5 hours with a concentration of 34 μg/L, and 78% of the active product is deposited in the oropharynx. As measured in different studies, the pharmacokinetic parameters after a single inhaled dose of 10 mg were area under curve (AUC), 247 μg/L · hour; t_{max}, 0.75 hours; $t_{1/2}$, 3.56 hours; C_{max}, 39 μg/L; and Cl_{ren}, 6.45 L/hour. Zanamivir is not metabolized, and 90% is eliminated unmetabolized in the urine.

Oseltamivir is given by mouth. Oseltamivir phosphate is an ethyl ester prodrug that is hydrolyzed by hepatic esterases to its active form, oseltamivir, specifically, oseltamivir carboxylate (see Fig. 11.8). Absolute bioavailability is approximately 80%, with an elimination half-life of oseltamivir carboxylate of 6.7 to 8.2 hours. The prodrug is

absorbed at 75%, with this form bound to serum proteins at 43%. Studies in healthy volunteers who received oral oseltamivir, 150 mg, and an intravenous infusion of oseltamivir, 150 mg, showed that the absolute bioavailability of oseltamivir (prodrug) was 79%, with a t_{max} of 5 hours and a maximum concentration of 456 μg/L. The metabolite (active drug) had an AUC of 6,834 μg/L · hour, t_{max} of 2.88 hours, V_d of 25.6 liters, $t_{1/2}$ of 1.79 hours, C_{max} of 2,091 μg/L, Cl of 6.67 L/hour, and a Cl_{ren} of 18.8 L/hour, with approximately 93% excreted in the urine. Pharmacokinetics of the active metabolite appeared to be linear up to dose of 500 mg oseltamivir orally twice daily (283).

Peramivir is the only intravenous (IV) option used for the treatment of severe influenza. Given its IV formulation, peramivir is quite useful for patients with oseltamivir-resistant strains but who are unable to use inhaled zanamivir due to preexisting asthma. In October 2009, during the pandemic, the FDA gave an emergency use authorization (EUA) to allow administration of peramivir based on safety data from phase 1, 2, and 3 clinical trials. The EUA for peramivir use in the United States expired in June 2010. It should be noted that peramivir is in clinical use in Japan and South Korea (259,272).

Both zanamivir and oseltamivir are well tolerated, with only minor side effects (284). However, because of the rare report of exacerbation of asthma in some young asthmatic patients, oseltamivir is not indicated in children with chronic asthma.

Other Antiinfluenza Agents and Approaches

The high rate of mutation of the influenza virus, combined with its ability to intermix its multiple RNA gene segments, allow for rapid development of new strains. This allows the virus to resist vaccination as well as standard therapies. Hence, there is an ongoing need to seek and develop new antiinfluenza agents using innovative strategies. There are several new inhibitors that attack traditional and also novel targets of influenza virus replication (see Fig. 11.6).

Laninamivir is a long-acting NA inhibitor that is effective against oseltamivir-resistant viruses (259). Laninamivir is available as a single-dose inhalation therapy. Another investigational drug against NA is favipiravir (6-fluoro-3-hydroxy-2-pyrazinecarboxamide). As this drug is metabolized, it gains nucleoside activity and inhibits influenza-specific RNA polymerase but does not inhibit human polymerases. This agent is effective against seasonal influenza viruses as well as oseltamivir-sensitive or oseltamivir-resistant highly pathogenic H5N1 strains and adamantine-resistant strains of influenza. Favipiravir is undergoing clinical trials in Japan (285).

New therapies based on pathogenic mechanisms of influenza viral life cycle and infectivity, similar to the work on ARVs in the HIV section, includes efforts to produce entry blocker, or EB. This is derived from fibroblast growth factor 4, which specifically binds to influenza viral HA protein. This drug exhibited broad antiviral activity against influenza viruses and also prevented reinfection (259).

DAS181 (Fludase) is a fungal sialidase chimeric protein that is fused to a cell surface–binding domain. This molecule functions like viral NA and destroys surface receptors required for host cell sialic acid binding. In studies, DAS181 (Fludase) inhibited both human and avian influenza (259).

Ribavirin is a synthetic nucleoside analog used most often in the treatment of HCV and has in vitro antiviral activity against influenza A and B viruses (246,286,287). It inhibits cellular inosine-5′-monophosphate dehydrogenase activity, thereby depleting intracellular pools of guanosine 5′-triphosphate. The phosphorylated ribavirin has a direct inhibitory effect on viral RNA-dependent RNA polymerase activity. However, studies focused on the role of ribavirin, either intravenous or inhaled, showed no definitive clinical benefit. Although ribavirin does have in vitro activity against influenza, the risks of side effects such as hemolytic anemia and teratogenicity belie its potential benefit and make this agent unsuitable for the treatment of influenza (244).

Testing Methodology for Influenza Therapies and Resistance

The rapid emergence of amantadine/rimantadine resistance in the late 1990s (275) and the recent observations of rapidly developing resistance to NAI during the 2007 to 2008 flu season (281) focused on the necessity to monitor susceptibility to influenza therapies. During 2007 to 2008, oseltamivir-resistant seasonal influenza A (H1N1) emerged, wherein the viruses carrying the H275Y mutation in NA did not respond to this therapy. By the 2008 to 2009 season, more than 95% of seasonal influenza A (H1N1) carried this resistance gene (279,280). Potential for the development and spread of resistant variants to each new therapy reinforces this stance.

Testing of Anti-M2 Products

The initial assay described was a PRA, which depended on incubation interval and showed great variability in results (288). Hence, alternative methods that can be easily standardized have been developed (289,290). These techniques are rapid, as compared with PRAs, and use an automated colorimetric assay with antibodies that detect virus growth in the inoculated cells (290). Briefly, virus stocks of the tested strains are prepared in cells to obtain a virus titer of approximately 10^4 per milliliter. Each virus stock is subsequently prepared in serial dilutions ranging from 10^{-1} to 10^{-5}; these dilutions are tested against six antiviral concentrations ranging from 40 to 0.0026 µg/mL in five-fold dilutions. The assay is performed in a 96-well microtiter plate and uses a chess-board titration technique that allows simultaneous titration of the virus both in the absence and the presence of increasing antiviral doses (amantadine or rimantadine). Vero or MDCK cells can be used; the results obtained with both cells are similar.

The titrated virus (i.e., 10^4 per milliliter) is used for cell inoculation in 96-well microtiter plates. The microtiter plate is prepared by inoculating 15,000 cells per well. The plates are incubated for 2 days at 35°C with 5% CO_2. Following incubation, culture medium is removed and 25 µL of the antiviral dilution, 25 µL of the calibrated virus suspension, and 200 µL of EMEM plus trypsine (final concentration, 2 µg/mL) are added to each well. Each test is performed in duplicate. After inoculation, the plates are centrifuged at 225 × g for 30 minutes at room temperature. The plates are subsequently incubated at 35°C in a 5% CO_2 atmosphere for 20 hours for MDCK cells and 44 hours for Vero cells. Subsequently, the medium is removed from each well and the cells are fixed with 200 µL of 0.1% glutaraldehyde prepared in PBS. The fixation is performed for 15 minutes at 20°C. The wells are then washed with 500 µL of PBS. Virus protein detection is performed with a rabbit polyclonal antiserum to the A or B strain and is used to detect a wide range of influenza proteins. Briefly, 50 µL of rabbit antisera prepared in PBS plus 0.5% bovine serum albumin (BSA) is added in each well and incubated for 90 minutes at 35°C. The wells are then washed with 500 µL of PBS. Next, 50 µL of protein A horseradish peroxidase conjugate is added and the

mixture is incubated for 60 minutes at 35°C. The wells are subsequently washed with PBS and 100 µL of the substrate solution is added to reveal the reaction. The substrate is a 2,2-azino-di-(3-ethylbenzthiazoline) sulfonic acid prepared in ABTS buffer. The incubation is performed at 20°C for 60 minutes. The optical densities are read at 405 nm by using a multichannel spectrophotometer; the data provided are analyzed with a microcomputer. For each antiviral concentration, a curve is drawn with the optical density values obtained with the different virus concentrations. This curve is compared with the control without antiviral agents. The antiviral concentration providing a 50% reduction in the production of antigenic material as determined at the optimal virus suspension is the IC_{50} value. This value is calculated from the data provided with the tested antiviral concentrations.

For strains sensitive to rimantadine, the IC_{50} range is from 0.02 to 1 µg/mL. The resistant strains have an IC_{50} ranging from 4 to 28 µg/mL.

Testing of Neuraminidase Inhibitors

Several assays are available and have been evaluated for testing NA inhibitors (Table 11.19). Cell-based assays are not convenient because of

Table 11.19

Summary of the Influenza Virus Neuraminidase Inhibitor Assays		
	Chemiluminescent Assay	**Fluorometric Assay**
Virus titration		
Volume of virus and buffer	50	20
Substrate	5 µL of NA-Star (100 µM)	50 µL of MUNANA (100 µL)
Titration conditions	15 min at 37°C, shaking	1 h at 37°C
Inhibition assay		
Signal-to-noise ratio	40:1	2:1
Volume of virus	40	25
Volume of inhibitor	40	25
Inhibitor concentration	0.028–550	0.0038–1,000
Inhibitor preincubation	30 min at room temperature	15 min at 37°C
Substrate	5 µL of NA-Star (100 µM)	50 µL of MUNANA (100 µL)
Incubation	15 min at 37°C, shaking	1 h at 37°C
Stop solution	55 µL of Sapphire II enhancer	150 µL of 50 mM glycin adjusted to pH 10.4 with NaOH
Substrate half-life	5 min	Hours
Assay duration	1 h	2 h, 15 min

the presence of alternative virus receptors to the α-2,6–linked sugar that is exclusively observed in human cells (291). Enzyme inhibition assays that are not subject to receptor specificity have been developed to determine enzyme inhibition with a substrate that mimics sialic acids. The most widely used substrate is the fluorogenic reagent 2'MUNANA (methyl umbelliferone *N*-acetyl aquaminic acid), initially described by Potier et al. (291).

The drawback of using fluorescent enzymatic assays is that evaluation of strains with poor enzymatic activity can be difficult. Therefore, an alternative chemiluminescent assay has been developed to overcome this problem (292), with a 1,2-dioxetane derivative of sialic acid. Both assays must be performed with the active antivirals zanamivir and oseltamivir carboxylate. Both procedures are summarized in Figure 11.9.

Fluorometric Neuraminidase Assay Method. The fluorometric assay was first described by Potier et al. (291). The input virus used for the assay must be titrated by making serial twofold dilutions and then graphically determining the virus and enzyme concentrations, which fall into the linear part of the curve for the inhibition assay. A signal-to-noise ratio of 2 or more is considered optimal for use in the inhibition assay. Equal volumes of drug and the appropriate virus dilution are mixed and incubated for 15 minutes at room temperature on 96-well microtiter plates. The final drug concentration uses ranges from 0.0033 to 30,000 nM in serial 1:10 dilutions. The reaction is initiated by the addition of 100 μM MUNANA substrate solution prepared in 2-(*N*- morpholino) ethanesulfonic acid (MES) buffer $CaCl_2$ (32.5 mM MES, pH 6.5, 4 mM $CaC1_2$). After 1 hour of incubation (37°C, with shaking), the reaction is stopped by the addition of 150 μL of a freshly prepared 50 mM glycin solution whose pH has been equilibrated to 10.4 with NaOH. This buffer is preferred to an alternative 0.14 M NaOH buffer prepared in 83% ethanol, which can result in precipitates in the reacting well.

Influenza virus NA activity is assayed in the fluorometric test by using a modification of the technique described by Potier et al. (291). The MUN, 2'-(4-methylumbelliferyl)-α-D-*N*-acetylneuraminic acid, sodium salt (MW, 489.4), was used as substrate, and 32.5 mM MES [2-(*N*-morpholino) ethanesulfonic acid, sodium salt (MW, 217.2), pH 5.8, 4 mM $CaC1_2$] was chosen for the buffer. The 100-μM working solution of MUN was prepared in MES.

Detailed Neuraminidase Activity Assay. Reaction mixtures containing 25 μL of calibrated virus obtained by twofold dilutions, 25 μL of MES $CaCl_2$, and 50 μL of 100 μM MUN working solution are incubated in flat-bottom plates for 1 hour at 37°C. The reaction is terminated by the addition of 150 μL of 50 mM glycine buffer, pH 10.4.

Fluorescence was quantified in a fluorometer with an excitation wavelength of 355 nm and an emission wavelength of 460 nm. Relative fluorescent units of sample were measured and corrected using the mean value of blank controls obtained when carrying out the reaction in the absence of virus.

The quantitation of NA activity was deduced from comparison of sample values with a standard curve established by using 4-methylumbelliferone (4-Mu) sodium salt. The equation establishing the correlation between free 4-Mu concentration and the amount of fluorescence is written as follows:

$$A \text{ (nmol 4} - \text{Mu/hour/mL)} = 22.7 \ 10^{-3} \times \Delta \text{ Fluorescence} \times \text{Dilution}^{-1}$$

(The constant value derived from the slope of the line.)

Detailed Neuraminidase Activity Inhibition Assay. A standard dose of virus (10 nmol/hour/mL) in 25 μL of MES buffer is preincubated with 25 μL of inhibitor dilution for 15 minutes at 37°C with shaking. After addition of 50 μL of 100 μM MUN working solution, the reaction mixture was incubated for 60 minutes at 37°C, with shaking. Finally, the reaction was terminated by adding 150 μL of 50 mM glycine buffer, pH 10.4. The IC_{50} values of inhibitors were further calculated as the inhibitor concentration required for reducing NA activity by 50%.

When used to determine NA activity inhibition assay, the values obtained with sensitive and resistant isolates were easy to interpret (see Fig. 11.9). Values of IC_{50} are between 0.05 and 2 nM, with the resistant isolates displaying IC_{50} values beyond 50 nM.

Chemiluminescent Assay. The chemiluminescent assay was developed as an alternative to the fluorometric assay. It is described by Buxton et al. (292). It requires the growth of cells and virus in phenol red–free media, since residual phenol red can interfere with the assay. The virus is initially titrated in twofold dilutions in 32.5 MES (pH 6.0)-4 mM $CaCl_2$, and the signal-to-noise ratio of 40 is used for the dilution. Final drug concentrations ranged from 0.028 to 550 nM

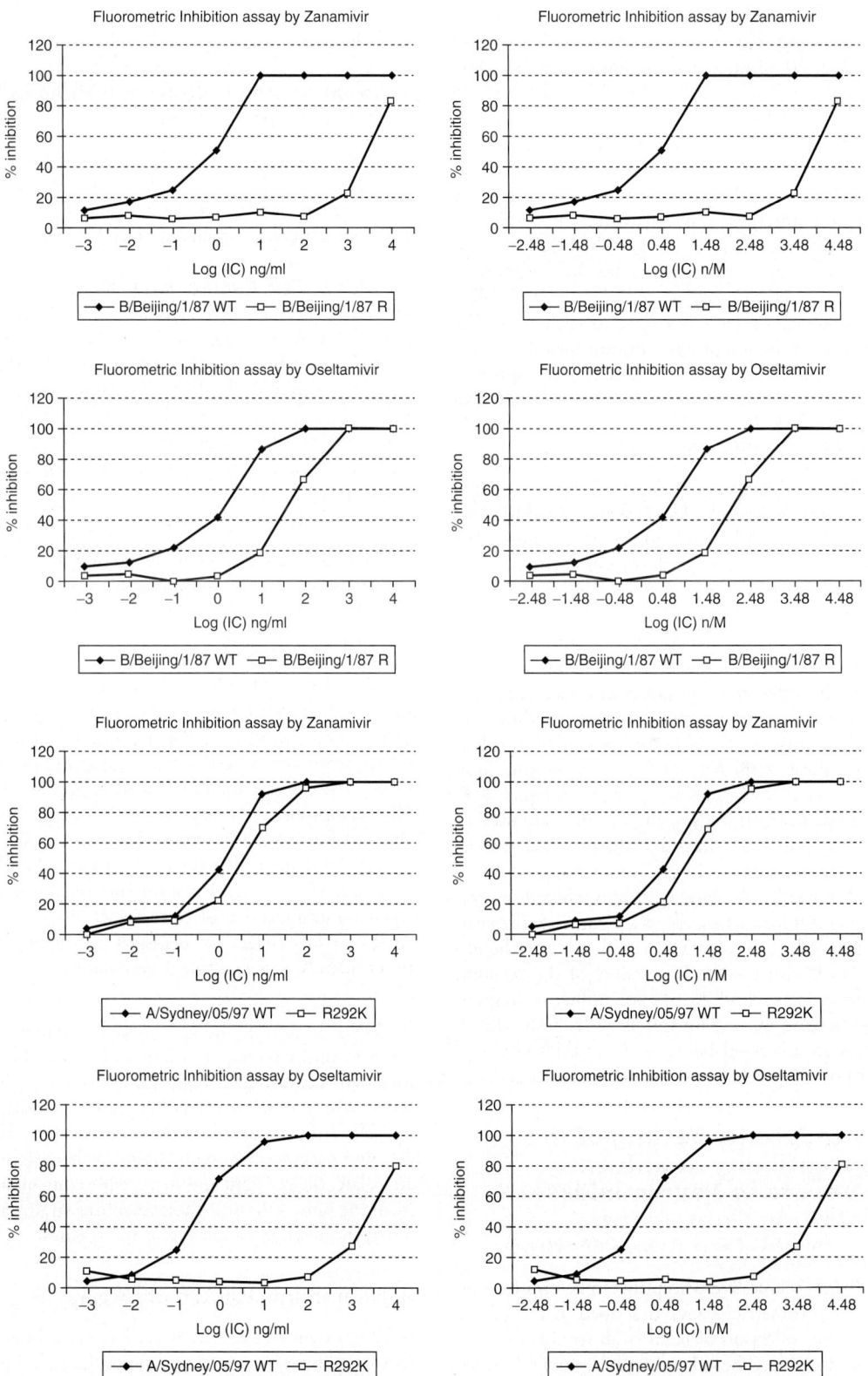

Figure 11.9 ■ Neuraminidase activity inhibition assay.

in serial 1:3 dilutions. The appropriate viral NA dilution (40 μL) was preincubated with 10 μL of drug for 30 minutes at room temperature on white Optiplates (Packard, Meridan, CT). The reaction was started by the addition of 5 μL of a 1:9 dilution of NA-Star prepared in 32.5 mM MES (pH 6.0)-4 mM $CaCl_2$. The final concentration of substrate used in the assay was 100 μM. The reaction mixture was incubated at 37°C for 15 minutes, with shaking. Chemiluminescent light emission was triggered by the addition of 55 μL of Light Emmission Accelerator II (Applied Biosystems, Foster City, CA) to each well. The half-life of the mixture is 5 minutes, which means that rapid automation is required to optimize sensitivity. All assay results were immediately read with an Applied Biosystems' (Foster City, CA) NORTHSTAR Luminometer.

IC$_{50}$ values were calculated by using the Robosage Microsoft Excel software add-in for curve fitting and calculation of IC$_{50}$ values. The equation used for the calculation of IC$_{50}$ values was $y = V_{max} \times (1 - [x/K + x])$. This equation describes a simple hyperbolic inhibition curve with a zero baseline. In this equation, x is the inhibitor concentration, y is the response being inhibited (i.e., the velocity of an enzymatic reaction), and V_{max} is the limiting response as x approaches zero. As x increases without bound, y tends toward its lower limit, zero. K is the IC$_{50}$ for the inhibition curve; that is, y is 50% V_{max} when x is equal to K. Graphic presentations of the raw data are used to identify possible sources of variability and to characterize any patterns in the data (see Fig. 11.9).

The results obtained with both chemiluminescent and fluorometric assays are consistent regarding the values for resistance thresholds in influenza A and B viruses. The IC$_{50}$ values of the resistant isolates are beyond 20 nM for influenza A stains and beyond 40 nM for influenza B. Some differences are observed between IC$_{50}$ values obtained with oseltamivir carboxylate and zanamivir.

Procedure for Testing of the Susceptibility of Influenza A Viruses to Neuraminidase Inhibition Fluorometric Neuraminidase Assay Method

Influenza viruses are susceptible to NA inhibition. The fluorometric assay, described here, begins with the collection of nasal swab specimens. This procedure may be adapted to begin with nasal

washes or throat swab specimens. Virus isolation must be performed on MDCK cells.

A. Isolation and Culture of Influenza Virus from Clinical Specimens

Clinical isolates are obtained by the culture of virus from clinical specimens on MDCK cells. Alternative culture systems for virus detection that have been proposed are less efficient than the MDCK cell system.

1. MDCK Cell Culture. MDCK cells can be purchased (ATCC, CCL34). Cells can be routinely passaged twice weekly in serum-free Ultra-MDCK medium (Cambrex Bioscience, Walkersville, MD) supplemented with 2 mM L-glutamine, penicillin (225 U/mL), and streptomycin (225 μg/mL). Alternatively, the passage medium can be EMEM with the same supplementation and with 2 μg/mL trypsin.

2. Virus Isolates. Swab samples are removed from the transport tube and expressed in 2.5 mL of EMEM, which has been supplemented with the antibiotic mix (penicillin plus streptomycin). The transport medium is then added. This suspension is inoculated onto MDCK subconfluent monolayers in 24-well microtiter plates. To promote growth of the influenza viruses, the microtiter plates are subsequently centrifuged at 300× g for 30 minutes (293). The cells are then incubated at 33°C in 5% CO_2 atmosphere. At day 4, the monolayers are checked for cytopathic effect. The supernatant is collected and may be tested for HA activity or blindly passaged. The HA activity of the supernatant must reach a minimum titer of 16 to detect NA activity. At least two passages are necessary to obtain this titer on MDCK cell culture supernatants.

3. Virus Controls. In each assay, a reference-sensitive and reference-resistant isolate should be included. The resistant isolate should have a specific resistant mutation in the NA gene (i.e., position R152). The susceptible isolates used were the ongoing vaccine prototype strains. When testing an isolate, the resistant and susceptible controls are from the same subtype. These reference strains are tested in the same conditions as the isolates.

B. Neuraminidase Activity Assay

Influenza virus NA activity is assayed in the fluorometric test by using a modification of the technique previously described by Potier et al. (291). The assay measures 4-methylumbelliferone released from the fluorogenic substrate 2′-MUN by the influenza virus NA.

1. Reagents. The *buffer* is 32.5 mL of 100 mM MES sodium salt, pH 5.8, and 4 mL of 100 mM $CaCl_2$ made up to a 100-mL final volume with sterile water. Store at 4°C.

The *substrate mix* is 100-μM working solution of MUN prepared in 32.5 mM MES, pH 5.8, 4-mM $CaCl_2$ buffer. Store 500-μL aliquots of 5 mM MUN at −20°C and dilute 1:50 in 32.5 mM MES, pH 5.8, 4 mM $CaCl_2$ buffer immediately prior to assay. This substrate mix must be stored in the dark (wrapped in aluminum foil).

The *stop solution* is 50 mM glycine, pH 10.4. Store at 4°C.

2. Titration of Neuraminidase Activity. The assay is performed in 96-well flat-bottom plates to allow optical reading from the bottom. Prior to performing the titration, creation of a standard curve is necessary to control the linearity of the assay within the concentration range used. This is also performed in a 96-well flat-bottom plate.

Standard Curve
Free 4-methylumbelliferone can be used to generate a standard curve and to verify the linearity of the assay. The reagents are 4-methylumbelliferone, sodium salt, and a stop solution of 50 mM glycine, pH 10.4. Store at 4°C.

For the reagent preparation of 5 mM of 4-methylumbelliferone stock solution, dissolve 9.91 mg in 10 mL of water. Store at 4°C in the dark for up to 2 months. For the preparation of 10 μM of 4-methylumbelliferone standard solution, dissolve 20 μL of stock solution into 10 mL of 50 mM glycine buffer, pH 10.4. Store at 4°C in the dark for up to 2 months. With the standard stock solution, prepare the dilution from 0.2 to 5 μM. Fluorescence is quantified with a fluorometer with an excitation wavelength of 355 nm and an emission wavelength of 460 nm.

Testing of Isolates
The isolate testing is done in 96-well flat-bottom plates. The reagents are added as follows: 25 μL of serial twofold dilutions (from 1/2 to 1/2,048) of culture supernatant of the controls and the tested isolates (HA titer above 16) prepared in 32.5 mM MES, pH 5.8; 4 mM $CaCl_2$ buffer are added in columns 2 to 12. Then 25 μL of 32.5 mM MES,

pH 5.8, and 4 mM $CaCl_2$ buffer are added to each well, except for the well of column 1 where the volume is 50 μL (reaction control). Fifty microliters of substrate are then added in every well to start the reaction. (A freshly made 100-μM working solution of MUN must be prepared in 32.5 mM MES, pH 5.8, and 4 mM $CaCl_2$ buffer.)

The contents of the plates are mixed gently on a mechanical vibrator. The plates are incubated for 1 hour at 37°C. The reaction is then stopped by adding 150 μL of 50 mM glycine buffer, pH 10.4, in each well. Fluorescence can be measured with a fluorometer with an excitation wavelength of 355 nm and an emission wavelength of 460 nm. If the measure is delayed, the plate must be stored in the dark.

Relative fluorescent units of a sample are measured and corrected using the mean value of blank controls obtained when performing the reaction in the absence of the virus (column 1). The quantification of NA activity is deduced from comparison of sample values with a standard curve established by using 4-Mu sodium salt. The equation establishing the correlation between free 4-Mu concentration and the amount of fluorescence is as follows:

$$A \text{ (nmol } 4 - \text{Mu/hour/mL)} = 22.7 \ 10^{-3} \times \Delta \text{ Fluorescence} \times \text{Dilution}^{-1}$$

(The constant value is derived from the slope of the line.) The A value obtained by this calculation is used to determine the input of the virus in the NA activity inhibition assay. This input must be 10 nmoL/hour/mL.

3. Neuraminidase Activity Inhibition Assay. The assay is done in 96-well flat-bottom plates to allow optical reading from the bottom. Reagents are added as described:

Twenty-five microliters of 10-fold dilutions of NA inhibitors prepared in 32.5 mM MES, pH 5.8, 4 mM $CaCl_2$ buffer (from 30,000 to 0.003 nM) are added in the wells from columns 1 to 8. Column 9 is used to determine the blank value and contains 50 μL of 32.5 mM MES, pH 5.8, and 4 mM $CaCl_2$ buffer. Twenty-five microliters of a standard dose of virus or control (10 nmoL/hour/mL, as determined in the titration of NA activity) prepared in 32.5 mM MES, pH 5.8, 4 mM $CaCl_2$ buffer is added to each well except well 9. Wells 10 to 12 are used as a control of the standard dose.

The contents of the plates are gently mixed on a mechanical vibrator. The plates are incubated for 15 minutes at 37°C. Then 50 μL of substrate is added in each well to start the reaction. (A freshly made 100-μM working solution of MUN is prepared in 32.5 mM MES, pH 5.8, and 4 mM $CaCl_2$ buffer.) The contents of the plates are gently mixed on a mechanical vibrator and the plates are incubated for 1 hour at 37°C. The reaction is then stopped by adding 150 μL of 50 mM glycine buffer, pH 10.4, in all wells. Fluorescence is immediately quantified by using a fluorometer with an excitation wavelength of 355 nm and an emission wavelength of 460 nm.

If this measurement is delayed, the plates must be stored in the dark. The IC_{50} values of antiviral agents are calculated according to the concentration required for reducing NA activity by 50%.

Phenotypic Assays

In general, genotypic assays are largely replaced by phenotypic assays for the detection of resistance to adamantine derivatives, amantadine and rimantadine. Complete cross-resistance between these antivirals is associated with amino acid substitution at position 26, 27, 30, 31, or 34 in the transmembrane region of the M2 protein of influenza A viruses (289). Conventional (Sanger) sequencing and pyrosequencing of the NA gene has also been used (294). The most frequently reported mutation with oseltamivir H1N1 resistance is H274Y (295). Mutations for E19V, R292K, and N294S were associated with oseltamivir resistance in N2NA (294).

CONCLUSIONS AND OUTLOOK

It is crucial to develop new agents/approaches to increase the global antiinfluenza armamentarium (259,285). There are five ongoing antiinfluenza approaches being used.

1. First is the development of new drugs that are directed against well-known viral proteins, such as NA, HA, the NS1 (e.g., laninamivir), and new agents directed against M2 ion channels.
2. Identification of effective compounds (see Fig. 11.6) that reduce virus growth has been identified that utilize small interfering RNA (siRNA) sequences to target influenza genes and limit viral protein synthesis. Investigational siRNA products targeting various influenza viral genes have been tested over the last few years but concerns regarding compound delivery and agent stability have yet to be resolved (259).
3. The third approach includes innovative treatments that target host factors, which are essential for virus replication, such as the host sialic

acid receptor using DAS181 (Fludase) as noted earlier (259,285).
4. Fourth, multidrug combination therapies that target several viral functions at once are being studied (285). Triple therapy with oseltamivir, amantadine, and ribavirin has demonstrated increased effectiveness against influenza A in high-risk populations; randomized clinical trials are underway to confirm these preliminary data. Other combinations of antiinfluenza agents will likely be studied as well given these preliminary observations.
5. Finally, the fifth possibility for new antiinfluenza regimens is to target naturally occurring innate peptides and other host immunologic factors, such as defensins, antibodies, and interferons, to maximize their antiinfluenza effects (259,285). Nitazoxanide, originally used as an antiparasitic agent, has been found to upregulate interferon response to influenza but also to exhibit specific inhibitory effect on the maturation of the HA protein (285). Defensins, also called retrocyclins, convey glycoprotein-binding inhibition, preventing fusion of other viruses, such as HIV, with host cells, revealing a novel antiviral mechanism. Another defensin may inhibit HA-mediated influenza viral fusion as well. Recently, retrocyclin synthetic analogs have been able to block influenza infection, suggesting that modification of defensins may produce new therapeutic agents to treat influenza (259). Antibody infusions derived from convalescent plasma have been used. Specific monoclonal antibodies (MABs) have also been developed. These MABs block HA from binding to its receptor, limiting the conformational change of the cell membrane, hence preventing infection. Several nonrandomized studies using antibodies have demonstrated decreased mortality in patients with complicated influenza (285). Clinical trials are under development to make use of these varied immunologic approaches.

Influenza remains a significant pathogen, which is the focus of global public health efforts. The rapid mutability of this virus and development of resistance genes has made worldwide control a challenge. Innovative therapies relying on both viral and host mechanisms are in use in some countries and other novel approaches are in development. Careful monitoring of viral resistance patterns and drug sensitivities will continue to be an important effort in the coming years to prevent and manage future pandemics.

REFERENCES

1. National Committee on Clinical Laboratory Standards. *Antiviral susceptibility testing: herpes simplex virus by plaque reduction assay; approved standard.* M11-A4. Wayne, PA: National Committee for Clinical Laboratory Standards, 2004.

2. Harmenberg J, Wahren B, Oberg B. Influence of cells and virus multiplicity on the inhibition of herpesviruses with acycloguanosine. *Intervirology* 1980;14(5-6):239–244.

3. Baldanti F, Underwood, MR, Talarico CL, et al. The Cys 607→Tyr change in the UL97 phosphotransferase confers ganciclovir resistance to two human cytomegalovirus strains recovered from two immunocompromised patients. *Antimicrob Agents Chemother* 1998;42:444–446.

4. Richman DD, Guatelli JC, Grimes J, et al. Detection of mutations associated with zidovudine resistance in human immunodeficiency virus utilizing the polymerase chain reaction. *J Infect Dis* 1991;164:1073–1081.

5. St. Clair MH, Martin JL, Tudor-Williams G, et al. Resistance to ddI and sensitivity to AZT induced by a mutation in HIV-1 reverse transcriptase. *Science* 1991;253:1557–1559.

6. Biron KK, Fyfe JA, Stanat SC, et al. A human cytomegalovirus mutant resistant to the nucleoside analog 9-{[2-hydroxy-1-(hydroxymethyl) ethoxy]} guanine (BW B579U) induces reduced levels of BW B759U triphosphate. *Proc Natl Acad Sci USA* 1986;83:8769–8773.

7. Gadler H. Nucleic acid hybridization for measurement of effects of antiviral compounds on human cytomegalovirus DNA replication. *Antimicrob Agents Chemother* 1983;24:370–374.

8. Belshe RB, Burk B, Newman F, et al. Resistance of influenza A virus to amantadine and rimantadine: results of one decade of surveillance. *J Infect Dis* 1989;159:430–435.

9. Bright RA, Medina MJ, Xu X, et al. Incidence of adamantine resistance among influenza A (H3N2) viruses isolated worldwide from 1994-2005: a cause for concern. *Lancet* 2005;366:1175–1181.

10. Deyde VM, Xu X, Bright RA, et al. Surveillance of resistance to adamantanes among influenza A(H3N2) and A(H1N1) viruses isolated worldwide. *J Infect Dis* 2007;196:249–257.

11. Durant J, Clevenbergh P, Halfon P, et al. Drug-resistance genotyping in HIV-1 therapy: the VIRADAPT randomised controlled trial. *Lancet* 1999; 353(9171):2195–2199.

12. Hirsch MS, Brun-Vezinet F, Clotet B, et al. Antiretroviral drug resistance testing in adults infected with human immunodeficiency virus type 1: 2003 Recommendations of an International AIDS Society–USA Panel. *Clin Infect Dis* 2003;37:113–128

13. The Euroguidelines Group for HIV resistance. Clinical and laboratory guidelines for the use of HIV-1 drug resistance testing as part of treatment management: recommendations for the European setting. *AIDS* 2001;15:309–320.

14. Demeter L, Haubrich RJ. Phenotypic and genotypic resistance assays: methodology, reliability, and interpretations. *J Acquir Immune Defic Syndr* 2001;26(Suppl 1):S3–S9.

15. Shafer RW. Genotypic testing for human immunodeficiency virus type 1 drug resistance. *Clin Microbiol Rev* 2002;2:247–277.

16. Vandamme AM, Houyez F, Banhegyi D, et al. Laboratory guidelines for the practical use of HIV drug resistance tests in patient follow-up. *Antivir Ther* 2001;6:21–39.

17. Shafer RW, Warford A, Winters MA, et al. Reproducibility of human immunodeficiency virus type 1 (HIV-1) protease and reverse transcriptase sequencing of plasma samples from heavily treated HIV-1 infected individuals. *J Virol Methods* 2000;86:143–153.

18. Japour AJ, Fiscus SA, Arduino JM, et al. Standardized microtiter assay for determination of syncytium-inducing phenotypes of clinical human immunodeficiency virus type 1 isolates. *J Clin Microbiol* 1994;32:2291–2294.

19. Brun-Vézinet F, Ingrand D, Deforges L, et al. HIV-1–1 sensitivity to zidovudine: a consensus culture technique validated by genotypic analysis of the reverse transcriptase. *J Virol Methods* 1992;37:177–188.

20. Kellam P, Larder BA. Recombinant virus assay: a rapid, phenotypic assay for assessment of drug susceptibility of human immunodeficiency virus type 1 isolates. *Antimicrob Agents Chemother* 1994;38:23–30.

21. Petropoulos CJ, Parkin NT, Limoli KL, et al. A novel phenotypic drug susceptibility assay for human immunodeficiency virus type 1. *Antimicrob Agents Chemother* 2000;44:920–928.

22. Whitcomb JM, Huang W, Fransen S, et al. Analysis of baseline Enfuvirtide (T20) susceptibility and co-receptor tropism in two-phase III study populations. *Proceedings of 10th conference on retrovirus and opportunistic infections*, Boston, MA, Feb 10–14, 2003; Abstract 557.

23. Qari SH, Respess R, Weinstock H, et al. Comparative analysis of two commercial phenotypic assays for drug susceptibility testing of human immunodeficiency virus type 1. *J Clin Microbiol* 2002;40:31–35.

24. Japour AJ, Mayers DL, Johnson VA, et al. Standardized peripheral blood mononuclear cell culture assay for determination of drug susceptibilities of clinical human immunodeficiency virus type 1 isolates. *Antimicrob Agents Chemother* 1993;37:1095–1101

25. Hertogs K, DeBethune MP, Miller V, et al. A rapid method for simultaneous detection of phenotypic resistance to inhibitors of protease and reverse transcriptase in recombinant human immunodeficiency virus type 1 isolates in patients treated with antiretroviral drugs. *Antimicrob Agents Chemother* 1998;42:269–276.

26. Kempf DJ, Isaacson JD, King MS, et al. Analysis of the virological response with respect to baseline viral phenotype and genotype in protease inhibitor-experienced HIV-1-infected patients receiving lopinavir/ritonavir therapy. *Antivir Ther* 2002;7:165–174.

27. Lanier ER, Hellmann N, Scott J, et al. Determination of a clinically relevant phenotypic resistance cut-off for abacavir using the PhenoSense assay. In: Proceedings of the 8th Conference on Retrovirus and Opportunistic Infections; February 4–8, 2001; Chicago, IL. Abstract 254.

28. Margot NA, Isaacson E, McGowan I, et al. Genotypic and phenotypic analyses of HIV-1 in antiretroviral-experienced patients treated with tenofovir DF. *AIDS* 2002;16:1227–1235.

29. Katzenstein DA, Bosch RJ, Wang N, et al. Baseline phenotypic susceptibility and virological failure over 144 weeks among NRTI experienced subjects in ACTG 364.

In: Proceedings of the 9th Conference on Retrovirus and Opportunistic Infections; February 24–28, 2002; Seattle, WA. Abstract 591.

30. Shulman NS, Hughes MD, Winters MA, et al. Subtle decreases in stavudine phenotypic susceptibility predict poor virologic response to stavudine monotherapy in zidovudine-experienced patients. *J Acquir Immune Defic Syndr* 2002;31:121–127.

31. Whitcomb JM, Huang W, Limoli K, et al. Hypersusceptibility to nonnucleoside reverse transcriptase inhibitors in HIV-1: clinical, phenotypic and genotypic correlates. *AIDS* 2002;16:F41–F47.

32. Katzenstein DA, Bosch RJ, Hellmann N, et al. Phenotypic susceptibility and virological outcome in nucleoside-experienced patients receiving three or four antiretroviral drugs. *AIDS* 2003;17:821–830.

33. Haubrich R, Keiser P, Kemper C, et al. CCTG 575: a randomised, prospective study of phenotype versus standard of care for patients failing antiretroviral therapy. *Antivir Ther* 2001;6(Suppl 1):63.

34. Sanger F, Nicklen S, Coulson AR. DNA sequencing with chain terminating inhibitors. *Proc Natl Acad Sci USA* 1977;74:5463–5467.

35. Meynard JL, Vray M, Morand-Joubert L, et al. Phenotypic or genotypic resistance testing for choosing antiretroviral therapy after treatment failure: a randomized trial. *AIDS* 2002;16:727–736.

36. Brun-Vézinet F, Descamps D, Ruffault A, et al. Clinically relevant interpretation of genotype for resistance to abacavir. *AIDS* 2003;17:1795–1802.

37. Calvez V, Costagliola D, Descamps D, et al. Impact of stavudine phenotype and thymidine analogue mutations on viral response to stavudine plus lamivudine in ALTIS 2 ANRS trial. *Antivir Ther* 2002;7:211–218.

38. Shulman NS, Machekano RA, Shafer RW, et al. Genotypic correlates of a virologic response to stavudine after zidovudine monotherapy. *J Acquir Immune Defic Syndr* 2001; 27:377–380.

39. Descamps D, Masquelier B, Mamet JP, et al. A genotypic sensitivity score for amprenavir based on genotype at baseline and virological response. *Antivir Ther* 2001; 6:S59.

40. Masquelier B, Breilh D, Neau D, et al. Human immunodeficiency virus type 1 genotypic and pharmacokinetic determinants of the virological response to lopinavir-ritonavir-containing therapy in protease inhibitor-experienced patients. *Antimicrob Agents Chemother* 2002; 46:2926–2932.

41. Calvez V, Cohen-Codar I, Marcelin AG, et al. Identification of individual mutations in HIV protease associated with virological response to lopinavir/ritonavir therapy. *Antivir Ther* 2001;6 (Suppl 1):64.

42. Van Laethem K, De Luca A, Antinori A, et al. A genotypic drug resistance interpretation algorithm that significantly predicts therapy response in HIV-1-infected patients. *Antivir Ther* 2002;7:123–129.

43. Tural C, Ruiz L, Holtzer C, et al. Clinical utility of HIV-1 genotyping and expert advice: the Havana trial. *AIDS* 2002;216:209–218.

44. Ravela J, Betts BJ, Brun-Vezinet F, et al. HIV-1 protease and reverse transcriptase mutation patterns responsible for discordances between genotypic drug resistance interpretation algorithms. *J Acquir Immune Defic Syndr* 2003; 33:8–14.

45. De Luca A, Cingolani A, Di Giambenedetto S, et al. Variable prediction of antiretroviral treatment outcome by different systems for interpreting genotypic human immunodeficiency virus type 1 drug resistance. *J Infect Dis* 2003;187:1934–1943.

46. Schmidt B, Walter H, Schwingel E, et al. Comparison of different interpretation systems for genotypic HIV-1 drug resistance data. *Antivir Ther* 2001;6(Suppl 1):102.

47. Larder BA, Kemp SD, Hertogs K. Quantitative prediction of HIV-1 phenotypic drug resistance from genotypes: the virtual phenotype (*Virtual* Phenotype). *Antivir Ther* 2000;5(Suppl 3):49–50.

48. Perez-Elias MJ, Garcia I, Munoz V. A randomized prospective study of phenotype (P) versus virtual phenotype (virtualP) testing for patients failing antiretroviral therapy. In: Proceedings of the 42nd Interscience Conference on Antimicrobial Agents; September 27–30, 2002; San Diego, CA. Abstract H-1079.

49. Parkin N, Chappey C, Maroldo L, et al. Phenotypic and genotypic HIV-1 drug resistance assays provide complementary information. *J Acquir Immune Defic Syndr* 2002; 31:128–136.

50. Brun-Vézinet F, Race E, Descamps D, et al. Difference between genotype and phenotype in the Narval trial, ANRS 088. *Antivir Ther* 2000;5(Suppl 3):78.

51. Bacheler L, Jeffrey S, Hanna G, et al. Genotypic correlates of phenotypic resistance to efavirenz in virus isolates from patients failing nonnucleoside reverse transcriptase inhibitor therapy. *J Virol* 2001;75:4999–5008.

52. Falloon J, Ait-Khaled M, Thomas DA, et al. HIV-1 genotype and phenotype correlate with virological response to abacavir, amprenavir and efavirenz in treatment-experienced patients. *AIDS* 2002;16:387–396.

53. Hsu A, Isaacson J, Brun S, et al. Pharmacokinetic-pharmacodynamic analysis of lopinavir-ritonavir in combination with efavirenz and two nucleoside reverse transcriptase inhibitors in extensively pretreated human immunodeficiency virus-infected patients. *Antimicrob Agents Chemother* 2003;47:350–359.

54. Shulman N, Zolopa A, Havlir D, et al. Virtual inhibitory quotient predicts response to ritonavir boosting of indinavir-based therapy in human immunodeficiency virus-infected patients with ongoing viremia. *Antimicrob Agents Chemother* 2002;46:3907–3916.

55. Marcelin AG, Lamotte C, Delaugerre C, et al. Genotypic inhibitory quotient as predictor of virological response to ritonavir-amprenavir in human immunodeficiency virus type 1 protease inhibitor-experienced patients. *Antimicrob Agents Chemother* 2003;47:594–600.

56. Perelson AS, Neumann AU, Markovitz M, et al. HIV-1 dynamics in vivo: virion clearance rate, infected cell life-span, and viral generation time. *Science* 1996;271: 1582–1586.

57. Weinstein MC, Goldie SJ, Losina E, et al. Use of genotypic resistance testing to guide HIV therapy: clinical impact and cost effectiveness. *Ann Intern Med* 2001; 134:440–450.

58. Schuurman R, Demeter L, Reichelderfer P, et al. Worldwide evaluation of DNA sequencing approaches for identification of drug resistance mutations in the human immunodeficiency virus type 1 reverse transcriptase. *Clin Microbiol* 1999;37:2291–2296.

59. Larder BA, Kohli A, Kellam P, et al. Quantitative detection of HIV-1 drug resistance mutations by automated DNA sequencing. *Nature* 1993;365:671–673.

60. Gunthard HF, Wong JK, Ignacio CC, et al. Comparative performance of high density oligonucleotide sequencing and dideoxynucleotide sequencing of HIV type 1

pol from clinical samples. *AIDS Res Hum Retroviruses* 1998;14:869–876.

61. D'Aquila RT. Limits of resistance testing. *Antivir Ther* 2000;5:71–76.

62. Charpentier C, Dwyer DE, Lecossier D, et al. Co-evolution and competition of viral populations with distinct resistance genotypes in patients failing treatment with protease inhibitors. *Antivir Ther* 2002;7:S42.

63. Moser MJ, Sharma PL, Nurpeisov V, et al. Using GENE-CODE technology to detect early emerging populations of drug-resistant human immunodeficiency virus Type 1. In: Proceedings of the XII International HIV Drug Resistance Workshop: Basic Principles and Clinical Implications; June 10–14, 2003; Los Cabos, Mexico. Abstract 89.

64. Simmonds P, Zhang LQ, McOmish F, et al. Discontinuous sequence change of human immunodeficiency virus (HIV) type 1 env sequences in plasma viral and lymphocyte-associated proviral populations in vivo: implications for models of HIV pathogenesis. *J Virol* 1991;65: 6266–6276.

65. Smith MS, Koerber KL, Pagano JS. Zidovudine-resistant human immunodeficiency virus type 1 genomes detected in plasma distinct from viral genomes in peripheral blood mononuclear cells. *J Infect Dis* 1993;167:445–448.

66. Wei X, Ghosh SK, Taylor ME, et al. Viral dynamics in human immunodeficiency virus type 1 infection. *Nature* 1995;373:117–122.

67. Koch N, Yahi N, Ariasi F, et al. Comparison of human immunodeficiency virus type 1 (HIV-1) protease mutations in HIV-1 genomes detected in plasma and in peripheral blood mononuclear cells from patients receiving combination drug therapy. *J Clin Microbiol* 1999;37:1595–1597.

68. Tashima KT, Flanigan TP, Kurpewski J, et al. Discordant human immunodeficiency virus type 1 drug resistance, including K103N, observed in cerebrospinal fluid and plasma. *Clin Infect Dis* 2002;35:82–83.

69. Ghosn J, Viard JP, De Almeida M, et al. HIV-1 resistance pattern may be frequently different than in blood in the male genital compartment of patients with therapeutic failure. *Antivir Ther* 2002;7:S46.

70. Solas C, Lafeuillade A, Halfon P, et al. Discrepancies between protease inhibitor concentrations and viral load in reservoirs and sanctuary sites in human immunodeficiency virus-infected patients. *Antimicrob Agents Chemother* 2003;47:238–243.

71. Marlowe N, Swanson P, Drews B, et al. Performance of Celera Diagnostics ViroSeq HIV-1 genotyping system on genetically diverse HIV-1 strains. In: Proceedings of the 10th Conference on Retroviruses and Opportunistic Infections; February 10–14, 2003; Boston, MA. Abstract 582.

72. Jagodzinski LL, Cooley JD, Weber M, et al. Performance characteristics of human immunodeficiency virus type 1 (HIV-1) genotyping systems in sequence-based analysis of subtypes other than HIV-1 subtype B. *J Clin Microbiol* 2003;41:998–1003.

73. Beddows S, Galpin S, Kazmi SH, et al. Performance of two commercially available sequence-based HIV-1 genotyping systems for the detection of drug resistance against HIV type 1 group M subtypes. *J Med Virol* 2003;70:337–342.

74. Kantor R, Katzenstein DA, Efron B, et al. Impact of HIV-1 subtype and antiviral therapy on protease and reverse transcriptase genotype: results of a global collaboration. *PLoS Med* 2005;2:325–337.

75. Beasley RP, Lin C-C, Hwang LY, et al. Hepatocellular carcinoma and hepatitis B virus: a prospective study of 22,707 men in Taiwan. *Lancet* 1981;2:1129–1133.

76. Rehermann B, Fowler P, Sidney J, et al. The cytotoxic T lymphocyte response to multiple hepatitis B virus polymerase epitopes during and after acute viral hepatitis. *J Exp Med* 1995;181:1047–1058.

77. Rehermann B, Lau D, Hoofnagle JH, et al. Cytotoxic T lymphocyte responsiveness after resolution of chronic hepatitis B virus infection. *J Clin Invest* 1996;97: 1655–1665.

78. Guidotti LG, Chisari FV. To kill or to cure: options in host defense against viral infection. *Curr Opin Immunol* 1996;8:478–483.

79. Ganem D, Schneider R. Hepadnaviridae: the viruses and their replication. In: Knipe DM, Howley PM, eds. *Fields virology*. Philadelphia: Lippincott Williams & Wilkins, 2001;2923–2970.

80. Kann M, Gerlich W. Hepadnaviridae: structure and molecular virology. In: Zuckerman A, Thomas H, eds. *Viral hepatitis*. London: Churchill Livingstone, 1998;77–105.

81. Kao JH. Clinical relevance of hepatitis B viral genotypes: a case of déjà vu? *J Gastroenterol Hepatol* 2002;17: 113–115.

82. Kao JH. Hepatitis B viral genotypes: clinical relevance and molecular characteristics. *J Gastroenterol Hepatol* 2002;17:643–650.

83. Kao JH, Liu CJ, Chen DS. Hepatitis B viral genotypes and lamivudine resistance. *J Hepatol* 2002;36:303–304.

84. Sugauchi F, Orito E, Ichida T, et al. Hepatitis B virus of genotype B with or without recombination with genotype C over the precore region plus the core gene. *J Virol* 2002;76:5985–5992.

85. Owiredu WK, Kramvis A, Kew MC. Hepatitis B virus DNA in serum of healthy black African adults positive for hepatitis B surface alone: possible association with recombination between genotypes A and D. *J Med Virol* 2001;64: 441–454.

86. Will H, Reiser W, Weimer T, et al. Replication strategy of human hepatitis B virus. *J Virol* 1987;61:904–911.

87. Okamoto H, Imai M, Kametani M, et al. Genomic heterogeneity of hepatitis B virus in a 54-year-old woman who contracted the infection through maternal fetal transmission. *Jpn J Exp Med* 1987;57:231–236.

88. Gunther S, Fischer L, Pult I, et al. Naturally occurring variants of hepatitis B virus. *Adv Virus Res* 1999;52: 25–137.

89. Zhang YY, Summers J. Enrichment of a precore-minus mutant of duck hepatitis B virus in experimental mixed infections. *J Virol* 1999;73:3616–3622.

90. Zhang YY, Summers J. Low dynamic state of viral competition in a chronic avian hepadnavirus infection. *J Virol* 2000;74:5257–5265.

91. Doo E, Liang TJ. Molecular anatomy and pathophysiologic implications of drug resistance in hepatitis B virus infection. *Gastroenterology* 2001;120:1000–1008.

92. Seeger C, Mason WS. Hepatitis B virus biology. *Microbiol Mol Biol Rev* 2000;64:51–68.

93. Lok AS, Akarca U, Greene S. Mutations in the pre-core region of hepatitis B virus serve to enhance the stability of the secondary structure of the pre-genome encapsidation signal. *Proc Natl Acad Sci USA* 1994;91:4077–4081.

94. Liang TJ, Hasegawa K, Rimon N, et al. A hepatitis B virus mutant associated with an epidemic of fulminant hepatitis. *N Engl J Med* 1991;324:1705–1709.

95. Omata M, Ehata T, Yokosuka O, et al. Mutations in the precore region of hepatitis B virus DNA in patients with fulminant and severe hepatitis. *N Engl J Med* 1991; 324:1699–1704.

96. Okamoto H, Yotsumoto S, Akahane Y, et al. Hepatitis B viruses with precore region defects prevail in persistently infected hosts along with seroconversion to the antibody against e antigen. *J Virol* 1990;64:1298–1303.

97. Hunt CM, McGill JM, Allen MI, et al. Clinical relevance of hepatitis B viral mutations. *Hepatology* 2000;31: 1037–1044.

98. Akarca U, Lok AS. Naturally occurring hepatitis B virus core gene mutations. *Hepatology* 1995;31:1037–1044.

99. Sirma H, Gianninni C, Poussin K, et al. Hepatitis B virus X mutants, present in hepatocellular carcinoma tissue abrogate both the antiproliferative and transactivation effects of HBx. *Oncogene* 1999;18:4848–4859.

100. Carman WF, Zanetti AR, Karayiannis P, et al. Vaccine-induced escape mutant of hepatitis B virus. *Lancet* 1990; 336:325–329.

101. Carman WF, Trautwein C, Van Deursen FJ, et al. Hepatitis B virus envelope variation after transplantation with and without hepatitis B immune globulin prophylaxis. *Hepatology* 1996;24:489–493.

102. Tavis J. The replication strategy of the hepadnaviruses. *Viral Hepatitis Rev* 1996;2:205–218.

103. Nassal M, Schaller H. Hepatitis B virus replication. *J Viral Hepatitis* 1996;3:217–226.

104. Hu J, Toft D, Seeger C. Hepadnavirus assembly and reverse transcription require a multi-component chaperone complex which is incorporated into nucleocapsids. *EMBO* 1997;16:59–68.

105. Von Weizacker F, Kock J, Weiland S, et al. Cis-preferential recruitment of duck hepatitis B virus core protein to the RNA/polymerase preassembly complex. *Hepatology* 2002;35:209–216.

106. Lok AS, Heathcote EJ, Hoofnagle JH. Management of hepatitis B: summary of a workshop. *Gastroenterology* 2001;120:1828–1853.

107. Guidotti LG, Rochford R, Chung J, et al. Viral clearance without destruction of infected cells during acute HBV infection. *Science* 1999;284:825–829.

108. Thimme R, Wieland S, Steiger C, et al. CD8+ T cells mediate viral clerance and disease pathogenesis during acute hepatitis B virus infection. *J Virol* 2003;77: 68–76.

109. Guo JT, Zhou H, Liu C, et al. Apoptosis and regeneration of hepatocytes during recovery from transient hepadnavirus infections. *J Virol* 2000;74:1495–505.

110. Kajino K, Jilbert AR, Saputelli J, et al. Woodchuck hepatitis virus infections: very rapid recovery after a prolonged viremia and infection of virtually every hepatocyte. *J Virol* 1994;68:5792–5803.

111. Boni C, Bertoletti A, Penna A, et al. Lamivudine treatment can restore T cell responsiveness in chronic hepatitis B. *J Clin Invest* 1998;102:968–975.

112. Valsamakis A. Molecular testing in the diagnosis and management of chronic hepatitis B. *Clin Microbiol Rev* 2007;20:426–439.

113. Chevaliez S, Rodriguez C, Pawlotsky JM. New virologic tools for management of chronic hepatitis B and C. *Gastroenterology* 2012;142:1303–1313.

114. Shaw T, Bartholomeusz A, Locarnini S. HBV drug resistance: mechanisms, detection and interpretation. *J Hepatol* 2006;44:593–606.

115. Chao DC, Hu KQ. Update on rescue therapies in patients with lamivudine-resistant chronic hepatitis B. *Drug Design Develop Ther* 2013;7:777–788.

116. Doong SL, Tsai CH, Schinazi RF, et al. Inhibition of the replication of hepatitis B virus in vitro by 2,′ 3′-di-deoxy-3′-thiacytidine and related analogues. *Proc Natl Acad Sci USA* 1991;88:8495–8499.

117. Liaw YF, Leung NW, Chang TT, et al. Effects of extended lamivudine therapy in Asian patients with chronic hepatitis B. Asia Hepatitis Lamivudine Study Group. *Gastroenterology* 2000;119:172–180.

118. Leung NW, Lai CL, Chang TT, et al. Extended lamivudine treatment in patients with chronic hepatitis B enhances hepatitis e antigen seroconversion rates: results after 3 years of therapy. *Hepatology* 2001;33:1527–1532.

119. Lewin SR, Ribeiro RM, Walters T, et al. Analysis of hepatitis B viral load decline under potent therapy: complex decay profiles observed. *Hepatology* 2001;34:1012–1020.

120. Ono SK, Kato N, Shiratori Y, et al. The polymerase L528M mutation cooperates with nucleotide binding-site mutations, increasing hepatitis B virus replication and drug resistance. *J Clin Invest* 2001;107:449–455.

121. Das K, Xiong X, Yang H, et al. Molecular modeling and biochemical characterization reveal the mechanism of hepatitis B virus polymerase resistance to lamivudine (3TC) and emtricitabine. *J Virol* 2001;75:4771–4779.

122. Allen MI, Gauthier J, DesLauriers M, et al. Two sensitive PCR-based methods for detection of hepatitis B virus variants associated with reduced susceptibility to lamivudine. *J Clin Microbiol* 1999;37:3338–3347.

123. Lau DTY, Khokhar F, Doo E, et al. Long-term therapy of chronic hepatitis B with lamivudine. *Hepatology* 2000;32:828–834.

124. Naesens L, Snoeck R, Andrei G, et al. HPMPC (cidofovir), PMEA (adefovir) and related acyclic nucleoside phosphonate analogues: a review of their pharmacology and clinical potential in the treatment of viral infections. *Antiviral Chem Chemother* 1997;8:1–23.

125. Heijtink RA, De Wilde GA, Kruining J, Berk L, et al. Inhibitory effect of 9-(2-phosphonylmethoxyethyl) adenine (PMEA) on human and duck hepatitis B virus infection. *Antiviral Res* 1993;21:141–153.

126. Del Gobbo V, Foli A, Balzarini J, et al. Immunomodulatory activity of 9-(2-phosphonylmethoxyethyl) adenine (PMEA), a potent anti-HIV nucleoside analogue, on in vivo murine models. *Antiviral Res* 1991;16:65–75.

127. Calio R, Villani N, Balestra E, et al. Enhancement of natural killer activity and interferon induction by different acyclic nucleoside phosphonates. *Antiviral Res* 1994;23:77–89.

128. Westland CE, Yang H, Delaney IV WE, et al. Week 48 resistance surveillance in two phase 3 clinical studies of adefovir dipivoxil for chronic hepatitis B. *Hepatology* 2003;38:96–103.

129. Angus P, Vaughan R, Xiong S, et al. Resistance to adefovir dipivoxil therapy associated with the selection of a novel mutation in the HBV polymerase. *Gastroenterology* 2003;125:292–297.

130. Westland CE, Villeneuve JP, Terrault N, et al. Resistance surveillance of liver transplantation patients with lamivudine-resistant hepatitis B virus after 96 weeks of adefovir dipivoxil treatment. *Hepatology* 2003;38:160A.

131. Balfour HHJ. Antiviral drugs. *N Engl J Med* 1999;340: 1255–1268.

132. Honkoop P, De Man RA. Entecavir: a potent new antiviral drug for hepatitis B. *Expert Opin Investig Drugs* 2003;12:683–688.

133. Yamanaka G, Wilson T, Innaimo S, et al. Metabolic studies on BMS-200475, a new antiviral compound active against hepatitis B virus. *Antimicrob Agents Chemother* 1999;43:190–193.

134. Levine S, Hernandez D, Yamanaka G, et al. Efficacies of entecavir against lamivudine-resistant hepatitis B virus replication and recombinant polymerases in vitro. *Antimicrob Agents Chemother* 2002;46:2525–2532.

135. Marion PL, Salazar FH, Winters MA, et al. Potent efficacy of entecavir (BMS-200475) in a duck model of hepatitis B virus replication. *Antimicrob Agents Chemother* 2002;46:82–88.

136. Colonno RJ, Genovesi EV, Medina I. Long term entecavir treatment results in sustained antiviral efficacy and prolonged life span in the woodchuck model of chronic hepatitis infection. *J Infect Dis* 2001;184:1236–1245.

137. Wolters LMM, Hansen BE, Niesters HGM. Viral dynamics during and after entecavir therapy in patients with chronic hepatitis B. *J Hepatol* 2002;37:137–144.

138. Tassopoulos NC, Hadziyannis SJ, Cianciara J, et al. Entecavir is effective in treating patients with chronic hepatitis B who failed lamivudine therapy. *Hepatology* 2001;34:340A.

139. Hayden FG. Antimicrobial agents (continued) antiviral agents (Nonretroviral). In: Hardman JG, Limbird LE, eds, Gilman AG, consulting ed. *Goodman & Gilman's: the pharmacological basis of therapeutics*, 10th ed. New York: McGraw-Hill, 2001:1313–1347.

140. James JS. Tenofovir approved: broad indication. *AIDS Treat News* 2001;(373):2–3.

141. Van Bommel F, Wunsche T, Schurmann D, et al. Tenofovir treatment in patients with lamivudine-resistant hepatitis B mutants strongly affects viral replication. *Hepatology* 2002;36:507–508.

142. Le Guerhier F, Pichoud C, Guerret S, et al. Characterization of the antiviral effect of 2'3'-dideoxy-2'-3' didehydro-beta-L-5-fluorocytidine in the duck hepatitis B virus infection model. *Antimicrob Agents Chemother* 2000;44:111–122.

143. Balakrishna PSS, Liu H, Zhu YL. Inhibition of hepatitis B virus by a novel L-nucleoside, 2' fluoro-5-methyl-beta-L-arabinofuranosyl uracil. *Antimicrob Agents Chemother* 1998;40:380–386.

144. Aguesse-Germon S, Liu H, Chevalier M, et al. Inhibitory effect of 2' fluoro-5-methyl-beta-L-arabinofuranosyl uracil on duck hepatitis B virus replication. *Antimicrob Agents Chemother* 1998;42:369–376.

145. Pierra C, Imbach JL, De Clercq E, et al. Synthesis and antiviral evaluation of some beta-L-2'-3' dideoxy-5-chloropyrimidine nucleosides and pronucleotides. *Antiviral Res* 2000;45:169–183.

146. Zhou XJ, Lim SG, Lai CL, et al. Phase 1 dose escalation pharmacokinetics of L-deoxithymidine in patients with chronic hepatitis B virus infection. *Hepatology* 2001;34:629A.

147. King RW, Ladner SK, Miller TJ, et al. Inhibition of human hepatitis B virus replication by AT-61, a phenylpropenamide derivative, alone and in combination with (−)beta-L-2,' 3'-dideoxy-3'thiacytidine. *Antimicrob Agents Chemother* 1998;42:3179–3186.

148. Delaney WE IV, Edwards R, Colledge D, et al. The phenylpropenamide derivatives AT-61 and AT-130 inhibit replication of both wild-type and lamivudine resistant strains of hepatitis B virus *in vitro*. *Antimicrob Agents Chemother* 2002;46:3057–3060.

149. Feld J, Colledge D, Sozzi T, et al. The phenylpropenamide derivative AT-130 inhibits HBV replication at viral encapsidation and packaging. *Hepatology* 2002;36:300A.

150. Deres K, Schroder CH, Paessens A, et al. Inhibition of hepatitis B virus replication by drug-induced depletion of nucleocapsids. *Science* 2003;299:893–896.

151. Kamiya N, Kubota A, Iwase Y, et al. Antiviral activities of MCC-478, a novel and specific inhibitor of hepatitis B virus. *Antimicrob Agents Chemother* 2002;46:2872–2877.

152. Ono-Nita SK, Kato N, Shiratori Y, et al. Novel nucleoside analogue MCC-478 (LY582563) is effective against wild-type or lamivudine-resistant hepatitis B virus. *Antimicrob Agents Chemother* 2002;46:2302–2605.

153. The European Association for the Study of Liver Jury. EASL international consensus conference on hepatitis B, 13–14 September, 2002, consensus statement. *J Hepatol* 2003;38:533–540.

154. Blum HE. Gene therapy of viral hepatitis. In: Tsuji T, Higashi T, Zeniya M, et al, eds. *Molecular biology and immunology in hepatology*. Freiburg, Germany: Elsevier Science, 2002;97–109.

155. Branch A. A hitchhiker's guide to antisense and nonantisense biochemical pathways. *Hepatology* 1996;24:1517–1529.

156. Hannon GJ. RNA interference. *Nature* 2002;41:244–251.

157. Shlomai A, Shaul Y. Inhibition of hepatitis B virus expression and replication by RNA interference. *Hepatology* 2003;37:764–770.

158. Lauer GM, Walker BD, MD. Hepatitis C virus infection. *N Engl J Med* 2001;345:41–52.

159. Colombo M. Natural history and pathogenesis of hepatitis C virus related hepatocellular carcinoma. *J Hepatol* 1999;31:25–30.

160. Penin F. Structural biology of hepatitis C virus. *Clin Liver Dis* 2003;7:1–21.

161. Glue P, Rouzier-Panis R, Raffanel C, et al. A dose-ranging study of pegylated interferon alfa-2b and ribavirin in chronic hepatitis C. The Hepatitis C Intervention Therapy Group. *Hepatology* 2000;32:647–653.

162. Fried MW, Shiffman ML, Reddy KR, et al. Peginterferon alfa-2a plus ribavirin for chronic hepatitis C virus infection. *N Engl J Med* 2002;347:975–982.

163. Jensen DM, Marcellin B, Freilich B, et al. Re-treatment of patients with chronic hepatitis C who do not respond to peginterferon-alpha2b: a randomized trial. *Ann Intern Med* 2009;150:528–540.

164. Jacobson IM, Gonzalez SA, Ahmed F, et al. A randomized trial of pegylated interferon alpha-2b plus ribavirin in the retreatment of chronic hepatitis C. *Am J Gastroenterol* 2005;100:2453–2462.

165. Heathcote EJ, Shiffman ML, Cooksley WG, et al. Peginterferon alfa-2a in patients with chronic hepatitis C and cirrhosis. *N Engl J Med* 2000;343:1673–1680.

166. Bressanelli S, Tomei L, Roussel A, et al. Crystal structure of the RNA-dependent RNA polymerase of hepatitis C virus. *Proc Natl Acad Sci USA* 1999;96:13034–13039.

167. Tellinghuisen TL, Foss KL, Treadaway JC, et al. Identification of residues required for RNA replication in domain II and III of the hepatitis C virus NS5A protein. *J Virol* 2008;82:1073–1083.

168. Kim JL, Morgenstern KA, Lin C, et al. Crystal structure of the hepatitis C virus NS3 protease domain complexed with a synthetic NS4A cofactor peptide. *Cell* 1996;87:343–355.

169. Fox AN, Jacobsen IM. Recent successes and noteworthy future prospects in the treatment of chronic hepatitis C. *Clin Infect Dis* 2012;55(Suppl 1):S16–S24.

170. Choo QL, Kuo G, Weiner AJ, et al. Isolation of a cDNA clone derived from a blood-borne non-A, non-B viral hepatitis genome. *Science* 1989;244:359–362.

171. Robertson B, Myers G, Howard C, et al. Classification, nomenclature, and database development for hepatitis C virus (HCV) and related viruses: proposals for standardization. International Committee on Virus Taxonomy. *Arch Virol* 1998;143:2493–2503.

172. Bantef H, Schulze-Ostoff K. Apoptosis in hepatitis C virus infection. *Cell Death Differ* 2003;10(Suppl 1): S48–S58.

173. Pawlotsky JM, Germanidis G, Frainais PO, et al. Evolution of the hepatitis C virus second envelope protein hypervariable region in chronically infected patients receiving alpha interferon therapy. *J Virol* 1999;73:6490–6499.

174. Simmonds P, Alberti A, Alter HJ, et al. A proposed system for the nomenclature of hepatitis C viral genotypes. *Hepatology* 1994;19:1321–1324.

175. Wasley A, Alter MJ. Epidemiology of hepatitis C: geographic differences and temporal trends. *Semin Liver Dis* 2000;20:1–16.

176. Martell M, Esteban JI, Quer J, et al. Hepatitis C virus (HCV) circulates as a population of different but closely related genomes: quasispecies nature of HCV genome distribution. *J Virol* 1992;66:3225–3229.

177. Giannini C, Bréchot C. Hepatitis C virus biology. *Cell Death Differ* 2003;10:27–38.

178. Pawlotsky JM. Hepatitis C virus resistance to antiviral therapy. *Hepatology* 2000;32:889–896.

179. Bartenschlager R, Lohmarm V. Novel cell culture systems for the hepatitis C virus. *Antiviral Res* 2001;52:1–17.

180. Griffin SD, Beales LP, Clarke DS, et al. The p7 protein of hepatitis C virus forms an ion channel that is blocked by the antiviral drug, amantadine. *FEBS Lett* 2003;535: 34–38.

181. Kaito M, Watanabe S, Tsukiyama-Kohara K, et al. Hepatitis C virus particle detected by immunoelectron microscopic study. *J Gen Virol* 1994;75:1755–1760.

182. Thomssen R, Bonk S, Thiele A. Density heterogeneities of hepatitis C virus in human sera due to the binding of beta-lipoproteins and immunoglobulins. *Med Microbiol Immunol* 1993;182:329–334.

183. Loriot MA, Bronowicki JP, Lagorce D, et al. Permissiveness of human biliary epithelial cells to infection by hepatitis C virus. *Hepatology* 1999;29:1587–1595.

184. Moldvay J, Deny P, Pot S, et al. Detection of hepatitis C virus RNA in peripheral blood mononuclear cells of infected patients by in situ hybridization. *Blood* 1994; 83:269–273.

185. Pileri P, Uematsu Y, Campagnoli S, et al. Binding of hepatitis C virus to CD81. *Science* 1998;282:938–941.

186. Meola A, Sbardellati A, Bruni Ercole B, et al. Binding of hepatitis C virus E2 glycoprotein to CD81 does not correlate with species permissiveness to infection. *J Virol* 2000;74:5933–5938.

187. Flint M, Quinn ER, Levy S. In search of hepatitis C virus receptor(s). *Clin Liver Dis* 2001;5:873–893.

188. Cocquerel L, Wychowski C, Minner F, et al. Charged residues in the transmembrane domains of hepatitis C virus glycoproteins play a major role in the processing, subcellular localization, and assembly of these envelope proteins. *J Virol* 2000;74:3623–3633.

189. Cocquerel L, Op de Beeck A, Lambot M, et al. Topological changes in the transmembrane domains of hepatitis C virus envelope glycoproteins. *EMBO J* 2002;21: 2893–2902.

190. Beales LP, Rowlands DJ, Holzenburg A. The internal ribosome entry site (IRES) of hepatitis C virus visualized by electron microscopy. *RNA* 2001;7:661–670.

191. Reed KE, Rice CM. Overview of hepatitis C virus genome structure, polyprotein processing, and protein properties. *Curr Top Microbiol Immunol* 2000;242:55–84.

192. Kunkel M, Lorinczi M, Rijnbrand R, et al. Self-assembly of nucleocapsid-like particles from recombinant hepatitis C virus core protein. *J Virol* 2001;75(5):2119–2129.

193. Fried MW, Shiffman ML, Reddy KR, et al. Peg interferon alfa-2a plus ribavirin for chronic hepatitis C virus infection. *N Engl J Med* 2002;347:975–982.

194. Hay AJ, Wolstenholme AJ, Skehel JJ, et al. The molecular basis of the specific anti-influenza action of amantadine. *EMBO J* 1985;4:3021–3024.

195. Lau JY, Tam RC, Liang TJ, et al. Mechanism of action of ribavirin in the combination treatment of chronic HCV infection. *Hepatology* 2002;35:1002–1009.

196. Dellamonica P, Calvez V, Marcelin AG, et al. The Antivirogram and the modes of action of antiviral agents, HIV, hepatitis, influenza and CMV. In: Lorian V, ed. *Antibiotics in Laboratory Medicine*. Philadelphia: Lippincott Williams & Wilkins, 2005;564–614

197. Mercer DF, Schiller DE, Elliott JF, et al. Hepatitis C virus replication in mice with chimeric human livers. *Nat Med* 2001;7:927–933.

198. Castet V, Fournier C, Soulier A, et al. Alpha interferon inhibits hepatitis C virus replication in primary human hepatocytes infected in vitro. *J Virol* 2002;76:189–199.

199. Rumin S, Berthillon P, Tanaka E, et al. Dynamic analysis of hepatitis C virus replication and quasispecies selection in long-term cultures of adult human hepatocytes infected in vitro. *J Gen Virol* 1999;80:3007–3018.

200. Lohmann V, Komer F, Koch J, et al. Replication of subgenomic hepatitis C virus RNAs in a hepatoma cell line. *Science* 1999;285:110–113.

201. Blight KJ, Kolykhalov AA, Rice CM. Efficient initiation of HCV RNA replication in cell culture. *Science* 2000 Dec 8;290:1972–1974.

202. Piertschmann T, Lohmann V, Rutter G, et al. Characterization of cell lines carrying self-replicating hepatitis C virus RNAs. *J Virol* 2001;75:1252–1264.

203. Pawlotsky JM. Mechanisms of antiviral treatment efficacy and failure in chronic hepatitis C. *Antiviral Res* 2003;59:1–11.

204. Lamarre D, Anderson PC, Bailey M, et al. An NS3 protease inhibitor with antiviral effects in humans infected with hepatitis C virus. *Nature* 2003;426:186–189.

205. Harrington PR, Zeng W, Neger LK. Clinical relevance of detectable but quantifiable hepatitic C virus RNA during boceprevir or telaprevir treatment. *Hepatology* 2012; 55:1048–1057.

206. Perlman BL, Traub N. Sustained virologic response to antiviral therapy for chronic hepatitis C virus infection: a cure and so much more. *Clin Infect Dis* 2011;52:889–900.

207. U.S. Food and Drug Administration. Chronic hepatitis C virus infection: developing direct-acting antiviral agents for treatment. Draft guidance for industry. September, 2010.

208. Ferenci P, Laferl H, Scherzer TM, et al. PEG-interferon alfa-2a and ribavirin for 24 weeks in hepatitis C type 1 and 4 patients with rapid virological response. *Gastroenterology* 2008;135:451–458.

209. Ghany MG, Strader DB, Thomas DL, et al. Diagnosis, management, and treatment of hepatitis C: an update. *Hepatology* 2009;49:1335–1374.

210. Bowen EF, Emery VC, Wilson P, et al. Cytomegalovirus polymerase chain reaction viraemia in patients receiving ganciclovir maintenance therapy for retinitis. *AIDS* 1998;12:605–611.

211. Boivin G, Gilbert C, Gaudreau A, et al. Rate of emergence of cytomegalovirus (CMV) mutations in leukocytes of patients with acquired immunodeficiency syndrome who are receiving valganciclovir as induction and maintenance therapy for CMV retinitis. *J Infect Dis* 2001; 184:1598–1602.

212. Weinberg A, Jabs DA, Chou S, et al. for the cytomegalovirus retinitis and viral resistance study group and the adult AIDS clinical trials group cytomegalovirus laboratories. Mutations conferring foscarnet resistance in a cohort of patients with acquired immunodeficiency syndrome and cytomegalovirus retinitis. *J Infect Dis* 2003; 187:777–784.

213. Limaye AP, Corey L, Koelle DM, et al. Emergence of ganciclovir-resistant cytomegalovirus disease among recipients of solid-organ transplants. *Lancet* 2000; 356:645–649.

214. Ducancelle A, Belloc S, Alain S, et al. Comparison of sequential cytomegalovirus isolates in a patient with lymphoma and failing antiviral therapy. *J Clin Virol* 2004; 29:241–247.

215. Lurain NS, Weinberg A, Crumpacker CS, et al. Sequencing of cytomegalovirus UL97 gene for genotypic antiviral resistance testing. *Antimicrob Agents Chemother* 2001;45:2775–2780.

216. Landry ML, Stanat S, Biron K, et al. A standardized plaque reduction assay for determination of drug susceptibilities of cytomegalovirus clinical isolates. *Antimicrob Agents Chemother* 2000;44:688–692.

217. Dankner WM, Scholl D, Stanat SC, et al. Rapid antiviral DNA-DNA hybridization assay for human cytomegalovirus. *J Virol Methods* 1990;28:293–298.

218. McSharry JM, Lurain NS, Drusano GL, et al. Flow cytometric determination of ganciclovir susceptibilities of human cytomegalovirus clinical isolates. *J Clin Microbiol* 1998;36:958–964.

219. Tatarowicz WA, Lurain NS, Thompson KD. In situ ELISA for the evaluation of antiviral compounds effective against human cytomegalovirus. *J Virol Methods* 1991;35:207–215.

220. Pépin JM, Simon F, Dussault A, et al. Rapid determination of human cytomegalovirus susceptibility to ganciclovir directly from clinical specimens primocultures. *J Clin Microbiol* 1992;30:2917–2920.

221. Gerna G, Sarasini A, Percivalle E, et al. Rapid screening for resistance to ganciclovir and foscarnet of primary isolates of human cytomegalovirus from culture-positive blood samples. *J Clin Microbiol* 1995;33:738–741.

222. Eckle T, Prix L, Jahn G, et al. Drug-resistant human cytomegalovirus infection in children after allogeneic stem cell transplantation may have different clinical outcomes. *Blood* 2000;96:3286–3289.

223. Chou E, Lurain NS, Thompson KD, et al. Viral DNA polymerase mutations associated with drug resistance in human cytomegalovirus. *J Infect Dis* 2003;188:32–39.

224. Baldanti F, Michel D, Simoncini L, et al. Mutations in the UL97 ORF of ganciclovir-resistant clinical cytomegalovirus isolates differentially affect GCV phosphorylation as determined in a recombinant vaccinia virus system. *Antiviral Res* 2002;54:59–67.

225. Sullivan V, Talarico CL, Stanat SC, et al. A protein kinase homologue controls phosphorylation of ganciclovir

in human cytomegalovirus-infected cells. *Nature* 1992; 358:162–164.

226. Smith IL, Cherrington JM, Jiles RE, et al. High-level resistance of cytomegalovirus to ganciclovir is associated with alterations in both the UL97 and DNA polymerase genes. *J Infect Dis* 1997;176:69–77.

227. Chou E, Marousek G, Guentzel S, et al. Evolution of mutations conferring multidrug resistance during prophylaxis and therapy for cytomegalovirus disease. *J Infect Dis* 1997;176:786–789.

228. Chou E, Marousek G, Parenti DM, et al. Mutation in region III of the DNA polymerase gene conferring foscarnet resistance in cytomegalovirus isolates from three subjects receiving prolonged antiviral therapy. *J Infect Dis* 1998;178:526–530.

229. Cihlar T, Fuller MD, Cherrington J. Characterization of drug resistance-associated mutations in the human cytomegalovirus DNA polymerase gene by using recombinant mutant viruses generated from overlapping DNA fragments. *J Virol* 1998;72:5927–5936.

230. Erice A. Resistance of human cytomegalovirus to antiviral drugs. *Clin Microbiol Rev* 1999;12(Suppl 2):S286–S297.

231. Sullivan V, Biron KK, Talarico CL, et al. A point mutation in the human cytomegalovirus DNA polymerase gene confers resistance to ganciclovir and phosphonylmethoxyalkyl derivatives. *Antimicrob Agents Chemother* 1993;37:19–25.

232. Hirt B. Selective extraction of polyoma DNA from infected mouse cell cultures. *J Mol Biol* 1967;26:365–369.

233. Alain S, Mazeron MC, Pepin JM, et al. Rapid detection of cytomegalovirus strains resistant to ganciclovir through mutations within the gene UL 97. *Mol Cell Probes* 1993;7:487–495.

234. Chou S, Guentzel S, Michels KR, et al. Frequency of UL97 phosphotransferase mutations related to ganciclovir resistance in clinical cytomegalovirus isolates. *J Infect Dis* 1995;172:239–242.

235. Chou S, Erice A, Jordan MC, et al. Analysis of the UL97 phosphotransferase coding sequence in clinical cytomegalovirus isolates and identification of mutations conferring ganciclovir resistance. *J Infect Dis* 1995; 171:576–583.

236. Hanson MH, Preheim LC, Chou S, et al. Novel mutation in the UL97 gene of a clinical cytomegalovirus strain conferring resistance to ganciclovir. *Antimicrob Agents Chemother* 1995;39:1204–1205.

237. Harada K, Eizuru Y, Isashiki Y, et al. Genetic analysis of a clinical isolate of human cytomegalovirus exhibiting resistance against both ganciclovir and cidofovir. *Arch Virol* 1997;142:215–225.

238. Chou S, Lurain NS, Weinberg A, et al. Interstrain variation in the human cytomegalovirus DNA polymerase sequence and its effect on genotypic diagnosis of antiviral drug resistance. *Antimicrob Agents Chemother* 1999; 43:1500–1502.

239. Fillet AM, Auray L, Alain S, et al. Natural polymorphism of cytomegalovirus DNA polymerase lies in two non-conserved regions spanning between domains delta-C and II and between domains III and I. *Antimicrob Agents Chemother* 2004;48:1865–1868.

240. Kotton CN, Kumar D, Caliendo AM, et al. Updated international consensus guidelines on the management of cytomegalovirus in solid-organ transplantation. *Transplantation* 2013;96:333–360.

241. Zambon MC. Epidemiology and pathogenesis of influenza. *J Antimicrobial Chemother* 1999;44:3–9.

242. World Health Organization. Influenza virus infections in humans. http://www.who.int/influenza /GIP_Influenza VirusInfectionsHumans_Jul13.pdf?ua=1. Accessed December 15, 2013.

243. Scholtissek C. Source for influenza pandemics. *Eur J Epidemiol* 1994;10:455–458.

244. Labella AM, Merel SE. Influenza. *Med Clin North Am* 2013;97:621–645.

245. Reid AH, Fanning TG, Hultin JV, et al. Origin and evolution of the 1918 "Spanish" influenza gene. *Proc Natl Acad Sci USA* 1999;96:1651–1656.

246. Stuart-Harris CH, Schild GC, Oxford JS, eds. *Influenza. The virus and the disease*. London: Edward Arnold, 1985:103–117.

247. Aymard M, Valette M, Lina B, et al. Surveillance and impact of influenza in Europe. *Vaccine* 1999;17: S30–S41.

248. Schrauwen EJ, de Graaf M, Herfst S, et al. Determinants of virulence of influenza A virus. *Eur J Clin Microbiol Infect Dis* 2013; Sep: 29.

249. Fiore AE, Fry A, Shay D, et al. Antiviral agents for the treatment and chemoprophylaxis of influenza—recommendation for the Advisory Committee on Immunization Practices (ACIP). *MMWR Recomm Rep* 2011; 60:1–24.

250. Murphy BR, Webster RG. Orthomyxoviruses. In: Fields BN, Knipe DM, Howley PM, eds. *Virology*. 3rd ed. Lippincott-Raven: Philadelphia, 1996:1397–1446.

251. Samji T. Influenza A: understanding the viral life cycle. *Yale J of Biol and Med* 2009;82:153–159.

252. Farrukee R, Mosse J, Hurt AC. Review of the clinical effectiveness of neuraminidase inhibitors against influenza B viruses. *Expert Rev Anti Infect Ther* 2013;11: 1135–1145.

253. Towers S, Chowell G, Hameed R, et al. Climate change and influenza: the likelihood of early and severe influenza seasons following warmer than average winters. *PLoS Curr* 2013;5.

254. Zambon MC. The pathogenesis of influenza in humans. *Rev Med Virol* 2001;11:227–241.

255. Tong HH, Long JP, Shannon A, et al. Expression of cytokine and chemokine genes by human middle ear epithelial cells induced by influenza A virus and *Streptococcus pneumoniae* opacity variants. *Infect Immun* 2003; 71:4289–4296.

256. Joseph C, Togawa Y, Shindo N. Bacterial and viral infections associated with influenza. *Influenza Other Respir Viruses* 2013;7(Suppl 2):105–113.

257. Harper SA, Bradley JS, Englund JA, et al. Seasonal influenza in adults and children—diagnosis, treatment, chemoprophylaxis and institutional outbreak management: clinical practice guidelines of the Infectious Diseases Society of America. *Clin Infect Dis* 2009;48:1003–1032.

258. Centers for Disease Control and Prevention. Influenza antiviral medications: summary for clinicians. http://www.cdc.gov/flu/pdf/professionals/antivirals/antiviral-summary-clinicians.pdf. Accessed December 15, 2013.

259. Barik S. New treatments for influenza. *BMC Med* 2012; 10:104.

260. Prevention and control of influenza with vaccines: recommendations of the Advisory Committee on Immunization Practices (ACIP)—United States, 2012–13 influenza season. http://www.cdc.gov/mmwr/preview/ mmwrhtml/. Accessed December 15, 2013.

261. Pielak RM, Chou JJ. Influenza M2 proton channels. *Biochim Biophys Acta* 2011;1808:522–529.

262. Holsinger LJ, Nichari D, Pinto LH, et al. Influenza A virus M2 ion channel protein: a structure-function analysis. *J Virol* 1994;68:1551–1563.

263. Whiley DC, Skehel JJ. The structure and function of the hemagglutinin membrane glycoprotein of influenza virus. *Annu Rev Biochem* 1987;56:365–394.

264. Skehel JJ, Wiley DC. Receptor binding and membrane fusion in virus entry: the influenza hemagglutinin. *Annu Rev Biochem* 2000;69:531–569.

265. Voeten JTM, Bestebroer TM, Nieuwkoop NJ, et al. Antigenic drift in the influenza A virus (H3N2) nucleoprotein and escape from recognition by cytotoxic T lymphocytes. *J Virol* 2000;74:6800–6807.

266. Wiley DC, Wilson IA, Skehel JJ. Structural identification of the antibody-binding sites of Hong Kong influenza haemagglutinin and their involvement in antigenic variation. *Nature* 1981;289:373–378.

267. Zhirnov OP, Ikizler MR, Wright PF. Cleavage of influenza A virus hemagglutinin in human respiratory epithelium is cell associated and sensitive to exogenous antiproteases. *J Virol* 2002;76:8682–8689.

268. Coleman PM. Influenza virus neuraminidase: structure, antibodies, and inhibitors. *Protein Sci* 1994;3: 1687–1696.

269. Barman S, Ali A, Hui EK, et al. Transport of viral proteins to the apical membranes and interaction of matrix protein with glycoproteins in the assembly of influenza viruses. *Virus Res* 2001;77:61–69.

270. Kawoka J. Enigmas of influenza. S4–2. Paper presented at: Fifth Annual Options for the control of Influenza Conference; October 7–11, 2003; Okinawa, Japan.

271. Blick TJ, Sahasrabudhe A, Mcdonald M, et al. The interaction of neuraminidase and haemagglutinin mutations in the influenza virus in resistance to 4-guanadino-Neu5Ac2en. *Virology* 1998;246:95–103.

272. Thorlund K, Awad T, Boivin G, et al. Systematic review of influenza resistance to the neuraminidase inhibitors. *BMC Infectious Dis* 2011;11:134–147.

273. Dolin R, Reichmein RC, Madore HP, et al. A controlled trial of amantadine and rimantadine in the prophylaxis of influenza A infection. *N Engl J Med* 1982;307: 580–584.

274. McKimm-Breschkin JL. Influenza neuraminidase inhibitors: antiviral action and mechanisms of resistance. *Influenza Other Respir Viruses* 2013;7(Suppl 1):25–36.

275. Bright RA, Shay DK, Shu B, et al. Adamantane resistance among influenza A viruses isolated early during the 2005-2006 influenza season in the United States. *JAMA* 2006;295:891–894.

276. Palese P, Compans RW. Inhibition of influenza virus replication in tissue culture by 2-deoxy-2,3-dehydro-N-trifluoro-acetylneuraminic acid (FANA): mechanism of action. *J Gen Virol* 1976;33:159–163.

277. McKimm-Breschin JL. Resistance of influenza viruses to neuraminidase inhibitors: a review. *Antiviral Res* 2000; 47:1–17.

278. Wetherall NT, Trivedi T, Zeller J, et al. Evaluation of neuraminidase enzyme assays using different substrates to measure susceptibility of influenza virus clinical isolates to neuraminidase inhibitors: report of the neuraminidase inhibitor susceptibility network. *J Clin Microbiol* 2003;41:742–750.

279. Pizzorno A, Bouhy X, Abed Y, et al. Generation and characterization of recombinant pandemic influenza A (H1N1) viruses resistant to neuraminidase inhibitors. *J Infect Dis* 2011;203:25–31.

280. Okomo-Adhiambo M, Sheu TG, Gubareva LV. Assays for monitoring susceptibility of influenza viruses to neuraminidase inhibitors. *Influenza Other Respir Viruses* 2013;7(Suppl 1):44–49.

281. Dharan NJ, Gubareva LV, Meyer JJ, et al. Infections with osltamivir-resistant influenza A (H1N1) in the United States. *JAMA* 2009;301:1034–1041.

282. Hsu J, Santesso N, Mustafa R, et al. Antivirals for treatment of influenza: a systematic review and meta-analysis of observational studies. *Ann Intern Med* 2012;156:512–524.

283. McNicholl IR, McNicholl JJ. Neuraminidase inhibitors: zanamivir and oseltamivir. *Ann Pharmacother* 2001; 35:57–70.

284. Gubareva LV, Kaiser L, Hayden FG. Influenza virus neuraminidase inhibitors. *Lancet* 2000;355:827–35.

285. Hayden FG. Newer influenza antivirals, biotherapeutics and combinations. *Influenza Other Resp Viruses* 2013; 7(Suppl 1):63–75.

286. Stiver G. The treatment of influenza with antiviral drugs. *CMAJ* 2003;168:49–56.

287. Shigeta S. Targets of anti-influenza chemotherapy other than neuraminidase and proton pump. *Antivir Chem Chemother* 2001;12(Supp 1):179–88.

288. Hayden FG, Cote KM, Douglas GJR. Plaque inhibition assay for drug susceptibility testing of influenza virus. *Antimicrob Agents Chemother* 1980;17:865–870.

289. Belshe RB, Smith MH, Hall CB, et al. Genetic basis of resistance to rimantidine emerging during treatment of influenza virus infection. *J Virol* 1988;62:1508–1512.

290. Valette M, Allard JP, Aymard M, et al. Susceptibilities to rimantadine of influenza A/H1N1 and A/H3N2 viruses isolated during the epidemics of 1988 to 1989 and 1989 to 1990. *Antimicrob Agents Chemother* 1993;37: 2239–2240.

291. Potier M, Mameli L, Bélisle M, et al. Fluorometric assay of neuraminidase with a sodium (4-methylumbel liferyl-D-N-acetylneuraminate) substrate. *Anal Biochem* 1979;94:287–296.

292. Buxton RC, Edwards B, Juo RR, et al. Development of a sensitive chemiluminescent neuraminidase assay for the detection of influenza virus susceptibility to zanamivir. *Anal Biochem* 2000;280:291–300.

293. Chonel JJ, Pardon D, Thouvenot D, et al. Comparison between three rapid methods for direct diagnosis of influenza and the conventional isolation procedure. *Biologicals* 1991;19:287–292.

294. Deyde VM, Okomo-Adhiambo M, Sheu TG, et al. Pyrosequencing as a tool to detect molecular markers of resistance to neuraminidase inhibitors in seasonal influenza A viruses. *Antivir Res* 2009;81:16–24.

295. Moscona A. Global transmission of oseltamivir resistant influenza. *N Engl J Med* 2009;360:953–956.

Disinfectants and Antiseptics: Modes of Action, Mechanisms of Resistance, and Testing Regimens

Daniel Amsterdam and Barbara E. Ostrov

This chapter describes biocides that serve as sterilants, disinfectants, and antiseptics, with emphasis on their use in health care facilities. Prevention of hospital-acquired infections is a national priority affirmed by the Institute for Healthcare Improvement (IHI) (1). These agents are key for prevention and are part of current standard infection control practices (2). An overview of the most widely used products, their active ingredients, their mechanism of action and spectrum of activity, and issues concerning resistance to these chemicals are addressed.

DEFINITIONS

In health care facilities, disinfectants are typically used in several different settings: by housekeeping to clean floors, walls, and other environmental surfaces; in laboratories, to decontaminate instruments and work surfaces; and in areas where instruments do not need sterilization but do require cleaning prior to reuse. As a group, these chemicals are referred to as *instrument or environmental surface disinfectants*. *Antiseptics* are used to reduce the microbial burden on skin or mucosal membranes.

Generally, a number of steps are required to properly achieve disinfection. These steps include cleaning, decontamination, low-level to high-level disinfection, and sterilization. *Cleaning* refers to the removal of organic material from an instrument or environmental surface. *Decontamination* is defined by the Occupational Safety and Health Administration (OSHA) as the removal, inactivation, and/or destruction of pathogens on a surface so they are no longer able to transmit infections and the surface is safe for handling, use, or disposal (3).

Cleaning and decontamination are usually achieved by use of both enzymatic and nonenzymatic detergents and are primarily used to prepare devices or surfaces for subsequent disinfection or sterilization. *Low- or intermediate-level disinfection* is a process using chemical agents that will kill most pathogenic bacteria and fungi and nonenveloped viruses in a reasonable period of exposure time (≤ 10 minutes); typically, spores are not killed by these products. *High-level disinfection* is characterized by the product's ability to kill or inactivate pathogenic bacteria and fungi and nonenveloped viruses as well as *Mycobacterium tuberculosis*; enveloped viruses; and, with prolonged exposure time, bacterial spores. The U.S. Food and Drug Administration (FDA) definition of high-level disinfection is an agent used for a defined contact time in order to achieve a $-6 \log_{10}$ reduction of *Mycobacterium* species (4); several products on the market are capable of this level of disinfection. The primary active ingredients of such products belong to the chemical class aldehydes or oxidizing agents; however, some quaternary ammonium compounds and phenolics can serve as high-level disinfectants (Tables 12.1 and 12.2).

Sterilization processes must render surfaces and devices free of all living microorganisms, including spores. The sterility assurance level (SAL) defines the probability of survival of any viable organisms after sterilization treatment and is typically a $-6 \log_{10}$ or less than one in a million. Nonsterilization processes, although highly effective, produce instruments and surfaces that may yet contain some residual organisms and/or spores. It is important to appreciate that the use of chemical sterilants with shorter exposure periods will kill

Table 12.1

Class and Mechanism of Action of Common Antiseptic and Disinfectant Ingredients

Class (References)	Structure of Common Examples	Targets and Mechanisms
Biguanides (45–47)	Chlorhexidine	Alters integrity of cytoplasmic membrane, leading to damage of cytoplasm Biphasic effects: – Low dose causes leakage of cellular constituents – High dose causes precipitation of nucleic acids and proteins with coagulation of intracellular contents
Halogen releasers (84,88)	Povidone-iodine	Inhibits synthesis of DNA by disrupting disulfide bonds Causes oxidation of bonds, leading to degradation and destruction of cellular proteins and DNA Inhibits DNA synthesis and degrades RNA Oxidizes cell wall and membrane
Alcohols (110–112,116,117)	Ethanol Isopropanol	Membrane damage leads to coagulation and denaturation of proteins Coagulation leads to loss of enzymatic function and cell lysis
Aldehydes (145,286,295)	Glutaraldehyde	Damages cell membrane envelop
	ortho-Phthalaldehyde	Causes cross-linking of macromolecules, leading to damage of DNA, RNA, and proteins

(Continued)

Table 12.1 *(Continued)*

Class and Mechanism of Action of Common Antiseptic and Disinfectant Ingredients

Class (References)	Structure of Common Examples	Targets and Mechanisms
Peroxygens (4,25,204,205)	Hydrogen peroxide	Causes DNA strand breakage
	Peracetic acid	Oxidizing effects of these agents form free radicals and disrupt cellular enzymatic function
Phenols (213, 218,227,228, 237,240)	Phenol	Damages cytoplasmic membrane, leading to leakage of intracellular constituents
	Triclosan	Damages cytoplasmic membrane fatty acids. Inhibits cellular respiration and leads to cell lysis
Quaternary ammonium compounds (112,259,262)	Benzalkonium chloride	Damages cytoplasmic membrane, leading to damage of phospholipid bilayers. Causes cellular membrane destruction. Leads to leakage of intracellular contents

Adapted from McDonnell GE. *Antisepsis, disinfection and sterilization. Types, action and resistance.* Washington, DC: ASM Press, 2007.

most microorganisms except large amounts of bacterial spores. Hence, sterilizing agents perform as high-level disinfectants in such situations. Unfortunately, some publications erroneously equate "disinfection" and "sterilization" or claim that items treated with short exposure times are "partially sterile." The claim of chemical sterilization must be used to refer to absolute eradication of all types of microbes (4). Some agents that function as chemical sterilants include greater than or equal to 2.4% glutaraldehyde-based formulations, 0.95%

glutaraldehyde with 1.64% phenol, 7.5% hydrogen peroxide, 7.35% hydrogen peroxide with 0.23% peracetic acid, 0.2% peracetic acid, and 0.08% peracetic acid with 1.0% hydrogen peroxide (see Table 12.2). These agents are most effective when cleaning precedes sterilization treatment and when standards for concentration, contact time, temperature, and pH are closely followed (4).

Antiseptics possess antimicrobial activity and may be used on living tissue to remove, inhibit the growth of, or inactivate microorganisms. The

Table 12.2

Microbial Resistance and Approaches to Treatment

	Microbial Group Examples	Susceptibility to Chemical Germicides	Treatment Required	Recommended Germicides
Least Resistant	Mycoplasma: *Urea-plasma, Mycoplasma*	Highly susceptible	Low or intermediate disinfection	Alcohols, aldehydes, biguanides, halogens, ozone, peroxide, phenols, QACs
	Gram-negative bacteria: *Pseudomonas, Escherichia*			
	Gram-positive bacteria: MRSA, MSSA, strep-tococci, enterococci, *Legionella*	Susceptible	Intermediate disinfection	Alcohols, aldehydes, biguanides, halogens, ozone, peroxide, some phenols, some QACs
	Enveloped viruses: HIV, HBV, HSV Adenovirus, rotavirus, influenza			
	Vegetative fungi: *Aspergillus, Candida*	Susceptible	Intermediate disinfection	Alcohols, aldehydes, biguanides, halogens, ozone, peroxide, some phenols, some QACs
	Fungal spores: *Aspergillus, Penicillium*	Susceptible to resistant	High-level disinfection	Some alcohols, aldehydes, biguanides, halogens, peroxide, some phenols
	Nonenveloped viruses: Parvovirus, HPV, Norovirus	Resistant to highly resistant	High-level disinfection	Aldehydes, halogens, ozone, peroxides
	Mycobacteria: MTB, *M. chelonae*			Aldehydes, halogens, some peroxides, some phenols
	Bacterial spores: *Bacillus, Clostridium*	Highly resistant	High-level disinfection; sterilization	Aldehydes, high-concentration halogens, peroxides (prolonged exposure time)
Most resistant	Prions: Scrapie, JCD	Extremely resistant	Special sterilization techniques	High-concentration sodium hypochlorite and/or heated sodium hydroxide

QACs, quaternary ammonium compounds; MRSA, methicillin-resistant *Staphylococcus aureus*; MSSA, methicillin-sensitive *Staphylococcus aureus*; HBV, hepatitis B virus; HSV, herpes simplex virus; HPV, human papillomavirus; MTB, mycobacteria tuberculosis; JCD, Jakob-Creutzfeld disease.
Adapted from McDonnell G, Burke P. Disinfection: is it time to reconsider Spaulding? *J Hosp Infect* 2011;78:163–170; McDonnell GE. *Antisepsis, disinfection and sterilization. Types, action and resistance.* Washington, DC: ASM Press, 2007; Fanning S. Altered tolerance to biocides: links to antibiotic resistance? Paper presented at: International Association of Food Protection (IAFP), European Symposium on Food Safety; 2011; The Netherlands. http://www.foodprotection.org/events/european-symposia/11Ede/Fanning.pdf. Accessed November 15, 2012; Rutala W, Weber D. Guideline for disinfection and sterilization of prion contaminated medical instruments. SHEA guidelines. *Infect Control Hosp Epidemiol* 2010;31:107–117.

distinction between an antiseptic and a disinfectant is frequently ignored. However, the differences between a disinfectant and an antiseptic are important, and their applications are significantly different. A *disinfectant* is a chemical biocide used solely on inanimate objects or surfaces such as medical instruments or environmental surfaces; an *antiseptic* is to be used for living tissues. Some chemical agents, such as iodophors, can be active ingredients in either disinfectants or antiseptics. However, the precise formulations, patterns of use, and efficacy differ substantially. Consequently, products categorized as disinfectants should never be used as antiseptics and vice versa. Active ingredients used in antiseptics, including the iodine/iodophor group, biguanides (chlorhexidine), alcohols (usually ethanol or isopropanol), and phenolics (phenol and triclosan) have unique features, benefits, and drawbacks addressed in the remainder of this chapter.

SPAULDING CLASSIFICATION

The requirements for disinfection or sterilization of medical instruments, devices, or equipment can be more easily understood if these items are categorized based on the risk of infectivity involved with their use, as first suggested by Spaulding (5). The Spaulding classification system (Table 12.3) has been used since the 1950s by epidemiologists and microbiologists when discussing or planning strategies for disinfection and sterilization. The Centers for Disease Control and Prevention (CDC) has endorsed this system and has supported its use nationally and internationally (6).

Spaulding (5) defined three surface categories for treatment: critical, semicritical, and noncritical. Critical instruments or devices present the greatest risk of acquiring infection if the item is contaminated with microorganisms at the time of use. These are instruments or objects that are

Table 12.3

Spaulding Classification

Category	Description	Examples	Treatment
Critical devices	Substantial risk of infection due to instruments coming in direct contact with normally sterile body areas	Needles, scalps, forceps, cardiac catheters, implants, internal components of dialyzers, and extracorporeal blood flow devices	Must be sterilized by heat, ethylene oxide, hydrogen peroxide gas plasma, other low-temperature sterilization methods, and/or liquid sterilants
Semicritical devices	Lower risk of infection transmission due to items in contact with mucosa but usually do not penetrate sterile body areas	Fiber-optic endoscopes, endotracheal tubes, bronchoscopes, laryngoscopes, cystoscopes, vaginal specula, and urinary catheters	Sterilization with heat, or cleaning followed by use of germicide with high-level disinfection
Noncritical devices	Lower risk of infection as items usually contact only unbroken skin	Face masks, blood pressure cuffs, neurologic or cardiac electrodes, and surfaces of X-ray machines	Simple washing and cleaning with detergent; germicide using quaternary ammonium and phenolic chemical classes; proper handwashing techniques
Environmental surfaces	Lowest risk of infection transmission as items have indirect contact with unbroken skin	Medical equipment such as knobs or handles; Housekeeping surfaces	Simple washing and cleaning with detergent; use of germicide using quaternary ammonium and phenolic chemical classes; proper handwashing techniques

Modified from Spaulding EH. Chemical disinfection of medical and surgical disinfection of medical and surgical materials. In: Lawrence CA, Block SS, eds. *Disinfection, sterilization and preservation*. Philadelphia, Lea & Febiger, 1968:517–531; Ascenzi J, Favero M. Disinfectants and antiseptics: modes of action, mechanisms of resistance and testing. In: Lorian V, ed. *Antibiotics in laboratory medicine*. 5th ed. Philadelphia: Lippincott Williams & Wilkins, 2005:615–653.

introduced directly into normally sterile areas of the human body. Examples include needles, scalpels, forceps, cardiac catheters, implants, and also the inner surface components of extracorporeal blood flow devices such as of the heart–lung oxygenator and the blood-side of hemodialyzers. Critical instruments must be sterilized by heat (such as steam autoclave or dry heat), ethylene oxide, hydrogen peroxide gas plasma, other low-temperature sterilization methods, and/or liquid sterilants between patient procedures.

Instruments or devices classified as "semicritical" have a lower risk of infection. Examples include flexible fiber-optic endoscopes, endotracheal tubes, bronchoscopes, laryngoscopes, respiratory therapy equipment, cystoscopes, vaginal specula, and urinary catheters. This category of devices comes in contact with mucous membranes and do not ordinarily penetrate body surfaces. Sterilization of many of these items, although desirable and often cost-effective if steam autoclaves can be used, is not absolutely essential. Semicritical instruments or devices should, at a minimum, be subjected to high-level disinfection using a product, usually a liquid chemical germicide, available for use as a sterilant but applied for a shorter exposure time so as to function as a high-level disinfectant. This approach has broad-spectrum efficacy and can destroy some bacterial spores, most fungal spores, all ordinary vegetative bacteria, mycobacteria, small or nonlipid viruses, and medium-sized or lipid viruses. In practice, good cleaning followed by high-level disinfection provides the medical practitioner assurance that these semicritical items are relatively free of pathogenic microorganisms.

"Noncritical" instruments or devices come into direct contact with the patient but usually only with intact skin. This category includes face masks, blood pressure cuffs, most diagnostic electrodes, and certain surfaces of X-ray machines. Depending on the particular item and the nature and degree of contamination during prior use, simple washing or scrubbing with a detergent and warm water may be sufficient to safely allow reuse. Transmission of infectious agents to patients from environmental surfaces typically involves a vector, commonly hospital personnel (7–10). Studies have indicated that skin surfaces harbor organisms such as *Clostridium difficile* (11–14), methicillin-resistant *Staphylococcus aureus* (MRSA) (7–9), and antibiotic-resistant *Enterococcus* strains. Controlling transmission of these pathogens can be accomplished by disinfection of environmental surfaces and use of proper handwashing with

products employing an effective active ingredient. Thorough handwashing, along with the use of effective antiseptics, is one of the most important facets of the current overall infection control strategy (15,16). Beginning with the work of Semmelweis in the 1840s and confirmed by the World Health Organization (17), effective handwashing alone reduces the transmission of infectious agents. When successful handwashing is achieved and paired with effective biocide(s), transmission of microbes can be further reduced (18).

Housekeeping surfaces have very low potential for cross-contamination between health care personnel, patients, and medical equipment and/or instruments. Safe levels of microbes can be achieved by keeping these surfaces clean by using water and detergent or a hospital-grade disinfectant. A detergent designed for general housekeeping purposes (as indicated on the product label) would be adequate as well. In instances of spilled blood or a potentially infectious body fluid or culture specimen, an intermediate-level chemical disinfectant should be considered to render the environmental surface "safe."

Spaulding's original classification may be modified to include additional environmental surfaces, which carry the least risk of disease transmission (19). These additional environmental surfaces may contribute to secondary cross-contamination by the hands of health care workers or by contact with medical instruments that will subsequently come into contact with patients. Surfaces in this category encompass only those that come into direct contact with intact patient skin. These environmental surfaces may be further divided into (a) medical equipment surfaces such as adjustment knobs or handles on hemodialysis equipment, X-ray machines, instrument carts, or dental units, and (b) housekeeping surfaces such as floors, walls, tabletops, curtains between hospital beds, window sills, and so forth. As with noncritical medical instruments, adequate levels of safety for environmental surfaces may be achieved by simple cleaning with a detergent and warm water, cleaning with soap and water, or application of an intermediate- to low-level chemical germicide. Controlling the level of contaminant on environmental surfaces is usually accomplished with agents belonging to the quaternary ammonium and phenolic chemical classes.

In current hospital disinfection practice, antimicrobial wipes are used both to clean and to disinfect environmental surfaces. Some antimicrobial wipes remove a large proportion of microorganisms from environmental surfaces. However, germicidal activity associated with wipes might be limited due to brief application times and repeated use on multiple surfaces (20). Inadvertently, wipes may transfer microbial contaminants to other surfaces after multiple wipings (20). Studies assessing the effectiveness of germicide-containing wipes have revealed variable benefit as biocides (21). For example, the crucial eradication of *C. difficile* spores was established using hypochlorite-soaked wipes; peroxide-, biguanide-, and ammonium chloride–soaked wipes were not effective (21).

Additional factors may also influence the efficacy of the disinfection and sterilization processes. These include prior cleaning of the item; amount of organic and inorganic material present on the item; type and amount of microorganisms present on the item; exposure time to the germicide and the concentration of the germicide used; the physical features of the item to be treated, that is, the presence of difficult-to-reach cracks and crevices that need to be reached during treatment; the existence of biofilms; and the importance of temperature and pH of the disinfection or sterilization product and the item(s) to be treated (4).

Recently, the Spaulding classification has been reaffirmed to be as useful today as when first developed in 1957. However, this schema may be an oversimplification as it does not consider problems noted earlier nor issues such as complicated medical equipment that may require unique considerations, such as heat sensitivity, and it does not address the concerns about killing certain difficult-to-treat infectious organisms (e.g., prions) (see Table 12.2). Therefore, in some situations, selecting the best method of disinfection is challenging, even after evaluating Spaulding's criteria. The efficacy and testing for the required levels of disinfectants and sterilants needs to constantly be reassessed in current times to address newly identified and changing pathogens as well as newer environmental surfaces or items that are used in the health care setting (4,22).

REGULATION AND TESTING OF PRODUCT CLAIMS

In the United States, disinfectants are regulated by the Environmental Protection Agency (EPA) and the FDA under the Federal Insecticide, Fungicide, and Rodenticide Act (FIFRA) (4). Some states have additional regulations. Under FIFRA, any product must be registered following approval of its claim of safety and effectiveness. The EPA regulates low- and intermediate-level disinfectants, and the FDA regulates high-level disinfectants. This division of regulatory responsibility parallels the use of the products, that is, the EPA controls environmental surfaces and the FDA controls medical devices. Antiseptics are regulated solely by the FDA as drugs. In the European Union (EU), in 2013, an updated directive regulating biocides was implemented, establishing a two-step process of evaluation at the EU level and product authorization at the member state level (23).

Regulatory Agencies

Testing regimens used for product claims are defined by the EPA and FDA in the United States. In the EU, requirements are defined by directives for biocides, disinfectants, and antiseptics. The European Committee for Standardization Technical Committee (CEN/TC) sets the standards for products in the EU. In the United States, test procedures used for meeting data requirements for disinfectants generally are those formulated by the Association of Official Analytical Chemists (AOAC), the American Society for Testing and Materials (ASTM), and the International Organization for Standardization (ISO). Internationally, regulatory agencies in some countries (e.g., Canada, Australia, and Brazil) use these or similar test methods. In the United States, historically, hospital disinfectants, whether used for noncritical; semicritical; or critical devices, were regulated by the EPA under the authority of FIFRA (4). Additionally, some regulatory agencies have adapted different end points that one must meet to make a claim. For instance, in the United States, the quantitative tuberculocidal test requires a 6 log reduction to make a claim for tuberculocidal activity, whereas in the EU, using the same procedure, a 5 log reduction is required. Hence, the same product marketed in the United States and the EU may have differing requirements needed to claim activity.

Testing Regimens

Test procedures have been established for disinfectants and antiseptics under the auspices of AOAC. The test protocols are primarily for determining the effectiveness of these agents against bacterial spores, fungi, vegetative bacteria, and mycobacteria, and they serve to determine accurate product claims. In addition, potency of ingredients must be verified periodically due to potential impact of continued use as well as mixing with organic material, such as blood or soil, on product efficacy (24). Various approaches are available, ranging from simple laboratory evaluation to assessment under actual clinical conditions. These approaches allow not only for evaluation of biocide activity but also new product development, regulatory approval, labeling of products, and standardization. Efficacy claims as reported in the literature have validity under described test conditions. However, one must keep in mind the potential impact of environmental and institutional variability when generalizing these results to one's local hospital practice.

The effectiveness of a disinfectant or antiseptic is assessed by testing in three stages. The first stage verifies whether a chemical has adequate antimicrobial activity; *suspension tests* are typically used (Table 12.4). The second stage is performed using methods that simulate real-life conditions. Ingredient activity with testing using standardized conditions, such as duration of contact time and temperature, are determined (e.g., *surface testing*). The third phase is "real life" or *in-use tests*. In-use tests also verify disinfectant effectiveness after employment for a typical period of time. These tests are discussed in detail in the following text.

Laboratory test methods include determination of chemical uptake into cells, lysis of microorganisms and release of intracellular contents, alteration of cell wall permeability, alterations of cell membrane and metabolic function, enzymatic activity, disruption of biochemical pathways, and observation of microbial cell changes via microscopic visualization (25). Antimicrobial activity of the active ingredients is measured by determining the minimum inhibitory concentration (MIC), lowest concentration of the biocide that inhibits the growth of the microorganism, and minimal bactericidal concentration (MBC), the lowest concentration of the germicide that kills the organism. These test assays are modeled after those used for evaluating antimicrobial activity (see Chapter 3). Table 12.5 lists the MIC for several common microbes and germicide ingredients (26). Investigators often express the effectiveness of disinfectants in terms of decimal reduction time, or D-value, which is a commonly used measure of product efficacy. The D-value represents the time it takes, while at a constant temperature, to measure a predetermined significant reduction, usually 90% or greater, of the microbial load following treatment with a biocide (27). The microbicidal effect (ME) can also be determined for a product by subtracting the log number of microbes before and after treatment. The ME of 1 means there was 90%

reduction of initial bacteria numbers, and ME of 2 equates to 99% killing. It is generally preferred that the ME is greater than or equal to 5, or that at least 99.999% microbes have been killed (24).

Ideally, a test protocol should simulate the conditions for which the product is intended. In vivo systems, involving human tissues or equivalent experimental models, and in situ systems, testing in real conditions, should be used when assessing antiseptics and disinfectants. For measuring in vivo or in situ activity, there are several protocols used to test formulations and preparations (see Table 12.4).

Suspension testing is a commonly used technique for assessment of efficacy of biocides (28). In this method, the test microbes are exposed to a series of chemical germicide dilutions and the MIC and/or MBC is determined. This method may be limited due to germicide interactions with organic or inorganic constituents in the growth media (e.g., halogens and aldehydes) or chemical agent interactions with the surface (e.g., chlorhexidine with certain fibers) (28). Analysis of the exposure time and the concentration of the biocide, along with other physical factors such as pH, temperature, and interfering substances (examples are organic materials such as serum or blood and inorganic materials such as hard water and soil), are crucial to determine the MBC and are practical considerations for use of the products in hospital settings.

Surface testing is necessary to assess the efficacy of the germicide on the surfaces for which they will be used. This is important for products to be used in hospital surfaces, including antiseptics, disinfectants, and sterilants. Typical methods used are *carrier tests*, *simulated-use tests*, and *in-use testing*. In the United States, stainless steel and porcelain surface items are used to perform carrier testing of products. The microbes are placed onto the item, with or without interfering substances such as soil, and then exposed to the germicide product. The test microbes are then assessed for survival via standard culture techniques. *Simulated-use tests* apply a sample inoculum of microorganisms to a surface to mimic actual use of the item and then wipe the surface with germicide. Recovery and culture then determines the survivability of the microbe. *In-use testing* is similar except that the assessment is performed in actual situations and conditions. This testing method may be recommended to evaluate the success of a product over time when used in hospital settings. The germicides must be assessed in-use with the most resistant organisms, such as spores, ("worst-case scenario") to ensure actual sterilization is

Table 12.4

Regimens for Evaluating the Efficacy of Disinfectants and Antiseptics

Method/Test	Procedure/Description	Features
Phenol coefficient (PC)	1. Bacterial inocula (e.g., *S. aureus* and *S. typhi*) used 2. Dilutions of test chemical compared to equivalent dilutions of phenol 3. PC >1.0 indicates chemical effectiveness greater than phenol. 4. PC <1.0 indicates chemical less effective than phenol.	Evaluates effectiveness of disinfectant or antiseptic by comparison to industry standard, phenol
Decimal reduction time (D-value)	1. Initial microbial inoculum concentration determined by culture and enumeration 2. Inoculum treated with disinfectant for varied times at constant temperature 3. After elapsed treatment time, surviving microbes cultured and enumerated. 4. D-value calculated as time to achieve predetermined significant reduction of microbes (usually ≥90%), following treatment	Excellent measure of comparative efficacy of products by contrasting calculated D-values
Surface testing	1. Microbial inocula placed on several sterile test surfaces. 2. Initial microbial concentrations determined by culture and enumeration. 3. Inoculated test surfaces treated with product for varied times. 4. After elapsed treatment time, test surfaces placed into neutralizing solution; surviving microbes cultured and enumerated.	Assesses efficacy of product on surfaces for which it will be used. Result a function of microbial concentration versus treatment time exposed to disinfectant.

Carrier method	1. Carrier surface contaminated with test organism, dried, then exposed to disinfectant for predetermined times.
	2. Carrier subcultured in nutrient broth:
	  - No microbial growth indicates disinfectant effectiveness
	  - Presence of microbial growth indicates disinfectant failure
		Oldest test as developed by Koch
		Difficult to standardize dried bacterial concentration on carrier
		Multiple concentrations and varying contact times develop concentration-time relationship of disinfectant efficacy.

Quantitative carrier test (QCT)	1. Carrier method variation; surface contaminated with test organisms then exposed to product for predetermined times. 2. QCT-1 uses glass surface without organic material. 3. QCT-2 uses stainless steel surface with organic challenge. 4. Microbes cultured and enumerated 5. Log reduction of surviving microbes measures effectiveness of germicide.	QCT avoids limitations noted in carrier method and increases reliability of results.
Suspension test (Rideal-Walker test)	1. Inoculum suspended in disinfectant solution. 2. Solution subcultured to determine degree of killing. 3. Qualitative suspension test results expressed as "growth" or "no growth" 4. Quantitative suspension test: ratio of number of surviving organisms compared to original inocula; decimal log reduction (DLR) or microbicidal effect (ME) calculated. Generally, ME ≥5; that is, at least 99.999% microbes killed, considered acceptable.	Bacterial inoculum uniformly exposed to disinfectant Quantitative end point, DLR or ME, used to compare products' efficacy

(Continued)

Table 12.4 (Continued)

Regimens for Evaluating the Efficacy of Disinfectants and Antiseptics

Method/Test	Procedure/Description	Features
Surface disinfection test	1. Test surface (often a small tile) contaminated with standardized inoculum and dried. 2. Predetermined volume of disinfectant added 3. After preset exposure time, number of microbial survivors determined by rinsing technique: - Carrier rinsed in diluent - Number of surviving bacteria determined by culture of rinsing fluid 4. Control plate using distilled water similarly tested; number of microbes surviving in control compared with disinfectant-treated plate. 5. Reduction of microbes by treatment quantified	Assesses quantitative effectiveness of disinfectant against surface-adhered microorganisms
In-use testing	1. Samples of 1:10 dilution of disinfectant containing neutralizer placed on two agar plates 2. One incubated at 37°C for 3 days; the other at room temperature for 7 days. 3. Five or more colonies on either plate indicate microbial contamination of disinfectant.	Simulates "real-life" conditions of disinfectant use Can detect disinfectant contamination
Capacity test (Kelsey-Sykes)	1. Four test organisms (usually *S. aureus*, *E. coli*, *Pseudomonas aeruginosa*, and *Proteus vulgaris*) added to disinfectant. 2. Dilutions of disinfectant put in hard water for "clean" and in yeast suspension for "dirty" conditions. 3. Test organism—with or without yeast—added at 0-, 10-, and 20-min intervals to disinfectant dilutions for 8-min contact time. 4. Disinfectant evaluated on ability to kill, "pass," or not kill, "fail," test organisms	Qualitative test to assess ability of chemical to inhibit microbial growth under clean or dirty (with organic material) conditions.
Disinfectant kill time test	1. Disinfectant placed into water bath and allowed to equilibrate for temperature control. 2. Once tube has reached temperature, inoculated with 10^6 CFU/mL. 3. At predetermined times (generally 0 to 5 points), aliquots removed and plated onto agar and subcultured. 4. Colonies enumerated and DLR of microbes calculated.	Fully quantitative test designed to demonstrate DLR over time for disinfectant against selected microbes.

Adapted from Sharma BK, Shamim A, Lalia A, et al. Chemical agents as disinfectants and antiseptics: a review. *The Global J of Pharmaceutical Res* 2012;1:795–803; Mazzola P, Jozala A, Lencastre Novaes L, et al. Choice of sterilizing/disinfecting agent—determination of the Decimal Reduction Time (D-Value). *Braz J Pharm Sci* 2009;45:701–718; McDonnell GE. *Antisepsis, disinfection and sterilization. Types, action and resistance.* Washington, DC: ASM Press, 2007; Sattar SA, Springthorpe VS. New methods for efficacy testing of disinfectants and antiseptics. In: Rutala WA, ed. *Disinfection, sterilization and antisepsis: principles and practices in healthcare facilities.* Washington, DC: Association for Professionals in Infection Control and Epidemiology, 2001:173–186; Ascenzi JM, Ezzell JM, Wendt TM. A more specific method for measurement of tuberculocidal activity of disinfectants. *Appl Environ Microbiol* 1987;53:2189–2192; Springthorpe VS, Sattar SA. Application of a quantitative carrier test to evaluate microbiocides against mycobacteria. *J AOAC Int* 2007;90:817–824.

achieved. Detailed test methods, guidelines, and standards can be reviewed in McDonnell (28).

In-use testing for antiseptics requires in vivo assessment of products. Comparing in vivo studies is complicated because methods used vary greatly. For example, when studying different alcohol-based waterless antiseptic handrubs, methodologies vary as to (a) whether or not hands are purposely contaminated, (b) the volume of test substance used, (c) the time period the solution is in contact with the skin, (d) the methods used to recover organisms, and (e) the method of

Table 12.5

Minimum Inhibitory Concentration of Biocides Tested with Microorganism Suspensions Greater than 6 log$_{10}$

Bacteria Biocide	B. stearo- thermophilus mg/L	B. subtilis mg/L	E. cloacae mg/L	E. coli mg/L	S. marcescens mg/L	S. aureus mg/L
QACs	156	117	78	59	59	59
Chlorhexidine	[a]	10,000	71	71	141	71
Glutaraldehyde	1,875	3,250	3,250	3,250	1,375	1,875
Ethanol	87,500	87,500	87,500	65,650	43,750	87,500
Ethanol + glycerin	[a]	[a]	87,500	87,500	87,500	87,500
Ethanol + iodine 1%	87,500	87,500	87,500	43,750	43,750	43,750
Ethanol + iodine 10%	[a]	43,750	43,750	[a]	[a]	21,870
PVP-I soap	6,250	50,000	6,250	6,250	6,250	6,250
Alcoholic PVP-I	12,500	25,000	3,125	1,560	3,125	3,125
CRA 1% pH >9	4,491	4,491	420	1,129	474	945
CRA 1% pH 7	621	621	150	150	150	150
H2O2	1,875	1,875	1,250	2,505	625	938

QAC, quaternary ammonium compounds; H2O2, hydrogen peroxide; PVP-I, polyvinylpyrrolidone iodine; CRA, chlorine-releasing agents.
[a]Without efficacy.
Modified from Mazzola P, Jozala A, Lencastre Novaes L, et al. Minimal inhibitory concentration (MIC) determination of disinfectant and/or sterilizing agents. *Braz J Pharm Sci* 2009;45:241–248.

expressing efficacy. Several protocols have been used for determining the effectiveness of such antiseptics (29). Recent approaches have included a two-step process of in vitro testing followed by in vivo treatment evaluation (30). Alternatively, sequential in vivo application of two different antiseptics has been found to be highly effective (31). Product efficacy can be determined in vivo by using volunteers. In the Vienna test model, a variant of in-use testing, for example, a product is compared to standard disinfection assessed during parallel use with the same volunteers (32). This standardized approach allows for comparison of efficacy, by using experimental contamination of volunteers, and assessment of the survivability of the bacteria before and after disinfection. An exhaustive review of additional methodologic designs is provided by Hobson and Bolsen (33).

Numerous concerns about the traditional approaches to product testing have been posited (34–36). These concerns include lack of standardization of inocula, organisms' resistance patterns, variations of the porcelain carriers used in the sporicidal tests, variations in the number of times the carriers are reused and processed, and

uncertain relationship between the tested carrier surfaces and the surfaces to be disinfected in real-life situations. In response to these criticisms, alternative procedures have been proposed and adopted. The EPA adopted the use of a *quantitative suspension test* for measuring tuberculocidal activity of disinfectants (37) and modification of this methodology was adopted by ASTM (29). Further refinements have been developed to improve test reliability claims against mycobacteria (38). The updated *quantitative carrier test* (QCT) method has the following advantages: fully quantitative; minimizes the potential for false positives; measures kill under ideal and stringent conditions; increases the reliability of the results; can be applied to a wide variety of microorganisms, vegetative and spore forming; and eliminates the potential loss of organisms from wash-off during the exposure period. The QCT encompasses two separate parts, QCT-1 and QCT-2, which differ in the hard surface used (glass vs. stainless steel) and the type of organic soil challenge incorporated into the test. QCT-1 tests the disinfectant under more ideal conditions, using a glass surface, and without including organic soil, while QCT-2 tests the disinfectant under less ideal conditions. The latter is achieved by use of stainless steel (a surface that can have more variability), less disinfectant, and an organic challenge added to the suspension. QCT-1 has been validated for use with vegetative bacteria, including mycobacteria, bacterial spores, and fungi, whereas QCT-2 has been validated for use with viruses and protozoans in addition to vegetative bacteria, mycobacteria, bacterial spores, and fungi. The data obtained from these procedures allows one to calculate a log reduction value for the potency of the germicide. Each regulatory agency may choose to set their end point, the SAL, for determining product efficacy.

EPA developed a method for evaluating chemical germicides for virucidal activity, a method also accepted by the FDA for those products under its authority. Claims made based on testing against specific viruses, such as norovirus and hepatitis B and hepatitis C viruses, have been allowed based on testing using the surrogate viruses feline calicivirus, duck hepatitis virus, and bovine diarrhea virus, respectively (39).

Although some chemical germicides maybe labeled as sterilants, guidelines from the CDC, FDA, Association for Professionals in Infection Control and Epidemiology (APIC), and other professional organizations do not recommend the use of these germicides for sterilization unless there are no other available products. Unlike terminal sterilization processes (such as steam, ethylene oxide, and peroxide gas plasma), where the items can be maintained in a microorganism-free state by packaging after sterilization, items so treated using liquid processes cannot be maintained in a sterile state when they are removed from the solution. Sterilization claims can be obtained for the liquid processed products using the AOAC sporicidal test (40). Humphreys' (41) report identifies the currently available methodologies and standards for sporicidal products.

ACTIVE INGREDIENTS

The active ingredients in antiseptics and disinfectants achieve their effects through interactions with the microorganism cell surface followed by penetration into the cytoplasm and action on cellular targets. The variable response to these products may be due to composition of the cell surface, change in the environment, and increasingly identified resistance to germicides. The following sections describe mechanisms of action and indications for commonly used products (summarized in Table 12.1; Fig. 12.1) (25,42).

BIGUANIDES

Chlorhexidine

Biguanides are compounds that contain the $C_2H_5N_7$ component. Chlorhexidine, a substituted biguanide, has a high degree of antimicrobial activity, low mammalian toxicity, and the ability to bind to the stratum corneum layer of the skin and to mucous membranes (43). The bactericidal activity of chlorhexidine is more potent than that of monomeric biguanides, hence is the only biguanide discussed in detail in the following text (44). These unique characteristics make it particularly attractive as an active ingredient in antimicrobial skin preparations. Chlorhexidine's general chemical structure is shown in Table 12.1.

Practically insoluble in water, chlorhexidine reacts with acids to form salts with varying degrees of solubility. Recognized as an effective antimicrobial, chlorhexidine is the active ingredient in a number of products: preoperative skin preparations, surgical hand scrubs, health care personnel handwash products, skin cleansers, acne creams, oral products (such as mouthwashes), burn ointments, and wound protectants; it has also been incorporated into products as a preservative.

Mechanism of Action

The activity of chlorhexidine relates to the interaction of the germicide with the cell surface (see Table 12.1 and Fig. 12.1), causing changes in the lipids in the cell membrane (45–47). Changes in the integrity of the membrane result in loss of membrane function. Experiments using ^{14}C-chlorhexidine indicate that chlorhexidine rapidly enters the cells of both bacteria and yeasts (48,49). The bacterial cell wall is generally negatively charged and is rapidly neutralized in the presence of chlorhexidine (43), indicating the reaction of chlorhexidine with the cell membrane. The outer membrane structure in gram-negative bacteria is stabilized by the interaction of divalent cations and the negative charges associated with lipid A of the lipopolysaccharide (LPS) in the cell membrane. It is hypothesized that polycationic molecules, such as chlorhexidine, can promote their own uptake by displacement of divalent cations associated with the LPS. Alterations in the LPS can lead to changes in susceptibility to antimicrobials (50), whereas disruption of the cell membrane results in leakage of cellular material from the cell. The leakage in *Escherichia coli* and *S. aureus* is biphasic, depending on chlorhexidine concentration (47).

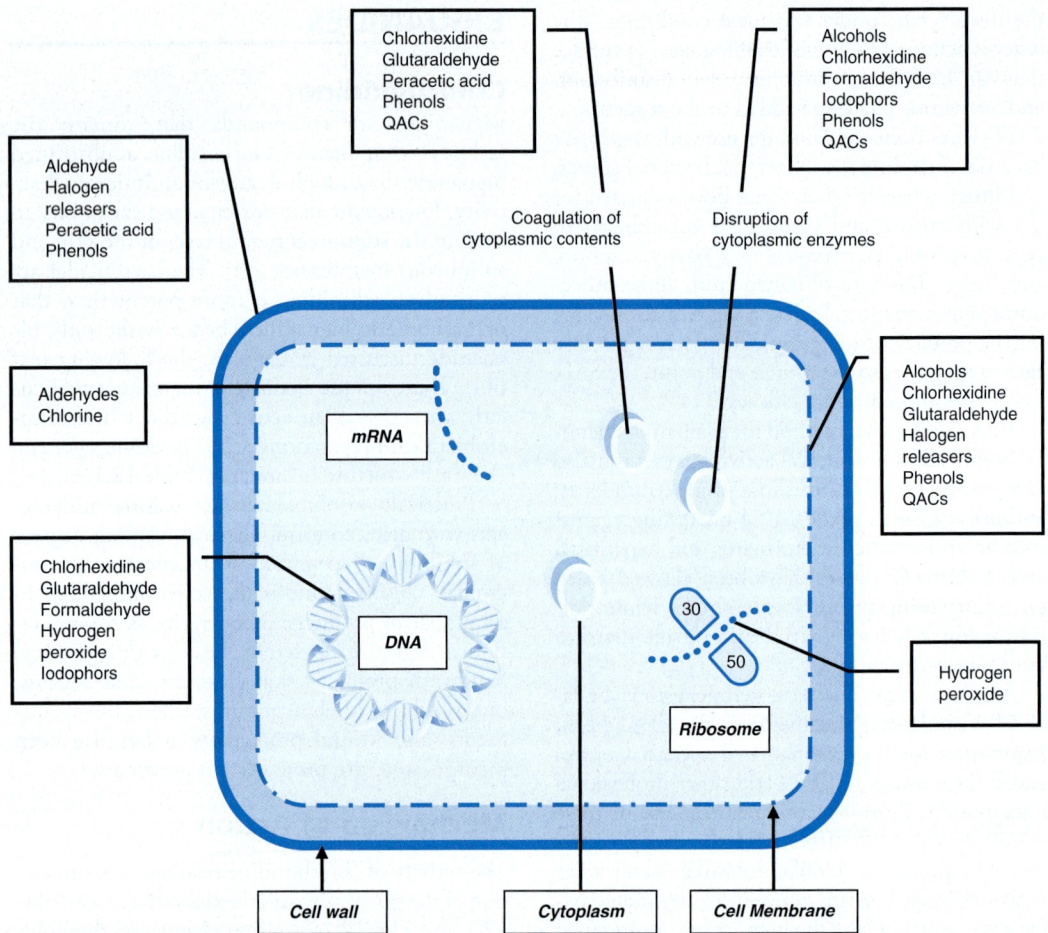

Figure 12.1 ■ Cellular targets of biocidal agents. (Adapted from Fanning S. Altered tolerance to biocides: links to antibiotic resistance? Paper presented at: International Association of Food Protection (IAFP), European Symposium on Food Safety; 2011; The Netherlands. http://www.foodprotection.org/events/european-symposia/11Ede/Fanning.pdf. Accessed November 15, 2012.)

At low concentrations (up to 200 μg/mL), chlorhexidine inhibits membrane enzymes and promotes leakage of cellular constituents. Cells treated with bacteriostatic concentrations lost up to 50% of their K⁺ but can recover upon neutralization of excess chlorhexidine (43,51). At higher concentrations, cytoplasmic contents are coagulated (52) and cells begin to leak higher molecular weight molecules such as nucleotides (43). Uptake of bis-(1,3-dibutylbarturic acid) trimethane oxonal and propidium iodide, which reflect membrane potential and membrane integrity, respectively, was directly related to chlorhexidine concentrations (0.003 to 0.3 mmol⁻¹), indicating changes in membrane structure with increasing concentrations of chlorhexidine (53).

The effect of chlorhexidine on mycobacterial cells is bacteriostatic, not bactericidal. The treatment of mycobacterial cells with ethambutol (an antituberculosis drug known to inhibit the synthesis of specific components of the mycobacterial cell wall) potentiates the activity of chlorhexidine against *Mycobacterium* spp, indicating that chlorhexidine needs access through the cell membrane to exert its activity (54).

For yeast, chlorhexidine can similarly damage the cytoplasmic membrane. Treatment of *Saccharomyces cerevisiae* cells with chlorhexidine resulted in the release of pentose indicating increased oxidative stress and cellular leakage from these organisms (55). In *Candida albicans*, sublethal concentrations of chlorhexidine resulted in loss of cytoplasmic components and coagulation of nucleoproteins (56) and prevented the outgrowth but not the germination of spores (57).

The general mechanisms of chlorhexidine can be summarized as follows:

- Damage to cell membrane by interaction with lipid layer
- Leakage of cellular constituents at low-level exposure
- Precipitation of nucleic acids and proteins at high-level exposure
- Coagulation of intracellular and disruption of enzymatic pathways at high-level exposure

Spectrum of Activity

A comprehensive review of in vivo and in vitro effectiveness of chlorhexidine activity has been reported (43). MICs for bacteria and fungi are presented in Tables 12.6 and 12.7, respectively. These data indicate the broad spectrum of activity of this ingredient, which is effective against gram-positive and gram-negative bacteria, yeasts, and molds.

Studies of a 0.05% chlorhexidine solution confirm the rapid inactivation of gram-positive and gram-negative bacteria, yeasts, and molds (43). Following a 10-minute exposure to this solution at 18°C to 21°C, only resistant microorganisms, such as *Pseudomonas stuartii*, *Streptococcus faecalis*, *Bacillus subtilis*, and *C. difficile*, did not show substantial reduction. The MIC values for *B. subtilis* and *Clostridium spp* (see Table 12.6) are relatively low, indicating the bacteriostatic effect on these organisms. All of the other bacterial species tested showed a greater than 2 $\log_{10}$ reduction in 10 minutes. Gram-negative bacteria were generally more susceptible (4.0 to 6.7 $\log_{10}$ reduction) than gram-positive bacteria (2.1 to 5.8 $\log_{10}$ reduction) under the conditions tested (58). Treatment of *E. coli* and *Klebsiella pneumoniae* with sublethal concentrations of chlorhexidine resulted in lower pathogenicity of these organisms when injected into mice (58). With the exception of the more resistant organisms listed earlier, among the gram-positive bacteria, the cocci (2.1 to 5.8 $\log_{10}$ reduction) were generally more resistant than the gram-negative bacilli (3.6 to 4.8 $\log_{10}$ reduction).

Data indicate that chlorhexidine may be capable of inhibiting spore growth and germination but that it does not kill the spores. As shown in Table 12.6, the MIC for spores is quite low. Data indicate that both *B. subtilis* and *C. difficile* spores show less than 1 $\log_{10}$ reduction when exposed to a 0.05% solution of chlorhexidine. Sporicidal activity can be achieved with chlorhexidine at higher temperatures (57).

Chlorhexidine has antiviral effects due to its interaction with viral membrane lipids. Viruses can be grouped into those with an outer lipid membrane composed of lipoproteins and glycoproteins around the protein coat (enveloped viruses) and those that are nonenveloped (i.e., lack a lipid membrane). Due to its solubility characteristics, chlorhexidine is more active against enveloped viruses with a lipid membrane (Table 12.8), such as HIV. Studies confirm the effectiveness of chlorhexidine against HIV. Preparations containing chlorhexidine (a 4% and a 0.5% solution in 70% alcohol) were completely effective against HIV-1 after 15 seconds of contact. An aqueous solution of 0.05% was equally effective in 1 minute (59). Aqueous chlorhexidine gluconate at 0.2% was effective but at 0.02% was not effective (60).

In vivo studies using chlorhexidine formulations provide further evidence of the activity of this germicide. The chemical components and the solubility of various chlorhexidine salts can make a difference in the activity of the formulation. When used in the presence of organic ions such as soaps, sodium lauryl sulfate, sodium carboxymethyl cellulose, alginates, and some dyes, chlorhexidine may be less effective. Many of these compounds are commonly used in formulations for antiseptic preparations. Although there may be no visual evidence of incompatibility, the chlorhexidine can be incorporated into micelles and not be readily available to interact with microorganisms (43). The addition of anionic thickeners or emulsifiers also serves to inactivate the long-lasting antibacterial activity (persistence) of chlorhexidine (61).

Chlorhexidine has been incorporated into detergent and alcohol preparations, powders, mouthwashes, and polymeric preparations for a variety of uses. Given its ability to bind to the stratum corneum layer of the epidermis, chlorhexidine exhibits persistence and substantivity; that is, it exerts its effect long after it has been used, and the more it is used, the greater the reduction in the resident flora of the skin. This activity is especially relevant for its use as a surgical scrub and in surgical site preparation.

As a surgical scrub, chlorhexidine has been prepared as 4% and 2% aqueous solutions as well as alcohol-based formulations of different concentrations. Chlorhexidine is effective in removing transient microflora from artificially contaminated hands (62). The effects are immediate and long-term (persistent or residual) on resident microflora (63). A study examining the difference between aqueous and alcohol preparations found that a

Table 12.6

Bacteriostatic Activity of Chlorhexidine Gluconate

Test Organism	No. of Strains	MIC (mg/L) Mean	Range
Gram-positive cocci			
Staphylococcus aureus	16	1.6	1–4
Staphylococcus epidermidis	41	1.8	0.25–8.0
Streptococcus faecalis	5	38.0	32–64
Streptococcus mutans	2	2.5	
Streptococcus pneumonia	5	11.0	8–16
Streptococcus pyogenes	9	3.0	1–8
Streptococcus sanguis	3	9.0	4–16
Streptococcus viridians	5	25.0	2–32
Gram-positive bacilli			
Bacillus cereus	1	8.0	
Bacillus subtilis	2	1.0	
Clostridium difficile	7	16.0	8–32
Clostridium welchii	5	14.0	4–32
Corynebacterium spp	8	1.6	0.5–8.0
Lactobacillus casei	1	128.0	
Listeria monocytogenes	1	4.0	
Propionibacterium acnes	2	8.0	
Gram-negative bacilli			
Acinetobacter anitratus	3	32.0	16–64
Alkaligenes faecalis	1	64.0	
Bacteroides disastonis	4	16.0	
Bacteroides fragilis	11	34.0	8–64
Burkholderia (Pseudomonas) cepacia	1	16.0	
Campylobacter pyloridis	5	17.0	8–32
Citrobacter freundii	10	18.0	4–32
Enterobacter cloacae	12	45.0	16–64
Escherichia coli	14	4.0	2–32
Gardnerella vaginalis	1	8.0	
Haemophilus influenza	10	5.0	2–8
Klebsiella aerogenes	5	25.0	16–64
Klebsiella pneumonia	5	64.0	82–128
Proteus mirabilis	5	115.0	64–128
Proteus vulgaris	5	57.0	32–128
Providencia stuartii	5	102.0	64–128
Pseudomonas aeruginosa	15	20.0	16–32
Pseudomonas fluorescens	1	4.0	
Salmonella bredeney	1	16.0	
Salmonella Dublin	1	4.0	

(Continued)

Table 12.6 *(Continued)*

Bacteriostatic Activity of Chlorhexidine Gluconate			
		MIC (mg/L)	
Test Organism	**No. of Strains**	**Mean**	**Range**
Salmonella galinarum	1	8.0	
Salmonella montivideo	1	8.0	
Salmonella typhimurium	4	13.0	8–16
Salmonella vichow	1	8.0	
Serratia marcescens	10	30.0	16–64

Reprinted from Denton GW. Chlorhexidine. In: Block SS, ed. *Disinfection, sterilization and preservation.* 5th ed. Philadelphia: Lippincott Williams & Wilkins, 2001:321–336.

Table 12.7

Fungistatic Activity of Chlorhexidine		
Organism	**No. of Strains**	**Mean MIC (mg/L)**
Mold fungi		
Aspergillus flavus	1	64
Aspergillus fumigates	1	32
Aspergillus niger	1	16
Penicillium notatum	1	16
Rhizopus sp	1	8
Scopulariopsis spp	1	8
Yeasts		
Candida albicans	2	9
Candida guillermondii	1	4
Candida parapsilosis	2	4
Candida pseudotorpicalis	1	3
Cryptococcus neoformans	1	1
Prototheca zopfii	1	6
Saccharomyces cerevisiae	1	1
Torulopsis glabrata	1	6
Dermatophytes		
Epidermophyton floccosum	1	4
Microsporum canis	2	4
Microsporum fulvum	1	6
Microsporum gypseum	1	6
Trichophyton equinum	1	4
Trichophyton interdigitale	2	3
Trichophyton mentagrophytes	1	3
Trichophyton quinkeanum	1	3
Trichophyton rubrum	2	3
Trichophyton tonsurans	1	3

Reprinted from Denton GW. Chlorhexidine. In: Block SS, ed. *Disinfection, sterilization and preservation.* 5th ed. Philadelphia: Lippincott Williams & Wilkins, 2001:321–336.

Table 12.8

Virucidal Activity of Chlorhexidine Gluconate

Virus	Viral Family	Activity[a]	Conc. (%)
Respiratory syncytial virus	Paramyxovirus	+	0.25
Herpes hominis/simplex	Herpesvirus	+	0.02
Poliovirus type 2	Enterovirus	–	0.02
Adenovirus type 2	Adenovirus	–	0.02
Equine infectious anemia virus	Retrovirus	+	2.0
Variola virus (smallpox)	Poxvirus	+	2.0
Herpes simplex types 1 and 2	Herpesvirus	+	0.02
Equine influenza virus	Orthomyxovirus	+	0.001
Hog cholera virus	Togavirus	+	0.001
Bovine viral diarrhea	Togavirus	+	0.001
Parainfluenza virus	Paramyxovirus	+	0.001
Transmissible gastroenteritis virus	Coronavirus	+	0.001
Rabies virus	Rhabdovirus	+	0.001
Canine distemper virus	Paramyxovirus	+	0.01
Infectious bronchitis virus	Coronavirus	+	0.01
Newcastle virus	Paramyxovirus	+	0.01
Pseudorabies virus	Herpesvirus	+	0.01
Cytomegalovirus	Herpesvirus	+	0.1
Coxsackievirus	Picornavirus	–	0.4
Echovirus	Picornavirus	–	0.4
Human rotavirus	Reovirus	–	1.5
HIV type 1	Retrovirus	+	0.2

[a] + indicates activity at concentration stated; – indicates activity not established at concentration stated.
Reprinted from Denton GW. Chlorhexidine. In: Block SS, ed. *Disinfection, sterilization and preservation*. 5th ed. Philadelphia: Lippincott Williams & Wilkins, 2001:321–336.

formulation containing 1% chlorhexidine in 61% ethanol resulted in significantly greater microbial reduction than a 4% aqueous solution or the 61% ethanol vehicle alone (64). When used as a health care personnel handwash, chlorhexidine has typically been employed as the active ingredient in aqueous or alcohol-based solutions. Comparison of four chlorhexidine formulations (two 4% aqueous formulations, a 2% aqueous chlorhexidine formulation, and an alcoholic 0.5% chlorhexidine formulation) versus a nonantiseptic soap revealed that after the initial wash with each, there was no difference in microbial reductions. However, as more washes were performed, there was a significant difference between the four chlorhexidine-containing formulations as compared to the soap,

although there was no difference between the chlorhexidine formulations (65).

Incorporation of chlorhexidine into surgical skin prep (2% chlorhexidine in 70% isopropyl alcohol) has proven to be effective. The chlorhexidine solution significantly reduced abdominal and inguinal microbial counts from baseline for up to 24 hours. It was more persistent in the abdominal region than were two other preparations containing isopropyl alcohol or chlorhexidine alone (66).

Chlorhexidine-containing powders used in routine umbilical decontamination in a neonatal unit controlled MRSA (67). Several studies have been done comparing infection rates when chlorhexidine gluconate and povidone-iodine were used as skin preparations in patients with central venous catheters. Comparison of catheter-related bloodstream infections indicates that chlorhexidine gluconate was superior; however, all the studies were limited by the small numbers of subjects (68–70). A meta-analysis indicates that chlorhexidine reduced the risk of catheter-related bloodstream infections by 50% (71). Several studies have assessed whether catheters impregnated with chlorhexidine and silver sulfadiazine (CHX-SS) reduced catheter-related bloodstream infections. When comparing patients with short-term indwelling catheters (median duration of 6 days) and those with long-term indwelling catheters (median duration of 12 days), a meta-analysis indicated that those in the short-duration group using CHX-SS catheters had a significant reduction in the incidence of catheter-related bloodstream infections, whereas the longer duration use group showed no difference between the CHX-SS catheters and standard catheters (72). In vitro studies with CHX-SS supported the data from the in vivo studies (73).

The incorporation of chlorhexidine into oral solutions goes back over 30 years (74), including mouthwash, varnish, and slow-release dental treatments. Chlorhexidine in varnish used on orthodontic patients helps prevent caries. Newer techniques such as epifluorescence microscopy can verify the dental effectiveness of chlorhexidine and other antimicrobial ingredients (75). Data indicate that there is a significant reduction in the level of *Streptococcus mutans* 1 week after the application of a sustained-release varnish. The decrease in *S. mutans* was measured for up to 3 weeks after the application. However, chlorhexidine-coated toothbrushes used for 30 days did not exhibit less bacterial contamination than untreated toothbrushes (76). A recent study compared the efficacy of chlorhexidine and a garlic extract in reducing colony-forming units of *S. mutans*. Although the chlorhexidine was beneficial, the garlic extract was more effective. It seems unlikely that the general public would be willing to perform regular garlic extract rinses, however (77). Studies have also shown high activity against typical oral flora when exposed for 1 minute to chlorhexidine digluconate 0.01% to 0.5% and no evidence of significant antimicrobial resistance was detected (78). Chlorhexidine may reduce ventilator-associated pneumonia (79) and possibly postdental implant bacteremia (80). Even with this known effect, current literature does not support a role for chlorhexidine rinses to prevent endocarditis in high-risk patients but instead recommend consistent comprehensive oral hygiene (81).

HALOGEN RELEASERS

Halogen releasers function as oxidizing agents, with bromine, chlorine, and iodine commonly used as disinfectants and antiseptics. Only certain halogen-containing species with iodine and chlorine are active antimicrobials due to their solvency and chemistry. Only these halogen releasers will be reviewed in this section.

Iodine and Iodophors

Iodine in the form of a tincture (alcohol extract of a low volatility substance) has been used since the early 1900s as a preoperative skin preparation. Cutaneous toxicity limited the use of iodine, whether in an aqueous or tincture preparation. The use of iodophors, which are complexes of iodine with a carrier such as polyvinylpyrrolidone (PVP) (see Table 12.1), allows for the slow release of free iodine, the active species, thereby reducing the preparation's toxicity and staining without limiting the antimicrobial activity. Iodophors have been used as both antiseptics and disinfectants in the form of solutions, ointments, and aerosols. Iodophors are classified as low- or intermediate-level disinfectants (82) because they are not sufficiently sporicidal in an appropriate short application time. The amount of free iodine present in iodophors is difficult to determine. Concentrated solutions contain less free iodine than those that are diluted (83), and free iodine is the active species, whereas the PVP or other molecules with which the iodine is complexed act as carriers. A comparison of several commercial formulations of 10% polyvinylpyrrolidone iodine (PVP-I) had two orders of magnitude range of free iodine, hence a wide range of antimicrobial activity (84). Improperly diluted ionophore formulations allow for less free iodine and lower antimicrobial effects (85). This was the presumed cause of the outbreak of bacteremia associated with *Pseudomonas aeruginosa* when using a contaminated 10% PVP-I solution (86). Today, the primary use of iodophors is as an antiseptic for surgical scrubs and skin preparations.

Mechanism of Action

The killing effect of iodine and iodophors is related to the concentration of the free molecular iodine, whose concentration correlates with antimicrobial activity (83,87). The exact mechanism of action of iodine is not known. Its ability to penetrate the cell wall rapidly may be the primary mode by which it exerts its antimicrobial activity (see Table 12.1 and

Fig. 12.1). Iodine can cause disruption of cells or cellular components as follows:

- Reactions with N–H groups of amino acids during which N-iodo compounds are formed, resulting in destruction of proteins
- Irreversible oxidation of -SH groups of cysteine, leading to loss of protein disulfide bonds (84,88)
- Iodination of phenolic and imidazolic groups of the amino acids tyrosine and histidine and iodination of the pyrimidine derivatives of cytosine and uracil, leading to steric hindrances in hydrogen bonds and denaturation of DNA
- Iodine binding to unsaturated fatty acids, altering the physical properties of lipids and hence lipid-containing membranes

For a more detailed description of the biochemical properties of these agents, the reader is referred to Gottardi (84).

Chlorine

The antiseptic- and disinfectant-oxidized chlorine compounds are formed in water. These include elemental chlorine, hypochlorous acid, and hypochlorite ion; the latter being the most widely used form. The antimicrobial action of available chlorine depends on the concentration, temperature, and pH of the solution; higher pH solutions have diminished antimicrobial activity. Many chlorine products have an irritating and corrosive nature, limiting their clinical use.

Disinfection of water is a common use of chlorine products and historically has controlled widespread waterborne diseases such as cholera and typhoid. Hypochlorites are used as environmental surface disinfectants but residual chlorine may need to be removed to prevent corrosion (28).

Mechanism of Action

Chlorine causes oxidation of proteins and lipids, thereby damaging the cell wall and membrane. Hypochlorous acid is the most active product and even at a neutral pH penetrates the outer cell layers. The moiety disrupts oxidative phosphorylation and other enzymatic activities of the cell. This germicide affects membrane-bound as well as cellular functional proteins, particularly those with sulfhydryl bonds (28), similar to the iodophors. Hypochlorous acid suppressed *E. coli* growth via complete inhibition of DNA synthesis and viral RNA is degraded into fragments (89). Increased bacterial spore and fungal cell wall permeability

has been observed, which causes better biocide penetration and microbe killing (89).

The general mechanisms of chlorine can be summarized as follows:

- Damage to cell membrane by oxidation of proteins and lipids
- Inhibition and degradation of DNA and RNA
- Increased spore and fungal cell wall permeability and subsequent microbe death

Spectrum of Activity

The antimicrobial activity of the halogen releasers and iodine and iodine-containing formulations is similar to chlorine-releasing compounds; these formulations have broad-spectrum activity against gram-positive and gram-negative bacteria, mycobacteria, fungi, and viruses (88). As with most chemical germicides, the activity of iodine and chlorine are dependent on their concentration, the formulation, the temperature, the growth conditions of the microorganism, and the presence of organic and inorganic material.

The sporicidal activity of iodine compounds is significantly less than chlorine-releasing compounds. A concentration of 2,000 to 5,000 ppm potassium iodine is necessary to produce a $5 \log_{10}$ reduction in *B. subtilis* spores within 5 minutes. Iodine solutions are somewhat effective in destroying spores of *Bacillus anthracis, B. subtilis, Bacillus megaterium, Bacillus mesentericus, Clostridium tetani,* and *Clostridium welchii* (90–92) with prolonged application. Generally, disinfectant formulations of iodophors are weakly sporicidal with prolonged application, whereas antiseptic-containing iodophors are not sporicidal (93).

The activity of iodine against *Pseudomonas* spp and *Legionella pneumophila* isolates from a water system was dramatically different if the organisms were grown in water versus rich medium. Water-grown organisms proved more resistant to the iodine (94,95). Studies have also shown that iodine-containing formulations are more effective against vegetative organisms than are chlorine-based formulations (88).

Antimycobactericidal activity of iodine and iodophors are inconsistent (96–98). The following data exemplify the lack of consistency regarding the tuberculocidal activity of iodine and iodophors; hence, these compounds are not considered high-level disinfectants. Some tests showed that very low concentration of free iodine (<0.1%) killed *M. tuberculosis* with a 5-minute exposure at room temperature (96). In other tests, however, several commercially available iodophor formulations were not effective in killing two strains of *M. tuberculosis* after a 30-minute exposure (97). A comparison of two different iodine formulations, povidone-iodine (1% titratable iodine) and an iodophor (0.008% titratable iodine), demonstrated that the iodophor was ineffective in killing greater than a 3 $\log_{10}$ CFU *M. tuberculosis* after 1-minute contact in suspension or dried on a carrier. The povidine-iodine was effective in producing more than a 3 $\log_{10}$ reduction in a suspension test but not when the organism was dried on carriers in the presence of sputum (98). The iodophor product was also ineffective against *Mycobacterium smegmatis* (99). As a result of these inconsistent tuberculocidal effects, these compounds are not classified as high-level disinfectants.

Chlorine, iodine, and iodine-containing products have good fungicidal and fungistatic properties. They are effective against species of *Trichophyton, Monilia, Epidermophyton, Torula*, and other genera (88,100).

Iodine and iodophors are effective against a wide range of viruses, including enteroviruses and polio, herpes, vaccinia, rabies, and tobacco mosaic viruses (101–103), with inactivation concentrations of 75 to 150 ppm for polio type 1, coxsackie B_1, adenovirus 2, vaccinia, herpes, influenza A, and HIV-1 viruses and 5,000 ppm for feline parvovirus. Complete inactivation of cell-free HIV was accomplished using 0.5% PVP-I with a 30- to 60-second exposure. Quantitative suspension testing has shown virucidal efficacy of povidone-iodine disinfectants against vaccinia, polyomavirus SV40, adenovirus and poliovirus, although more than 60 minutes of exposure was required for the most resistant poliovirus species (104). Some preparations of PVP-I have proven to be active against hepatitis B virus and enteroviruses as measured by the morphologic alteration test, while other preparations had no activity at all (105). In accord with the observation for *Pseudomonas* spp, this variability may be attributable to the amount of free iodine in the preparation.

Iodine-containing solutions have been primarily used as skin preparation/degerming solutions and surgical hand scrubs. Chlorine antiseptics are not used commonly due to skin irritation. In general, most iodine-containing skin prep and surgical scrubs show rapid reduction in the resident flora of the skin; however, they do not show residual activity. Studies have shown them to be inferior to chlorhexidine gluconate (106). Utilizing the Vienna test method, a 3 $\log_{10}$ reduction was achieved after a 2-minute wash with PVP-I; the same effect

was achieved with chlorhexidine gluconate after a 1-minute wash (32). These results were confirmed comparing 14 different iodine preparations (107). In general, PVP-I solutions are more negatively affected by the presence of organic material than are chlorhexidine formulations (108,109).

ALCOHOLS

Alcohols have been used for disinfection of both skin and surface since antiquity (110). In Europe, the use of ethanol as a skin antiseptic has been the standard (110), while in the United States, ethanol is often replaced by antiseptic chemicals such as chlorhexidine, povidone-iodine, and triclosan. Alcohol preparations have been used as hygienic hand disinfectants, surgical hand disinfectants, and skin disinfectants, each having its own set of requirements. In addition, alcohol is often a constituent of combination skin disinfectants. Health care workers should be aware that anionic additives in hand disinfectants containing alcohol may inactivate antibacterial activity and persistence of chlorhexidine (61).

Alcohols have the general chemical formula R–OH, where R can be any organic structure such as an alkyl or benzyl molecule (see Table 12.1). The –OH group is the reactive species and its reactivity is influenced by the attached R group.

Alcohols have been commonly used as hard-surface disinfectants because of their general antimicrobial properties. However, volatility and flammability can be an issue when using alcohols in this manner. The flash points of ethanol and propanols are below 15°C, requiring caution in their use. On the other hand, short-chain alcohols can be suitable as disinfectants because they have unlimited solubility in water, have low toxicity, are fast acting, and are microbicidal. Low-weight alcohols possess less surface tension than water and thus have better wetting characteristics. This is important for antiseptics used on skin or for surface disinfectants used on nonuniform surfaces (110).

Regardless of the application, the order of antibacterial effect of alcohol isomers is *n*-primary > *iso*-primary > secondary > tertiary. This review is confined to the use of alcohols as antiseptics (i.e., their use on skin), as that is the primary use in health care today.

Mechanism of Action

It is generally believed that alcohols, like most chemical germicides, act at multiple sites of the cell. The primary mode of action is related to coagulation/denaturation of proteins and solubility of the alcohols in lipids (111,112) (see Table 12.1, Fig. 12.1). In the absence of water, coagulation will not occur. For example, 70% ethanol is more effective than 95% ethanol as a germicide because higher concentrations of alcohol may deprive the bacterial cell of water, thereby inducing an impermeable cell membrane. This activity prevents the penetration of alcohol into the cell (110). Hence, with dry cells, water is needed for antimicrobial activity, though this is not true for moist cells.

Coagulation of cell wall and cytoplasmic proteins occurs after exposure to alcohol disinfectants but does not appear to affect nucleoproteins (113). Coagulation of enzymatic proteins leads to loss of cellular function but there is no specificity with regard to which enzymes are affected. In addition, as the chain length of the alcohol increases, there is further impact on diminishing enzyme function (114).

Bacterial enzymes in the cell wall are more easily inactivated than intracellular enzymes (115). Microbe cell lysis following alcohol exposure is likely due to disruption of the cell membrane (110,116,117).

The general mechanisms of alcohols can be summarized as follows:

- Coagulation/denaturation of proteins and lipids
- Water-dependent activity due to water requirement to achieve cell membrane permeability
- Cytoplasmic components coagulate after intracellular concentration
- Disruption of cell membrane followed by cell lysis

Spectrum of Activity

A review of the in vitro activity against bacterial spores indicates that alcohols are considered to have little killing effect. As a matter of routine procedure, spore preparations are often kept in 95%

Table 12.9

Comparison of Minimum Microbicidal Concentrations of Various Alcohols in Suspension Tests

Alcohol		Minimum Effective Concentrations (% v/v)					
		S. aureus			*E. coli*		
	Exposure (min)	1	2	10	1	2	12
Methanol		65	67[a]		60–65		
Ethanol		50	58[a]		40–50		
Propan-1-ol		20	23[a]		17		
Propan-2-ol		45	46[a]		26		
Butan-1-ol		9	11[a]		5		
Isobutanol		16			6.5		
sec-Butanol		15			11		
tert-Butanol			26–46[b]			14	
Pentan-1-ol				3	2		
Isopentanol			4		2.75		
sec-Pentanol		7.5		4			
tert-Pentanol		15			9		
Hexan-1-ol		0.6[b]	5[b]	0.7			
Heptan-1-ol		0.12[c]					0.12
Octan-1-ol		0.06[c]			0.06		

[a]Converted from % w/w.
[b]In 30 minutes.
[c]In >30 minutes.
Adapted from Rotter ML. Alcohols for antisepsis of hands and skin. In: Ascenzi JM, ed. *Handbook of disinfectants and antiseptics*. New York: Marcel Dekker, 1996:177–233.

ethanol to prevent them from contamination by other vegetative organisms. However, other data indicate that some sporicidal activity may be found and is related to the alcohol itself, its concentration, and the species of microorganism (110).

A number of studies document the activity of alcohols against gram-positive and gram-negative organisms (118–120) and against multidrug-resistant pathogens (121–123). Tables 12.9 and 12.10 summarize the antimicrobial activity of a variety of alcohols against common microorganisms using carrier and suspension testing methods.

Ethanol is bacteriostatic and inhibits spore growth at concentrations around 10%, is bactericidal at 30% or more, but loses its activity at 90% or more, indicating the need for water for biocidal activity to kill *S. aureus* as well as other bacterial species (118,124).

Alcohol has in vitro activity against *M. tuberculosis* and a variety of fungi (110,119,125). Clinical isolates of *Mycobacterium* have been shown to be resistant to 75% alcohol (the alcohol type was not identified). *Mycobacterium chelonae* and *Mycobacterium nonchromogenicum* showed prolonged survival in 75% alcohol (126). Water content is necessary for the effectiveness of this antiseptic (Table 12.11).

The fungicidal activity of short-chain alcohols, mainly ethanol, is well established (110). Most are killed within short exposure periods (5 to

60 minutes) at concentrations ranging from 35% to 96%. *Candida* spp and *Aspergillus niger* appear to be very susceptible, with a minimum effective concentration of 35% at an exposure time of 1 minute.

As with other chemical agents, the virucidal activity of alcohols is generally related to the presence or absence of a lipophilic envelope. Among the enveloped viruses, methanol, at concentrations of 20% to 80%, inactivates viruses in 15 minutes to 24 hours (127,128). Ethanol at concentrations ranging from 50% to 60% inactivates the same viruses in 1 hour (110). The propanols seem more active, since they require lower concentrations to have the same effect with similar exposure times (110,129,130).

The nonenveloped viruses such as picornaviruses, however, are more difficult to kill with longer chain alcohols than with ethanol. Seventy percent ethanol was effective in 2 minutes against poliovirus type 1 (131), though at 25% concentration, a 240-minute exposure was necessary for killing. Ninety-five percent 2-propanol was not effective after exposure for 10 minutes against this virus. Coxsackievirus type B was not killed by 95% 2-propanol after 10 minutes of exposure (130). Echovirus type 6 was inactivated with 50% ethanol in 10 minutes, whereas 90% 2-propanol was not effective. Seventy percent ethanol and 45% 2-propanol were not effective against hepatitis A after 1 minute of exposure (132) but hepatitis B,

Table 12.10

Comparison of Minimum Bactericidal Concentrations (% v/v) of Various Alcohols in Carrier Tests

Alcohol	S. aureus 2 min[a]	S. aureus 30 min	S. aureus 30 min	E. coli 0.25–15 s	E. coli 10[b] min	E. coli 10[b] min	M. tuberculosis 15 min	M. tuberculosis 30 min	M. tuberculosis 120 min
Methanol		57[c]	70	95					90
Ethanol	80	43[c]	60	80	96	80		80	
Propan-2-ol	50		50	50	60			20	
Propan-1-ol		23[c]	30	20	50	50		20	
Butan-1-ol								5	
Isobutanol									10
Propen(1)-ol(3)								20	
Benzyl alcohol							~4		

[a]Length of exposure.
[b]Dried in sputum on glass.
[c]Converted from % w/w.
Adapted from Rotter ML. Alcohols for antisepsis of hands and skin. In: Ascenzi JM, ed. *Handbook of disinfectants and antiseptics.* New York: Marcel Dekker, 1996:177–233.

Table 12.11

Efficiency of Short-Chain Alcohols to Reduce Release of Test Bacteria from Artificially Contaminated Hands at Various Concentrations and Exposure Times in Hygienic Handrubs[a] (Mean Log Reduction)

Alcohol	Conc. (% w/v)	Test Organism	Exposure Time (Min)			
			0.5	1.0	2.0	4.0
Ethanol	60	*Escherichia coli*		3.8		
	70	*E. coli*	2.6–3.6	3.8–4.3	4.5–5.1	5.4
		Staphylococcus saprophyticus	3.5	4.0		
		Staphylococcus aureus	2.6–3.7			
	80	*E. coli*		4.5		
2-Propanol	50	*E. coli*	3.4	3.9	4.4	
	60	*E. coli*		4.0–4.7		
		Serratia marcescens		4.1		
	70	*E. coli*	3.4–3.5	4.8–4.9		
1-Propanol	40	*E. coli*		4.3		
	50	*E. coli*	3.7	4.7–5.0	4.9	
	60	*E. coli*		5.5		
	100	*E. coli*		5.8		

[a]Tested with comparable methods.
Adapted from Rotter ML. Alcohols for antisepsis of hands and skin. In: Ascenzi JM, ed. *Handbook of disinfectants and antiseptics*. New York: Marcel Dekker, 1996:177–233.

which is normally considered resistant to many chemical germicides, was relatively sensitive to both alcohols (133,134).

The microflora of the skin can be divided into two groups: the resident flora (more difficult to remove) and the transient flora (easily removed). The resident microflora also replicate on the skin. Health care personnel handwash preparations are designed primarily to remove the transient organisms, whereas surgical scrubs and skin prepping formulations are directed more at reducing the resident flora. It has been demonstrated that although bacteria on a patient's skin are the main cause of surgical site infections, it is important for health care personnel to further reduce the risk of infection by careful hand hygiene (110). Studies demonstrate that alcohol rubbed on the skin reduce the microbial flora as effectively as a 6-minute scrub with water. Unlike other antiseptics (e.g., chlorhexidine and triclosan), alcohols do not have any residual or substantive properties. Mixtures of alcohols and agents such as chlorhexidine combine the rapid effect of the alcohol with an ingredient with substantive activity (110).

Alcohols have a sublethal effect on skin microflora and allow very slow bacterial regrowth (25,110). Table 12.11 summarizes the data demonstrating the efficiency of short-chain alcohols for reducing bacteria from artificially contaminated hands at various concentrations and exposure times in a hygienic handwash study (110). The data indicate that alcohols are quickly able to reduce bacteria from hands by 2.6 to 5.8 $\log_{10}$, depending on the type of alcohol and the concentration. Concentration and exposure time are critical for both immediate and residual activity. The greatest residual activity is noted when 2-propanol is combined with chlorhexidine.

Health care workers are less likely to transfer gram-negative bacilli to urinary catheters when they use 2-propanol as a handrub rather than washing with soap (135). The data for rhinoviruses is less striking. Seventy percent ethanol impregnated into towels was only slightly more effective than 10% ethanol. Ethanol-2-propanol and 3% benzyl alcohol were only slightly better than 70% ethanol alone (136). Single treatment with an ethanol handwash was ineffective against rhinovirus (137);

however, soap and water was effective. Against influenza H1N1, killing was achieved with up to 70% alcohol-based handrubs, with or without chlorhexidine, although soap and water hand hygiene was slightly more effective (138).

ALDEHYDES

Glutaraldehyde and ortho-Phthalaldehyde

Formaldehyde and glutaraldehyde have been used for sterilization and disinfection of medical devices since the 1960s (139). Although formaldehyde is an excellent biocide, its toxicity has limited its use. Glutaraldehyde is used for routine disinfection of medical devices, especially flexible fiber-optic endoscopes and heat-sensitive medical devices. It has excellent biocidal activity and materials compatibility. ortho-Phthalaldehyde (OPA) is a high-level disinfectant. It has the same materials' compatibility characteristics of glutaraldehyde and enhanced antimicrobial properties. The structure of these agents is shown in Table 12.1. Many other aldehydes have antimicrobial activity but have not been developed into commercial products and hence will not be discussed here.

Mechanism of Action

Several aldehydes have antimicrobial properties, but the most widely used are glutaraldehyde and formaldehyde. Benzaldehyde, succinaldehyde, malonaldehyde, glyoxal, and several of the β-unsaturated aldehydes (e.g., cinnamaldehyde) also have antimicrobial activity.

The antimicrobial activity of aldehydes in general is based on the reactivity of the aldehyde group (140) and its ability to undergo alkylation reactions. Reactivity of this group can be changed by other functional groups on the molecule. Aldehydes tend to become hydrated in aqueous solutions and in equilibrium with the free aldehyde form, which is believed to be the active moiety. In the case of glutaraldehyde, the monomeric-free aldehyde molecule is in equilibrium with the cyclic hemiacetal and acetal polymers, together coexisting with smaller quantities of mono- and dihydrates. This equilibrium appears to be temperature sensitive, since at higher temperatures, there is a shift to the more active monomeric form. The effect of pH on aldehydes is well described. The reaction of glutaraldehyde with protein increases as the pH rises from 4 to 9 (141). Glutaraldehyde activity is greater at a basic pH of 9 to 10, possibly because condensation reactions are catalyzed better at an alkaline pH (141).

Amines and sulfhydryl groups react most strongly with aldehydes. Cellular constituents involved most often are both enzymes and structural proteins and nucleic acids. Treatment of *Micrococcus lysodeikticus* cells with glutaraldehyde prevented the release of selective enzymes from the periplasmic space, indicating interaction of glutaraldehyde with the outer cell surface (142). In poliovirus type 1 and echovirus type 25, glutaraldehyde reacts with lysine residues in the protein capsid (143). Enzymatic function via DNA polymerase was affected when the virus was exposed to a glutaraldehyde disinfectant (144). Formaldehyde is known to react with amino groups to bring about intermolecular cross-linking (145) and although it reacts with both RNA and DNA, its reaction with RNA is stronger (146). Glutaraldehyde, like formaldehyde, can cause intramolecular and intermolecular cross-linking of molecules. Antimicrobial properties of OPA involve binding to membrane receptors followed by entrance of the biocide into the cell through the permeable membrane. OPA then compromises cell cycle function through disruption of DNA and RNA (147). Transport of low-molecular-weight amino acids in glutaraldehyde-treated *E. coli* was reduced about 50%. One would expect much less transport if this was the only mechanism of action (148). In a comparative study of mechanism of action of glutaraldehyde and of OPA on mycobacterial cells, the data suggest that the cross-linking effect of glutaraldehyde on the cell membrane is the mechanism by which glutaraldehyde exerts its antimicrobial action and that the more lipophilic OPA molecule is more efficient at crossing the lipid-rich cell surface of the mycobacterial cell and exerting its action internally (149).

Investigations into the sporicidal activity of glutaraldehyde indicate that the spore coat is protective and that the glutaraldehyde must be alkalinized in order to penetrate this protective barrier (150–152).

The general mechanisms of aldehydes can be summarized as follows:

- Interaction with cell membrane and cytoplasmic proteins, especially those with sulfhydryl moieties
- Penetration into cells is pH dependent, with aldehydes working better at basic pH
- Intramolecular and intermolecular cross-linking of molecules
- Compromise of cellular function by disrupting DNA and RNA

Spectrum of Activity

Glutaraldehyde was first proposed as an antimicrobial in 1962 (139) as an alternative to formaldehyde sterilization of sutures. The sporicidal properties of alkaline glutaraldehyde were demonstrated in 1963 (153), making this form preferable as a chemical sterilant. OPA is a commercially available high-level disinfectant. Since the only aldehydes commercially available for hospital use in the United States are glutaraldehyde and OPA, the spectrum of activity of other aldehydes, although of interest, is not dealt with here.

The literature describes the effectiveness of glutaraldehyde against gram-positive and gram-negative bacteria. Rubo et al. (154) demonstrated the rapid bactericidal activity of 0.02% glutaraldehyde against *Staphylococcus aureus*, *E. coli*, and *Pseudomonas aeruginosa*. In a 20-minute exposure to this low concentration, inactivation of 10^4 cells or more was observed. *Pseudomonas aeruginosa* appeared to be the most resistant of the three organisms tested. Additional work by Borick (155) demonstrated rapid kill (less than 1 minute) of *E. coli*, *Pseudomonas aeruginosa*, *Serratia marcescens*, *Proteus vulgaris*, and *K. pneumonia* by 2% glutaraldehyde. *Helicobacter pylori* was rapidly killed by 0.5% glutaraldehyde with exposure as short as 15 seconds (156). OPA has been shown to be effective against both vancomycin-resistant enterococci (VRE) and MRSA (157).

Several strains of atypical mycobacteria (158–162) were assessed for susceptibility to glutaraldehyde. In evaluating a modified in-use method, it was shown that exposure of strains of *Mycobacterium avium-intracellulare*, *Mycobacterium gordonae*, *Mycobacterium fortuitum*, and *M. chelonae* to 1% glutaraldehyde for 15 minutes resulted in a 4 $\log_{10}$ reduction, and exposure to a 2% solution for 1 minute resulted in 100% kill (160). In another study, 2% glutaraldehyde tested against several of the same species in a quantitative suspension and carrier test was shown to reduce their populations 5 $\log_{10}$ within 30 minutes in the presence of organic soil and hard water (161). Further work by the same group showed that endoscopes artificially contaminated with *M. tuberculosis* and *M. avium-intracellulare* in sputum and endoscopes precleaned using a neutral soap could be disinfected with 2% glutaraldehyde in 10 and 20 minutes, respectively (162). The data indicate that there is a range of times for the inactivation of the various species. Collins (160) found that the most resistant species to glutaraldehyde were *M. gordonae*

and members of the *M. avium-intracellulare* group (Table 12.12).

Microorganisms isolated from water systems or grown in water are much more resistant to the action of disinfectants than bacteria grown in laboratory media (163,164). Studies have evaluated a variety of disinfectants against several strains of atypical mycobacteria, including glutaraldehyde-resistant strains isolated from washer disinfectors. As expected, the washer disinfector isolates were extremely resistant to glutaraldehyde but notably, both acidic OPA and alkaline OPA, under dirty and clean conditions, were effective (158). The mycobacteria are a heterogeneous group of organisms but the one thing they have in common is a cell wall with high lipid content. This makes them less susceptible to hydrophilic molecules, hence less vulnerable to many disinfectants. The surrogate organism used to determine tuberculocidal activity is *Mycobacterium bovis* var BCG. Collins and Montalbine (159) examined the activity of glutaraldehyde against a variety of mycobacteria, including the virulent strain *M. tuberculosis* H37Rv.

OPA has several advantages over glutaraldehyde, including its superior activity against mycobacteria. Based on the claims for high-level disinfection, a 0.55% solution of OPA is effective within 5 minutes, whereas a 2.5% glutaraldehyde solution requires 45 minutes to achieve the same 6 $\log_{10}$ reduction in *M. bovis* (158).

In general, aldehydes are less effective against bacterial spores than vegetative forms of the same organism and other vegetative organisms. Glutaraldehyde is the only aldehyde with substantial activity against spores. A 2% alkaline glutaraldehyde solution has the same activity as an 8% formaldehyde solution (153,165) and 10 times the activity of a small aldehyde, glyoxal (ethanedial) (139). The sporicidal activity is directly related to the pH of the solution; alkaline solutions have been shown to be more sporicidal. When bicarbonate is added to glutaraldehyde, substantial increases in the sporicidal activity result (139). It appears that bicarbonate affects the spore and not the glutaraldehyde molecule, as pretreatment of spores with bicarbonate renders them sensitive to acidic glutaraldehyde (166).

C. difficile is a clinically important spore-forming bacterium, especially in hospitalized patients and following the use of certain antibiotic therapies (167–170). Data indicate an in vitro susceptibility of *C. difficile* spores to glutaraldehyde with short exposure periods of 5 to 30 minutes for 0.1% to 2.0% glutaraldehyde. Longer exposure times are required to kill *B. subtilis* and *Bacillus stearothermophilus* spores (171).

A study evaluating the performance of 2% glutaraldehyde against *C. difficile* in situ corroborates the in vitro data (172). Endoscopes contaminated with *C. difficile* were effectively disinfected in 5 minutes. A comparison of glutaraldehyde and of OPA indicates that glutaraldehyde is considerably more sporicidal. Two percent and 3% glutaraldehyde solutions achieved a 6 $\log_{10}$ reduction in spores of *B. subtilis* in 6 and 3 hours, respectively, while 0.3% and 0.55% OPA required 72 and 48 hours, respectively. With spores of *C. tetani*, 2% and 3% glutaraldehyde achieved a 2 $\log_{10}$ reduction in 2 minutes, and 0.3% and 0.55% OPA achieved the same results in 20 minutes and 5 minutes, respectively. For spores of *C. difficile*, 2% and 3% glutaraldehyde achieved a 3 $\log_{10}$ reduction in 15 seconds, whereas 0.3% and 0.55% OPA achieved the same level of sporicidal activity at 2 minutes and 1 minute, respectively (173).

Fungi, as yeasts and molds, are generally susceptible to glutaraldehyde at concentrations marketed as high-level disinfectants. The effect of pH again has been demonstrated. A 0.5% solution of alkaline glutaraldehyde was shown to be more effective than an acidic solution at the same concentration at inhibiting spore production and growth of *A. niger* (174). A 2% acidic glutaraldehyde solution, however, was found to be effective in 15 minutes at 25°C against a wide variety of fungi except *A. niger*, which required 30 minutes for complete kill. The MIC for acidic glutaraldehyde was five times higher than for alkaline glutaraldehyde in inhibiting the growth of *S. cerevisiae* (175). Other work has shown glutaraldehyde to be potent against a wide variety of fungi, including *Trichophyton interdigitale*, *Microsporum gypseum*, *C. albicans*, *Mucor hiemalis*, *Rhizopus stolonifer*, *Penicillium chrysogenum*, and *Byssochlamys fulva* (176). A 10% alkaline glutaraldehyde solution was shown in vitro to eradicate *Trichophyton mentagrophytes* and *Cephalosporium* and *Fusarium* spp (177). In vivo activity of glutaraldehyde was demonstrated in the treatment of onychomycoses (178). Isenberg et al. (179) demonstrated the

Table 12.12

Mycobactericidal Activity of 2% Alkaline Glutaraldehyde Solution Tested at 20°C against a Number of Mycobacterial Species			
Organism	**Inoculum Size (log)**	**Rate of Kill (logs per 10 min)**	**ETS[a] (min)**
M. tuberculosis TMC 102[b]	6.10	2.41	25
M. tuberculosis BCG Pasteur TMC 1011	5.92	1.74	30
M. kansasii TMC 1201	4.80	2.50	15
M. kansasii TMC 1203	5.25	2.38	15
M. kansasii TMC 1204	5.35	2.44	15
M. simiae TMC 1226	6.25	2.22	20
M. marinum TMC 1218	5.05	4.33	10
M. avium TMC 706	6.15	1.54	35
M. avium TMC 724	6.21	1.28	40
M. intracellulare TMC 673	6.38	0.44	>60
M. intracellulare TMC 1406	5.75	0.80	60
M. scrofulaceum TMC 1306	6.38	4.05	12
M. gordonae TMC 1327	5.97	0.59	60
M. szulgae TMC 1328	6.24	2.12	20
M. smegmatis TMC 1546	4.86	4.55	10
M. fortuitum TMC 1529	5.70	5.00	10

[a]Estimated time to sterility (<50 CFU/mL).
[b]TMC, Trudeau Mycobacterium Culture Collection number.
Adapted from Collins FM. Bactericidal activity of alkaline glutaraldehyde solution against a number of atypical mycobacterial species. *J Appl Bacteriol* 1986;61:247–251.

effectiveness of 2% alkaline glutaraldehyde against *Candida albicans* in normal hospital practice. The data in Table 12.13 indicate that, with normal hospital use of a commercially available glutaraldehyde, the activity of the solution was maintained for 2 to 4 weeks following in-use stress.

Glutaraldehyde has proven virucidal activity. Glutaraldehyde is active against enveloped and nonenveloped viruses, the former being more susceptible. Poliovirus type 1, coxsackievirus type B1, and echovirus type 6 were more difficult to inactivate, requiring greater than 1% glutaraldehyde, than were herpes simplex virus, vaccinia virus, Asian influenza virus, and adenovirus. (Although adenovirus is classified as a nonenveloped virus, it does contain lipids absorbed to its protein surface and they are considered an integral part of the virus structure, as with enveloped viruses.) The enveloped viruses and adenovirus required 0.2% or more glutaraldehyde with a 1-minute exposure at room temperature for inactivation (143). Isolates of echovirus showed differences in susceptibility to glutaraldehyde. Table 12.14 lists the viruses susceptible to glutaraldehyde (180–196).

After an exposure for 5 minutes at 20°C, OPA is effective against bovine viral diarrhea virus, a surrogate test organism for hepatitis C virus (197), and against duck hepatitis B virus, a surrogate test virus for human hepatitis B virus (198). Organic material, which affects the activity of many chemical germicides, has little effect on the virucidal activity of glutaraldehyde (181,182,189,190,195). Saitanu and Lund (181) present data that indicate improved activity of glutaraldehyde in the presence of organic material (10% horse serum and 20% mouse droppings). Glutaraldehyde was also shown to retain its activity against cell-associated HIV in the presence of blood (187).

PEROXYGEN COMPOUNDS: HYDROGEN PEROXIDE AND PERACETIC ACID

The two peracids that are the most commonly used for the purposes of disinfection and/or sterilization are hydrogen peroxide and peracetic acid. Both of these compounds belong to the group known as peracids or peroxygen compounds.

Table 12.13

Dilution of Glutaraldehyde Solution Required to Inactivate 90% and 99.9% Fast-Growing Non–Spore-Forming Microorganisms

Microorganism	Disinfectant	Condition	10 min 90% (24 h)	10 min 99.9% (72 h)	60 min 90% (24 h)	60 min 99.9% (72 h)
Staphylococcus aureus	2% glutaraldehyde	S	32	32	64	64
		U	64	64	128	128
	3.4% glutaraldehyde	S	64	32	128	64
		U	128	64	256	256
Pseudomonas aeruginosa	2% glutaraldehyde	S	128	64	128	128
		U	256	128	1024	256
	3.4% glutaraldehyde	S	128	64	512	256
		U	256	128	1024	512
Mycobacterium spp	2% glutaraldehyde	S	8	4	8	4
		U	16	16	16	16
	3.4% glutaraldehyde	S	4	4	8	8
		U	32	32	32	32
Candida albicans	2% glutaraldehyde	S	512	8	512	8
		U	>1024	8	>1024	16
	3.4% glutaraldehyde	S	16	8	16	8
		U	32	16	64	32

S, stressed; U, fresh disinfectant.
Modified from Isenberg HD, Giugliano ER, France K, et al. Evaluation of three disinfectants after in-use stress. *J Hosp Infect* 1988;11:278–285.

Table 12.14

Viruses Shown to Be Susceptible to Glutaraldehyde

Virus	Reference
Coxsackievirus B1	180
Coxsackievirus B3	181,182
Human immunodeficiency	183–185
virus type 1	186,187
Herpes simplex virus type 2	188,189
Yellow fever virus	190
Influenza virus PR-8	190
Aphthovirus	182
Pestivirus	182
Iridovirus	182
Hepatitis B virus	133,134,191,192
Hepatitis A virus	132,193
Duck hepatitis virus	194
Poliovirus type 1	180
Echovirus	180
Rotavirus	195
Feline calcivirus	196

Hydrogen peroxide has been used for its antiseptic properties since the 1800s. It is most useful for applications where breakdown into nontoxic by-products is crucial (199). Originally, hydrogen peroxide was used for the preservation of milk and water and for the sterilization of certain beverages. As an antiseptic, it has been used in the treatment of periodontal disease and endodontic therapy as well as for oral topical applications. As a disinfectant, it is used at various concentrations to disinfect materials such as drinking water, medical equipment, and septic tank waste. It was the first nonthermal disinfectant cleared by the FDA for use on contact lenses (200). The general structure of these agents is shown in Table 12.1.

Mechanism of Action

Hydrogen peroxide is produced in phagocytes, where it kills bacteria. The activity of commercially produced hydrogen peroxide is less affected by pH than that of many other disinfectants such as phenols, organic acids, and glutaraldehyde (201).

Peracetic acid may be a more potent antimicrobial than hydrogen peroxide. Peracetic acid has the added advantage of being more lipid soluble and not susceptible to decomposition by catalase and peroxidase (202), which effectively neutralize the action of hydrogen peroxide. Like hydrogen peroxide, it has been used for the disinfection and sterilization of medical devices (e.g., hemodialyzers) and environmental surfaces. It is more resistant than hydrogen peroxide to the neutralizing effect of organic material (25).

The hydroxyl radical is an extremely potent oxidant and is responsible for the killing action of peroxide (203). The free hydroxyl radical reacts with essential components of the cell such as lipids, proteins, and nucleic acids. Antimicrobial properties of hydrogen peroxide may be due to the oxidation of double bonds in proteins, lipids, and surface membranes. However, it has other known effects, such as dissociation of 70S ribosomal subunits (see Fig. 12.1). These effects cause cell surface changes and cleavage of the DNA backbone and hence damage to spore DNA (204). Investigations suggest that the oxidizing radical is the ferryl radical formed from DNA-associated iron. Research also suggests that selective oxidation of certain proteins occurs and that vapor-phase hydrogen peroxide is a more potent oxidizer of protein than liquid-phase hydrogen peroxide (199).

The mechanism of action of peracetic acid is not as well studied but it functions as an oxidizing agent. Therefore, its mechanisms include denaturing proteins, disrupting cell membrane permeability, and oxidizing sulfhydral bonds in proteins and enzymes (4,25,205). Decomposition of peracetic acid produces the highly reactive molecule singlet oxygen and it has been proposed that this moiety is responsible for peracetic acid's activity (206). Malachesky (207) reviewed the chemical reactions of peracetic acid. Many of the groups that peracetic acid reacts with are present throughout living cells; therefore, the mechanism of action is probably not specific to any one cell structure.

The general mechanisms of peroxides can be summarized as follows:

- Free hydroxyl radical reacts with essential components of the cell such as lipids, proteins, and nucleic acids
- Dissociation of 70S ribosomal subunits
- Cell surface changes and cleavage of the DNA backbone
- Oxidation causing denaturation of proteins, disruption of cell membrane permeability, and sulfhydral bonds in proteins and enzymes

Spectrum of Activity

A number of investigators have looked at the activity and disinfecting properties of 3% hydrogen peroxide expressed as D-values. Table 12.15 lists

Table 12.15

D-Values for 3% Hydrogen Peroxide against a Variety of Microorganisms		
Organism	H₂O₂ Conc. (%)	D-value (min)
Staphylococcus epidermidis	3	1.7
Pseudomonas aeruginosa	3	1.7
Serratia marcescens	3	3.1
	3	2.8
Aspergillus fumigates	3	25.1
Candida albicans	3	27.9

Adapted from Lever AM, Sutton SVW. Antimicrobial effects of hydrogen peroxide as an antiseptic and disinfectant. In: Ascenzi JM, ed. *Handbook of disinfectants and antiseptics*. New York: Marcel Dekker, 1996:159–176.

these values. Bacteria show rapid disinfection; however, the two fungal species tested show more resistance to 3% peroxide. The data reveal discrepancies between the two studies with regard to the resistance. *C. albicans* was very resistant in both studies, indicating that longer disinfection times would be required for this organism. D-values for organisms on the surfaces of contact lenses were lower (201). Tables 12.16 and 12.17 indicate the lethality of peroxide at concentrations less than 3% toward a number of bacteria, fungi, viruses, and spores.

Peroxide has a wide spectrum of activity. Its activity is generally better against gram-negative than gram-positive organisms. In addition, viruses are extremely susceptible, being inactivated at concentrations of 30 ppm or less, although some viruses required extended periods of contact. Higher concentrations or temperature would presumably speed the action. Most bacteria are easily killed with relatively low concentrations of peroxide and in a relatively short period of time. Anaerobes are even more susceptible because they lack the enzymes catalase, peroxidase, and superoxide dismutase. However, to kill spore-forming bacteria such as *B. subtilis* and *C. sporogenes*, 6% hydrogen peroxide or 2% glutaraldehyde solutions applied for 6 and 10 hours, respectively, are needed for effective sporicidal activity. However, at lower dilutions, even such prolonged hours of exposure are not efficacious (208). Alternatively, a dilution of 0.2% peracetic acid at 50°C in the presence of 5% serum and hard water shows

rapid activity against vegetative bacteria, fungi, and spores (207).

Peracetic acid is effective against *M. tuberculosis*, *M. smegmatis* (207), and a variety of clinical isolates of *Mycobacterium* and *Cryptosporidium* spp (209). Table 12.18 presents a comparison between peracetic acid and two other disinfectants commonly used on environmental surfaces, chlorine and benzalkonium chloride. The two other disinfectants require a much longer duration of exposure to achieve the same result as peracetic acid. Combinations with other biocides may also have synergistic effects against various microorganisms (28).

New trends in peroxide disinfectants include low-temperature sterilization technology, hydrogen peroxide gas plasma, vaporized hydrogen peroxide, and ozone. Ozone as a disinfectant has increasing applicability in hospital settings. Newer generators permit maintenance of adequate ozone concentrations and temperature control which improve its functionality in hospital disinfection. Ozone often plays a role in improving the efficacy of mixed products, which contain chlorine, for example, thereby exerting increased antimicrobial action (28).

Both hydrogen peroxide and peracetic acid have been commercialized in liquid and vapor forms. It is generally accepted that the vapor phase of each compound possesses great antimicrobial activity. Low-temperature sterilizing systems using vaporized hydrogen peroxide has been shown to be very effective (210). The difference in effectiveness may be due to oxidative structural changes in the gaseous as compared to the liquid forms of hydrogen peroxide (205). In the liquid phase, each compound is unstable and requires careful handling and storage to ensure it maintains its level of antimicrobial activity. Prions may be sterilized more readily by vaporized hydrogen peroxide generators (211). These generators produce gas, which has greater antimicrobial activity at lower concentration than the liquid form of hydrogen peroxide. Vaporized products can be used for cleaning critical environments and rooms.

PHENOLS: PHENOLS, TRICLOSAN, AND HEXACHLOROPHENE

Phenol use as antiseptics and disinfectants dates to the application of coal tar poultices. However, it was the use of carbolic acid (currently referred to as *phenol*) by Lister as an antiseptic during surgery that demonstrated this compound's antimicrobial potential. The phenolic group comprise

Table 12.16

Antimicrobial Activity of Hydrogen Peroxide on Bacteria, Yeasts, and Viruses			
Organism	**Conc. (ppm)**	**Lethality (min)**	**Temp. (°C)**
Bacteria			
Staphylococcus aureus	1,000	60	NS
Staphylococcus aureus	25.8×10^4	0.2	24
Escherichia coli	1,000	60	NS
Escherichia coli	500	10–30	37
Eberthella typhi	1,000	60	NS
Aerobacter aerogenes	500	10–30	37
Sarcina spp	500	150	37
Streptococcus lactis	500	150	37
Streptococcus liquifaciens	500	240	37
Micrococcus spp	30	10	NS
Staphylococcus epidermidis	30	10	NS
Yeasts			
Torula spp	500	180–210	37
Oidium spp	500	180–210	37
Viruses			
Orthinosis virus	30	180	NS
Rhinovirus types 1A, 1B, 7	7.5	50–60	37
Rhinovirus types 1A, 1B, 7	15	18–20	37
Rhinovirus types 1A, 1B, 7	30	6–8	37
Poliovirus type 1	15	75	20
Poliovirus type 1	30	75	20

NS, not stated.
Modified from Block SS. Peroxygen compounds. In: Block SS, ed. *Disinfection, sterilization and preservation*. 5th ed. Philadelphia: Lippincott Williams & Wilkins, 2001:185–204.

compounds whose basic structure is phenol. Phenol itself is the simplest of the group. The more complex compounds include *p-tert*-amylphenol and phenylphenols such as hexachlorophene and triclosan (2,4,4′-trichloro-2′-hydroxydiphenyl ether) (see Table 12.1). In general, phenolic compounds are used in the hospital setting as low- to intermediate-level disinfectants. Effectiveness of other disinfectant is compared to phenol as an industry standard (phenol coefficient method; see Table 12.4). They are primarily used on environmental surfaces. Other phenolics have been used in skin antiseptic formulations. Triclosan is commonly used in home products (toys, kitchen utensils, etc.), cosmetics, oral hygiene, and dermatologic preparations as well as health care personnel handwashes. Phenolic disinfectants should not be used to disinfect critical instruments because they are not sporicides and exhibit inadequate tuberculocidal activity. Treatment of semicritical devices is also limited because of the difficulty rinsing them from many materials as well as patient tissue irritation caused by residuals (82).

Mechanism of Action

The mechanism by which phenolic compounds exert their antimicrobial actions is not fully elucidated.

Table 12.17

Sporicidal Activity of Hydrogen Peroxide toward Spore-Forming Bacteria and Bacterial Spores

Organism	Conc. (ppm)	Lethality (min)	Temp. (°C)	Comment
Bacillus subtilis	500	420–1,080	37	bc
Bacillus cereus	500	420–1,080	37	bc
Bacillus megaterium	500	420–1,080	37	bc
Bacillus subtilis ATCC 15411[a]	30	1,440	37	Spores
Bacillus subtilis SA22	25.8×10^4	7.3	24	ss
Bacillus coagulaus	25.8×10^4	1.8	24	ss
Bacillus stearothermophilus	25.8×10^4	1.5	24	ss
Clostridium sporogenes	25.8×10^4	0.8	24	ss
	25.8×10^4	2.0	24	ss
Bacillus subtilis var globigii	35×10^4	1.5	24	ss
	41×10^4	0.75	24	ss
	17.7×10^4	9.4	20	ss
	17.7×10^4	0.53	45	ss
	29.5×10^4	3.6	20	ss
Bacillus subtilis SA 22	29.5×10^4	0.35	45	ss
	35.4×10^4	2.3	20	ss
	35.4×10^4	0.19	45	ss

bc, bacterial culture; ss, spore suspension.
Carrier Test.
Adapted from Block SS. Peroxygen compounds. In: Block SS, ed. *Disinfection, sterilization and preservation*. 5th ed. Philadelphia: Lippincott Williams & Wilkins, 2001:185–204.

Table 12.18

Comparison of Peracetic Acid with Other Disinfectants: Effect of Temperature and Concentration in PPM to Obtain Lethality in 5 Minutes

Organism	Peracetic Acid	Active Chlorine	Benzalkonium Chloride
At 20°C			
Listeria monocytogenes	45	100	200
Staphylococcus aureus ATCC 6538	90	860	500
Enterococcus faecium DSM 2918	45	300	250
At 5°C			
Listeria monocytogenes	90	860	500
Staphylococcus aureus ATCC 6538	90	1100	750
Enterococcus faecium DSM 2918	90	450	500

Reprinted from Block SS. Peroxygen compounds. In: Block SS, ed. *Disinfection, sterilization and preservation*. 5th ed. Philadelphia: Lippincott Williams & Wilkins, 2001:185–204.

The free hydroxyl group is the reactive site of the molecule. Alkyl or halogen substitution affects the reactivity of the hydroxyl group. The hydrophobic nature of the polar group contributes to the membrane-active properties of phenolic compounds.

In general, phenolics exert their biocidal activity by binding to the cell surface, targeting the cell membrane. Subsequent to binding, interference with membrane-associated functions takes place (212). It is hypothesized that binding to the membrane results in inhibition of respiratory activity, substrate oxidation, and transport processes (213). Hexachlorophene inhibits the membrane-bound part of electron transport near the terminal acceptor (214). Uncoupling of oxidative phosphorylation is supported by studies on the effects of 4-ethylphenol on *E. coli* and of fentichlor on *E. coli* and *S. aureus* (212,215–218).

Phenolic compounds affect cell membrane permeability. A strong correlation exists between the loss of K^+ and cell viability in *Serratia marcescens* exposed to phenol (219). Treatment of *Streptococcus faecalis* with 1% phenol produced leakage of amino acids consistent with cell lysis (220). Leakage of ^{14}C-labeled glutamate, ^{14}C-adenosine, and ^{32}P-phosphate from cells exposed to several phenolic compounds further substantiates this observation (221–224). The extent of release directly correlates with the concentration of the biocide. Early events were shown to be reversible, but ultimately, leakage led to cell death. The high lipid content of the mycobacterial cell wall is thought to be this organism's target for phenols. In mycobacteria, phenols are not particularly sporicidal but have been shown to be sporostatic, inhibiting germination and outgrowth (225). Phenol appears to bind loosely to sites on the spore surface, exerting its inhibitory but reversible effects (226). Inhibition of cellular systems by phenolic compounds has also been reported, suggesting that after penetrating the cell membrane and entering the cytoplasm, a secondary site of action may be cytoplasmic enzymes. This is further suggested by the observation of coagulation of cytoplasmic proteins in phenol-treated cells (227,228). Treatment of *Staphylococcus aureus* with a 1:1,000 dilution of phenol also inhibited activation of several enzymatic pathways, although to varying degrees (229,230). Succinate dehydrogenase, a cytoplasmic enzyme, was inactivated by 4-butyl phenol and hexylresorcinol at concentrations higher than those required for microbicidal activity (114).

The phenol triclosan also interferes with the function of the cellular membrane. It inhibits uptake of certain amino acids (231). Activity of triclosan is also related to its effect on fatty acid synthesis (FAS). Bacteria utilize dissociative FAS or type II FAS (FAS-II), as opposed to the single multifunctional enzyme system in associative FAS or type I FAS (FAS-I) present in animal cells and fungi. McMurray et al. (232,233) showed that a mutation in the gene responsible for NADH-dependent *trans*-2-enoyl-acyl carrier protein reductase of bacterial FAS resulted in an increase in the tolerance of *M. smegmatis* and *E. coli* to triclosan. The *fabI* gene encodes this enzyme, which catalyzes the last step in the elongation of fatty acid biosynthesis. Triclosan is known to be very effective against *S. aureus*, including MRSA, by also inhibiting de novo fatty acid biosynthesis (234). The *fabI* gene product is also the biocide target in this organism (235,236). Additionally, the FAS-II system has been identified in *Plasmodium falciparum* (237). Triclosan analogs were shown to bind to the protein encoded for by the enoyl acyl carrier protein reductase gene from *P. falciparum*. Inhibition is thought to occur by mimicking the natural substrate of the reductase enzyme. The three-dimensional structure of this enzyme binds to triclosan, which further substantiates this observation (238). These studies suggest mechanisms other than cell membrane damage are involved with triclosan activity. At higher concentrations, as available in commercial products, cell membrane disruption may be the primary mechanism of action. Very little information appears in the literature concerning the specific mechanism of action of phenols against fungi and viruses.

An analysis and review of the structure–activity relationship of phenolic compounds reveals the general mechanisms of phenols, which can be summarized (220) as follows:

- Halogen substitution intensifies the microbicidal activity.
- Introduction of aliphatic or aromatic groups into the nucleus further increases bactericidal activity.
- Aliphatic chains intensify the bactericidal activity to a greater degree than branched chains or 2-alkyl groups of the same total number of carbon atoms.
- 2-Alkyl derivatives of 4-chlorophenol are more germicidal that 4-alkyl derivatives of 2-chlorophenol.

Spectrum of Activity

Most commercially available phenolic products are a mixture of two or more phenolic chemicals. Substitution of the ring structure of phenol changes the reactivity and activity of that base compound. Table 12.19 shows the activity of commonly used phenolic compounds. Based on this table, it appears that *Pseudomonas* is more resistant than other organisms, whereas the other gram-negative and gram-positive bacteria and fungi are inhibited at relatively low concentrations. Studies with parachlorometaxylenol (PCMX) used in topical preparations confirm this (239). However, higher resistance, as demonstrated by MIC and MBC data, may not be important, as most commercially available products are formulated at much higher concentrations.

Improved antimicrobial activity has been achieved with the combination of *ortho*-phenylphenol and *ortho*-benzyl-*para*-chlorophenol,

Table 12.19

Minimum Inhibitory Concentration of Phenol Derivatives in Nutrient Agar

Organism	OPP	BP	OBPCP	PCMC	PCMX	DC	PCP
Aeromonas punctata	200	100	10	200	100	50	10
Bacillus subtilis	100	100	10	150	75	100	10
Escherichia coli	200	500	3,500	250	200	100	500
Leuconostoc mesenteroides	100	100	10	200	100	5	35
Proteus vulgaris	200	200	100	200	200	50	100
Pseudomonas aeruginosa	1,500	5,000	5,000	800	1,000	>5,000	500
Pseudomonas fluorescens	1,500	5,000	>5,000	800	500	3,500	500
Staphylococcus aureus	100	100	20	200	100	5	10
Desulfovibrio desulfuricans	50	100	50	35	50	20	35
Candida albicans	100	100	50	200	75	50	35
Torula rubra	100	100	50	50	100	50	100
Alternaria tenuis	100	75	20	200	75	50	1
Aspergillus flavus	85	200	75	100	100	50	100
Aspergillus niger	75	100	100	100	100	100	50
Aureobasidium pullulans	35	100	20	30	50	35	20
Chaetomium globosum	60	50	20	80	50	20	20
Cladosporium herbarum	60	200	100	200	100	200	50
Coniophora puteana	50	35	5	100	35	2	35
Lentinus tigrinus	100	75	20	3,500	75	5	10
Paecilomyces variotii	100	100	50	200	100	50	50
Penicillium citrinum	35	100	75	100	50	50	50
Penicillium glaucum	80	100	50	100	35	50	50
Polyporus versicolor	65	100	50	5,000	75	50	20
Rhizopus nigricans	50	100	50	100	100	35	15
Sclerophoma pityophila	100	100	20	100	75	20	10
Stachybotrys atracorda	50	35	20	100	35	15	15
Tricoderma viride	75	200	100	140	100	50	200
Trichophyton pedis	20	20	10	100	50	10	10

OPP, 2-phenylphenol; BP, benzylphenol; OBPCP, 2-benzyl-4-chlorophenol; PCMC, 4-chloro-3-methylphenol; PCMX, 4-chloro-3,5-dimethylphenol; DC, 5,5'-dichloro-2,2'-dihydroxy-diphenyl methane; PCP, pentachlorophenol.
From Goddard PA, McCue KA. Phenolic compounds. In: Block SS, ed. *Disinfection, sterilization and preservation.* 5th ed. Philadelphia: Lippincott Williams & Wilkins, 2001:255–281.

which is commonly used in hospital disinfectants. There is still little evidence to suggest that these compounds have substantial activity against mycobacteria, including *M. tuberculosis* and *M. smegmatis* (98,99,240). For this reason, they are generally not classified as high-level disinfectants. Commercially available phenolic disinfectants completely inactivated cell-free HIV and cell-associated HIV in culture medium, but when suspended in blood, this virus was not completely inactivated when exposed to the same formulations (241,242). Phenolic compounds generally require long exposure times and high concentrations to be effective against hepatitis B virus (105).

Triclosan has been shown to have activity against a wide variety of microorganisms, including anaerobic bacteria including multidrug-resistant *S. aureus*, and fungi (243). Determination of MIC with clinical strains of *S. aureus* indicated that these strains were highly susceptible ($MIC_{90} = 0.12$ μg/mL) compared with *S. epidermidis* ($MIC_{90} = 8$ μg/mL) (244). Triclosan was recommended for the control of MRSA outbreaks after publication of several reports of its successful use in a neonatal nursery and cardiothoracic surgical unit (245). The daily use of triclosan in patient baths resulted in MRSA with significantly higher MIC to the germicide. The transfer of resistance was associated with plasmid-mediated mupirocin resistance (246). When 1% triclosan was introduced into hospital units, there was a reduction in MRSA infections over a 7-week period, from 3.4 to 0.14 cases per week, but there was no change in the control (triclosan-free) hospital units (247).

Like chlorhexidine, triclosan binds to the skin and exhibits moderate substantivity, hence its use in surgical preparation formulations and health care personnel handwash preparations (248,249). Triclosan, along with PCMX, was shown to be less effective as a skin antiseptic than formulations containing chlorhexidine.

Studies on oral preparations containing triclosan indicate that in an in vitro system simulating a periodontal disease–like state, exposure of organisms to triclosan or triclosan monophosphate (a more soluble form) caused gram-negative anaerobic organisms to be inhibited to a greater extent than gram-positive organisms (250,251). In studies utilizing pure cultures of oral microorganisms, the results indicate the same trend, with streptococci and lactobacilli being the least susceptible and the organisms *Neisseria subflava*, *Prevotella nigrescens*, and *Porphyromonas gingivalis* being highly susceptible to 0.6 mg/mL triclosan (252).

QUATERNARY AMMONIUM COMPOUNDS

Quaternary ammonium compounds (QACs) are widely used as disinfectants. However, by the 1990s, the CDC advised elimination of QACs as antiseptics because of several outbreaks of infection associated with in-use contamination (253,254). As with several other products (e.g., phenolics and iodophors), disinfectant-resistant gram-negative bacteria have been found to survive or grow in QAC (255). Several reports have documented the association of nosocomial infections associated with contaminated QAC used to disinfect patient care supplies or equipment such as cystoscopes or cardiac catheters (256,257). The quaternaries are good cleaning agents, but use with hard water can influence their antimicrobial effectiveness. Materials used to apply the QAC, such as cotton and gauze pads, can make them less microbicidal, as these materials absorb the active ingredients.

Chemically, the quaternaries are organically substituted ammonium compounds in which the nitrogen atom has a valence of five (see Table 12.1). Four of the substituted radicals (R1–R4) are alkyl or heterocyclic radicals of a given size or chain length, and the fifth (X^-) is a halide, sulfate, or similar radical. Each compound exhibits its own antimicrobial characteristics. The chemical names of QACs used in hospitals include *alkyl dimethyl benzyl ammonium chloride*, *alkyl didecyl dimethyl ammonium chloride*, and *dialkyl dimethyl ammonium chloride*. Fourth-generation QACs, referred to as *twin-chain* or *dialkyl quaternaries* (e.g., didecyl dimethyl ammonium bromide and dioctyl dimethyl ammonium bromide), purportedly remain active in hard water and are tolerant of anionic residues (258).

Mechanism of Action

The bactericidal action of the quaternaries has been attributed to the inactivation of energy-producing enzymes, denaturation of essential cell proteins, and disruption of the cell membrane. In bacteria, QACs may cause structural and functional changes in the cell wall, release of wall components, cell lysis, inhibition of membrane ATPase, and interactions with negatively charged polar groups of phospholipids (259). The general mechanism of action of QAC compounds are summarized as follows:

- Penetration through the cell wall
- Binding to cell membrane lipids and proteins

- Disruption of cell membranes and, with higher concentrations, cellular leakage
- Intracellular damage to proteins and DNA
- Lysis of cell wall components by autoenzymes
- Loss of structural organization of the microbial cell (112,258,259)

Spectrum of Activity

The quaternaries are commonly used in ordinary environmental sanitation of noncritical surfaces such as floors, furniture, and walls. Manufacturers' data sheets and results from published studies indicate that the quaternaries sold as hospital disinfectants are generally fungicidal, bactericidal, and virucidal against lipophilic viruses; they are not sporicidal and generally not tuberculocidal or virucidal against hydrophilic viruses. Gram-positive bacteria are generally more susceptible than gram-negative bacteria, thought to be due to the outer membrane of gram-negative bacteria, absent in gram-positive organisms. QACs are effective against *S. aureus* and protozoa, plasmodia in particular (259). Best et al. (98) demonstrated the low level of effectiveness of QACs against mycobacteria.

Attempts to reproduce the bactericidal and tuberculocidal results claimed by manufacturers using the AOAC tests with a limited number of QACs have not demonstrated consistent microbe killing (260,261). QACs exhibit significant antimicrobial activities but to varying degrees based

Table 12.20

Mechanisms and Examples of Resistance

Resistance Feature	Example	Mechanism
Impermeability		
- Gram-positive bacteria - Gram-negative bacteria	QACs, triclosan	Intrinsic: Outer membrane (gram-negative more than gram-positive) may prevent uptake of antiseptic or disinfectant Acquired plasmid can change outer membrane protein permeability to biocides
	Chlorhexidine	Mucopolysaccharide associated with reduced penetration of antiseptic
- Mycobacteria	Chlorhexidine, QACs Glutaraldehyde	Intrinsic lipid cell wall of mycobacteria prevents entry Acquired resistance prevents uptake of glutaraldehyde by *M. chelonae*
- Bacterial spores	Chlorhexidine, QACs, phenolics	Spore coat and cortex prevent penetration of biocides
- Extracellular matrices	Glutaraldehyde	Biofilm barriers form; Prevented penetration of biocide in *M. chelonae*
Inactivation	Chlorhexidine Peroxides	Intrinsic or acquired plasmid-associated enzymes break down and neutralize chemical molecules responsible
Efflux pumps	Chlorhexidine, triclosan QACs	Exit of biocides from the cell due to intrinsic efflux pump mechanisms; Acquired: genes encode for upregulated efflux pumps
Decreased target susceptibility	Triclosan	Acquired mutations decrease affinity for some cellular targets

QACs, quaternary ammonium compounds.
Modified from McDonnell GE. *Antisepsis, disinfection and sterilization. Types, action and resistance.* Washington, DC: ASM Press, 2007; Gershenfeld L. Iodine as a virucidal agent. *J Am Pharm Assoc* 1995;44:177–182; Nye K, Chadha DK, Hodgkin P, et al. *Mycobacterium chelonei* isolation from broncholalveolar lavage fluid and its practical implications. *J Hosp Infect* 1990;16:257–261.

on the hydrophobic group at the 4-amino side chain position. QACs having larger hydrophobic groups are significantly more effective against *E. coli* and *S. aureus* (262).

RESISTANCE

Mechanisms of resistance to antibiotics are well understood. The mechanisms generally fall into one of three categories: (a) altered targets, (b) production of enzyme(s) that degrade the active molecule, and/or (c) decreased ability to take up the compound. Resistance to many antibiotics is linked to the cell's chromosomes or a plasmid (263,264). However, the actions of chemical antiseptics or disinfectants are, in most instances, not specific for a target molecule. In fact, these biocides may act at several sites in the cell (see Fig. 12.1; Table 12.20). The response of cells to disinfectants is not likely to be as specific as the response to antibiotics. Organisms may develop resistance to various chemicals following heavy use and then revert to normal responsiveness after removal of the active ingredient. There is some evidence that there is an association between plasmid-linked antibiotic resistance and resistance

to disinfectants (265–267) (Table 12.21). While some researchers are not convinced that the use of germicides has significantly increased the resistance of microorganisms to antibiotic therapies (268,269), others have pointed to disinfectants and antiseptics as a cause of antibiotic resistance (270). Increased resistance to germicides used in the sanitization of environmental surfaces has, at times, been implicated, as in the outbreak of antibiotic-resistant *Listeria monocytogenes* in food processing plants (271).

McDonnell and Russell (25) emphasized that resistance to disinfectants and germicides does not necessarily result in inadequate germicidal action. Unlike antibiotics, where an increase in an MIC can have a significant negative therapeutic impact, increased MIC values for antiseptics and disinfectants may not have a noticeable effect. This is because antibiotics work on specific targets within the cell yet antiseptics and disinfectants generally work on the principles of chemical reactions (e.g., oxidation, alkylation, and detergency), hence many cell components may be susceptible to the action of these germicides.

Resistance of microorganisms to chemical germicides can be the result of *intrinsic* or *acquired*

Table 12.21

Microbial Genes: Acquired Resistance to Germicides and Antibiotics

Microbe	Gene Identified	Mechanism	Antibiotic Resistance	Germicide Resistance	References
Staphylococcus aureus	QacA, QacB	Efflux and drug extrusion	Fluoroquinolones	QACs	275, 306, 314
	NorA, BlaZ, Tetk	β-lactamase Multidrug-resistant efflux pumps	Methicillin Tetracycline	QACs Chlorhexidine	
Klebsiella pneumonia	CepA	Cephalosporinase	Cephalosporin	Chlorhexidine	317
Pseudomonas aeruginosa	nfxB	Efflux pump and drug extrusion	Tetracycline Erythromycin Trimethoprim	Triclosan	301 28, 269
Listeria monocytogenes	MdrL	Efflux and drug extrusion	Macrolides Cefotaxime	QACs	271 101, 274
Escherichia coli	AcrAB-TolC	Efflux and drug extrusion	β-lactams Fluoroquinolones Tetracycline	Phenolics, triclosan, QACs, chlorhexidine	28
Mycobacteria smegmatis	inhA	Mutation of enoyl-ACP reductase	Isoniazid	Triclosan, QACs, Chlorhexidine	269

QACs, quaternary ammonium compounds.

resistance. Acquired resistance develops through a change in the genetic makeup of the cell, either by mutation or by acquisition of plasmids. Intrinsic resistance is demonstrated in naturally occurring isolates. This is genetically controlled and may be constitutive (i.e., the normal state of the cell) or inducible or adaptive (i.e., in response to an agent).

Intrinsic Resistance

Intrinsic resistance may represent adaptive changes in the cell wall and/or outer membrane structure in response to exposure to germicides. Intrinsic resistance to chemical germicides may occur as a result of several different mechanisms (see Table 12.20). One prominent mechanism is reduced permeability to the agent due to changes in the exterior of the cell or spore (cell wall and/or outer membrane) (272). Intrinsic resistance in this scenario may be due to the natural state of the organism, as with the impenetrable high lipid content in the cell wall of some organisms, making them resistant to antibiotics and germicides (273). Efflux mechanisms (274–277) that prohibit or reduce internal concentrating capability of the germicide are another potential and relatively common pathway of resistance. A third mechanism, degradation of the germicide by enzymatic activity and rendering of the active ingredient ineffective, has occasionally been reported as a mechanism (278). Finally, increased microbe resiliency due to phenotype switching when living in certain growth conditions, an intrinsic virulence factor for some organisms, may also change susceptibility to some disinfectants such as for *Candida* species to chlorhexidine (100).

Biofilm production has been associated with intrinsic resistance of organisms to germicides. Biofilm production is usually associated with adherence of microorganisms to a surface and production of extensive layers of polysaccharide exopolymer (279,280). Biofilms have been found on devices and are a major component of dental plaque. However, there is no evidence that cells form biofilms in response to germicides. The resistance due to biofilms is primarily a physical phenomenon in which cells are protected from chemical germicides by the extracellular material, which either inhibits access of the biocide to the cells or interact with the biocide to effectively neutralize it. Although the biofilm formed by microorganisms may be resistant to a given germicide, once the biofilm is disrupted and the cells are subcultured, they do not show the same level of resistance. This indicates the mechanism of resistance of biofilm to be primarily physical (281). There have been reports of glutaraldehyde-resistant strains of *M. chelonae* isolated from automated endoscope reprocessors and processed scopes (282–284). This was due to the formation of biofilms on the surfaces of the tubing in the machines. The strain, which had never been exposed to disinfectants, was very sensitive to all the disinfectants tested, with the exception of the peroxygen. The isolates from the scope disinfector, however, were less susceptible to the peroxygen- and chlorine-releasing compounds and were very resistant to glutaraldehyde, with some strains showing a less than 1 $\log_{10}$ reduction with a 60-minute exposure to 2% glutaraldehyde (285). It was suggested that glutaraldehyde may have selected for the growth of resistant strains of *M. chelonae* (284).

Bacterial spores, known to be resistant to many chemical and physical agents, exemplify intrinsic resistance by impermeability. The spore coat has also been shown to be the structure responsible for resistance to OPA, for example (286). *Bacillus* and *Clostridium* spores are known to be the most resistant to antiseptics and disinfectants (25) and, as stated earlier, resistant *C. difficile* is a major cause of infections in hospitals and other health care facilities. Some chemical germicides are known to be sporicidal (glutaraldehyde, peracetic acid, and peroxide), but they require high concentrations and/or long periods of contact and/or high temperatures to be effective (Table 12.22) (287). Russell and collaborators have elucidated the development of resistance to a number of germicides during sporulation (57,288,289). As sporulation proceeds (developmental stages 0 through VI), spores become increasingly resistant to germicides in the following order: formaldehyde, sodium lauryl sulfate, phenol, *m*-cresol, chlorocresol, chlorhexidine gluconate, cetylpyridinium chloride, sodium dichloroisocyanurate, and glutaraldehyde. Resistance to germicides develops primarily during stages IV through VII, correlating with the start of cortex development, coat synthesis, maturation, and release of mature spores. Spore coat formation plays a significant role in the resistance to chlorine-containing compounds (290–292) and formaldehyde. Cortex formation is critical in conferring resistance to QACs, chlorhexidine, and glutaraldehyde (289,293). Other factors involved in the resistance of spores to chemical agents include conformational changes in the inner cell membrane conferred by small multi-drug resistance proteins (294).

Mycobacteria as a group are more resistant than other vegetative bacteria and less resistant than bacterial spores. *Mycobacterium* spp represent a unique class of bacteria having high lipid content in their cell walls. It has been proposed that these lipids interfere with the uptake or penetration of hydrophilic molecules into the cell. Support for this hypothesis can be found in the relative sensitivity of mycobacteria to disinfectants with varying hydrophilic properties. Two aldehydes, glutaraldehyde and OPA, have vastly different effectiveness against mycobacteria. Glutaraldehyde is a highly water-soluble compound, with solubility approaching 50% in water, whereas OPA is hydrophobic in nature, with water solubility reaching a maximum at 5%, though it is highly soluble in alcohol and other organic solvents. *OPA* is at least five to eight times more active against mycobacteria than is glutaraldehyde when tested under the same conditions (295). Increased activity may be attributable to the hydrophobicity of the OPA molecule and its ability to penetrate the lipid cell wall layer. Phenol and phenolic compounds also exhibit better activity against the mycobacteria than more hydrophilic compounds. Several studies evaluating the role of the mycobacterial cell wall support the cell wall barrier hypothesis. The treatment of *M. avium* and *M. tuberculosis* with ethambutol, which acts by inhibiting a component of the mycobacterial cell wall, renders these organisms more susceptible to the activity of chlorhexidine and QACs (54).

Gram-negative organisms in general are less susceptible to germicides than are gram-positive bacteria. This is most likely due to the protective outer membrane in gram-negative organisms, which limits penetration of chemicals into the cell (25). It has been demonstrated that changes in the composition of the cell surface, especially the LPSs and lipids, can reduce or prevent the penetration of QACs into gram-negative cells (296). The cell wall of gram-positive bacteria may sometimes act as an important mechanism in the resistance of these bacteria to chemical agents, although this mechanism is not uniform across all species (297,298). In addition, the role of extracellular material in the protection of cells is further supported by the existence of mucoid and nonmucoid strains of *S. aureus*: The nonmucoid cells are more susceptible to several commonly used germicidal agents (299).

Studies on the adaptive resistance of *Salmonella enterica* and *E. coli* 0157 and cross-resistance to antimicrobial agents reported that *E. coli* 0157 exhibited a high level of resistance to triclosan after exposure to just two sublethal doses. This was accompanied by decreased susceptibility to a number of antibiotics, including chloramphenicol, erythromycin, tetracycline, trimethoprim, and imipenem. Cross-resistance in *S. enterica* was also demonstrated (300).

P. aeruginosa exhibits both intrinsic and acquired resistance. This organism is intrinsically resistant to many germicides and antibiotics. Within *P. aeruginosa*, a chromosomal DNA fragment conferring triclosan resistance has been isolated. The *mexJK* operon is responsible for the efflux mechanism required for triclosan effectiveness and, in conjunction with the outer membrane channel protein OprM, the mechanism required for erythromycin activity. Triclosan can select for mutants that are cross-resistant to antibiotics (301). Growth of *Pseudomonas fluorescences* in gradually higher concentrations of the QAC didecyl dimethylammonium chloride resulted in higher resistance and cross-resistance to several antibacterial agents. Microscopic observation of cells revealed slime formation as well as loss of flagella. Removal of the slime layer (a biofilm or a physical mechanism of resistance) resulted in loss of resistance (302).

Acquired Resistance

Acquired resistance to germicidal agents may occur through mutation or by acquisition of extrachromosomal DNA (plasmids or transposons). The role of plasmids in antibiotic resistance has been known for some time. In the past, it was thought that resistance to chemical germicides was not mediated through plasmids. A number of studies have indicated that plasmids do play a role in resistance to chemical germicides.

Acquired staphylococcal resistance to QACs has been reported extensively (303–306). Several genes involved in resistance to QACs have been isolated from strains of *S. aureus* and coagulase-negative staphylococcus (*qac A*, *qacB*, and *qacC* [*smr*]) (307–309) found in humans. Additionally, two genes, *qacG* and *qacH*, have been isolated from coagulase-negative staphylococcus identified by the food industry (303,304). A fifth gene encoding for resistance to QACs, *qacJ*, has been

Table 12.22

Minimum Sporicidal Concentration of Agents with Product Dilutions for Effective Treatment of *Clostridium difficile* Strains Using Different Exposure Times						
Agent(s)		**Test Dilutions with Effective Sporicidal Activity against *C. difficile* Strain**				
Recommended Standard Product Dilution (Brand Name)	**Exposure Time (min)**	**630**	**VPI 10463**	**Ribotype 027**	**Ribotype 001**	**Ribotype 106**
Chlorine: sodium dichloroisocyanurate	2	<1:5	<1:5	1:2	<1:5	1:2
1,000 ppm dilution	10	<1:5	<1:5	<1:5	<1:5	<1:5
(Antichlor [Ecolab])	30	<1:5	<1:5	<1:5	<1:5	<1:5
Anionic and nonanionic surfactants	2	1	1:2	1:2	1	1:2
1:10 dilution	10	1:2	<1:5	<1:5	1:2	<1:5
(Decon 90 [Decon Labs])	30	<1:5	<1:5	<1:5	<1:5	<1:5
Peroxide: potassium peroxymonosulfate	2	1	1	1	1	1
1:100 dilution	10	1	<1:5	1	<1:5	<1:5
(Virkon [AntecInternational])	30	1	<1:5	1	<1:5	<1:5
QAC and alylamine	2	<1:5	<1:5	<1:5	<1:5	<1:5
1:10 dilution	10	<1:5	<1:5	<1:5	<1:5	<1:5
(Microsol 3+ [Anachem])	30	<1:5	<1:5	<1:5	<1:5	<1:5
QAC and biguanide	2	<1:5	<1:5	<1:5	<1:5	<1:5
1:100 dilution	10	<1:5	<1:5	<1:5	<1:5	<1:5
(TriGene Advance [Medichem International])	30	<1:5	<1:5	<1:5	<1:5	<1:5

Suspension testing using 100 mL spore suspension was added to 900 mL of each dilution (full strength, 1; 1:2 dilution; 1:5 dilution). After 2 minutes, 10 minutes, and 30 minutes of disinfectant exposure, 100 mL of the test was inoculated into 900 mL of medium and incubated at 37°C for 5 days.

Agents were sporicidal at commercially available concentrations. When diluted further, optimal sporicidal activity for ribotypes 027 and 106 required a greater concentration of sodium dichloroisocyanurate for destruction of spores. For potassium peroxymonosulfate, any dilution below manufacturer's recommended concentration was not sporicidal at 2 minutes, making it less effective than sodium dichloroisocyanurate. QAC combination products were sporicidal at a fivefold dilution of commercially available products. See Vohra P, Poxton I. Efficacy of decontaminants and disinfectants against *Clostridium difficile*. *J Med Microbiol* 2011;60:1218–1224.

identified in several species of *Staphylococcus* isolated from horses (310). In addition, resistance of *S. aureus* to triclosan by a novel mechanism, sh-fabI derived from *Staphylococcus haemolyticus*, revealed the potential for horizontal gene transfer. This demonstrated that a biocide could spread resistance in a human pathogen (311).

Concern has been expressed over emerging cross-resistance or coresistance to widely used disinfectants and antibiotics (269). The *qac* genes have been found near antibiotic resistance genes for several antibiotics (gentamicin, kanamycin, tobramycin, trimethoprim, and penicillin) on several plasmids (pST6, pSK4, pSK410) and transposons (Tn*552* and Tn*4002*) (305,307,312,313). In a survey of 522 clinical strains of *S. aureus* in Japanese hospitals, 32.6% of the MRSA strains and 7.5% of the methicillin-sensitive *S. aureus* strains also contained the *qacA* and *qacB* genes. The *qacC* (*smr*) gene was noted at a much lower frequency (314). Clinical isolates of staphylococci were resistant to a QAC, and benzalkonium chloride in 50% of cases (306). In those QAC-resistant strains, there was a high frequency of organisms also resistant to a range of antibiotics. The plasmid DNA of most isolates hybridized with one or more of the *qac* genes as well as *blaZ* (which codes for β-lactamase) and *tetK* (which codes for the tetracycline efflux pump). Approximately 34% of the plasmids had both the *qac A/B* and *blaZ* genes. One isolate had a multiresistant plasmid (pMS62) that contained the *qacA/B*, *blaZ*, and *tetK* genes.

Resistance to other antiseptics may also be found in some of these strains. Approximately 25% of the benzalkonium chloride–resistant strains also showed low-level resistance to the antiseptic chlorhexidine (314). A correlation between resistance to QACs and resistance to antibiotics in *L. monocytogenes* has also been reported (271). The genes responsible for this resistance can be plasmid-acquired (315) or chromosomal, similar to that found in *S. aureus*. The *mdrL* gene in *L. monocytogenes* forms a protein that is similar to efflux mechanism proteins in *B. subtilis* (316). Originally, *mdrL* was reported to be a chromosomal gene (317), that is, intrinsic resistance. However, further work demonstrated that it may be chromosomal or plasmid-acquired. Chlorhexidine resistance in *K. pneumoniae* has been linked to the *cepA* gene (associated with the production of cephalosporinase). Transformation of the *cepA* to the *E. coli* XLOLR resulted in chlorhexidine sensitivity, and retransformation resulted in chlorhexidine-sensitive *K. pneumonia*. It is hypothesized that the gene product CepA may act as a cation efflux pump. The incorporation of triclosan in many household products may contribute to the problem of increased antibiotic resistance (270), yet evidence collected in environmental samples (318,319) and human skin flora (320) does not support this supposition. The accumulated data suggest that resistance to antiseptics and disinfectants may impart antibiotic resistance in some instances (321,322). Table 12.21 reviews genes that may be responsible for shared resistance to both antibiotics and disinfectants. Consideration of these important potential interactions must be addressed when assessing isolates from clinical human samples.

Anticipated Role of Disinfectants and Antiseptics in the Health Care Environment

Hospital-acquired or nosocomial infections are the major cause of morbidity and mortality in patients contributing to health care costs and prolonged lengths of hospitalization (1). As medical practice extends beyond inpatient hospital settings, with an increasing outpatient presence, including at-home care, the more inclusive phrase "health care–acquired infection" should be used (323). The IHI (1) has focused the medical community on the need to control and prevent such infections. This chapter has addressed the commonly used disinfectants and antiseptics; however, many issues remain regarding health care–acquired infections and the health care environment (1,268,322,323).

- There are continued concerns regarding multiresistant microorganisms in the environment (e.g., MRSA and VRE).
- Data continue to reveal inadequate handwashing by health care workers and the contribution to contamination of the health care environment.
- Concerns remain regarding prior hospital or institutional room utilization by an infected patient and the risk of contamination to a new room occupant.
- The mandate to identify and incorporate updated methods of terminal cleaning of hospital or institutional rooms, such as ultraviolet light treatment and vaporized hydrogen peroxide generators (211,324,325) continues.
- There is an ongoing need to perform continuous surveillance of the health care environment to assess microorganism burden and changing patterns of resistance.
- Perform frequent updates and education for health care and environmental health services, as well as patients and visitors, about the risk of health-care acquired infections.

Innovative approaches supported by laboratory methods using antiseptics and disinfectants in creative ways, such as vaporization and ingredient combinations, will further minimize the risk of microorganism transmission. These tactics will enhance health care institutions' efforts to achieve The Joint Commission's 2013 National Patient Safety Goals, including improved hand hygiene and decrease/reduce surgical site infections, catheter-associated line infections, and urinary tract infections (326). Fewer health care–acquired infections will ultimately reduce morbidity and mortality, coming closer to achieving the crucial goals set by the IHI. It is likely that these goals will be incorporated into the Centers for Medicare & Medicaid Services (CMS) "value-based purchasing" initiatives that will tie diagnosis-related group (DRG) and medical reimbursement schema to performance in the coming years.

REFERENCES

1. Institute for Healthcare Improvement. 5 million lives campaign. 2008. http://www.ihi.org/offerings/Initiatives/PastStrategicInitiatives/5MillionLivesCampaign. Accessed November 15, 2012.
2. Ducel G, Fabry J, Nicolle L, eds. *World Health Organization Prevention of hospital-acquired infections. A practical guide.* 2nd ed. Geneva: World Health Organization, 2002:1–3.
3. Occupational Safety and Health Administration. U.S. Department of Labor compliance with the OSHA bloodborne pathogens standard 29 CFR 1910.1030. http://www.osha.gov/pls/oshaweb/owadisp. Accessed November 15, 2012.
4. Rutala W, Weber D; Healthcare Infection Control Practices Advisory Committee, Centers for Disease Control and Prevention. Guideline for disinfection and sterilization in healthcare facilities 2008. http://www.cdc.gov/hicpac/Disinfection_Sterilization/table. Accessed November 15, 2012.
5. Spaulding EH. Chemical disinfection of medical and surgical disinfection of medical and surgical materials. In: Lawrence CA, Block SS, eds. *Disinfection, sterilization and preservation.* Philadelphia: Lea & Febiger, 1968:517–531.
6. Garner JS, Favero MS. Guidelines for handwashing and hospital environmental control, 1985. *Am J Infect Control* 1986;14:110–126.
7. Boyce JM. Methicillin-resistant *Staphylococcus aureus* in hospitals and long-term care facilities: microbiology, epidemiology, and preventive measures. *Infect Control Hosp Epidemiol* 1992;13:725–737.
8. Boyce JM, Jackson MM, Pugliese G, et al. Methicillin-resistant *Staphylococcus aureus* (MRSA): a briefing for acute care hospitals and nursing facilities. *Infect Control Hosp Epidemiol* 1994;15:105–115.
9. Mulligan ME, Murray-Leisure KA, Ribner BS, et al. Methicillin-resistant *Staphylococcus aureus*: a consensus review of the microbiology, pathogenesis, and epidemiology with implications for prevention and management. *Am J Med* 1993;94:311–328.
10. Weber DJ, Rutala WA. Environmental issues and nosocomial infections. In: Wenzel RP, ed. *Prevention and control of nosocomial infections.* 3rd ed. Baltimore: Lippincott Williams & Wilkins, 1997:491–514.
11. Kim KH, Fekety R, Batts DH, et al. Isolation of *Clostridium difficile* from the environment and contacts of patients with antibiotic-associated colitis. *J Infect Dis* 1981;143:42–50.
12. Larson HE, Barclay FE, Honour P, et al. Epidemiology of *Clostridium difficile* in infants. *J Infect Dis* 1982;146:727–733.
13. Malamou-Ladas H, O'Farrell S, Nash JQ, et al. Isolation of *Clostridium difficile* in hospitalized children: a prospective study. *Acta Paediatr Scand* 1990;79:292–299.
14. Kaatz GW, Gitlin SD, Schaberg DR, et al. Acquisition of *Clostridium difficile* from the hospital environment. *Am J Epidemiol* 1988;127:1289–1294.
15. Boyce JM. Scientific basis for hand washing with alcohol and other waterless antiseptic agents. In: Rutala WA, ed. *Disinfection, sterilization and antisepsis: principles and practices in healthcare facilities.* Washington, DC: Association for Professionals in Infection Control and Epidemiology, 2001:140–150.
16. Longtin Y, Sax H, Allegranzi B, et al. Hand hygiene. *N Engl J Med* 2011;364:13–17.
17. Sax H, Allegranzi B, Chraiti MN, et al. The WHO hand hygiene observation method. *Am J Infect Control* 2009;37:827–834.
18. Rotter ML. Hand washing, hand disinfection and skin disinfection. In: Wenzel RP, ed. *Prevention and control of nosocomial infections.* 3rd ed. Baltimore: Lippincott Williams & Wilkins, 1997:691–709.
19. Ascenzi J, Favero M. Disinfectants and antiseptics: modes of action, mechanisms of resistance and testing. In: Lorian V, ed. *Antibiotics in laboratory medicine.* 5th ed. Philadelphia: Lippincott Williams & Wilkins, 2005:615–653.
20. Williams G, Denyer S, Hosein I, et al. The development of a new three-step protocol to determine the efficacy of disinfectant wipes on surfaces contaminated with *S. aureus*. *J Hosp Infect* 2007;67:329–335.
21. Siani H, Cooper C, Maillard JY. Efficacy of "sporicidal" wipes against *Clostridium difficile*. *Am J Infect Control* 2011;39:212–218.
22. McDonnell G, Burke P. Disinfection: is it time to reconsider Spaulding? *J Hosp Infect* 2011;78:163–170.
23. European Union. Regulation (EU) No 528/2012 of the European Parliament and of the Council of 22 May 2012 concerning the making available on the market and use of biocidal products. *Official J of EU* 2012;1–123. http://eur-lex.europa.eu/LexUriServ/LexUriServ.do. Accessed November 15, 2012.
24. Sharma BK, Shamim A, Lalia A, et al. Chemical agents as disinfectants and antiseptics: a review. *The Global J of Pharmaceutical Res* 2012;1:795–803.
25. McDonnell G, Russell AD. Antiseptics and disinfectants: activity, action, and resistance. *Clin Microbiol Rev* 1999;12:147–179.
26. Mazzola P, Jozala A, Lencastre Novaes L, et al. Minimal inhibitory concentration (MIC) determination of disinfectant and/or sterilizing agents. *Braz J Pharm Sci* 2009;45:241–248.
27. Mazzola P, Jozala A, Lencastre Novaes L, et al. Choice of sterilizing/disinfecting agent—determination of the Decimal Reduction Time (D-Value). *Braz J Pharm Sci* 2009;45:701–718.
28. McDonnell GE. *Antisepsis, disinfection and sterilization. Types, action and resistance.* Washington, DC: ASM Press, 2007.
29. Sattar SA, Springthorpe VS. New methods for efficacy testing of disinfectants and antiseptics. In: Rutala WA, ed. *Disinfection, sterilization and antisepsis: principles and practices in healthcare facilities.* Washington, DC: Association for Professionals in Infection Control and Epidemiology, 2001:173–186.
30. Herruzo R, Vizcaino MJ, Herruzo I. In vitro-in vivo sequence studies as a method of selecting the most efficacious alcohol-based solution for hygienic hand disinfection. *Clin Microbiol Infect* 2010;16:518–523.
31. Ramirez-Arcos S, Goldman M. Skin disinfection methods: prospective evaluation and postimplementation results. *Transfusion* 2010;50:59–64.
32. Rotter ML, Koller W, Wewalka G. Povidone-iodine and chlorhexidine gluconate–containing detergents for disinfection of hands. *J Hosp Infect* 1980;1:149–158.
33. Hobson DW, Bolsen K. Methods of testing oral and topical antiseptics and antimicrobials. In: Block SS, ed. *Disinfection, sterilization and preservation.* 5th ed. Philadelphia: Lippincott Williams & Wilkins, 2001:1329–1359.

34. Sattar SA, Springthorpe VS. Methods under development for evaluating the antimicrobial activity of chemical germicides. In: Rutala WA, ed. *Chemical germicides in health-care*. 3rd ed. Morin Heights, Canada: Polyscience and Association for Professionals in Infection Control and Epidemiology, 1994:237–254.

35. Sattar SA. Microbiocidal: testing of germicides: an update. In: Rutala WA, ed. *Disinfection, sterilization, and antisepsis in healthcare*. Washington, DC: Association for Professionals in Infection Control and Epidemiology, 1998:227–240.

36. Miner NA, Mulberry GK, Starks AN, et al. Identification of possible artifacts in the Association of Official Analytical Chemists sporicidal test. *Appl Environ Microbiol* 1995;61:1658–1660.

37. Ascenzi JM, Ezzell JM, Wendt TM. A more specific method for measurement of tuberculocidal activity of disinfectants. *Appl Environ Microbiol* 1987;53:2189–2192.

38. Springthorpe VS, Sattar SA. Application of a quantitative carrier test to evaluate microbiocides against mycobacteria. *J AOAC Int* 2007;90:817–824.

39. Steinmann J. Surrogate viruses for testing virucidal efficacy of chemical disinfectants. *J Hosp Infect* 2004;56:549–554.

40. Association of Official Analytical Chemists International. *Disinfectants: sporicidal activity of disinfectants*. Washington, DC: Association of Official Analytical Chemists, Official Methods of Analysis, 1998.

41. Humphreys PN. Testing standards for sporicides. *J Hosp Infect* 2011;77:193–198.

42. Beyth N, Redlich M, Harari D, et al. Effect of sustained-release chlorhexidine varnish of *Streptococcus mutans* and *Actinomyces viscosus* in orthodontic patients. *Am J Orthod Dentofacial Orthop* 2003;123:345–348.

43. Denton GW. Chlorhexidine. In: Block SS, ed. *Disinfection, sterilization and preservation*. 5th ed. Philadelphia: Lippincott Williams & Wilkins, 2001:321–336.

44. Davies GE, Field BS. Action of biguanides, phenols, and detergents on *E. coli* and its spheroplasts. *J Appl Bacteriol* 1969;32:233–243.

45. Hugo WB, Longworth AR. Some aspects of mode of action of chlorhexidine. *J Pharm Pharmacol* 1964;16:655–662.

46. Hugo WB, Longworth AR. Cytological aspects of the mode of action of chlorhexidine. *J Pharm Pharmacol* 1965;17:28–32.

47. Hugo WB, Longworth AR. The effect of chlorhexidine on the electrophoretic mobility, cytoplasmic constituents, dehydrogenase activity and cell walls of *E. coli* and *S. aureus*. *J Pharm Pharmacol* 1966;18:569–578.

48. Fitzgerald KA, Davies A, Russell AD. Uptake of ^{14}C-chlorhexidine diacetate to *Escherichia coli* and *Pseudomonas aeruginosa* and its release by azolectin. *FEMS Microbiol Lett* 1989;60:327–332.

49. Hiom SJ, Furr JR, Russell AD. Effects of chlorhexidine diacetate on *Candida albicans*, *C. glabrata*, and *Saccharomyces cerevisiae*. *J Appl Bacteriol* 1992;72:335–340.

50. Tattawasart U, Maillard J-Y, Furr JR, et al. Outer membrane changes in *Pseudomonas stutzeri* resistant to chlorhexidine diacetate and cetylpyridinium chloride. *Int J Antimicrob Agents* 2000;16:233–238.

51. Tattawasart U, Hann AC, Maillard JY, et al. Cytological changes in chlorhexidine-resistant isolates of *Pseudomonas stutzeri*. *J Antimicrob Chemother* 2000;45:145–152.

52. Ranganathan NS. Chlorhexidine. In: Ascenzi JM, ed. *Handbook of disinfectants and antiseptics*. New York: Marcel Dekker, 1996:235–264.

53. Sheppard FC, Mason DJ, Bloomfield SF, et al. Flow cytometric analysis of chlorhexidine action. *FEMS Mircobiol Lett* 1997;2:283–288.

54. Broadley SJ, Jenkins PA, Furr JR, et al. Potentiation of effects of chlorhexidine diacetate and cetylpyridinium chloride on mycobacteria by ethambutol. *J Med Microbiol* 1995;43:458–460.

55. Walters TH, Furr JR, Russell AD. Antifungal action of chlorhexidine. *Microbios* 1983;38:195–204.

56. Bobichon H, Bouchet P. Action of chlorhexidine on budding of *Candida albicans*: scanning and transmission electron microscopic study. *Mycopathologia* 1987;100:27–35.

57. Shaker LA, Russell AD, Furr JR. Aspects of the action of chlorhexidine on bacterial spores. *Int J Pharm* 1986;34:51–56.

58. Holloway PM, Bucknall RA, Denton GW. The effect of sub-lethal concentrations of chlorhexidine on bacterial pathogenicity. *J Hosp Infect* 1986;8:39–46.

59. Montefiori DC, Robinson WE, Modliszewski A, et al. Effective inactivation of human immunodeficiency virus with chlorhexidine antiseptics containing detergents and alcohol. *J Hosp Infect* 1990;15:279–282.

60. Harbison MA, Hammer SM. Inactivation of human immunodeficiency virus by Betadine and chlorhexidine. *J AIDS* 1989;2:16–20.

61. Kaiser N, Klein D, Karanja P, et al. Inactivation of chlorhexidine gluconate on skin by incompatible alcohol hand sanitizing gels. *J Infect Control* 2009;37:569–573.

62. Peterson AF, Rosenberg A, Alatary SD. Comparative evaluation of surgical scrub preparations. *Surg Gynecol Obstet* 1978;146:63–65.

63. Wade JJ, Casewell MW. The evaluation of residual antimicrobial activity on hands and its clinical relevance. *J Hosp Infect* 1991;18(Suppl B):23–28.

64. Mulberry G, Snyder AT, Heilman J, et al. Evaluation of a waterless, scrubless chlorhexidine gluconate/ethanol scrub for antimicrobial efficacy. *Am J Infect Control* 2001;29:377–382.

65. Larson EL, Laughon BE. Comparison of four antiseptic products containing chlorhexidine gluconate. *Antimicrob Agents Chemother* 1987;31:1572–1574.

66. Hibbard JS, Mulberry GK, Brady AR. A clinical study comparing the skin antisepsis and safety of ChloraPrep, 70% isopropyl alcohol, and 2% aqueous chlorhexidine. *J Infus Nurs* 2002;25:244–249.

67. Wilcox MH, Hall J, Gill AB, et al. Effectiveness of topical chlorhexidine powder as an alternative to hexachlorophene for the control of *Staphylococcus aureus* in neonates. *J Hosp Infect* 2004;56:156–159.

68. Maki DG, Ringer M, Alvarado CJ. Prospective randomized trial of povidone-iodine, alcohol, and chlorhexidine for prevention of infection associated with central venous and arterial catheters. *Lancet* 1991;228:339–343.

69. Clemence MA, Walker D, Farr BM. Central venous catheter practices: results of a survey. *Am J Infect Control* 1995;23:5–12.

70. Mimoz O, Pieroni L, Lawerence C, et al. Prospective randomized trial of two antiseptic solutions for prevention of central venous or arterial catheter colonization and infection in intensive care unit patients. *Crit Care Med* 1996;24:1818–1823.

71. Rubinson L, Diette GB. Best practices for insertion of central venous catheters in intensive-care units to prevent catheter-related bloodstream infections. *J Lab Clin Med* 2004;143:5–13.

72. Walder B, Pittet D, Tramer MR. Prevention of blood-stream infections with central venous catheters treated with anti-infective agents depends on catheter type and insertion time: evidence from a meta-analysis. *Infect Control Hosp Epidemiol* 2002;23:748–756.

73. Heard O, Wagle M, Vijayakumar E, et al. Influence of triple lumen catheter venous catheters coated with chlorhexidine and silver sulfadiazine on the incidence of catheter-related bacteremia. *Arch Intern Med* 1998;158:81–87.

74. Magnusson I. Local delivery of antimicrobial agents for the treatment of periodontitis. *Compend Contin Educ Dent* 1998;19:953–956.

75. Tomás I, García-Caballero L, Cousido MC, et al. Evaluation of chlorhexidine substantivity on salivary flora by epifluorescence microscopy. *Oral Dis* 2009;15:428–433.

76. Turner LA, McCombs GB, Hynes WL, et al. A novel approach to controlling bacterial contamination on toothbrushes: chlorhexidine coating. *Int J Dent Hyg* 2009;7:241–245.

77. Chavan SD, Shetty NL, Kanuri M. Comparative evaluation of garlic extract mouthwash and chlorhexidine mouthwash on salivary *Streptococcus mutans* count—an in vitro study. *Oral Health Prev Dent* 2010;8:369–374.

78. Eick S, Goltz S, Nietzsche S, et al. The efficacy of chlorhexidine digluconate containing formulations and other mouth rinses against periodontopathogenic microorganisms. *Quintessence Int* 2011;42:687–700.

79. Labeau SO, Van de Vyver K, Brusselaers N, et al. Prevention of ventilator-associated pneumonia with oral antiseptics: a systematic review and meta-analysis. *Lancet Infect Dis* 2011;11:845–854.

80. Piñeiro A, Tomás I, Blanco J, et al. Bacteremia following dental implant placement. *Clin Oral Implants Res* 2010;21:913–918.

81. Stokes T, Richey R, Wrayon D. Prophylaxis against endocarditis: summary of NICE guidelines. *Heart* 2008;94:930–931.

82. Favero MS, Bond WW. Chemical disinfection of medical and surgical materials. In: Block SS, ed. *Disinfection, sterilization and preservation*. 5th ed. Philadelphia: Lippincott Williams & Wilkins, 2001:881–918.

83. Berkelmann RI, Holland BW, Anderson RI. Increased bactericidal activity of dilute preparations of povidone-iodine solution. *J Clin Microbiol* 1982;15:635–639.

84. Gottardi W. Iodine and iodine compounds. In: Block SS, ed. *Disinfection, sterilization and preservation*. 5th ed. Philadelphia: Lippincott Williams & Wilkins, 2001:159–183.

85. Weber D, Rutala W, Sickert-Bennett E. Outbreaks associated with contaminants of antiseptics and disinfectants. *Antimicrob Agents Chemother*. 2007;51:4217–4224.

86. Craven DE, Moody B, Connolly BS, et al. Pseudobacteremia caused by povidone-iodine solution contaminated with *Pseudomonas aeruginosa*. *N Eng J Med* 1981;305:621–623.

87. Gottardi W, Puritscher M. Degerming experiments with aqueous povidone-iodine containing disinfecting solutions: influence of the concentration of free iodine on the bactericidal reaction against *Staphylococcus aureus*. *Zentralbl Bakteriol* 1986;182:372–380.

88. Bloomfield SA. Chlorine and iodine formulations. In: Ascenzi JM, ed. *Handbook of disinfectants and antiseptics*. New York: Marcel Dekker, 1996:133–158.

89. Wei MK, Wu QP, Huang Q, et al. Plasma membrane damage to *Candida albicans* caused by chlorine dioxide (ClO2). *Lett Appl Microbiol* 2008;47:67–73.

90. Gershenfeld L, Witlin B. Iodine solution as a sporicidal agent. *J Am Pharm Assoc* 1952;41:451–452.

91. Bartlett PG, Schmidt W. Disinfectant iodine complexes as germicides. *J Appl Microbiol* 1957;5:355–359.

92. Sykes G. The sporicidal properties of chemical disinfectants. *J Appl Bacteriol* 1970;33:147–156.

93. Russell AD. Chemical sporicidal and sporostatic agents. In: Block SS, ed. *Disinfection, sterilization and preservation*. 5th ed. Philadelphia: Lippincott Williams & Wilkins, 2001:529–541.

94. Pyle BH, McFeters GA. Iodine sensitivity of bacteria isolated from iodinated water systems. *Can J Microbiol* 1989;35:520–523.

95. Cargill KL, Pyle BH, Sauer RL, et al. Effects of culture conditions and biofilm formation on iodine susceptibility of *Legionella pneumophila*. *Can J Microbiol* 1992;38:423–429.

96. Gershenfeld L, Flagg W, Witlin B. Iodine as a tuberculocidal agent. *Mil Surg* 1954;114:172–183.

97. Nelson KE, Larson PA, Schraufnagel DE, et al. Transmission of tuberculosis by flexible fiberbronchoscopes. *Am Rev Respir Dis* 1983;127:97–100.

98. Best M, Sattar SA, Springthorpe VS, et al. Efficacies of selected disinfectants against *Mycobacterium tuberculosis*. *J Clin Microbiol* 1990;28:2234–2239.

99. Best M, Sattar SA, Springthorpe VS, et al. Comparative mycobactericidal efficacy of chemical disinfectants in suspension and carrier tests. *Appl Environ Microbiol* 1988;54:2856–2858.

100. Arzmi MH, Abdul R, Yusoff M, et al. Effect of phenotype switching on the biological properties and susceptibility to chlorhexidine in *Candida krusei*. *FEMS Yeast Res* 2012;12:351–358.

101. Berg G, Chang SL, Harris EK. Devitalization of microorganisms by iodine. *Virology* 1964;22:469–481.

102. Gershenfeld L. Iodine as a virucidal agent. *J Am Pharm Assoc* 1955;44:177–182.

103. Prince HN, Prince DL. Principles of viral control and transmission. In: Block SS, ed. *Disinfection, sterilization and preservation*. 5th ed. Philadelphia: Lippincott Williams & Wilkins, 2001:543–571.

104. Sauerbrei A, Wutzler P. Virucidal efficacy of povidone iodine containing disinfectants. *Letters Applied Microbiol* 2010;51:158–163.

105. Thraenhart O, Jursch C. Measures for disinfection and control of viral hepatitis. In: Block SS, ed. *Disinfection, sterilization and preservation*. 5th ed. Philadelphia: Lippincott Williams & Wilkins, 2001:585–615.

106. Crabtree TD, Pelletier SJ, Pruett TL. Surgical antisepsis. In: Block SS, ed. *Disinfection, sterilization and preservation*. 5th ed. Philadelphia: Lippincott Williams & Wilkins, 2001:919–934.

107. Ayliffe GA, Babb JR, Davies JG, et al. Hand disinfection: a comparison of various agents in laboratory and ward studies. *J Hosp Infect* 1988;11:226–243.

108. Lowbury EJ, Lilly HA. The effect of blood on disinfection of surgeons' hands. *Br Surg J* 1974;61:19–21.

109. Ally R, Maibach H. Comparative evaluation of chlorhexidine gluconate (Hibiclens) and povidone-iodine (E-Z Scrub) sponge/brushes for presurgical hand scrubbing. *Curr Ther Res* 1983;34:740–745.

110. Rotter ML. Alcohols for antisepsis of hands and skin. In: Ascenzi JM, ed. *Handbook of disinfectants and antiseptics*. New York: Marcel Dekker, 1996:177–233.

111. Kamm O. The relation between structure and physiological action of the alcohols. *J Am Pharm Assoc* 1921;10:87–92.

112. Sykes G. *Disinfection and sterilization*. 2nd ed. London: E & FN Spon Ltd, 1965:362–376.

113. Soberheim G. Alkohol als Disinfektionsmittel. *Schweiz Med Wochenschr* 1943;73:1280–1333.

114. Sykes G. Influence of germicides on dehydrogenase of *Bacterium coli*: succinic acid dehydrogenase of *Bacterium coli*. *J Hyg* 1939;59:463–469.

115. Kirschhoff H. Wirkungmechanismem chemischer Desinfektionsmittel. I. Allgemeiner Reaktionsablauf. *Gesundheitwes Desinfekt* 1974;66:125–130.

116. Pulvertaft RJV, Lumb GD. Bacterial lysis and antiseptics. *J Hyg* (London) 1948;46:62–64.

117. Razin S, Argaman M. Lysis of Mycoplasma, bacterial protoplasts, spheroplasts and L-forms by various agents. *J Gen Microbiol* 1963;30:155–172.

118. Harrington C, Walker H. The germicidal activity of alcohol. *Boston Med Surg J* 1903;148:548–552.

119. Coulthard CE, Sykes G. The germicidal effect of alcohol with special reference to its action on bacterial spores. *Pharm J* 1936;137:79–81.

120. Pohle WD, Stuart LS. The germicidal action of cleaning agents: a study of a modification of Price's procedure. *J Infect Dis* 1940; 67:275–281.

121. Sakuragi T, Yanagisawa K, Dan K. Bactericidal activity of skin disinfectants on methicillin-resistant *Staphylococcus aureus*. *Anesth Analg* 1995;81:555–558.

122. Kampf G, Jarosch R, Ruden H. Limited effectiveness of chlorhexidine based hand disinfectants against methicillin resistant *Staphylococcus aureus* (MRSA). *J Hosp Infect* 1998;38:297–303.

123. Kampf G, Hofer M, Wendt C. Efficacy of hand disinfectants against vancomycin resistant enterococci. *J Hosp Infect* 1999;42:143–150.

124. Morton HW. Relationship of concentration and germicidal efficacy of ethyl alcohol. *Ann NY Acad Sci* 1950;532:191–196.

125. Ali Y, Dolan MJ, Fendler EJ, et al. Alcohols. In: Block SS, ed. *Disinfection, sterilization and preservation*. 5th ed. Philadelphia: Lippincott Williams & Wilkins, 2001:229–254.

126. Woo PCY, Leung K-W, Wong SSY, et al. Relatively alcohol-resistant Mycobacteria are emerging pathogens in patients receiving acupuncture treatment. *J Clin Microbiol* 2002;40;1219–1224.

127. Gordon MH. *Studies on viruses of vaccinia and variola*. Privy Council Medical Research Council, Special Reports 1925; Series 98.

128. Kuwert EK, Thraendhardt O. Theoretische, Methodische und praktische Probleme der Virusdesinfektion in der Hummanmedizin. *Immun Infekt* 1977;4:125–130.

129. Groupe V, Engle CG, Gaffney PE, et al. Virucidal activity of representative anti-infective agents against influenza A and vaccinia viruses. *Appl Microbiol* 1955;3: 333–339.

130. Klein M, Deforest A. The inactivation of virus by germicides. *Proc Chem Spec Manuf* 1963:116–118.

131. Kewitsch A, Weuffen W. Wirkung chemischer Desinfektionsmittel gegenuber Influenza-Vacciniaund Poliomyelitisvirus. *Med Welt* 1966;17:76–81.

132. Mbithi JN, Springthorpe VS, Sattar SA. Chemical disinfection of hepatitis A virus on environmental surfaces. *Appl Env Microbiol* 1990;56:3601–3604.

133. Bond WW, Favero MS, Petersen NJ, et al. Inactivation of hepatitis B virus by intermediate-to-high level disinfectant chemicals. *J Clin Microbiol* 1983;18: 535–538.

134. Kobayashi H, Tsuzuki M, Koshimizu K, et al. Susceptibility of hepatitis B virus to disinfectants or heat. *J Clin Microbiol* 1984;20:214–216.

135. Ehrenkranz HN, Alfonso BC. Failure of hand washing to prevent hand transfer of patient bacteria to urethral catheters. *Infect Control Hosp Epidemiol* 1991;12: 654–658.

136. Handley JO, Mika LA, Gwaltney JM. Evaluation of virucidal compounds for inactivation of rhinovirus on hands. *Antimicrob Agents Chemother* 1978;14:690–694.

137. Savolainen-Kopra C, Korpela T, Simonen-Tikka ML, et al. Single treatment with ethanol hand rub is ineffective against human rhinovirus—hand washing with soap and water removes the virus efficiently. *J Med Virol* 2012;84:543–547.

138. Grayson ML, Melvani S, Druce J, et al. Efficacy of soap and water and alcohol-based hand-rub preparations against live H1N1 influenza virus on the hands of human volunteers. *Clin Infect Dis* 2009;48:285–291.

139. Pepper RE, Lieberman ER. Dialdehyde alcoholic sporicidal composition. US Patent 3,016,328. January 9, 1962.

140. Rehn D, Nolte H. Zur antimikrobiellen wirksamkeit substituierter aromatischer aldehyde und alkohole. *Zentrabl Bakteriol Hyg Abt I Orig B* 1979;168:506–516.

141. Hopewood D, Allen CR, McCabe C. The reactions between glutaraldehyde and various proteins: an investigation of their kinetics. *Histochem J* 1970; 2:137–150.

142. Ellar DJ, Munoz E, Salton MRJ. The effect of low concentrations of glutaraldehyde on *Micrococcus lysodeikticus* membranes. *Biochim Biophys Acta* 1971;225:140–150.

143. Chambon M, Jallat-Archimbaud C, Bailly JL, et al. Comparative sensitivities of Sabin and Mahoney poliovirus type 1 prototype strains and two recent isolates to low concentrations of glutaraldehyde. *Appl Environ Microbiol* 1997;63:3199–3204.

144. Howard CR, Dixon JL, Young P, et al. Chemical inactivation of hepatitis B virus: the effect of disinfectants on virus associated DNA polymerase activity, morphology and infectivity. *J Virol Methods* 1983;7:135–148.

145. Fraenkel-Conrat H, Cooper M, Olcott HS. The reaction of formaldehyde with proteins. *J Am Chem Soc* 1945;67:950–954.

146. Staehlin M. Reaction of tobacco mosaic virus nucleic acid with formaldehyde. *Biochim Biophys Acta* 1958;29:410–417.

147. Simoes M, Simoes LC, Cleto S, et al. Antimicrobial mechanisms of ortho-phthalaldehyde action. *J Basic Microbiol* 2007;47:230–242.

148. Gorman SP, Scott EM. Transport capacity, alkaline phosphatase activity and protein content of glutaraldehyde-treated cell forms of *Escherichia coli*. *Microbios* 1977;19:205–212.

149. Fraud S, Hann AC, Maillard J-Y, et al. Effect of *ortho*-phthalaldehyde, glutaraldehyde and chlorhexidine diacetate on *Mycobacterium chelonae* and *Mycobacterium abscessus* strains with modified permeability. *J Antimicrob Chemother* 2003;51:575–584.

150. McErlean EP, Gorman SP, Scott EM. Physical and chemical resistance of ion-exchange and coat defective spores of *Bacillus subtilis*. *J Pharm Pharmacol* 1980;32:32P.

151. Gorman SP, Scott EM, Hutchinson EP. Interaction of *Bacillus subtilis* spore protoplast, cortex, ion-exchange and coatless forms with glutaraldehyde. *J Appl Bacteriol* 1984;56:95–102.

152. Gorman SP, Hutchison EP, Scott EM, et al. Death, injury and revival of chemically treated *Bacillus subtilis* spores. *J Appl Bacteriol* 1983;54:91–99.

153. Stonehill AA, Krop S, Borick PM. Buffered glutaraldehyde, a new chemical sterilizing solution. *Am J Hosp Pharm* 1963;20:458–465.

154. Rubo SD, Gardner JF, Webb RL. Biological activities of glutaraldehyde and related compounds. *J Appl Bacteriol* 1967;30:78–87.

155. Borick PM. Chemical sterilizers. *Adv Appl Microbiol* 1968;10:291–312.

156. Akamatsu T, Tabata K, Hironga M, et al. Transmission of *Helicobacter pylori* infection via flexible fiberoptic endoscopy. *Am J Infect Control* 1996;24:396–401.

157. Chan-Myers H, Roberts C, Ascenzi J. Virucidal activity of *o*-phthalaldehyde solutions against drug resistant bacteria. Abstracts of American Society for Microbiology Meeting 2001; Q64:595

158. Fraud S, Hann AC, Maillard J-Y, et al. Comparison of the mycobacteriocidal activity of *ortho*-phthalaldehyde, glutaraldehyde and other dialdehydes by a quantitative suspension test. *J Hosp Infect* 2001;48: 214–221.

159. Collins FM, Montalbine V. Mycobacteriocidal activity of glutaraldehyde solutions. *J Clin Microbiol* 1976;4:408–412.

160. Collins FM. Bactericidal activity of alkaline glutaraldehyde solution against a number of atypical mycobacterial species. *J Appl Bacteriol* 1986;61:247–251.

161. Hernandez A, Martró E, Matas L, et al. In-vitro evaluation of Persafe compared with 2% alkaline glutaraldehyde against *Mycobacterium* spp. *J Hosp Infect* 2003;54:52–56.

162. Hernandez A, Martró E, Puzo C, et al. In-use evaluation of Persafe compared with Cidex in fiberoptic bronchoscope disinfection. *J Hosp Infect* 2003;54:46–51.

163. Carson LA, Favero MS, Bond WW, et al. Factors affecting comparative resistance of naturally occurring and subcultured *Pseudomonas aeruginosa* to disinfectants. *Appl Microbiol Biotechnol* 1972;23:863–869.

164. Carson LA, Petersen NJ, Favero MS, et al. Growth characteristics of atypical mycobacteria in water and their comparative resistance to disinfectants. *Appl Env Microbiol* 1978;36:839–846.

165. Sagripanti J-L, Bonafacino A. Comparative sporicidal effects of liquid chemical agents. *Appl Environ Microbiol* 1996;62:545–551.

166. Gorman SP, Scott EM. Effect of alkalination of the bacterial cell and glutaraldehyde molecule. *Microbio Lett* 1977;6:39–44.

167. Bartlett JG, Onderdonk AB, Cisneros RL, et al. Clindamycin-associated colitis due to toxin-producing species of Clostridium in hamsters. *J Infect Dis* 1977;136: 701–705.

168. Bartlett JG, Chang TW, Gurwith M, et al. Antibiotic-associated pseudo-membranous colitis due to toxin producing clostridia. *N Engl J Med* 1978;298:531.

169. Larson HE, Price AB, Honour P, et al. *Clostridium difficile* and the etiology of pseudomembranous colitis. *Lancet* 1978;1:1063–1066.

170. Teasley DG, Gerding DN, Olson MM. Prospective randomized trial of metronidazole versus vancomycin for *Clostridium difficile*–associated diarrhea and colitis. *Lancet* 1983;2:1043–1046.

171. Dyas A, Das BC. The activity of glutaraldehyde against *Clostridium difficile*. *J Hosp Infect* 1985;6:41–45.

172. Hughes CE, Gerhard RL, Petersen LR, et al. Efficacy of routine fiberoptic endoscope cleaning and disinfection for killing *Clostridium difficile*. *Gastrointest Endosc* 1986;32:7–9.

173. Oie S, Kamiya A. Sporicidal activity of aldehyde disinfectants. *Env Infect* 2003;18:1–9.

174. Gorman SP, Scott EM. A quantitative evaluation of the antifungal activity of glutaraldehyde. *J Pharm Pharmacol* 1977;43:83–89.

175. Terleckyj B, Axler DA. Quantitative neutralization assay of fungicidal properties of disinfectants. *Antimicrob Agents Chemother* 1987;31:794–798.

176. Scott EM, Gorman SP. Glutaraldehyde. In: Block SS, ed. *Disinfection, sterilization and preservation*. 5th ed. Philadelphia: Lippincott Williams & Wilkins, 2001:361–381.

177. Dabrowa N, Landau JW, Newcomer VD. Antifungal activity of glutaraldehyde in vitro. *Arch Dermatol* 1972;105:555–557.

178. Suringa DWR. Treatment of superficial onychomycoses with topically applied glutaraldehyde. *Arch Dermatol* 1970;102:163–167.

179. Isenberg HD, Giugliano ER, France K, et al. Evaluation of three disinfectants after in-use stress. *J Hosp Infect* 1988;11:278–285.

180. Narang HK, Codd AA. Action of commonly used disinfectants against enteroviruses. *J Hosp Infect* 1983;4: 209–212.

181. Saitanu K, Lund E. Inactivation of enterovirus by glutaraldehyde. *Appl Microbiol* 1975;29:571–574.

182. Cunliffe HR, Blackwell JH, Walker JS. Glutaraldehyde inactivation of exotic animal viruses in swine heart tissue. *Appl Env Microbiol* 1979; 37:1044–1046.

183. Spire B, Montagnier L, Barre-Sinoussi F, et al. Inactivation of lymphadenopathy associated virus by chemical disinfectants. *Lancet* 1984;2:899–901.

184. Hanson PJV, Gor D, Jefferies DJ, et al. Chemical inactivation of HIV on surfaces. *Br Med J* 1989;298:862–864.

185. Hanson PJV, Gor D, Clarke JR, et al. Contamination of endoscopes used in patients with AIDS. *Lancet* 1989;2:86–88.

186. Hanson PJV, Gor D, Jefferies DJ, et al. Elimination if high titer HIV from fiberoptic endoscopes. *Gut* 1990; 31:657–660.

187. Druce JD, Jardine D, Locarnini SA, et al. Susceptibility of HIV to inactivation by disinfectants and ultraviolet light. *J Hosp Infect* 1995;30:167–180.

188. Blackwell JH, Chen JHS. Effects of various germicidal chemicals on HEp 2 cell culture and herpes simplex virus. *J Assoc Off Anal Chem* 1970; 53:1229–1236.

189. Prince DL, Prince RN, Prince HN. Inactivation of human immunodeficiency virus type 1 and herpes simplex virus type 2 by commercial hospital disinfection. *Chem Times Trends* 1990:13–16.

190. Sable FL, Hellman A, McDade J. Glutaraldehyde inactivation of virus in tissue. *Appl Microbiol* 1969;17:645–646.

191. Seefeld U, Bansky G, Jaeger M, et al. Prevention of hepatitis B virus transmission by gastrointestinal fiberscope: successful disinfection with an aldehyde liquid. *Endoscopy* 1981;13:238–239.

192. Adler-Storthz K, Sehulster LM, Dreesman GR, et al. Effect of alkaline glutaraldehyde on hepatitis B virus antigen. *Eur J Clin Microbiol* 1983;2:316–320.

193. Passagot J, Crance JM, Biziagos E, et al. Effect of glutaraldehyde on the antigenicity and infectivity of hepatitis A virus. *J Virol Methods* 1987;16:21–28.

194. Deva AK, Vickery K, Zou J, et al. Evaluation of an in-use testing method for evaluating disinfection of surgical instruments using the duck hepatitis B model. *J Hosp Infect* 1996;33:119–130.

195. Sattar AS, Raphael RA, Lochman H, et al. Rotavirus inactivation by chemical disinfectants and antiseptics used in hospitals. *Can J Microbiol* 1983;29:1464–1469.

196. Doultree JC, Druce JD, Birch CJ. Inactivation of feline calcivirus, a Norwalk surrogate virus. *J Hosp Infect* 1999;41:51–57.

197. Chan Myers H, Roberts C. Virucidal activity of *o*-phthalaldehyde solution against bovine viral diarrhea virus (BVDV). Paper presented at: The Association for Professionals in Infection Control and Epidemiology Conference; May 2002; Nashville, TN.

198. Roberts C, Chan Myers H. Virucidal activity of *o*-phthalaldehyde solution against duck hepatitis B virus. Paper presented at: The Association for Professionals in Infection Control and Epidemiology Conference; June 2001; Seattle, WA.

199. Linley E, Denyer S, McDonnell G. Use of hydrogen peroxide as a biocide: new consideration of its mechanism. *J Antimicrob Chemother* 2012;67:1589–1596.

200. Lever AM, Sutton SVW. Antimicrobial effects of hydrogen peroxide as an antiseptic and disinfectant. In: Ascenzi JM, ed. *Handbook of disinfectants and antiseptics*. New York: Marcel Dekker, 1996:159–176.

201. Block SS. Peroxygen compounds. In: Block SS, ed. *Disinfection, sterilization and preservation*. 5th ed. Philadelphia: Lippincott Williams & Wilkins, 2001:185–204.

202. Klopotek BB. Peracetic acid methods for preparation and properties. *Chimica Oggi* 1998;16:33–37.

203. Fridovich I. The biology of oxygen radicals. *Science* 1978;201:875–879.

204. Russell AD. Similarities and differences in the response of microorganism to biocides. *J Antimicrob Chemother* 2003;52:750–763.

205. Finnegan M, Linley L, Denyer SP, et al. Mode of action of H2O2 and other oxidizing agents: differences between liquid and gas forms. *J Antimicrob Chemother* 2010;65:2108–2115.

206. Hofmann J, Jusdt G, Pritzkow W, et al. Bleaching activators and mechanism of bleaching activation. *J Prakt Chem* 1992;334:293–297.

207. Malchesky PS. Medical applications of peracetic acid. In: Block SS, ed. *Disinfection, sterilization and preservation*. 5th ed. Philadelphia: Lippincott Williams & Wilkins, 2001:979–996.

208. Rutala WA, Gergen MF, Weber DJ. Sporicidal activity of chemical sterilants used in hospitals. *Infect Control Hosp Epidemiol* 1993;14:713–718

209. Holton J, McDonald V. Efficacy of selected disinfectants against *Mycobacteria* and *Cryptosporidium*. *J Hosp Infect* 1994;27:105–115.

210. Rutala W, Weber D. Sterilization, high level disinfection and environmental cleaning. *Infect Dis Clin North Am* 2011;25:45–76.

211. Rogez-Kreuz C, Yousfir R, Soufflet C, et al. Inactivation of animal and human prions by hydrogen peroxide gas plasma sterilization. *Infect Control Hosp Epidemiol* 2009;30:769–777.

212. Commager H, Judis J. Mechanism of action of phenolic disinfectants. VI. Effects on glucose and succinate metabolism of *Escherichia coli*. *J Pharm Sci* 1965;54:1436–1439.

213. Denyer SP. Mechanism of action of biocides. *Int Biodeterior Biodegradation* 1990;26:89–100.

214. Fredrick JJ, Corner TR, Gerhardt P. Antimicrobial actions of hexachlorophene: inhibition of respiration in *Bacillus megaterium*. *Antimicrob Agents Chemother* 1974;6:712–721.

215. Hugo WB, Bowen JG. Studies on the mode of action of 4-ethylphenol on *Escherichia coli*. *Microbios* 1973;8:189–197.

216. Hugo WB, Bloomfield SF. Studies on the mode of action of the phenolic antibacterial agent fentichlor against *Staphylococcus aureus* and *Escherichia coli*. III. The effect of fentichlor on the metabolic activities of *Staphylococcus aureus* and *Escherichia coli*. *J Appl Bacteriol* 1971;34:579–591.

217. Bloomfield SF. The effect of the phenolic antibacterial agent fentichlor on energy coupling in *Staphylococcus aureus*. *J Appl Bacteriol* 1974;37:117–131.

218. Goddard PA, McCue KA. Phenolic compounds. In: Block SS, ed. *Disinfection, sterilization and preservation*. 5th ed. Philadelphia: Lippincott Williams & Wilkins, 2001:255–281.

219. Kroll RG, Anagnostopoulos GD. Potassium leakage as a lethality index of phenol and the effect of solute and water activity. *J Appl Bacteriol* 1981;50:139–147.

220. Gale EF, Taylor ES. Action of tyrocidin and some detergent substances in releasing amino acids from the internal environment of *Streptococcus faecalis*. *J Gen Microbiol* 1947;1:77–84.

221. Judis J. Studies on the mechanism of action of phenolic disinfectants. I. Release of radioactivity from ^{14}C-labelled *Escherichia coli*. *J Pharm Sci* 1962;51:261–265.

222. Judis J. Studies on the mechanism of action of phenolic disinfectants. II. Patterns of release of radioactivity from *Escherichia coli* labeled by growth on various compounds. *J Pharm Sci* 1963;52:126–131.

223. Joswick HL, Corner TR, Silvernale JN, et al. Antimicrobial action of hexachlorophene: release of cytoplasmic materials. *J Bacteriol* 1971;108:492–500.

224. Hugo WB, Bloomfield SF. Studies on the mode of action of the phenolic antibacterial agent fentichlor against *Staphylococcus aureus* and *Escherichia coli*. II. The effect of fentichlor on the bacterial membrane and the cytoplasmic constituents of the cell. *J Appl Bacteriol* 1971;34:569–578.

225. Rubin J. Mycobacteriocidal disinfection and control. In: Block SS, ed. *Disinfection, sterilization, and preservation*. 4th ed. Philadelphia: Lea & Febiger, 1991:331–384.

226. Russell AD, Chopra I. Sporostatic and sporicidal agents: their properties and mechanism of action. In: *Understanding antibacterial action and resistance*. 2nd ed. London: Ellis Horwood, 1996:150–171.

227. Bancroft WD, Richter GH. The chemistry of disinfection. *J Phys Chem* 1931;35:511–530.

228. Hugo WB. Disinfection mechanisms. In: Russell AD, Hugo WB, Ayliffe GA, eds. *Principles and practices of disinfection, preservation and sterilization*. 3rd ed. Oxford: Blackwell Scientific Publications, 1999:258–283.

229. Bach D, Lambert J. Action de quelques antiseptiques sur les dehydrogenase du staphylocoque dore. *Compt Rend Soc Biol (Paris)* 1937;126:298–300.

230. Bach D, Lambert J. Action de quelques antiseptiques sur les dehydrogenase du staphylocoque dore; activants le glucose, l'acide formique et un certain nombre d'autres substrates. *Compt Rend Soc Biol (Paris)* 1937;126:300–302.

231. Regos J, Hitz HR. Investigations on the mode of action of triclosan, a broad spectrum antimicrobial agent. *Zentralbl Bakteriol* 1974;226:390–401.

232. McMurray LA, Oethinger M, Levy SB. Triclosan targets lipid synthesis. *Nature* 1998;394:531–532.

233. McMurray LA, McDermott PT, Levy SB. Genetic evidence that *inhA* of *Mycobacterium smegmatis* is a target for triclosan. *Antimicrob Agents Chemother* 1999;43:711–713.

234. Slater-Radosti C, Van Aller G, Greenwood R. Biochemical and genetic characterization of the action of triclosan on *Staphylococcus aureus*. *J Biol Chem* 2001;48:1–6.

235. Heath RJ, Yu Y-T, Shapiro MA, et al. Broad spectrum antimicrobial biocides target the FABI component of fatty acid synthesis. *J Biol Chem* 1998;46:30316–30320.

236. Heath RJ, Ronald JR, Holland DR, et al. Mechanism of triclosan inhibition of bacterial fatty acid synthesis. *J Biol Chem* 1999;274:11110–11114.

237. Waller RF, Keeling PJ, Donald RG, et al. Nuclear-encoded proteins target the plasmid in *Toxoplasma gondii* and *Plasmodium falciparum*. *Proc Natl Acad Sci USA* 1998;95:12352–12357.

238. Perozzo R, Kuo M, Sidhu A. Structural elucidation of the specificity of the antibacterial agent triclosan for malarial enoyl acyl carrier protein reductase. *J Biol Chem* 2002; 277:13106–13114.

239. Bruch M. Chlorxylenol: an old-new chemical. In: Ascenzi JM, ed. *Handbook of disinfectants and antiseptics*. New York: Marcel Dekker, 1996:265–294.

240. Rutala WA, Clontz EP, Weber DI, et al. Disinfection practices for endoscopes and other semicritical items. *Infect Control Hosp Epidemiol* 1991;12:282–288.

241. Martin LS, et al. Disinfection and inactivation of human T-lymphotropic virus type III/lymphadenopathy-associated virus. *J Infect Dis* 1985;2:400–403.

242. Druce JD, Jardine D, Locarnini SA, et al. Syringe cleaning techniques and transmission of HIV. *AIDS* 1995;9:1105–1107

243. Regos J, Zak O, Solf R, et al. Antimicrobial spectrum of triclosan, a broad-spectrum antimicrobial agent for topical applications. II. Comparison with some other antimicrobial agents. *Dermatologica* 1979;158:72–79.

244. Schmid MB, Kaplan M. Reduced triclosan susceptibility in methicillin resistant *Staphylococcus epidermidis*. *Antimicrob Agents Chemother* 2004;48:1397–1399.

245. Suller MTE, Russell AD. Triclosan and antibiotic resistance in *Staphylococcus aureus*. *J Antimicrob Chemother* 2000;46:11–18.

246. Cookson BD, Farrelly H, Stapleton P, et al. Transferable resistance to triclosan in MRSA. *Lancet* 1991;337:1548–1549.

247. Webster J. Handwashing in a neonatal intensive care nursery: product acceptability and effectiveness of chlorhexidine gluconate and triclosan 1%. *J Hosp Infect* 1992;21:137–141.

248. Bhargava HN, Leonard PA. Triclosan: applications and safety. *Am J Infect Control* 1996;24:209–218.

249. Larson EL. Guidelines for the use of topical antimicrobial agents. *Am J Infect Control* 1988;8:253–266.

250. Sharma S, Ramya TNC, Surolia A, et al. Triclosan as a systemic antibacterial agent in a mouse model of acute bacterial challenge. *Antimicrob Agents Chemother* 2003;47:3859–3866.

251. Saunders KA, Greenman J, McKenzie C. Ecological effects of triclosan and triclosan monophosphate on defined mixed cultures of oral species grown in continuous culture. *J Antimicrob Chemother* 2000;48:447–452.

252. McBain AJ, Bartolo RG, Catrenich CF, et al. Effects of triclosan-containing rinse on the dynamics and antimicrobial susceptibility of in vitro plaque ecosystems. *Antimicrob Agents Chemother* 2003;11:3531–3538.

253. Simmons BP. Guideline for hospital environmental control. *Am J Infect Control* 1983;11:97–115.

254. Boyce JM, Pittet D. Guideline for hand hygiene in health care settings. *MMWR Recomm Rep* 2002;51:1–44.

255. Rutala WA, Cole EC. Antiseptics and disinfectants—safe and effective? *Infect Control* 1984;5:215–218.

256. Shickman MD, Guze LB, Pearce ML. Bacteremia following cardiac catheterization. *N Engl J Med* 1959;260:1164–1166.

257. Ehrenkranz NJ, Bolyard EA, Wiener M, et al. Antibiotic-sensitive *Serratia marcescens* infections complicating cardiopulmonary operations: contaminated disinfectant as a reservoir. *Lancet* 1980;2:1289–1292.

258. Merianos JJ. Surface-active agents. In: Block SS, ed. *Disinfection, sterilization and preservation*. 5th ed. Philadelphia: Lippincott Williams & Wilkins, 2001:283–320.

259. Tischer M, Pradel G, Ohlsen K, et al. Quaternary ammonium salts and their antimicrobial potential: targets or nonspecific interactions. *Chem Med Chem* 2012;7:22–31.

260. Rutala WA, Cole EC. Ineffectiveness of hospital disinfectants against bacteria: a collaborative study. *Infect Control* 1987;8:501–506.

261. Cole EC, Rutala WA, Samsa GP. Disinfectant testing using a modified use-dilution method: collaborative study. *J Assoc Off Anal Chem* 1988;71:1187–1194.

262. Zhao T, Sun G. Hydrophobicity and antimicrobiology and activity of quaternary ammonium compounds. *J Applied Micro* 2008;104:824–830.

263. Sasatsu M, Shibata Y, Noguchi N, et al. High-level resistance to ethidium bromide and antiseptics in *Staphylococcus aureus*. *FEMS Microbiol Lett* 1992;93:109–114.

264. Russell AD. Plasmid and bacterial resistance to biocides. *J Appl Microbiol* 1997;82:155–165.

265. Russell AD. The role of plasmids in bacterial resistance to antiseptics, disinfectants and preservatives. *J Hosp Infect* 1985;6:9–19.

266. Moken MC, McMurray LM, Levy SB. Selection of multiple-antibiotic-resistant (mar) mutants of *Escherichia coli* by using the disinfectant pine oil: roles of the *mar* and *acr* AB loci. *Antimicrob Agents Chemother* 1997;41:2770–2772.

267. Price CTD, Singh VK, Jayaswal RK, et al. Pine oil cleaner resistant *Staphylococcus aureus:* reduced susceptibility for vancomycin and oxicillin and involvement of SigB. *Appl Env Microbiol* 2002;68:5417–5421.

268. Rutala W. Elaine L. Larson Lectureship. Disinfection and sterilization: from benchtop to bedside. Association for Professionals in Infection Control and Epidemiology (APIC) Annual Education 2012 Conference. http://www.unc.edu/depts/spice/dis/LarsonLect12NP. Accessed November 15, 2012.

269. Sheldon AT. Antiseptic "resistance": real or perceived threat? *Clin Infect Dis* 2005;40:1650–1656.

270. Levy SB. Antimicrobial household products: cause for concern. *Emerg Infect Dis* 2001;7:512–515.

271. Romanova N, Favrin S, Griffiths MW. Sensitivity of *Listeria monocytogenes* to sanitizers used in the meat processing industry. *Appl Environ Microbiol* 2002;68:6405–6409.

272. Tumah HN. Bacterial biocide resistance. *J Chemother* 2009;21:5–15.

273. Jalier V, Nikaido H. Mycobacterial cell wall: structure and role in natural resistance to antibiotics. *FEMS Microbiol Lett* 1994;123:11–18.

274. Romanova NA, Wolffs PF, Brovko LY, et al. Role of efflux pumps in adaptation and resistance of *Listeria monocytogenes* to benzalkonium chloride. *Appl Environ Microbiol* 2006;72:3498–3503.

275. Huet AA, Raygada JL, Mendiratta K, et al. Multidrug efflux pump overexpression in Staphylococcus aureus after single and multiple in vitro exposures to biocides and dyes. *Microbiology* 2008;154:3144–3153.

276. Russell AD. Mechanism of bacterial resistance to biocides. *Int Biodeterior Biodegradation* 1995;36:247–265.

277. To MS, Favrin S, Romanova N, et al. Post-adaptational resistance to benzalkonium chloride and subsequent physiochemical modifications of *Listeria monocytogenes*. *Appl Env Microbiol* 2002; 68:5258–5264.

278. Ogase HI, Nigai I, Kameda K, et al. Identification and quantitative analysis of degradation products of chlorhexidine and chlorhexidine-resistant bacteria with three-dimensional high performance liquid chromatography. *J Appl Bacteriol* 1992;73:71–78.

279. Costerton JW, Cheng KJ, Geesey GG, et al. Bacterial biofilms in nature and disease. *Ann Rev Microbiol* 1987;41:435–464.

280. Costerton JD, Lewandowski Z, DeBeer D, et al. Biofilms, the customized niche. *J Bacteriol* 1994;176: 2137–2142.

281. Brown MRW, Gilbert P. Sensitivity of biofilms to antimicrobial agents. *J Appl Bacteriol Symp Suppl* 1993;74:87S–97S.

282. Nye K, Chadha DK, Hodgkin P, et al. *Mycobacterium chelonei* isolation from bronchoalveolar lavage fluid and its practical implications. *J Hosp Infect* 1990;16: 257–261.

283. Fraser VJ, Jones M, Murray PR, et al. Contamination of flexible fiberoptic bronchoscopes with *Mycobacterium chelonae* linked to an automated bronchoscope disinfection machine. *Am Rev Resp Dis* 1992;145: 853–855.

284. Griffiths PA, Babb JR, Bradley CR, et al. Glutaraldehyde-resistant *Mycobacterium chelonae* from endoscope washer disinfectors. *J Appl Bacteriol* 1997;82: 519–526.

285. Lynam P, Babb JR, Fraise AP. Comparison of the mycobacteriocidal activity of 2% alkaline glutaraldehyde and "Nu-Cidex" (0.35% peracetic acid). *J Hosp Infect* 1995;30:237–240.

286. Cabrera-Martinez R-M, Setlow B, Setlow P. Studies on the mechanism of the sporicidal action of *ortho*-phthalaldehyde. *J Appl Bacteriol* 2002;92:675–680.

287. Vohra P, Poxton I. Efficacy of decontaminants and disinfectants against *Clostridium difficile*. *J Med Microbiol* 2011;60:1218–1224.

288. Powers EGM, Dancer BN, Russell AD. Emergence of resistance to glutaraldehyde in spores of *Bacillus subtilis*. *FEMS Microbiol Lett* 1988;50:223–226.

289. Knott AG, Russell AD, Dancer BN. Development of resistance to biocides during sporulation of *Bacillus subtilis*. *J Appl Bacteriol* 1995;79:492–498.

290. Bloomfield SF, Arthur M. Interaction of *Bacillus subtilis* spores with sodium hypochlorite, sodium dichloroisocynaurate. *J Appl Bacteriol* 1992;72:166–172.

291. Bloomfield SF, Arthur M. Mechanism of inactivation and resistance of spores to chemical biocides. *J Appl Bacteriol Symp Suppl* 1994;76:91S–104S.

292. Setlow B, Setlow P. Binding of small, acid-soluble spore proteins to DNA plays a significant role in the resistance of *Bacillus subtilis* spores to hydrogen peroxide. *Appl Environ Microbiol* 1993;59:3418–3423.

293. Sabli MZH, Setlow P, Waites WM. The effect of hypochlorite on spores of *Bacillus subtilis* lacking small acid-soluble proteins. *Lett Appl Microbiol* 1996;22:405–507.

294. Bay D, Turner R. Spectroscopic analysis of the intrinsic chromophores within small resistance protein SugE. *Biochem Biophys Acta* 2011;1808:2233–2244.

295. Walsh SE, Maillard JY, Russell AD. *Ortho*-phthalaldehyde: a possible alternative to glutaraldehyde for high level disinfection. *J Appl Microbiol* 1999;86:1039–1046.

296. Guerin-Mechin L, Dubois-Brissonnet F, Heyd B, et al. Quaternary ammonium compound stress induces specific variation in fatty acid composition of *Pseudomonas aeruginosa*. *Int J Food Microbiol* 2000;55:157–159.

297. Bridier A, Briandet R, Thomas V, et al. Comparative biocidal activity of paracetic acid, benzalkonium chloride and OPA on 77 bacterial strains. *J Hosp Infect* 2011;78:208–213.

298. Gilbert P, Brown MRW. Some perspectives on preservation and disinfection in the present day. *Int Biodeterior Biodegradation* 1995;36:219–226.

299. Kolawole DO. Resistance mechanism of mucoid-grown *Staphylococcus aureus* to the antibacterial action of some disinfectants and antiseptics. *FEMS Microbiol Lett* 1984;25:205–209.

300. Braoudaki M, Hilton AC. Adaptive resistance to biocides in *Salmonella* and *Escherichia coli* 0157 and cross-resistance to antimicrobial agents. *J Clin Microbiol* 2004;42:73–78.

301. Chuanchuen R, Narasaki CT, Schweizer HP. The MexJK efflux pump of *Pseudomonas aeruginosa* requires OprM for antibiotic efflux but not for efflux of triclosan. *J Bacteriol* 2002;184:5036–5044.

302. Langsrud S, Sundheim G, Borgman-Strahsen R. Intrinsic and acquired resistance to quaternary ammonium compounds in food related *Pseudomonas* spp. *J Appl Microbiol* 2003;95:874–882.

303. Heir E, Sundheim G, Holck AL. The *Staphylococcus qacH* gene product: a new member of the SMR family encoding multidrug resistance. *FEMS Microbiol Lett* 1998;163:49–56.

304. Heir E, Sundheim G, Holck AL. The *qacG* gene on plasmid pST94 confers resistance to quaternary ammonium compounds in staphylococci isolated from the food industry. *J Appl Microbiol* 1999;86:378–388.

305. Sidhu MS, Heir WE, Sørum H, et al. Genetic linkage between resistance to quaternary ammonium compounds and β-lactam antibiotics in food-related *Staphylococcus* spp. *Microb Drug Resist* 2001;7:363–371.

306. Sidhu MS, Heir E, Leegaard T, et al. Frequency of disinfectant resistance genes and genetic linkage with β-lactamase transposon Tn552 among clinical staphylococci. *Antimicrob Agents Chemother* 2002;46:2797–2803.

307. Leelaporn A, Firth N, Paulsen IT, et al. Multidrug resistance plasmid pSK108 from coagulase-negative staphylococci; relationship to *Staphylococcus aureus qacC* plasmids. *Plasmid* 1995;34:62–67.

308. Littlejohn TG, DiBerardino D, Messerotti LJ, et al. Structure and evolution of a family of genes encoding antiseptic and disinfectant resistance in *Staphylococcus aureus*. *Gene* 1991;101:59–66.

309. Paulsen IT, Brown MH, Littlejohn TG, et al. Multidrug resistance proteins QacA and QacB from *Staphylococcus aureus*: membrane topology and identification of residues involved in substance specificity. *Proc Natl Acad Sci USA* 1996;93:3630–3635.

310. Bjorland J, Steinum T, Sunde M, et al. Novel plasmid-borne *qacJ* mediates resistance to quaternary ammonium compounds in equine *Staphylococcus aureus*, *Staphylococcus simulans*, and *Staphylococcus intermedius*. *Antimicrob Agents Chemother* 2003;47:3046–3052.

311. Ciusa ML, Furi L, Knight D, et al. A novel resistance mechanism to triclosan that suggests horizontal gene transfer and demonstrates a potential selective pressure for reduced biocide susceptibility in clinical strains of *S. aureus*. *Int J Antimicrob Agents* 2012;40:210–220.

312. Lyon BR, Skurray RA. Antimicrobial resistance of *Staphylococcus aureus*: genetic basis. *Microbiol Rev* 1987;51:88–134.

313. Berq T, Firth N, Apisirdiej S, et al. Complete nucleotide sequence of pSK41: evolution of staphylococcal conjugative multiresistance plasmids. *J Bacteriol* 1998;180:4350–4359.

314. Alam MM, Kobayashi N, Uehara N, et al. Analysis of distribution and genomic diversity of high-level antiseptic resistance genes *qacA* and *qacB* in human clinical isolates of *Staphylococcus aureus*. *Microb Drug Res* 2003;9:109–121.

315. Lemaitre JP, Echchannaoui H, Michaut G, et al. Plasmid-mediated resistance to antimicrobial agents among listerae. *J Food Prot* 1998;61:1459–1464.

316. Huillet E, Larin S, Pardon P, et al. Identification of a new locus in *Listeria monocytogenes* involved in cellobiose dependent repression of *hly* expression. *FEMS Microbiol Lett* 1999;174:265–272.

317. Mereghetti L, Quentin R, Marquet-Van Der Mee N, et al. Low sensitivity of *Listeria monocytogenes* to quaternary ammonium compounds. *Appl Env Microbiol* 2000;66:5083–5086.

318. Rutala WA, Stergel MM, Sarubbi FA, et al. Susceptibility of antibiotic-susceptible and antibiotic-resistant hospital bacteria to disinfectants. *Infect Control Hosp Epidemiol* 1997;18:417–421.

319. Cole EC, Addison RM, Rubino JR, et al. Investigation of antibiotic and antibacterial agent cross-resistance in target bacteria from homes of antibacterial users and nonusers. *J Appl Microbiol* 2003;95:664–676.

320. Jones RD. Bacterial resistance and topical antimicrobial wash products. *Am J Infect Control* 1999;27:351–363.

321. Russell AD. Do biocides select for antibiotic resistance? *J Pharm Pharmacol* 2000;52:227–233.

322. Fanning S. Altered tolerance to biocides: links to antibiotic resistance? Paper presented at: International Association of Food Protection (IAFP), European Symposium on Food Safety; 2011; The Netherlands. http://www.foodprotection.org/events/european-symposia/11Ede/Fanning.pdf. Accessed November 15, 2012.

323. Alexander L. Nosocomial infections. http://www.netce-groups.com/372/course_9447.pdf. Accessed November 15, 2012.

324. Andersen B, Banrud H, Boe E, et al. Comparison of UV C light and chemicals for disinfection of surfaces in hospital isolation units. *Infect Control Hosp Epidemiol* 2006;27:729–734.

325. Rutala W, Weber D. Guideline for disinfection and sterilization of prion contaminated medical instruments. SHEA guidelines. *Infect Control Hosp Epidemiol* 2010;31:107–117.

326. The Joint Commission. Joint Commission 2013 National Patient Safety Goals. January 2013. http://www.jointcommission.org/hap_2013_npsg/. Accessed November 15, 2012.

Chapter 13

Evaluation of Antimicrobials in Experimental Animal Infections

David R. Andes, Alexander J. Lepak, Niels Frimodt-Møller

In vitro studies provide important information on the potency and spectrum of activity of new antimicrobials, but animal models form the link between in vitro testing and anticipated clinical results. The results of animal studies suggest appropriate indications and clinical trials, uncover potential toxicity problems, and provide insight into the pharmacokinetics (PKs) of new agents in relation to those of known agents. Furthermore in recent years, animal studies have become crucial in evaluating the importance of bacterial resistance mechanisms and which antibiotics to use against them. Thus, it is essential that new and old agents shown to be of interest following in vitro evaluation exhibit sufficient activity in vivo to justify their continued clinical development. Clinical evaluation guidelines for antiinfective drugs place experimental evaluation of new compounds (or novel combinations or therapeutic modalities) in animals as a prerequisite for clinical trials (1). Specifically, indications of the PKs of new molecules, including their metabolism and pharmacodynamics (PDs) (e.g., the effects of the interaction of drug, host, and infecting microbe, including postantibiotic effects [PAEs] and the efficacy of the drug in animal models mimicking human disease), are required and indeed may assist in the planning of clinical trials of new antibiotics (1).

Due to restrictions of space we have in the present text deliberately focused on experimental animal models, which test some aspect of antimicrobial drugs (antibiotics, antifungals, etc.), that is, PK, PD, or effect, which means that we excluded parts only describing virulence factors of microorganisms, immunologic treatment, or host factors. The reader is referred to the extensive specialized literature concerning such subjects. Further, we have not included nonvertebrate models, because these models in our view cannot evaluate a true humanlike in vivo approach for the effect of antimicrobials incorporating a sensible PK/PD analysis. Following a previous edition of the book by Zak and Sande (3), a subsequent "how-to" book was commissioned (4) that covers the technical aspects of almost every major animal model used in infection research.

ETHICAL ASPECTS OF THE USE OF ANIMALS IN ANTIMICROBIAL DRUG DISCOVERY AND DEVELOPMENT

When considering in vitro tests, the challenge is to consider whether they are really sufficient indicators of the efficacy and safety of a compound. When considering in vivo tests, the challenges include not only assessing whether such tests are reliable indicators of efficacy and safety but also considering the morality of exploitation of animals in research (5). A "practical-minded" discussion of ethics of animal use is available (6). In any discussion of the ethics of animal experimentation, it is critical to expand the discussion to consider the rights of the afflicted, whose suffering may be alleviated based on information gained through animal experimentation (7,8); there is a certain "cost" involved in not using animals, just as there is a cost in their use. Although open and direct discussion between proponents of each view is apparently scarce, it is the key to resolution of this conflict. However, because the goal of the animal rights or animal liberation activists is the complete discontinuation of animal experimentation (9–11), the opposing positions appear fundamentally irreconcilable. What remains clear is that individual researchers remain responsible for their own conduct. In light of this, readers are urged to carefully consider both points of view in order to resolve, as far as possible, this issue for themselves, as well as to provide for themselves a basis for intelligent discussion with fellow biomedical researchers, the general public, and those opposed to vivisection.

Acceptance of the position that it is ethically justified to perform animal experiments does not solve all of the ethical problems associated with such research (8). In answering these questions, it is clear that the bulk of the responsibility again lies with the individual researchers, but the questions should not be decided in isolation. Ethics committees need to be consulted prior to embarking on any experimentation. In brief, the other questions include the following:

- Is this experiment necessary and can it answer the proposed questions? (12)
- Is the welfare of the animals being used in this experiment given due consideration?
- Are the data gained by such experiments being utilized to best advantage?

Perhaps the most difficult issue is the degree of pain and suffering that animals experience during the course of infection. An excellent review of the recognition of pain and distress in animals and the physiologic basis and consequences of pain has been published (13).

Most governments have passed legislation concerning the use of animals in experiments and require that certain basic requirements be met before such experiments can be carried out. The European Union (EU) has in 2010 renewed and expanded on the recommendations for the use of animals for research (14), which appear to be stricter than the Animals Welfare Act imposed in the United States (15). There has, in Europe, been a general trend toward considerably stricter rules for animal research in the wake of very active animal rights organizations and thereby higher public interest in this issue. The EU directive is based on the three Rs—replacement, reduction, and refinement—and encompasses ruling within the following list of headings:

- Relevance and justification of the following:
  a. Use of animals including their origin, estimated numbers, species, and life stages
  b. Procedures

- Application of methods to replace, reduce, and refine the use of animals in procedures
- The planned use of anesthesia, analgesia, and other pain relieving methods
- Reduction, avoidance, and alleviation of any form of animal suffering, from birth to death where appropriate
- Use of humane end points
- Experimental or observational strategy and statistical design to minimize animal numbers, pain, suffering, distress, and environmental impact where appropriate
- Reuse of animals and the accumulative effect thereof on the animals
- The proposed severity classification of procedures
- Avoidance of unjustified duplication of procedures where appropriate
- Housing, husbandry, and care conditions for the animals
- Methods of killing
- Competence of persons involved in the project

Examples include the restriction in using death as an end point, where the text reads as follows: "The methods selected should avoid, as far as possible, death as an end point due to the severe suffering experienced during the period before death. Where possible, it should be substituted by more humane end points using clinical signs that determine the impending death, thereby allowing the animal to be killed without any further suffering." The directive includes rules for the methods used for killing of each category of animals used. Death as end point is not allowed for LD- or ED50 determination purposes.

Important issues of reporting of animal studies have recently been raised (16,17). Detailed and relevant reporting is essential for peer review and to inform future research, both to be able to repeat experiments but also to avoid redundant use of animals. Thus, there is also a responsibility of the peer reviewers of studies to impose such rules and demand that missing details are provided. Ideally, scientific publications should present sufficient information to allow a knowledgeable reader to understand what was done, why, and how, and to assess the biologic relevance of the study and the reliability and validity of the findings. A review of animal welfare issues in studies on murine tuberculosis from 1997 to 2009 (17) found that although the quality of the studies had improved in the way of focus on handling of the animals, avoiding mice being unduly exposed to serious, debilitating disease and dying from infection, they found that 80% of papers did not report the method for euthanasia, and information on the sex of the animals used was not available in 34% of the studies. Further, spontaneous death was the chosen end point for 66% of so-called lethal studies. Kilkenny et al. (16) and others (18) have suggested guidelines for publication of animal research, which is a good step forward in this field, although the list is not comprehensive enough (17). The next step forward is for scientific journals to impose such guidelines as a minimal requirement for authors to have their results published.

PRINCIPLES OF ANIMAL CARE

Standards for animal care differ in their details, and various governments have issued guidelines that are periodically updated. Controlling the factors that contribute to animal health will lead to more uniform experimental results (19). The impact of animal health on the outcomes of experiments using infection models has been reviewed (20,21). Key factors to monitor and control are the environmental conditions the animals are housed under, the adequacy and consistency of the animals' nutrition, and restriction of access to animal rooms in order to protect the animals and minimize risk to the investigator, particularly when animals are experimentally infected.

PRINCIPLES OF PLANNING EXPERIMENTS INVOLVING ANIMAL TESTING

Selecting an Animal Model of Infection

The objectives of a particular study form the basis for model selection, but as complete an understanding of the model as possible is needed to ascertain that the model is appropriate to meet these objectives. Furthermore, at least in testing antimicrobial agents, the choice of model may be dependent on the nature of the compound, the quantities available (in the case of medicinal chemistry programs, the compound supply is limiting at the early stages), and the extent of information available (e.g., the spectrum of action, the PKs). For example, medicinal chemistry programs aimed at discovering a new chemical entity effective against a novel target would normally use a mouse screening model (e.g., thigh infection or

peritoneally initiated sepsis with parenteral and oral compound administration to answer the question: Which of the many newly synthesized compounds that are active in vitro are orally active in vivo?) early in the program to select compounds for later profiling using the more complex discriminative models needed to provide a basis for clinical trial design (e.g., to determine the PK/PD relationships and demonstrate efficacy in a model closely mimicking a clinical indication so as to discover the best treatment regimen using the selected compound to treat, say, endocarditis alone and in combination with other antibiotics). Therefore, the "ideal" model varies depending on the questions asked. However, the preferred models will be similar to humans in terms of tolerability, drug absorption, distribution, metabolism, and excretion and if possible will demonstrate a pathophysiology of infection similar to that observed in humans. Lastly, using the model should be technically feasible.

Categories of Animal Models of Infection

Animal models of infection have been classified according to the complexity of the model (22). Basic screening models, *ex vivo* models (where implants such as fibrin clots are infected and subsequently removed for further analysis), monoparametric/polyparametric models (which are similar to screening models but where a single parameter or, preferably, many parameters are examined during the experiment), and discriminative models are models designed to simulate human infection as closely as possible. A discriminative model is ideal if there is a simple technique of infection; the causative organism, the route of entry, and the spread in the body are identical or at least similar to the human equivalents; the tissue involvement and the severity, course, and duration of the disease should be predictable, reproducible, and amenable to analysis; and the response of the model to chemotherapy should be measurable and reproducible.

Reproducibility of Animal Models

The response (e.g., the rate and extent of bacterial growth or the onset of clinical signs) observed in the control group has to be in the same range every time the experiment is performed. Furthermore, the response to reference compounds should be reliable and dose-dependent. It is difficult and potentially misleading to uncategorically rely on response ranges found in the literature for the interpretation of data collected in a new experiment. For this reason, investigators should establish in-house reference ranges, and these should be periodically reconfirmed. There are many other sources of variation that can affect the results of individual animal experiments and thereby complicate data interpretation. Mainly, these are strain and gender differences, age-related changes, animal well-being, and the mode and nature of infection initiation and compound administration.

Limitations of Animal Models

Differences in adsorption, distribution, metabolism, and excretion can be profoundly different, and care has to be taken to study drug doses that are "reasonable" so that the effective dose found in the model is similar to one envisioned for patients; despite the general trend of longer drug half-lives in larger animals, the requirement of large doses in mice is normally a sign that the compound is too weakly active. Ideally, drug exposure should utilize regimens that produce humanlike PK profiles. However, what such a regimen would be is obviously not known for experimental drugs at the preclinical stage. The resulting limitations can be profound and must be taken seriously when performing an animal experiment and interpreting the data obtained. Animal models should be used cautiously, their limitations should be recognized, and only those questions that the models can answer should be asked.

Model Validation

Once the most appropriate model is selected, the next step is to validate model, that is, to establish its suitability mostly in terms of responsiveness to chemotherapeutic intervention (therapy or prophylaxis). The results of the validation tests must delineate the similarities and differences between the disease as it occurs in the model and in humans. As will be discussed later, redefining or modifying the animal model to better reflect the clinical situation, particularly in terms of response to treatment, apparently seldom occurs but can produce dramatic improvements in the predictive value of the model (see Eichaker et al. [23]). Standard drugs are usually marketed drugs with proven efficacy in patients. Due consideration should be given to devising an appropriate therapeutic regimen so that the outcome in the model is similar to outcome clinically (e.g., creating a severity of infection and devising a treatment regimen that results in a "cure" rate that is similar to the clinical cure rate [see reference 23]).

Validation should be seen as a continuous process. This implies that a positive control (reference compound) should be included as an internal standard every time the model is used. A negative control (vehicle treatment) is almost always needed to account for time-related changes or other "hard-to-control" variables during the experiment.

The nature and extent of variability depends on the homogeneity of the experimental animals used and to a lesser extent on the variability of the analytical methods used. Therefore, experimental animals, especially small rodents, are often derived from inbred populations in order to reduce this variability. Moreover, individual variability due to the physical status of the animals or the procedure itself can occur. Adaptation or acclimatization times may vary depending on the animals used and the time of day of the experiment (many indicators of a disease process are subject to individual circadian rhythms). Differences may be in part controlled by stratifying the treatment groups. In the process of stratification, animals are placed into groups (blocks) based on criteria defined before the experiment, and then the groups are randomized with respect to treatments. However, stratification, though it is likely to reduce variability between groups, may increase variability within groups.

Finally, the use of the most appropriate statistical test to analyze the data is critical to successfully conclude an in vivo study. The sizes of the groups of experimental subjects and the exact statistical tests should be chosen based on the expected or desired minimal responses to therapy and the inherent variability of the groups. The downside of these fully justified efforts to minimize variability is that such experiments give no hints of the variability to be expected under clinical conditions, where many factors (e.g., pharmacogenomics, the time of the disease presentation, and the presence of underlying diseases) render extrapolation of preclinical data to the clinical situation more difficult.

Statistics and Experimental Design

The following is extensively based on previous publications (24–27).

Experimental Design

Any experiment comprises experimental units or subjects, questions posed, experimental design, facilities for performing the experiment, and the logistics of material supply and labor, all of which need to be considered carefully. For several reasons, both ethical and cost-related, in vivo pharmacologists have an obligation to consistently use the best possible experimental design. A good experimental design should make efficient use of resources and extract the maximum amount of information from the available material, and the number of animals per group should be neither so small that treatment effects remain undetected and incorrect conclusions are reached nor so large that animals and other resources are wasted. However, it is important to state that if an animal experiment is embarked on, care should be taken to include so many animals in the experiment that a statistically valid answer to the research question can be delivered.

Experimental design involves the following:

■ The question(s) to be answered must be clearly formulated (but the researchers must be prepared to analyze unexpected observations). The researchers must also recognize the constraints that the model possesses in terms of "relevance" (i.e., they must limit the questions to those that the model can really address).

■ Sources of bias must be minimized, normally by including randomization steps.

■ The natural subdivisions of experimental subjects (or the treatments) must be accounted for. This is normally accomplished by using specialized experimental designs.

■ Whenever possible, the numbers of experimental subjects should be the same in each group to facilitate statistical analysis. Plans for dealing with "dropouts" that reduce the number in a group or cause the loss of data (i.e., censored data) should be in place.

■ The researchers must take into account the chronobiologic aspects (e.g., orally administered treatments at night will likely be administered to mice with full stomachs).

■ They must weigh feasibility versus perfection and the logistics of carrying out the experiment.

■ They must plan statistical analyses prior to initiation of the experiment and include questions indicating how large a difference between groups is expected (or desired) and the likely variability of data, both of which are used in estimating the experimental group sizes.

■ The researchers must consider the final display of the data. Complex experiments are not easily amenable to graphic display (normally more than four to five lines on a single graph are difficult to follow, especially during oral presentations), and therefore, it may be necessary to break a single experiment into several parts for effective display of the data.

In a typical experiment, only one set of treatments are administered in order to isolate a single variable. However, whenever possible, the design should allow several independent variables (or factors) to be considered simultaneously. Further, the design should be such that each combination of variables is represented in the form of treatments, preferably with replicates in a single experiment. Experimental designs of this type can be used to look at the effect of individual variables but also at possible interactions between the variables. Such "multifactorial" designs clearly require built-in statistical analysis plans (e.g., two-way or three-way analysis of variance [ANOVA]). Essential to good experimental design is the inclusion of appropriate controls. Vehicle controls and, if needed, separate controls for each treatment formulation (e.g., saline groups as well as an ethanol group if the test compounds are formulated in saline or ethanol) or each route of administration (e.g., intravenous administration and oral administration) should be included. Controls for the ageing of the experimental animals during long-term experiments are often overlooked.

Prevention of bias and appropriate randomization are also important factors to consider. Bias occurs when interfering factors have dissimilar effects on different groups, with the end result that the data are unreliable. The main ways of reducing this are through randomization and elimination of investigator bias through use of blinded treatment and observations. Animals or stratified groups can be assigned to treatments randomly (using random number tables or a computer program). Although somewhat laborious, blinding investigators to treatments by the coding of compounds is recommended, particularly when clinical observation or (histo)pathology is used for the evaluation of effects.

Statistical Analyses

The main purpose of statistical evaluation of animal experiments is to ensure that any findings are not due to chance variation within or between the experimental groups. However, statistical evaluation should also be used to illuminate the data, helping to uncover effects that might otherwise be overlooked. It is critical to understand that statistical analyses do not prove biologic "cause and effect" hypotheses nor do they necessarily prove the biologic relevance of an effect of the compound in question. Although statistical significance may be shown, the effect may be so small as to be of little interest biologically (or clinically). A second purpose of statistical analyses is to show that the experiment was carried out so as to be free from the kind of experimental errors that may compromise the data (e.g., placement of all animals having the highest body weight in one group). Statistical analyses should demonstrate that before beginning of the treatment, the groups were balanced and that during the course of the experiment, no detectable unwanted bias occurred (e.g., high mortality in a treatment group in which the survivors were cured of the disease).

IN VITRO CHARACTERIZATION BEFORE EVALUATING A SUBSTANCE USING ANIMAL MODELS

Owing to both the ethical aspects of animal experimentation and the costs involved in performing an in vivo experiment, it behooves researchers to obtain results characterizing the substance(s) in vitro. Tests to consider include the following.

Determination of In Vitro Antimicrobial Properties

The minimum inhibitory concentration (MIC) and minimal bactericidal concentration (MBC) of a substance used against a particular microorganism indicate the inherent susceptibility of the microorganism to that substance. When combinations are proposed, potential interactions (interference or antagonism, indifference, additivity, or synergy) should be evaluated by the use of checkerboard titrations or time kill studies. Determination of the MIC and MBC should be considered the minimum prerequisite before proceeding to in vivo evaluations. Also, the goal should be to test the in vitro activity of antibiotics under conditions likely to exist in vivo because environmental factors (e.g., pH, pO_2, and pCO_2) can dramatically affect antibiotic activity.

Although requiring specialized equipment that is not always available, the following supplemental experiments may be considered. The activity of antimicrobials against intracellular microorganisms should be determined in specialized models of intracellular growth (e.g., *Mycobacterium avium* growing in J774A cells). Because biofilms

have been proposed to be an essential part of the in vivo situation (28–30), and the activity of antibiotics against adherent bacteria can differ from their activity against planktonic bacteria (31), determination of antimicrobial activity against adherent bacteria using the "Robbins device" (32) or other procedures (33–38) may yield insight into the effectiveness of a particular agent. Furthermore, microorganisms may grow at slower rates in vivo than in vitro (29,34), and this may affect their susceptibility to antimicrobial agents (30,34,39,40); this can be appropriately determined by evaluation of antimicrobial activity in chemostats, where the growth rate of bacteria can be controlled. Lastly, in vitro PK models (41,42) may assist in planning dosing schedules, for such models can be used to predict critical parameters of antimicrobial drug concentration and effectiveness (e.g., time above MIC or peak area). However, a problem with in vitro kinetic models is that it is often difficult to create so low elimination half-lives in the in vitro models as found in small animals such as mice. Therefore, extrapolations from dose-kinetic studies may be tested, or multiple dosing in the mice can better simulate the in vitro kinetics.

Preparation of Suitable Formulations for Administration of Antimicrobial Agents to Animals

The formulation of compounds may have a profound effect on the activity of antimicrobials. Practical reviews of formulations are available (43). Although generally not a problem with well-characterized antiinfective agents, the solubility of novel agents may dictate the routes of administration and the in vivo pharmacologic activity of an agent. Generally, the substance should be prepared so that it is in the most soluble form possible. However, specialized delivery systems such as liposomes, depot formulations, or formulations for topical administration may not require highly soluble substances. The choice of formulation ultimately affects the bioavailability and PK attributes of any particular substance, and this should be carefully considered when making comparisons of different chemical classes. In particular, formulations can dramatically affect the oral absorption of compounds and also tissue distribution. Note, however, that formulation effects can differ between species (44), and subtle differences can occur between animal strains (45).

Some formulations can also reduce the toxicity of compounds (e.g., cyclodextrin [46]).

When considering oral administration of substances, it is important to recognize that the degree of uptake of antibiotics from the gastrointestinal tract varies between species. For example, in vitro tests using intestinal brush-border vesicles to study the kinetics and inhibition of cephalosporin uptake have indicated that the characteristics of transport of β-lactams by brush-border membranes are similar for rat and human tissues but that rabbit tissues possess distinct properties (47). The plasma PKs of amoxicillin are nonlinear in both humans and rats, but rats have lower oral bioavailability (48,49). These studies showed that mathematical modeling could result in false predictions of human PKs of amoxicillin in humans from rat plasma profiles (48,49) and also showed that precipitation of a portion of the total orally administered dose in rats may occur in proximal gastrointestinal areas, complicating prediction of human oral bioavailability from data obtained from rats. Furthermore, the lower amoxicillin bioavailability in rats is in part owing to degradation within the intestine (50).

In general, however, use of formulations acceptable for use in humans is recommended whenever possible. When used parenterally, some formulations may provide more of a depot of active substance rather than resulting in immediate high blood levels of the antimicrobial. When comparing a few antimicrobials, the best strategy is to use the best formulation for each compound in order to ensure maximal bioavailability. However, this approach may not be useful for large-scale screening. In this case, a standard formulation optimized for the class of substances to be compared should be used; however, one must accept that some substances may fail due to poor formulation and will be considered poorly active in vivo. Adequate formulation of novel antimicrobials is often neglected during in vivo evaluations, and following are suggestions that should be considered prior to performing animal experiments. Aqueous solvents are preferred, and poorly soluble substances can be formed into fine suspensions by sonication. At least in initial evaluations, a fine precipitate, if kept in even suspension, can be well tolerated, particularly with oral application. Note, however, that particulate material, especially when administered parenterally, has altered PKs and bioavailability compared with soluble compounds, and this may complicate the interpretation of the findings. Suspensions intended for intravenous application need to consist of nanoparticles (<100 nm in diameter), and because this requires specialized technology, suspensions made by sonication should generally not be administered intravenously. Poorly soluble compounds can be prepared using a variety of mixed solvent systems. In these cases, the substance is first dissolved in an organic solvent and then carefully diluted in an aqueous solvent system. For example, a widely suitable method for preparing compounds is to dissolve the substance in N-methylpyrrolidine (NMP) and add PEG300 to a final 90% v/v. This procedure can use ethanol (10% v/v) or benzyl alcohol (6% v/v). Mixed solvents may additionally contain tetraglycol (polyethylene glycol monotetrahydrofurfuryl ether), polyethylene glycol 400, or propylene glycol (50% w/v, maximum final concentration). Substances can be dissolved in these solutions (sometimes adding Tween 80 initially) and then diluted in aqueous solutions (e.g., dissolution in PEG300 and then dilution with 0.9% saline to a final 30% PEG30). In all cases, the aqueous solvent should not contain high concentrations of salts, and often, physiologic saline is the best cosolvent. Specialized formulations in cyclodextrins, chemically modified celluloses, Gelucire, liposomes, and so on, have been described previously (51). Due to such constraints in solubility is of paramount importance, that PK studies are performed with different doses in order to evaluate the dosages needed to obtain a possible effect in vivo, that is, serum antimicrobial concentrations need to surpass the MIC for a certain period for the drug to show antimicrobial activity in vivo. In this context, the degree of serum protein binding should be determined prior to PK studies, because only free, unbound drug is active in vivo. Intelligent pilot studies of the PK in the animal to be tested should be performed also for the purpose of avoiding senseless use of animals for useless effect studies.

Stability of Dissolved or Formulated Compounds

Although generally not a problem if compounds are prepared immediately before use, the stability of the compound in solution may become a problem when continuous dosing or prolonged fractional dosing is proposed as an administration technique. Although variations in the biologic activity (MIC/MBC) of the substance when it is stored for varying lengths of time may indicate severe stability problems, chemical assay of the substance (normally by high-performance liquid chromatography [HPLC] or combined with mass spectrum analysis) is perhaps best, given the crude activity estimates achievable by in vitro activity assessments. Determination of biologic activity may not be appropriate for some formulations (e.g., Gelucire), because this would require rescue of the compound from fine suspensions, which may be incomplete.

ADMINISTRATION OF SUBSTANCES TO ANIMALS

Administration of infectious agents, antimicrobial compounds, or other substances to animals is the central technique in experimental chemotherapy. Excellent introductions to these procedures are available (52,53). Substances are routinely administered subcutaneously (s.c.), intraperitoneally (i.p.), intramuscularly (i.m.), intravenously (i.v.), orally (p.o.), or topically (e.g., on the skin or in a wound). More specialized methods include intranasal, intratracheal, and intragastric administration and injection directly into the cerebrospinal fluid (CSF) or into the vitreous humor of the eye.

The administration of the antimicrobial compound should take into consideration that the purpose of testing the compound in vivo is to study the process of the compound reaching the infectious site via the bloodstream and subsequent diffusion or transport out of the blood vessels. Therefore, intraperitoneal injection of the drug for treatment of a peritonitis infection is more a direct treatment than a systemic treatment, whereas i.p. administration of a drug for treatment of a thigh infection can simulate i.v. or s.c. administration, because the drug is taken up in the peritoneum to the blood and then distributed to the infectious site.

ANESTHESIA AND ANALGESIA

This subject has been thoroughly covered previously (13,54). Anesthetics and analgesics can be of variable duration of action, and care should be taken to provide a suitable period of anesthesia (neither too long nor too short). Postoperative pain relief should be administered, with compensation made in planning the experiment to allow a degree of "washout" of the substance prior to initiation of the experiment, because analgesics

may alter normal host responses to infection or provide a source of unwanted drug interaction. However, in certain cases (e.g., models of infection associated with surgery), the use of analgesics may serve to make the models better reflect the clinical situation.

Certain anesthetics may not be applicable to all types of surgical interventions involved in experimental infections, and this should be considered and experimentally tested prior to widespread application. For example, agents that strongly depress respiratory rates (e.g., pentobarbital) are not suitable for pulmonary infection models involving tracheal exposure, and another anesthetic should be used. Furthermore, due consideration should be given to the stress placed on an animal due to anesthesia (long-term depression of normal body function and disorientation of the animal during recovery) versus the stress placed on the animal by not using anesthetics. For example, most routes of compound administration do not require anesthetics, and their use may place additional stress on the animal.

PHARMACOKINETIC PARAMETERS OF ANTIBIOTICS IN ANIMAL MODELS OF INFECTIOUS DISEASE

In vitro activity of a drug, as measured by MIC or MBC, provides a means of comparing potency for antibacterial drugs; however, PK measurements are necessary to ensure an agent will be active at a given site of infection in a mammalian host. The integration of PK, MIC, and outcome gave birth to the science of PD. The main goal of these studies is to examine relationships between antimicrobial concentration at the site of infection and drug activity over time (56–60). PK, as it relates to PD, is primarily measured in terms of elimination half-life ($t_{1/2}$), area under the drug concentration curve (AUC), and maximal concentrations achieved (C_{max}). Practically, this is performed by administering a group of mice the same concentration of drug by the same route and sampling serum or plasma at regular time intervals to determine drug concentration. From this information, the PK parameters of interest can be determined. A further step can then be performed by modeling the relationship of drug concentration and efficacy to determine which PK/PD index best correlates with outcome (for a general review of PK/PD principles, see references 56–59,61–67).

PHARMACOKINETIC EXPERIMENTS

General Considerations

Analytical Method

The analytical method must be both reliable and accurate, thus balancing sensitivity of detection, precision of measurement, and reproducibility of results. Currently, HPLC and mass spectroscopy measurement methods have largely supplanted traditional methods such as bioassay. One caveat that deserves recognition with these newer methods is that they measure the presence and amount of a chemical. They do not necessarily indicate biologic activity, which is included in the bioassay. Appropriate controls should be performed to ensure sample matrices (blood, plasma, serum, or tissue) do not interfere with the analysis and that an appropriate extraction method is available and validated.

Experimental Design

The experimental design must balance the potential use of large numbers of animals, the logistics of completing the experiment, and the PK information that is deemed necessary. In general, pilot studies with a small number of animals are useful to identify optimal sampling approaches. It is important to note the frequency and number of samples can greatly influence the accuracy of results. For example, if a drug has a very short half-life such that PK measurements are planned at 10-minute intervals over an hour, this would prove very difficult in terms of accuracy if one or two lab technicians are responsible for drawing serum on a large number of animals at each time point.

In addition to determining the appropriate time points for sampling and number of animals, one must also determine the dose range and route of administration. The dose range employed for PK studies often utilizes at least three different doses that vary from each other by two- to fourfold. The route is usually determined by the intended route of administration should the drug make it to human trials and is usually oral or subcutaneous in most animal models. The administration of oral drug does bring up the potential influence of food on PK and therefore it must be decided whether animals need to be fasted or not. Again, a small pilot study to determine food effect is often helpful to determine whether or not this consideration is necessary for a full PK study.

Organ Tissue Sampling

Although bloodstream (whole blood, serum, or plasma) measurements of drug concentration are most common, there are situations in which tissue or target-organ drug concentration measurement is necessary. This can include determination antimicrobial activity or drug-related toxicity in specific tissues. Traditionally, antimicrobial activity has been evaluated based on plasma or serum drug concentration levels unless the site of infection is considered sequestered (e.g., brain, CSF, urine, eye, placenta) or for pathogens that are primarily intracellular. In the absence of these aforementioned scenarios, plasma drug concentrations have correlated well with outcome at many infection sites (68–70). However, there is still debate on the merits of tissue-specific drug concentration sampling (68,70). For example, many preclinical PK investigations now include measurement of drug concentration in the epithelial lining fluid (ELF) compartment for investigational compounds in development for pulmonary infections. However, in most studies, the plasma PK concentration-effect relationships (PK/PD) accurately predict the outcome in animal model pulmonary infections. Thus, it is not clear whether ELF PK/PD relationships offer a clear advantage over serum PK/PD. An additional limitation to tissue sampling is in the processing tissue samples. The most common method of processing tissue samples for drug concentration measurement is tissue homogenization (71,72). However, tissues have two distinct fluid components consisting of the interstitial and intracellular compartments. When homogenized, these two compartments are irrevocably mixed. Since the intracellular compartment is usually of larger volume, drugs that concentrate more in the interstitial compartment will appear to be much lower in total concentration than drugs that accumulate in the intracellular compartment (e.g., β-lactams vs. fluoroquinolones). More recently, a technique to determine tissue-specific drug concentrations via microdialysis has been developed (73,74).

Pharmacokinetics Parameters

Several informative reviews on PK parameters have been previously published (75,76). In general, there are five parameters of interest including elimination half-life ($t^{1/2}$), apparent volume of distribution (V), total plasma clearance (C_L), absolute bioavailability (BAV) (relative bioavailability can also be useful), and free fraction of drug (nonprotein bound). With the exception of the last, these PK parameters can all be calculated using the plasma or serum drug concentration measurements. Most calculations are now performed with the aid of powerful computer programs that can provide the parameters of interest from the input of raw PK data. As mentioned earlier, separate parameter estimates should ideally be performed for tissue sites when relevant (i.e., sequestered sites of infection).

Free Fraction of Drug

Protein constituents in blood and tissues (chiefly albumin) can, and often do, have a high capacity to bind antimicrobial agents (77,78). Generally, drugs are pharmacologically active, metabolized, or excreted only in their nonprotein-bound state (i.e., free fraction). Therefore, it is often critical to know the level of protein binding in the animal model to determine relative total and free concentrations of drug. It is important to note that the relative amount of protein in circulation and the degree of protein binding can change under certain disease states (79,80). Protein binding can also markedly slow clearance of drugs that undergo glomerular filtration (81) and protein binding can change depending on the host animal model. Therefore, the extent of protein binding should be determined for an antimicrobial agent in each animal model used.

Factors Affecting the Pharmacokinetics of Antibiotics in Animals

Effect of Animal Species on Antibiotic Pharmacokinetics

The host animal species can have profound effects on the PK of a drug. It is often noted that smaller mammals (i.e., rodents) possess much more rapid routes of metabolism and elimination, and therefore, half-lives in these models can be considerably shorter than in larger mammals such as humans (81). Even among rodents, though, PK parameters can differ. For example, moxifloxacin PK profiles differ between mice and rats (T_{max} 0.25 vs. 0.08 hour, C_{max} 0.137 vs. 0.312 mg/L, AUC 0.184 vs. 0.305 mg × h/L, respectively) following administration of 9.2 mg/kg p.o. (82). The route of administration can also affect drug PK in different animal species, as demonstrated by rifampicin where the $t^{1/2}$ in rats was 4.72 hours following i.v. administration, but

increased to 9.31 hours following oral administration of the same drug dose (83). This same increase was not evident in mice. Finally, even the strain of animal can affect the PK. For example, BALB/c mice and DBA/2 mice display markedly different serum drug concentrations of itraconazole over time in multiple administration experiments (84). In sum, the aforementioned examples highlight the need to measure PK in each animal model used for preclinical antimicrobial evaluation.

Effect of Infection on Antibiotic Pharmacokinetics

The infection process can have a dramatic effect on the PK of a drug. Perhaps, the most well-known clinical scenario that has long been recognized to demonstrate this effect is bacterial meningitis, where bacterial and host inflammatory-induced damage to the blood–brain barrier produces profound changes in the penetration of antibiotics into this otherwise privileged site (85–87). For example, one of the most commonly relied upon drugs to treat gram-positive bacterial meningitis is vancomycin, which penetrates poorly through an intact blood–brain barrier due to the presence of tight junctions (86,88). However, significant damage occurs to the tight junctions during bacterial meningitis leading to increased permeability. In a study using rabbits, there was a near fourfold increase in CSF vancomycin levels in animals with meningitis versus healthy controls (86). Sepsis can also alter drug PK via a variety of mechanisms including increased volume of distribution and organ dysfunction leading to altered metabolism and elimination (89–91). The translatability of preclinical animal model PK to patients therefore usually includes both uninfected and infected animal PK to determine if the disease state significantly alters drug PK.

Effect of Fever on Antibiotic Pharmacokinetics

The physiologic effects of fever could potentially alter PK of a drug although this is not well studied (92). The reasons for this are likely related to confounders in the febrile model. For example, most febrile models use sepsis or endotoxemia to stimulate the febrile response (93–96). However, PK changes in this disease state may be due to vascular and/or organ dysfunction associated with the sepsis/endotoxemia and not necessarily attributable to fever itself. One PK parameter that is likely affected at higher body temperatures is protein binding, which has been shown to be reduced at higher temperatures (97). Thus, fever could potentially increase the free fraction of drug, which could enhance distribution and microbiologic activity, although could also hasten metabolism and excretion. Outside of protein binding, the effects of fever on drug PK are largely unknown in animal models due to difficulty in the ability to dissociate fever from other confounders induced in the febrile state.

Effect of Animal Age on Antibiotic Pharmacokinetics

As would be expected, age can have a profound effect on drug PK. Recognition of these differences is important; however, the clinical applicability of using age-related PK in an animal model and correlating it to age-related PK in a human is limited. The main reason for this is the need to prove age-related changes in the animal model mimic those noted in humans. For example, plasma PK of five β-lactam antibiotics are markedly different in neonatal versus adult mice (98). Without a study in neonatal humans, it is unknown whether these differences are applicable from the animal model. When differences do occur in the animal model, it can provide the stimulus to study the PK in the age groups the antibiotic is being developed for in humans. However, when age-related differences do not occur in the animal model, it does not necessarily indicate that there are no significant clinical differences in drug PK in different aged humans. With this caveat aside, there are examples of age-related changes in antimicrobial PK in animal models (99,100).

Effects of Various Factors on Antibiotic Pharmacokinetics

Many other factors may affect antibiotic PK. A number of notable examples include animal gender, administration of concomitant drugs, timing of administration in regard to circadian rhythm, presence of organ dysfunction, and genetic background. Each of these may or may not affect a specific antibiotic's PK properties, and unfortunately, it is not always predictable which antibiotic may possess one or more of these less common influences on PK. Oftentimes, these less common factors are investigated in animal models only after significant differences in PK are noted in different populations of humans.

PHARMACOKINETICS/ PHARMACODYNAMICS OF ANTIBIOTICS: RELATIONSHIP OF EXPERIMENTAL ANIMALS AND HUMANS

Pharmacodynamics

One advantage of experimental animal infections is the ability to monitor drug effect over time in an in vivo system. A variety of questions can be addressed in these preclinical models to help direct clinical dosing regimens as well as address clinical problems such as toxicity or drug resistance. The principal analysis tool in most of these studies is PD. There are too numerous to cite examples of how informative and predictive PD animal studies can be. The reader is directed to the many insightful reviews cited here (53,56–59,61,63–67,81) for further information.

PD examines the relationships between an antimicrobial agent and the target pathogen over time. Drug effect can be concentration-independent or concentration-dependent and time-independent or time-dependent. Consideration of these concentration- and time-related activities lead to three common PK/PD indices used to describe optimal drug concentration-effect relationships. They include the 24-hour area under the serum concentration time curve (AUC) over the minimum inhibitory concentration (MIC) ratio (AUC/MIC), the peak serum drug concentration level over MIC ratio (C_{max}/MIC), or the time that serum drug levels remain above the MIC (T>MIC) over a defined period (usually 24 hours; often, the total T>MIC of several doses during 24 hours is calculated as the percentage covered of the dosing intervals, %T>MIC). Determining which of the three PD indices is predictive of efficacy provides a framework for dosing regimen design. For example, concentration-dependent antimicrobials demonstrate enhanced effect as the drug concentration increases over the MIC. The dosing design that optimizes this activity is administration of large doses infrequently. The concentration-dependent indices, C_{max}/MIC and AUC/MIC, are the PD indices associated with optimal treatment effect for this dosing design. Conversely, drugs that exhibit optimal efficacy at concentrations near the MIC but lack increased effect as concentrations exceed the MIC are considered time-dependent killing. These agents therefore exert optimal effect when smaller doses are given frequently to keep the concentration relatively stable just above the MIC. The predictive index in this case is T>MIC.

Dose Fractionation

Two common experimental approaches are used to find the predictive PD index of an antimicrobial agent and include dose escalation and dose fractionation. The former examines two important aspects of concentration-effect. The first is the impact of escalating drug concentrations on the extent and rate of organism killing or growth inhibition over time. The second outcome considered is the antimicrobial effect after the drug concentration has fallen below the MIC. The phenomenon of growth suppression following antimicrobial exposure is called the postantibiotic effect. For some compounds, organism growth suppression persists for prolonged periods of time after drug exposure, allowing for lengthening of the dosing interval. The PAE is usually concentration-dependent (i.e., the duration and effect usually increase with higher concentrations or doses). Thus, the activity of drugs exhibiting prolonged postantifungal effects (PAFEs) is best described by the C_{max}/MIC or AUC/MIC indices.

Dose fractionation is performed by administering the same total dose level while changing the interval of administration. For example, a total 24-hour antimicrobial dose of 100 mg/kg can be fractionated as follows: 100mg/kg q24h, 50 mg/kg q12h, 25 mg/kg q6h, and 12.5 mg/kg q3h. In this situation, each group of animals is receiving the same total daily dose, thus the AUC for each regimen is similar; however, the peak level and T>MIC will vary dramatically. Using this scheme, one can investigate which dosing interval results in optimal efficacy. If regimens using higher, infrequent dosing result in lower burdens, then the PD index predictive of efficacy is related to peak concentrations (C_{max}). If regimens using frequent, small doses result in lower burdens, then the PD index predictive of efficacy is the %T>MIC. If efficacy is similar in each of the dosing fractionations, then outcome depends on total drug exposure (AUC/MIC). Table 13.1 lists predictive PK/PD indices for commonly used antimicrobial drug classes.

The crucial step to making animal model PD studies clinically relevant, and thus translatable, is to study dosing regimens that mimic human drug concentrations over time at the site of infection. This can be more problematic than it first appears. The first issue is accounting for differences in PK of a drug from animals to humans, which at times can vary dramatically. For example, small mammals, such as rodents, often have much more rapid me-

Table 13.1

Pharmacokinetics/Pharmacodynamics Index Associated with Optimal Treatment Outcome for Selected Antimicrobial Drug Classes

Antimicrobial Drug Class	Pharmacokinetics/ Pharmacodynamics Index
β-Lactams (penicillins, cephalosporins, carbapenems, aztreonam)	Time above MIC
Fluoroquinolones	AUC/MIC and C_{max}/MIC
Aminoglycosides	AUC/MIC and C_{max}/MIC
Glycopeptides (vancomycin)	AUC/MIC
Oxazolidinones	AUC/MIC
Lipopeptide (daptomycin)	AUC/MIC or C_{max}/MIC
Echinocandins	AUC/MIC or C_{max}/MIC
Azoles	AUC/MIC

MIC, minimal inhibitory concentration; AUC, area under the drug concentration curve; C_{max}, maximal concentration.

tabolism and elimination of antimicrobial agents. This can usually be accounted for by adjusting the dosing regimen to more closely approximate drug concentration profiles in humans, for example, by more frequent administration of drug or increased concentration on a milligram per kilogram basis. Other strategies include attempting to slow the metabolism or rate of elimination. The second potential difficulty is that human PK, concentration profiles over time, and potential dosing strategy in humans may not be known at the time of preclinical animal model studies. Thus, it can be difficult to predict what dosing strategy or drug exposure is best to use in the animal model to mimic human drug exposures.

Strategies to Prolong Drug Concentrations in Animal Models

The two most common strategies to attempt to mimic human PK in an animal model where there is rapid metabolism or clearance of the drug is to either directly alter the clearance or provide a means of very rapid drug replenishment by frequent or continuous dosing systems. Impairment in renal function can result in slower elimination of antimicrobials if this mechanism is the major clearance organ (e.g., cephalexin [101]). In mice, this has been accomplished by a single subcutaneous injection of uranyl nitrate (10 mg/kg) 3 days prior to animal infection (102). Uranyl nitrate produces acute tubular necrosis and subsequent stable but decreased renal glomerulofiltration for a duration of 7 days (103–105). As shown by Craig and colleagues (104), the administration of uranyl nitrate to mice in the study of amikacin increased the half-life of the drug, the peak concentration for each dose, and the AUC for each dose when compared to non–renally impaired mice. The resultant PK parameters and concentration-time curves more appropriately simulated human PK. It also led to a 10-fold greater potency (as measured by total daily dose required to reduce 1 log CFU/g tissue) in renally impaired mice. Thus, human-simulated PK in this model was more effective than dosing more frequently in renally sufficient mice. Antimicrobial agents actively secreted by renal tubular cells can be competitively blocked by other compounds that use the same excretion process. An example of this is probenicid, a weak organic acid which blocks the secretion of penicillin and other cephalosporins that are excreted by renal tubular cells (105).

A variety of renal impairment mechanisms have also been reported for rats (101). This includes proximal tubular necrosis induced by cisplatin (one dose at 5 mg/kg IP), papillary necrosis induced by 2-bromoethylamine hydrobromide (one dose at 75 mg/kg IV), glomerulonephritis induced by sodium aurothiomalate (six weekly injections of 0.05 mg/kg IV) or anti–rabbit antibodies to rat glomerular basement membrane (single IV injection).

Continuous dosing of antimicrobials has been used to counteract the effect of rapid antimicrobial clearance that can be marked in small rodents. There are a number of systems that have achieved continuous antimicrobial levels and include tissue cage infusion (106), a variety of pump techniques (107–111), and more recently, sophisticated computer programmable pumps (112). These systems work best from an efficacy standpoint for time-dependent drugs in which the time above MIC is the driving PD index. Roosendaal and colleagues (109) demonstrated an example of this approach and correlation with PD indices. They examined the efficacy of intermittent versus continuous administration of ceftazidime, gentamicin, and ciprofloxacin in a rat endobronchial *Klebsiella pneumoniae* infection model. Despite subinhibitory serum concentrations, continuous dosing of ceftazidime was more effective than intermittent dosing, in which serum levels exceeded the inhibitory concentration with each dose. The converse was true for gentamicin and less so ciprofloxacin.

Osmotic pumps are advantageous as they can provide a constant release of drug over periods of several days to weeks. They can also overcome interspecies differences in antibiotic elimination. However, limitations involve many prerequisite factors, including the compound must be prepared in a fully soluble and highly concentrated solution, dosing times need to be limited, surgical implant of the device, and necessary stability of drug for days to weeks at 37°C. Additional requirements include the compatibility of the solvent system with the pump, confirmation of consistency in the release of active drug over time, and that no precipitation of the compound occurs on the outside of the pump after coming into contact with biologic fluids. These latter requirements can be determined by immersing a filled pump in a suitable isotonic buffer containing 5% to 50% fetal bovine serum and incubating it at 37°C followed by periodic sampling.

Continuous Dosing to Mimic Human Pharmacokinetic Profiles

This subject has been thoroughly reviewed by Mizen (113). Continuous- or variable-rate infusion of antibiotics into animals has been used to obtain plasma antibiotic clearance similar to that found in humans administered bolus or drip infusions. Based on careful determination of temocillin PKs in both humans and rabbits, a continuous-rate infusion system was developed to deliver temocillin to rabbits with meningitis due to *K. pneumoniae* in such a manner that human plasma elimination rates following a 2-g dose were obtained (114). The femoral artery was cannulated to allow continuous infusion of antibiotic. Rabbits received first a bolus dose (82 mg/kg) to mimic the temocillin distribution phase and then an infusion of continuously diluted temocillin to mimic the β-elimination phase observed in humans. Phosphate-buffered saline was administered at a constant rate (equivalent to the human temocillin elimination rate corrected for the rate of temocillin elimination by rabbits) into a fixed-volume, stirred reservoir containing temocillin such that the concentration of temocillin infused into the animal was constantly declining. Rabbits receiving infusions were treated with a total of 758 mg/kg temocillin over 12 hours at 2.0 mL/hour. Compared to bolus dosing (82 mg/kg), infusion dosing resulted in a dramatically prolonged temocillin half-life and larger AUC values without altering the percent penetration into the CSF. Note that, after a 2-g dose to humans, the plasma half-life was 5.0 ± 0.2 hours and the AUC was 784.5 ± 47.1 μg × h/mL. However, considering the serum binding of temocillin (60% to 85% in human serum, depending on the temocillin concentration; 35% in rabbit serum, concentration independent), this mode of temocillin administration to rabbits would result in free temocillin concentrations similar to that observed after a 4-g dose to humans. Humanlike PKs resulted in a dramatically improved therapeutic outcome, in that *K. pneumoniae* was rapidly removed from the CSF (to less than log 2 CFU/mL within 6 hours) during infusion but remained essentially unaltered during bolus dosing. The authors did not evaluate the effect of the same total temocillin dose in bolus infusion (114).

This infusion method was adapted to rats in order to mimic the human plasma PKs of cefazolin, piperacillin, and the β-lactamase inhibitor BRL 42715 (115). Rats were infected intraperitoneally with either *Escherichia coli* or *Serratia marcescens*, and treatment began 1 hour after infection; both microorganisms demonstrated susceptibility to cefazolin or piperacillin only in the presence of BRL 42715 (concentrations more than ~0.1 μg/mL). Simulation of human plasma PKs was obtained. The half-lives for BRL 42715, cefazolin, and piperacillin in humans were 0.6, 1.6, and 1.1 hours, respectively, considerably different from those in rats (0.1, 0.51, and 0.33 hours, respectively). Despite the plasma concentration of the β-lactamase inhibitor falling below the level predicted to be effective within 3 hours, coadministration of BRL 42715 with piperacillin (*E. coli* infection) or cefazolin (*S. marcescens* infection) dramatically improved efficacy in terms of survival and bacterial counts in blood and peritoneal fluid (115); these results indicate that β-lactamase inhibitors need not have plasma PKs identical to those of their partner antibiotics in order to have synergistic effects. Comparison of the effectiveness of human-simulated PKs and the efficacy of these combinations in bolus administration (rat PK) was not reported (115).

A similar approach was used to mimic the PK of 3- and 0.1-g doses of ticarcillin/clavulanic acid and a 2-g dose of ceftazidime administered to humans (116) in rabbits with meningitis due to *K. pneumoniae*. The infusion system was modified to include two pumps, one infusing a constant dose of agent for a short time (to produce a

peak serum concentration similar to that seen in humans) and the other constantly infusing a continuously diluted solution of drug (to mimic the serum elimination PKs manifest in humans). This system was successful in overriding the more rapid elimination of ticarcillin, clavulanic acid, and ceftazidime by rabbits. Single doses of ticarcillin/clavulanic acid were able to reduce (by 99% at 4 hours) but not eliminate the drug combination–susceptible *K. pneumoniae* present in the CSF due to regrowth of the organisms after clavulanic acid levels fell below the MBC. Multiple dosing of ticarcillin/clavulanic acid (three doses every 4 hours) according to simulated human PKs resulted in higher AUCs in both plasma and CSF (without altering the CSF penetration) and correspondingly greater antibacterial efficacy (99.99% reduction of colony-forming units [CFU] per milliliter in the CSF). Two ceftazidime doses (every 8 hours) reduced the counts of the drug-susceptible microbe below the limit of detectability and sterilized the CSF in two of three rabbits at 12 hours. The efficacy of bolus doses of these drugs (rabbit PKs) was not reported (116).

A computer-controlled, variable-speed pump was used to mimic human serum concentrations of amoxicillin in a study to determine the effectiveness of amoxicillin prophylaxis in preventing streptococcal endocarditis (117). Sterile aortic vegetations were produced by placement of a polyethylene catheter through the right carotid artery across the aortic valve. Amoxicillin was administered by infusion through a Silastic catheter placed into the jugular vein and brought through the skin of the intercapsular region. Intravenous infection with *Streptococcus intermedius* or *Streptococcus sanguis* (1, 10, or 100 × the 90% inhibitory dose) occurred 1 hour after administration of 40 mg/kg amoxicillin (rat PKs) or amoxicillin dosage to mimic human PKs following a 3-g oral dose. At the time of bacterial challenge, the serum antibiotic levels were similar (bolus dose, 18 ± 0.3 μg/mL; infusion, 16 ± 5 μg/mL), but the durations of detectable amoxicillin levels were different (bolus, 4.5 hours; infusion, 9 hours). Simulation of human serum PKs was decidedly more effective than bolus dosing in the protection of rats from developing endocarditis (117). A similar procedure was used to deliver ceftriaxone to obtain humanlike PKs in rats with *Streptococcus sanguis* or *Streptococcus mitis* (118) or methicillin-resistant *Staphylococcus epidermidis* (119) endocarditis.

EVALUATION OF ANTIBIOTICS IN ANIMAL MODELS OF INFECTION

Use of animal models in the evaluation of antimicrobial compounds is considered when a clinical study involving humans is not possible because (a) the toxicity of the compound is unknown, (b) its antibacterial ability in vivo is unknown, (c) the type of infection under consideration is rarely encountered or impossible to encounter in humans, or (d) the effect parameters needed (e.g., bacterial counts in tissues or fluids) cannot easily be obtained in patients. Otherwise, a clinical study will be the optimal method for studying any drug for clinical use, since it automatically answers the question (which is always asked after an experimental animal study), "Can the results be extrapolated to the clinic?" Animals are always used when new compounds have shown relevant antimicrobial activity in vitro and their in vivo effects are questioned. Furthermore, experimental animal infections are considered when other important issues need to be solved prior to clinical studies, such as the advantages or disadvantages of the compound in activity, its PK profile (i.e., its dosing advantage), the best mode of administration (i.e., oral or parenteral), and potential toxicity problems (diarrhea, nephrotoxicity, etc.). Given the ethical considerations and government legislation involved, the testing of novel compounds, or novel combinations of known compounds, requires comparative testing in animal experiments in order to indicate efficacy in vivo. As in the evaluation of antimicrobials from known classes (e.g., new cephalosporins), the questions include not just whether the agent will be active in vivo but how it will compare in spectrum and potency to other antibiotics. β-Lactamase inactivation seen in vitro might not occur in vivo. In many instances, very low MIC values in vitro are not reflected by the in vivo results. Thus, for new compounds or derivatives of known antibiotics, the in vivo test is also a tool for selecting the potentially best candidate from a number of active agents. The following discussion mostly concerns the evaluation of antibacterial or antifungal substances in animal models, although the evaluation of antiviral compounds is not covered. Furthermore, for purpose of simplicity and because they can be obtained elsewhere (3,4), details on the establishment of models have been reduced to a minimum.

General considerations for working safely with infectious agents have been summarized in Richmond and Quimby (121), and readers are encouraged to read this review prior to embarking on establishing animal models of infection in their laboratory.

Factors Influencing Antimicrobial Activity in the In Vivo Tests

A number of the factors can influence the activity of antimicrobial agents in vivo (e.g., see 122):

- Inoculum size and vehicle. If the inoculum is too small, an infection will not be established; if it is too large, overwhelming endotoxemia can occur.
- Virulence or pathogenicity of the infecting strain. Highly virulent strains may produce rapidly fatal disease, necessitating early treatment initiation.
- Generation time in vivo. Slow-growing bacteria in vivo are phenotypically very different from fast-growing bacteria in vitro. Similarly, biofilm growth in vivo is different from planktonic growth in vitro.
- Timing of treatment. A delay in treatment initiation often results in greater difficulty curing the infection. This is often related to the inoculum, see the following text.
- Method of antimicrobial administration. The lack of oral uptake of a drug highly active in vitro may render it inactive in vivo.
- The PK/PD of the antimicrobial. Generally, more rapidly eliminated drugs need to be administered more frequently.
- The development of resistance in vivo. Unique resistance patterns in vivo may render a drug highly active in vitro inactive in vivo.
- In vivo growth of an intracellular compartment that the drug cannot penetrate.
- Inactivation of the compound in vivo. The host metabolism may render a drug that is highly active in vitro inactive in vivo.

Inoculum size has a major influence on the in vivo activity of antimicrobials. An increase of 1 log unit or even less in the challenge bacterial dose can render an antibacterial ineffective. In addition, virulence or pathogenicity is closely connected to the inoculum size, since high virulence to a particular animal species often leads to lower inocula being used in order not to induce an overwhelming infection. On the other hand, higher doses are still needed to achieve an effect against a highly virulent strain, compared with strains with lower virulence. For example, the heavily capsulated *Streptococcus pneumoniae* serotype 3 (penicillin

MIC, 0.01 mg/L) has an LD_{50} of 10^2 CFU for intraperitoneal infection in CF1 mice, in comparison with 10^7 CFU for *S. pneumoniae* serotype 6B (penicillin MIC, 0.01 mg/L). Still, the ED_{50} for single-dose benzylpenicillin against serotype 3 is 180 mg/kg, in comparison with 0.8 to 2 mg/kg against serotype 6B strains (123,124).

For *Streptococcus pyogenes*, increasing the in vitro starting inoculum (from log 3 to 7 CFU/mL) had no effect on the MIC of cefoxitin (0.5 μg/mL) and mezlocillin (0.05 μg/mL). In contrast, increasing the inoculum of *K. pneumoniae* from log 5 to log 8 CFU/mL had no effect on the MIC of cefoxitin (4 μg/mL) but dramatically altered the MIC of mezlocillin (4 μg/mL at log 5 or 6 CFU/mL, 32 μg/mL at log 7 CFU/mL, and >128 μg/mL at log 9 CFU/mL).

Preparation of the microorganism for inoculation in animal experiments can dramatically affect the results obtained, and this fact is often overlooked. Fundamentally, the microbe should be at maximal viability, and care should be taken to obtain suitable cultures for inoculum preparation. Whether the microbe should be taken from the in vitro culture in lag phase, log phase, or stationary phase has to our knowledge never been validated. The use of overnight broth cultures may be problematic for bacteria such as *S. pneumoniae* or *Haemophilus influenzae*, which undergo autolysis shortly after reaching the stationary phase (125). Agar plate cultures have the advantage that they can be directly studied to determine if any contamination has occurred and whether loss of potential capsule has occurred. Many investigators prefer to bring the microbe into the exponential growth phase in a broth culture prior to its use or inoculation. None has proven, however, that the bacteria will stay in this exponential phase after the procedures used (e.g., washing) to achieve the exact inoculum needed.

An increase in the virulence of certain microorganisms can be achieved in various ways. In vitro growth in specialized media can alter virulence. For example, growth of *Neisseria meningitidis* under conditions of low pH and low growth medium iron content increases the virulence of this organism 1,200-fold, relative to bacteria grown in neutral-pH, iron-replete medium (126). Growth of uropathogenic *Escherichia coli* in human urine increased siderophore production and renal pathogenicity in ascending pyelonephritis in mice (127). Furthermore, virulence-associated gene expression by *Enterococcus faecalis* is modulated during the growth phase and affected by the growth medium (128). Using the guinea pig subcutaneous chamber model as a test system, iron-limited gonococci were found to be extremely virulent, whereas cystine-limited (iron-replete) gonococci did not survive in the chambers despite retention of pili. Loss of piliation also occurred during the shift from iron-limited to glucose-limited growth, but the bacteria remained virulent. No change in susceptibility to normal human serum killing occurred, and the lipooligosaccharide composition remained similar despite varied culture conditions. Some membrane proteins traditionally associated with iron limitation were produced by cystine- or glucose-limited bacteria (129). Note, however, that iron restriction apparently does not affect all bacteria. The rate and extent of in vitro growth of *Salmonella typhimurium* are unaffected by the addition of deferoxamine, and treatment of mice with deferoxime prior to infectious challenge exacerbates *Salmonella typhimurium* infection (130). Virulence can also be enhanced by serial passage in animals; for example, intraperitoneal inoculation with subsequent subculture from peritoneal wash, blood, or organs such as the liver or spleen and use of this growth either directly or after subculture will enhance the virulence of *Streptococcus pneumoniae*, *Streptococcus pyogenes*, or *H. influenzae*. In spite of great care taken to standardize the inoculum, one of the major problems encountered in animal experiments is the variation in the virulence and growth of organisms. This problem highlights the need for control groups for every new infection experiment considered rather than relying on historical controls.

Generation time (rate of bacterial cell division) is also a factor of major importance that differs between in vivo and in vitro test conditions. In vivo, the generation time seems to increase progressively during the course of infection and, depending on the site of infection, may last up to 20 hours. Little is known about nutrient limitations on bacterial growth in infected tissues, with the exception of iron, which has been found to limit bacterial growth in serum. It has been demonstrated that prolonged lag phase as well as prolonged generation time may adversely affect the clinical activity of antimicrobials (especially β-lactams) that are most effective against bacterial cells that are rapidly dividing (31,34,39,118). The nature of bacterial growth in vivo in tissues is not well studied. Good evidence is available indicating that bacteria grow as biofilms in many urinary tract infections (131,132), cases of otitis media (133), catheter-related infections (134–136), and pulmonary infections

(131,137–139). For a review, see Costerton et al. (28,29). Further, bacteria growing as biofilm have a dramatically different physiology and antibiotic sensitivity (30). A set of genes are specifically activated during the establishment of a biofilm, both in vitro and in vivo (140). However, not all bacterial growth in vivo occurs as biofilms (141). Multicolor fluorescence microscopy has been used to delineate the nature of *Salmonella enterica* in the livers of infected mice (142). The growth of *Salmonella* occurred by the formation of new foci of infection from initial ones as well as by the expansion of each focus. Each focus consisted of phagocytes containing low numbers of bacteria and of independently segregating bacterial populations. The net increase in bacteria paralleled the increase in the number of infected phagocytes in the tissues (142).

BASIC SCREENING TESTS

Mouse Protection Test

The animal models most frequently used in the evaluation of antibacterials may be categorized as basic screening, *ex vivo*, monoparametric, or discriminative (143,144). For the preliminary evaluation of new agents, the basic screening system is usually employed. The *ex vivo* and monoparametric models are used to measure specific variables (e.g., dosage schedule, serum binding, or penetration into extravascular spaces). The discriminative systems are employed to differentiate the new agents from related or unrelated active agents. Screening models involve simple one-step infections, simple techniques and schedules of treatment, short-duration experiments, reproducible courses of infection, simple evaluation (all-or-nothing models), economy of test drugs, and low costs. These requirements are best met by the mouse protection test, which is the most widely used in vivo screening model in antibacterial research. The mouse protection test is suitable for determining the efficacy and toxicity of new antibacterials, and it can indicate whether a drug is likely to be active orally or parenterally. The features and use of the mouse protection test have been previously reviewed (145–147).

Various mouse strains are the primary hosts used for the following reasons: (a) good correlation between the clinical response to an antimicrobial agent and the agent's activity in mice; (b) the ease of obtaining large numbers; (c) the economy of the compound to be tested; (d) the relatively small cost per unit test; and (e) normal use of an outbred strain of mice, which provides a heterogenous population and allows for immunologic and other host factor variations (however, in special situations [e.g., *Mycobacterium* infection models], inbred, genetically defined strains may be required in order to provide a suitably susceptible host). It should be clearly recognized, though, that the mouse protection model represents an unnatural infection in which the host is usually subjected to an overwhelming challenge (148).

Correlation of In Vitro and In Vivo Results

This subject—the correlation of in vitro and in vivo activity—has a long history (149) and is critical for a medicinal chemistry program, given the costs of in vivo screening.

Many substances that are active in vivo are also active in vitro; however, the converse is not always true. Many antibacterials that are active in vitro either are inactive when tested against systemic infections in vivo or are only active in the more sensitive topical infections. Zak and Sande (150) reported a correlation of in vitro and in vivo activity in only 14.8% of 2,000 compounds randomly screened for antimicrobial activity. Of the 2,000 compounds, 45.3% were inactive in vitro and in vivo. Of those inactive in vitro, 0.3% showed in vivo activity. Of those active in vitro, 36.6% were inactive in vivo. Of the total, 14.8% displayed activity both in vitro and in vivo. Given that currently only compounds with in vitro activity are tested in vivo, recalculation based only on those having in vitro activity would change the figures to 73% for in vitro activity only and 27% for activity in both tests. The latter percentage is typical of those noted by investigators. Furthermore, a major problem in correlating in vitro and in vivo results occurs when the agent being tested is very active in vitro but inactive or moderately active in vivo. Because in vitro and in vivo tests differ in their general characteristics and specific variables, discrepancies are likely to occur. However, they may be understood and interpreted if the limitations of the tests are taken into account. Causes of missing activity in animal experiments in spite of good activity in vitro can include PK factors, such as minimal distribution in the host due to poor uptake and rapid metabolism or other inactivation (e.g., high protein binding) of the drug, resulting in insufficient dosing. Differences in the pharmacology of compounds between humans and animals commonly used for experimentation can lead to effective drugs being wasted because their potential clinical effect is never tested. Beneficial effects of drugs other than their antimicrobial activity (e.g., immunostimulative behavior) have a risk of being overlooked if they do not reach in vivo testing (e.g., the potential immunity-stimulating activity of the macrolides has only recently been detected using experimental animal testing).

Commonly used in vitro tests do appear to fail to predict outcome in certain types of infections, especially device-related infections (151). Characteristically, bacteria involved in device-related infections are adherent, slow-growing bacteria that are phenotypically distinct from the rapidly multiplying bacteria that grow during in vitro susceptibility testing (see reference 30). Consequently, specialized in vitro techniques are needed to obtain a better correlation between in vitro and in vivo (experimental or clinical) activity. Using a model of S. aureus device-related infections (subcutaneous chamber implant) in guinea pigs, Zimmerli et al. (151) found that, as a single agent, only rifampicin was active, in contrast to vancomycin, teicoplanin, ciprofloxacin, and fleroxacin, despite the fact that the S. aureus strain was sensitive to all compounds in vitro using standard tests. Determination of peak and trough drug levels in tissue cage fluid showed that, at the doses given, the drug levels of rifampicin, vancomycin, and teicoplanin exceeded the MIC constantly throughout the 4-day experiment. Further experimentation demonstrated a dramatic loss of drug activity against stationary phase bacteria (the minimal loss occurring with rifampicin) and that testing the killing effect of antibiotics and their combinations against bacteria adherent to glass beads at drug levels achieved in vivo did provide an accurate prediction of treatment effect in vivo.

Anaissie et al. (152) and Rex et al. (153) have studied the correlation between in vitro susceptibility and in vivo activity in a Candida sepsis model in mice. Lack of in vitro susceptibility in a microbroth dilution test correlated well with fungal kidney colonization 4 days postinfection and with prolongation of survival (152). Follow-up studies indicated that MICs determined at 24 hours (as opposed to 48 hours) correlated better with in vivo outcomes (153).

Acute Toxicity Assays to Determine Tolerated Doses

Important technical issues that must be considered include the amount of drug administered during a primary screening program and the most suitable route of administration. If possible, some measure of toxicity should be obtained in vitro. Although more often done only if anomalous results are obtained, before use in the treatment of infected animals, the maximum tolerated dose of a substance should be determined by administering single injections of the substance to groups of mice ($N = 3$ to 6) by oral, subcutaneous, and intraperitoneal routes. The animals are then observed for survival for periods from 24 hours to 7 days. Care should be taken to observe the mice continuously after drug administration and note their clinical condition in order to kill them in a humane way before they die from the toxic activity. Such killed mice are still counted as dead from toxicity. These acute toxicity studies establish for each route the 100% toxic dose (LD_{100}), the 50% lethal dose (LD_{50}), and the maximum tolerated dose (LD_0)—the dose at which all animals survive. Various methods of determining the LD_{50} (or infectious dose) have been previously reviewed (154). Approximately one-fifth of the maximum tolerated dose of a substance can be well tolerated when treatments are given once daily for 5 days or longer. For 1 to 3 days of treatment, one-half of the maximum dose can usually be given. When using these crude guidelines, it would be reasonable to assume that animals dying after multiple treatments succumb to the effects of the particular infection rather than to drug toxicity. The use of LD_{50} models is currently under debate regarding the mortality in the high-dose groups (14). Toxicity models where toxic effects are analyzed by histology or other means should be preferred to simple LD_0 experiments, because this may decrease unnecessary harm to the animals (14).

In addition to initial information on toxicity, some information on oral bioavailability may also be obtained. For example, if a substance is tolerated at 1,000 mg/kg when given orally but is toxic when given at a dose of 50 mg/kg intraperitoneally or intravenously, the lack of toxicity by the oral route probably reflects poor oral absorption.

Choice of Organism

In developing an experimental mouse model for in vivo testing, it is desirable to use human pathogens whenever possible. It is also desirable to infect with strains of microorganisms that are sufficiently virulent so that conditioning procedures to lower the host's resistance are unnecessary. Natural infections typically result from inoculation with

Streptococcus pneumoniae, Streptococcus pyogenes, certain strains of *K. pneumoniae, Salmonella typhi, Salmonella typhimurium, Mycobacterium tuberculosis,* and *Cryptococcus neoformans.* When reproducible infections cannot be achieved by inoculation of the organisms alone, it is necessary to reduce the resistance of the animal. A common procedure is to suspend the organism in 3% to 10% hog gastric mucin and to administer 0.5 mL amounts by the intraperitoneal route. In the case of infections with *Candida albicans* and *Histoplasma capsulatum,* the animals are infected intravenously with virulent strains; for less virulent strains, the animals are conditioned by injection of 0.1 mL of a 1% suspension of cortisone in saline twice daily by the intramuscular route before the introduction of the organisms. Alternatively, immunosuppression can be achieved by rendering the mice leukopenic by administering cyclophosphamide.

Preparation of Inoculum for Infection: Virulence Titration

In order to obtain reproducible infections, it is necessary to determine the degree of virulence of each strain to be studied. To carry out virulence tests, suitable broth cultures (where high viability of the culture is maintained) are serially diluted in broth to obtain 10-fold decreases in the number of organisms. If mucin is to be used, one part of each broth dilution is combined with nine parts of mucin. Groups of four to six mice are injected intraperitoneally with 0.5 mL of each dilution. Samples are taken from peritoneum, blood, or organs such as liver and spleen and bacteria quantified in order to construct in vivo growth curves. Concomitantly and before sampling, mice (or control groups of mice) are evaluated for symptoms and signs of systemic infection (for rating schemes, see reference 14). When animals are considered to progress to clinical stages, which will lead to death of the animals, the animals are killed and quantification of bacteria in vivo ascertained and compared to the in vivo growth curves. In this manner, a surrogate LD_{50} (or LD_{100}) can be determined, which will enable an intelligent choice of the inoculation strategy for that pathogen/mouse combination. The original calculation of an LD_{50} from mortality of mice has increasingly been replaced by bacterial quantification studies (154).

The virulence of many organisms is so low for an unnatural animal host that some type of stressing agent or adjuvant is usually required to achieve a reproducible infection. As previously stated, mucin is usually required to provide reproducible bacterial infections in mice. Without mucin, infections would require the large numbers of organisms provided by cultures that are undiluted or only marginally diluted. Such an inoculum may be overwhelming, either because of toxic effects (e.g., endotoxic shock or the introduction of toxic components of spent culture broth) or because the antibacterial would not be able to inhibit the large numbers of organisms (see reference 155). We have found in the past that mucin, at a concentration of 5%, gives consistent results with few deaths directly attributable to the effect of mucin, although with certain batches of mucin, an 8% to 10% concentration may be required to give consistent results. The quality of the mucin available is variable, and thus the mucin used should be evaluated in separate experiments. One problem often encountered is contamination of the commercial hog gastric mucin powder. The mucin can be autoclaved without loosing its macrophage-inhibiting abilities. Furthermore, in all experiments, or at least periodically, a group of uninfected animals should receive mucin alone to ensure that deaths are not due to the stressing effects of this adjuvant.

Previous studies (156) clearly show the enhancing effect of mucin on the proliferation of bacteria in the murine host. Mice were infected intraperitoneally with 0.5 mL of an overnight broth culture of *E. coli* either as a saline suspension or in 3% gastric mucin. Groups of five mice were killed, samples of blood were collected from the axillary region at 10 minutes and at hourly intervals after infection, peritoneal lavage was performed, and CFU/mL determinations were made of both fluids. A count of 10^5 CFU/mL was obtained from intraperitoneal washings immediately after infection with bacteria suspended in saline. The count dropped to approximately 10^3 CFU/mL within 10 minutes and remained in this range for the next 7 hours. The viable count in the blood rose to approximately 50 CFU/mL within 10 minutes and then showed little increase over the next 7 hours (approximately 100 CFU/mL). In contrast, when 3% mucin was used as an adjuvant, the initial count in the peritoneal washings of 10^5 CFU/mL increased stepwise with time to a count in excess of 10^9 CFU/mL by the end of 8 hours. The viable count in the blood closely paralleled that seen in the peritoneal washings (increasing from 5×10^3 CFU/mL after 1 hour to 7×10^8 CFU/mL at 8 hours).

For certain slowly growing, fastidious organisms (e.g., *S. pyogenes* and *S. pneumoniae*), mucin is not required in order to obtain a reproducibly virulent infection. The virulence of these organisms can be maintained by passage of the cultures in mice. One or two mice are infected intraperitoneally with 1 mL of an overnight broth culture. After 6 to 8 hours, when the animals show signs of illness, they are anesthetized, the hearts are removed aseptically, and several drops of heart blood are added to a tube of appropriate broth medium. For *S. pyogenes* and *S. pneumoniae*, trypticase soy broth containing 10% serum is suitable. The serum of any animal species is suitable. At the same time, the blood is also streaked on blood agar plates. After overnight incubation, serial 10-fold dilutions of the broth cultures are prepared for use as the infecting inoculum. The blood agar plates are used for confirmation of the purity and identity of the infecting inoculum. The quellung reaction can be used to type the pneumococci, and standard procedures are used to confirm the identity of group A streptococci. In vivo passage can dramatically affect the virulence of many other pathogens (e.g., some strains of *H. influenzae*), and this method should be considered for all strains proposed to be used for many experiments. Following in vivo passage, stocks of the organisms should be made from exponential-phase cultures of low passage and then stored frozen. If available, liquid nitrogen is preferred; otherwise, a −80°C freezer provides sufficient stability, while storage at −40°C can lead to loss of virulence in *S. pneumoniae* strains often used for animal experiments.

If there is doubt whether animals died from drug toxicity rather than infection, samples of blood from the hearts of dead animals as well as from some of the survivors should be inoculated onto agar plates. The cultures from the dead animals should show the infecting organism, whereas the cultures from surviving animals should be sterile.

The three methods most frequently used for calculating the 50% dose parameter are the method of Reed and Muench (157), the probit method (158), and method of the sigmoidal dose-response (variable slope), also known as the Hill equation (159).

Treatment Routes and Times

By altering the treatment route or schedule, differences in activity can be demonstrated. In addition, the relative efficacy of oral and subcutaneous administration of a substance can be compared (as discussed earlier).

Studies in which mice infected with *S. pneumoniae* serotypes 1 and 2 were treated once, orally or subcutaneously, with doses of ampicillin or amoxicillin demonstrate the influence of the treatment route (160). Treatment by the subcutaneous route was more effective than treatment by the oral route. When administered orally, amoxicillin was more active against the type 1 *S. pneumoniae* than was ampicillin. Otherwise, the two agents were equivalent in activity (160).

Tests with ampicillin and amdinocillin (mecillinam) in which the antibacterials were administered to mice subcutaneously immediately (0 hour) or at 1, 2, or 4 hours after infection indicate the potential problems with delay in treatment initiation (160). With treatment 4 hours after inoculation, the regimens were considerably less effective than when administered immediately or at 1 hour (160). Similarly, multiple-dose regimens were more effective than single-dose regimens, which are typical for all β-lactam antibiotics. This can be explained by the importance of T>MIC (i.e., the duration the antibiotic concentration remains above the MIC). Interestingly, the greater effectiveness of multiple dosing was also apparent for ampicillin against enterobacteria resistant toward the drug (160).

For drugs such as the aminoglycosides or the fluoroquinolones, single-dose regimens would result in lower PD_{50}s than those of multiple-dose regimens due to the importance of the AUC/MIC ratio for these types of compounds (e.g., reference 149). In this manner, PK/PD relationships can be demonstrated by relatively simple dosing experiments using the mouse protection test.

Differences in the PK patterns of various agents may also be determined by prophylactic-type experiments (i.e., treatment before infection). The activities of ceftriaxone and cefotaxime were similar when treatment was administered immediately (0 hour) after treatment (161). However, when treatment was administered at 24 or 8 hours before infection, the activity of ceftriaxone was clearly superior against the gram-negative bacteria. No such differences were seen against *S. aureus* in this model.

Duration of treatment can affect the outcome (for reviews, see references 51 and 162). For example, extending ciprofloxacin treatment (p.o., 20 mg/kg twice a day.) of systemic *S. typhimurium*–infected mice from 17 to 28 days improved the outcome (163).

Synergy or Antagonism In Vivo in Screening Models

In order to study interaction between two antibiotics in vivo, graded doses of the combined agents and the single agents are administered to groups of four to six mice after infection. The PD_{50} can be calculated for the combination and compared to the 50% doses for the single agents. A fractional index (FIC) can be calculated for the combination doses by dividing the PD_{50} value for each of the components in the combination by the PD_{50} value obtained for each component alone and adding the two quotients. Synergy can then be defined using the FIC (e.g., a value of ≤0.5–0.6), similar to the method of studying synergy in vitro (164). Delay of treatment causes loss of synergistic activity.

Setting the PD_{50} value of the combination at one-fourth that of the most active single agent is perhaps an easier way of evaluating the results of the experiments. Combining different dosing regimens over a 24-hour dosing period after inoculation will further allow estimation of the importance of different PK parameters for synergy in vivo. This approach has been studied in the neutropenic mouse thigh model (160,165,166) but could also be used in the mouse peritonitis model.

Antagonism between antibiotics in vivo has been studied in the mouse peritonitis model (167). The combination of erythromycin and penicillin against *S. pneumoniae* in vivo resulted in the same mortality as erythromycin alone and significantly higher mortality than penicillin alone. The inhibiting effect of erythromycin on the activity of penicillin could also be demonstrated by in vivo time-kill curves of bacterial counts in peritoneal wash. This apparent antagonism between erythromycin and penicillin has been contested by others, at least in vitro (168). The use of animal models and PK/PD relationships in determining in vivo antibiotic synergy has been reviewed (160,164,166,169–171).

Den Hollander et al. (172) used in vitro–derived FIC determinations to attain PD parameters of the combination of tobramycin and ceftazidime. They first determined the MICcombi, which is the MIC of tobramycin in the presence of ceftazidime. Using humanlike PK profiles, they then divided the tobramycin and ceftazidime concentrations at each time point along the dosing interval to construct FIC over time curves, which were used to derive PD parameters. $T_{>FICI}$ (time above a specified FIC value during the dosing interval) appears to be the key PD parameter for this combination. Although difficult, to date, little application of this methodology has occurred with in vivo data.

Mouse Peritonitis Model for the Study of Antibiotic Activity against Intracellular Bacteria

The mouse peritonitis model has for many years been used to harvest leukocytes for in vitro purposes (173). The extravasation into the peritoneal fluid of leukocytes can be stimulated by microbiologic or chemical means. Although in vitro cell culture has long been in use for the study of antibiotic activity against intracellular bacteria (174), few have extended this to the in vivo situation. Sandberg et al. (175–179) studied the mouse peritonitis model with i.p. inoculation with *Staphylococcus aureus* and used peritoneal wash to enumerate extra- and intracellular staphylococci after a series of centrifugation steps and washing, addition of lysozyme to remove extracellular bacteria, and lysing of the leukocytes in plain, sterile water. Enumeration of colony counts in the supernatant, without cells, and the lysed pellet with cells resulted in reasonable estimates of extra- and intracellular staphylococcal cells, which were validated by electron microscopy. Treatment with various antibiotics showed slower killing effect intracellularly, which correlated with slower intracellular growth and the the theoretical penetrability of the antibiotics (175). PK/PD analyses of dicloxacillin and linezolid showed surprisingly good effect of the former, which is standard treatment of staphylococcal infections in many European countries, whereas the latter drug showed almost no intracellular activity (176,177). Similar studies have been performed with *Salmonella* sp revealing excellent both extra- and intracellular activity of ceftriaxone but less so of carbapenems (180).

Thigh Lesion (Selbie) Model

The rodent thigh lesion model was originally described by Selbie and Simon in 1952 (181) and continues to be a fundamental experimental method in animal model antimicrobial efficacy studies. This model is commonly employed in the development of new antimicrobial agents given its relative simplicity compared to other sites of infection. It can also allow for more limited numbers of animals as each thigh can represent one biologic replicate in the infection model (i.e., An investigator only needs to use two mice, four thighs, to achieve statistically evaluable data). Note, however, that using both thighs from same mice for infection is not allowed by all animal ethics committees in Europe. In general, the model involves intramuscular injection of an inoculum into the dorsal thighs of the animal. Mice are then treated with an antimicrobial agent for a defined period, euthanized at study end point, and CFU enumerated from each thigh. In order to make the data most meaningful, 0-hour control mice are necessary to determine the viable burden at the start of therapy, which allows one to determine whether infectious burden increased, decreased, or remained stable over time. Untreated controls are also necessary to prove fitness in the animal model. Most studies use a neutropenic mouse model. There are a number of reasons for this but two are likely the most important. First, an unconfounded evaluation of drug–pathogen effect can be performed if the immune system is removed or significantly inhibited from affecting the outcome. Secondly, many animals are inherently resistant to some types of infection and/or species, or the organism has limited fitness, unless the immune system is compromised. While CFU determination of pathogen abundance is most commonly performed, novel techniques such as fluorescent protein markers, serum biomarkers of infection, image scoring, quantitative polymerase chain reaction (qPCR), and antigen/antibody testing have been developed for certain pathogens as a means to monitor infectious burden in animals.

FUNGAL INFECTIONS

Animal model research using fungal pathogens has increased dramatically in the past decade. Similar to bacteria, fungal pathogens have the ability to cause localized disease (e.g., esophageal candidiasis or dermatophytosis), disseminated disease (e.g., invasive candidiasis), or a combination of the two (e.g., invasive aspergillosis or cryptococcosis). Therefore, models have been developed to mimic either site-specific inoculation routes or disseminated routes (e.g., intravenous inoculation). A comprehensive review and practical descriptions of many of these models is presented in the following citations (4,150,182,183). Important differences from bacterial models do require consideration and include the inoculum size and immune suppression. Many fungal pathogens require a high inoculum to produce disease, most commonly on the order of 7 to 9 $\log_{10}$. Given a very high inoculum, at times, this

can lead to relatively small growth in end organ burden prior to study end point or animal death (i.e., 1 $\log_{10}$ or less) (184). Additionally, although many bacterial studies use a neutropenic host animal, it is almost universally employed for fungal studies. This is required as most fungal infections cannot be established in the animal host without significant immune suppression, which is likely intuitive as a major risk factor to these pathogens in humans is significant immune suppression. An often-employed additional step in immune suppression in pulmonary mold infection models is the use of high doses of corticosteroids (185–190). A few investigations have employed rodents deficient in specific immune components (191,192). For example, severe combined immunodeficient (SCID) mice devoid of B- or T-cell immunity have been used for a mucosal candidiasis model to mimic infection in patients with HIV (192). Finally, a murine model of diabetic ketoacidosis, a major risk factor for disseminated and cerebral zygomycosis, has been successfully described and used to examine antifungal therapy in this setting (193,194).

Animal model investigation for fungal pathogens is most robust for *Candida* species and includes oropharyngeal and esophageal candidiasis (195,196), vaginitis (49), and invasive candidiasis (too numerous to cite examples, however, representative studies are referenced here [84,182,190,197–237]). The most common model used in the study of antifungal agents in murine models is disseminated infection. This is achieved through direct intravenous injection of the organism inoculum into the tail vein of a mouse. Provided a large enough inoculum is introduced (6 to 7 log), *C. albicans* disseminated infection in the neutropenic mouse model will rapidly progress to death in 24 to 72 hours (209). If one wishes to study organism growth or decline over longer treatment periods, this can be accomplished using a lower starting inoculum (18). For other *Candida* spp (such as *Candida glabrata*), severe infection is more difficult to establish and often requires longer experimental durations to find discernable differences in treatment groups (199,200,211,238). Nonetheless, the disseminated candidiasis model continues to be one of the most commonly used fungal models for drug development and dosing regimen refinement.

A relatively clinical complication of invasive candidiasis is dissemination to the eye with subsequent endophthalmitis. Animal models examining drug efficacy in animal models of endophthalmitis have been developed (239–247). These models have provided important guidance on therapeutic options for which drug and immune system penetration is limited. Models mimicking human fungal keratitis have also been described (248–259).

Filamentous fungal pathogen models (most commonly *Aspergillus*) have also undergone significant experimental refinement. Many of these pathogens are acquired via inhalation and therefore primary pulmonary infection models with dissemination most closely mimic human disease (189). However, disseminated models via intravenous injection of the organism inoculum have also been used (260). As stated previously, these models often employ significant immune suppression in the form of a combination of chemotherapy-induced neutropenia and corticosteroid treatment. Treatment durations of 7 days or longer are often required as in general, despite the immunosuppression, filamentous fungi require longer incubation periods to grow to significant levels and/or disseminate via a pulmonary infection route. A previous limitation to robust filamentous fungal pathogen investigation has been difficulty in quantitation, as filamentous fungi do not grow in discrete colonies as do bacteria and yeast. Additionally, concern has been raised that homogenization can fracture a filament into multiple pieces leading to overestimation of organism burden. Current molecular surrogates of organism burden have largely alleviated this limitation. The most common methods of organism burden include galactomannan measurement (185) or real-time qPCR (261,186,262). For example, a recent publication evaluated whether qPCR was a good surrogate marker for disease progression, treatment outcome, and animal mortality in a 7-day study of invasive pulmonary aspergillosis (IPA) in a murine model using numerous *Aspergillus fumigatus* isolates (186). The authors demonstrated a very strong relationship between qPCR result and treatment efficacy. In fact, every 1-log increased growth of organism based on qPCR resulted in a 17% increase in mortality. Additionally, the increase in survival was most profound at the dose exposure that was associated with net stasis (static dose) of organism burden. Thus, stasis or net cidal drug activity based on qPCR is a very strong predictor of clinical survival in this model. Other measures of organism viability and abundance have also been used such as XTT, DiBAC staining, chitin measurement, histopathology grading, lung weights, and pulmonary infarct scoring (263,264). These types of models have also been

recently expanded to examine less common filamentous fungal pathogens including *Zygomycetes* (194,265–268).

Models mimicking fungal meningitis for pathogens that commonly cause primary central nervous system (CNS) infection or have a high likelihood of dissemination to the CNS have been developed for a number of pathogens (e.g., *Cryptococcus*, *Aspergillus*, and dimorphic pathogens *Blastomyces*, *Histoplasma*, and *Coccidioides*). Infection is induced by either intravenous or intracisternal injection of a defined inoculum and organism burden is quantified in the CSF and brain parenchyma to determine outcome. One of the more common pathogens examined in animal models given its predilection to cause CNS infection is *Cryptococcus* sp (269–278). Animal hosts in these experiments have included rabbits, mice, and guinea pigs. Animal models of CNS aspergillosis, many developed by Clemons and Stevens, have been described and used to determine therapeutic efficacy of various antifungal agents (279–286). Additionally, CNS models of invasive candidiasis have been developed to better understand treatment strategies for this rare pediatric complication (287–289).

Dimorphic fungal pathogens are acquired via the pulmonary route but can also disseminate to involve the CNS. This is not uncommon for *Coccidioides* sp and a number of investigations have examined antifungal therapy in animal models of CNS coccioidomycosis (290–296). For reference, a thorough review of dimorphic fungal animal models is provided by Sorensen et al. (297). Finally, animal models of CNS phaeohyphomycosis have been described for this rare but severe infectious entity (298–300).

The efficacy of agents directed at dermatophytes has been evaluated in animal models with cutaneous infection (301–305). Most commonly, the site of infection (skin, foot pad, or nail) is mechanically abraded prior to topical inoculation to predispose the tissue to infection. The infection often takes several days or weeks to establish and therefore initiation of systemic or local topical therapy is delayed. After therapy, which may also require a prolonged period of time, tissue samples are cultured and examined by histopathology to determine drug efficacy.

Rare fungal infections that can occur in patients with severe or prolonged immunosuppression have also been studied to a limited extent. Some examples include and blastoschizomycosis (306–308), fusariosis (309–312), scedosporiosis (313–315), and trichosporonosis (316,317).

DISCRIMINATIVE ANIMAL MODELS OF INFECTION

Animal Models of Urinary Tract Infections

The models for experimental acute urinary tract infections (UTIs) that are commonly used to evaluate antibacterials produce either hematogenous or ascending infections, depending on whether the inoculum is administered intravenously or intravesically, with or without the addition of a foreign body (318). Mice and rats are the most common species used in experimental UTIs, and they have been used to determine the pathogenesis of this infection as well as test experimental chemotherapy. Note, however, that naturally occurring vesicoureteral reflux (backflow of the urine from the bladder to the kidneys) normally occurs in rodents but only infrequently in humans (319). Although some bacteria have a trophism for the urinary tract, even when inoculated intraperitoneally (e.g., *Borrelia burgdorferi* [320]), and some models of UTIs utilize bloodstream inoculation with bacteria to generate pyelonephritis (321), normally, manipulation of the urinary tract of rodents is a prerequisite for establishing infection. Some of the bacterial virulence factors necessary to establish UTI in humans (e.g., type 1 and type P fimbriae of *E. coli*) are also required to establish ascending UTI in mice and rats with the same binding mechanisms to the epithelium of the urinary tract. With focus on these virulence factors in strains used for inoculation, little manipulation of the urinary tract is actually needed for creating ascending infection in these rodents. In addition to testing antimicrobials, these models have been used to evaluate adjunct antiinflammatory agents (e.g., pentoxifylline [322]). Previous reviews (144,321,323,324) describe additional models for establishing UTI, in particular, pyelonephritis.

Ascending Obstructive Pyelonephritis

The original model for pyelonephritis (325) was further developed (323). Rats are operated on and bacteria are inoculated directly into the bladder, whereafter one of the ureters is obstructed by ligation, which is removed 18 to 24 hours later. This model has been used to demonstrate that, following acute infection, inflammation leading to chronic pyelonephritis is the major contributor to renal damage. Early antibiotic therapy suppresses renal damage (326) by rapid eradication of bacterial infection, but antiinflammatory treatment with dexamethasone failed to suppress renal damage (327). This model has also been used to compare the efficacy of various antibiotics (328).

Chronic Cystitis and Subacute Pyelonephritis

A model of persistent bladder infection has been described that requires placement of a foreign body into the bladder (329). A small cylinder of polyurethane foam (4 × 2 mm) was introduced into the bladder via a needle pushed bluntly into the bladder via the urethra. Two weeks later, the surgically exposed bladder was inoculated directly with *E. coli*. Chronic bacteriuria ensued for as long as 8 weeks after infection, leading to focal and diffuse inflammation of the bladder wall. Furthermore, bilateral pyelonephritis developed in the majority of the animals. The model is amenable to antimicrobial therapy (329). Several drugs have been tested for 7 days duration, and the effect was measured as reduction of CFU in the bladder wall and kidney homogenates (329).

Acute and Subclinical Pyelonephritis by Intrarenal Infection

This procedure is commonly used to establish kidney infections for the evaluation of antimicrobial agents, usually in rats. The kidney is surgically exposed, and the inoculum (50 to 100 CFU/μL) is injected directly into one (330,331) or both poles (332) of the kidney. Usually, only one of the kidneys is used, but infection of the contralateral kidney can ensue (332). The passive infection of the contralateral kidney has been used to study subclinical pyelonephritis in comparison with the acute infection in the directly inoculated kidney (332).

The model has been used to study the effect as well as toxicity of gentamicin (330,331) and the importance of duration of therapy in pyelonephritis (330). Several different antibiotics have been compared in this model (329,330). The most effective drugs have been gentamicin, ceftriaxone, and various fluoroquinolones, while ampicillin and co-trimoxazole have shown lower efficacy (329,330).

Ascending Pyelonephritis following Direct Bladder Inoculation

Direct inoculation of surgically exposed bladders has long been used to induce experimental UTI. Rodents generally do not need to be water deprived. The urethra is clamped and the bladder exposed by surgical intervention. Bacteria (50 to 200 CFU/μL) are slowly injected into the bladder, and the urethra remains clamped for 2 to 4 hours in order to avoid discharge of the inoculum. Ascending infection with development of bilateral pyelonephritis will follow. Renal scarring for up to 6 weeks later has been used as a parameter to study interventional therapy (333). Early quinolone treatment eliminated the incidence of renal scarring, while delayed treatment resulted in renal damage in approximately 50% of the animals (333). Reduction as compared to untreated controls of CFU of *E. coli* after homogenizing the kidneys was used to study the effect of nemonoxacin, a novel nonfluorinated quinolone, as compared to common fluoroquionlones as part of screening for in vivo efficacy of this compound in several animal models (334).

Ascending Urinary Tract Infection by Bladder Inoculation via Urethral Catheter

During the last 10 to 15 years, this model in mice has been the most widely used to study virulence factors and host resistance in UTI. With this model, detailed knowledge of the binding mechanisms between bacteria harboring various virulence traits and epithelial cells in the urinary tract has been discovered, and it has further been utilized to reveal the various facets of the host mechanisms of resistance to infection, both in the bladder and in the kidney. A detailed review of this literature is beyond the scope of this chapter, and the reader is referred to recent reviews (335–338).

The model is probably by far the easiest to use for the study of UTI when the technique of bladder cauterization has been learned, since no other surgical manipulation is needed. With the correct bacterial strain harboring the virulence factors needed (i.e., type 1 or type P fimbriae of *E. coli* or other enterobacteria), UTI with moderate to high bacterial counts in the urine, bladder wall, and kidneys (40% to 70% of the infected mice) will ensue (339–341). The presence of type 1 fimbriae in *E. coli* can easily be tested for by agglutination with bakers yeast cells or with sheep erythrocytes (342). CFUs appear to decrease after 2 to 3 weeks, which is why antibiotic treatment studies should preferably be performed 1 to 8 days after inoculation. Higher colony counts can be obtained by pretreating the mice with 5% glucose in the drinking water starting 3 days prior to infection (341,342).

Antibiotic concentrations can be measured simultaneously in serum, urine, and renal tissue, and these can be related to the effect of the antibiotics according to the MICs of the infecting strains (340,342). PD relationships for dosing of antibiotics in UTI can be studied with this model (343), which has also been used to study antibiotic effect against UTI caused by *Enterococcus faecalis* and *Pseudomonas aeruginosa* (344). The model has been used to show effect of different antibiotics and has revealed that no antibiotics are able to eradicate bacteria in the bladder wall because the bacteria are situated intracellularly in bacterial colonies, perhaps in a kind of biologic biofilm, which renders the bacteria resistant to antibiotics present both in blood and urine (340). Bacteria in the urine and in the kidneys are more easily removed, as long as urine and serum antibiotic concentrations lie above the MIC, while resistance correlates with missing antibiotic effect even for lowly ciprofloxacin-resistant *Escherichia coli* bearing the qnr-genes (345,346).

Models of Urinary Tract Infections Associated with Indwelling Catheters

Models of short-term and long-term indwelling catheter infections have been described (347,348). Both long (25-mm) and short (4-mm) segments of tubing have been used in mice; the short not secured and therefore expelled, with 3 to 7 days serving as a short-term model. When the longer segment has been secured to the bladder, it has been left for up to 12 months, thus mimicking a long-term indwelling urinary catheter (348). Spontaneous bacteriuria (>10^2 CFU/mL urine) was not reported in the mice with unsecured tubing but occurred intermittently in 44% of the animals with secured bladder catheters and was predominantly due to *Proteus mirabilis*. Apparently, no colonization of the kidneys occurred unless the infection was persistent and of high density (10^5 CFU/mL). Postsurgery ampicillin treatment for 7 days and housing on wire platforms reduced the incidence of bacteriuria to 7% over 12 months.

Placing a catheter precolonized with *P. aeruginosa* in the rat bladder with subsequent 3-day treatment showed higher reduction of catheter biofilm counts with a combination of fosfomycin and a novel fluoroquinolone, prulifloxacine, than with the latter drug alone (349). A bladder cathether model in mice for the study of *Candida* biofilm on catheters with or without silver coating was introduced by Wang and Fries (350). A rabbit indwelling bladder catheter model was used to show that silver-coated catheters significantly reduced bacteriruia as compared to noncoated catheters (351).

Models of Urinary Tract Infection Resulting from Bloodstream Inoculation

Hematogenous infection has been long used to establish UTI (321,352). Normally, no manipulations of the animals are required, but strain selection is essential in order to have selective colonization of the kidneys. Examples of this model have used *E. faecalis* (353–355) or *S. aureus* or *K. pneumoniae* (356). Trovafloxacin and rifampin alone or in combination were compared in a rat model against *E. faecalis* pyelonephritis (354). Although antagonism is usually considered the result of combining these two types of antibiotics, no such effect was evident from the reduction in renal colony counts found, which was similar to those achieved with the two drugs given alone. A new cephalosporin with gram-positive activity was compared with ampicillin and vancomycin against *E. faecalis* in the hematogenous model in mice (353). With the higher doses used, the cephalosporin was as effective as the two other antibiotics.

Animal Models of Foreign Body Infections

Advances in the development of prostheses and a variety of vascular grafts and permanently residing catheters have been limited by problems of bacterial infections, which are exceedingly difficult to cure and often necessitate removal of the device. Reviews of animal models of foreign body infections have appeared (357–360), prompting review of strategies for dealing with such infections clinically (361,362). Foreign bodies and bone and joint infections are discussed in "Animal Models of Osteomyelitis" section.

One of the most common foreign body infection models utilizes the subcutaneous implantation of a perforated plastic cylinder (363). Although commonly used in guinea pigs and rats, this model can also be used in mice. This model is suitable for evaluation of antibiotic treatment, although the infections are difficult to treat. For example, one study demonstrated that only triple therapy with 50 mg/kg vancomycin, 50 mg/kg fleroxacin, and 25 mg/kg rifampin (i.p. every 12 hours for 21 days) provided an adequate response (364). The same model has recently been used to study the effect of vancomycin, gentamicin, and daptomycin against

E. faecalis (365); daptomycin against methicillin-resistant *Staphylococcus aureus* (MRSA) (366); and levofloxacin and rifampicin, alone or in combination, against methicillin-susceptible *Staphylococcus aureus* (MSSA) (367). In an effort to study infections related to artificial vascular devices, Artini et al. (368) studied the antimicrobial properties of two kinds of vascular prosthesis to prevent early-onset infections and the efficacy of the concomitant action of a systemic antibiotic treatment. In adult male Wistar, they subcutaneously implanted in four groups a silver-coated prosthesis fragment, and a rifampicin-soaked prosthesis fragment in the remaining four groups. They inoculated the site of implant with *S. aureus* and administered systemic levofloxacin for 7 days in four groups representing the two kinds of prosthesis; after 21 days, the rats were sacrificed, prosthesis fragments were sonicated, and the corresponding supernatants were plated for bacterial counts. The rifampicin-soaked prostheses explanted from rats treated with levofloxacin were sterile, regardless of the bacterial inoculum. In other groups, some prostheses were colonized (368). Jean-Baptiste et al. (369) studied the efficacy, safety, and healing properties of polyester vascular prostheses coated with a hydroxypropyl-β-cyclodextrin (HPβCD)–based polymer (PVP-CD) and loaded with one or two antibiotics in vitro and in an experimental model in dogs. The study end points included hemolysis, platelet aggregation, antibacterial efficacy, polymer biodegradation, acute toxicity, and chronic tolerance and PVP-CD was proved safe and demonstrated excellent biocompatibility, healing, and degradation properties. Effective antimicrobial activity was achieved with PVP-CD in conditions consistent with a sustained-release mechanism (369).

Infected Sutures

Intramuscular implantation of infected sutures into the thighs of mice has been described (370). Lengths of cotton 2–0 suture are sterilized in broth, which is subsequently inoculated (in this example, with *K. pneumoniae*). The contaminated suture is then attached to a sterile needle and drawn through the thigh muscle of a mouse, the exposed ends are trimmed flush with the skin, and the ends are buried under the skin. Culture of homogenized suture material facilitates determination of the infecting CFU. The infection spreads from the suture to the surrounding muscle, and subsequently, a sepsis develops. This model is amenable to antibiotic intervention (371); continuous infusion of 180 mg/kg/day cefazolin by use of intraperitoneally implanted osmotic pumps was superior to an equal amount of antibiotic given by intramuscular bolus dosing (every 8 hours).

Animal Models of Skin, Burn, and Surgical Wound Infections

Several models of infection associated with surgical intervention (in the absence of foreign bodies) have been described and utilized for experimental evaluation of antimicrobial chemotherapy. These models rely on direct inoculation of the wound site and generally achieve simulated prophylaxis of postsurgical infection by administering antibiotics at the time of infection, or just before, and ascertain efficacy of treatment by determining infection remaining at the inoculation site as well as dissemination to internal organs. These models can be used to evaluate oral, parenteral, or topical antibiotic administration. Several reviews of postsurgical infectious complications and burn wound infection are available (361,372). A model of clean wound infections has been described (373).

Surgical wounds in mice infected with either MSSA or MRSA have been used to study the effect of teicoplanin, antimicrobial peptides, and hyaluronic acid (374,375). Ozcan et al. (376) induced sternal wound infection with MRSA and compared topical, systemic, or combination of topical and systemic vancomycin with untreated controls and found best effect of the combination as measured by reduction of bacteria in the wound. Mihu and coworkers (377) examined the capacity of a nitric oxide–releasing nanoparticle (NO-np) to treat wounds in mice infected with *Acinetobacter baumannii*. They demonstrated that NO-np treatment reduced suppurative inflammation, decreased microbial burden, reduced the degradation of collagen, and altered the local cytokine milieu.

Models of Infected Burn Wounds

Infections following burns are difficult to treat and have been modeled in several systems. Typically, partial-thickness or full-thickness burn wounds are made on the shaved skin of anesthetized animals by using a metal stamp or by partially immersing the animals in heated water; a minimum of about 30% of the skin area of the animal needs to be damaged. Normally, the burn wound is then directly inoculated, but translocation of normal intestinal bacteria often follows; interestingly, animal models have demonstrated

that infection of a skin burn apparently promotes translocation of intestinal bacteria, compared with that occurring when wounds are kept sterile (378,379). Experimental burn-induced wound infections for the study of antimicrobial treatment have been performed in rats or mice with MRSA (380,381), MSSA (382), *K. pneumoniae* (383), and *C. albicans* (384). Treatment modalities investigated have ranged from topical agents, systemic antibiotics, phage therapy, and photodynamic therapy.

Research in this area has also evaluated promotion of host resistance to infection by use of cytokines, whose expression in some cases also occurs as part of the normal healing process. In experimental full-thickness murine wounds, the expression of inducible nitric oxide synthase (iNOS) by infiltrating inflammatory cells is not a part of normal repair processes but is a response to bacterial colonization due to *S. aureus* (385).

Skin Infection Models

Skin infection models in guinea pigs and mice have recently been developed and used for treatment effect studies with topical and systemic antibiotic treatment (304,386,387). In both animal species, the skin is prepared under anesthesia by first removal of hair, then scraping the skin with, for example, fine sand paper until the superficial corneal skin layers are removed. Bacteria (*Staphylococcus aureus* or *Streptococcus pyogenes*) or dermatophytes are then inoculated directly on the denuded skin, which creates a skin infection spreading only to the fascia but shows up as a red, inflamed, and edematous lesion (386,387). Usually, the infection remains localized to the skin without signs of systemic infection and the animals appear healthy apart from the local infection. After treatment, a skin biopsy is taken from the infected skin and homogenated, from which bacteria or fungi can be quantified. Both topical and systemic treatments have shown significant reduction in bacterial or fungal counts as compared to untreated controls (387).

Animal Models of Pneumonia

Rodent Models of Acute Pneumonia

A useful model for production of pneumococcal pneumonia in rats has been described by Ansfield et al. (388). Lung bacterial counts progressively increased, reaching 10^7 CFU per lung within 48 hours. This increase was associated with localized atelectasis and consolidation. Bacterial multiplication could be inhibited with 50 mg/kg tetracycline given once intraperitoneally prior to infection or at 4 or 12 hours after infection. Viable pneumococci were rapidly killed by lung defenses if bacterial multiplication was inhibited within 12 hours of the onset of infection. No change occurred in the bacterial population if tetracycline treatment was delayed until 24 hours after infection.

A similar rat model of pneumococcal pneumonia was used to determine the role of the host defense system in antimicrobial therapy by impairing the phagocytic system by complement depletion using cobra venom factor (389). There was a consistent decrease in body weight with time (approximately 15% to 20% loss by 108 hours postinfection). The temperature was initially elevated (approximately 1°C to 2°C, up from normal levels of 37°C to 37.4°C), but by 108 hours, it was depressed (by as much as 4°C). The weight of the left lung increased (from about 0.6 ± 0.15 g to 3 to 4 g) with the involvement of the lung tissue in the infectious process. Pulmonary lesions were very extensive in the left lung by 108 hours, and the number of pneumococci increased from 6×10^7 CFU to approximately 10^9 CFU per lung. By the end of 108 hours, the infectious process had spread, so that both the blood (approximately 10^3 to 10^6 CFU/mL) and the pleural fluid were positive for pneumococci. Treatment of infected rats with 2 mg/kg penicillin G every 12 hours starting from 36 hours postinfection was very effective in preventing weight loss (only a transient 6% to 8% loss by 36 hours, 0% to 5% by 132 hours), normalizing the temperature (approximately 38°C to 39°C at 36 hours and within normal range from 84 hours onward), and maintaining the weight of the left lung near normal (a transient rise up to 2 g at 36 hours, within the normal range from 84 hours onward). By 84 hours, there was a significant but highly variable fall in the number of viable pneumococci, and by 132 hours, all lung, blood, and pleural fluid cultures were sterile. After treatment with cobra venom factor, the whole complement hemolytic activity was decreased to less than 2% of normal values. When cobra venom factor–treated rats were also administered penicillin, the results very closely paralleled the course of infection seen in normal untreated infected rats, indicating the importance of an intact innate immune system for the outcome of antimicrobial therapy (389).

Rat models have also been used to demonstrate that chronic alcohol ingestion increases susceptibility to infection (390), as does liver cirrhosis (391) and neutropenia (392). Intratracheal injection of soft agar (0.7%) encased penicillin-resistant

S. pneumoniae to create an acute pneumonia model in immunocompetent rats (393). Lung CFU and mortalities were dependent on the size of the infectious challenge (inocula of 2.9×10^8 or 4.2×10^9 were uniformly fatal, but only the higher inocula produced stable lung CFU of approximately 10^9 CFU/g over 3 days). Despite an in vitro MIC of 2 μg/mL for penicillin, 100,000 IU/kg penicillin G every 2 hours for eight administrations reduced lung CFU (the change was approximately log 2/g vs. controls) and promoted survival (13% mortality vs. 33% for controls), whereas 250,000 IU/kg reduced the mortality to 7% and the change in CFU/g was approximately log 3. Similar activity was seen with cefpirome (200 mg/kg) and cefotaxime (100 mg/kg). With the latter, the lung CFU/g was similar to that resulting from the penicillin G treatment, but the mortality was apparently higher (19%). Two administrations of 50 mg/kg vancomycin every 8 hours produced a change in CFU/g of log 4 and 7% mortality.

Murine models of acute pneumonia are increasingly incorporated into drug development and PK/PD studies. An early description published in 1981 by Beskid and colleagues (394) examined a novel cephalosporin (ceftriaxone) efficacy in a murine model of pneumococcal pneumonia. Mice were infected by intranasal instillation of the inoculum and treated with either ceftriaxone or another comparator antibiotic (cefotaxime, ampicillin, piperacillin, cefamandole, and carbenicillin). After 48 hours, the mice were sacrificed and lungs aseptically harvested and a touch prep culture of a freshly sectioned area of lung was performed on blood agar plates. Overall, ceftriaxone was superior to the comparators in terms of PD_{50} (mg/kg): ceftriaxone, 0.88; ampicillin, 11; cefotaxime, 16; piperacillin, 79; cefamandole, 79; and carbenicillin, 84. This is a prime example of the use of preclinical animal model studies as ceftriaxone is now a cornerstone antimicrobial agent in community-acquired pneumonia.

Many contemporary models have also been described and a thorough review of murine models to mimic human pneumonia is provided (395). The models have been adapted to include common community pulmonary pathogens including *S. pneumoniae*, *H. influenzae*, *Chlamydia pneumoniae*, and *Mycoplasma pneumoniae*. Important considerations in the model include host immune dysfunction, organism pathogenicity in mice, route of infection, inoculum size, experimental duration, and end point (e.g., mortality, organism burden, etc.). Mice are usually made neutropenic by methods previously described in this chapter.

This allows for the most accurate evaluation of drug efficacy by removing immune function as a confounder on treatment effect. Additionally, many bacterial organisms will not produce disease in the model without some level of immune suppression. For a few organisms, even with immune suppression, it is difficult to obtain reproducible results in biologic replicates. One strategy to overcome this has been to use pulmonary administration of a chemical irritant (1% formalin) just prior to organism inoculation (396). A decreased ability to cause infection (i.e., decreased fitness) has also been noted in drug-resistant isolates, where presumably the loss of fitness is due to genetic changes in the isolate (397). Therefore, it is important at the outset to ensure all organisms used have similar degrees of fitness and pathogenesis in the animal model if one is attempting to compare efficacy against resistant strains.

The routes of infection used for production of murine pneumonia vary and include aerosolization of the inoculum, intranasal instillation with subsequent aspiration, injection into the trachea via percutaneous puncture with a fine needle, or direct instillation into the lungs by tracheal intubation. One advantage of aerosolized inoculation is the ability to infect large numbers of animals in large chambers at the same time with similar inoculum burden. For example, nebulization of 10^8 CFU/mL of *K. pneumoniae* via a Collison nebulizer for 45 minutes produced a similar degree of pneumonia in up to 100 mice at the same time (398). Experiment duration can vary depending on pathogenicity of the infecting organism but usually does not need to be prolonged more than 24 to 48 hours. Finally, determination of organism burden is most commonly performed by quantitative culture techniques (CFU determination).

The earlier mentioned techniques are now increasingly used for hospital-/health care–acquired pneumonia including multiple drug–resistant (MDR) organisms, difficult-to-treat gram-negative organisms, and MRSA. For example, *A. baumannii* is an increasingly recognized respiratory pathogen in patients who are mechanically ventilated and develop hospital-acquired pneumonia. Many of these isolates have limited therapeutic options and therefore animal models have been helpful to delineate treatment strategies (399–408). Dudhani and colleagues (399) examined the predictive PD index for colistin in treatment of experimentally infected mice. The free drug AUC/MIC correlated best with efficacy ($R^2 = 0.80$). The PD drug target in the pneumonia model was a free drug AUC/MIC of 1.57 to 6.52 for net stasis.

This was essentially identical to the PD target in a murine thigh model with the same organism. Unfortunately, drug resistance emergence was detected in subpopulations. Many other common health care–associated pulmonary pathogens have also been studied in rodent models such as MRSA (409–417), *P. aeruginosa* (418–426), and *K. pneumoniae* (427–434). Additionally, anthrax models have been actively pursued in recent years given the continued threat of bioterrorism in the United States and other parts of the world (435–442). These models are particularly relevant as clinical studies are not possible.

Chronic Pneumonia Models

Many chronic pneumonia models are based on the premise of preexisting lung conditions, such as chronic obstructive pulmonary disease (COPD) and cystic fibrosis (CF), which produce intermittent obstruction and subsequent risk for chronic infection. These preexisting conditions are difficult to mimic in rodents and bacteria are inherently rapidly cleared from the airways in these animals (443–445). Therefore, strategies to mimic periodic obstruction and prevent bacterial clearance have been developed. To date, the most common method is the use of agarose or alginate beads (444,446). This method successfully resulted in a persistent *P. aeruginosa* infection in rats for up to 35 days (444).

Most commonly, *P. aeruginosa* is the pathogen of choice for studies of chronic pneumonia as it is not only one of the most common isolates found in colonization and infection in COPD and CF patients but is also particularly difficult to treat and has high propensity of acquiring drug resistance. One of the earliest studies examined antimicrobial therapy in a guinea pig model of chronic *P. aeruginosa* pneumonia (447). Infection was established using agar bead–encased bacteria and the compounds tested included ticarcillin (120 mg/kg), ciprofloxacin (10 mg/kg), and tobramycin (1.7 mg/kg). Three days after infection, the drugs were administered as monotherapy for 5 days. Ciprofloxacin was judged to be most effective, followed by tobramycin and ticarcillin, which was ineffective, based on CFU counts. Notably, no single drug treatment was able to eradicate the infecting organism completely. Rodent models more recently have been used to examine antimicrobial therapy in chronic *P. aeruginosa* pneumonia (448–452). For example, Macia and colleagues (449) examined ciprofloxacin and tobramycin monotherapy and combination therapy in a murine model of chronic pneumonia using a reference strain and its hypermutable derivative. After exposure to cipro-floxacin, the hypermutable isolate of *P. aeruginosa* demonstrated a profound and rapid increase in drug-resistant subpopulations despite having the same in vitro susceptibility as the reference strain, which did not show any resistant subpopulations after drug exposure. This effect was not observed with tobramycin monotherapy. Finally, the combination of the two drugs appeared synergistic against the hypermutable isolate. Inhaled therapeutics are an additional area of investigation garnering more interest for chronic pneumonia (448,453–457). The advantage of this method is directly targeting antimicrobial therapy at the site of infection as well as limiting systemic toxicity that can be problematic for certain antimicrobial agents.

Animal Models of Otitis Media

Otitis media, an infection of the middle ear, is largely a childhood infection that apparently very few people avoid contracting. Caused chiefly by *H. influenzae* and *S. pneumoniae*, the infection, despite being painful, is often self-resolving, and although antibiotic therapy hastens its resolution, recurrence is common. Spread of the infection from the ear to produce sepsis and/or meningitis can occur, as can damage to the ear, suggesting that antibiotics still have a role in its treatment. Antibiotic treatment often results in the transformation of acute otitis media (AOM) into sterile otitis media with effusion (OME). However, culture-negative OME fluid may contain viable bacteria (458–460), likely due to the growth of bacteria as biofilm (133,458–460), which conveys different physiologic character to the bacteria, including antibiotic sensitivity.

Excellent technical descriptions of the models are available for the chinchilla (461), guinea pig (462), gerbil (463), and rat (464,465). Briefly, anesthetized animals have their ear canals thoroughly cleaned and are infected by direct administration of bacteria into the ear canal, normally by injection through the thin bone structures of the cephalad bulla. A thorough review of the histopathology and pathophysiology of experimental models of AOM is available (465).

A gerbil model of bilateral AOM induced by either penicillin-resistant or penicillin-sensitive *S. pneumoniae*, combined with the measurement of ear fluid CFU and drug levels, was used to establish PK/PD parameters for linezolid (466). Following intrabullar injection of *S. pneumoniae*,

peak infection occurred at day 2 for the penicillin-resistant strain and at day 3 for the penicillin-sensitive strain. Linezolid, amoxicillin, or vehicle was administered twice per day over 4.5 days. Amoxicillin was effective only against the sensitive strain, whereas linezolid doses of 10 mg/kg or greater produced cure rates above 72% versus both strains. A similar study (467) demonstrated that, for penicillin-sensitive *S. pneumoniae*, doses of amoxicillin (>2.5 mg/kg) resulting in ear fluid concentrations = 1.4 µg/mL or serum concentrations greater than the MIC for = 14% of the dosing interval were effective in resolving clinical signs and reducing bacterial CFU.

Using a model of mixed infection with *S. pneumoniae* and *H. influenzae* (468), amoxicillin/clavulanate and cefuroxime were evaluated as treatment by stratifying the gerbils according to the presence of effusions. Mixed infections had lower effusion rates than AOM due just to *H. influenzae*, and treatment of OME was more difficult. Additionally, the mixed infection model was treatable, but more than 80% of the animals developed culture-negative OME. Furthermore, AOM models have been used to demonstrate the potential of antibiotic treatment to promote a protective immune response (469) and immunization (483). Initiation of penicillin treatment early in *S. pneumoniae* infection in chinchillas produced greater inflammation than late treatment (470). The importance of delay of treatment was studied in the gerbil model for amoxicillin against *S. pneumoniae* with varying susceptibility to penicillin (471). Independent of penicillin susceptibility delay of amoxicillin therapy resulted in lower effect, which was considered due to changes in metabolic activity of the pathogens. The same group showed the same lack of effect with delay of treatment with erythromycin (472).

The addition of dexamethasone to antibiotic treatment reduced the structural damage associated with this infection as compared with antibiotics alone (473). However, treatment of experimental AOM in gerbils with antibiotics plus acetaminophen delayed eradication of *H. influenzae* as compared with antibiotics alone, possibly due to a reduction of phagocyte recruitment to the site caused by the antiinflammatory agent (474). Addition of ibuprofen therapy to amoxicillin or erythromycin against experimental pneumococcal infection also in the gerbil model did not interfere with antibiotic therapy (475). In comparing mixed *S. pneumoniae* and *H. influenzae* with monoinfection by *H. influenzae*, it was demonstrated that the exact characteristics of AOM or OME in models depends, at least in part, on the time from the appearance of clinical symptoms until the diagnosis/intervention, on the bacteria involved, and on previous antibiotic treatment. Furthermore, poorer eradication rates occurred with lower levels of inflammation, and PK/PD relationships in middle ear fluid provide better predictive value than serum PK/PD parameters (468). These models have also used β-lactamase–positive *H. influenzae* (476), and in one study, this pathogen did not protect *S. pneumoniae* against the activity of amoxicillin (477).

Animal Models of Meningitis

Animal models of bacterial meningitis have been considered extremely useful in delineating the pathophysiology of meningitis and elucidating optimal antibiotic and adjunct therapies.

Mouse Models of Meningitis

An increasing number of studies using mouse models of meningitis have been performed recently, in particular, with the use of gene-modulated knockout mice. Mice have been infected with various pathogens (e.g., *S. pneumoniae, N. meningitidis*, group B streptococci [GBS], *E. coli, H. influenzae*, and *C. neoformans*) and using three different routes of inoculation (systemic [478], intracisternal [479–481], and intracerebral [482]). These models primarily involve evaluating survival and to some degree brain histopathologic alterations and have been useful in the study of antibiotic therapy efficacy, adjunctive therapy, and the pathophysiology of meningitis.

Rat Models of Meningitis

A model for the induction of *H. influenzae* type b meningitis in infant rats, which appears to be both simple and reproducible, has been described (483). Five-day-old rats were inoculated intranasally with *H. influenzae* type b, and bacteremic rats and rats with meningitis were identified by sampling of the CSF. The rats were sacrificed, the skin and soft tissue over the cisterna magna were removed by dissection for exposure of the dura, and the cisterna magna was entered by puncturing the dura with a sterile dissecting needle. This model system provides a simple method for determining the effectiveness of antibacterials in an acute meningitis infection similar to that seen in human infants (483). The infant rat pneumococcal meningitis

model was used to investigate the importance of bacteriolytical properties of daptomycin (nonbacteriolytic) and ceftriaxone (bacteriolytic) on inflammation and brain damage. Daptomycin treatment resulted in more rapid bacterial killing, lower CSF inflammation, and less brain damage than ceftriaxone treatment as measured by lower CSF concentrations of interleukin (IL)-1β, IL-10, IL-18, monocyte chemoattractant protein-1 (MCP-1), and macrophage inflammatory protein (MIP)-1α (484).

An excellent infant rat model for studying survival, brain damage, and learning deficiency has been described (485). This model, which uses intracisternal inoculation of GBS and *S. pneumoniae*, seems to be able to induce histopathologic alterations that mimic the findings in human meningitis and has provided significant knowledge about the pathophysiology of meningitis. Less brain damage seems to develop in the adult rat model of pneumococcal meningitis, but it has been very useful in the study of cerebrovascular alterations, CSF and brain tissue cytochemistry, and hearing loss (486).

Meningitis in adult rats can be induced via cisterna magna tap with a 23-gauge needle (487). The animals received either 10 μL of sterile saline as a placebo or an equivalent volume of *S. pneumoniae* suspension and treatment for 7 days with daptomycin or ceftriaxone was compared (487). Apart from spinal taps for efficacy, the animals underwent separately to four behavioral tasks: habituation to an open field, step-down inhibitory avoidance task, continuous multiple trials step-down inhibitory avoidance task and object recognition. Although both antibiotics were effective in clearing the infection, the investigators found evidence suggesting the potential alternative of the treatment with daptomycin in preventing learning and memory impairments caused by pneumococcal meningitis. In the same model, the same group showed that early ceftriaxone (8 hours vs. 16 hours) administration was an effective strategy to prevent long-term cognitive impairment (488).

The adult rat model has also been used to study hearing loss and cochlear damage as related to pneumococcal meningitis. Hearing loss and cochlear damage were assessed by distortion product otoacoustic emission (DPOAE), auditory brainstem response (ABR), and histopathology in rats treated with ceftriaxone 28 hours after infection. Furthermore, rats were treated with granulocyte colony-stimulating factor (G-CSF) initiated prior to infection, 28 hours after infection or with ceftriaxone only. Rats were followed for 7 days, and assessment of hearing was performed before infection and 24 hours and day 8 after infection. Pretreatment with G-CSF increased hearing loss 24 hours after infection and on day 8 compared to untreated rats and this was associated with significantly decreased spiral ganglion cell counts, increased damage to the organ of Corti, increased areas of inflammatory infiltrates and increased white blood cell (WBC) counts in CSF on day 8 after infection. Initiation of G-CSF 28 hours after infection did not significantly affect hearing loss or cochlear pathology compared to controls (489).

Because of the limited access for repetitive CSF sampling, the rat meningitis model and the mouse meningitis model have only been used sporadically for the study of antibacterial PKs (490). Excellent technically orientated reviews of the infant rat (491) and adult rat (492) meningitis models are available.

Guinea Pig Model of Meningitis

Force and coworkers (493) used both the guinea pig and the rabbit model of meningitis to evaluate the efficacy of meropenem against cephalosporin-susceptible and cephalosporin-resistant pneumococcal infection. Results with meropenem in the experimental rabbit model of penumococcal meningitis have been controversial perhaps due to the possible role of renal dehydropeptidase I in meropenem efficacy, why the investigators wanted to determine the efficacy of meropenem in two meningitis models, and the possible influence of the animal model over results. Meropenem was bactericidal at 6 hours in the guinea pig model against both strains with a reduction of greater than 4 log CFU/mL. In the rabbit model, it was bactericidal at 6 hours against the susceptible strain, but against the resistant, 3/8 therapeutical failures were recorded at 6 hours, being bactericidal at 24 hours. The authors concluded that meropenem showed bactericidal activity in both experimental models and that the guinea pig should be considered the best choice among laboratory animal species when assessing meropenem efficacy (493).

Rabbit Model of Meningitis

The optimal model for studying the PKs and PDs of antibiotics in CNS infections seems to be the rabbit meningitis model, which provides a controlled system for testing antibacterial penetration and efficacy in inflamed and normal CSF (494). Rabbits have been challenged with various pathogens (e.g., *Streptococcus pneumoniae*,

N. meningitidis, *Staphylococcus aureus* including in later years MRSA, *H. influenzae*, *Listeria monocytogenes*, and enterobacteria). The rabbit model allows simultaneous and repetitive sampling of CSF and blood, and it is therefore very useful in kinetic studies of CSF bacterial killing and CSF cytochemistry (495), though less useful in the study of brain damage and survival. For more than 20 years, the rabbit model has yielded considerable information about the PKs and efficacy of antibacterials as well as the pathophysiology of meningitis. The efficacy of antifungals has also been studied using a rabbit model of *C. neoformans* (496); an excellent technical review of this model has appeared previously (497). Surgical intervention is required to attach prosthesis to the rabbit's skull, facilitating immobilization of the deeply anesthetized animal. Blood samples (normally 1 to 3 mL) and simultaneous CSF samples (normally 0.1 to 0.2 mL) can be collected at frequent intervals (e.g., 0, 2, 4, 6, and 8 hours after initiation of therapy). The rate of removal of CSF should not exceed the rate of its synthesis (approximately 0.4 mL/hour [498]). In this manner, the antibacterial levels in both the blood and CSF and the bactericidal or bacteriostatic titers were determined. This model provides a controlled system for testing antibacterial penetration and efficacy in inflamed and normal meninges (499).

This model yields considerable information about the PKs and efficacy of antibacterials. In one study (500) using the basic model system described, the PK profile and bacteriologic efficacy of a single dose or continuous infusion of six antibacterials (penicillin, cefoperazone, ceftriaxone, cefuroxime, moxalactam, and chloramphenicol) were determined in two infections (*S. pneumoniae* and *H. influenzae*). The PK results following continuous infusion allow a comparative determination of the penetration of the antibacterial into the CSF of infected animals. It is evident that the rabbit meningitis model system can provide a great deal of information about the activity of different agents in a very difficult infection. Antibiotic–pathogen combinations tested in the rabbit model in later years have included daptomycin, vancomycin, and linezolid against MRSA (501); daptomycin, ceftriaxone, and vancomycin against *S. pneumoniae* (503); moxifloxacin, ampicillin, and gentamicin against *L. monocytogenes* (504); and doripenem against *E.coli* and *K. pneumoniae* (505).

The extrapolation of the results in rabbits to efficacy in humans has generally been good, with one or two exceptions (506).

Animal Models of Brain Abscess

The mortality associated with brain abscesses ranges from 0% to 24%, with neurologic sequellae in 30% to 55% of survivors and the incidence of brain abscess appears to be increasing, likely due to an increase in the population of immunosuppressed patients. A rat model of brain abscess/cerebritis was developed by Nathan and Scheld (507) and used to determine the relative efficacy of trovafloxacin as compared to ceftriaxone in animals infected with *S. aureus*. Very slowly, 10^5 CFU of *S. aureus* in 1 μL was injected with a Hamilton syringe, through a 2-mm burr hole created with a spherical carbide drill just posterior to the coronal suture and 4-mm lateral to the midline. Eighteen hours later, treatment was initiated and continued for 4 days three times a day with ceftriaxone, trovafloxacin, or saline for controls. The brains were removed and the entire injected hemisphere was homogenized and quantitative cultures performed. Both ceftriaxone and trovafloxacin reduced bacterial counts with a factor 1,000, with no significant difference between the two drugs. The authors concluded that trovafloxacin or other quinolones may provide a viable alternative to intravenous antibiotics in patients with brain abscess/cerebritis (507).

Animal Models of Infectious Endocarditis

Experimental endocarditis in rabbits and rats has been well studied and been shown to be reliable for the evaluation of the pathogenesis of the disease and the effectiveness of antibacterials (508–512); it is considered highly predictive of the clinical situation. Technical aspects of the rabbit model and some examples of the type of data that can be obtained have been well described (513). Essentially, a polyethylene catheter is inserted into the right carotid artery and advanced toward the heart; after it crosses the aortic valve, it is secured in place by suturing at the site of insertion. The presence of a catheter in the heart results in the development of sterile vegetations consisting of small, rough, whitish nodules 1 to 2 mm in size, usually at points of contact between the catheter and the endocardium. The sterile vegetations were infected by a single injection of bacteria into an ear vein; *S. epidermidis*, *S. aureus*, *C. albicans*, *Proteus mirabilis*, and *Pseudomonas aeruginosa*, among many other strains, have been used in this model. This basic approach has also been applied to rats (511,514).

Combinations of antibiotics in most cases are required to effectively treat endocarditis clinically, and this has been largely predicted by animal models (515). In the study by Batard et al. (516), in vitro checkerboard assays and time-kill curves showed an indifferent response by various *Staphylococcus aureus* strains (with different antibiotic resistance mechanisms) to the combination of quinupristin-dalfopristin and gentamicin. Using a rabbit endocarditis model and simulated human PK, the authors found no benefit from the combination in vivo, a result predicted by the in vitro testing. An in vitro infection model, which uses simulated endocardial vegetations, has been shown to produce results similar to these of the rabbit model when the PK parameters are known (517). Recent studies have used animal models for evaluating prophylaxis, including the use of azithromycin or ampicillin (518) and trovafloxacin or ampicillin (519) for *Streptococcus oralis* infection and azithromycin or vancomycin for MRSA (520).

Inflammation of the heart valves occurs in human and experimental endocarditis. The rabbit model was used to evaluate possible benefits of adjunctive dexamethasone regarding the course of experimental aortic valve endocarditis and the degree of valve tissue damage. Using a methicillin-resistant strain of *S. aureus*, researchers found that combining low-dose dexamethasone with an effective dose of vancomycin had no effect on survival, the blood culture sterilization rate, or the valve bacterial CFU. Dexamethasone adjunct treatment did reduce the inflammation and structural damage to the valves; this study also was able to demonstrate an inverse correlation between neutrophil number in vegetations and degree of tissue damage (520).

A number of studies have evaluated treatment of MRSA and glycopeptide nonsusceptible MRSA aortic endocarditis in rabbits or rats with a range of antibiotics including vancomycin and generics, teicoplanin, daptomycin, telavancin, linezolid, rifampicin, gentamicin, ceftobiprole, tigecycline, garenoxacin, levofloxacin, quinopristin/dalfopristin, and the experimental antimicrobial peptide, plectasin (521–535). Generally, combination treatment was more active than single drugs and daptomycin was more active than vancomycin, which was more bactericidal than linezolid. Two studies evaluated treatment of daptomycin-resistant MRSA isolates in the rabbit aortic endocarditis model and found that either telavancin (531) or a combination of oxacillin with daptomycin (537) was effective.

Several studies have evaluated the optimal treatment for *E. faecalis* endocarditis in rabbit or rat aortic endocarditis models (537–542). An interesting result was the effect of ceftriaxone in combination with ampicillin for vancomycin-susceptible *E. faecalis*; however, daptomycin showed superior effect against all types of strains, both vancomycin-susceptible *E. faecalis* and vancomycin-resistant *Enterococcus faecium* (540). In a study by Boutoille and coworkers (543), the in vivo impact of the MexAB-OprM efflux system in *P. aeruginosa* on antipseudomonal β-lactam efficacy (ticarcillin, piperacillin/tazobactam, and ceftazidime) was investigated in the aortic endocarditis model in rabbits comparing two isogenic strains with and without the resistance mechanism. Against the resistant strain, only the high-dose regimens of ceftazidime were effective, with the most significant effect being achieved by continuous infusion. In contrast, all the tested regimens were effective against the susceptible wild-type. In the same model, with a susceptible *P. aeruginosa*, Navas and coworkers (544) showed that constant infusion with cefepime or imipenem at plasma concentrations three to four times the MIC was sufficient for effect and that addition of tobramycin did not add to the killing effect of the β-lactams.

Colistin's effect against *A. baumannii* aortic endocarditis in rabbits was studied by Rodríguez-Hernández et al. (545), who found that although colistin cleared the bloodstream, it could not sterilize the aortic vegetations. Thus, endocarditis models are used extensively to support clinical decisions how to treat endocarditis caused by the rapidly appearing and troublesome antibiotic-resistant pathogens.

Animal Models of Eye Infections

Experimental eye infections have received much attention for the evaluation of antiinfective therapy. Animal models of keratitis, endophthalmitis, and eye injury and conjunctivitis are available (546). Technical descriptions of the rabbit model of conjunctivitis (547) and the mouse model of bacterial keratitis (548) have been provided.

Experimental Keratitis

Keratitis can be established by inoculation of the surface of an eye of an anesthetized animal damaged by scratching the surface with a syringe needle

(e.g., a 26-gauge needle) or by direct injection into the cornea. The rabbit is used most often due to the size of its eye also for clinical, macroscopic evaluation, but rats and mice have also been studied. For therapeutic studies, antibacterial therapies by a parenteral or topical (or combined) route are started at different times, but usually within 24 hours after infection. Topical treatment usually is frequently applied to the surface of the eye or administered by less frequent (often only once) intravitreal injection. Normally, the concentration of antibiotic in the aqueous humor correlates more closely with therapeutic efficacy than does the concentration in the cornea. Although many antibacterials can extensively reduce the number of bacteria in the cornea, typically by more than 99% in the first 24 hours of therapy, sterilization of the cornea is difficult and may require several additional days of continuous therapy (548).

P. aeruginosa mutants with a lipopolysaccharide (LPS) core and O antigen defects exhibit reduced viability after internalization by corneal epithelial cells, and a complete core LPS is required for full epithelial invasion (549). Despite effective antibacterial therapy, disease resolution can be delayed with respect to the time of bacterial eradication (550). Ofloxacin (mammalian cell penetrable) and tobramycin (less cell permeable) have been tested against invasive and noninvasive *P. aeruginosa* in a mouse model of keratitis. Topical ofloxacin and tobramycin, with or without prednisolone acetate, were administered hourly as eye drops for 12 hours postinfection. Tobramycin was less effective than ofloxacin against the invasive strain, but in the other groups, antibiotic treatment was effective against both strains. However, despite effective antibacterial treatment, disease progression continued in all groups, and differences in responses to treatment were not manifest until day 7 (550).

The rabbit keratitis model has been used to study antimicrobial treatment, in most cases by topical application of antimicrobial solutions, for infections caused by *Staphylococcus aureus*, both methicillin susceptible and resistant (551–560), *Staphylococcus epidermidis* (555), *P. aeruginosa* (559–564), *Serratia marcescens* (562,563), *Mycobacterium chelonae* (565,566), *C. albicans* (248), *Fusarium* sp (567,568), and *Acanthamoeba* sp (569). The following drug–pathogen combinations have been studied: MSSA and methicillin-susceptible *Staphylococcus epidermidis* (MSSE): cefazolin, vancomycin, tobramycin, chlorohexidine, benzalkonium, and a number of fluoroquinolones (ciprofloxacin,

ofloxacin, levofloxacin, moxifloxacin, gatifloxacin, gemifloxacin, and besifloxacin) (551–560); *P. aeruginosa*: gentamicin, tobramycin, ciprofloxacin, ofloxacin, moxifloxacin, levofloxacin, gatifloxacin, and chlorhexidine (559–564); *M. chelonae*: amikacin, clarithromycin, ciprofloxacin, levofloxacin, and gatifloxacin (565,566); *C. albicans*: amphotericin B, natamycin, and caspofungin (248); *Fusarium* sp: amphotericin B, caspofungi, itraconazole, and voriconazole (567,568); and for *Acanthamoeba* sp: chlorhexidine and neosporin (569). In general terms, most antimicrobials administered topically show effect in reducing pathogen CFUs significantly as compared to controls if the pathogens are susceptible to the drugs in vitro and doses are high enough. Furthermore, early treatment is better than late treatment (553). Even chlorhexidine showed effect against MRSA and *P. aeruginosa* (560).

Experimental Intraocular Infections

Several methods to obtain reproducible intraocular infections in laboratory animals have been described and many are modifications of the method discussed here (570). In this method, *S. aureus, E. coli,* or *P. aeruginosa* is inoculated into the center of the rabbit cornea, the anterior chamber, or the vitreous of the eye, and samples of the vitreous humor, irises, and anterior chamber as well as the retina are used to determine the progress of the infection. The authors (570) found that, when 3 $\times$ 10^6 CFU/0.2 mL of broth were inoculated into the corneas, anterior chamber, and vitreous of rabbit eyes, a virulent panophthalmitis was produced within 24 to 48 hours, and destruction of the eye took place within 72 hours regardless of the site of inoculation. When 5 $\times$ 10^3 CFU/0.2 mL were inoculated into the corneas, anterior chambers, and vitreous, a panophthalmitis resulted in 72 hours. The infections were most severe following intravitreal inoculations and less intense when the anterior chamber was the site of inoculation. When 7 $\times$ 10^2 CFU/0.02 mL were used as the inoculum, the infections were eliminated in the corneas and anterior chambers within 24 hours but not in the vitreous. The anterior chambers were most resistant, the cornea slightly less, and the vitreous the least resistant to virulent infection.

Infectious endophthalmitis is characterized by an inflammatory reaction in a sensitive, normally immune-privileged or protected tissue. Depletion of circulating neutrophils by i.v. administration of specific antibody at 6 or 12 hours after intravitreal injection of *S. aureus* into rats resulted in diminished neutrophil influx, lower and delayed clinical and histopathologic evidence of disease, but also a reduction in bacterial clearance from the eye (571). The inflammatory response appears to lag behind bacterial growth of either *S. epidermidis* or *P. aeruginosa*, for a maximum in the number of microorganisms was reached earlier than the influx of leukocytes (572). In *S. epidermidis* endophthalmitis, the number of microorganisms reached a maximum at day 2 after intraviteral inoculation and then declined spontaneously; clinical scores were the worst on day 5 but poor scores persisted in the absence of detectable bacteria. In *P. aeruginosa* endophthalmitis, the number of microorganisms reached a maximum 36 hours after inoculation, and bacteria were detectable for 15 days.

Ravindranath et al. (573) measured the immune response during endophthalmitis. Rats received an intravitreal injection of viable *S. epidermidis* that resolved by day 14. The inflammatory cell content of the vitreous switched from neutrophilic to monocytic-macrophagic/lymphocytic by day 3 postinfection. B cells (CD45+/CD3−) were also detected, and IgM and IgG antibodies but not IgA antibodies to glycerol teichoic acid were found in the vitreous of injected eyes; IgM antibodies declined by day 7 postinfection. Anti-GTA IgM was observed in vitreous and serum, anti-GTA IgM antibodies were significantly elevated, but a weak IgG response and no IgA response were observed in serum *S. epidermidis*–infected rats (573).

The use of adjunct antiinflammatory agents in endophthalmitis is controversial. Intravitreal vancomycin once plus 7 days of i.m. methylprednisolone was not as effective as vancomycin alone in reducing ocular inflammation and improving retinal function in experimental *S. aureus* endophthalmitis (574). Using a variety of antibiotics in an animal model of *S. aureus* endophthalmitis, researchers found that the combination of vitrectomy and injection of intraocular vancomycin was the most effective regimen and that no improvement resulted from administering adjunct i.v. corticosteroids (575). The timing of dexamethasone treatment appears to influence outcome (576). Bilateral eye *S. aureus* infection in rabbits was treated once with vancomycin in one eye and vancomycin plus dexamethasone in the other at 24, 36, 48, or 72 hours after intravitreal infection. Early combination treatment (at 24 or 36 hours) produced reduced ocular inflammation as compared with antibiotic alone, but only when treated at 36 hours postinfection did the combination group preserve retinal function better than vancomycin alone; no treatment was able to eradicate infection. However, dexamethasone has improved antibacterial and antifungal effect and reduced inflammation in several subsequent studies of endophthalmitis (577–582).

Many studies have evaluated the PK of antibiotics in eye tissue. PK modeling of antibiotic eye-blood barrier penetration data has been used to compare different formulations (583) and explain in part why eye penetration in rodents may overestimate antibiotic penetration due to the dependence of larger species on convective fluid flow (584). A single intravenous administration of 5 or 20 mg/kg moxifloxacin demonstrated good penetration into the vitreous, but apparently, the penetration was dose-independent and increased when inflammation was present (585). Microdialysis has been used to both measure drugs (e.g., ceftazidime [586] and vancomycin [587]) and dispense drugs (588). Inflammation or eye trauma appears to increase the penetration and residency of many topically applied antibiotics (e.g., levofloxacin [579], ofloxacin [589], ciprofloxacin [590], and vancomycin [575]), but apparently not ceftazidime, whose half-life is decreased by inflammation and eye surgery (575). A 1% vancomycin hydrochloride ophthalmic ointment was administered to the corners of the eyes of rabbits with *Bacillus subtilis* infection. Vancomycin reached effective concentrations in the aqueous humor and extraocular tissues but was not detected in the aqueous humor, iris-ciliary body, vitreous, or serum in uninfected animals; nonetheless, the presence of inflammation permitted concentrations to reach potentially therapeutic levels in these tissues (591).

Systemic treatment with moxifloxacin demonstrated effectiveness against MRSA and MSSA (585), as did treatment with trovafloxacin against *S. epidermidis* (592); this is somewhat surprising, as most antibiotics show poor ocular penetration. Despite inflamed eyes demonstrating improved penetration of i.v. gentamicin or amikacin, aminoglycoside levels in the eye failed to reach therapeutic concentrations sufficient for either *Pseudomonas* spp or *S. epidermidis* (593). However, systemic administration of sparfloxacin, pefloxacin, or imipenem (though not vancomycin or amikacin) was effective as a prophylaxis against intravitreal *S. aureus* challenge (594). Combined topical and oral ofloxacin (590) or ciprofloxacin (589) increased the ocular levels of the drug in a model of posttraumatic endophthalmitis due to

S. aureus infection (590). Topical treatment with liposomal formulation increased the half-life of fluconazole (595) but was inferior to free fluconazole in the treatment of *C. albicans* endophthalmitis (596; see also 597). Intravitreal treatment with vancomycin plus amikacin was effective against vancomycin-sensitive *E. faecalis*, and intravitreal ampicillin plus gentamicin was effective against vancomycin-resistant *E. faecalis* endophthalmitis (598). Gatifloxacin or ofloxacin ophthalmic ointments prevented *E. faecalis* endophthalmitis when administered 1-hour postinfection, but this effect decreased with application of antibiotics with longer intervals after infection (599). Intravitreal treatment has been shown to reduce pathogen counts significantly for vancomycin and moxifloxacin against *Bacillus cereus* (600), linezolid, vancomycin, imipenem, ceftazidime, amikacin, moxifloxacin, and other fluorquinolones against MSSA (601–603); levofloxacin, piperacillin/tazobactam, and ceftazidime against *P. aeruginosa* (604,605); tigecycline against *A. baumannii* (606); and amphotericin B and caspofungin but not itraconazole or voriconazole against *C. albicans* (243).

Animal Models of Osteomyelitis

Although of relatively low incidence, bone and joint infections are difficult to cure, largely due to limited penetration of antibiotics, coupled with the fact that slow-growing or adherent bacteria are likely to be more resistant to antibiotics. Furthermore, designing and executing clinical trials is difficult due to the likelihood of low recruitment, the heterogeneity of the disease, and the many hard-to-control factors influencing treatment outcome. Consequently, advances in clinical management have heavily relied on the contribution of animal models (607).

The experimental conditions for the rabbit model initially described by Norden (608,609) have recently been reviewed (610). In one study using this procedure, 89% or more of the animals developed osteomyelitis (608,609). The infecting organism was recovered from 91% of rabbits sacrificed 60 to 180 days after infection. If blood samples were taken 6 hours after infection, more than 80% were positive for the infecting organism, but by 24 hours, less than 20% were positive. Injection of a bacterial suspension or sodium morrhuate alone did not cause osteomyelitis, as evidenced by radiologic examination or culture of the bone. Antibacterial therapy was initiated

1 to 14 days after infection. Because the radiologic changes of chronic osteomyelitis were present at day 14, treatment at this time was considered to represent therapy of chronic osteomyelitis.

The rabbit model has also been used to study treatment of MRSA osteomyelitis with ceftaroline as compared to linezolid and vancomycin and tigecycline or vancomycin in combination with or without rifampicin (611).

The rat is another commonly used animal for osteomyelitis (612). This model is widely used for experimental chemotherapy, and the practical aspects of this model have been previously described (613). Occasionally overlooked, it is critical to culture at least some remaining crushed bone, initially in broth with subculture on agar plates, in order estimate bone sterility. Typically, single agents are weakly active, and combination chemotherapy generally produces superior results (614). More thorough determinations of PK/PD relationships for osteomyelitis are warranted. The rat tibia osteomyelitis model has been used to study the effect of fosfomycin (615) and tigecycline as compared to teicoplanin (616) against MRSA-induced infection, all drugs showing significant effect as compared to untreated controls.

These models have also been used to evaluate various drug delivery systems (e.g., a sulbactam-cefoperazone polyhydroxybutyrate-co-hydroxyvalerate depot formulation [617], several depot formulations [618], tobramycin pellets [619], tobramycin fibrin sealant [620], and anti-biotic-impregnated hydroxyapatite [621]), hyperbaric oxygen combined with antibiotics (622), and adjuvant treatment with granulocyte-macrophage colony-stimulating factor (GM-CSF) (623). Further, recent studies have used vancomycin-loaded borate glass or calcium sulfate (624), vancomycin-coated titanium plates (625), vancomycin or daptomycin-loaded beads (626), polyelectrolyte multilayers with gentamicin (627), biodegradable dilactide polymer releasing ciprofloxacin (628), a synthetic semihydrate form of calcium sulphate impregnated with moxifloxacin (629), gentamicin-vancomycin–impregnated polymethylmethacrylate (PMMA) coating nail (630), and calcium-deficient apatites with linezolid (631), in all cases with preventive effect on staphylococcal infections.

An interesting study performed by Nijhof et al. (632) demonstrated that combined tobramycin bone cement and systemic cefazolin was superior to monotherapies, suggesting that combining local and systemic treatments might be a useful approach to treatment of osteomyelitis. Furthermore, this study demonstrated the utility of measuring bacterial DNA, as persistence of DNA may occur despite effective treatment.

Osteomyelitis models with precontaminated (methicillin-susceptible or resistant *S. aureus* or *S. epidermidis*) foreign bodies inserted into the medulla of either tibia or femur of rabbits or rats have been used to study treatment effect with various systemically administered antibiotics or even electric current (633–636). Various treatment durations from 7 to 28 days were used, why comparisons among studies are difficult.

Animal Models of Mycobacterium Infections

Models of Disseminated *Mycobacterium avium* Infections

Models of disseminated *M. avium* infection have usually used beige mice (bearing an *Nramp1* mutation), although alternatives include C57BL/6 mice (637); hamsters (638); and immunosuppressed, cyclosporine-treated rats (approximately 0.03 mg cyclosporine/kg [639]). Reviews of the technical aspects of the beige mouse model of *M. avium* infection have been published (640,641).

Several details of the model have been described (e.g., the influence of the route of infection) (641,642). Infections are initiated by intravenous injection of large inocula (10^7 to 10^8 CFU). Although the disease is usually nonfatal, high numbers of *M. avium* are found in the liver, spleen, and lung, and determination of the efficacy of treatment is accomplished by ascertaining the organ bacteria loads. Furthermore, mild chronic CNS infection develops in the mice during sustained systemic *M. avium* infection, similar to what has been reported in most human cases. In one study, *M. avium* was detected initially in the parenchyma of the choroid plexus but also in the ventricles and meninges. However, the mice did not develop clinical signs nor did they die due to CNS involvement (643). Iron restriction inhibits the in vitro and intramacrophagic growth of *M. avium*, and mice fed an iron-poor diet experienced reduced *M. avium* proliferation; administration of iron chelators had small effects, as they impacted little on the iron status of mice (644).

In some studies, the beige mouse model demonstrated poor outcome against *M. avium* in the testing of marketed antibiotics (645). Note that in vitro tests do not always accurately predict in vivo susceptibility (646). Although previous reports indicated a benefit to infected mice, administration of recombinant G-CSF failed to improve the course of *M. avium* infection in C57Bl/6 or beige mice and did not enhance the activity of the combination of clarithromycin plus ethambutol plus rifabutin (647). A rather extensive combination of antimicrobials was tested by Fattorini et al. (648). The activity of 18 anti–*M. avium* regimens was evaluated. Mice were treated with clarithromycin, ethambutol, amikacin, rifabutin, ciprofloxacin, or clofazimine alone or in combination. Monotherapies were less effective than combinations, and resistant *M. avium* emerged. Some two-drug combinations were active, but none more than clarithromycin alone. The triple combination of clarithromycin, amikacin, and ethambutol was the most effective (648). Moxifloxacin is active against *M. avium* in combination with other agents (649).

Animal Models of *Mycobacterium tuberculosis* Infections

Animal models have been used to model tuberculosis since Robert Koch started his pioneering work on the infecting pathogen, *M. tuberculosis*. The use of *M. tuberculosis*–infected animals for testing antituberculosis drugs date back to the start of the 19th century, but have gained broad and increased importance in later years due to better understanding of the PK/PD of available drugs as well as for testing a range of novel drugs or other treatment strategies in the era of multi- of pan-resistant *M. tuberculosis* (650). In 2012, a group of experts, funded by the Bill and Melinda Gates Foundation, published a comprehensive review on the analysis of methods used for the evaluation of compounds against *M. tuberculosis* (651). In addition to in vitro methods, the review presents a detailed discussion of the available animal models based on the literature as well as personal visits and interviews with most of the pharmaceutical and academic investigators working with these models. This review is highly recommended for both the interested infectious disease specialist as well as the researcher who intends to embark on an animal model for the study of treatment of experimental tuberculosis (651). The availability of this review also precludes the need for a detailed review of animal tuberculosis models in this book. In short, although a range of animals have been used for experimental tuberculosis including non-human primates, guinea pigs, hamsters, rabbits, rats, and mice, the guinea pig as the historic model for *M. tuberculosis* infections has largely been supplanted by mice (in- and outbred) models which

now remain the most commonly used (651). Among the many explanations for its popularity are small size, ease of handling, low prize, small volumes only needed for expensive drugs, ease of inoculation, similarity to humans of pulmonary infection induced and proven predictability of treatment of human infections. On the negative side are factors such as variability in response to infection and tolerance to drugs of different mouse strains, PK behavior of drugs different from humans, and many others. Further adding to problems with animal tuberculosis models are major differences in virulence of and host response to the *M. tuberculosis* strains generally used for animal studies, size (1 to 4 aerosolized bacilli up to 10^6 CFU installed intratracheally) and route of inoculum (inhalation, intratracheal installation, nasal application, intravenous injection), type of infectious processes occurring in lungs and other organs (extra- or intracellular bacteria, silent or latent infection, biofilm), relapse, re- or superinfection, etc. The review called for standardization and comparison among models which has already resulted in published studies on these issues (652). Most of the discussion on the earlier mentioned issues is extremely relevant and pertinent for all animal models discussed in this chapter, why the review is recommended reading for all scientists working with experimental animal models.

Animal Models of Sexually Transmitted Diseases

Animal models of human sexually transmitted infections (STIs) can be problematic owing to high-level specificity many of the STI pathogens display for a human host. Despite this, a number of models have been successfully developed. In some cases, investigators have used a microbial species that is distinct from that which causes human disease but is related and specific for the urogenital tract of the animal model used.

Disseminated Gonococcal Infection in Mice

Mice were traditionally considered resistant to disseminated gonococcal infection (653) despite some initial descriptions by Corbeil and colleagues (654). Many early studies used an infection route with subcutaneous chambers to study pathogenicity and therapeutic effects of antimicrobial therapy (655–658). However, more recently, a murine model has been developed and used by a number of investigators (659,660). Mice are made susceptible to colonization and infection with *Neisseria gonorrhoeae* via the combination of pretreatment with antibiotics (e.g., vancomycin and TMP-sulfa) and estradiol (659,661). A recent interesting finding was a functioning MtrCDE multidrug efflux system enhanced experimental genital tract infection in female mice (662). This discovery has led to additional studies on delineating the genetic mechanisms of regulating expression for the efflux system and its effect on in vivo fitness (663,664). The model has also been used recently to examine the effects of fluoroquinolone resistance mutation development and associated compensatory mutations to restore wild-type fitness (665).

Syphilis

Animal models examining antimicrobial efficacy in syphilis have been developed for localized disease (i.e., dermal), genitourinary tract disease, CNS/disseminated disease, and congenital disease. Most models use rabbits as the animal host; however, a model in the hamster has also been well described (666).

Localized dermal infection models were the first to be developed in rabbits. Localized infection is induced by intradermal injection of live spirochetes. Antimicrobial therapy is usually withheld until signs of an active syphilitic lesion are present and confirmed by dark-field microscopic analysis of a skin scraping. Once active infection is confirmed, antimicrobial therapy is administered to the rabbits. Representative examples of the use of this protocol to test antimicrobial efficacy for localized disease includes study of penicillin G (667), aztreonam (668), cefetamet (669), cefmetazole (670), an investigational penem (667), ceftriaxone (671), and azithromycin (672). A similar hamster model of intradermal infection has been employed for study of clarithromycin efficacy (673).

Genitourinary tract disease models have primarily been limited to orchitis infection models. In this model, the rabbits receive an inoculum of syphilis spirochetes directly into the testes. It has been used on a limited basis to determine drug efficacy, with encouraging results from a study of ceftriaxone, ceftizoxime, and penicillin G (674,675).

Disseminated disease can be induced by intravenous or intraperitoneal inoculation, although there has been limited use of this model for examining antimicrobial therapy (667). More commonly disseminated disease that includes CNS infection is used. CNS infection with syphilis can be achieved by direct intracisternal injection of *Treponema pallidum*. Marra and colleagues (676)

used this procedure to develop a rabbit model of CNS syphilis that very closely mimicked human disease including a 6% rate of uveitis in the animal model (676). A year later, the same group of authors demonstrated enhanced efficacy for penicillin G versus ceftriaxone in the rabbit model (677). The model has also been used to examine whether certain strains of *T. pallidum* exhibit increased neuroinvasion (678).

Finally, congenital syphilis has been described in a rabbit and hamster model (679–681). However, antimicrobial therapy in congenital syphilis models has not been well explored.

Chlamydia Genital Tract Infections

Chlamydia trachomatis is a major cause of STI worldwide and remains the most common STI in the United States. Despite its long history and medical importance, attempts at developing an animal model have proved difficult (682). Reproducible establishment of infection of the upper genital tract in female mice with human isolates of *C. trachomatis* requires hormonal manipulation, inbred animals, and surgical intervention to place the organisms directly into the site (i.e., to produce salpingitis) (683). However, in 1994, Beale and Upshon (683) developed a novel upper genital tract infection model in mice. They used *C. trachomatis* MoPN (primarily a mouse respiratory pathogen) and were able to demonstrate upper genital tract disease in progesterone-treated mice administered the inoculum by intravaginal injection. Treatment studies with minocycline, doxycycline, amoxicillin-clavulanate, and azithromycin each demonstrated efficacy when initiated 1 or 7 days postinfection. Both doxycycline and azithromycin were highly effective in restoring animal fertility. A study of azithromycin efficacy in female mice demonstrated the antimicrobial agent could reverse chlamydial-induced damage and restore fertility if administered within 2 or 7 days of infection (684). Conversely, if administered 12 or more days after infection, even at very high doses, antimicrobial therapy failed to prevent infertility. A male murine model of genital tract disease caused by *C. trachomatis* MoPN has also been described (685) that also closely mimics disease in human males. However, evaluation of antimicrobial therapy in this model has not been performed. Another strategy to circumvent problems with establishing genital tract disease with human isolates of *C. trachomatis* is to utilize a microbial species that does cause intrinsic genital tract infection in the animal host. This has been accomplished using the isolate *Chlamydia muridarum* to infect the urogenital tract of mice (686–691) and *Chlamydophila caviae* in guinea pigs (692–694).

Animal Models of Peritonitis

Peritonitis can be established in animals either by direct intraperitoneal infection of fecal material (often encased in gelatin capsules) or by puncture of the cecum to provide a focus of infection. These models have been reviewed previously (695).

Intraperitoneal Inoculation

A rat model for simulating intraabdominal sepsis, either with known organisms or with mixed fecal flora cultures, has been developed by Weinstein et al. (696). A uniform inoculum was prepared from the pooled cecal and large bowel contents of 15 rats that had been maintained on a diet of lean ground meat and water for 2 weeks. The value of this mixed infection model for evaluating agents for effectiveness in preventing mortality and the formation of intraabdominal abscesses was confirmed as follows. A clindamycin–gentamicin combination reduced mortality rates and the formation of the abscesses, whereas either drug alone reduced mortality rates (gentamicin) or abscess formation (clindamycin) but not both (696).

Cecal Ligation and Puncture

The cecal ligation and puncture (CLP) model has been described for both mice (697), rats (698), and rabbits (699). The description given by Hyde et al. (700) is typical of this approach to induction of lethal peritonitis in animals as a model of postsurgical sepsis. By measurement of bacterial counts in peritoneum, blood, and various organs, as well as antigens and immunologic factors in peritoneum and blood (LPS, TNF-α, ILs, etc.), the model has been used to study pathogenicity and effect of antimicrobial agents and biologic response modifiers (701). Combination immunotherapy with soluble tumor necrosis factor receptors plus IL-1 receptor antagonist decreases mortality in the CLP model (702). Similarly, a range of different antimicrobial peptides (tachyplesin III, pexiganan, cathelicidine [LL-37], S-thanatin, tritrpticin, indolicidin) have been shown to both have antibacterial effect in vivo as well as reducing unwanted immunologic responses, and these effects have shown reduced mortality when combining with various antibiotics (703–708).

However, the cautionary suggestions by Eichaker and associates (23) need to be heeded when using this model, as it is apparent that more severe sepsis, which is usual for the model, benefits best from chemotherapeutic intervention but may not represent a typical clinical presentation.

The CLP model has been used to evaluate some parameters concerning the differential sensitivity of internal organs to damage during sepsis (709). Increases in microcirculatory permeability were greater in the lung than in the liver 12 hours after CLP, and increases in water mass fraction were greater and occurred earlier in the lung than in the liver. The CLP model has been used to evaluate cardiovascular responses during sepsis characterized by an early hyperdynamic phase followed by a late hypodynamic phase (710). Mice made septic by CLP demonstrated hypotension and a hyperdynamic state that could be monitored using manometric catheters and echocardiography and could be modulated with fluid resuscitation and antibiotics (711).

The administration of the antioxidant phenyl N-tert-butyl nitrone (PBN) (150 mg/kg 30 minutes after CLP), followed by the antibiotic imipenem (10 mg/kg 1 hour after CLP), significantly increased survival compared with other single treatment groups. However, the increase in survival found in the PBN plus imipenem-treated group was abrogated by anti–IL-10 antibody, indicating that endogenous IL-10 is an effective protective factor (712).

Animal Models of Infected Abscesses

The technical aspects of intraabdominal abscess models have been presented previously (713). As an example of the formation of abscesses by anaerobes, a model of subcutaneous abscesses in mice caused by *Bacteroides fragilis* has been described (714). Among the advantages of this model are that host factors involved in abscess formation can be studied and that the PK properties of the antimicrobial agents, especially penetration of the abscess, can be assessed. Both the inoculum size and the time of treatment significantly altered the effectiveness of both clindamycin and cefoxitin. In a larger experiment, the rank order of antibiotic efficacy could clearly be determined and related to the peak levels of antimicrobials in serum and abscesses (714).

A model of intraperitoneal abscess formation by *S. aureus* has been described (715).

Animal Models of Gastrointestinal Infections

As with sexually transmitted diseases, animal models of gastrointestinal tract infections are hampered because of the apparent specificity of the causative pathogens for humans, particularly in the case of *Helicobacter* infections.

Clostridium difficile Enterocolitis

Diarrhea following antibiotic chemotherapy can be caused by *Clostridium difficile* and is referred to as *pseudomembranous colitis* or *antibiotic-associated colitis* (716). Proliferation of *C. difficile* following suppression of normal gastrointestinal flora results in an enteric intoxication owing to the release of exotoxins TcdA and TcdB from *C. difficile*. Current standard treatments include vancomycin (125 to 200 mg/kg orally four times per day) or metronidazole (250 to 500 mg/kg orally four times per day) (717). *C. difficile* infection has been studied in a number of animal models, including hamsters, guinea pigs, rabbits, germ-free piglets, germ-free mice, and conventional mice (718–723).

Inoculation of experimental animals can be done either with spore preparations via the oral route or direct instillation into the colon, or by instillation of toxin preparations into the lumen of the colon. Typically, antibiotics (e.g., mixtures of aminoglycosides, colistin, metronidazole, and vancomycin) are administered prior to inoculation in order to change the intestinal flora, which renders the animals more susceptible to *C. difficile* infection.

Golden Syrian hamsters are widely used to model this disease because they have the causative organism as part of their normal flora, are known to succumb to antibiotic-induced colitis (724,725), and are sensitive to the activity of *C. difficile* toxins (726). Typically, clindamycin (0.8 to 100 mg/kg intraperitoneally or subcutaneously once) is administered, and death attributed to *C. difficile* (by virtue of culture and detection of toxins) ensues rapidly (up to 100% mortality within 1 week), though it is dependent on the clindamycin dose. Modifications of this model include the orogastric infection of clindamycin-treated hamsters with axenic *C. difficile* (4×10^5 spores/clindamycin-treated hamster [727]). Modulation of the diet of hamsters can alter the extent of *C. difficile* disease. As compared with hamsters fed a normal fat and cholesterol diet, hamsters fed an atherogenic (defined high-fat) diet have increased susceptibility to *C. difficile* (728).

Peptidic antibiotics (e.g., vancomycin) appear to be efficacious in this model, but most must be given continuously because regrowth of *C. difficile* occurs following cessation of treatment (729). Following p.o. clindamycin treatment and inoculation with a toxigenic *C. difficile* strain, hamsters developed *C. difficile*–associated ileocecitis and 3 days later were treated with intragastric nitazoxanide (30 to 150 mg/kg), vancomycin (50 mg/kg), or metronidazole (150 mg/kg). All three compounds inhibited the appearance of *C. difficile* gastroenteritis symptoms, but upon treatment cessation, the hamsters relapsed, indicating failure to eradicate *C. difficile*. In a prophylactic mode, only nitazoxanide produced hamsters free of clinical symptoms, histopathology, or residual bacteria (730). *C. difficile* is affected in vitro by sub-MIC levels of antibiotics that establish conditions that precipitate disease (e.g., amoxicillin, clindamycin, cefoxitin, and ceftriaxone) and those antibiotics used for treatment of established infection (vancomycin and metronidazole). The sub-MIC effects are, however, complex, strain-dependent and affect both bacterial growth (increasing lag time and overall growth rate) and the timing of initiation of toxin production (faster initiation of production). These effects were observed with clindamycin, metronidazole, and amoxicillin, rarely with vancomycin, and never with cefoxitin (731). However, the in vivo significance of the sub-MIC effects remains to be determined.

The hamster model has been criticized for being too sensitive to *C. difficile* developing clinical signs of disease already after 2 to 3 days and thereafter showing high mortality with death in a few days (732). Mice models have gained increasing interest due to more closely resembling the disease seen in humans (733). Although true relapses do not occur in hamsters due to the acute infection, a relapse model has been developed in conventional mice (733). Using the mouse models, several investigators have shown that vancomycin treatment only delays disease occurrence, while, for example, antibodies against the two exotoxins do protect animals against relapse (733,735). One of the reasons for the missing posttreatment effect of vancomycin is its lack of activity against *C. difficile* spores (736). Other glycol- or lipopeptides such as ramoplanin or oritavancin do not appear to induce germination of *C. difficile* (736,737). The mouse model has also shown the importance of antibiotic-induced reduction of the anaerobic gram-negative flora for promoting colonization and infection with *C. difficile* (738,739).

Models of *Helicobacter* Gastric Infection

The association of *Helicobacter pylori* with gastric ulcers and gastritis has dramatically altered approaches to gastroduodenal disease to now include antimicrobial chemotherapy as a therapeutic modality (740). Normal laboratory animals apparently are difficult to colonize with *H. pylori* but are more susceptible to the related species *Helicobacter felis* and *Helicobacter mustelae*. Development of a suitable animal model has delayed evaluation of novel antibacterial strategies because in vitro antimicrobial susceptibility is apparently not consistently predictive of in vivo efficacy (740). Some models have used predisposition of the animals with acetic acid to induce a gastric ulcer, followed by orogastric inoculation; *H. pylori* is capable of efficiently colonizing these heavily damaged areas. Marchetti et al. (741) presented evidence suggesting that passage of clinical *H. pylori* isolates in the gastrointestinal tracts of mice selects for those bacteria with increased colonizing ability while maintaining several of the features of the disease in humans.

Various models have demonstrated that combination chemotherapy is more effective than monotherapy in eradicating *Helicobacter* organisms from gastric tissues. Except for treatment with metronidazole, monotherapy and dual therapies involving amoxicillin, bismuth subcitrate, and clarithromycin (with or without the proton pump inhibitor omeprazole) did not cure mice bearing *H. pylori* Sydney strain gastric infection (742). The triple therapies of OMC (omeprazole, metronidazole, clarithromycin) and BMT (bismuth subcitrate, metronidazole, tetracycline) were more successful in eradicating infection. However, these treatments also produced a different pattern of stomach colonization, suggesting the antrum-body transitional zone is a "sanctuary site" harboring *H. pylori* in cases of treatment failure. The authors concluded that there was good correlation between the Sydney strain mouse model and antibiotic therapy outcome in humans (except for metronidazole monotherapy and OAC triple therapy).

Combination treatments involving proton pump inhibitors or antiulcer agents have been evaluated in animal models. The apparent synergic anti–*H. pylori* effects of the proton pump inhibitor lansoprazole are apparently due to enhanced penetration of orally administered amoxicillin in gastric mucus and tissue by lansoprazole-produced increased intragastric pH. Supplemental treatment of rats with clarithromycin did not affect this drug interaction (743). Using a C57BL/6 mouse model, the cytoprotective antiulcer agent plaunotol was shown to enhance the activity of clarithromycin or amoxicillin in the treatment of *H. pylori* infection (744). In the same model hyperimmune bovine colostrum with N-acetylcysteine and zinc in combination with amoxicillin in high-dose eradicated *H. pylori* in all mice treated for 10 days (745).

Animal Models for Determining the Effect of Age on Susceptibility to Infection

Host susceptibility and response to infection change dramatically based on age. It has been well established that very young (i.e., neonates) and elderly humans are more susceptible to certain infectious diseases, and this can often be attributed to changes in immune function at the extremes of age. Neonatal animal models have been established to study common infectious diseases noted in this group including GBS infection (746,747), staphylococcal infection (748–751), and invasive candidiasis (287,751). A limited number of these studies also included an evaluation of antimicrobial therapy. Conversely, advanced age animal models have focused primarily on specific immune function such as studying innate immune responses (e.g., cytokine response and neutrophil function) as well as adaptive immune responses (e.g., T- and B-cell specific responses). For example, Boyd and colleagues (692) studied the toll-like receptor (TLR)-2 responses in mature and aged mice infected with pneumococcal pneumonia. In a previous study, they demonstrated senescent mice were more susceptible to pneumococcal pneumonia through potential priming effect of chronic inflammation and TLR dysfunction (60). In a more recent study, they were able to show that aged macrophages exhibit impaired TLR-2–dependent recognition of pneumococcus and this was associated with a delayed proinflammatory cytokine response in vivo along with enhanced susceptibility to pneumococcal pneumonia. Other common infections noted in elderly humans have also been modeled in aged animals including bacterial peritonitis, intraabdominal abscess and sepsis via cecal ligation, invasive candidiasis, and *C. difficile* (752–756). Unfortunately, while susceptibility to infection has been examined in aged animal models, study of antimicrobial efficacy in these models has been limited.

TOLERABILITY OF ANTIBIOTICS IN LABORATORY ANIMALS

In comparison with other disease areas (e.g., cancer), antiinfectives are generally exceedingly well tolerated within a wide therapeutic window (the difference between the dosage required for maximal desired pharmacologic effect and the dosage at which unwanted effects become apparent). This is likely in part due to the drug substance being directed to targets unique to microorganisms or distinct from mammalian counterparts. Preclinical in vitro and in vivo toxicity/tolerability testing of novel antibiotics is required prior to initiating clinical trials (757), and although this will reveal toxic effects, they generally occur at doses far in excess of those required for efficacy studies in animal models. There are five main types of toxicity associated with antimicrobials (758): direct effects, where the molecule acts against the host tissues (e.g., anemia caused by chloramphenicol is inhibition of mitochondrial protein synthesis); hypersensitivity, which can include allergic responses (e.g., anaphylactic reaction) or other nonallergic reactions such as diarrhea; disorders resulting from antibiotic-produced changes in bacterial flora (e.g., vaginal yeast infections); drug interactions, where coadministered drugs interact deleteriously together (e.g., ketoconazole interference with cytochrome P450–mediated drug metabolism); and microbial lysis, with the associated massive release of proinflammatory bacterial products that can cause widespread tissue damage, as occurs in bacterial meningitis.

An excellent overview of the use and tolerability of some older (but still clinically used) antibiotics in laboratory animals has been prepared by Morris (759). Experience has indicated that guinea pigs and, to a lesser extent, rabbits tolerate antibiotic treatment much less well than mice or rats. There are species and strain differences in tolerability to antibiotics (760). Strain is critical to the tolerance of certain compounds; for example, tobramycin is more toxic to Fischer rats than to Sprague-Dawley rats (759). Mice show strain differences in susceptibility to the toxic effects of chloramphenicol (761). Qualitative and quantitative strain differences were observed in the hematologic response to chloramphenicol succinate (500 to 2,500 mg/kg administered orally for 7 days). When administered to several inbred mice strains (C3H/He, CBA/Ca, BALB/c, and C57BL/6) and one outbred strain (CD-1), the inbred strains were more susceptible to the toxic effects and produced more variable results. Only the inbred strain developed leukopenia, despite the fact that all strains displayed reticulocytopenia and anemia. The toxicity of chloramphenicol is apparently due to minor metabolites, which may vary due to subtle differences in the metabolism of chloramphenicol, and the levels of antioxidants (e.g., glutathione and vitamin E) may account in part for the differences in tolerability (762).

In a broad sense, animals tolerate drugs better than humans, and in most efficacy studies, tolerability issues are not revealed; often relevant effects are simply not observed by the experimenter or the study plan does not facilitate their being observed. This may partly be due to inherent physiologic properties of the animal that result in faster elimination of the compound (or deleterious metabolites) from the body, generally short treatment courses because of the fulminant nature of the infection, and the masking of tolerability problems by the symptoms of the infection. Additionally, the psychobehavioral nature of the animal may mask the toxicity of the antibiotic. Anatomic and physiologic differences—for example, differences in the gastrointestinal tract resulting in different degrees of exposure, rates of absorption and total fraction of drug absorbed, and drug transit time—may affect tolerability as well as efficacy (763). Antibiotic treatment of rats will change the gastrointestinal bacterial flora and/or composition of the feces but may have little effect on transit time (764). Due to their coprophilic nature, antibiotic treatment of pregnant rats and the resultant changes in intestinal microflora lead to abnormal gastrointestinal flora in suckling rats along with the establishment of potential pathogens in the gastrointestinal tract (765); the same study also found that antibiotic treatment had less impact on skin and vaginal microflora than on gastrointestinal tract microflora (765).

The nephrotoxicity of antiinfectives in animals is often the result of proximal tubule damage, which is related to its relative size and the drug concentration-time profile, the latter being the sum of the effects of drug movement across the lumen and the contraluminal secretory transport processes (766). These processes can be profoundly different in different species. Enhanced renal excretion by rats with streptozotocin-induced diabetes reduces cephaloridine renal toxicity due to higher renal excretion rates (producing lower kidney cephaloridine levels) than normal rats (767); serum PK profiles were similar.

Macrolides possess potential arrhythmogenic properties. The PKS/PDS of the prolongation of the Q-T interval by clarithromycin, roxithromycin, erythromycin, and azithromycin has been determined from electrocardiograms (ECGs) in rats (768). Compounds were administered by infusion in order to override the different PK properties of these compounds and produce controlled serum levels. The data for clarithromycin and erythromycin fit an E_{max} model, whereas the data for roxithromycin and azithromycin fit better a linear model. The order of potency of the compounds was erythromycin > clarithromycin > azithromycin > roxithromycin. Futher, the Q-T–prolonging activity of erythromycin and clarithromycin occurred at serum concentrations required for antibacterial effect, whereas such activity occurred only at supraantibacterial levels for azithromycin and roxithromycin.

Norfloxacin was also tested for CNS effects in rats. The PK/PD profile was monitored using an electroencephalogram (EEG) in order to arrive at a PK/PD relationship for norfloxacin (769). Rats received 5 mg/kg norfloxacin over 30 minutes, and the EEG demonstrated a pattern suggestive of eliptogenic potential; in addition, PK/PD modeling indicated that longer diffusion times have a greater eliptogenic potential (769).

Many factors contribute to the tolerability of animals to antimicrobial agents (759). Age, which affects metabolic enzymes and renal function, is another factor. Given that most laboratory animals are nocturnal, time-related functions, such as metabolic rates, food and water intake, and sleep time/activity, may also alter the tolerability (and effectiveness) of antibiotics; for example, exercise can alter the PK profile of mice. The single most important mechanism of antibiotic toxicity in small animals is disruption of the normal bacterial flora. In guinea pigs and hamsters, antibiotic toxicity leading to death is very often due to overgrowth of *C. difficile* and consequent toxin release (759), although *L. monocytogenes*, *Clostridium perfringens*, and *Clostridium spiroforme* have all been implicated as mediators of toxicity. Induction of overgrowth appears to be most prominent with some macrolides, notably clindamycin and lincomycin. Allergic reactions sensu stricto do not readily occur in lab animals, and the typical "allergic response" of guinea pigs to penicillin is likely due to enteric overgrowth. Newborn and germ-free guinea pigs are not susceptible to enterocolitis, suggesting the lack of a true allergic response (759). This may also be the case with many of the antibiotics given to laboratory animals.

Commonly, tolerability to compounds is reported without data presentation. Occasionally, some objective measure of tolerability is included. For example, Van Etten et al. (770) reported the maximally tolerated dose of amphotericin B in different formulations and determined renal and liver toxicity based on blood chemistry measurements. Additionally, in rats with subcutaneous staphylococcal abscesses, daptomycin was superior to vancomycin in treating both MSSA and MRSA. No detectable renal damage was elicited by daptomycin. The combination of daptomycin and tobramycin produced less renal injury (as determined by function tests and histology) than tobramycin alone (771). Rarely has observation of the extent of well-being of the experimental animal (i.e., the sum of illness due to infection, toxicity due to the drug substance, and relief from symptoms of infection due to antimicrobial effect) been included in the study design. Radiotelemetry was used to monitor a panel of physiologic indices to devise a "sickness behavior" index, which was then applied by Bauhofer et al. (772,773) to monitor the response to antibiotics with or without G-CSF in parallel with more classic indicators of the CLP model such as fever and mortality. Their study indicated a mild improvement from combined treatment over antibiotics alone, prompting their suggestion that the sickness behavior index could serve as the equivalent of a human quality-of-life index.

DETERMINATION OF THE IN VIVO POSTANTIBIOTIC EFFECT

PD parameters such as the rate of bactericidal activity with increasing drug concentrations, the PAE, sub-MIC effects, postantibiotic leukocyte enhancement, and the first-exposure effect more accurately describe the time course of antimicrobial activity than the MIC and MBC (62). The PAE is the persistent inhibition of bacterial growth after a brief exposure to an antibiotic. Most easily demonstrated in the in vitro systems, this effect is observable in vivo (104,774–782), although it is complicated by compounding sub-MIC effects (e.g., the postantibiotic sub-MIC effect [PASME]; 783–785) and by the enhancement of the phagocytic activity of leukocytes that occurs during the PAE phase and is partially due to sub-MIC effects on bacteria; this effect is termed the postantibiotic leukocyte effect (PALE) (e.g., aminoglycosides and quinolones demonstrate a longer in vivo PAE in the presence of neutrophils [104,774,775]).

The PAE may be nonexistent or of varying duration depending on the compound class and target bacterium (62,774). Typically, β-lactams and cephalosporins produce a substantial PAE against streptococci, but a small PAE or none at all against gram-negative bacteria, although there are exceptions (e.g., imipenem against *P. aeruginosa*) (786). Nucleic acid synthesis inhibitors and protein synthesis inhibitors (notably the aminoglycosides) produce an in vivo PAE with many bacteria (e.g., streptococci and gram-negatives). An in vivo PAE occurs with staphylococci treated with many different antibiotics. Furthermore, the use of humanlike PK prolongs the duration of the PAE in vivo. Indeed, the expected duration of the PAE (in combination with sub-MIC effects or the PALE) can be incorporated into estimates of clinical treatment regimens (46,104,787). However, Fantin et al. (776) found neither the duration of the PAE in vitro nor the MIC nor bactericidal activity in vivo correlated with the duration of the in vivo PAE.

The following are critical for defining the presence and duration of a PAE: the specific microorganism–antimicrobial combination, the antimicrobial combination and the experimental conditions, including the antimicrobial concentration and the length of the antimicrobial exposure (788,789). The PAE is probably also affected by the density of bacteria, their growth rate and metabolic activity, and the extent of inflammation at the site of infection (230). Proposed mechanisms by which the PAE occurs include both nonlethal damage induced by the antimicrobial agent and a limited persistence of the antimicrobial agent at the bacterial binding site (788).

Determination of the PAE in vivo is complicated by sub-MIC effects on the bacteria, which can suppress growth and have other physiologic effects that contribute to a composite PAE in vivo (785). The PASME is the growth suppression that may occur when a low concentration of antibiotic (typically ≤0.3 × MIC) is in the presence of bacteria previously exposed to a suprainhibitory concentration. As low levels of antibiotic are likely still at the infection site at the time of the next treatment, the PASME probably reflects the in vivo situation more closely than the PAE (62,774).

Taken together, dissection of the various components of the protracted effects of drug near the end of the treatment interval, where drug levels fall to the sub-MIC level of activity and then fall still further to the "true" postantibiotic level, is complicated.

Required groups include immunocompromised (leukopenic) and immunocompetent animals (to control for the PALE), PK measurements of bloodstream and infected tissue (to determine the duration of the sub-MIC levels and identify the initiation of the true PAE phase) in both groups of animals (to control for the influence of neutrophil influx on PK properties), and perhaps a group treated with an antibiotic-inactivating enzyme to further control for sub-MIC effects. Furthermore, groups treated with antibiotic producing a humanlike PK profile would be desirable. With so many groups being followed over time, the mouse thigh infection model is most frequently used for determination of the PAE.

The capability of producing a long PAE facilitates therapy using those antibiotics (e.g., aminoglycosides) to be administered infrequently, and continuous or frequent administration is required for those compounds that lack an in vivo PAE (e.g., β-lactams) (789). Extending the dosing interval of an antimicrobial agent that has a PAE has several potential advantages, among them reduced cost, less toxicity, and better compliance among outpatients receiving antimicrobial therapy (62,66,774).

IMPACT OF PRETREATMENT INTERVAL ON ANTIMICROBIAL EFFICACY

It is fairly well established that severity of clinical infection, usually associated with a delay in presentation or diagnosis, is related to treatment failure, particularly in the case of neutropenic patients (791,792). Delay in beginning antimicrobial therapy, and hence, progression of infection, has been demonstrated to have profound effects on the outcome of antibiotic treatment of experimental infections; however, this issue has not yet been thoroughly studied.

Using the thigh infection model in both leukopenic and normal mice, Gerber et al. (793) found that the age of infection had a profound influence on the outcome of antibacterial therapy of *P. aeruginosa* infection using gentamicin, ticarcillin, and ceftazidime.

Several factors were proposed to account for these observations:

- Alteration of the physiology of the bacteria (e.g., alteration to nongrowing or slowly growing phenotypes typically more resistant to antibiotics or production of an extracellular matrix inhibitory to antibiotics). Note, however, that in the study by Gerber et al. (793), *P. aeruginosa* grew at a constant rate during the entire infection, and therefore, slow growth cannot be the only contributing factor.

■ The presence of an in vivo correlate of the inoculum effect observed in vitro. In this case, bacteria within clusters or microcolonies may be protected from the effects of antibiotics or antibiotics may poorly penetrate these foci.

■ Pathophysiology at the site of the lesion, resulting in reduction of the activity of antibiotics. For example, low pH and low oxygen at the infected site are nonoptimal for aminoglycosides, and there is reduced penetration of antibiotics in large cardiac vegetations in advanced endocarditis (794).

The effect of delay in treatment of experimental pneumonia due to *S. pneumoniae* with temafloxacin was studied in a mouse model (795). Whereas initiation of doxycycline (1.5 mg/kg intraperitoneally once) at 4 hours postinfection with anthrax spores in mice was effective (90% survival), initiation of treatment at 24 and 48 hours had no substantial effect on mortality rates, although the onset of death was delayed to 4 days in the 24-hour treatment group and to 2 to 3 days in the 48-hour treatment group and the control group (796). As death from anthrax infection occurs due to toxin production, it is not surprising that a delay in treatment initiation past a threshold point would have a very small impact on outcome.

IMAGING TECHNIQUES USED FOR THE EVALUATION OF EXPERIMENTAL INFECTIONS

Noninvasive imaging encompasses a rapidly developing palette of techniques that are continuing to set new standards for clinical diagnosis and disease monitoring. However, such techniques are only slowly becoming established for use in experimental animals and in particular models of infection (797–799); a general review of imaging techniques specifically for application in small animals has been published (800). An obvious advantage of the use of noninvasive imaging in animal models is the possibility of a direct comparison of response in animals with that of human patients. As compared with human and human systems, animals require machines with increased resolution before particular techniques can be used really successfully.

Imaging of the Host's Response to Infection

Many imaging techniques are available to noninvasively monitor disease states and their response to therapy. Difficulty in accessing the required equipment and designing of animal-specific imaging systems has perhaps hampered the use of these approaches. Access to specialized reagents may also be limiting (e.g., ^{18}F for use in PET imaging has a short half-life). Labeled cytokines have found use in a variety of imaging techniques for monitoring different leukocyte subsets in vivo during infection (801).

Magnetic Resonance Imaging

Using magnetic resonance imaging (MRI) and magnetic resonance spectroscopy (MRS), histopathology and segmentation maps were obtained by the mathematical processing of three-dimensional T2-weighted MRI data via a neural network. The MRI patterns varied according to the nature and extent of infection with *A. fumigatus*. The MRS results show a statistically significant increase in inorganic phosphate and a significant decrease in phosphocreatine levels in the inflamed region (802). MRI along with contrast agent gadolinium-diethylene-triamine-pentaacetic acid was used to monitor the transient modulation of the blood–brain barrier following intravenous injection of bacterial glycopeptides (803).

The *S. aureus* thigh infection model, including treatment with vancomycin and imipenem/cilastatin, showed that MRI images closely paralleled histologic changes occurring as the infection progressed or resolved with antibiotic therapy (804). Therefore, this noninvasive procedure could be used repeatedly on an individual animal to monitor at least some aspects of antimicrobial chemotherapy. Experimental *S. aureus* osteomyelitis in New Zealand white rabbits was examined by MRI, computed tomography (CT), and plain film radiography (PF). MRI detected periostitis despite the absence of periosteal ossification and was more sensitive than CT or PF (805).

Positron Emisson Tomography

Positron emisson tomography (PET) can be used for PK studies as long as the compound can be synthesized to contain the short-lived isotopes used in PET (806,807). In an elegant study of the dynamics of tubercle lesions in the rabbit lungs and effect of antituberculosis treatment PET was used to illustrate the lesions as well as quantify the development during antibiotic treatment (808).

Computed Tomography

Contrast material–enhanced CT and MRI were used on rabbits with osteomyelitic *S. aureus* lesions, and the detection rates were similar (809). Three-phase technetium-99m methylene diphosphonate gallium-67 MRI images were obtained from New Zealand rabbits with *S. aureus* osteomyelitis (810). There was no significant difference between radionuclide studies and MRI images in the detection of osteomyelitis, but MRI was significantly more sensitive in the detection of soft tissue infection, including cellulitis and abscesses. Arthritic knee joints of rabbits have been monitored using CT. The use of the perfluorocarbon macrophage-labeling contrast agent perfluoroctylbromide facilitated discerning the response of rabbits aseptic or septic to tetracycline therapy (811). Microcomputed tomography has been used to study bone formation within and adjacent to the defect around implanted polyacetyl plates and Kirchner wires in rats infected with *S. aureus* (812).

Echocardiography

Serial transthoracic echocardiography, during and after treatment of experimental *S. aureus* endocarditis in rabbits, was used as a physiologic indicator of the relative benefits of different antibiotic regimens (813). It has also been used with murine CLP models (711).

As for emerging technologies, fluorescence-mediated molecular tomography (FMT) can three-dimensionally image gene expression by resolving fluorescence activation in deep tissues (814).

DETECTION OF BACTERIAL ACTIVITY BY USE OF BIOLUMINESCENCE

Detection of Bacterial Activity by Use of Bacterial Labeling with *lux* Genes

General reviews of the use of cellular labeling by luciferase expression have been published (798,815), and a review of the use of bioluminescence techniques to study gene expression is available (816).

Use of bioluminescence to detect bacteria in vivo provides a noninvasive way of monitoring the progress of infection and the response to antiinfective therapies (for reviews, see 797–799,817). First described by Contag et al. (818), construction of virulent bacteria bearing lux operons constitutes a sensitive marker of bacterial viability, as the bioluminescence reaction is adenosine triphosphate (ATP)–dependent. The article by Contag et al. (798) describes the construction and use of this technique in detail.

A thorough description of this approach has been presented by Rocchetta et al. (819), who used *lux*-transformed *E. coli* and a neutropenic mouse thigh infection model. The incorporation of an intensified charge-coupled device (ICCD) camera system facilitated the determination of light emission and therefore the sequential evaluation of individual mice. Dose-dependent bacterial CFU and light emission values were obtained in vitro and in vivo for controls and the bacteria exposed to ceftazidime, tetracycline, or ciprofloxacin. The detection methods were found to be highly correlated. Similar results were obtained with murine lung infections due to *S. pneumoniae* (820).

Given the extreme differences in the nature of bacterial growth as biofilms or planktonic cultures, bioluminescence may help in understanding the chemotherapy of device-related infections. *lux*-Transposed *S. aureus* and *P. aeruginosa* were used to establish Teflon catheter biofilm infection model mice, with either precolonized or postimplant-infected catheters being used (134). The effectiveness of various antibiotics, the determination of the in vivo PAE, and the monitoring of the emergence of antibiotic resistance in this model have also been discussed (135). Seven days after subcutaneous implantation of catheters precolonized with *S. aureus*, treatment with rifampin, tobramycin, or ciprofloxacin was initiated. Tobramycin and ciprofloxacin were poorly active, but rifampin led to an initial decline of bacterial CFU, after which resistance developed as expected.

Bioluminiscense imaging has been evaluated for in vivo illustration as well as quantification of antibiotic effect in *S. aureus*–infected skin wounds in mice (821).

Detection of Bacterial Activity by Use of Bacterial Labeling with Green Fluorescent Protein

Green fluorescent protein, a 31-kDa gene product of the jellyfish *Aequorea victoria*, has been extensively used to label mammalian and microbial cells. It is capable of "nonspecifically" labeling bacteria (822,823) and of being inserted to act as a reporter gene system (e.g., in organisms [824], *Salmonella* and *Pseudomonas* spp and an *Alcaligenes* sp [825], a *Yersinia* sp [826], *Legionella pneumophila* [824], *Streptococcus pneumoniae* [827], *Yersina pseudotuberculosis* [828], *C. neoformans* [829], and a *Helicobacter* sp [830]). Care must be taken in the construction of such cell lines in order to optimize the system for in vivo activity (831). This technology is advancing, and color variants are being developed (simulation of gene expression [832], profiling of a genetically modified gfp [831], and profiling of a genetically modified gfp [828]). Single-copy gene insertion has been noted for *P. aeruginosa* (824), salmonellae (268), and *Streptococcus pneumoniae* (1). Improved data processing (833) and the ability to see single cells have contributed to enhancing this technology. The GFP expression levels of 7,000 to 200,000 copies per cell have been viewed as nondeleterious to the virulence of *Salmonella typhimurium* (834).

PHARMACOGENOMICS IN ANIMAL MODELS OF INFECTION

Genomic approaches utilizing animal models of infection fall into two distinct categories: (a) bacterial genomics, whose goal is to identify bacterial genes involved in the initiation, survival, and propagation of bacteria during pathogenic infection and to uncover the genetic basis of sensitivity (or resistance) to antibiotics; and (b) pharmacogenomics, which in the specialized case of infection, concerns itself with understanding the genetics of differences in antibiotic metabolism and disposition and their toxic effects without considering the effects of the drugs on the host physiology as the drugs are targeted to the microorganism. A good overview of the study of microorganism and host genomics using DNA microarrays has been provided by Bryant et al. (835). They outline the use of DNA microarrays in studying the infectious process from the aspect of the pathogen (diagnostics, epidemiology, pathogenicity, and antimicrobial resistance), the host (innate immunity, adoptive or learned immunity, physiological differences related to susceptibility, and drug metabolism and toxicity), and the host–microbe interaction ("normal" and abnormal responses to infectious insult, pathogenic processes such as microbe-induced host cell apoptosis, responses to antibiotic treatment such as inflammatory responses to antibiotic-lysed bacteria, and vaccination).

Pharmacogenomics of Pathogens

Clearly, genomic investigation of the microorganisms' genotype/phenotype during infection will uncover novel genes, perhaps expressed only in vivo, that represent potential novel targets for antimicrobial therapy or the means of antimicrobial resistance (836–839). However, despite the sequencing of entire genomes of several bacteria, exploitation of this new knowledge especially in in vivo models has been slow. Despite this, there is great potential for genomics to "customize" clinical treatment of infection, providing information on both the pathogen and the host to aid in drug selection (838). De Backer and Van Dijck (840) have provided a review of the role pharmacogenomics might play in the development of novel antifungal chemotherapeutics.

Pharmacogenomics of the Infected Host

Pharmacogenomics focuses on the host, evaluating genetic-based differences in host drug transport and metabolism, both of which form the basis of PK and tolerability features of any antibiotic (841). For example, polymorphisms occur in P-glycoprotein, an ATP-binding cassette transporter that pumps drugs out of cells and thus affects drug uptake from the gastrointestinal tract as well as tissue distribution. Polymorphisms also occur in drug-metabolizing enzymes that are components of both the "phase I" metabolizing group (e.g., the cytochrome P450 family, which metabolize drugs through oxidation, reduction, or hydrolysis steps) and members of the "phase II" family (e.g., UDP glucuronosyltransferases, glutathione transferases, methyltransferase, and acetyl transferases) and that by conjugating the drug help to facilitate its elimination from the body. In addition to genetic predisposition to infection, inbred mouse strains also carry alterations in drug metabolism, such as the differences in tolerability of inbred strains to chloramphenicol toxicity (see reference 841). Genetic mapping of inbred strains to identify loci and eventually genes that are involved in drug metabolism and display polymorphisms will likely lead to the identification of human homologues. In addition, use of genetically modified mice will aid in identifying drug-metabolizing enzymes (842), and such information can be applied to medicinal chemistry programs to design antibiotics with better PK and metabolic/tolerability profiles. In this regard, the apparent failure or poor activity of antibiotics in some animal models may be due to differences in drug metabolism between different mouse strains or different species.

PREDICTABILITY OF ANIMAL MODELS OF INFECTION FOR HUMAN DISEASE

Perhaps the ultimate question that arises following the preclinical evaluation of an antiinfectives in an animal model of infectious disease is, what is the true utility of the data obtained from the animal model, namely, how predictive is the model for the clinical situation? The answer to this lies in understanding both the model and the clinical situation. In understanding the model, it is as important to know the limitations of the model as much as its advantages and to ask only those questions that the particular model can answer. Few studies have systematically reviewed the correlation of the effect of antibiotics in animal models and clinical outcome. One such a review (612) suggests that the rat osteomyelitis model does have a good measure of predictability. Although discriminative models of infection are designed to mimic the clinical situation more closely than screening models, all models can provide useful information. This is probably due to the mode of action of antibiotics, for they primarily target pathogens of another hierarchical kingdom (prokaryotes). Given this likelihood of high specificity of drug-target interaction, the infecting organism bearing the target remains "constant" irrespective of host, be it an experimental one (mouse, rat, etc.) or one that acquires the infection naturally (humans among other animals) (63). Therefore, the issue of predictability becomes an issue of PK/PD relationship: can the drug attain a sufficient PK profile (and be well tolerated) in the patient and satisfy the PD criteria established during the experimental evaluation (e.g., plasma concentration above the MIC for 80% of the administration interval). Allometry or physiologically based PK/PD modeling can be used to predict dosages for the target patient. But this serves only as a guide to aid decisions; it is on the basis of animal efficacy model data that clinical trials are most often initiated. Such a modeling exercise requires input from many different models to provide a database sufficient for making an educated prediction concerning clinical success.

However, in spite of careful experimentation, clinical failure of a compound effective in preclinical testing will sometimes occur. In such cases, the researchers will ask, "What went wrong?"

If only to provide a basis for discussion, consideration should be given to an excellent publication by Eichaker and associates (23). In this study, the authors review clinical data (from 22 trials) and preclinical data (from 95 "trials") concerning the testing of antiinflammatory agents in bacterial sepsis. They argue that the vast amount of preclinical data, do not reflect clinical experience. Using meta-regression techniques to pool the data, they test the hypothesis that a strong relationship exists between risk of death from disease and the effectiveness of antiinflammatory agents in treating disease. If preclinical studies show an exceedingly high risk of death and the clinical trials a more moderate one, then the preclinical data would be misleading; for the findings to be truly comparable, the disease outcomes should be similar in both the preclinical and the clinical trials. The authors show that the mortality rates of control animals (88% [79% to 96%]; median [25th to 75th quartiles]) were highly different from those of the clinical trials (39% [32% to 43%], $p = 0.0001$). Regression analysis of the animal data indicated that, of the factors evaluated, 70% of the variability of the effect of antiinflammatory agents could be attributed to the risk of death. Normally, the clinical trials did not categorize the patients regarding risk of death, but in two trials that did, the greatest benefit of the antiinflammatory agents was to those at the highest risk of death, similar to the preclinical studies. Plotting the control odds ratio of dying and the odds ratio of the treated group dying for both animal and human studies shows a clustering of the human trial data at a lower risk than in the majority of the animal trials. The authors then modified their animal model to have a range of severity of disease when testing antiinflammatory agents in sepsis and produced data yielding an odds ratio plot very similar to that obtained from the clinical trials. In a reiterative process, the animal model was modified to produce data that better fit the spectrum of disease observed clinically, thus obtaining an animal model of greater predictive quality.

In some cases, definitive clinical trials are difficult, if not impossible, to perform. In such cases, reliance on animal model data is extensive, if not exclusive. For example, endocarditis is a severe, costly infection, and therefore identification of situations invoking prophylaxis against this infection is clearly warranted. Prophylaxis requires the ability to identify clinical procedures that might result in bacteremia, identify the patients at risk, and determine the optimal prophylactic antibiotic regimen, one that maximizes effectiveness and minimizes the risk of side effects. Owing to the difficulty of performing appropriate clinical studies, Moreillon (844) summarized the information obtained from animal studies of endocarditis and used it as a basis for a proposal regarding guidelines for clinical prophylaxis of endocarditis.

In the comprehensive review of animal models used for the study of antibiotic treatment of tuberculosis, Franzblau et al. (651) discuss the predictability of the models for human disease in detail. Although mouse models have been fairly useful in predicting multidrug treatment effect for humans, the lack of standardization of the models and effect parameters may be seen as an obstacle to such evaluation. In the quest for the future collaborative efforts in standardizing animal tuberculosis models researchers should take a cautionary note from the advice on animal welfare issues connected with murine tuberculosis models (17).

In summary, there is a vast amount of information on animal models of infection, but it is likely that only when the models are used wisely and modified to better reflect the clinical situation can predictions based on them be relied upon.

ACKNOWLEDGMENT

The authors would like to acknowledge the contributions of Terry O'Reilly, PhD, made to the 5th edition of this book.

REFERENCES

1. Beam TR, Gilbert DN, Kunin CM. General guidelines for the clinical evaluation of anti-infective drug products. *Clin Infect Dis* 1992;15(Suppl 1):S5–S32.
2. O'Reilly T, Andes DA, Østergaard C, et al. Evaluation of antimicrobials in experimental animal infections. In: Lorian V, ed. *Antibiotics in laboratory medicine*. 5th ed. New York: Lippincott Williams & Wilkins, 2005:654–718.
3. Zak O, Sande MA, eds. *Experimental models in antimicrobial chemotherapy*. London: Academic Press, 1986.
4. Zak O, Sande MA, eds. *Handbook of animal models of infection*. San Diego, CA: Academic Press, 1999.
5. Zak O, O'Reilly T. Animal infection models and ethics: the perfect infection model. *J Antimicrob Chemother* 1993;31(Suppl D):193–205.
6. Morton DB. Ethical aspects of the use of animal models of infection. In: Zak O, Sande MA, eds. *Handbook of animal models of infection*. San Diego, CA: Academic Press, 1999:29–48.
7. Cohen C. The case for use of animals in biomedical research. *N Engl J Med* 1986;315:865–870.
8. Obrink KJ. Animal models and ethics. In: Keusch G, Wadstrom T, eds. *Experimental bacterial and parasitic infections*. New York: Elsevier Biomedical, 1982:3–10.
9. Regan T. The case for animal rights. In: Singer P, ed. *Defense of animals*. New York: Harper & Row, 1985:13–26.
10. Regan T. *The case for animal rights*. London: Routledge, 1988.
11. Singer P. *Animal liberation*. New York: Avon Books, 1990.
12. Bateson P. Do animals feel pain? *New Sci* 1992;134 (1818):30–33.
13. Flecknall P, Waterman-Pearson A. *Pain management in animals*. London: WB Saunders, 2000.
14. European Union. Directive 2010/63/EU of the European parliament and of the council of 22 September 2010 on the protection of animlas used for scientific purposes. *Official Journal of the European Union*. September 22, 2010:33–79.
15. Cowan T. The Animal Welfare Act: background and selected legislation. http://nationalaglawcenter.org/wp-content/uploads/assets/crs/RS22493.pdf. Congressional Research Service RS22493. Published June 2013.
16. Kilkenny C, Browne WJ, Cuthill IC, et al. Improving bioscience research reporting: the ARRIVE guidelines for reporting animal research. *PLos Biol* 2010;8:e1000412.
17. Franco NH, Correia-Neves M, Olsson AS. Animal welfare in studies of murine tuberculosis: assessing progress over a 12-year period and the need for further improvement. *PLos One* 2012;7:e47723.
18. Hooijmanns CR, Leenaars M, Ritskes-Hoitinga M. A gold standard publicatin checklist to improve the quality of animal studies, to fully integrate the three Rs, and to make systematic reviews more feasible. *Altern Lab Anim* 2010;38:167–182.
19. van Zutphen LFM, Baumans V, Beyen AC, eds. *Principles of laboratory animal science*. Amsterdam: Elsevier, 1993.
20. Hansen AK. The impact of general laboratory animal health on experimental models in antimicrobial chemotherapy. In: Zak O, Sande MA, eds. *Handbook of animal models of infection*. San Diego, CA: Academic Press, 1999:49–59.
21. Torres-Molina F, Peris-Ribera JE, Garcia-Carbonell MC, et al. Nonlinearities in amoxicillin pharmacokinetics. II. Absorption studies in the rat. *Biopharm Drug Dispos* 1992;13:39–53.
22. Harter DH, Petersdorf RG. A consideration of the pathogenesis of bacterial meningitis: review of experimental and clinical studies. *Yale J Biol Med* 1960;32:280–309.
23. Eichacker PQ, Parent C, Kalil A, et al. Risk and the efficacy of antiinflammatory agents retrospective and confirmatory studies of sepsis. *Am J Respir Crit Care Med* 2002;166:1197–1205.
24. Beynen AC, Festing MFW. Phases in an animal experiment. In: van Zutphen LFM, Baumans V, Beyen AC, eds. *Principles of laboratory animal science*. Amsterdam: Elsevier, 1993:197–208.
25. Beynen AC, Festing MFW, van Montfort MAJ. Design of animal experiments. In: van Zutphen LFM, Baumans V, Beyen AC, eds. *Principles of laboratory animal science*. Amsterdam: Elsevier, 1993:209–240.
26. Hanfelt JJ. Statistical approaches to experimental design and data analysis of in vivo studies. *Breast Cancer Res Treat* 1997;46:279–302.

27. Hermans PGC, Fosse RT, van der Gulden WJI, et al. Organisation and management of animal experiments. In: van Zutphen LFM, Baumans V, Beyen AC, eds. *Principles of laboratory animal science.* Amsterdam: Elsevier, 1993:241–254.

28. Costerton JW, Cheng K-J, Geesey GG, et al. Bacterial biofilms in nature and disease. *Annu Rev Microbiol* 1987;41:435–464.

29. Costerton JW, Veeh R, Shirtliff M, et al. The application of biofilm science to the study and control of chronic bacterial infections. *J Clin Invest* 2003;112:1466–1477.

30. Foley I, Brown MRW. Activity of antibiotics against adherent/slow-growing bacteria reflecting the situation in vivo. In: Zak O, Sande MA, eds. *Handbook of animal models of infection.* San Diego, CA: Academic Press, 1999:117–123.

31. Schwank S, Rajacic Z, Zimmerli W, et al. Impact of bacterial biofilm formation on in vitro and in vivo activities of antibiotics. *Antimicrob Agents Chemother* 1998;42:895–898.

32. Domingue G, Ellis B, Dasgupta M, et al. Testing antimicrobial susceptibilities of adherent bacteria by a method that incorporates guidelines of the National Committee for Clinical Laboratory Standards. *J Clin Microbiol* 1994;32:2564–2568.

33. Anwar H, Strap JL, Chen K, et al. Dynamic interactions of biofilms of mucoid *Pseudomonas aeruginosa* with tobramycin and piperacillin. *Antimicrob Agents Chemother* 1992;36:1208–1214.

34. Brown MRW, Collier PJ, Gilbert P. Influence of growth rate on susceptibility to antimicrobial agents: modification of the cell envelope and batch and continuous culture studies. *Antimicrob Agents Chemother* 1990;34:1623–1628.

35. Dalhoff A, Matuat S, Ullmann U. Effect of quinolones against slowly growing bacteria. *Chemotherapy* 1995;41:92–99.

36. Duguid IG, Evans E, Brown MRW, et al. Growth-rate–independent killing by ciprofloxacin of biofilm-derived *Staphylococcus epidermidis*: evidence for cell-cycle dependency. *J Antimicrob Chemother* 1992;30:791–802.

37. Eng RHK, Hsieh A, Smith SM. Antibiotic killing of bacteria: comparison of bacteria on surfaces and in liquid, growing and nongrowing. *Chemotherapy* 1995;41:113–120.

38. Vergeres P, Blaser J. Amikacin, ceftazidime, and flucloxacillin against suspended and adherent *Pseudomonas aeruginosa* and *Staphylococcus epidermidis* in an in vitro model of infection. *J Infect Dis* 1992;165:281–289.

39. Cozens RM, Tuomanen E, Tosch W, et al. Evaluation of the bactericidal activity of β-lactam antibiotics on slowly growing bacteria cultured in the chemostat. *Antimicrob Agents Chemother* 1986;29:797–802.

40. Davey PG, Renneberg J, Speller DCE, eds. Bacterial infection models in antimicrobial chemotherapy. *J Antimicrobial Chemother* 1993(Suppl D);31:1–205.

41. Blaser J, Zinner SH. In vitro models for the study of antibiotic activities. *Prog Drug Res* 1987;31:349–381.

42. Dudley MN, Blaser J, Gilbert D, et al. Combination therapy with ciprofloxacin plus azlocillin against *Pseudomonas aeruginosa*: effect of simultaneous versus staggered administration in an in vitro model of infection. *J Infect Dis* 1991;164:499–506.

43. Cozens RM. Formulation of compounds and determination of pharmacokinetic parameters. In: Zak O, Sande MA, eds. *Handbook of animal models of infection.* San Diego, CA: Academic Press, 1999:83–92.

44. Martinez MN, Pedersoli WM, Ravis WR, et al. Feasibility of interspecies extrapolation in determining the bioequivalence of animal products intended for intramuscular administration. *J Vet Pharmacol Ther* 2001;24:125–135.

45. Perkins RJ, Liu W, Drusano G, et al. Pharmacokinetics of ofloxacin in serum and vitreous humor of albino and pigmented rabbits. *Antimicrob Agents Chemother* 1995;39:1493–1498.

46. Bhardwaj R, Dorr RT, Blanchard J. Approaches to reducing toxicity of parenteral anticancer drug formulations using cyclodextrins. *PDA J Pharm Sci Technol* 2000;54:233–239.

47. Sugawara M, Toda T, Iseki K, et al. Transport characteristics of cephalosporin antibiotics across intestinal brush-border membrane in man, rat and rabbit. *J Pharm Pharmacol* 1992;44:968–972.

48. Torres-Molina F, Peris-Ribera JE, Garcia-Carbonell MC, et al. Nonlinearities in amoxicillin pharmacokinetics. I. Disposition studies in the rat. *Biopharm Drug Dispos* 1992;13:23–38.

49. Torres-Molina F, Peris-Ribera JE, Garcia-Carbonell MC, et al. Nonlinearities in amoxicillin pharmacokinetics. II. Absorption studies in the rat. *Biopharm Drug Dispos* 1992;13:39–53.

50. Chesa-Jimenez J, Peris JE, Torres-Molina F, et al. Low bioavailablity of amoxicillin in rats as a consequence of presystematic degradation in the intestine. *Antimicrob Agents Chemother* 1994;38:842–847.

51. O'Reilly T, Cleeland R, Squires E. Evaluation of antimicrobials in experimental animal infections. In: Lorian V, ed. *Antibiotics in laboratory medicine.* 4th ed. Baltimore: Williams & Wilkins, 1996:599–759.

52. Baumans V, ten Berg RGM, Beterns APMG, et al. Experimental procedures. In: van Zutphen LFM, Baumans V, Beyen AC, eds. *Principles of laboratory animal science.* Amsterdam: Elsevier, 1993:299–318.

53. Van Dongen JJ, Remie R, Rensema JW, et al. *Manual of microsurgery on the laboratory rat.* Part 1. *General information and experimental techniques.* Amsterdam: Elsevier, 1990.

54. Beterns APMG, Booij LHDJ, Flecknell PA, et al. Anaesthesia, analgesia and euthanasia. In: van Zutphen LFM, Baumans V, Beyen AC, eds. *Principles of laboratory animal science.* Amsterdam: Elsevier, 1993:267–298.

56. Ambrose PG, Bhavnani SM, Rubino CM, et al. Pharmacokinetics-pharmacodynamics of antimicrobial therapy: it's not just for mice anymore. *Clin Infect Dis* 2007;44:79–86.

57. Andes D. Clinical utility of antifungal pharmacokinetics and pharmacodynamics. *Curr Opin Infect Dis* 2004;17:533–540.

58. Craig WA. Pharmacokinetic/pharmacodynamic parameters: rationale for antibacterial dosing of mice and men. *Clin Infect Dis* 1998;26:1–10;quiz 11–12.

59. Drusano GL. Pharmacokinetics and pharmacodynamics of antimicrobials. *Clin Infect Dis* 2007;45(Suppl 1):S89–S95.

60. Hinojosa E, Boyd AR, Orihuela CJ. Age-associated inflammation and toll-like receptor dysfunction prime the lungs for pneumococcal pneumonia. *J Infect Dis* 2009;200:546–554.

61. Andes D. Pharmacokinetics and pharmacodynamics of antifungals. *Infect Dis Clin North Am* 2006;20:679–697.

62. Craig W. Pharmacodynamics of antimicrobial agents as a basis for determining dosage regimens. *Europ J Clin Microbiol Infect Dis* 1993;12(Suppl 1):S6–S8.

63. Drusano GL. Antimicrobial pharmacodynamics: critical interactions of "bug and drug." *Nat Rev Microbiol* 2004;2:289–300.

64. Frimodt-Møller N. How predictive is PK/PD for antibacterial agents? *Int J Antimicrob Agents* 2002;19:333–339.

65. Hope W, Drusano GL. Antifungal pharmacokinetics and pharmacodynamics: bridging from the bench to bedside. *Clin Microbiol Infect* 2009;15:602–612.

66. Nicolau DP. Predicting antibacterial response from pharmacodynamic and pharmacokinetic profiles. *Infection* 2001;29(Suppl 2):11–15.

67. Schentag JJ, Gilliland KK, Paladino JA. What have we learned from pharmacokinetic and pharmacodynamic theories? *Clin Infect Dis* 2001;32(Suppl 1):S39–S46.

68. Barza M. 1993. Pharmacokinetics of antibiotics in shallow and deep compartments. *J Antimicrob Chemother* 1993;31(Suppl D):17–27.

69. Bergan T. Pharmacokinetic properties of the cephalosporins. *Drugs* 1987;34(Suppl 2):89–104.

70. Carbon C. Significance of tissue levels for prediction of antibiotic efficacy and determination of dosage. *Eur J Clin Microbiol Infect Dis* 1990;9:510–516.

71. Mouton JW, Theuretzbacher U, Craig WA, et al. Tissue concentrations: do we ever learn? *J Antimicrob Chemother* 2008;61:235–237.

72. Redington J, Ebert SC, Craig WA. Role of antimicrobial pharmacokinetics and pharmacodynamics in surgical prophylaxis. *Rev Infect Dis* 1991; 13(Suppl 10):S790–S799.

73. Brunner M, Derendorf H, Muller M. Microdialysis for in vivo pharmacokinetic/pharmacodynamic characterization of anti-infective drugs. *Curr Opin Pharmacol* 2005;5:495–499.

74. Liu P, Muller M, Derendorf H. Rational dosing of antibiotics: the use of plasma concentrations versus tissue concentrations. *Int J Antimicrob Agents* 2002;19:285–290.

75. Clark B, Smith D. *An introduction to pharmacokinetics.* 2nd ed. Oxford: Blackwell Scientific Publications, 1986.

76. Rowland M, Tozer T. *Clinical pharmacokinetics: concepts and applications.* 3rd ed. Philadelphia: Lippincott Williams & Wilkins, 1995.

77. Craig WA, Ebert SC. Protein binding and its significance in antibacterial therapy. *Infect Dis Clin North Am* 1989;3:407–414.

78. Zeitlinger MA, Derendorf H, Mouton JW, et al. Protein binding: do we ever learn? *Antimicrob Agents Chemother* 2011;55:3067–3074.

79. Zini R, Riant P, Barre J, et al. Disease-induced variations in plasma protein levels. Implications for drug dosage regimens (Part I). *Clin Pharmacokinet* 1990;19:147–159.

80. Zini R, Riant P, Barre J, et al. Disease-induced variations in plasma protein levels. Implications for drug dosage regimens (Part II). *Clin Pharmacokinet* 1990;19:218–229.

81. Andes D, Craig WA. Animal model pharmacokinetics and pharmacodynamics: a critical review. *Int J Antimicrob Agents* 2002;19:261–268.

82. Siefert HM, Domdey-Bette A, Henninger K, et al. Pharmacokinetics of the 8-methoxyquinolone, moxifloxacin: a comparison in humans and other mammalian species. *J Antimicrob Chemother* 1999;43(Suppl B):69–76.

83. Bruzzese T, Rimaroli C, Bonabello A, et al. Pharmacokinetics and tissue distribution of rifametane, a new 3-azinomethyl-rifamycin derivative, in several animal species. *Arzneimittelforschung* 2000;50:60–71.

84. MacCallum DM, Odds FC. Influence of grapefruit juice on itraconazole plasma levels in mice and guinea pigs. *J Antimicrob Chemother* 2002;50:219–224.

85. Andes DR, Craig WA. Pharmacokinetics and pharmacodynamics of antibiotics in meningitis. *Infect Dis Clin North Am* 1999;13:595–618.

86. Krontz DP, Strausbaugh LJ. Effect of meningitis and probenecid on the penetration of vancomycin into cerebrospinal fluid in rabbits. *Antimicrob Agents Chemother* 1980;18:882–886.

87. Scheld WM. Drug delivery to the central nervous system: general principles and relevance to therapy for infections of the central nervous system. *Rev Infect Dis* 1989;11(Suppl 7):S1669–S1690.

88. Levy RM, Gutin PH, Baskin DS, et al. Vancomycin penetration of a brain abscess: case report and review of the literature. *Neurosurgery* 1986;18:632–636.

89. Ganzinger U, Haslberger A. Pharmacokinetics of cephalosporins in normal and septicemic rabbits. *Antimicrob Agents Chemother* 1985;28:473–477.

90. Mimoz O, Jacolot A, Padoin C, et al. Influence of experimental rat model of multiple organ dysfunction on cefepime and amikacin pharmacokinetics. *Antimicrob Agents Chemother* 1996;40:819–821.

91. Ngeleka M, Auclair P, Tardif D, et al. Intrarenal distribution of vancomycin in endotoxemic rats. *Antimicrob Agents Chemother* 1989;33:1575–1579.

92. Mackowiak PA. Influence of fever on pharmacokinetics. *Rev Infect Dis* 1989;11:804–807.

93. Ahmad M, Raza H, Murtaza G, et al. Pharmacokinetic variations of ofloxacin in normal and febrile rabbits. *Pak Vet J* 2008;28:181–185.

94. Goudah A, Mounier SM, Shim JH, et al. Influence of endotoxin induced fever on the pharmacokinetics of intramuscularly administered cefepime in rabbits. *J Vet Sci* 2006;7:151–155.

95. Marier JF, Beaudry F, Ducharme MP, et al. A pharmacokinetic study of amoxycillin in febrile beagle dogs following repeated administrations of endotoxin. *J Vet Pharmacol Ther* 2001;24:379–383.

96. Pennington JE, Dale DC, Reynolds HY, et al. Gentamicin sulfate pharmacokinetics: lower levels of gentamicin in blood during fever. *J Infect Dis* 1975;132:270–275.

97. Sarwari AR, Mackowiak PA. The pharmacologic consequences of fever. *Infect Dis Clin North Am* 1996;10:21–32.

98. Morita E, Mizuno N, Nishikata M, et al. Comparison of the pharmacokinetics of five beta-lactam antibiotics between neonatal and adult rats. *Dev Pharmacol Ther* 1990;14:223–230.

99. Tanira MOM, Ali BH, Bashir AK. Effect of endotoxin on gentamicin pharmacokinetics in old and young adult rats. *Life Sci* 1997;60:413–424.

100. Thadepalli H, Reddy U, Chuah SK, et al. Evaluation of trovafloxacin in the treatment of *Klebsiella pneumoniae* lung infection in tumour-bearing mice. *J Antimicrob Chemother* 2005;45:69–75.

101. Maiza A, Daley-Yates PT. Variability in the renal clearance of cephalexin in experimental renal failure. *J Pharmacokinet Biopharm* 1993;21:19–30.

102. Giacomini KM, Roberts SM, Levy G. Evaluation of methods for producing renal dysfunction in rats. *J Pharm Sci* 1981;70:117–121.

103. Andes D, Craig WA. In vivo activities of amoxicillin and amoxicillin-clavulanate against *Streptococcus pneumoniae*: application to breakpoint determinations. *Antimicrob Agents Chemother* 1998;42:2375–2379.

104. Craig WA, Redington J, Ebert SC. Pharmacodynamics of amikacin in vitro and in mouse thigh and lung

infections. *J Antimicrob Chemother* 1991;27(Suppl C): 29–40.

105. Nierenberg DW. Drug inhibition of penicillin tubular secretion: concordance between in vitro and clinical findings. *J Pharmacol Exp Ther* 1987;240:712–716.

106. Thonus A, de Lange-Macdaniel AV, Otte CJ, et al. Tissue cage infusion: a technique for the achievement of prolonged steady state in experimental animals. *J Pharmacol Methods* 1979;2:63–69.

107. Astry Cl, Nelson S, Karam GH, et al. Interactions of clindamycin with antibacterial defenses of the lung. *Am Rev Respir Dis* 1987;135:1015–1019.

108. Naziri W, Cheadle WG, Trachtenberg LS, et al. Second place winner of the Conrad Jobst Award in the gold medal paper competition. Increased antibiotic effectiveness in a model of surgical infection through continuous infusion. *Am Surg* 1995;61:11–15.

109. Roosendaal R, Bakker-Woudenberg IAJM, van den Berghe-van Raffe M, et al. Impact of the dosage schedule on the efficacy of ceftazidime, gentamicin and ciprofloxacin in *Klebsiella pneumoniae* pneumonia and septicemia in leukopenic rats. *Eur J Clin Microbiol Infect Dis* 1989;8:878–887.

110. Thauvin C, Eliopoulos GM, Willey S, et al. Continuous-infusion ampicillin therapy of enterococcal endocarditis in rats. *Antimicrob Agents Chemother* 1987;31: 139–143.

111. Tran Ba Huy P, Meulemans A, Wassef M, et al. Gentamicin persistence in rat endolymph and perilymph after a two-day constant infusion. *Antimicrob Agents Chemother* 1983;23:344–346.

112. Robaux MA, Dube L, Caillon J, et al. In vivo efficacy of continuous infusion versus intermittent dosing of ceftazidime alone or in combination with amikacin relative to human kinetic profiles in a *Pseudomonas aeruginosa* rabbit endocarditis model. *J Antimicrob Chemother* 2001;47:617–622.

113. Mizen L. Methods for obtaining human-like pharmacokinetic patterns in experimental animals. In: Zak O, Sande MA, eds. *Handbook of animal models of infection.* San Diego, CA: Academic Press, 1999: 93–103.

114. Woodnutt G, Catherall EJ, Kernutt I, et al. Temocillin efficacy in experimental *Klebsiella pneumoniae* meningitis after infusion into rabbit plasma to simulate antibiotic concentrations in human serum. *Antimicrob Agents Chemother* 1988;32:1705–1709.

115. Woodnutt G, Berry V, Mizen L. Simulation of human serum pharmacokinetics of cefazolin, piperacillin, and BRL 42715 in rats and efficacy against experimental intraperitoneal infections. *Antimicrob Agents Chemother* 1992;36:1427–1431.

116. Mizen L, Woodnutt G, Kernutt I, et al. Simulation of human serum pharmacokinetics of ticarcillin-clavulanic acid and ceftazidime in rabbits, and efficacy against experimental *Klebsiella pneumoniae* meningitis. *Antimicrob Agents Chemother* 1989;33:693–699.

117. Fluckiger U, Moreillon P, Blaser J, et al. Simulation of amoxicillin pharmacokinetics in humans for the prevention of streptococcal endocarditis in rats. *Antimicrob Agents Chemother* 1994;38:2846–2849.

118. Entenza JM, Blatter M, Glauser MP, et al. Parenteral sparfloxacin compared with ceftriaxone in treatment of experimental endocarditis due to penicillin-susceptible and -resistant streptococci. *Antimicrob Agents Chemother* 1994;38:2638–2688.

119. Entenza JM, Fluckiger U, Glauser MP, et al. Antibiotic treatment of experimental endocarditis due to methicillin-resistant *Staphylococcus epidermidis. J Infect Dis* 1994;170:100–109.

121. Richmond JY, Quimby F. Considerations for working safely with infectious disease agents in research animals. In: Zak O, Sande MA, eds. *Handbook of animal models of infection.* San Diego, CA: Academic Press, 1999: 69–73.

122. Frimodt Møller N, Thomsen VF. The pneumococcus and the mouse protection test: inoculum, dosage and timing. *Acta Path Microbiol Immunol Scand* 1986;94:33–37.

123. Frimodt-Møller N, Thomsen VF. Interaction between beta-lactam antibiotics and gentamicin against *Streptococcus pneumoniae* in vitro and in vivo. *APMIS* 1987;95:269–275.

124. Knudsen JD, Odenholt I, Erlendsdottir H, et al. Selection of resistant *Streptococcus pneumoniae* during penicillin treatment in vitro and in three animal models. *Antimicrob Agents Chemother* 2003;47:2499–2506.

125. O'Reilly T, Niven DF. Tryptone-yeast extract broth as a culture medium for *Haemophilus pleuropneumoniae* and *Haemophilus parasuis* to be used as challenge inocula. *Can J Vet Res* 1986;50:441–443.

126. Brenner D, DeVoe IW, Holbein BE. Increased virulence of *Neisseria meningitidis* after in vitro iron-limited growth at low pH. *Infect Immun* 1981;33:59–66.

127. Sharma S, Harjai K, Mittal R. Enhanced siderophore production and mouse kidney pathogenicity in *Escherichia coli* grown in urine. *J Med Microbiol* 1991;35: 325–329

128. Shepard BD, Gilmore MS. Differential expression of virulence-related genes in *Enterococcus faecalis* in response to biological cues in serum and urine. *Infect Immun* 2002;70:4344–4352.

129. Keevil CW, Davies DB, Spillane BJ, et al. Influence of iron-limited and replete continuous culture on the physiology and virulence of *Neisseria gonorrhoeae. J Gen Microbiol* 1989;135:851–863.

130. Collins HL, Kaufmann SHE, Schaible UE. Iron chelation via deferoxamine exacerbates experimental salmonellosis via inhibition of the nicotinamide adenine dinucleotide phosphate oxidase-dependent respiratory burst. *J Immunol* 2002;168:3456–3463.

131. Bagge N, Ciofu O, Skovgaard LT, et al. Rapid development in vitro and in vivo of resistance to ceftazidime in biofilm-growing *Pseudomonas aeruginosa* due to chromosomal beta-lactamase. *APMIS* 2000;108:589–600.

132. Li X, Zhao H, Lockatell CV, et al. Visualization of *Proteus mirabilis* within the matrix of urease-induced bladder stones during experimental urinary tract infection. *Infect Immun* 2002;70:389–394.

133. Ehrlich GD, Veeh R, Wang X, et al. Mucosal biofilm formation on middle-ear mucosa in the chinchilla model of otitis media. *JAMA* 2002;287:1710–1715.

134. Kadurugamuwa JL, Sin L, Albert E, et al. Direct continuous method for monitoring biofilm infection in a mouse model. *Infect Immun* 2003;71:882–890.

135. Kadurugamuwa JL, Sin LV, Yu J, et al. Rapid direct method for monitoring antibiotics in a mouse model of bacterial biofilm infection. *Antimicrob Agents Chemother* 2003;47:3130–3137.

136. Saint S, Chenoweth CE. Biofilms and catheter-associated urinary tract infections. *Infect Dis Clin North Am* 2003;17:411–432.

137. Chmiel JF, Davis PB. State of the art: why do the lungs of patients with cystic fibrosis become infected and why can't they clear the infection? *Respir Res* 2003;4:8.

138. Ciofu O, Bagge N, Hoiby N. Antibodies against beta-lactamase can improve ceftazidime treatment of lung infection with beta-lactam-resistant *Pseudomonas aeruginosa* in a rat model of chronic lung Infection. *APMIS* 2002;110:881–891.

139. Mongodin E, Bajolet O, Cutrona J, et al. Fibronectin-binding proteins of *Staphylococcus aureus* are involved in adherence to human airway epithelium. *Infect Immun* 2002;70:620–630.

140. Vandecasteele SJ, Peetermans WE, Merckx R, et al. Expression of biofilm-associated genes in *Staphylococcus epidermidis* during in vitro and in vivo foreign body infections. *J Infect Dis* 2003;188:730–737.

141. Francois P, Tu Quoc PH, Bisognano C, et al. Lack of biofilm contribution to bacterial colonisation in an experimental model of foreign body infection by *Staphylococcus aureus* and *Staphylococcus epidermidis*. *FEMS Immunol Med Microbiol* 2003;35:135–140.

142. Sheppard M, Webb C, Heath F, et al. Dynamics of bacterial growth and distribution within the liver during Salmonella infection. *Cell Microbiol* 2003;5:593–600.

143. Peterson LR. Animal models: the in vivo evaluation of ciprofloxacin. *J Antimicrob Chemother* 1986;18(Suppl D):55–64.

144. Zak O. Scope and limitations of experimental chemotherapy. *Expertmentia* 1980;36:479–483.

145. Frimodt-Møller N. Correlation of in vitro activity and pharmacokinetic parameters with effect in vivo for antibiotics: observations from experimental pneumococcus infection. *Dan Med Bull* 1988;35:422–437.

146. Frimodt-Møller N. The mouse peritonitis model: present and future use. *J Antimicrob Chemother* 1993; 31(Suppl D):55–60.

147. Frimodt Møller N, Knudsen JD, Espersen F. The mouse peritonitis/sepsis model. In: Zak O, Sande MA, eds. *Handbook of animal models of infection*. San Diego, CA: Academic Press, 1999:127–136.

148. Cross AS, Opal SM, Sadoff JC, et al. Choice of bacteria in animal models of sepsis. *Infect Immun* 1993;61:2741–2747.

149. Fantin B, Legget J, Ebert S, et al. Correlation between in vitro and in vivo activity of antimicrobial agents against Gram-negative bacilli in a murine infection model. *Antimicrob Agents Chemother* 1991;35:1413–1422.

150. Zak O, Sande MA. Correlation of in vitro antimicrobial activity of antibiotics with results of treatment in experimental animal models and human infection In: Sabath LD, ed. *Action of antibiotics in patients*. Bern, Switzerland: Hans Huber Publishers, 1982:55–67.

151. Zimmerli W, Frei R, Widmer AF, et al. Microbiologic tests to predict treatment outcome in experimental device-related infections due to *Staphyloccus aureus*. *J Antimicrob Chemother* 1994;33:959–967.

152. Anaissie EJ, Karyotakis NC, Hachem R, et al. Correlation between in vitro and in vivo activity of antifungal agents against *Candida* species. *J Infect Dis* 1994;170:384–389.

153. Rex JH, Nelson PW, Paetznick VL, et al. Optimizing the correlation between results of testing in vitro and therapeutic outcome in vivo for fluconazole by testing critical isolates in a murine model of invasive candidiasis. *Antimicrob Agents Chemother* 1998;42:129–134.

154. Welkos S, O'Brien A. Determination of median lethal and infectious doses in animal model systems. *Methods Enzymol* 1994;235:29–39.

155. Johnson JA, Lau BH, Nutter RL, et al. Effect of L1210 leukemia on the susceptibility of mice to *Candida albicans* infections. *Infect Immun* 1978;19:146–151.

156. Comber KR, Osborne CD, Sutherland R. Comparative effects of amoxicillin and ampicillin in the treatment of experimental mouse infections. *Antimicrob Agents Chemother* 1975;7:179–185.

157. Reed LJ, Muench H. A simple method of estimating fifty percent endpoints. *Am J Hyg* 1938;27:4934–4997.

158. Finney DJ. *Probit analysis*. Cambridge: Cambridge University Press, 1971.

159. Hoogeterp JJ, Mattie H, Krul AM, et al. The efficacy of rifampicin against *Staphylococcus aureus* in vitro and in an experimental infection in normal and granulocytopenic mice. *Scand J Infect Dis* 1988;20:649–656.

160. Isenberg HD, Sampson-Scherer J, Cleeland R, et al. Correlation of the results of antibiotic synergy and susceptibility testing in vitro with results in experimental mouse infections. *Crit Rev Microbiol* 1982;10:1–76.

161. Beskid G, Christenson JG, Cleeland R, et al. In vivo activity of ceftriaxone (Ro 13–9904), a new broad-spectrum semisynthetic cephalosporin. *Antimicrob Agents Chemother* 1981;20:159–167.

162. Norrby SR, O'Reilly T, Zak O. Efficacy of antimicrobial agent treatment in relation to treatment regimen: experimental models and clinical evaluation. *J Antimicrob Chemother* 1993;31(Suppl D):41–54.

163. Brunner H, Zeiler HJ. Oral ciprofloxacin treatment for *Salmonella typhimurium* infection of normal and immunocompromised mice. *Antimicrob Agents Chemother* 1988;32:57–62.

164. Grunberg E, Cleeland R. In vivo activity of the 6-amidino-penicillanic acid derivative, mecillinam, chemically linked or combined in varying ratios with 6-aminopenicillanic acid derivatives. *J Antimicrob Chemother* 1977;3(Suppl B):59–68.

165. Mouton JW, Punt N. Use of the t>MIC to choose between different dosing regimens of β-lactam antibiotics. *J Antimicrobial Chemother* 2001;47:500–501.

166. Mouton JW, van Ogtrop ML, Andes D, et al. Use of pharmacodynamic indices to predict efficacy of combination therapy in vivo. *Antimicrob Agents Chemother* 1999;43:2473–2478.

167. Johansen HK, Jensen TG, Dessau RB, et al. Antagonism between penicillin and erythromycin against *Streptococcus pneumoniae* in vitro and in vivo. *J Antimicrob Chemother* 2000;46:973–980.

168. Deshpande LM, Jones RN. Antagonism between penicillin and erythromycin against *Streptococcus pneumoniae*: does it exist? *Diagn Microbiol Infect Dis* 2003;46:223–225.

169. Fantin B, Carbon C. In vivo antibiotic synergism: contribution of animal models. *Antimicrob Agents Chemother* 1992;36:907–912.

170. Grunberg E. The effect of trimethoprim on the activity of sulfonamides and antibiotics in experimental infections. *J Infect Dis* 1973;128(Suppl):S478–S485.

171. Schentag JJ, Strenkoski-Nix LC, Nix DE, et al. Pharmacodynamic interactions of antibiotics alone and in combination. *Clin Infect Dis* 1998;27:40–46.

172. den Hollander JG, Mouton JW, Verbrugh HA. Use of pharmacodynamic parameters to predict efficacy of combination therapy by using fractional inhibitory

concentration kinetics. *Antimicrob Agents Chemother* 1998;42:744–748.

173. Nishi Y, Hasegawa MM, Ohkawa Y, et al. Mouse peritoneal lymphocytes, a new target for analyzing induction of sister chromatid exchanges on in vivo exposure to a genotoxic agent. *Cancer Res* 1986;46:3341–3347.

174. Barcia-Macay M, Seral C, Mingeot-Leclerq MP, et al. Pharmacodynamic evaluation of the intracellular activities of antibiotics against *Staphylococcus aureus* in a model of THP-1 macrophages. *Antimicrob Agents Chemother* 2006;50:841–851.

175. Sandberg A, Hessler JHR, Skov RL, et al. Intracellular activity of antibiotics against *Staphylococcus aureus* in a mouse peritonitis model. *Antimicrob Agents Chemother* 2009;53:1874–1883.

176. Sandberg A, Jensen KS, Baudoux P, et al. Intra- and extracellular activities of dicloxacillin against *Staphylococcus aureus* in vivo and in vitro. *Antimicrob Agents Chemother* 2010;54:2391–2400.

177. Sandberg A, Jensen KS, Baudoux P, et al. Intra- and extracellular activity of linezolid against *Staphylococcus aureus* in vivo and in vitro. *J Antimicrob Chemother* 2010;65:962–973.

178. Brinch KS, Sandberg A, Baudoux P, et al. Plectasin shows intracellular activity against *Staphylococcus aureus* in human THP-1 monocytes and in a mouse peritonitis model. *Antimicrob Agents Chemother* 2009;53:4801–4808.

179. Sandberg A, Lemaire S, Van Bambeke F, et al. Intra- and extracellular activities of dicloxacillin and linezolid against a clinical *Staphylococcus aureus* strain with a small-colony-variant phenotype in an in vitro model of THP-1 macrophages and an in vivo mouse peritonitis model. *Antimicrob Agents Chemother* 2011;55:1443–1452.

180. Tang H, Chen C-C, Zhang C-C, et al. Use of carbapenems against clinical, nontyphoid *Salmonella* isolates: results from in vitro and in vivo animal studies. *Antimicrob Agents Chemother* 2012;56:2916–2922.

181. Selbie FR, Simon RD. Virulence to mice of *Staphylococcus pyogenes*: its measurement and its relation to certain in vitro properties. *Br J Exp Pathol* 1952;33:315–326.

182. Capilla J, Clemons KV, Stevens DA. Animal models: an important tool in mycology. *Med Mycol* 2007;45: 657–684.

183. Guarro J. Lessons from animal studies for the treatment of invasive human infections due to uncommon fungi. *J Antimicrob Chemother* 2011;66:1447–1466.

184. Dannaoui E, Mouton JW, Meis JFGM, et al. Efficacy of antifungal therapy in a nonneutropenic murine model of zygomycosis. *Antimicrob Agents Chemother* 2002;46:1953–1959.

185. Howard SJ, Lestner JM, Sharp A, et al. Pharmacokinetics and pharmacodynamics of posaconazole for invasive pulmonary aspergillosis: clinical implications for antifungal therapy. *J Infect Dis* 2011;203:1324–1332.

186. Lepak AJ, Marchillo K, Vanhecker J, et al. Posaconazole pharmacodynamic target determination against wild-type and Cyp51 mutant isolates of *Aspergillus fumigatus* in an in vivo model of invasive pulmonary aspergillosis. *Antimicrob Agents Chemother* 2013;57:579–585.

187. Lewis RE, Prince RA, Chi J, et al. Itraconazole preexposure attenuates the efficacy of subsequent amphotericin B therapy in a murine model of acute invasive pulmonary aspergillosis. *Antimicrob Agents Chemother* 2002;46:3208–3214.

188. Patterson TF, George D, Ingersoll R, et al. Efficacy of SCH 39304 in treatment of experimental invasive aspergillosis. *Antimicrob Agents Chemother* 1991;35: 1985–1988.

189. Sheppard DC, Rieg G, Chiang LY, et al. Novel inhalational murine model of invasive pulmonary aspergillosis. *Antimicrob Agents Chemother* 2004;48:1908–1911.

190. Wiederhold NP, Kontoyiannis DP, Chi J, et al. Pharmacodynamics of caspofungin in a murine model of invasive pulmonary aspergillosis: evidence of concentration-dependent activity. *J Infect Dis* 2004;190:1464–1471.

191. Clemons KV, Stevens DA. Efficacy of ravuconazole in treatment of mucosal candidosis in SCID mice. *Antimicrob Agents Chemother* 2001;45:3433–3436.

192. Ju JY, Polhamus C, Marr KA, et al. Efficacies of fluconazole, caspofungin, and amphotericin B in *Candida glabrata*-infected p47phox-/- knockout mice. *Antimicrob Agents Chemother* 2002;46:1240–1245.

193. Ibrahim AS, Avanessian V, Spellberg B, et al. Liposomal amphotericin B, and not amphotericin B deoxycholate, improves survival of diabetic mice infected with Rhizopus oryzae. *Antimicrob Agents Chemother* 2003;47:3343–3344.

194. Luo GT, Gebremariam T, Lee H, et al. Efficacy of liposomal amphotericin B and posaconazole in intratracheal models of murine mucormycosis. *Antimicrob Agents Chemother* 2013l;57:3340–3347.

195. Foldvari M, Jaafari MR, Radhi J, et al. Efficacy of the antiadhesin octyl O-(2-acetamido-2-deoxy-beta-D-galacto pyranosyl)-(1-4)-2-O-propyl-beta-D-galactopy ranoside (Fimbrigal-P) in a rat oral candidiasis model. *Antimicrob Agents Chemother* 2005;49:2887–2894.

196. Takakura N, Sato Y, Ishibashi H, et al. A novel murine model of oral candidiasis with local symptoms characteristic of oral thrush. *Microbiol Immunol* 2003;47:321–326.

197. Andes D. Use of an animal model of disseminated candidiasis in the evaluation of antifungal therapy. *Methods Mol Med* 2005;118:111–128.

198. Andes D, Ambrose PG, Hammel JP, et al. Use of pharmacokinetic-pharmacodynamic analyses to optimize therapy with the systemic antifungal micafungin for invasive candidiasis or candidemia. *Antimicrob Agents Chemother* 2011;55:2113–2121.

199. Andes D, Diekema DJ, Pfaller MA, et al. In vivo comparison of the pharmacodynamic targets for echinocandin drugs against *Candida* species. *Antimicrob Agents Chemother* 2010;54:2497–2506.

200. Andes D, Diekema DJ, Pfaller MA, et al. In vivo pharmacodynamic characterization of anidulafungin in a neutropenic murine candidiasis model. *Antimicrob Agents Chemother* 2008;52:539–550.

201. Andes D, Forrest A, Lepak A, et al. Impact of antimicrobial dosing regimen on evolution of drug resistance in vivo: fluconazole and *Candida albicans*. *Antimicrob Agents Chemother* 2006;50:2374–2383.

202. Andes D, Lepak A, Nett J, et al. In vivo fluconazole pharmacodynamics and resistance development in a previously susceptible *Candida albicans* population examined by microbiologic and transcriptional profiling. *Antimicrob Agents Chemother* 2006;50:2384–2394.

203. Andes D, Marchillo K, Conklin R, et al. Pharmacodynamics of a new triazole, posaconazole, in a murine model of disseminated candidiasis. *Antimicrob Agents Chemother* 2004;48:137–142.

204. Andes DK, Marchillo K, Lowther J, et al. In vivo pharmacodynamics of HMR 3270, a glucan synthase inhibitor, in a murine candidiasis model. *Antimicrob Agents Chemother* 2003;47:1187–1192.

205. Andes D, Marchillo K, Stamstad T, et al. In vivo pharmacodynamics of a new triazole, ravuconazole, in a murine candidiasis model. *Antimicrob Agents Chemother* 2003;47:1193–1199.

206. Andes D, Marchillo K, Stamstad T, et al. In vivo pharmacokinetics and pharmacodynamics of a new triazole, voriconazole, in a murine candidiasis model. *Antimicrob Agents Chemother* 2003;47:3165–3169.

207. Andes D, Safdar N, Marchillo K, et al. Pharmacokinetic-pharmacodynamic comparison of amphotericin B (AMB) and two lipid-associated AMB preparations, liposomal AMB and AMB lipid complex, in murine candidiasis models. *Antimicrob Agents Chemother* 2006;50:674–684.

208. Andes D, Stamsted T, Conklin R. Pharmacodynamics of amphotericin B in a neutropenic-mouse disseminated-candidiasis model. *Antimicrob Agents Chemother* 2001;45:922–926.

209. Andes D, van Ogtrop M. Characterization and quantitation of the pharmacodynamics of fluconazole in a neutropenic murine disseminated candidiasis infection model. *Antimicrob Agents Chemother* 1999;43:2116–2120.

210. Andes D, van Ogtrop M, et al. In vivo characterization of the pharmacodynamics of flucytosine in a neutropenic murine disseminated candidiasis model. *Antimicrob Agents Chemother* 2000;44:938–942.

211. Andes DR, Diekema DJ, Pfaller MA, et al. In vivo pharmacodynamic target investigation for micafungin against *Candida albicans* and *C. glabrata* in a neutropenic murine candidiasis model. *Antimicrob Agents Chemother* 2008;52:3497–3503.

212. Arendrup MC, Perlin DS, Jensen RH, et al. Differential in vivo activities of anidulafungin, caspofungin, and micafungin against *Candida glabrata* isolates with and without FKS resistance mutations. *Antimicrob Agents Chemother* 2012;56:2435–2442.

213. Clancy CJ, Cheng S, Nguyen MH. Animal models of candidiasis. *Methods Mol Biol* 2009;499:65–76.

214. Gumbo T, Drusano GL, Liu W, et al. Once-weekly micafungin therapy is as effective as daily therapy for disseminated candidiasis in mice with persistent neutropenia. *Antimicrob Agents Chemother* 2007;51:968–974.

215. Gumbo T, Drusano GL, Liu W, et al. Anidulafungin pharmacokinetics and microbial response in neutropenic mice with disseminated candidiasis. *Antimicrob Agents Chemother* 2006;50:3695–3700.

216. Hope WW, Drusano GL, Moore CB, et al. Effect of neutropenia and treatment delay on the response to antifungal agents in experimental disseminated candidiasis. *Antimicrob Agents Chemother* 2007;51:285–295

217. Hope WW, Mickiene D, Petraitis V, et al. The pharmacokinetics and pharmacodynamics of micafungin in experimental hematogenous Candida meningoencephalitis: implications for echinocandin therapy in neonates. *J Infect Dis* 2008;197:163–171.

218. Hope WW, Warn PA, Sharp A, et al. Derivation of an in vivo drug exposure breakpoint for flucytosine against *Candida albicans* and impact of the MIC, growth rate, and resistance genotype on the antifungal effect. *Antimicrob Agents Chemother* 2006;50:3680–6388.

219. Howard SJ, Livermore J, Sharp A, et al. Pharmacodynamics of echinocandins against *Candida glabrata*: requirement for dosage escalation to achieve maximal antifungal activity in neutropenic hosts. *Antimicrob Agents Chemother* 2011;55:4880–4887.

220. Lepak A, Castanheira M, Diekema D, et al. Optimizing Echinocandin dosing and susceptibility breakpoint determination via in vivo pharmacodynamic evaluation against *Candida glabrata* with and without fks mutations. *Antimicrob Agents Chemother* 2012;56:5875–5882.

221. Lepak A, Nett J, Lincoln L, et al. Time course of microbiologic outcome and gene expression in *Candida albicans* during and following in vitro and in vivo exposure to fluconazole. *Antimicrob Agents Chemother* 2006;50:1311–1319.

222. Louie A, Banarjee P, Drusano GL, et al. Interaction between fluconazole and amphotericin B in mice with systemic infection due to fluconazole-susceptible or -resistant strains of *Candida albicans*. *Antimicrob Agents Chemother* 1999;43:2841–2847.

223. Louie A, Deziel M, Liu W, et al. Pharmacodynamics of caspofungin in a murine model of systemic candidiasis: importance of persistence of caspofungin in tissues to understanding drug activity. *Antimicrob Agents Chemother* 2005;49:5058–5068.

224. Louie A, Drusano GL, Banerjee P, et al. Pharmacodynamics of fluconazole in a murine model of systemic candidiasis. *Antimicrob Agents Chemother* 1998;42:1105–1109.

225. MacCallum DM, Coster A, Ischer A, et al. Genetic dissection of azole resistance mechanisms in *Candida albicans* and their validation in a mouse model of disseminated infection. *Antimicrob Agents Chemother* 2010;54:1476–1483.

226. Marine M, Pastor FJ, Guarro J, et al. Efficacy of posaconazole in a murine disseminated infection by *Candida tropicalis*. *Antimicrob Agents Chemother* 2010;54:530–532.

228. Sanati H, Ramos CF, Bayer AS, et al. Combination therapy with amphotericin B and fluconazole against invasive candidiasis in neutropenic-mouse and infective-endocarditis rabbit models. *Antimicrob Agents Chemother* 1997;41:1345–1348.

229. Spellberg B, Fu Y, Edwards JE Jr, et al. Combination therapy with amphotericin B lipid complex and caspofungin acetate of disseminated zygomycosis in diabetic ketoacidotic mice. *Antimicrob Agents Chemother* 2005;49:830–832.

230. Spellberg B, Ibrahim AS, Edwards JE Jr, et al. Mice with disseminated candidiasis die of progressive sepsis. *J Infect Dis* 2005;192:336–343.

231. Sugar AM. Interactions of amphotericin B and SCH 39304 in the treatment of experimental murine candidiasis: lack of antagonism of a polyene-azole combination. *Antimicrob Agents Chemother* 1991;35:1669–1671.

232. Sugar AM, Goldani LZ, Picard M. Treatment of murine invasive candidiasis with amphotericin B and cilofungin: evidence for enhanced activity with combination therapy. *Antimicrob Agents Chemother* 1991;35:2128–2130.

233. Sugar AM, Hitchcock CA, Troke PF, et al. Combination therapy of murine invasive candidiasis with fluconazole and amphotericin B. *Antimicrob Agents Chemother* 1995;39:598–601.

234. Sugar AM, Liu XP. Interactions of itraconazole with amphotericin B in the treatment of murine invasive candidiasis. *J Infect Dis* 1998;177:1660–1663.

235. Wiederhold NP, Najvar LK, Bocanegra R, et al. Comparison of anidulafungin's and fluconazole's in vivo activity in neutropenic and non-neutropenic models of invasive candidiasis. *Clin Microbiol Infect* 2012;18:E20–E23.

236. Wiederhold NP, Najvar LK, Bocanegra R, et al. In vivo efficacy of anidulafungin and caspofungin against *Candida glabrata* and association with in vitro potency in the presence of sera. *Antimicrob Agents Chemother* 2007;51:1616–1620.

237. Wiederhold NP, Najvar LK, Bocanegra RA, et al. Caspofungin dose escalation for invasive candidiasis due to resistant *Candida albicans. Antimicrob Agents Chemother* 2011;55:3254–3260.

238. Brieland J, Essig D, Jackson C, et al. Comparison of pathogenesis and host immune responses to *Candida glabrata* and *Candida albicans* in systemically infected immunocompetent mice. *Infect Immun* 2001;69:5046–5055.

239. Demant E, Easterbrook M. An experimental model of candida endophthalmitis. *Can J Ophthalmol* 1977;12:304–307.

240. Deren YT, Ozdek S, Kalkanci A, et al. Comparison of antifungal efficacies of moxifloxacin, liposomal amphotericin B, and combination treatment in experimental *Candida albicans* endophthalmitis in rabbits. *Can J Microbiol* 2010;56:1–7.

241. Edwards JE Jr, Montgomerie JZ, Foos RY, et al. Experimental hematogenous endophthalmitis caused by *Candida albicans. J Infect Dis* 1975;131:649–657.

242. Gupta SK, Dhingra N, Velpandian T, et al. Efficacy of fluconazole and liposome entrapped fluconazole for C. *albicans* induced experimental mycotic endophthalmitis in rabbit eyes. *Acta Ophthalmol Scand* 2000;75:448–450.

243. Kusbeci T, Avci B, Cetinkaya Z, et al. The effects of caspofungin and voriconazole in experimental Candida endophthalmitis. *Curr Eye Res* 2007;57:64.

244. Livermore JL, Felton TW, Abbott J, et al. Pharmacokinetics and pharmacodynamics of anidulafungin for experimental Candida endophthalmitis: insights into the utility of echinocandins for treatment of a potentially sight-threatening infection. *Antimicrob Agents Chemother* 2013;57:281–282.

245. Louie A, Liu W, Miller DA, et al. Efficacies of high-dose fluconazole plus amphotericin B and high-dose fluconazole plus 5-fluorocytosine versus amphotericin B, fluconazole, and 5-fluorocytosine monotherapies in treatment of experimental endocarditis, endophthalmitis, and pyelonephritis due to *Candida albicans. Antimicrob Agents Chemother* 1999;43:2831–2840.

246. Omuta J, Uchida K, Yamaguchi H, et al. Histopathological study on experimental endophthalmitis induced by bloodstream infection with *Candida albicans. Jpn J Infect Dis* 2007;60:33–39.

247. Savani DV, Perfect JR, Cobo LM, et al. Penetration of new azole compounds into the eye and efficacy in experimental Candida endophthalmitis. *Antimicrob Agents Chemother* 1987;31:6–10

248. Goldblum D, Frueh BE, Sarra GM, et al. Topical caspofungin for treatment of keratitis caused by *Candida albicans* in a rabbit model. *Antimicrob Agents Chemother* 2005;49:1359–1363.

249. Hu J, Wang Y, Xie L. Potential role of macrophages in experimental keratomycosis. *Invest Ophthalmol Vis Sci* 2009;50:2087–2094.

250. Ishibashi Y, Kaufman HE. Topical ketoconazole for experimental Candida keratitis in rabbits. *Am J Ophthalmol* 1986;102:522–526.

251. Mitchell BM, Wu TG, Jackson BE, et al. *Candida albicans* strain-dependent virulence and Rim13p-mediated filamentation in experimental keratomycosis. *Invest Ophthalmol Vis Sci* 2007;48:774–780.

252. O'Day DM, Head WS, Csank C, et al. Differences in virulence between two *Candida albicans* strains in experimental keratitis. *Invest Ophthalmol Vis Sci* 2000;41:1116–1121.

253. Ohno S, Fuerst DJ, Okumoto M, et al. The effect of K-582, a new antifungal agent, on experimental Candida keratitis. *Invest Ophthalmol Vis Sci* 1983;24:1626–1629.

254. Pleyer U, Legmann A, Mondino BJ, et al. Use of collagen shields containing amphotericin B in the treatment of experimental *Candida albicans*-induced keratomycosis in rabbits. *Am J Ophthalmol* 1992;113:303–308.

255. Ray WA, O'Day DM, Head WS, et al. Variability in isolate recovery rates from multiple and single breeds of outbred pigmented rabbits in an experimental model of Candida keratitis. *Curr Eye Res* 1984;3:949–953.

256. Wu TG, Wilhelmus KR, Mitchell BM. Experimental keratomycosis in a mouse model. *Invest Ophthalmol Vis Sci* 2003;44:210–216.

257. Yuan X, Hua X, Wilhelmus KR. The corneal expression of antimicrobial peptides during experimental fungal keratitis. *Curr Eye Res* 2010;35:872–879.

258. Yuan X, Mitchell BM, Wilhelmus KR. Gene profiling and signaling pathways of *Candida albicans* keratitis. *Mol Vis* 2008;14:1792–1798.

259. Zhong W, Yin H, Xie L. Expression and potential role of major inflammatory cytokines in experimental keratomycosis. *Mol Vis* 2009;15:1303–1311.

260. Mavridou E, Bruggeman RJ, Melchers WJ, et al. Efficacy of posaconazole against three clinical *Aspergillus fumigatus* isolates with mutations in the cyp51A gene. *Antimicrob Agents Chemother* 2010;54:860–865.

261. Bowman JC, Abruzzo GK, Anderson JW, et al. Quantitative PCR assay to measure *Aspergillus fumigatus* burden in a murine model of disseminated aspergillosis: demonstration of efficacy of caspofungin acetate. *Antimicrob Agents Chemother* 2001;3474–3481.

262. Vallor AC, Kirkpatrick WR, Navjar LK, et al. Assessment of *Aspergillus fumigatus* burden in pulmonary tissue of guinea pigs by quantitative PCR, galactomannan enzyme immunoassay, and quantitative culture. *Antimicrob Agents Chemother* 2008;52:2593–2598.

263. Hope WW, V Petraitis, Petraitiene R, et al. The initial 96 hours of invasive pulmonary aspergillosis: histopathology, comparative kinetics of galactomannan and (1->3) beta-d-glucan and consequences of delayed antifungal therapy. *Antimicrob Agents Chemother* 2010;54:4879–4886.

264. Lewis RE, Ben-Ami R, Best L, et al. Tacrolimus enhances the potency of posaconazole against Rhizopus oryzae in vitro and in an experimental model of mucormycosis. *J Infect Dis* 2013;207:834–841.

265. Ibrahim AS, Bowman SJC, Avanessian V, et al. Caspofungin inhibits Rhizopus oryzae 1,3-beta-D-glucan synthase, lowers burden in brain measured by quantitative PCR, and improves survival at a low but not a high dose during murine disseminated zygomycosis. *Antimicrob Agents Chemother* 2005;49:721–727.

266. Lamaris GA, Ben-Ami R, Lewis RE, et al. Increased virulence of Zygomycetes organisms following exposure to voriconazole: a study involving fly and murine models of zygomycosis. *J Infect Dis* 2009;199:1399–1406.

267. Lewis RE, Albert ND, Liao G, et al. Comparative pharmacodynamics of amphotericin B lipid complex and

liposomal amphotericin B in a murine model of pulmonary mucormycosis. *Antimicrob Agents Chemother* 2010;54:1298–1304.

268. Rodriguez MM, Serena C, Marine M, et al. Posaconazole combined with amphotericin B, an effective therapy for a murine disseminated infection caused by Rhizopus oryzae. *Antimicrob Agents Chemother* 2008;52:3786–3788.

269. Calvo E, Pastor FJ, Rodriguez MM, et al. Antifungal therapy in a murine model of disseminated infection by Cryptococcus gattii. *Antimicrob Agents Chemother* 2010;54:4074–4077.

270. Clemons KV, Stevens DA. Comparison of fungizone, Amphotec, AmBisome, and Abelcet for treatment of systemic murine cryptococcosis. *Antimicrob Agents Chemother* 1998;42:899–902.

271. Larsen RA, Bauer M, Thomas AM, et al. Correspondence of in vitro and in vivo fluconazole dose-response curves for *Cryptococcus neoformans*. *Antimicrob Agents Chemother* 2005;49:3297–3301.

272. Lengerova M, Kocmanova I, Racil K, et al. Detection and measurement of fungal burden in a guinea pig model of invasive pulmonary aspergillosis by novel quantitative nested real-time PCR compared with galactomannan and (1,3)-beta-D-glucan detection. *J Clin Microbiol* 2012;50:602–608.

273. Schwarz P, Dromer F, Lortholary O, et al. Efficacy of amphotericin B in combination with flucytosine against flucytosine-susceptible or flucytosine-resistant isolates of *Cryptococcus neoformans* during disseminated murine cryptococcosis. *Antimicrob Agents Chemother* 2006;50:113–120.

274. Serena C, Pastor FJ, Marine M, et al. Efficacy of voriconazole in a murine model of cryptococcal central nervous system infection. *J Antimicrob Chemother* 2007;60:162–165.

275. Thompson GR 3rd, Wiederhold NP, Najvar R, et al. A murine model of Cryptococcus gattii meningoencephalitis. *J Antimicrob Chemother* 2012;67:1432–1438.

276. Widmer F, Wright LC, Obando D, et al. Hexadecylphosphocholine (miltefosine) has broad-spectrum fungicidal activity and is efficacious in a mouse model of cryptococcosis. *Antimicrob Agents Chemother* 2006;50:414–421.

277. Wiederhold NP, Navjar LK, Bocanegra R, et al. Limited activity of miltefosine in murine models of cryptococcal meningoencephalitis and disseminated cryptococcosis. *Antimicrob Agents Chemother* 2013;57:745–750.

278. Zaragoza O, Mihu C, Casadevall A, et al. Effect of amphotericin B on capsule and cell size in *Cryptococcus neoformans* during murine infection. *Antimicrob Agents Chemother* 2005;49:4358–4361.

279. Chiller TM, Sobel RA, Luque JC, et al. Efficacy of amphotericin B or itraconazole in a murine model of central nervous system *Aspergillus* infection. *Antimicrob Agents Chemother* 2003;47:813–815.

280. Clemons KV, Espiritu M, Parmar R, et al. Comparative efficacies of conventional amphotericin b, liposomal amphotericin B (AmBisome), caspofungin, micafungin, and voriconazole alone and in combination against experimental murine central nervous system aspergillosis. *Antimicrob Agents Chemother* 2005;49:4867–4875.

281. Clemons KV, Parmar R, Martinez M, et al. Efficacy of Abelcet alone, or in combination therapy, against experimental central nervous system aspergillosis. *J Antimicrob Chemother* 2006;58:466–469.

282. Clemons KV, Schwartz JA, Stevens DA. Experimental central nervous system aspergillosis therapy: efficacy, drug levels and localization, immunohistopathology, and toxicity. *Antimicrob Agents Chemother* 2012;56:4439–4449.

283. Clemons KV, Stevens DA. The contribution of animal models of aspergillosis to understanding pathogenesis, therapy and virulence. *Med Mycol* 2005;43(Suppl 1):S101–S110.

284. Imai J, Singh G, Fernandez B, et al. Efficacy of Abelcet and caspofungin, alone or in combination, against CNS aspergillosis in a murine model. *J Antimicrob Chemother* 2005;56:166–171.

285. Imai JK, Singh G, Clemons KV, et al. Efficacy of posaconazole in a murine model of central nervous system aspergillosis. *Antimicrob Agents Chemother* 2004;48:4063–4066.

286. Singh G, Imai J, Clemons KV, et al. Efficacy of caspofungin against central nervous system *Aspergillus fumigatus* infection in mice determined by TaqMan PCR and CFU methods. *Antimicrob Agents Chemother* 2005;49:1369–1376.

287. Flattery AM, Hickey E, Gill CJ, et al. Efficacy of caspofungin in a juvenile mouse model of central nervous system candidiasis. *Antimicrob Agents Chemother* 2011;55:3491–3497.

288. Kang CI, Rouse MS, Mandrekar JN, et al. Anidulafungin treatment of candidal central nervous system infection in a murine model. *Antimicrob Agents Chemother* 2009;53:3576–3578.

289. Warn PA, Livermore J, Howard S, et al. Anidulafungin for neonatal hematogenous Candida meningoencephalitis: identification of candidate regimens for humans using a translational pharmacological approach. *Antimicrob Agents Chemother* 2012;56:708–714.

290. Capilla J, Clemons KV, Sobel RA, et al. Efficacy of amphotericin B lipid complex in a rabbit model of coccidioidal meningitis. *J Antimicrob Chemother* 2007;60:673–676.

291. Clemons KV, Capilla J, Sobel RA, et al. Comparative efficacies of lipid-complexed amphotericin B and liposomal amphotericin B against coccidioidal meningitis in rabbits. *Antimicrob Agents Chemother* 2009;53:1858–1862.

292. Gonzalez GM, Gonzalez G, Najvar LK, et al Therapeutic efficacy of caspofungin alone and in combination with amphotericin B deoxycholate for coccidioidomycosis in a mouse model. *J Antimicrob Chemother* 2007;60:1341–1346.

293. Kamberi P, Sobel RA, Clemons A, et al. Comparison of itraconazole and fluconazole treatments in a murine model of coccidioidal meningitis. *Antimicrob Agents Chemother* 2007;51:998–1003.

294. Sorensen KN, Sobel RA, Clemons KV, et al. Comparative efficacies of terbinafine and fluconazole in treatment of experimental coccidioidal meningitis in a rabbit model. *Antimicrobial Agents Chemother* 2000;44:3087–3091.

295. Sorensen KN, Sobel RA, Clemons KV, et al. Comparison of fluconazole and itraconazole in a rabbit model of coccidioidal meningitis. *Antimicrob Agents Chemother* 2000;44:1512–1517.

296. Williams PL, Sobel RA, Sorensen KN, et al. A model of coccidioidal meningoencephalitis and cerebrospinal vasculitis in the rabbit. *J Infect Dis* 1998;178:1217–1221.

297. Sorensen KN, Clemons KV, Stevens DA. Murine models of blastomycosis, coccidioidomycosis, and histoplasmosis. *Mycopathologia* 1999;146:53–65.

298. Al-Abdely HM, Najvar LK, Bocanegra R, et al. Antifungal therapy of experimental cerebral phaeohyphomycosis due to Cladophialophora bantiana. *Antimicrob Agents Chemother* 2005;49:1701–1707.

299. Calvo E, Pastor FJ, Guarro J. Antifungal therapies in murine disseminated phaeohyphomycoses caused by Exophiala species. *J Antimicrob Chemother* 2010;65:1455–1459.

300. Calvo E, Pastor FJ, Rodriguez MM, et al. Murine model of a disseminated infection by the novel fungus Fonsecaea monophora and successful treatment with posaconazole. *Antimicrob Agents Chemother* 2010;54:919–923.

301. Itoyama T, Uchida K, Yamaguchi H. Therapeutic effects of omoconazole nitrate on guinea-pigs experimentally infected with *Trichophyton mentagrophytes*. *J Antimicrob Chemother* 1997;39:825–827.

302. Itoyama T, Uchida K, Yamaguchi H, et al. Therapeutic effects of omoconazole nitrate on experimental tinea pedis, an intractable dermatophytosis, in guinea-pigs. *J Antimicrob Chemother* 1997;40:441–444.

303. Koga H, Nanjoh Y, Kaneda H, et al. Short-term therapy with luliconazole, a novel topical antifungal imidazole, in guinea pig models of tinea corporis and tinea pedis. *Antimicrob Agents Chemother* 2012;56:3138–3143.

304. Saunte DM, Simmel F, Frimodt-Møller N, et al. In vivo efficacy and pharmacokinetics of voriconazole in an animal model of dermatophytosis. *Antimicrob Agents Chemother* 2007;51:3317–3321.

305. Shimamura T, Kobota N, Nagasaka S, et al. Establishment of a novel model of onychomycosis in rabbits for evaluation of antifungal agents. *Antimicrob Agents Chemother* 2011;55:3150–3155.

306. Serena C, Marine M, Marimon R, et al. Effect of antifungal treatment in a murine model of blastoschizomycosis. *Int J Antimicrob Agents* 2007;29:79–83.

307. Serena C, Rodriguez MM, Marine M, et al. Combined therapies in a murine model of blastoschizomycosis. *Antimicrob Agents Chemother* 2007;51:2608–2610.

308. Serena C, Rodriguez MM, Marine M, et al. Micafungin combined with fluconazole, an effective therapy for murine blastoschizomycosis. *J Antimicrob Chemother* 2008;61:877–879.

309. Lionakis MS, Chamilos G, Lewis RE, et al. Pentamidine is active in a neutropenic murine model of acute invasive pulmonary fusariosis. Antimicrobial agents and chemotherapy 50:294-297.

310. Ruiz-Cendoya M, Marine M, Guarro J. Combined therapy in treatment of murine infection by Fusarium solani. *J Antimicrob Chemother* 2008;62:543–546.

311. Ruiz-Cendoya M, Marine M, Rodriguez MM, et al. Interactions between triazoles and amphotericin B in treatment of disseminated murine infection by Fusarium oxysporum. *Antimicrob Agents Chemother* 2009;53:1705–1708.

312. Wiederhold NP, Najvar LK, Bocanegra R, et al. Efficacy of posaconazole as treatment and prophylaxis against Fusarium solani. *Antimicrob Agents Chemother* 2010;54:1055–1059.

313. Bocanegra R, Najvar LK, Hernandez S, et al. Caspofungin and liposomal amphotericin B therapy of experimental murine scedosporiosis. *Antimicrob Agents Chemother* 2005;49:5139–5141.

314. Rodriguez MM, Calvo E, Serena C, et al. Effects of double and triple combinations of antifungal drugs in a murine model of disseminated infection by Scedosporium prolificans. *Antimicrob Agents Chemother* 2009;53:2153–2155.

315. Rodriguez MM, Pastor FJ, Salas V, et al. Experimental murine scedosporiosis: histopathology and azole treatment. *Antimicrob Agents Chemother* 2010;54:3480–3984.

316. Serena C, Gilgado M, Marine M, et al. Efficacy of voriconazole in a guinea pig model of invasive trichosporonosis. *Antimicrob Agents Chemother* 2006;50:2240–2243.

317. Serena C, Pastor FJ, Gilgado F, et al. Efficacy of micafungin in combination with other drugs in a murine model of disseminated trichosporonosis. *Antimicrob Agents Chemother* 2005;49:497–502.

318. Ryan DM. The usefulness of experimental models of urinary tract infections in the assessment of chemotherapeutic compounds. In: Williams JD, Gedes AM, eds. *Chemotherapy*. Vol. 2. New York: Plenum, 1976:205–215.

319. Roberts JA. Vesicoureteral reflux and pyelonephritis in the monkey: a review. *J Urol* 1992;148:1721–1725.

320. Goodman JL, Jurkovich P, Kodner C, et al. Persistent cardiac and urinary tract infections with *Borrelia burgdorferi* in experimentally infected Syrian hamsters. *J Clin Microbiol* 1991;29:894–896.

321. Kaijser B, Larsson P. Experimental acute pyelonephritis caused by enterobacteria in animals: a review. *J Urol* 1982;127:786–790.

322. Yagmurlu A, Boleken ME, Ertoy D, et al. Preventive effect of pentoxifylline on renal scarring in rat model of pyelonephritis. *Urology* 2003;61:1037–1041.

323. Glauser MP, Ransley P, Bille J. Urinary tract infections, pyelonephritic scars, and chemotherapy. In: Zak O, Sande MA, eds. *Experimental models in antimicrobial chemotherapy*. Vol. 1. London: Academic Press, 1986:319–346.

324. Rank RG. Animal models for urogenital infections. *Methods Enzymol* 1994;235:83–93.

325. Brooks SJD, Lyons JM, Braude AL. Immunization against retrograde pyelonephritis. I. Production of an experimental model of severe ascending *Escherichia coli* pyelonephritis without bacteremia in rats. *Am J Pathol* 1974;74:345–358.

326. Glauser MP, Lyons JM, Braude AI. Synergism of ampicillin and gentamicin against obtructive pyelonephritis due to *Escherichia coli* in rats. *J Infect Dis* 1979;139:133–140.

327. Meylan PR, Glauser MP. Failure of dexamethasone to prevent polymorphonuclear leukocyte infiltration during experimental acute exudative pyelonephritis and to reduce subsequent chronic scarring. *J Infect Dis* 1988;157:480–485.

328. Glauser MP, Bonard M. Treatment of experimental ascending *Escherichia coli* pyelonephritis with ceftriaxone alone and in combination with gentamicin. *Chemotherapy* 1982;28:410–416.

329. Lecamwasam JP, Miller TE. Antimicrobial agents in the management of urinary tract infection: an experimental evaluation. *J Lab Clin Med* 1989;114:510–519.

330. Bergeron MG, Marois Y. Benefit from high intrarenal levels of gentamicin in the treatment of E. coli pyelonephritis. *Kidney Int* 1986;30:481–487.

331. LeBrun M, Grenier L, Gourde P, et al. Effectiveness and toxicity of gentamicin in an experimental model of pye-

lonephritis: effect of time of administration. *Antimicrob Agents Chemother* 1999;43:1020–1026.

332. Miller TE, Findon G, Rainer SP, et al. The pathobiology of subclinical pyelonephritis: an experimental evaluation. *Kidney Int* 1992;41:1356–1365.

333. Haraoka M, Matsumoto T, Takashi K, et al. Suppression of renal scarring by prednisolone combined with ciprofloxacin in ascending pyelonephritis in rats. *J Urol* 1994;151:1078–1080.

334. Li C-R, Li Y, Li G-Q et al. In vivo antibacterial activity of nemonoxacin, a novel non-fluorinated quinolone. *J Antimicrob Chemother* 2010;65:2411–2415.

335. Anderson GG, Palermo JJ, Schilling JD, et al. Intracellular bacterial biofilm-like pods in urinary tract infections. *Science* 2003;301:105–107.

336. Mulvey MA, Schilling JD, Hultgren SJ. Establishment of a persistent *Escherichia coli* reservoir during the acute phase of a bladder infection. *Infect Immun* 2001;69:4572–4579.

337. Mulvey MA, Schilling JD, Martinez JJ, et al. Bad bugs and beleaguered bladders: interplay between uropathogenic *Escherichia coli* and innate host defenses. *Proc Natl Acad Sci USA* 2000;97:8829–8835.

338. Schilling JD, Martin SM, Hung CS, et al. Toll-like receptor 4 on stromal and hematopoietic cells mediates innate resistance to uropathogenic *Escherichia coli*. *Proc Natl Acad Sci USA* 2003;100:4203–4208.

339. Hagberg L, Engberg I, Freter R, et al. Ascending unobstructed urinary tract infection in mice caused by pyelonephritogenic *Escherichia coli* of human origin. *Infect Immun* 1983;40:273–283.

340. Hvidberg H, Struve C, Krogfelt KA, et al. Development of a long-term ascending urinary tract infection mouse model for antibiotic treatment studies. *Antimicrob Agents Chemother* 2000;44:156–163.

341. Johnson JR, Brown JJ. Defining inoculation conditions for the mouse model of ascending urinary tract infection that avoid immediate vesicoureteral reflux yet produce renal and bladder infection. *J Infect Dis* 1996;173:1306–1311.

342. Kerrn MB, Frimodt-Møller N, Espersen F. Effects of sulfamethizole and amdinocillin against *Escherichia coli* strains (with various susceptibilities) in an ascending urinary tract infection mouse model. *Antimicrob Agents Chemother* 2003;47:1002–1009.

343. Frimodt-Møller N. Correlation between pharmacokinetic/pharmacodynamic parameters and efficacy for antibiotics in the treatment of urinary tract infection. *Int J Antimicrob Agents* 2002;19:546–553.

344. Tsuchimori N, Yamasaki T, Okonogi K. Therapeutic effects of cefozopran against experimental mixed urinary tract infection with *Enterococcus faecalis* and *Pseudomonas aeruginosa* in mice. *J Antimicrob Chemother* 1997;39:423–425.

345. Allou N, Cambau E, Massias L, et al. Impact of low-level resistance to fluoroquinolones due to qnrA1 and qnrS1 genes or a gyrA mutation on ciprofloxacin bactericidal activity in a murine model of *Escherichia coli* urinary tract infection. *Antimicrob Agents Chemother* 2009;53:4292–4297.

346. Jakobsen L, Cattoir V, Jensen KS, et al. Impact of low-level fluoroquinolone resistance genes qnrA1, qnrB19 and qnrS1 on ciprofloxacin treatment of isogenic *Escherichia coli* strains in a murine urinary tract infection model. *J Antimicrob Chemother* 2012;67:2438–2444.

347. Johnson DE, Lockatell CV. Mouse model of ascending UTI involving short- and long-term indwelling catheters. In: Zak O, Sande MA, eds. *Handbook of animal models of infection*. San Diego, CA: Academic Press, 1999:441–445.

348. Johnson DE, Lockatell CV, Hall-Craggs M, et al. Mouse models of short- and long-term foreign body in the urinary bladder: analogies to the bladder segment of urinary catheters. *Lab Anim Sci* 1991;41:451–455.

349. Mikuniya T, Kato Y, Ida T, et al. Treatment of *Pseudomonas aeruginosa* biofilms with a combination of fluoroquinolones and fosfomycin in a rat urinary tract infection model. *J Infect Chemother* 2007;13:285–290.

350. Wang X, Fries BC. A murine model for catheter-associated candiduria. *J Med Microbiol* 2011;60:1523–1529.

351. Evliyaoğlu Y, Kobaner M, Celebi H, et al. The efficacy of a novel antibacterial hydroxyapatite nanoparticle-coated indwelling urinary catheter in preventing biofilm formation and catheter-associated urinary tract infection in rabbits. *Urol Res* 2011;39:443–449.

352. Yuste J, Jado I, Fenoll A, et al. β-lactam modification of the bacteraemic profile and its relationship with mortality in a pneumococcal mouse sepsis model. *J Antimicrob Chemother* 2002;49:331–335.

353. Griffith DC, Harford L, Williams R, et al. In vivo antibacterial activity of RWJ-54428, a new cephalosporin with activity against Gram-positive bacteria. *Antimicrob Agents Chemother* 2003;47:43–47.

354. Montgomerie JZ, Schick DG. Treatment of enterococcal pyelonephritis with trovafloxacin and rifampin: in vitro in vivo contrast. *Antimicrob Agents Chemother* 1998;42:188–189.

355. Sapico FL, Ginunas VJ, Montgomerie JZ, et al. Cefpirome, alone and in combination with gentamicin, for enterococcal pyelonephritis in the rodent model. *Diagn Microbiol Infect Dis* 1991;14:297–300.

356. Fu KP, Foleno BD, Lafredo SC, et al. In vitro and in vivo antibacterial activities of FK037, a novel parenteral broad-spectrum cephalosporin. *Antimicrob Agents Chemother* 1993;37:301–307.

357. Attardo Genco C, Arko RJ. Animal chamber models for study of host-parasite interactions. *Methods Enzymol* 1994;235:120–140.

358. Espersen F, Frimodt-Møller N, Corneliussen L, et al. Experimental foreign body infection in mice. *J Antimicrob Chemother* 1993;31(Suppl D):103–111.

359. Zimmerli W. Experimental models in the investigation of device-related infections. *J Antimicrob Chemother* 1993;31(Suppl D):97–102.

360. Zimmerli W. Tissue cage infection model. In: Zak O, Sande MA, eds. *Handbook of animal models of infection*. San Diego, CA: Academic Press, 1999:409–417.

361. de Lalla F. Antimicrobial chemotherapy in the control of surgical infectious complications. *J Chemother* 1999;11:440–445

362. Pascual A. Pathogenesis of catheter-related infections: lessons for new designs. *Clin Microbiol Infect* 2002;8:256–264.

363. Zimmerli W, Waldvogel FA, Vaudaux P, et al. Pathogenesis of foreign body infection: description and characteristics of an animal model. *J Infect Dis* 1982;146:487–497.

364. Chuard C, Vaudaux P, Waldvogel FA, et al. Susceptibility of *Staphylococcus aureus* growing on fibronectin-coated surfaces to bactericidal antibiotics. *Antimicrob Agents Chemother* 1993;37:625–632.

365. Furustrand Tafin U, Majic I, Zalila Belkhodja, et al. Gentamicin improves the activities of daptomycin and vancomycin against *Enterococcus faecalis* in vitro and in an experimental foreign-body infection model. *Antimicrob Agents Chemother* 2011;55(10):4281–4827.

366. John A-K, Schmaler M, Khanna N, et al. Reversible daptomycin tolerance of adherent staphylococci in an implant infection model. *Antimicrob Agents Chemother* 2011;55(7):3510–3516.

367. Murillo O, Pachon ME, Euba G, et al. Antagonistic effect of rifampin on the efficacy of levofloxacin at high doses in staphylococcal experimental foreign-body infection. *Antimicrob Agents Chemother* 2008;52(10):3681–3686.

368. Artini M, Scoarughi GL, Papa R, et al. Comparison of anti-bacterial prophylactic properties of two different vascular grafts: action of anti-bacterial graft coating and systemic antibiotic treatment. *Int J Immunopathol Pharmacol* 2010;23:383–386.

369. Jean-Baptiste E, Blanchemain N, Martel B, et al. Safety, healing, and efficacy of vascular prostheses coated with hydroxypropyl-β-cyclodextrin polymer: experimental in vitro and animal studies. *Eur J Vasc Endovasc Surg* 2012;43:188–197.

370. Polk HC, Lamont PM, Galland RB. Containment as a mechanism of nonspecific enhancement of defenses against bacterial infection. *Infect Immun* 1990;58:1807–1811.

371. Naziri W, Cheadle WG, Trachtenberg LS, et al. Increased antibiotic effectivness in a model of surgical infection through continuous infusion. *Am Surg* 1995;61:11–15.

372. Dai T, Kharkwal GB, Tanaka M, et al. Animal models of external traumatic wound infections. *Virulence* 2011;2,296–315.

373. Kaiser AB, Kernodle DS. Low-inoculum model of clean wound infection. In: Zak O, Sande MA, eds. *Handbook of animal models of infection*. San Diego, CA: Academic Press, 1999:205–211.

374. Simonetti O, Cirioni O, Goteri G, et al. Temporin A is effective in MRSA-infected wounds through bactericidal activity and acceleration of wound repair in a murine model. *Peptides* 2008;29:520–528.

375. Zaleski KJ, Kolodka T, Cywes-Bentley C, et al. Hyaluronic acid binding peptides prevent experimental staphylococcal wound infection. *Antimicrob Agents Chemother* 2006;50:3856–3860.

376. Ozcan AV, Demir M, Onem G, et al. Topical versus systemic vancomycin for deep sternal wound infection caused by methicillin-resistant *Staphylococcus aureus* in a rodent experimental model. *Tex Heart Inst J* 2006;33:107–110.

377. Mihu MR, Sandkovsky U, Han G, et al. The use of nitric oxide releasing nanoparticles as a treatment against *Acinetobacter baumannii* in wound infections. *Virulence* 2010;1:62–67.

378. Dijkstra HM, Manson WL, Klasen HJ, et al. Effect of polymixin B on intestinal bacterial translocation in *Pseudomonas aeruginosa* wound-colonized burned mice. *Eur Surg Res* 1992;24:69–76.

379. Manson WL, Coenen JMFH, Klasen HJ, et al. Intestinal bacterial transolcation in experimentally burned mice with wounds colonized by *Pseudomonas aeruginosa*. *J Trauma* 1992;33:654–658.

380. Simonetti O, Cirioni O, Orlando F, et al. Effectiveness of antimicrobial photodynamic therapy with a single treatment of RLP068/Cl in an experimental model of *Staphylococcus aureus* wound infection. *Br J Dermatol* 2011;164:987–995.

381. Ulkür E, Oncul O, Karagoz H et al. Comparison of silver-coated dressing (Acticoat), chlorhexidine acetate 0.5% (Bactigrass), and fusidic acid 2% (Fucidin) for topical antibacterial effect in methicillin-resistant Staphylococci-contaminated, full-skin thickness rat burn wounds. *Burns* 2005;31:874–877.

382. Simonetti O, Cirioni O, Lucarini G et al. Tigecycline accelerates staphylococcal-infected burn wound healing through matrix metalloproteinase-9 modulation. *J Antimicrob Chemother* 2012;67:191–201.

383. Kumari S, Harjai K, Chhibber S. Evidence to support the therapeutic potential of bacteriophage Kpn5 in burn wound infection caused by Klebsiella pneumoniae in BALB/c mice. *J Microbiol Biotechnol* 2010;20: 935–941.

384. Acar A, Uygur F, Diktaş H et al. Comparison of silver-coated dressing (Acticoat®), chlorhexidine acetate 0.5% (Bactigrass®) and nystatin for topical antifungal effect in *Candida albicans*-contaminated, full-skin-thickness rat burn wounds. *Burns* 2011;37:882–885.

385. Mahoney E, Reichner J, Bostom LR, et al. Bacterial colonization and the expression of inducible nitric oxide synthase in murine wounds. *Am J Pathol* 2002;161:2143–2152.

386. Kugelberg E, Norström T, Petersen TK, et al. Establishment of a superficial skin infection model in mice by using *Staphylococcus aureus* and *Streptococcus pyogenes*. *Antimicrob Agents Chemother* 2005;49:3435–3441.

387. Vingsbo Lundberg C, Frimodt-Møller N. Efficacy of topical and systemic antibiotic treatment of methicillin-resistant *Staphylococcus aureus* in a murine superficial skin wound infection model. *Int J Antimicrob Agents* 2013;42:272–275.

388. Ansfield MJ, Woods DE, Johanson WG. Lung bacterial clearance in murine pneumococcal pneumonia. *Infect Immun* 1977;17:195–204.

389. Bakker-Woudenberg IAJM, Jong-Hoenderop YT, Michel MF. Efficacy of antimicrobial therapy in experimental rat pneumonia: effects of impaired phagocytosis. *Infect Immun* 1979;25:366–375.

390. Davis CC, Mellencamp MA, Preheim LC. A model of pneumococcal pneumonia in chronically intoxicated rats. *J Infect Dis* 1991;163:799–805.

391. Mellencamp MA, Preheim LC. Pneumococcal pneumonia in a rat model of cirrhosis: effects of cirrhosis on pulmonary defense mechanisms against *Streptococcus pneumoniae*. *J Infect Dis* 1991;163:102–108.

392. Wakebe H, Imada T, Yoneda H, et al. Evaluation of OPC-17116 against important pathogens that cause respiratory tract infections. *Antimicrob Agents Chemother* 1994;38:2340–2345.

393. Gavalda J, Capdevila JA, Almirante B, et al. Treatment of experimental pneumonia due to penicillin-resistant *Streptococcus pneumoniae* in immunocompetent rats. *Antimicrob Agents Chemother* 1997;41:795–801.

394. Beskid G, Christenson JG, Cleeland R, et al. In vivo activity of ceftriaxone (Ro 13-9904), a new broad-spectrum semisynthetic cephalosporin. *Antimicrob Agents Chemother* 1981;20:159–167.

395. Mizgerd JP, Skerrett SJ. Animal models of human pneumonia. American journal of physiology. *Lung Cell Mol Physiol* 2008;294:L387–L398.

396. Miyazaki S, Nunoya T, Matsumoto T, et al. New murine model of bronchopneumonia due to cell-bound *Haemophilus influenzae*. *J Infect Dis* 1997;175: 205–209.

397. Fukuoka T, Kawada H, Kitayama A, et al. Efficacy of CS-834 against experimental pneumonia caused by penicillin-susceptible and -resistant *Streptococcus pneumoniae* in mice. *Antimicrob Agents Chemother* 1998;42:23–27.

398. Leggett J. *Murine models of pneumonia using aerosol infection.* San Diego, CA: Academic Press, 1999.

399. Dudhani RV, Turnidge JD, Nation RL, et al. fAUC/MIC is the most predictive pharmacokinetic/pharmacodynamic index of colistin against *Acinetobacter baumannii* in murine thigh and lung infection models. *J Antimicrob Chemother* 2010;65:1984–1990.

400. Harris G, Kuo Lee R, Lam CK, et al. A mouse model of *Acinetobacter baumannii* associated pneumonia using a clinically isolated hypervirulent strain. *Antimicrob Agents Chemother* 2013;57:3601–3613.

401. Koomanachai P, Kim A, Nicolau DP. Pharmacodynamic evaluation of tigecycline against *Acinetobacter baumannii* in a murine pneumonia model. *J Antimicrob Chemother* 2009;63:982–987.

402. Mutlu Yilmaz E, Sunbul M, Aksoy A, et al. Efficacy of tigecycline/colistin combination in a pneumonia model caused by extensively drug-resistant *Acinetobacter baumannii*. *Int J Antimicrob Agents* 2012;40:332–336.

403. Pachon-Ibanez ME, Docobo-Perez F, Jimenez-Mejias ME, et al. Efficacy of rifampin, in monotherapy and in combinations, in an experimental murine pneumonia model caused by panresistant *Acinetobacter baumannii* strains. *Eur J Clin Microbiol Infect Dis* 2011;30:895–901.

404. Pachon-Ibanez ME, Dacobo-Perez F, Lopez-Rojas R, et al. Efficacy of rifampin and its combinations with imipenem, sulbactam, and colistin in experimental models of infection caused by imipenem-resistant *Acinetobacter baumannii*. *Antimicrob Agents Chemother* 2010;54:1165–1172.

405. Pichardo C, Pachon-Ibanez ME, Docobo-Perez F, et al. Efficacy of tigecycline vs. imipenem in the treatment of experimental *Acinetobacter baumannii* murine pneumonia. *Eur J Clin Microbiol Infect Dis* 2010;29:527–531.

406. Song JY, Cheong HJ, Lee J, et al. Efficacy of monotherapy and combined antibiotic therapy for carbapenem-resistant *Acinetobacter baumannii* pneumonia in an immunosuppressed mouse model. *Int J Antimicrob Agents* 2009;33:33–39.

407. Tang HJ, Chuang YC, Ko WC, et al. Comparative evaluation of intratracheal colistimethate sodium, imipenem, and meropenem in BALB/c mice with carbapenem-resistant *Acinetobacter baumannii* pneumonia. *Int J Infect Dis* 2012;16:e34–e40.

408. Yuan Z, Ledesma KR, Singh R, et al. Quantitative assessment of combination antimicrobial therapy against multidrug-resistant bacteria in a murine pneumonia model. *J Infect Dis* 2010;201:889–897.

409. Bhalodi AA, Crandon JL, Biek D, et al. Efficacy of ceftaroline fosamil in a staphylococcal murine pneumonia model. *Antimicrob Agents Chemother* 2012;56:6160–6165.

410. Crandon JL, Kuti JL, Nicolau DP. Comparative efficacies of human simulated exposures of telavancin and vancomycin against methicillin-resistant *Staphylococcus aureus* with a range of vancomycin MICs in a murine pneumonia model. *Antimicrob Agents Chemother* 2010;54:5115–5119.

411. Docobo-Perez F, Lopez-Rojas R, Dominguez-Herrera J, et al. Efficacy of linezolid versus a pharmacodynamically optimized vancomycin therapy in an experimental pneumonia model caused by methicillin-resistant *Staphylococcus aureus*. *J Antimicrob Chemother* 2012;67:1961–1967.

412. Karau MJ, Tilahun AY, Schmidt SM, et al. Linezolid is superior to vancomycin in experimental pneumonia caused by Superantigen-Producing *Staphylococcus aureus* in HLA class II transgenic mice. *Antimicrob Agents Chemother* 2012;56:5401–5405.

413. Koomanachai P, Crandon JL, Banevicius L, et al. Pharmacodynamic profile of tigecycline against methicillin-resistant *Staphylococcus aureus* in an experimental pneumonia model. *Antimicrob Agents Chemother* 2009;53:5060–5063.

414. Laohavaleeson S, Tessier PR, Nicolau DP. Pharmacodynamic characterization of ceftobiprole in experimental pneumonia caused by phenotypically diverse *Staphylococcus aureus* strains. *Antimicrob Agents Chemother* 2008;52:2389–2394.

415. Lepak AJ, Marchillo K, Pichereau S, et al. Comparative pharmacodynamics of the new oxazolidinone tedizolid phosphate and linezolid in a neutropenic murine *Staphylococcus aureus* pneumonia model. *Antimicrob Agents Chemother* 2012;56:5916–5922.

416. Reyes N, Skinner R, Kaniga K, et al. Efficacy of telavancin (TD-6424), a rapidly bactericidal lipoglycopeptide with multiple mechanisms of action, in a murine model of pneumonia induced by methicillin-resistant *Staphylococcus aureus*. *Antimicrob Agents Chemother* 2005;49:4344–4346.

417. Tessier PR, Keel RA, Hagihara M, et al. Comparative in vivo efficacies of epithelial lining fluid exposures of tedizolid, linezolid, and vancomycin for methicillin-resistant *Staphylococcus aureus* in a mouse pneumonia model. *Antimicrob Agents Chemother* 2012;56:2342–2346.

418. Aoki N, Tateda K, Kikuchi Y, et al. Efficacy of colistin combination therapy in a mouse model of pneumonia caused by multidrug-resistant *Pseudomonas aeruginosa*. *J Antimicrob Chemother* 2009;63:534–542.

419. Bretonniere C, Jacqueline C, Caillon J, et al. Efficacy of doripenem in the treatment of *Pseudomonas aeruginosa* experimental pneumonia versus imipenem and meropenem. *J Antimicrob Chemother* 2010;65:2423–2427.

420. Crandon JL, Nicolau DP. Human stimulated studies of aztreonam and aztreonam-avibactam to evaluate activity against challenging gram-negative organisms, including metallo-beta-lactamase producers. *Antimicrob Agents Chemother* 2013;57:3299–3306.

421. Crandon JL, Schuck VJ, Banevicius MA, et al. Comparative in vitro and in vivo efficacies of human simulated doses of ceftazidime and ceftazidime-avibactam against *Pseudomonas aeruginosa*. *Antimicrob Agents Chemother* 2012;56:6137–6146.

422. Hagihara M, Crandon JL, Urban CM, et al. KPC presence in *Pseudomonas aeruginosa* has minimal impact on the in vivo efficacy of carbapenem therapy. *Antimicrob Agents Chemother* 2013;57:1086–1088.

423. Jacqueline C, Roquilly A, Desessard C, et al. Efficacy of ceftolozane in a murine model of Pseudomonas aeruginosa acute pneumonia: in vivo antimicrobial activity and impact on host inflammatory response. *J Antimicrob Chemother* 2013;68:177–183.

424. Louie A, Fregeau C, Liu W, et al. Pharmacodynamics of levofloxacin in a murine pneumonia model of *Pseudomonas aeruginosa* infection: determination of epithelial lining fluid targets. *Antimicrob Agents Chemother* 2009;53:3325–3330.

425. Morinaga Y, Yanagihara K, Nakamura S, et al. In vivo efficacy and pharmacokinetics of tomopenem (CS-023), a novel carbapenem, against *Pseudomonas aeruginosa* in a murine chronic respiratory tract infection model. *J Antimicrob Chemother* 2008;62:1326–1331.

426. Sabet M, Miller CE, Nolan TG, et al. Efficacy of aerosol MP-376, a levofloxacin inhalation solution, in models of mouse lung infection due to *Pseudomonas aeruginosa. Antimicrob Agents Chemother* 2009;53:3923–3928.

427. Bakker-Woudenberg IA, ten Kate MT, Goessens WH, et al. Effect of treatment duration on pharmacokinetic/pharmacodynamic indices correlating with therapeutic efficacy of ceftazidime in experimental *Klebsiella pneumoniae* lung infection. *Antimicrob Agents Chemother* 2006;50:2919–2925..

428. Docobo-Perez F, Nordmann P, Dominguez-Herrera J, et al. Efficacies of colistin and tigecycline in mice with experimental pneumonia due to NDM-1-producing strains of *Klebsiella pneumoniae* and *Escherichia coli. Int J Antimicrob Agents* 2012;39:251–254.

429. Goessens WH, Mouton JW, ten Kate MT, et al. The therapeutic effect of tigecycline, unlike that of Ceftazidime, is not influenced by whether the *Klebsiella pneumoniae* strain produces extended-spectrum beta-lactamases in experimental pneumonia in rats. *Antimicrob Agents Chemother* 2013;57:643–646.

430. Hilliard JJ, Melton JL, Hall L, et al. Comparative effects of carbapenems on bacterial load and host immune response in a *Klebsiella pneumoniae* murine pneumonia model. *Antimicrob Agents Chemother* 2011;55:836–544.

431. Hirsch EB, Guo B, Chang KT, et al. Assessment of antimicrobial combinations for *Klebsiella pneumoniae* carbapenemase-producing *K. pneumoniae. J Infect Dis* 2013;207:786–793.

432. Padilla E, Alonso D, Domenech-Sanchez A, et al. Effect of porins and plasmid-mediated AmpC beta-lactamases on the efficacy of beta-lactams in rat pneumonia caused by *Klebsiella pneumoniae. Antimicrob Agents Chemother* 2006;50:2285–2260.

433. Pichardo C, del Carmen Conejo M, Bernabeu-Wittel M, et al. Activity of cefepime and carbapenems in experimental pneumonia caused by porin-deficient *Klebsiella pneumoniae* producing FOX-5 beta-lactamase. *Clin Microbiol Infect* 2005;11:31–38.

434. Pichardo C, Rodriguez-Martinez JM, Pachon-Ibanez ME, et al. Efficacy of cefepime and imipenem in experimental murine pneumonia caused by porin-deficient *Klebsiella pneumoniae* producing CMY-2 beta-Lactamase. *Antimicrob Agents Chemother* 2005;49:3311–3316.

435. Ambrose PG, Forest A, Craig WA, et al. Pharmacokinetics-pharmacodynamics of gatifloxacin in a lethal murine *Bacillus anthracis* inhalation infection model. *Antimicrob Agents Chemother* 2007;51:4351–4355.

436. Deziel MR, Heine H, Louie A, et al. Effective antimicrobial regimens for use in humans for therapy of *Bacillus anthracis* infections and postexposure prophylaxis. *Antimicrob Agents Chemother* 2005;49:5099–5106.

437. Gill SC, Rubino CM, Bassett J, et al. Pharmacokinetic-pharmacodynamic assessment of faropenem in a lethal murine *Bacillus anthracis* inhalation postexposure prophylaxis model. *Antimicrob Agents Chemother* 2010;54:1678–1683.

438. Heine HS, Bassett J, Miller L, et al. Efficacy of oritavancin in a murine model of *Bacillus anthracis* spore inhalation anthrax. *Antimicrob Agents Chemother* 2008;52:3350–3357.

439. Heine HS, Bassett J, Miller L, et al. Determination of antibiotic efficacy against Bacillus anthracis in a mouse aerosol challenge model. *Antimicrob Agents Chemother* 2007;51:1373–1379.

440. Heine HS, Bassett J, Miller L, et al. Efficacy of Daptomycin against *Bacillus anthracis* in a murine model of anthrax spore inhalation. *Antimicrob Agents Chemother* 2010;54:4471–4473.

441. Heine HS, Purcell BK, Bassett J, et al. Activity of dalbavancin against *Bacillus anthracis* in vitro and in a mouse inhalation anthrax model. *Antimicrob Agents Chemother* 2010;54:991–996.

442. Kao LM, Bush K, Barnewall R, et al. Pharmacokinetic considerations and efficacy of levofloxacin in an inhalational anthrax (postexposure) rhesus monkey model. *Antimicrob Agents Chemother* 2006;50:3535–3542.

443. Hansen EJ, Toews GB. Animal models for the study of noninvasive *Haemophilus influenzae* disease: pulmonary clearance systems. *J Infect Dis* 1992;165(Suppl 1): S185–S187.

444. O'Reilly T. Relevance of animal models for chronic bacterial airway infections in humans. *Am J Respir Crit Care Med* 1995;151:2101–2107; discussion 2107–2108.

445. Toews GB, Gross GN, Pierce AK. The relationship of inoculum size to lung bacterial clearance and phagocytic cell response in mice. *Am Rev Respir Dis* 1979;120:559–566.

446. Johansen HK, Høiby N. Rat model of chronic *Pseudomonas aeruginosa.* In: Zak O, Sande MA, eds. *Handbook of animal models of infection.* San Diego, CA: Academic Press, 1999:517–532.

447. Schiff JB, Small GJ, Pennington JE. Comparative activities of ciprofloxacin, ticarcillin, and tobramycin against experimental *Pseudomonas aeruginosa* pneumonia. *Antimicrob Agents Chemother* 1984;26:1–4.

448. Hraiech S, Bregeon F, Brunel JM, et al. Antibacterial efficacy of inhaled squalamine in a rat model of chronic *Pseudomonas aeruginosa* pneumonia. *J Antimicrob Chemother* 2012;67:2452–2458.

449. Macia MD, Borrell N, Segura M, et al. Efficacy and potential for resistance selection of antipseudomonal treatments in a mouse model of lung infection by hypermutable *Pseudomonas aeruginosa. Antimicrob Agents Chemother* 2006;50:975–983.

450. Moser C, Van Gennip M, Bjarnsholt T, et al. Novel experimental *Pseudomonas aeruginosa* lung infection model mimicking long-term host-pathogen interactions in cystic fibrosis. *APMIS* 2009;117:95–107.

451. Song Z, Wu H, Mygind P, et al. Effects of intratracheal administration of novispirin G10 on a rat model of mucoid *Pseudomonas aeruginosa* lung infection. *Antimicrob Agents Chemother* 2005;49:3868–3874.

452. van Gennip M, Moser C, Christensen LD, et al. Augmented effect of early antibiotic treatment in mice with experimental lung infections due to sequentially adapted mucoid strains of *Pseudomonas aeruginosa. J Antimicrob Chemother* 2009;64:1241–1250.

453. Beaulac C, Sachetelli S, Lagace J. Aerosolization of low phase transition temperature liposomal tobramycin as a dry powder in an animal model of chronic pulmonary infection caused by *Pseudomonas aeruginosa. J Drug Target* 1999;7:33–41.

454. Cannon CL, Hogue LA, Vajravelu RK, et al. In vitro and murine efficacy and toxicity studies of nebulized SCC1, a methylated caffeine-silver(I) complex, for treatment of pulmonary infections. *Antimicrob Agents Chemother* 2009;53:3285–3293.

455. Ferrari F, Lu Q, Girardi C, et al. Nebulized ceftazidime in experimental pneumonia caused by partially resistant *Pseudomonas aeruginosa. Intensive Care Med* 2009;35:1792–1800.

456. Goldstein I, Wallet F, Nicolas-Robin A, et al. Lung deposition and efficiency of nebulized amikacin during

Escherichia coli pneumonia in ventilated piglets. *Am J Respir Crit Care Med* 2002;166:1375–1381.

457. Lu Q, Girardi C, Zhang M, et al. Nebulized and intravenous colistin in experimental pneumonia caused by *Pseudomonas aeruginosa*. *Intensive Care Med* 2010;36: 1147–1155.

458. Post JC. Direct evidence of bacterial biofilms in otitis media. *Laryngoscope* 2001;111:2083–2094.

459. Post JC, Aul JJ, White GJ, et al. PCR-based detection of bacterial DNA after antimicrobial treatment is indicative of persistent, viable bacteria in the chinchilla model of otitis media. *Am J Otolaryngol* 1996;17:106–111.

460. Post JC, Preston RA, Aul JJ, et al. Molecular analysis of bacterial pathogens in otitis media with effusion. *JAMA* 1995;273:1598–1604.

461. Hajek DM, Yuan Z, Quartey MK, et al. Otitis media: the chinchilla model. In: Zak O, Sande MA, eds. *Handbook of animal models of infection*. San Diego, CA: Academic Press, 1999:389–401.

462. Estrem SA. Bacterial otitis externa in the guinea-pig model. In: Zak O, Sande MA, eds. *Handbook of animal models of infection*. San Diego, CA: Academic Press, 1999:385–387.

463. Barry B, Muffat-Joly M. Gerbil model of acute otitis media. In: Zak O, Sande MA, eds. *Handbook of animal models of infection*. San Diego, CA: Academic Press, 1999:375–384.

464. Lim DJ, Hermansson A, Hellström SO, et al. Recent advances in otitis media. 3. Animal models; anatomy and pathology; pathogenesis; cell biology and genetics. *Ann Otol Rhinol Laryngol Suppl* 2005;194:31–41.

465. Caye-Thomasen P, Hermansson A, Tos M, et al. Effect of penicillin on experimental acute otitis media: a histopathological study of goblet cell density, bone modelling dynamics, polyp and adhesion formation. *Acta Otolaryngol [Suppl] (Stockh)* 2000;543:56–57.

466. Humphrey WR, Shattuck MH, Zielinski RJ, et al. Pharmacokinetics and efficacy of linezolid in a gerbil model of *Streptococcus pneumoniae*-induced acute otitis media. *Antimicrob Agents Chemother* 2003;47:1355–1363.

467. Parra A, Ponte C, Cenjor C, et al. Optimal dose of amoxicillin in treatment of otitis media caused by a penicillin-resistant pneumococcus strain in the gerbil model. *Antimicrob Agents Chemother* 2002;46:859–862.

468. Soriano F, Parra A, Cenjor C, et al. Role of *Streptococcus pneumoniae* and *Haemophilus influenzae* in the development of acute otitis media and otitis media with effusion in a gerbil model. *J Infect Dis* 2000;181:646–652.

469. Westman E, Melhus A. The treatment of *Haemophilus influenzae* acute otitis media with amoxicillin protects against reinfection but not against structural changes. *J Antimicrob Chemother* 2002;49:141–147.

470. Sato K, Quartey MK, Liebeler CL, et al. Timing of penicillin treatment influences the course of *Streptococcus pneumoniae*–induced middle ear inflammation. *Antimicrob Agents Chemother* 1995;39:1896–1898.

471. Parra A, Ponte C, Cenjor C, et al. Effect of antibiotic treatment delay on therapeutic outcome of experimental acute otitis media caused by *Streptococcus pneumoniae* strains with different susceptibilities to amoxicillin. *Antimicrob Agents Chemother* 2004;48:860–866.

472. Martínez-Marín C, Huelves L, del Prado G, et al. Effect of erythromycin treatment delay on therapeutic outcome of experimental acute otitis media caused by *Streptococcus pneumoniae*. *J Antimicrob Chemother* 2005;56:783–786.

473. Park SN, Yeo SW. Effects of antibiotics and steroid on middle ear mucosa in rats with experimental acute otitis media. *Acta Otolaryngol* 2001;121:808–812.

474. Parra A, Ponte C, Cenjor C, et al. Is it possible to achieve bacterial eradication in otitis media with effusion by empirical antibiotic high doses and concomitant administration of acetaminophen? A microbiological and pharmacological study in the gerbil model. *Int J Antimicrob Agents* 2003;22:508–515.

475. del Prado G, Martínez-Marín C, Huelves L, et al. Impact of ibuprofen therapy in the outcome of experimental pneumococcal acute otitis media treated with amoxicillin or erythromycin. *Pediatr Res* 2006;60:555–559.

476. Ponte C, Cenjor C, Parra A, et al. Antimicrobial treatment of an experimental otitis media caused by a beta-lactamase positive isolate of *Haemophilus influenzae*. *J Antimicrob Chemother* 1999;44:85–90.

477. Westmann E, Lundin S, Hermansson A, et al. β-Lactamase-producing nontypeable *Haemophilus influenzae* fails to protect *Stretococcus pneumoniae* from amoxicillin during experimental acute otitis media. *Antimicrob Agents Chemother* 2004;48:3536–3542.

478. Zwijnenburg PJ, van der PT, Florquin S, et al. Experimental pneumococcal meningitis in mice: a model of intranasal infection. *J Infect Dis* 2001;183:1143–1146.

479. Echchannaoui H, Frei K, Schnell C, et al. Toll-like receptor 2-deficient mice are highly susceptible to *Streptococcus pneumoniae* meningitis because of reduced bacterial clearing and enhanced inflammation. *J Infect Dis* 2002;186:798–806.

480. Gazzoni AF, Capilla J, Mayayo E, et al. Efficacy of intrathecal administration of liposomal amphotericin B combined with voriconazole in a murine model of cryptococcal meningitis. *Int J Antimicrob Agents* 2012;39: 223–227.

481. Mook-Kanamori BB, Rouse MS, Kang C, et al. Daptomycin in experimental murine pneumococcal meningitis. *BMC Infect Dis* 2009;9:50.

482. Nau R, Wellmer A, Soto A, et al. Rifampin reduces early mortality in experimental *Streptococcus pneumoniae* meningitis. *J Infec Dis* 1999;179:1557–1560.

483. Moxon ER, Ostrow PT. *Haemophilus influenzae* meningitis in infant rats: role of bacteremia in pathogenesis of age-dependent inflammatory responses in cerebrospinal fluid. *J Infect Dis* 1977;135:303–307.

484. Grandgirard D, Oberson K, Bühlmann A, et al. Attenuation of cerebrospinal fluid inflammation by the nonbacteriolytic antibiotic daptomycin versus that by ceftriaxone in experimental pneumococcal meningitis. *Antimicrob Agents Chemother* 2010;54:1323–1326.

485. Leib SL, Heimgartner C, Bifrare YD, et al. Dexamethasone aggravates hippocampal apoptosis and learning deficiency in pneumococcal meningitis in infant rats. *Pediatr Res* 2003;54:353–357.

486. Klein M, Koedel U, Pfister HW, et al. Meningitis-associated hearing loss: protection by adjunctive antioxidant therapy. *Ann Neurol* 2003;54:451–458.

487. Barichello T, Gonçalves JCN, Generoso JJS, et al. Attenuation of cognitive impairment by the nonbacteriolytic antibiotic daptomycin in Wistar rats submitted to pneumococcal meningitis. *BMC Neurosci* 2013;14:42.

488. Barichello T, Silva GZ, Batista AL, et al. Early antibiotic administration prevents cognitive impairment induced by meningitis in rats. *Neurosci Lett* 2009;465:71–73.

489. Brandt CT, Cayé-Thomasen P, Lund SP, et al. Hearing loss and cochlear damage in experimental pneumococcal

meningitis, with special reference to the role of neutrophil granulocytes. *Neurobiol Dis* 2006;23:300–311.

490. Dupuis A, Limosin A, Paquereau J, et al. Pharmacokinetic-pharmacodynamic modeling of electroencephalogram effect of imipenem in rats with acute renal failure. *Antimicrob Agents Chemother* 2001;45:3607–3609.

491. Vogel U, Frosch M. Infant rat model of acute meningitis. In: Zak O, Sande MA, eds. *Handbook of animal models of infection*. San Diego, CA: Academic Press, 1999:619–626.

492. Townsend GC, Scheld WM. Adult rat model of bacterial meningitis. In: Zak O, Sande MA, eds. *Handbook of animal models of infection*. San Diego, CA: Academic Press, 1999:631–638.

493. Force E, Taberner F, Cabellos C, et al. Experimental study of meropenem in the therapy of cephalosporin-susceptible and -resistant pneumococcal meningitis. *Eur J Clin Microbiol Infect Dis* 2008;27:685–690.

494. Cottagnoud P, Pfister M, Cottagnoud M, et al. Activities of ertapenem, a new long-acting carbapenem, against penicillin-sensitive or -resistant pneumococci in experimental meningitis. *Antimicrob Agents Chemother* 2003;47:1943–1947.

495. Østergaard C, Benfield T, Gesser B, et al. Pretreatment with granulocyte colony–stimulating factor attenuates the inflammatory response but not the bacterial load in cerebrospinal fluid during experimental pneumococcal meningitis in rabbits. *Infect Immun* 1999;67:3430–3436.

496. Kartalija M, Kaye K, Tureen JH, et al. Treatment of experimental cryptococcal meningitis with fluconazole: impact of dose and addition of flucytosine on mycologic and pathophysiologic outcome. *J Infect Dis* 1996;173:1216–1221.

497. Tureen J, Tuomanen E. Rabbit model of bacterial meningitis. In: Zak O, Sande MA, eds. *Handbook of animal models of infection*. San Diego, CA: Academic Press, 1999:631–638.

498. Spector R, Lorenzo AV. Inhibition of penicillin transport from cerebral spinal fluid after intracisternal inoculation of bacteria. *J Clin Invest* 1974;54:316–325.

499. Scheld WM, Brown RS, Sande MA. Comparison of netilmicin with gentamicin in the therapy of experimental *Escherichia coli* meningitis. *Antimicrob Agents Chemother* 1978;13:899–904.

500. McCracken GH, Nelson JD, Grimm L. Pharmacokinetics and bacteriological efficacy of cefoperazone, cefuroxime, ceftriaxone, and moxalactam in experimental *Streptococcus pneumoniae* and *Haemophilus influenzae* meningitis. *Antimicrob Agents Chemother* 1982;21:262–267.

501. Bardal-Ozcem S, Turhan T, Sipahi OR, et al. Daptomycin versus vancomycin in treatment of methicillin-resistant *Staphylococcus aureus* meningitis in an experimental rabbit model. *Antimicrob Agents Chemother* 2013;57:1556–1558.

502. Bardak-Ozcem S, Turhan T, Sipahi OR, et al. Daptomycin versus vancomycin in treatment of methicillin-resistant *Staphylococcus aureus* meningitis in an experimental rabbit model. *Antimicrob Agents Chemother* 2013;57:1556–1558.

503. Egermann U, Stanga Z, Ramin A, et al. Combination of daptomycin plus ceftriaxone is more active than vancomycin plus ceftriaxone in experimental meningitis after addition of dexamethasone. *Antimicrob Agents Chemother* 2009;53:3030–3033.

504. Sipahi OR, Turhan T, Pullukcu H, et al. Moxifloxacin versus ampicillin + gentamicin in the therapy of experimental *Listeria monocytogenes* meningitis. *J Antimicrob Chemother* 2008;61;670–673.

505. Stucki A, Cottagnoud M, Acosta F, et al. Efficacy of doripenem against *Escherichia coli* and *Klebsiella pneumoniae* in experimental meningitis. *J Antimicrob Chemother* 2012;67:661–665.

506. Ernst JD, Sande MA. Selected examples of failure of in vitro testing to predict in vivo response to antibiotics. In: Sabath LD, ed. *Action of antibiotics in patients*. Bern, Switzerland: Hans Huber Publishers, 1982:68–73.

507. Nathan BR, Scheld WM. The efficacy of trovafloxacin versus ceftriaxone in the treatment of experimental brain abscess/cerebritis in the rat. *Life Sci* 2003;73:1773–1782.

508. Bayer AS, Greenberg DP, Yih J. Correlates of therapeutic efficacy in experimental methicillin-resistant *Staphylococcus aureus* endocarditis. *Chemotherapy* 1988;34:46–55.

509. Braddour LM. Virulence factors among Gram-positive bacteria in experimental endocarditis. *Infect Immun* 1994;62:2143–2148.

510. Carbon C. Experimental endocarditis: a review of its relevance to human endocarditis. *J Antimicrob Chemother* 1993;31(Suppl D):71–86.

511. Eliopoulos GM, Thauvin-Eliopoulos C, Moellering RC. Contribution of animal models in the search for effective therapy for endocarditis due to enterococci with high-level resistance to gentamicin. *Clin Infect Dis* 1992;15:58–62.

512. Gutschik E. The *Enterococcus endocarditis* model in experimental animals and its relevance to human infections. *J Antimicrob Chemother* 1993;31(Suppl D):87–96.

513. Lefort A, Fantin B. Rabbit model of bacterial endocarditis. In: Zak O, Sande MA, eds. *Handbook of animal models of infection*. San Diego, CA: Academic Press, 1999:611–618.

514. Santoro J, Levison ME. Rat model of experimental endocarditis. *Infect Immun* 1978;19:915–918.

515. Le T, Bayer AS. Combination antibiotic therapy for infective endocarditis. *Clin Infect Dis* 2003;36:615–621.

516. Batard E, Jacqueline C, Boutoille D, et al. Combination of quinupristin-dalfopristin and gentamicin against methicillin-resistant Staphylococcus aureus: experimental rabbit endocarditis study. *Antimicrob Agents Chemother* 2002;46:2174–2178.

517. Hershberger E, Coyle EA, Kaatz GW, et al. Comparison of a rabbit model of bacterial endocarditis and an in vitro infection model with simulated endocardial vegetations. *Antimicrob Agents Chemother* 2000;44:1921–1924.

518. Tsitsika A, Pefanis A, Perdikaris GS, et al. Single-oral-dose azithromycin prophylaxis against experimental streptococcal or staphylococcal aortic valve endocarditis. *Antimicrob Agents Chemother* 2000;44:1754–1756.

519. Katsarolis I, Pefanis A, Iliopoulos D, et al. Successful trovafloxacin prophylaxis against experimental streptococcal aortic valve endocarditis. *Antimicrob Agents Chemother* 2000;44:2564–2566.

520. Siaperas P, Pefanis A, Iliopoulos D, et al. Evidence of less severe aortic valve destruction after treatment of experimental staphylococcal endocarditis with vancomycin and dexamethasone. *Antimicrob Agents Chemother* 2001;45:3531–3537.

521. Galani L, Pefanis A, Sakka V, et al. Successful treatment with moxifloxacin of experimental aortic valve endocarditis due to methicillin-resistant *Staphylococcus aureus* (MRSA). *Int J Antimicrob Agents* 2009;33:65–69.

522. Jacqueline C, Amador G, Batard E et al. Comparison of ceftaroline fosamil, daptomycin and tigecycline in an experimental rabbit endocarditis model caused by methicillin-susceptible, methicillin-resistant and glycopeptide-intermediate *Staphylococcus aureus. J Antimicrob Chemother* 2011;66:863–866.

523. Jacqueline C, Caillon J, Grossi O, et al. In vitro and in vivo assessment of linezolid combined with ertapenem: a highly synergistic combination against methicillin-resistant *Staphylococcus aureus. Antimicrob Agents Chemother* 2006;50:2547–2549.

524. Miro JM, Garcia-de-la-Maria C, Armero Y, et al. Addition of gentamicin or rifampin does not enhance the effectiveness of daptomycin in treatment of experimental endocarditis due to methicillin-resistant *Staphylococcus aureus. Antimicrob Agents Chemother* 2009;53: 4172–4177.

525. Miró JM, García-de-la-Mària C, Armero Y, et al. Efficacy of telavancin in the treatment of experimental endocarditis due to glycopeptide-intermediate *Staphylococcus aureus. Antimicrob Agents Chemother* 2007;51: 2373–2377.

526. Sacar, M, Sacar S, Cevahir N, et al. Comparison of antimicrobial agents as therapy for experimental endocarditis caused by methicillin-resistant *Staphylococcus aureus. Tex Heart Inst J* 2010;37:400–404.

527. Seidl K, Chen L, Bayer A, et al. Relationship of agr expression and function with virulence and vancomycin treatment outcomes in experimental endocarditis due to methicillin-resistant *Staphylococcus aureus. Antimicrob Agents Chemother* 2011;55:5631–5639.

528. Tattevin P, Basuino L, Bauer D, et al. Evaluation of ceftobiprole in a rabbit model of aortic valve endocarditis due to methicillin-resistant and vancomycin-intermediate *Staphylococcus aureus. Antimicrob Agents Chemother* 2010;54:610–613.

529. Tattevin P, Saleh-Mghir A, Davido B, et al. Comparison of six generic vancomycin products for treatment of methicillin-resistant *Staphylococcus aureus* experimental endocarditis in rabbits. *Antimicrob Agents Chemother* 2013;57:1157–1162.

530. Tsaganos T, Skiadas I, Koutoukas P, et al. Efficacy and pharmacodynamics of linezolid, alone and in combination with rifampicin, in an experimental model of methicillin-resistant *Staphylococcus aureus* endocarditis. *J Antimicrob Chemother* 2008;62:381–383.

531. Xiong YQ, Hady WA, Bayer AS, et al. Telavancin in therapy of experimental aortic valve endocarditis in rabbits due to daptomycin-nonsusceptible methicillin-resistant *Staphylococcus aureus. Antimicrob Agents Chemother* 2012;56:5528–5533.

532. Entenza JM, Veloso TR, Vouillamoz J, et al. In vivo synergism of ceftobiprole and vancomycin against experimental endocarditis due to vancomycin-intermediate *Staphylococcus aureus. Antimicrob Agents Chemother* 2011;55:3977–3984.

533. Entenza JM, Vouillamoz J, Glauser MP, et al. Efficacy of garenoxacin in treatment of experimental endocarditis due to *Staphylococcus aureus* or viridans group streptococci. *Antimicrob Agents Chemother* 2004;48: 86–92.

534. Marco F, de la Mària CG, Armero Y, et al. Daptomycin is effective in treatment of experimental endocarditis due to methicillin-resistant and glycopeptide-intermediate *Staphylococcus aureus. Antimicrob Agents Chemother* 2008;52:2538–2543.

535. Fox PM, Lampen RJ, Stumpf KS, et al. Successful therapy of experimental endocarditis caused by vancomycin-resistant *Staphylococcus aureus* with a combination of vancomycin and beta-lactam antibiotics. *Antimicrob Agents Chemother* 2006;50:2951–2956.

537. Yang S-J, Xiong YQ, Boyle-Vavra S, et al. Daptomycin-oxacillin combinations in treatment of experimental endocarditis caused by daptomycin-nonsusceptible strains of methicillin-resistant *Staphylococcus aureus* with evolving oxacillin susceptibility (the "seesaw effect"). *Antimicrob Agents Chemother* 2010;54:3161–3169.

538. Dubé L, Caillon J, Jacqueline C, et al. The optimal aminoglycoside and its dosage for the treatment of severe *Enterococcus faecalis* infection. An experimental study in the rabbit endocarditis model. *Eur J Clin Microbiol Infect Dis* 2012;11:2545–2547.

539. Dubé L, Caillon J, Gras-Le Guen C, et al. Simulation of human gentamicin pharmacokinetics in an experimental *Enterococcus faecalis* endocarditis model. *Antimicrob Agents Chemother* 2003;47:3663–3666.

540. Gavaldá J, Onrubia PL, Gómez MTM, et al. Efficacy of ampicillin combined with ceftriaxone and gentamicin in the treatment of experimental endocarditis due to *Enterococcus faecalis* with no high-level resistance to aminoglycosides. *J Antimicrob Chemother* 2003;52:514–517.

541. Pavleas J, Skiada A, Daikos GL, et al. Efficacy of teicoplanin, administered in two different regimens, in the treatment of experimental endocarditis due to *Enterococcus faecalis. J Chemother* 2008;20:208–212.

542. Vouillamoz J, Moreillon P, Giddey M, et al. Efficacy of daptomycin in the treatment of experimental endocarditis due to susceptible and multidrug-resistant enterococci. *J Antimicrob Chemother* 2006;58:1208–1214.

543. Boutoille D, Jacqueline C, Le Mabecque V, et al. In vivo impact of the MexAB-OprM efflux system on beta-lactam efficacy in an experimental model of *Pseudomonas aeruginosa* infection. *Int J Antimicrob Agents* 2009;33: 417–420.

544. Navas D, Caillon J, Gras-Le Guen C, et al. Comparison of in vivo intrinsic activity of cefepime and imipenem in a *Pseudomonas aeruginosa* rabbit endocarditis model: effect of combination with tobramycin simulating human serum pharmacokinetics. *J Antimicrob Chemother* 2004; 54:767–771.

545. Rodríguez-Hernández M-J, Jiménez-Mejias ME, Pichardo C, et al. Colistin efficacy in an experimental model of *Acinetobacter baumannii* endocarditis. *Clin Microb Infect* 2004;10:581–584.

546. Rank RG, Whittum-Hudson JA. Animal models for ocular infections. *Methods Enzymol* 1994;235:69–83.

547. Motschmann M, Behrens Baumann W. Rabbit model of bacterial conjunctivitis. In: Zak O, Sande MA, eds. *Handbook of animal models of infection*. San Diego, CA: Academic Press, 1999:353–359.

548. Kernacki KA, Hobden JA, Hazlett LD. Murine model of bacterial keratitis. In: Zak O, Sande MA, eds. *Handbook of animal models of infection*. San Diego, CA: Academic Press, 1999:361–366.

549. Evans D, Kuo T, Kwong M, et al. *Pseudomonas aeruginosa* strains with lipopolysaccharide defects exhibit reduced intracellular viability after invasion of corneal epithelial cells. *Exp Eye Res* 2002;75:635–643.

550. Lee EJ, Truong TN, Mendoza MN, et al. A comparison of invasive and cytotoxic *Pseudomonas aeruginosa* strain-induced corneal disease responses to therapeutics. *Curr Eye Res* 2003;27:289–299.

551. Romanowski EG, Mah FS, Yates KA, et al. The successful treatment of gatifloxacin-resistant *Staphylococcus aureus* keratitis with Zymar (gatifloxacin 0.3%) in a NZW rabbit model. *Am J Ophthalmol* 2005;139:867–877.

552. Oguz H, Ozbilge H, Oguz E, et al. Effectiveness of topical taurolidine versus ciprofloxacin, ofloxacin, and fortified cefazolin in a rabbit *Staphylococcus aureus* keratitis model. *Curr Eye Res* 2005;30:155–161.

553. Wu X, Jiang H, Xu Y, et al. Efficacy of gemifloxacin for the treatment of experimental *Staphylococcus aureus* keratitis. *J Ocul Pharmacol Ther* 2012;28:420–427.

554. Wu XG, Xin M, Chen H, et al. Novel mucoadhesive polysaccharide isolated from *Bletilla striata* improves the intraocular penetration and efficacy of levofloxacin in the topical treatment of experimental bacterial keratitis. *J Pharm Pharmacol* 2010;62:1152–1157.

555. Romanowski EG, Mah FS, Kowalski RP, et al. Benzalkonium chloride enhances the antibacterial efficacy of gatifloxacin in an experimental rabbit model of intrastromal keratitis. *J Ocul Pharmacl Ther* 2008;24:380–384.

556. Sanders ME, Norcross EW, Moore QC 3rd, et al. Efficacy of besifloxacin in a rabbit model of methicillin-resistant *Staphylococcus aureus* keratitis. *Cornea* 2009;28:1055–1060.

557. Eguchi H, Shiota H, Oguro S, et al. The inhibitory effect of vancomycin ointment on the manifestation of MRSA keratitis in rabbits. *J Infect Chemother* 2009;15:279–283.

558. Balzli CL, McCormick CC, Caballero AR, et al. The effectiveness of an improved combination therapy for experimental *Staphylococcus aureus* keratitis. *Adv Ther* 2010;27:933–940.

559. Aliprandis E, Ciralsky J, Lai H, et al. Comparative efficacy of topical moxifloxacin versus ciprofloxacin and vancomycin in the treatment of *P. aeruginosa* and ciprofloxacin-resistant MRSA keratitis in rabbits. *Cornea* 2005;24:201–205.

560. Bu P, Riske PS, Zaya NE, et al. A comparison of topical chlorhexidine, ciprofloxacin, and fortified tobramycin/cefazolin in rabbit models of *Staphylococcus* and *Pseudomonas keratitis*. *J Ocul Pharmacol Ther* 2007;23:213–220.

561. McCormick C, Caballero A, Tang A, et al. Effectiveness of a new tobramycin (0.3%) and dexamethasone (0.05%) formulation in the treatment of experimental *Pseudomonas keratitis*. *Curr Med Res Opin* 2008;24:1569–1575.

562. Mah FS, Romanowski EG, Kowalski RP, et al. Zymar (Gatifloxacin 0.3%) shows excellent Gram-negative activity against *Serratia marcescens* and *Pseudomonas aeruginosa* in a New Zealand White rabbit keratitis model. *Cornea* 2007;26:585–588.

563. Thibodeaux BA, Dajcs JJ, Caballero AR, et al. Quantitative comparison of fluoroquinolone therapies of experimental gram-negative bacterial keratitis. *Curr Eye Res* 2004;28:337–342.

564. Frucht-Pery J, Raiskup F, Mechoulam H, et al. Iontophoretic treatment of experimental pseudomonas keratitis in rabbit eyes using gentamicin-loaded hydrogels. *Cornea* 2006;25:1182–1186.

565. Hyon JY, Joo MJ, Hose S, et al. Comparative efficacy of topical gatifloxacin with ciprofloxacin, amikacin, and clarithromycin in the treatment of experimental *Mycobacterium chelonae* keratitis. *Arch Ophthalmol* 2004;122:1166–1169.

566. Sarayba MA, Shamie N, Reiser BJ, et al. Fluoroquinolone therapy in *Mycobacterium chelonae* keratitis after lamellar keratectomy. *J Cataract Refract Surg* 2005;31:1396–1402.

567. Ozturk F, Yavas GF, Kusbeci T, et al. Efficacy of topical caspofungin in experimental fusarium keratitis. *Cornea* 2007;26:726–728.

568. Yavas GF, Ozturk F, Kusbeci T, et al. Antifungal efficacy of voriconazole, itraconazole and amphotericin b in experimental fusarium solani keratitis. *Graefes Arch Clin Exp Ophthalmol* 2008;246:275–279.

569. Polat ZA, Vural A. Effect of combined chlorhexidine gluconate and neosporin on experimental keratitis with two pathogenic strains of *Acanthamoeba*. *Parasitol Res* 2012;110:1945–1950.

570. Maylath FR, Leopold IH. Study of experimental intraocular infection I. The recoverability of organisms inoculated into ocular tissues and fluids. II. The influence of antibiotics and cortisone, alone and combined, on intraocular growth of these organisms. *Am J Ophthalmol* 1955;40:86–101.

571. Giese MJ, Rayner SA, Fardin B, et al. Mitigation of neutrophil infiltration in a rat model of early *Staphylococcus aureus* endophthalmitis. *Invest Ophthalmol Vis Sci* 2003;44:3077–3082.

572. Kim IT, Park SK, Lim JH. Inflammatory response in experimental *Staphylococcus* and *Pseudomonas endophthalmitis*. *Ophthalmologica* 1999;213:305–310.

573. Ravindranath RM, Hasan SA, Mondino BJ. Immunopathologic features of *Staphylococcus epidermidis*–induced endophthalmitis in the rat. *Curr Eye Res* 1997;16:1036–1043.

574. Yoshizumi MO, Kashani A, Palmer J, et al. High dose intramuscular methylprednisolone in experimental *Staphylococcus aureus* endophthalmitis. *J Ocul Pharmacol Ther* 1999;15:91–96.

575. Callegan MC, Hill JM, Insler MS, et al. Methicillin-resistant *Staphylococcus aureus* keratitis in the rabbit: therapy with ciprofloxacin, vancomycin and cefazolin. *Curr Eye Res* 1992;11:1111–1119.

576. Yoshizumi MO, Lee GC, Equi RA, et al. Timing of dexamethasone treatment in experimental *Staphylococcus aureus* endophthalmitis. *Retina* 1998;18:130–135.

577. Smith MA, Sorenson JA, D'Aversa G, et al. Treatment of experimental methicillin-resistant *Staphylococcus epidermidis* endophthalmitis with intravitreal vancomycin and intravitreal dexamethasone. *J Infect Dis* 1997;175:462–466.

578. Park SS, Samiy N, Ruoff K, et al. Effect of intravitreal dexamethasone in treatment of pneumococcal endophthalmitis in rabbits. *Arch Ophthalmol* 1995;113:1324–1329.

579. Yildirim O, Oz O, Aslan G, et al. The efficacy of intravitreal levofloxacin and intravitreal dexamethasone in experimental *Staphylococcus epidermidis* endophthalmitis. *Ophthalmic Res* 2002;34:349–356.

580. De Kaspar HM, Ta CN, Engelbert M, et al. Effects of intravitreal corticosteroid in the treatment of *Staphylococcus aureus*-induced experimental endophthalmitis. *Retina* 2008;28:326–332.

581. Ermis SS, Cetinkaya Z, Kiyici H, et al. Effects of intravitreal moxifloxacin and dexamethasone in experimental *Staphylococcus aureus* endophthalmitis. *Curr Eye Res* 2007;32:337–344.

582. Liu F, Kwok AK, Cheung BM. The efficacy of intravitreal vancomycin and dexamethasone in the treatment of experimental bacillus cereus endophthalmitis. *Curr Eye Res* 2008;33:761–768.

583. Fukuda M, Sasaki K. General purpose antimicrobial ophthalmic solutions evaluated using new pharmacokinetic parameter of maximum drug concentration in aqueous. *Jpn J Ophthalmol* 2002;46:384–390.

584. Xu J, Heys JJ, Barocas VH, et al. Permeability and diffusion in vitreous humor: implications for drug delivery. *Pharm Res* 2000;16:664–669.

585. Bronner S, Jehl F, Peter JD, et al. Moxifloxacin efficacy and vitreous penetration in a rabbit model of *Staphylococcus aureus* endophthalmitis and effect on gene expression of leucotoxins and virulence regulator factors. *Antimicrob Agents Chemother* 2003;47:1621–1629.

586. Waga J, Nilsson-Ehle I, Ljungberg B, et al. Microdialysis for pharmacokinetic studies of ceftazidime in rabbit vitreous. *J Ocul Pharmacol Ther* 1999;15:455–463.

587. Fernandez de Gatta MM, Fruns I, Calvo MV, et al. Influence of pharmacokinetic model on vancomycin peak concentration targets. *Ther Drug Monit* 1996;18:145–148.

588. Waga J, Ehinger B. Intravitreal concentrations of some drugs administered with microdialysis. *Acta Ophthalmol Scand* 1997;75:36–40.

589. Ozturk F, Kortunay S, Kurt E, et al. Effects of trauma and infection on ciprofloxacin levels in the vitreous cavity. *Retina* 1999;19:127–130.

590. Ozturk F, Kurt E, Inan UU, et al. Penetration of topical and oral ofloxacin into the aqueous and vitreous humor of inflamed rabbit eyes. *Int J Pharm* 2000;204:91–95.

591. Fukuda M, Hanazome I, Sasaki K. The intraocular dynamics of vancomycin hydrochloride ophthalmic ointment (TN-011) in rabbits. *J Infect Chemother* 2003;9:93–96.

592. Ng EW, Samiy N, Ruoff KL, et al. Treatment of experimental *Staphylococcus epidermidis* endophthalmitis with oral trovafloxacin. *Am J Ophthalmol* 1998;126:278–287.

593. el-Massry A, Meredith TA, Aguilar HE, et al. Aminoglycoside levels in the rabbit vitreous cavity after intravenous administration. *J Ophthalmol* 1996;122:684–689.

594. Marrakchi-Benjaafar S, Cochereau I, Pocidalo JJ, et al. Systemic treatment of experimental staphylococcal endophthalmitis: comparative efficacy of sparfloxacin, pefloxacin, imipenem, vancomycin, and amikacin. *J Infect Dis* 1995;172:1312–1316.

595. Gupta SK, Dhingra N, Velpandian T, et al. Efficacy of fluconazole and liposome entrapped fluconazole for *C. albicans* induced experimental mycotic endophthalmitis in rabbit eyes. *Acta Ophthalmol Scand* 2000;78:448–450.

596. Gupta SK, Velpandian T, Dhingra N, et al. Intravitreal pharmacokinetics of plain and liposome-entrapped fluconazole in rabbit eyes. *J Ocul Pharmacol Ther* 2000;16:511–518.

597. Park SS, D'Amico DJ, Paton B, et al. Treatment of exogenous *Candida endophthlamitis* in rabbits with oral fluconazole. *Antimicrob Agents Chemother* 1995;39:958–963.

598. Choi S, Hahn TW, Osterhout G, et al. Comparative intravitreal antibiotic therapy for experimental *Enterococcus faecalis* endophthalmitis. *Arch Ophthalmol* 1996;114:61–65.

599. Wada T, Kozai S, Tajika T, et al. Prophylactic efficacy of ophthalmic quinolones in expeimental endophthalmitis in rabbits. *J Ocul Pharmacol Ther* 2008;24:278–289.

600. Sakalar YB, Ozekinci S, Celen MK. Treatment of experimental *Bacillus cereus* endophthalmitis using intravitreal moxifloxacin with or without dexamethasone. *J Ocul Pharmacol Ther* 2011;27:593–598.

601. Saleh M, Lefèvre S, Acar N, et al. Efficacy of intravitreal administrations of linezolid in an experimental model of *S. aureus*-related endophthalmitis. *Invest Ophthalmol Vis Sci* 2012;53:4832–4841.

602. Engelbert M, Miño de Kaspar H, Thiel M, et al. Intravitreal vancomycin and amikacin versus intravenous imipenem in the treatment of experimental *Staphylococcus aureus* endophthalmitis. *Graefes Arch Clin Exp Ophthalmol* 2004;242:313–320.

603. Engelbert M, Miño de Kaspar H, Mette M, et al. Intravenous treatment of experimental Staphylococcus aureus endophthalmitis: imipenem versus the combination of ceftazidime and amikacin. *Graefes Arch Clin Exp Ophthalmol* 2003;241:1029–1036.

604. Ferrer C, Rodríguez A, Abad JL, et al. Bactericidal effect of intravitreal levofloxacin in an experimental model of endophthalmitis. *Br J Ophthalmol* 2008;92:672–682.

605. Ozkiriş A, Evereklioglu C, Akgün H, et al. A comparison of intravitreal piperacillin/tazobactam with ceftazidime in experimental *Pseudomonas aeruginosa* endophthalmitis. *Exp Eye Res* 2005;80:361–367.

606. Horozoglu F, Metan G, Sever O, et al. Intravitreal tigecycline treatment in experimental *Acinetobacter baumannii* endophthalmitis. *J Chemother* 2012;24:101–106.

607. Cremieux AC, Carbon C. Experimental models of bone and prosthetic joint infections. *Clin Infect Dis* 1997;25:1295–1302.

608. Norden CW. Experimental osteomyelitis. I. A description of the model. *J Infect Dis* 1970;122:410–418.

609. Norden CW. Experimental osteomyelitis. II. Therapeutic trials and measurement of antibiotic levels in bone. *J Infect Dis* 1971;124:565–571.

610. Lazzarini L, Overgaard KA, Conti E, et al. Experimental osteomyelitis: what have we learned from animal studies about the systemic treatment of osteomyelitis? *J Chemother* 2006;18:451–460.

611. Yin LY, Lazzarini L, Li F, et al. Comparative evaluation of tigecycline and vancomycin, with and without rifampicin, in the treatment of methicillin-resistant *Staphylococcus aureus* experimental osteomyelitis in a rabbit model. *J Antimicrob Chemother* 2005;55:995–1002.

612. O'Reilly T, Mader JT. Rat model of osteomyelitis of the tiba. In: Zak O, Sande MA, eds. *Handbook of animal models of infection*. San Diego, CA: Academic Press, 1999:561–576.

613. Rissing JP, Buxton TB, Weinstein RS, et al. Model of experimental osteomyelitis in rats. *Infect Immun* 1985;47:581–586.

614. Dworkin R, Modin G, Kunz S, et al. Comparative efficacies of ciprofloxacin, pefloxacin, and vancomycin in combination with rifampin in a rat model of methicillin-resistant *Staphylococcus aureus* chronic osteomyelitis. *Antimicrob Agents Chemother* 1990;34:1014–1016.

615. Poeppl W, Tobudic S, Lingscheid T, et al. Efficacy of fosfomycin in experimental osteomyelitis due to methicillin-resistant *Staphylococcus aureus*. *Antimicrob Agents Chemother* 2011;55:931–933.

616. Kandemir O, Oztuna V, Colak M, et al. Comparison of the efficacy of tigecycline and teicoplanin in an experimental methicillin-resistant *Staphylococcus aureus* osteomyelitis model. *J Chemother* 2008;20:53–57.

617. Yagmurlu MF, Korkusuz F, Gursel I, et al. Sulbactam-cefoperazone polyhydroxybutyrate-co-hydroxyvalerate (PHBV) local antibiotic delivery system: in vivo effectiveness and biocompatibility in the treatment of implant-related experimental osteomyelitis. *J Biomed Mater Res* 1999;46:494–503.

618. Korkusuz F, Korkusuz P, Eksioglu F, et al. In vivo response to biodegradable controlled antibiotic release systems. *J Biomed Mater Res* 2001;55:217–228.

619. Nelson CL, McLaren SG, Skinner RA, et al. The treatment of experimental osteomyelitis by surgical debridement and the implantation of calcium sulfate tobramycin pellets. *J Orthop Res* 2002;20:643–647.

620. Mader JT, Stevens CM, Stevens JH, et al. Treatment of experimental osteomyelitis with a fibrin sealant antibiotic implant. *Clin Orthop* 2002;403:58–72.

621. Shirtliff ME, Calhoun JH, Mader JT. Experimental osteomyelitis treatment with antibiotic-impregnated hydroxyapatite. *Clin Orthop* 2002;401:239–247.

622. Mimoz O, Leotard S, Jacolot A, et al. Efficacies of imipenem, meropenem, cefepime, and ceftazidime in rats with experimental pneumonia due to a carbapenemhydrolyzing β-lactamase–producing strain of *Enterobacter cloacae*. *Antimicrob Agents Chemother* 2000;44: 885–890.

623. Subasi M, Kapukaya A, Kesemenli C, et al. Effect of granulocyte-macrophage colony–stimulating factor on treatment of acute osteomyelitis: an experimental investigation in rats. *Arch Orthop Trauma Surg* 2001;121: 170–173.

624. Xie Z, Liu X, Jia W, et al. Treatment of osteomyelitis and repair of bone defect by degradable bioactive borate glass releasing vancomycin. *J Controlled Release* 2009;139:118–126.

625. Stewart S, Barr S, Engiles J, et al. Vancomycin-modified implant surface inhibits biofilm formation and supports bone-healing in an infected osteotomy model in sheep: a proof-of-concept study. *J Bone Joint Surg Am* 2012;94:1406–1415.

626. Rouse MS, Piper KE, Jacobson M, et al. Daptomycin treatment of *Staphylococcus aureus* experimental chronic osteomyelitis. *J Antimicrob Chemother* 2006;57: 301–305.

627. Moskowitz JS, Blaisse MR, Samuel RE, et al. The effectiveness of the controlled release of gentamicin from polyelectrolyte multilayers in the treatment of *Staphylococcus aureus* infection in a rabbit bone model. *Biomaterials* 2010;31:6019–6030.

628. Kanellakopoulou K, Thivaios GC, Kolia M, et al. First identification of *Pseudomonas aeruginosa* isolates producing a KPC-type carbapenem-hydrolyzing β-lactamase. *Antimicrob Agents Chemother* 2007;51:1553–1555.

629. Kanellakopoulou K, Galanopoulos I, Soranoglou V, et al. Treatment of experimental osteomyelitis caused by methicillin-resistant *Staphylococcus aureus* with a synthetic carrier of calcium sulphate (Stimulan) releasing moxifloxacin. *Int J Antimicrob Agents* 2009;33: 354–359.

630. Giavaresi G, Borsari V, Fini M, et al. Preliminary investigations on a new gentamicin and vancomycin-coated PMMA nail for the treatment of bone and intramedullary infections: an experimental study in the rabbit. *J Orthop Res* 2008;26:785–792.

631. Gaudin A, Jacqueline C, Gautier H, et al. A delivery system of linezolid to enhance the MRSA osteomyelitis prognosis: in vivo experimental assessment. *Eur J Clin Microbiol Infect Dis* 2013;32:195–198.

632. Nijhof MW, Fleer A, Hardus K, et al. Tobramycincontaining bone cement and systemic cefazolin in a onestage revision: treatment of infection in a rabbit model. *J Biomed Mater Res* 2001;58:747–753.

633. Del Pozo JL, Rouse MS, Euba G, et al. The electricidal effect is active in an experimental model of *Staphylococcus epidermidis* chronic foreign body osteomyelitis. *Antimicrob Agents Chemother* 2009;53:4064–4068.

634. Ozturan KE, Yucel I, Kocoglu E, et al. Efficacy of moxifloxacin compared to teicoplanin in the treatment of implant-related chronic osteomyelitis in rats. *J Orthop Res* 2010;28:1368–1372.

635. Vergidis P, Rouse MS, Euba G, et al. (2011). Treatment with linezolid or vancomycin in combination with rifampin is effective in an animal model of methicillinresistant Staphylococcus aureus foreign body osteomyelitis. *Antimicrob Agents Chemother* 2011;55:1182–1186.

636. Schroeder K, Simank H, Lorenz H, et al. Implant stability in the treatment of MRSA bone implant infections with linezolid versus vancomycin in a rabbit model. *J Orthop Res* 2012;30:190–195.

637. Cohen Y, Perronne C, Lazard T, et al. Use of normal C57BL/6 mice with established *Mycobacterium avium* infections as an alternative model for evaluation of antibiotic activity. *Antimicrob Agents Chemother* 1995;39:735–738.

638. Yangco BG, Lackman-Smith C, Espinoza CG, et al. The hamster model of chronic *Mycobacterium avium* complex infection. *J Infect Dis* 1989;159:556–561.

639. Brown ST, Edwards FF, Bernhard EM, et al. Azithromycin, rifabutin, and rifapentine for treatment and prophylaxis of *Mycobacterium avium* complex in rats treated with cyclosporine. *Antimicrob Agents Chemother* 1993;37:398–402.

640. Cynamon MH, DeStefano MS. Beige mouse model of disseminated Mycobacterium avium complex infection. In: Zak O, Sande MA, eds. *Handbook of animal models of infection*. San Diego, CA: Academic Press, 1999:321–330.

641. Gangadharam PRJ, Ashtekar DR, Flasher DL, et al. Therapy of *Mycobacterium avium* complex infections in beige mice with streptomycin encapsulated in sterically stabilized liposomes. *Antimicrob Agents Chemother* 1995;39:725–730.

642. Gangadharam PR. Beige mouse model for *Mycobacterium avium* complex disease. *Antimicrob Agents Chemother* 1995;30:1647–1654.

643. Wu HS, Kolonoski P, Chang YY, et al. Invasion of the brain and chronic central nervous system infection after systemic *Mycobacterium avium* complex infection in mice. *Infect Immun* 2000;68:2979–2984.

644. Gomes MS, Dom G, Pedrosa J, et al. Effects of iron deprivation on *Mycobacterium avium* growth. *Tuberc Lung Dis* 1999;79:321–328.

645. Siso JP, Yao Y, Klemper CA, et al. Treatment of *Mycobacterium avium* complex infection: does the beige mouse model predict therapeutic outcome in humans? *J Infect Dis* 1996;173:750–753.

646. Bermudez LE, Inderlied CB, Kolonoski P, et al. Telithromycin is active against *Mycobacterium avium* in mice despite lacking significant activity in standard in vitro and macrophage assays and is associated with low frequency of resistance during treatment. *Antimicrob Agents Chemother* 2001;45:2210–2214.

647. Goncalves AS, Appelberg R. Effects of recombinant granulocyte-colony stimulating factor administration during *Mycobacterium avium* infection in mice. *Clin Exp Immunol* 2001;124:239–247.

648. Fattorini L, Xiao Y, Mattei M, et al. Activities of eighteen antimicrobial regimens against *Mycobacterium avium* infection in beige mice. *Microb Drug Resist* 1999;5:227–233.

649. Bermudez LE, Inderlied CB, Kolonoski P, et al. Activity of moxifloxacin by itself and in combination with ethambutol, rifabutin, and azithromycin in vitro and in vivo against *Mycobacterium avium*. *Antimicrob Agents Chemother* 2001;45:217–222.

650. Nuermberger E. Using animal models to develop new treatments for tuberculosis. *Semin Respir Crit Care Med* 2008;29:542–551.

651. Franzblau SG, DeGroote MA, Cho SH, et al. Comprehensive analysis of methods used for the evaluation of compounds against *Mycobacterium tuberculosis*. *Tuberculosis* 2012;92:453–488.

652. De Groote MA, Gilliland JC, Wells CL, et al. Comparative studies evaluating mouse models used for efficacy testing of experimental drugs against *Mycobacterium tuberculosis*. *Antimicrob Agents Chemother* 2011;55:1237–1247.

653. Johnson AP, Tuffrey M, Taylor-Robinson D. Resistance of mice to genital infection with *Neisseria gonorrhoeae*. *J Med Microbiol* 1989;30:33–36.

654. Corbeil LB, Wunderlich AC, Corbeil RR, et al. Disseminated gonococcal infection in mice. *Infect Immun* 1979;26:984–990.

655. Arka RJ, Balows A. Animal models of experimental gonococcal infection. In: Zak O, Sande MA, eds. *Experimental models in antimicrobial chemotherapy*. Vol 1. London: Academic Press, 1986:355–369.

656. Demarco de Hormaeche R, Macpherson A, Bowe F, et al. Alterations of the LPS determine virulence of Neisseria gonorrhoeae in guinea-pig subcutaneous chambers. *Microb Pathog* 1991;11:159–170.

657. Elmros T, Holm SE, Kjellberg E, et al. Ampicillin treatment of Neisseria gonorrhoeae in vivo. An experimental study in rabbits. *Acta Pathol Microbiol Scand B* 1981;89:143–148.

658. Keevil CW, Davies DB, Spillane BJ, et al. Influence of iron-limited and replete continuous culture on the physiology and virulence of *Neisseria gonorrhoeae*. *J Gen Microbiol* 1989;135:851–863.

659. Jerse AE. Experimental gonococcal genital tract infection and opacity protein expression in estradiol-treated mice. *Infect Immun* 1999;67:5699–5708.

660. Kita E, Katsui N, Emoto M, et al. Virulence of transparent and opaque colony types of *Neisseria gonorrhoeae* for the genital tract of mice. *J Med Microbiol* 1991;34:355–362.

661. Song W, Condron S, Mocca BT, et al. Local and humoral immune responses against primary and repeat *Neisseria gonorrhoeae* genital tract infections of 17beta-estradiol-treated mice. *Vaccine* 2008;26:5741–5751.

662. Jerse AE, Sharma ND, Simms AN, et al. A gonococcal efflux pump system enhances bacterial survival in a female mouse model of genital tract infection. *Infect Immun* 2003;71:5576–5582.

663. Warner DM, Folster JP, Shafer WM, et al. Regulation of the MtrC-MtrD-MtrE efflux-pump system modulates the in vivo fitness of *Neisseria gonorrhoeae*. *J Infect Dis* 2007;196:1804–1812.

664. Warner DM, Shafer WM, Jerse AE. Clinically relevant mutations that cause derepression of the *Neisseria gonorrhoeae* MtrC-MtrD-MtrE Efflux pump system confer different levels of antimicrobial resistance and in vivo fitness. *Mol Microbiol* 2008;70:462–478.

665. Kunz AN, Begum AA, Wu H, et al. Impact of fluoroquinolone resistance mutations on gonococcal fitness and in vivo selection for compensatory mutations. *J Infect Dis* 2012;1821–1829.

666. Alder JD. The hamster model of syphilis. In: Zak O, Sande MA, eds. *Handbook of animal models of infection*. San Diego, CA: Academic Press, 1999:285–289.

667. Baughn RE, Adams C, Musher DM. Evaluation of Sch 29482 in experimental syphilis and comparison with penicillin G benzathine in disseminated disease and localized infection. *Antimicrob Agents Chemother* 1984;26:401–404.

668. Lukehart SA, Baker-Zander SA, Holmes KK. Efficacy of aztreonam in treatment of experimental syphilis in rabbits. *Antimicrob Agents Chemother* 1984;25:390–391.

669. Fitzgerald TJ. Effects of cefetamet (Ro 15-8074) on Treponema pallidum and experimental syphilis. *Antimicrob Agents Chemother* 1992;36:598–602.

670. Baker-Zander SA, Lukehart SA. Efficacy of cefmetazole in the treatment of active syphilis in the rabbit model. *Antimicrob Agents Chemother* 1989;33:1465–1469.

671. Johnson RC, Bey RF, Wolgamot SJ. Comparison of the activities of ceftriaxone and penicillin G against experimentally induced syphilis in rabbits. *Antimicrob Agents Chemother* 1982;21:984–989.

672. Lukehart SA, Fohn MJ, Baker-Zander SA. Efficacy of azithromycin for therapy of active syphilis in the rabbit model. *J Antimicrob Chemother* 1990;25(Suppl A):91–99.

673. Alder J, Jarvis K, Mitten M, et al. Clarithromycin therapy of experimental Treponema pallidum infections in hamsters. *Antimicrob Agents Chemother* 1993;37:864–867.

674. Korting HC, Haag R, Walter D, et al. Efficacy of ceftizoxime in the treatment of incubating syphilis in rabbits. *Chemotherapy* 1993;39:331–335.

675. Korting HC, Walther D, Riethmuller U, et al. Ceftriaxone given repeatedly cures manifest syphilis in the rabbit. *Chemotherapy* 1987;33:376–380.

676. Marra C, Baker-Zander SA, Hook EW 3rd, et al. An experimental model of early central nervous system syphilis. *J Infect Dis* 1991;163:825–829.

677. Marra CM, Slatter V, Tartaglione TA, et al. Evaluation of aqueous penicillin G and ceftriaxone for experimental neurosyphilis. *J Infect Dis* 1992;165:396–397.

678. Tantalo LC, Lukehart SA, Marra CM. Treponema pallidum strain-specific differences in neuroinvasion and clinical phenotype in a rabbit model. *J Infect Dis* 2005;191:75–80.

679. Kajdacsy-Balla A, Howeedy A, Bagasra O. Experimental model of congenital syphilis. *Infect Immun* 1993;61:3559–3561.

680. Kajdacsy-Balla A, Howeedy A, Bagasra O. Syphilis in the Syrian hamster. A model of human venereal and congenital syphilis. *Am J Pathol* 1987;126:599–601.

681. Wicher V, Wicher K. Guinea-pig model of acquired and congenital syphilis. In: Zak O, Sande MA, eds. *Handbook of animal models of infection*. San Diego, CA: Academic Press, 1999:291–301.

682. Moller BR, Mardh PA. Animal models for the study of chlamydial infections of the urogenital tract. *Scand J Infect Dis Suppl* 1982;32:103–108.

683. Beale AS, Upshon PA. Characteristics of murine model of genital infection with *Chlamydia trachomatis* and effects of therapy with tetracyclines, amoxicillin-clavulanic acid, or azithromycin. *Antimicrob Agents Chemother* 1994;38:1937–1943.

684. Tuffrey MC, Woods C, Inman C, et al. The effect of a single oral dose of azithromycin on chlamydial infertility and oviduct ultrastructure in mice. *J Antimicrob Chemother* 1994;34:989–999.

685. Pal S, Sarcon AK, de la Maza LM. A new murine model for testing vaccines against genital *Chlamydia trachomatis* infections in males. *Vaccine* 2010;28:7606–7612.

686. Carey A, Cunningham K, Andrew D, et al. A comparison of the effects of a chlamydial vaccine administered during or after a *C. muridarum* urogenital infection of female mice. *Vaccine* 2011;29:6505–6513.

687. Imtiaz MT, Schripsema JH, Sigar IM, et al. Inhibition of matrix metalloproteinases protects mice from ascending infection and chronic disease manifestations resulting from urogenital *Chlamydia muridarum* infection. *Infect Immun* 2006;74:5513–5521.

688. Imtiaz MT, Schripsema JH, Sigar IM, et al. Outcome of urogenital infection with Chlamydia muridarum in CD14 gene knockout mice. *BMC Infect Dis* 2006;6:144.

689. Johnson RM, Kerr MS, Slaven JE. Plac8-dependent and inducible NO synthase-dependent mechanisms clear *Chlamydia muridarum* infections from the genital tract. *J Immunol* 2012;188:1896–1904.

690. Johnson RM, Yu H, Kerr MS, et al. PmpG303-311, a protective vaccine epitope that elicits persistent cellular immune responses in *Chlamydia muridarum*-immune mice. *Infect Immun* 2012;80:2204–2211.

691. Reeves DM, Nagarajan U, O'Connell C, et al. Lack of an effect of antibiotic treatment on prolonged detection of chlamydial DNA in murine genital tract infection. *Antimicrob Agents Chemother* 2007;51:2646–2648.

692. Boyd AR, Shivshankar P, Jiang S, et al. Age-related defects in TLR2 signaling diminish the cytokine response by alveolar macrophages during murine pneumococcal pneumonia. *Exp Gerontol* 2012;47:507–518.

693. Frazer LC, Darville T, Chandra-Kuntal K, et al. Plasmid-cured Chlamydia caviae activates TLR2-dependent signaling and retains virulence in the guinea pig model of genital tract infection. *PLoS One* 2012;7:e30747.

694. Wang Y, Nagarajan U, Hennings L, et al. Local host response to chlamydial urethral infection in male guinea pigs. *Infect Immun* 2010;78:1670–1681.

695. Sayek I. Animal models for intra-abdominal infection. *Hepatogastroenterology* 1997;44:923–926.

696. Weinstein WM, Onderdonk AB, Bartlen JC, et al. Antimicrobial therapy of experimental intraabdominal sepsis. *J Infect Dis* 1975;132:282–286.

697. Su H, Morrison R, Messer R, et al. The effect of doxycycline treatment on the development of protective immunity in a murine model of chlamydial genital infection. *J Infect Dis* 1999;180:1252–1258.

698. Dupont H, Montravers P. Rat polymicrobial peritonitis infection model. In: Zak O, Sande MA, eds. *Handbook of animal models of infection*. San Diego, CA: Academic Press, 1999:189–194.

699. Atmatzidis S, Koutelidakis I, Chatzimavroudis G, et al. Clarithromycin modulates immune responses in experimental peritonitis. *Int J Antimicrob Agents* 2011;37: 347–351.

700. Hyde SR, Stitih RD, McCallum RE. Mortality and bacteriology of sepsis following cecal ligation and puncture in aged mice. *Infect Immun* 1990;58:619–624.

701. Vianna RC, Gomes RN, Bozza FA, et al. Antibiotic treatment in a murine model of sepsis: impact on cytokines and endotoxin release. *Shock* 2004;21:115–120.

702. Remick DG, Call DR, Ebong SJ, et al. Combination immunotherapy with soluble tumor necrosis factor receptors plus interleukin 1 receptor antagonist decreases sepsis mortality. *Crit Care Med* 2001;29:473–481.

703. Cirioni O, Ghiselli R, Kamysz W, et al. Tachyplesin III and granulocyte-colony stimulating factor enhance the efficacy of tazobactam/piperacillin in a neutropenic mouse model of polymicrobial peritonitis. *Peptides* 2008;29:31–38.

704. Cirioni O, Giacometti A, Ghiselli R, et al. LL-37 protects rats against lethal sepsis caused by gram-negative bacteria. *Antimicrob Agents Chemother* 2006;50:1672–1679.

705. Cirioni O, Wu G, Li L, et al. S-thanatin enhances the efficacy of tigecycline in an experimental rat model of polymicrobial peritonitis. *Peptides* 2010;31:1231–1236.

706. Ghiselli R, Cirioni O, Giacometti A, et al. The cathelicidin-derived tritrpticin enhances the efficacy of ertapenem in experimental rat models of septic shock. *Shock* 2006;26:195–200.

707. Ghiselli R, Giacometti A, Cirioni O, et al. Efficacy of the bovine antimicrobial peptide indolicidin combined with piperacillin/tazobactam in experimental rat models of polymicrobial peritonitis. *Crit Care Med* 2008;36:240–245.

708. Giacometti A, Cirioni O, Ghiselli R, et al. Effects of pexiganan alone and combined with betalactams in experimental endotoxic shock. *Peptides* 2005;26:207–216.

709. Wu RQ, Xu YX, Song XH, et al. Relationship between cytokine mRNA expression and organ damage following cecal ligation and puncture. *World J Gastroenterol* 2002;8:131–134.

710. Yang S, Chung CS, Ayala A, et al. Differential alterations in cardiovascular responses during the progression of polymicrobial sepsis in the mouse. *Shock* 2002;17: 55–60.

711. Hollenberg SM, Dumasius A, Easington C, et al. Characterization of a hyperdynamic murine model of resuscitated sepsis using echocardiography. *Am J Respir Crit Care Med* 2001;164:891–895.

712. Kotake Y, Moore DR, Vasquez-Walden A, et al. Antioxidant amplifies antibiotic protection in the cecal ligation and puncture model of microbial sepsis through interleukin-10 production. *Shock* 2003;19:252–256.

713. Brook I. Intra-abdominal abscess. In: Zak O, Sande MA, eds. *Handbook of animal models of infection*. San Diego, CA: Academic Press, 1999:163–172.

714. Joiner K, Lower B, Dzink J, et al. Comparative efficacy of 10 antimicrobial agents in experimental infections with *Bacteroides fragilis*. *J Infect Dis* 1982;145:561–568.

715. Kapral FA, Godwin JR, Dye ES. Formation of intraperitoneal abscesses by *Staphylococcus aureus*. *Infect Immun* 1980;30:204–211.

716. Stoddart B, Wilcox MH. *Clostridium difficile*. *Curr Opin Infect Dis* 2002;15:513–518

717. Tran MC, Claros MC, Goldstein EJ. Therapy of *Clostridium difficile* infection: perspectives on a changing paradigm. *Expert Opin Pharmacother* 2013;14: 2375–2386.

718. Abrams GD, Allo M, Rifkin GD, et al. Mucosal damage mediated by clostridial toxin in experimental clindamycin-associated colitis. *Gut* 1980;21:493–499.

719. Czuprynski CJ, Johnson WJ, Balish E, et al. Pseudomembranous colitis in *Clostridium difficile*-monoassociated rats. *Infect Immun* 1983;39:1368–1376.

720. Fekety R, Silva J, Toshniwal R, et al. Antibiotic-associated colitis: effects of antibiotics on *Clostridium difficile* and the disease in hamsters. *Rev Infect Dis* 1979;1: 386–397.

721. Knoop FC. Clindamycin-associated enterocolitis in guinea pigs: evidence for a bacterial toxin. *Infect Immun* 1979;23:31–33.

722. Pawlowski SW, Calabrese G, Kolling GL, et al. Murine model of Clostridium difficile infection with aged gnotobiotic C57BL/6 mice and a BI/NAP1 strain. *J Infect Dis* 2010;202:1708–1712.

723. Steele J, Feng H, Parry N, et al. Piglet models of acute or chronic *Clostridium difficile* illness. *J Infect Dis* 2010;201:428–434.

724. Bartlett JG, Chang TW, Onderdonk AB. Comparison of five regimens for treatment of experimental clindamycin-associated colitis. *J Infect Dis* 1977;136:81–86.

725. Bartlett JG, Onderdonk AB, Cisneros RL. Clindamycin-associated colitis due to a toxin-producing species of Clostridium in hamsters. *J Infect Dis* 1977;136:701–705.

726. Lyerly DM, Saum KE, MacDonald DK, et al. Effects of *Clostridium difficile* toxins given intragastrically to animals. *Infect Immun* 1985;47:349–352.

727. Wilson KH, Sheagren JN, Freter R. Population dynamics of infested *Clostridium difficile* in the gastrointestinal tract of the Syrian hamster. *J Infect Dis* 1985;151:355–361.

728. Blankenship-Paris TL, Walton BJ, Hayes YO, et al. Clostridium difficile infection in hamsters fed an atherogenic diet. *Vet Pathol* 1995;32:269–273.

729. Dong M-Y, Chang T-W, Gorbach SL. Treatment of *Clostridium difficile* colitis in hamsters with a lipopeptide antibiotic, LY146032. *Antimicrob Agents Chemother* 1987;31:1135–1136.

730. McVay CS, Rolfe RD. In vitro and in vivo activities of nitazoxanide against *Clostridium difficile*. *Antimicrob Agents Chemother* 2000;44:2254–2258.

731. Drummond LJ, Smith DG, Poxton IR. Effects of sub-MIC concentrations of antibiotics on growth of and toxin production by *Clostridium difficile*. *J Med Microbiol* 2003;52:1033–1038.

732. Sun X, Wang H, Zhang Y, et al. Mouse relapse model of *Clostridium difficile* infection. *Infect Immun* 2011;79:2856–2864.

733. Chen X, Katchar K, Goldsmith JD, et al. A mouse model of *Clostridium difficile*-associated disease. *Gastroenterology* 2008;135:1984–1992.

735. Li Y, Figler RA, Kolling G, et al. Adenosine A2A receptor activation reduces recurrence and mortality from *Clostridium difficile* infection in mice following vancomycin treatment. *BMC Infect Dis* 2012;12:342.

736. Freeman J, Baines SD, Jabes D, et al. Comparison of the efficacy of ramoplanin and vancomycin in both in vitro and in vivo models of clindamycin-induced *Clostridium difficile* infection. *J Antimicrob Chemother* 2005;56:717–725.

737. Freeman J, Marquis M, Crowther GS, et al. Oritavancin does not induce *Clostridium difficile* germination and toxin production in hamsters or a human gut model. *J Antimicrob Chemother* 2012;67:2919–2926.

738. Jump RL, Li Y, Pultz MJ, et al. Tigecycline exhibits inhibitory activity against *Clostridium difficile* in the colon of mice and does not promote growth or toxin production. *Antimicrob Agents Chemother* 2011;55:546–549.

739. Adams DA, Riggs MM, Donskey CJ. Effect of fluoroquinolone treatment on growth of and toxin production by epidemic and nonepidemic *Clostridium difficile* strains in the cecal contents of mice. *Antimicrob Agents Chemother* 2007;51:2674–2678.

740. Lee A, Fox J, Hazell S. Pathogenicity of *Helicobacter pylori*: a perspective. *Infect Immun* 1993;61:1601–1610.

741. Marchetti M, Arico B, Burroni D. Development of a mouse model of *Helicobacter pylori* infection that mimics human disease. *Science* 1995;267:1655–1658.

742. Van Zanten SJ, Kolesnikow T, Leung V, et al. Gastric transitional zones, areas where Helicobacter treatment fails: results of a treatment trial using the Sydney strain mouse model. *Antimicrob Agents Chemother* 2003;47:2249–2255.

743. Endo H, Yoshida H, Ohmi N, et al. Effects of lansoprazole, clarithromycin and pH gradient on uptake of [^{14}C] amoxicillin into rat gastric tissue. *J Antimicrob Chemother* 2001;47:405–410.

744. Koga T, Inoue H, Ishii C, et al. Effect of plaunotol in combination with clarithromycin or amoxicillin on *Helicobacter pylori* in vitro and in vivo. *J Antimicrob Chemother* 2002;50:133–136.

745. Tran CD, Kritas S, Campbell MA, et al. Novel combination therapy for the eradication of *Helicobacter pylori* infection in a mouse model. *Scand J Gastroenterol* 2010;45:1424–1430.

746. Madoff LC, Michel JL, Gong EW, et al. Protection of neonatal mice from group B streptococcal infection by maternal immunization with beta C protein. *Infect Immun* 1992;60:4989–4994.

747. Rodewald AK, Onderdonk AB, Warren HB, et al. Neonatal mouse model of group B streptococcal infection. *J Infect Dis* 1992;166:635–639.

748. Kronforst KD, Mancuso CJ, Pettengill M, et al. A neonatal model of intravenous *Staphylococcus epidermidis* infection in mice <24 h old enables characterization of early innate immune responses. *PLoS One* 2012;7:e43897.

749. Oluola O, Kong L, Fein M, et al. Lysostaphin in treatment of neonatal Staphylococcus aureus infection. *Antimicrob Agents Chemother* 2007;51:2198–2200.

750. Placencia FX, Kong L, Weisman LE. Treatment of methicillin-resistant *Staphylococcus aureus* in neonatal mice: lysostaphin versus vancomycin. *Pediatr Res* 2009;65:420–424.

751. Venkatesh MP, Pham D, Fein M, et al. Neonatal coinfection model of coagulase-negative Staphylococcus (*Staphylococcus epidermidis*) and *Candida albicans*: fluconazole prophylaxis enhances survival and growth. *Antimicrob Agents Chemother* 2007;51:1240–1245.

752. Ashman RB, Papadimitriou JM, Fulurija A. Acute susceptibility of aged mice to infection with *Candida albicans*. *J Med Microbiol* 1999;48:1095–1102.

754. Murciano C, Villamon E, Yanez A, et al. Impaired immune response to *Candida albicans* in aged mice. *J Med Microbiol* 2006;55:1649–1656.

755. Pawlowski SW, Calabrese G, Kolling GL, et al. Murine model of *Clostridium difficile* infection with aged gnotobiotic C57BL/6 mice and a BI/NAP1 strain. *J Infect Dis* 2010;202:1708–1712.

756. Turnbull IR, Wlzorek JJ, Osborne D, et al. Effects of age on mortality and antibiotic efficacy in cecal ligation and puncture. *Shock* 2003;19:310–313.

757. Bass R, Lehnert T. Basic requirements for the toxicity testing of antimicrobial agents. *Eur J Clin Microbiol Infect Dis* 1990;9:488–491.

758. Mandell LA, Ball P, Tillotson G. Antimicrobial safety and tolerability: differences and dilemmas. *Clin Infect Dis* 2001;32:S72–S75.

759. Morris TH. Antibiotic therapeutics in laboratory animals. *Lab Anim* 1995;29:16–36.

760. Kacew S, Festing MFW. Role of rat strain in the differential sensitivity to pharmaceutical agents and naturally occurring substances. *J Toxicol Environ Health* 1996;47:1–30.

761. Festing MF, Diamanti P, Turton JA. Strain differences in haematological response to chloramphenicol succinate in mice: implications for toxicological research. *Food Chem Toxicol* 2001;39:375–383.

762. Holt D, Harvey D, Hurley R. Chloramphenicol toxicity. *Adverse Drug React Toxicol Rev* 1993;12:83–95.

763. Kararli TT. Comparison of the gastrointestinal anatomy, physiology, and biochemistry of humans and commonly used laboratory animals. *Biopharm Drug Dispos* 1995;16:351–380.

764. Cherbut C, Ferre JP, Corpet DE, et al. Alterations of intestinal microflora by antibiotics: effects on fecal excretion, transit time, and colonic motility in rats. *Dig Dis Sci* 1991;36:1729–1734.

765. Brunel A, Gouet P. Influence of the destabilization of the maternal digestive microflora on that of the newborn. *Biol Neonate* 1993;63:236–245.

766. Tune BM. Renal tubular transport and nephrotoxicity of beta lactam antibiotics: structure-activity relationships. *Miner Electrolyte Metab* 1994;20:221–231.

767. Valentovic MA, Ball JG, Rogers BA. Comparison of renal accumulation and urinary excretion in normoglycemic and diabetic animals. *Toxicology* 1996;108:93–99.

768. Ohtani H, Taninaka C, Hanada E, et al. Comparative pharmacodynamic analysis of Q-T interval prolongation induced by the macrolides clarithromycin, roxithromycin, and azithromycin in rats. *Antimicrob Agents Chemother* 2000;44:2630–2637.

769. Chenel M, Barbot A, Dupuis A, et al. Pharmacokinetic-pharmacodynamic modeling of the electroencephalogram effect of norfloxacin in rats. *Antimicrob Agents Chemother* 2003;47:1952–1957.

770. Van Etten EWM, ten Kate MT, Stearne LET, et al. Amphotericin B liposomes with prolonged circulation in blood: in vitro antifungal activity, toxicity, nd efficacy in systemic candidiasis in leukopenic mice. *Antimicrob Agents Chemother* 1995;39:1954–1958.

771. Wood CA, Finkbeiner HC, Kohlhepp SJ, et al. Influence of daptomycin on staphylococcal abscesses and experimental tobramycin nephrotoxicity. *Antimicrob Agents Chemother* 1989;33:1280–1285.

772. Bauhofer A, Witte K, Celik I, et al. Sickness behaviour, an animal equivalent to human quality of life, is improved in septic rats by G-CSF and antibiotic prophylaxis. *Langenbecks Arch Surg* 2001;386:132–140.

773. Bauhofer A, Witte K, Lemmer B, et al. Quality of life in animals as a new outcome for surgical research: G-CSF as a quality of life improving factor. *Eur Surg Res* 2002;34:22–29.

774. Craig WA. Post-antibiotic effects in experimental infection models: relationship to in-vitro phenomena and to treatment of infections in man. *J Antimicrob Chemother* 1993;31(Suppl D):149–158.

775. Craig WA, Legget J, Totsuka K, et al. Key pharmacokinetic parameters of antibiotic efficacy in experimental animal infections. *J Drug Dev* 1988;1(Suppl 3):7–15.

776. Fantin B, Ebert S, Leggett J, et al. Factors affecting duration of in-vivo postantibiotic effect for aminoglycosides against Gram-negative bacilli. *J Antimicrob Chemother* 1991;27:829–836.

777. Gudmundsson S, Vogelman B, Craig WA. The in-vivo postantibiotic effect of imipenem and other new antimicrobials. *J Antimicrob Chemother* 1986;18(Suppl E): 67–73.

778. MacKenzie FM, Gould IM. The post-antibiotic effect. *J Antimicrob Chemother* 1993;32:519–537.

779. Minguez F, Izquierdo J, Caminero MM, et al. In vivo postantibiotic effect of isepamicin and other aminoglycosides in a thigh infection model in neutropenic mice. *Chemotherapy* 1992;38:179–184.

780. Vogelman B, Gudmundsson S, Leggett J, et al. Correlation of antimicrobial pharmacokinetic indices with therapeutic efficacy in an animal model. *J Infect Dis* 1988;158:831–847.

781. Vogelman B, Gudmundsson S, Tumidge J, et al. In vivo postantibiotic effect in a thigh infection in neutropenic mice. *J Infect Dis* 1988;157:287–298.

782. Zhanel GG, Craig WA. Pharmacokinetic contributions to postantibiotic effects: focus on aminoglycosides. *Clin Pharmacokinet* 1994;27:377–392.

783. Cars O, Odenholt-Tornqvist I. The post-antibiotic sub-MIC effect in vitro and in vivo. *J Antimicrob Chemother* 1993;31(Suppl D):159–166.

784. Odenholt-Tornqvist I. Pharmacodynamics of beta-lactam antibiotics: studies on the paradoxical and postantibiotic effects in vitro and in an animal model. *Scand J Infect Dis Suppl* 1989;58:1–55.

785. Oshida T, Onta T, Nakanishi N, et al. Activity of subminimal inhibitory concentrations of aspoxicillin in prolonging the postantibiotic effect against *Staphylococcus aureus*. *J Antimicrob Chemother* 1990;26:29–38.

786. Majcherczyk PA, Kunz S, Hattenberger M, et al. Isolation and in-vitro and in-vivo characterisation of a mutant of *Pseudomonas aeruginosa* PA01 that exhibited a reduced postantibiotic effect in response to imipenem. *J Antimicrob Chemother* 1994;34:485–505.

787. Andes D, Marchillo K, Lowther J, et al. In vivo pharmacodynamics of HMR 3270, a glucan synthase inhibitor, in a murine candidiasis model. *Antimicrob Agents Chemother* 2003;47:1187–1192.

788. Spivey JM. The postantibiotic effect. *Clin Pharm* 1992;11:865–875.

789. Zhanel GG, Hoban DJ, Harding GK. The postantibiotic effect: a review of in vitro and in vivo data. *DICP* 1991;25:153–163.

790. Hughes WT, Armstrong D, Bodey GP, et al. Guidelines for the use of antimicrobial agents in neutropenic patients with unexplained fever. *J Infect Dis* 1990;161:381–396.

792. Love LJ, Schimpff SC, Schiffer CA, et al. Improved prognosis for granulocytopenic patients with Gram-negative bacteremia. *Am J Med* 1980;68:643–647.

793. Gerber AU, Greter U, Segessenmann C, et al. The impact of pre-treatment interval on antimicrobial efficacy in a biological model. *J Antimicrob Chemother* 1993; 31(Suppl D):29–39.

794. Cremieux A-C, Saleh-Mghir A, Vallois J-M, et al. Influence of the pre-treatment duration of infection on the efficacies of various antibiotic regimens in experimental streptococcal endocarditis. *J Antimicrob Chemother* 1993;32:843–852.

795. Azoulay-Dupuis E, Bedos J-P, Vallee E, et al. Anti-pneumococcal activity of ciprofloxacin, ofloxacin, and temafloxacin in an experimental mouse pneumonia model at various stages of disease. *J Infect Dis* 1991;163:319–324.

796. Kalns J, Morris J, Eggers J, et al. Delayed treatment with doxycycline has limited effect on anthrax infection in BKL57/B6. *Biochem Biophys Res Commun* 2002;297:506–509.

797. Contag PR. Whole-animal cellular and molecular imaging to accelerate drug development. *Drug Discov Today* 2002;7:555–562.

798. Contag PR, Olomu AB, Contag CH. Non-invasive monitoring of infection and gene expression in living animal models. In: Zak O, Sande MA, eds. *Handbook of animal models of infection*. San Diego, CA: Academic Press, 1999:61–68.

799. Contag PR, Olomu IN, Stevenson DK, et al. Bioluminescent indicators in living mammals. *Nat Med* 1998;4:245–247.

800. Balaban RS, Hampshire VA. Challenges in small animal noninvasive imaging. *ILAR J* 2001;42:248–262.

801. Signore A, Procaccini E, Annovazzi A, et al. The developing role of cytokines for imaging inflammation and infection. *Cytokine* 2000;12:1445–1454.

802. Ruiz-Cabello J, Regadera J, Santisteban C, et al. Monitoring acute inflammatory processes in mouse muscle by MR imaging and spectroscopy: a comparison with pathological results. *NMR Biomed* 2002;15:204–214.

803. Spellerberg B, Prasad S, Cabellos C, et al. Penetration of the blood-brain barrier: enhancement of drug delivery and imaging by bacterial glycopeptides. *J Exp Med* 1995;182:1037–1043.

804. Marzola P, Nicolato E, Di Modugno E, et al. Comparison between MRI, microbiology and histology in evaluation of antibiotics in a murine model of thigh infection. *MAGMA* 1999;9:21–28.

805. Spaeth HJ, Chandnani VP, Beltran J, et al. Magnetic resonance imaging detection of early experimental periostitis: comparison of magnetic resonance imaging, computed tomography, and plain radiography with histopathologic correlation. *Invest Radiol* 1991;26:304–308.

806. Fischman AJ, Alpert NM, Babich JW, et al. The role of positron emission tomography in pharmacokinetic analysis. *Drug Metab Rev* 1997;29:923–956.

807. Fischman AJ, Babich JW, Alpert NM, et al. Pharmacokinetics of ^{18}F-labeled trovafloxacin in normal and *Escherichia coli*–infected rats and rabbits studied with positron emission tomography. *Clin Microbiol Infect* 1997;3:63–72.

808. Via LE, Schimel D, Weiner DM, et al. Infection dynamics and response to chemotherapy in a rabbit model of tuberculosis using ^{18}F-2-Fluoro-deoxy-D-glucose positron emission timographt and computed tomography. *Antimicrob Agents Chemother* 2012;56:4391–4402.

809. Chandnani VP, Beltran J, Morris CS, et al. Acute experimental osteomyelitis and abscesses: detection with MR imaging versus CT. *Radiology* 1990;174:233–236.

810. Beltran J, McGhee RB, Shaffer PB, et al. Experimental infections of the musculoskeletal system: evaluation with MR imaging and Tc-99m MDP and Ga-67 scintigraphy. *Radiology* 1988;167:167–172.

811. Sartoris DJ, Guerra J Jr, Mattrey RF, et al. Perfluorooctylbromide as a contrast agent for computed tomographic imaging of septic and aseptic arthritis. *Invest Radiol* 1986;21:49–55.

812. Chen X, Schmidt AH, Mahjouri S, et al. Union of a chronically infected internally stabilized segmental defect in the rat femur after debridement and application of rhBMP-2 and systemic antibiotics. *J Orthop Trauma.* 2007;21:693–700.

813. Xiong YQ, Kupferwasser LI, Zack PM, et al. Comparative efficacies of liposomal amikacin (MiKasome) plus oxacillin versus conventional amikacin plus oxacillin in experimental endocarditis induced by *Staphylococcus aureus*: microbiological and echocardiographic analyses. *Antimicrob Agents Chemother* 1999;43:1737–1742.

814. Ntziachristos V, Bremer C, Weissleder R. Fluorescence imaging with near-infrared light: new technological advances that enable in vivo molecular imaging. *Eur Radiol* 2003;13:195–208.

815. Greer LF 3rd, Szalay AA. Imaging of light emission from the expression of luciferases in living cells and organisms: a review. *Luminescence* 2002;17:43–74.

816. Contag CH, Bachmann MH. Advances in in vivo bioluminescence imaging of gene expression. *Annu Rev Biomed Eng* 2002;4:235–260.

817. Burns SM, Jon D, Francis KP, et al. Revealing the spatiotemporal patterns of bacterial infectious diseases using bioluminescent pathogens and whole body imaging. Animal testing in infectology. *Contrib Microbiol* 2001;9:71–88.

818. Contag CH, Contag PR, Mullins JI, et al. Photonic detection of bacterial pathogens in living hosts. *Mol Microbiol* 1995;18:593–603.

819. Rocchetta HL, Boylan CJ, Foley JW, et al. Validation of a noninvasive, real-time imaging technology using bioluminescent *Escherichia coli* in the neutropenic mouse thigh model of infection. *Antimicrob Agents Chemother* 2001;45:129–137.

820. Francis KP, Yu J, Bellinger-Kawahara C, et al. Visualizing pneumococcal infections in the lungs of live mice using bioluminescent *Streptococcus pneumoniae* transformed with a novel Gram-positive. *Infect Immun* 2001;69:3350–3358.

821. Guo Y, Ramos RI, Cho JS, et al. In vivo biolumiinscense imaging to evaluate systemic and topical antibiotics against commuity-acquired methicillin-resistant *Staphylococcus aureus*-infected skin wounds in mice. *Antimicrob Agents Chemother* 2013;57:855–863.

822. Valdevia RH, Falkow S. Probing bacterial gene expression within host cells. *Trends Microbiol* 1997;5:360–363.

823. Valdevia RH, Falkow S. Fluorescence-based isolation of bacterial genes expressed within host cells. *Science* 1997;26:2007–2011.

824. Suarez A, Guttler A, Stratz M, et al. Green fluorescent protein-based reporter systems for genetic analysis of bacteria including monocopy applications. *Gene* 1997;196:69–74.

825. Bongaerts RJ, Hautefort I, Sidebotham JM, et al. Green fluorescent protein as a marker for conditional gene expression in bacterial cells. *Methods Enzymol* 2002;358:43–66.

826. Jacobi CA, Roggenkamp A, Rakin A, et al. In vitro and in vivo expression studies of yopE from *Yersinia enterocolitica* using the gfp reporter gene. *Mol Microbiol* 1998;30:865–882.

827. Acebo P, Nieto C, Corrales MA, et al. Quantitative detection of *Streptococcus pneumoniae* cells harbouring single or multiple copies of the gene encoding the green fluorescent protein. *Microbiology* 2000;146:1267–1273.

828. Valdivia RH, Hromockyj AE, Monack D, et al. Applications for green fluorescent protein (GFP) in the study of host-pathogen interactions. *Gene* 1996;173(1 Spec No):47–52.

829. del Poeta M, Toffaletti DL, Rude TH, et al. *Cryptococcus neoformans* differential gene expression detected in vitro and in vivo with green fluorescent protein. *Infect Immun* 1999;67:1812–1820.

830. Josenhans C, Friedrich S, Suerbaum S. Green fluorescent protein as a novel marker and reporter system in *Helicobacter* sp. *FEMS Microbiol Lett* 1998;161:263–273.

831. Scholz O, Thiel A, Hillen W, et al. Quantitative analysis of gene expression with an improved green fluorescent protein, p6. *Eur J Biochem* 2000;267:1565–1570.

832. Maksimow M, Hakkila K, Karp M, et al. Simultaneous detection of bacteria expressing GFP and DsRed genes with a flow cytometer. *Cytometry* 2002;47:243–247.

833. Leveau JH, Lindow SE. Predictive and interpretive simulation of green fluorescent protein expression in reporter bacteria. *J Bacteriol* 2001;183:6752–6762.

834. Wendland M, Bumann D. Optimization of GFP levels for analyzing Salmonella gene expression during an infection. *FEBS Lett* 2002;521:105–108.

835. Bryant PA, Venter D, Robins-Browne R, et al. Chips with everything: DNA microarrays in infectious diseases. *Lancet Infect Dis* 2004;4:100–111.

836. Chalker AF, Lunsford RD. Rational identification of new antibacterial drug targets that are essential for viability using a genomics-based approach. *Pharmacol Ther* 2002;95:1–20.

837. Fritz B, Raczniak GA. Bacterial genomics: potential for antimicrobial drug discovery. *BioDrugs* 2002;16:331–337.

838. Hayney MS. Pharmacogenomics and infectious diseases: impact on drug response and applications to disease management. *Am J Health Syst Pharm* 2002;59:1626–1631.

839. Knowles DJ, King F. The impact of bacterial genomics on antibacterial discovery. *Adv Exp Med Biol* 1998;456:183–195.

840. De Backer MD, Van Dijck P. Progress in functional genomics approaches to antifungal drug target discovery. *Trends Microbiol* 2003;11:470–478.

841. Watters JW, McLeod HL. Using genome-wide mapping in the mouse to identify genes that influence drug response. *Trends Pharmacol Sci* 2003;24:55–58.

842. Kimura S, Gonzalez FJ. Applications of genetically manipulated mice in pharmacogenetics and pharmacogenomics. *Pharmacology* 2000;61:147–153.

843. Drusano GL. Antimicrobial pharmacodynamics: critical interactions of "bug and drug." *Nat Rev Microbiol* 2004;2:289–300.

844. Moreillon P. Endocarditis prophylaxis revisited: experimental evidence of efficacy and new Swiss recommendations. Swiss Working Group for Endocarditis Prophylaxis. *Schweiz Med Wochenschr* 2000;130:1013–1026.

Chapter 14

Extravascular Antimicrobial Distribution and the Respective Blood and Urine Concentrations in Humans

David M. Bamberger, John W. Foxworth, Michael A. Kallenberger, Brian S. Pepito, and Dale N. Gerding

Systemically administered antimicrobials enter the vascular circulation and diffuse or are secreted into a variety of sites in the human body, in widely differing concentrations. The concentration of antimicrobials eventually achieved in a body site is the result of a complex set of factors that includes drug concentration, half-life, protein binding, lipid solubility, ionization, passive diffusion and active transport, extravascular site geometry, and degree of inflammation. Considerable data have been accumulated in the literature about antimicrobial distribution in humans, far more than can be reviewed completely in this chapter. Our purpose is to discuss the principles, models, and methods of assessing antimicrobial distribution in humans and to catalog that distribution in a number of representative extravascular sites.

Parenthetically, the presumed basis for a treatise of this kind, that is, that the extravascular site antimicrobial concentration correlates with the cure of infection at that site, has been demonstrated for some, but by no means all, infection sites. The ultimate cure of an infection entails far more variables than attainment of a specific concentration of an antimicrobial agent at the site of infection. Despite a presumed adequate antimicrobial concentration, the inflammatory milieu at sites of infection may be inhibitory to antimicrobial function (1). Nevertheless, the topic is discussed and the data presented on the assumption that extravascular antimicrobial concentrations

within specific sites have at least some importance in the treatment of infection.

TYPES OF EXTRAVASCULAR SITES

Sites of extravascular antimicrobial distribution may be divided into four major categories (2), as shown in Table 14.1. Antibiotic concentrations vary greatly from category to category and from site to site within categories. In general, the highest drug concentrations are found in certain secretory fluids, such as urine or bile, and the lowest in cerebrospinal fluid (CSF) and glandular secretions, such as breast milk and saliva (2).

Fluid-Filled Spaces

These sites provide the most readily interpretable data on extravascular drug distribution. The drug accumulates by means of passive diffusion, specimens rarely are contaminated by blood, and repeated samples can be obtained to profile the drug distribution and determine equilibrium conditions. Sites such as ascitic fluid, joint effusions, pleural effusions, amniotic fluid, pericardial effusions, bursae, blisters, and abscesses are classified in this category. These sites are also characterized by having a relatively small surface area for diffusion, compared with their volume. This results in a slow accumulation of antibiotic with repeated

Table 14.1

Categories of Extravascular Sites in Humans that Have Been Evaluated for Antibiotic Distribution

1. Fluid-filled spaces of relatively large volume into which drug passively diffuses
   Examples: ascites, pleural effusion, joint effusion, pericardial effusion, amniotic fluid, bursae, blisters, abscesses

2. Fluids produced by the excretion or secretion of glands or organs
   Examples: urine, bile, sputum, saliva, tears, sweat, milk, middle ear fluid, sinus fluid, prostatic fluid, semen

3. Fluid-filled spaces with probable diffusion barriers or active excretory systems
   Examples: CSF, aqueous humor, vitreous humor

4. Whole-body tissues
   Examples: skeletal muscle, skin, bone, cardiac muscle, liver, gallbladder, brain, uterus, ovary, fat, colon, tonsil, adenoid, lung, kidney, prostate, thyroid

CSF, cerebrospinal fluid.

dosing, as well as lower peak and higher trough drug concentrations than those of serum (3,4). In humans, the need to perform an invasive procedure (needle aspiration) to obtain fluid limits the utility of these sites for routine sampling, but cutaneous blister models in humans and tissue cages and semipermeable implanted chambers in animals provide useful models of this type of extravascular site (5–7).

Excretory and Secretory Fluids

These fluids provide the greatest variability in achievable drug concentrations of all extravascular sites. Because many antimicrobials are actively secreted into urine or bile, tremendous concentration of drug is possible. In contrast, many glands and organs appear to pose a substantial barrier to penetration by antimicrobials (e.g., milk and prostatic fluid). Numerous glandular secretions have been studied for antimicrobial penetration, but bile, urine, sputum, and milk are the most frequently examined. Many of these fluids are readily obtained without the aid of invasive techniques (urine, sputum, milk, and saliva) and thus have been repetitively sampled over time to garner data on secretory rates. As with fluid-filled spaces, secretory fluids usually are free of blood contamination

and thus provide the opportunity to determine antimicrobial concentrations quite reliably.

Spaces with Diffusion Barriers

Two body sites, the eye and the CSF, have traditionally been treated as unique because of the low concentration of many antimicrobials achieved there. Other secretory organs, such as breast and prostate, also pose barriers to drug penetration but are included under secretory organs. Although referred to as *barriers to diffusion*, active transport from CSF to blood or removal, by bulk CSF flow, of certain compounds such as penicillins may be a major reason for the low concentrations in CSF (8). Again, these sites provide reliable data about drug penetration because of their usual lack of blood contamination. However, the invasive nature of procedures used to obtain these fluids limits the number of determinations that can be made in patients.

Whole-body Tissues

Concentrations of antimicrobials in whole tissues are frequently difficult to interpret because of contamination of the tissues by blood and body fluids. Tissues have distinct compartments including interstitial fluid and cells, and cells contain various subcellular organelles and cytosol. Antimicrobial concentrations vary among these compartments. Some antimicrobials such as quinolones and macrolides attain high intracellular concentrations, whereas β-lactams and aminoglycosides do not. Further, the site of the infection may vary from being primarily extracellular or intracellular, making the knowledge of total tissue concentrations of questionable value (9). Despite these interpretation difficulties, whole tissue samples are among the specimens most frequently obtained for antimicrobial assay. We have included in this chapter our recommendations for the preparation and assay of whole tissues in order to make these determinations more reliable.

MODELS OF EXTRAVASCULAR ANTIBIOTIC DISTRIBUTION IN HUMANS

The use of human experimental models for extravascular distribution of antimicrobial agents is a potentially important development because it allows the controlled investigation of complex pharmacokinetic relationships seen in humans as intact individuals (10). The proper use and interpretation of these models can lead to a clearer understanding of the nature of drug distribution to sites outside the extravascular space. The primary experimental models currently under investigation include so-called skin-window techniques (both disk and chamber), skin-blister models (created by suction and irritant cantharides), the implantation of subcutaneous threads, and the use of microdialysis probes inserted into muscle or adipose tissue. The most useful models are likely to be the skin-blister models and microdialysis probes. The use of skin blisters provide sufficient volume of locally produced extravascular fluid to enable enough samples to be taken both for evaluation of the chemical composition of the extravascular fluid and for multiple antimicrobial concentration determinations so that a complete drug area under the curve (AUC) for extravascular fluid can be measured. This complete evaluation makes comparison to intravascular kinetic data more meaningful and valid conclusions more likely. Similarly, the use of microdialysis probes is a minimally invasive technique that provides complete pharmacokinetic data, including AUC data, of non–protein-bound antimicrobial concentrations within the interstial space of a tissue.

Skin-Window Disk

This technique was described by Raeburn (10) as a modification of the skin-window method of Rebuck and Crowley (11). A 25-mm^2 area of skin is abraded using a 25,000-rpm motorized buffer. The abrasion is done (without bleeding) just prior to measurement of the antibiotic. A sterile paper antibiotic disk (6- or 12-mm diameter) is then applied directly to the abraded area and covered with a sterile glass slide, which is secured in position for a selected period of time (usually 1 hour). New applications are made for each additional 1 hour that tissue fluid is to be sampled. Assays are performed by the bioassay technique using paper disks. The amount of tissue fluid on the disk is quantitated by a comparison of disk weight before and after application. Antibiotic standards for the bioassay should contain the same weight of fluid as the unknown specimen (12), a problem of considerable difficulty because disks increase their absorptive capacity with increasing time in contact with fluid, even up to 24 hours (13). The standards should be prepared in a diluent with a protein content similar to that of the tissue fluid (14). The latter point is particularly important for the assay of highly protein-bound drugs and has not been addressed in published studies with this model (10,12). The method allows for measurement of fluid for a

relatively short time period at each site and appears to sample tissue fluid that is absorbed from the denuded dermis by the capillary action of the paper disk. However, the limited amount of fluid obtained makes analysis of its composition difficult.

Skin-Window Chamber

This method, described by Tan et al. (15) and used by Tan and Salstrom (16,17), is also a modification of the Rebuck and Crowley (11) skin-window technique. The dermis is exposed by scraping the epidermis with a scalpel blade and placing a tissue culture chamber, with one glass window removed, over the exposed dermis (18). The chamber is taped in place and filled with 1 mL of sterile saline under slightly negative pressure. During study of a drug, the chamber is periodically emptied and refilled (usually at hourly intervals). The method results in marked dilution of the tissue fluid by saline or buffer. The assumption that equilibration of chamber and tissue fluid occurs within a 1-hour period is likely erroneous, based on the limited diffusing surface area compared with chamber volume. Protein content of the saline fluid is low, as anticipated, and therefore, this method is likely to show an apparent reduced penetration of highly bound drugs, compared with systems containing higher levels of albumin (7).

Skin Blister by Suction

This method is based on work by Kiistala and Mustakallio (19), who demonstrated a noninflammatory separation of the epidermis from the dermis by the application of negative pressure. The method used a Perspex block with eight 8-mm holes drilled in it (17). The block is tightly applied to the skin and 0.3 kg/cm^2 of pressure is applied to each bore for approximately 2 hours. A block applied to each forearm yields 16 0.15-mL blisters. A different blister is available for evacuation at each sample time. Blisters differ from the skin-window chambers in having fluid with high, rather than low, protein levels. This fluid is produced by the host without the addition of extraneous buffer.

Skin Blister by Cantharides

Cutaneous blisters can also be formed by application of the skin irritant, cantharides, which is prepared from the dried Spanish fly (*Cantharis vesicatoria*) or blister bug. Cantharidin, the most important active ingredient in Spanish fly, has also been used. Simon and Malerczyk (20) were probably the first to use this method. A plaster of 0.2% cantharides (or cantharidin ointment) is applied to the forearms in a 1-cm^2 area 8 to 12 hours before study (21). After formation, the blisters are repeatedly sampled with a fine-bore needle and syringe or capillary tube and the integrity of the blister is maintained by spraying the puncture site with a plastic dressing. The total protein and albumin contents of this inflammatory blister model are the highest of the models currently in use (21).

Subcutaneous Threads

Another method for the study of cutaneous antibiotic penetration in humans (22–24) is the subcutaneous thread. An area of the skin is anesthetized locally with lidocaine and multiple umbilical tapes are threaded under the skin with a needle for a distance of 1 to 2 cm. Studies are begun 30 minutes after placement. Tapes are advanced 1 to 2 cm after each time interval to be measured (for long tapes) or removed completely (when multiple short tapes are implanted), and the subcutaneous segment is cut off and assayed. Assay is typically performed by cutting the tape into 1-cm lengths with different concentrations of antibiotic in each piece. Tapes may also be left in place 24 hours prior to antibiotic administration, but this results in a greater inflammatory response (24). The method allows only a limited time for diffusion of tissue fluid at the site when long tapes are continuously advanced, but this problem can be overcome by the implantation of multiple short lengths of umbilical tape. The umbilical tape has a very large surface area exposed for absorption because of the porous cotton weave of the thread. This model poses similar problems for standardization as seen with the paper disk models (13).

Microdialysis Probes

Muller et al. (25) first described the method of measuring antimicrobial concentrations by use of microdialysis probes. Antimicrobial concentrations within the free interstitial fluid of a tissue are measured by insertion of a microdialysis probe into tissue, usually muscle or subcutaneous adipose tissue. The probe has a semipermeable membrane at its tip and is constantly perfused with a physiologic solution at a flow rate of of 1.5 to 2.0 µL/minute. Antimicrobials within the tissue diffuse out of the extravascular fluid into the probe, resulting in a concentration in the perfusion medium. However, the diffusion may be incomplete and depend on flow rates, temperature,

membrane surface and porosity, and may not be constant over time (26). Therefore, calibration is required, usually using the retrodialysis method, which assumes that the process of diffusion is equal in both directions. The antimicrobial being studied is added to the perfusion medium and its disappearance rate through the membrane is calculated. In vivo percent recovery is then defined as

$$100 - [100 \bullet \text{(dialysate concentration out/} \\ \text{dialysate concentration in)}]$$

In vivo recovery differs markedly among differing antimicrobials (25). The absolute concentration in the interstitial space is calculated by the following equation:

$$100 \bullet \text{(concentration in the dialysate/} \\ \text{percent in vivo recovery)}$$

Since the semipermeable membrane excludes protein-bound drug, the technique measures free interstitial drug concentrations.

ANTIMICROBIAL ASSAY OF EXTRAVASCULAR FLUIDS AND TISSUE

The determination of antimicrobial agent concentrations contained in tissues can be accomplished by methods that are similar to those used for the determination of antibiotics in body fluids (see Chapter 8). The most readily available assay system at the present time is a microbiologic method. This system is based on an indicator organism that is very sensitive to the antibiotic under study and requires no special equipment. It allows for processing of large numbers of samples with minimal expense. An important aspect of this method is preparation of the standard concentration of antibiotic in the same tissue as the unknown sample (14,27). This is necessary so that drug binding to sample constituents is the same in both the unknown sample and the standard curve. Other methods also available for determination of antimicrobial concentrations include (high-pressure) liquid chromatography as well as many specific antibody-based systems such as radioimmunoassay (28) and enzyme immunoassay (29). These other methods, notably liquid chromatography and radioimmunoassay, require extraction of the antimicrobial agent from the specimen prior to assay. Use of these methods necessitates standardization with the tissue and antibiotic under study to ensure that all of the antimicrobial is extracted from the tissue sample or fluid prior to assay.

Microbiologic Assay

Antimicrobials can be determined using the bioassay method with only a limited number of organism species and a few selected media. The agar diffusion bioassay method described by Sabath (30) using *Bacillus subtilis* American Type Culture Collection strain 6633 is demonstrative of the technique for assay of antimicrobial compounds. The bioassay relies on an antibiotic-sensitive indicator organism seeded into an agar base on to which paper disks containing antibiotic are placed. Tissue homogenates or body fluids may also be placed on the agar in cylinders or in wells that have been cut into the agar. The cylinder and agar-well techniques usually provide increased sensitivity for the bioassay method. The antibiotic in the sample then diffuses into the agar and inhibits growth of the indicator organism. The diameter of the zone of inhibition is proportional to the concentration of antibiotic in the sample. Multiple variables can affect the diameter of the zone of inhibition. These variables include the indicator organism chosen, the agar base used, and the nature of the sample itself. Most of these variables can be eliminated by preparing the samples for the standard curve determination in the same type of tissue homogenate or body fluid as the specimen to be assayed.

Once the indicator organism and specific medium are selected, the microorganism is grown overnight and added to molten agar at 50°C. The microorganisms and agar are thoroughly mixed and this mixture is then poured into flat Petri dishes (15 × 100 mm) on a level surface. Each Petri dish contains a measured volume of 6 mL of the bacteria-seeded agar. The plates are left at room temperature on a level surface to harden and are then stored at 4°C until used. Plates should be stored for a maximum of 14 days under these conditions. The standard line is prepared by adding known concentrations of antibiotic to either tissue fluid or tissue homogenate and subsequently making serial dilutions. Samples of both known and unknown antibiotic-containing fluid are then placed on filter paper disks (usually 20 μL per disk) or pipetted (20 to 200 μL) into cylinders or wells cut in the agar surface. If wells or cylinders are used, the sample should be allowed to diffuse into the agar before movement of the plates to the incubator is attempted. The plates are incubated for 24 hours at 37°C and the diameter of the zone of inhibition is read with calipers to the nearest 0.1 mm. All samples should be assayed in triplicate to ensure an error rate of no more than 10%. The standard line is then plotted on semilogarithmic graph paper and the concentration of antimicrobial in the specimen is read from the standard line.

Occasionally, combinations of antimicrobials can be assayed using this method; however, it is not recommended because the influence of combined agents on indicator microorganisms is often unpredictable. Inactivation of aminoglycosides can be accomplished by lowering the agar pH to 5.5 or less. Also, penicillins or cephalosporins can be inactivated by the addition of β-lactamases to the specimen. When this is done, the same procedure should be performed on all standards to ensure the accuracy of the results.

Liquid Chromatography

Liquid chromatography for the measurement of antimicrobial agent concentrations is a specific method for assay of these drugs. The technique measures drugs in a liquid mobile phase by separating them from interferences on a column under high pressure and then using light absorption for agent detection. The technique is able to separate antimicrobials from other compounds in the sample as well as from both serum and tissue interferences. The method has been reviewed by Yoshikawa et al. (31). Extraction of antimicrobial compounds from the specimen is critical for this assay method. Because of the high protein content in most specimens, direct injection onto the liquid chromatography column is not recommended because the proteins plug the column, thus diminishing its efficiency and useful lifetime. Deproteination of samples can be accomplished by use of organic solvents or acids. Methanol, acetonitrile, and trichloroacetic acid are commonly used for this purpose.

After mixing the specimen with these agents, it is necessary to sediment the protein by centrifugation of the specimen and then inject the supernatant into the chromatographic equipment. Extraction has also been performed by adsorption of the specimen with silica gel and by ion-exchange chromatography for aminoglycosides. We have described a method using ion-exchange chromatography for extraction of penicillins and cephalosporins as well (32–34). Liquid chromatography has the advantage of specifically identifying the compounds under study by their pattern of retention on the chromatographic column. The disadvantages are that the extraction procedures and chromatography time required limit the number of specimens that can be assayed in one 24-hour period. The applicability of liquid chromatography for separation of antimicrobial drugs either singly or in combination is extensive. Once extraction techniques and detection methods have been standardized, this method can quantitate virtually any agent. Liquid chromatography is also very precise and highly reproducible, with coefficients of variation usually less than 5%. The sensitivity of liquid chromatography is similar to that of microbiologic assays and is satisfactory for both clinical and research use. Liquid chromatography with tandem mass spectrometry (LC-MS/MS) has the advantages of high sensitivity and specificity with short analysis time, which is advantageous in analysis of unstable drugs (35).

Antibody Methods

These methods of antimicrobial assay are based on the availability of specific antibody that binds the drug. The amount of drug bound is then measured either by radioactivity or by the availability for enzymatic reaction (28,29). Antimicrobial detection with radioimmunoassay is generally available for the aminoglycosides. The assays are rapid and specific and are as sensitive as microbiologic assays. The radioimmunoassay requires an extraction step; however, the enzyme immunoassay techniques are very rapid and have the advantage of not requiring an extraction. Their usefulness is limited by the availability of specific antisera and thus far, they have been applied to assays of aminoglycosides, vancomycin, and chloramphenicol. The antibody-based methods have been used little for antimicrobial assays of tissue homogenates and therefore require considerable standardization before being applied to assays of drugs in tissues.

PREPARATION AND INTERPRETATION OF SAMPLES COLLECTED FROM EXTRAVASCULAR FLUIDS AND TISSUES

The accurate determination and interpretation of antimicrobial assay results from extravascular sites are difficult and often confusing. The tables presented in this chapter illustrate the need for careful sample preparation and standardization in order to avoid conflicting results and possible misinterpretation of data.

Sampling of whole tissues for antibiotic assays in excised tissue should be performed in a carefully controlled manner. The area to be sampled should be identified at operation and easily visible. If possible, the arterial supply should be transiently clamped to allow blood to flow out of the prospective sample area. The specimen is then surgically removed and freed of adherent blood by gentle pressure with sterile gauze. Tissue samples should then be either immediately processed or stored at $-70°C$ until antibiotic assay can be performed. Tissue fluid can be obtained from the tissue sample by homogenization in a phosphate-buffered saline solution at neutral pH. It is usually necessary to dilute the specimen with three volumes of buffer for every one volume of sampled tissue. The homogenization should be done in a hand-homogenizer so that temperature in the specimen is not elevated, which may destroy some drugs. The resulting homogenate can then be assayed directly for antibiotic content as well as for markers of various tissue compartments and blood. The homogenate can also be centrifuged and the supernatant assayed. We suggest preparation of antibiotic solutions for the standard line at the same time as preparation of the unknown sample so that the standards and the unknown are exposed to the tissue for the same amount of time under the same conditions (27).

Rauws and Van Klingeren (36) and Bergan (37) have discussed the difficulty in interpretation of antimicrobial tissue concentrations obtained from homogenized whole tissues. The final amount of detected drug is the sum of the concentrations of the individual components of the tissue as given by:

$$C_T = C_p f_b(1 - Ht) + C_e f_b(Ht) + C_i f_i + C_c f_c + C_s f_s$$

where C is the concentration in whole tissue (C_T), plasma (C_p), erythrocytes (C_e), interstitial fluid (C_i), tissue cells (C_c), and specialized tissue components (C_s) such as secretory fluids, and f is the fraction of the homogenate contributed by blood (f_b), interstitial fluid (f_i), tissue cells (f_c), and specialized tissue components (f_s). Ht is the hematocrit level, a critical determination for most studies. The sum of the homogenate fractions is equal to 1, that is, $f_b + f_i + f_c + f_s = 1$. Because the contribution of antimicrobial agent in blood is one of the most important potential inaccuracies in the assay of tissue homogenates, correction for blood contamination is essential. We have indicated in the tables whenever this has been done. The formula of Plaue et al. (38) can be used for this correction. Their formula simply states that extravascular concentration = (tissue concentration − serum concentration)/(tissue water volume − blood volume).

Blood contamination can be estimated most simply by measurement of the hemoglobin content of the tissue homogenate and comparison of this with the hemoglobin content of the subject's circulating blood. If estimation of blood contamination is not possible, the significance of this factor can be minimized by obtaining the extravascular fluid or tissue sample at a time when the intravascular antibiotic concentration is expected to be low or at least lower than that in the extravascular site under study. Rinsing the specimen to remove blood should also be avoided because most antimicrobials at the low concentrations found in vivo are readily water-soluble and easily washed out. If desired, the extracellular or interstitial fluid in tissue can also be measured with high-molecular-weight dextran, sodium bromide, or sodium thiocyanate, which is excluded from intact cells (e.g., kidney, gallbladder, and prostate). Corrections for antibiotic concentrations of the secretory product also need to be considered because these fluids often contain high concentrations of antimicrobial agent and significantly contaminate tissue specimens. Most published work on tissue distribution of antibiotics fails to make even simple adjustments for blood contamination, making interpretation difficult or impossible.

Finally, because various body tissues bind antimicrobial agents with different capacities (39) and tissue fluid–antibiotic concentration is a combination of bound and unbound drug (40), it is necessary to know the protein binding of an antibiotic to both the tissue or body fluid and plasma or serum in order to interpret correctly the significance of the tissue concentration. Methods for measurement of protein binding to serum, tissues, and body fluids have been published (39,41,42) and measurements should be performed to optimally interpret extravascular fluid and tissue antimicrobial concentrations.

INTERPRETATION OF EXTRAVASCULAR ANTIMICROBIAL DISTRIBUTION

The proper interpretation of an extravascular antimicrobial concentration depends on a series of factors that are often overlooked or ignored (Table 14.2). These factors (with the possible exception of protein concentration) are independent of permeability barriers or effects of inflammation that may influence the amount of antimicrobial that reaches a given site. They also do not take into account the antimicrobial susceptibility of

Table 14.2

Factors that Influence the Interpretation of Extravascular Antimicrobial Concentrations

1. Antimicrobial administration method (oral, intravenous, intramuscular, constant infusion, bolus injection)
2. Single- or multiple-dosage administrations
3. Collection, processing, and assay of specimens
4. Protein (albumin) content of the extravascular site
5. Geometry (ratio of surface area to volume) of the extravascular site
6. Method used to compare serum and extravascular site concentrations
   a. Peak site-to-peak serum concentrations
   b. Simultaneous site and serum concentrations
   c. AUC site-to-AUC serum determination

AUC, area under the curve.

pathogens likely to be found within a given extravascular site. Such comparisons require a higher level of cognition and are left to readers who may wish to correlate minimal inhibitory concentrations for specific organisms found elsewhere in this text with extravascular site drug concentrations found at the end of this chapter (43). Readers who make such an effort are cautioned that expectations of clinical cure or failure should not be made with a high degree of confidence until more clinical studies on this subject are available (44,45).

Administration Method

The method used to administer an antimicrobial can result in marked differences in serum concentration. High concentrations in serum result rapidly from bolus injections and influence the rate at which antimicrobials enter an extravascular site (46,47). Similarly, intermittent administration results in more rapid attainment of high extravascular levels than does constant intravenous infusion (48,49). Furthermore, extravascular drug concentrations are frequently compared with peak serum concentrations. Rapid intravenous infusions can result in very high serum peaks that, when compared with extravascular concentrations, may give the erroneous perception of poor extravascular drug penetration.

Single or Multiple Dosages

The concentration of antimicrobial at an extravascular site is influenced by the number of doses administered, particularly if the administration frequency is short relative to the serum half-life of the drug (50). Multiple doses may result in considerably higher extravascular antibiotic concentrations than do single doses (51), as a drug accumulates over multiple half-lives depending on the dosing interval. This gradient may be reduced if a loading dose is administered, but the level achieved by a loading dose may not equal the result of the multiple half-lives of accumulation required to reach steady-state condition.

Specimen Handling

Different methods of processing and assaying specimens may lead to confusion in interpretation of extravascular levels, particularly in whole tissues. As previously discussed, the method used to remove blood from tissues, the assay method and standards, and blood contamination corrections are all important to the interpretation of extravascular antibiotic concentrations. Comparison of studies that use dissimilar handling methods is extremely difficult.

Extravascular Protein Content

Antibiotics often bind to proteins (usually albumin) at the extravascular site as well as in serum. For highly bound antimicrobials, the amount of drug that accumulates in an extravascular space depends on the protein content of the space. A site with high albumin content binds a substantial amount of a highly bound antibiotic, and the total (free plus protein-bound) antibiotic concentration in the site is greater at equilibrium than it would be for a site with low albumin content (7,40). In contrast, a site that contains little albumin may have a low total antibiotic concentration, but most of the antibiotic present is free (unbound) drug.

Site Geometry

The amount of antibiotic in a fluid-filled space largely depends on diffusion and, in turn, on the surface area available for diffusion compared with the volume of the space, the so-called surface area to volume (SA/V) ratio. It has been shown in experimental models that spaces with high SA/V ratios show fluctuations of antibiotic concentrations that parallel serum fluctuations, while spaces with low SA/V ratios show a damped response with lower peaks and higher troughs than in serum (52). Animal models that use tissue cages and chambers as extravascular sites and human blister models

of extravascular distribution are subject to variation in drug penetration because of differences in SA/V ratios (52). This simple ratio of SA/V is the major determinant of peak and trough drug levels in large-volume, fluid-filled spaces that fill mainly by passive diffusion. Experimental data for ascites in dogs clearly support this concept (53).

Method of Serum and Site Comparison

The method used to compare serum and extravascular site antibiotic concentrations can markedly influence the perception of how well a drug enters an extravascular site. Most antimicrobials are administered intermittently, yielding a rapid rise in serum concentration followed by a logarithmic decay in serum levels. Extravascular site concentrations follow a similar pattern but peak levels are usually lower and occur later than in serum, while trough levels are higher than those in serum (Fig. 14.1). Comparisons of serum and site concentrations are usually done in one of three ways: peak-to-peak comparison, simultaneous-time comparison, or AUC-to-AUC comparison. Peak-to-peak comparisons are difficult to obtain clinically because large numbers of specimens are

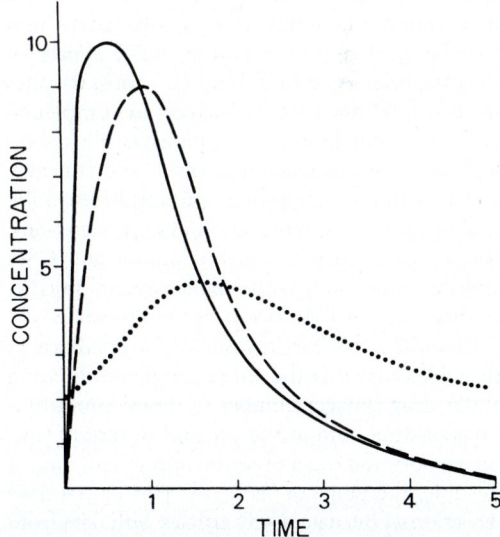

Figure 14.1 ■ Theoretical concentration versus time profile for an intermittently administered antimicrobial. Serum (——), interstitial fluid (– – –), and a large-volume site with limited surface area for diffusion (. . . .) are shown at equilibrium. AUC values are equal for all sites. (From Cunha BA, Ristuccia AM. *Antimicrobial therapy*. New York: Raven Press, 1984, with permission.)

required to ensure that the peak is obtained. In addition, serum peaks may be very high following rapid intravenous infusion, resulting in an inappropriately low ratio of site-to-serum concentrations. Simultaneous-time determinations are most often employed clinically because it is simpler to obtain a serum specimen at the same time that the site is sampled. Because serum levels are falling at the same time that site levels are rising, the perceived penetration of an antibiotic into an extravascular site may be low if specimens are taken shortly after administration (high serum level and low site level) but appear much higher if sampling is delayed until serum levels have fallen and site levels have risen. Perhaps the best way to compare serum and site antibiotic penetration is by means of AUC data. These studies also require multiple serum and site samples and thus are difficult to perform in certain sites in humans. They are best done following multiple antimicrobial doses to allow equilibrium to occur.

TABLES AND COMMENTS

General Comments

Tables 14.3 to 14.20 have been prepared from published literature for reference purposes to illustrate the concentrations of antimicrobials found in a variety of human extravascular sites. Sites have been selected to be representative of each of the categories listed in Table 14.1. Thus, the sites include fluid-filled spaces such as ascites, pleural effusions, joint fluids, and cutaneous blisters (as well as cutaneous chambers, disks, and threads); secretory fluids such as bile, sputum, breast milk, middle ear fluid, and prostate and sinus secretions; barrier spaces such as aqueous humor and CSF; and the whole-body tissues bone, skeletal muscle, cardiac tissue, gallbladder, lung, and prostate.

Requirements for inclusion of a reference in the tables were that the article supply information about drug dosage; number of doses; concentrations of drug both at the site and in serum; timing of both the site and serum specimens; and, if possible, the range or standard error or standard deviation of the data. Only articles with data from at least three subjects were included. Data from articles were frequently reorganized to include only information for specific sampling times in order to make interpretation easier. Extrapolation of graphical data was occasionally required. Many articles contained far more data than could be included in these concise tables. In such cases,

data from specific sampling times (e.g., 1, 2, or 3 hours) were arbitrarily selected to obtain simultaneous-time data for the tables. Certain antimicrobials have been studied numerous times at certain body sites. In these instances, no attempt was made to include every reference in the tables. Rather, emphasis was placed on inclusion of data about as many different drugs as possible.

Antimicrobials are grouped into aminoglycosides, cephalosporins and related β-lactams, penicillins, quinolones, tetracyclines, and other antimicrobials. Included under cephalosporins are cephamycins and related β-lactams such as moxalactam, monobactams, and carbapenems. All antimicrobials are listed alphabetically within categories. Method of administration, dose (in grams), and whether single or multiple doses were given are listed after the drug name. The number of subjects studied to obtain the data in the table is given in the column headed *n*. Serum half-life, if not supplied in the references, was obtained from standard tables (54). The remainder of the table gives the serum concentration (micrograms per milliliter or units per milliliter for penicillin) and time obtained, followed by the site concentration (micrograms per milliliter or micrograms per gram of tissue) and time obtained. The ratio of site concentration to serum concentration is given as a percentage. The "Notes" column includes special information about whether the site was infected or uninfected (if the information is known), whether site assays were corrected for blood contamination (a rarity), and any special information needed to interpret a given study. Specific comments regarding each table are included in the following sections.

Ascites

There are only limited data on antibiotic penetration into ascitic fluid. Data in Table 14.3 are limited to patients from whom ascitic fluid could be aspirated. Only studies that included fluid obtained by aspiration are included. Studies that obtained fluid by placing a paper disk under a loop of bowel at surgery or that measured peritoneal fluid samples from peritoneal drains after abdominal surgery or from patients undergoing peritoneal dialysis were not included. In the majority of studies, antibiotics penetrated into ascitic fluid well, although there was a lag in the ascitic fluid values compared with the serum values in the first few hours after the initial dose. AUC ratios of ascites to serum for several antimicrobial agents of different classes ranged from 30% to greater than 100% (55–61).

(continued on page 689)

Table 14.3

Antimicrobial Concentrations in Ascites

Reference	Antimicrobial	Administration Method[a]	Dose (g) (Multiple or Single)[b]	n	Serum Half-life (h)	Serum Concentration Mean (μg/mL) (Range)	Time Serum Obtained (h)	Site Concentration Mean (μg/mL) (Range)	Time Site Specimen Obtained (h)	Ratio of Site/Serum (%)	Notes[c]
Aminoglycosides											
170	Amikacin	IV	7.5 mg/kg (S)	8	2.5	9.5 (4.5–2.0)	4	4.15 (0.56–6.8)	5	58	U
171	Gentamicin	IV or IM	0.06 (M) 0.12 (S)	11	2.0	3.9 (0.6–10)	0.5–30	3.1 (0.7–8.2)	0.5–30	90	I
171	Tobramycin	IM	0.06 (M)	4	2.0	7.0 (2.5–13.6)	1–5	4.5 (1.3–10.8)	1–5	79	I
Cephalosporins and related β-lactams											
172	Aztreonam	IV	0.5 (S)	26	1.8	24.9 (12.6–38.4)	0.5	10.8 (3.4–19.6)	1	43	I
56	Cefdozime	IV	1.0 (S)	6	6.4	17.0	4	10.0	4	59	U
173	Cefepime	IV	1.0 (S)	8	2	96 ± 19	0.5	55.3 ± 11.7	0.9 ± 0.5	59 ± 15	I
174	Cefonicid	IV	2.0 (M)	9	8.9	83 (37–138)	1	23 (10–16)	1	28	I
61	Cefoperazone	IV	15 mg/kg (S)	7	3.8	25	4	10	4	40	U
175	Cefotaxime	IV	2.0 (S)	41	2.5	22 ± 18	6	23 ± 17	6	120	I
176	Cefotaxime	IM	1.0 (M)	6	2.5	20	2	10.0 (3.8–17.6)	2	50	U
177	Cefoxitin	IV	30 mg/kg (S)	8	1.36	28 (10.3–40.8)	2	32.8 (15.1–54.5)	2	117	U, R
55	Ceftazidime	IV	1.0 (S)	6	5.9	~21	2	9.4	2	45	U
55	Ceftriaxone	IV	1.0 (S)	6	13.6	~35	2	18.4	2	53	U
178	Cefuroxime	IV	2.0 (S)	5	0.8	18	3	16	3	89	U
179	Cephalothin	IV	1.0 (S)	5	0.5	10.22 (±2.46 SD)	1	3.22 (±0.71 SD)	1	31	U
180	Ertapenem	IV	1.0 (S)	8		80.1 ± 19.9	2 ± 0.25	41.1 ± 22.1	2 ± 0.25	56.4 ± 24.1	I
181	Meropenem	IV	0.5 (S)	8		46.2 ± 12.5	0.5	23.3 ± 7.9	0.5	52 ± 18	U
182	Imipenem/ cilastatin	IV	0.5 (S)	5	0.9	4.7 ± 2.2/3.5 ± 1.9	3	4.0 ± 1.7/2.8 ± 1.6	3	85/71	U

(Continued)

Table 14.3 (Continued)

Antimicrobial Concentrations in Ascites

Reference	Antimicrobial	Administration Method[a]	Dose (g) (Multiple or Single)[b]	n	Serum Half-life (h)	Serum Concentration Mean (μg/mL) (Range)	Time Serum Obtained (h)	Site Concentration Mean (μg/mL) (Range)	Time Site Specimen Obtained (h)	Ratio of Site/Serum (%)	Notes[c]
Penicillins											
57	Amoxicillin/clavulanic acid	IV	1.0 (S)/0.2 (S)	6	1.0	12/1.2	2	10/1	2	83/83	U
171	Ampicillin	IV	1–2 (M)	3	1.1	184 (27–313)	2–3.5	185 (27–313)	2–3.5	100	I
183	Penicillin V	Oral	1 × 10^6 units (M)	3	0.5	6.6 (4.2–8.3)	2	2.6 (0.9–4.7)	2	39	U
57	Piperacillin	IV	4.0 (S)	11	1.95	45	2.5	25	2.5	55	U
Quinolones											
184	Moxifloxacin	IV	0.4 (S)	10		2.29	2	3.32	2	145	U
44	Ofloxacin	IV	0.4	7	10.5	2.21	24	1.53	24	69	I
60	Ofloxacin	Oral	0.2 (S)	12	11.6	1.5	8	1.4	8	93	U
Others											
171	Clindamycin	IV	0.4–0.6 (M)	3	2.0	6.5 (5.9–7.6)	1–5.5	2.8 (2.3–3.2)	1–5.5	44	I
185	Lincomycin	Oral	1.0 (S)	7	4.5	5.7 (1.4–10.4)	4	22.0 (1.6–70)	4	528	U
77	Rifampin	Oral	0.15	4	2.5	1.3 (0.4–7.4)	4	0.3 (0.1–0.5)	4	23	U
186	Vancomycin	IV	0.5 (S)	11	6.0	6.9 (6.4–8.0)	1.4	3.6 (1.5–5.2)	1.5	52	U

[a]IV, intravenously; IM, intramuscularly.
[b]S, single dose; M, multiple dose.
[c]U, uninfected; I, infected; R, patients had renal impairment.

Pleural Fluid

The antibiotic levels in pleural fluid are listed as infected (i.e., empyema) or uninfected (Table 14.4). The uninfected groups consist of patients with congestive heart failure and malignant or parapneumonic effusions; some also included cases of nonpyogenic infection such as tuberculosis. When specified, most samples were collected by chest tube drainage. Few studies provided data on antibiotic penetration into pleural empyemas. It is notable that the aminoglycosides penetrated poorly into empyema fluid, compared with uninfected pleural fluid, as shown by the study of Thys et al. (62). The quinolones demonstrated good pleural fluid penetration, which appeared to be enhanced by the presence of empyema. Aztreonam also demonstrated excellent penetration into the pleural fluid.

Joint Fluid

In compiling this table of antimicrobial penetration into joint fluid spaces (Table 14.5), single-patient studies were combined when possible to give a better overall reflection of the penetration of individual agents. No attempt at correction for blood contamination was made, and only rarely was there an attempt made to correlate protein content or antimicrobial/tissue fluid protein binding with drug penetration (24). The reported fluid-to-serum antimicrobial concentration ratios are quite high for this group of studies, which is primarily due to the high protein content of the extravascular fluid plus the fact that many of these studies were performed after multiple systemic doses of the antimicrobial agent had been administered. Data from single infected patients treated with cephapirin (63) have not been included in Table 14.5.

Cutaneous Blister/Disks/Threads/Microdialysis Samples of Interstitial Fluid

Table 14.6 contains a summary of reports of antimicrobial distribution based on models in humans. All sites were done in uninfected patients except the studies done by Tegeder et al. (64) of imipenem. None of the studies have made any attempt to correct for blood contamination other than avoiding gross blood. Data are also available for penicillin (23) and pivampicillin (23) but are not included in Table 14.6 because fewer than three subjects were studied. While only a limited number of multiple-dose studies have been done,

even the single-dose studies often demonstrate high ratios of drug concentration in the extravascular site to that in serum, reflecting the small size of the extravascular space under study. One study attempted to correlate protein concentration to drug penetration and found a significant correlation at $r = 0.97$ (22). There was considerable variability in the ratio of extravascular to intravascular antimicrobial concentrations, reflected by ratios as low as 3% for nafcillin in the skin-window model (15) to 238% for FCE22101 in a cantharides blister study (65). Many articles supply data that can provide an AUC for the agent under study in both the intravascular and extravascular spaces. This is a notable achievement in the study of extravascular drug penetration, although more multiple-dose studies are needed as well as more attention to antimicrobial binding at extravascular sites.

Bile

Specimens of bile obtained by three methods are included in Table 14.7: aspirations of gallbladder or common duct bile at surgery, external bile drainage from T-tubes, or bile obtained by endoscopic retrograde cholangiopancreatography. Studies in which bile was obtained by duodenal aspiration were not included because of unknown specimen dilution by gastrointestinal fluids. Several studies in Table 14.7 confirm the observation that bile concentrations are lower or absent in the presence of cystic duct obstruction (66) or common bile duct obstruction (67–69). In general, T-tube and common duct bile levels seem to be somewhat higher than gallbladder bile levels (70–74) when comparably timed specimens are obtained. This may be related to partial obstruction of the cystic duct. Multiple antibiotic doses also result in higher bile levels than do single doses (74–76).

Ratios of site-to-serum levels are extremely variable, ranging from zero in the presence of obstruction to 18,400% for rifampin (77), with numerous examples of ratios greater than 100%. After relief of biliary obstruction, the excretion of antibiotics (aztreonam, piperacillin, and cefamandole) remains depressed for a prolonged period of time, which may exceed 28 days (67,78). Data on ratios of AUC in bile to AUC in serum were available for a limited number of drugs, and they also showed wide variation: 19% for cephacetrile (79); 38% to 44% for amoxicillin, penicillin G, and oral ampicillin (71,72); 46% for ceftazidime (80); 65% for amikacin (75); 96% for intravenous ampicillin (72); 100% for cefuroxime (81); and 2,089% for mezlocillin (82).

(continued on page 703)

Table 14.4

Antimicrobial Concentrations in Pleural Fluid

Reference	Antimicrobial	Administration Method[a]	Dose (g) (Multiple or Single)[b]	n	Serum Half-life (h)	Serum Concentration Mean (μg/mL) (Range)	Time Serum Obtained (h)	Site Concentration Mean (μg/mL) (Range)	Time Site Specimen Obtained (h)	Ratio of Site/ Serum (%)	Notes[c]
Aminoglycosides											
62	Amikacin	IV	7.5 mg/kg (S)	10	2.6	27.6 (±2.0)	0.5	11.0 (±3.1)	0–1	40	U, T, PD
62	Amikacin	IV	7.5 mg/kg (S)	5	2.6	27.6 (±2.0)	0.5	5.7 (±2.2)	7–8	21	I, T, PD
62	Gentamicin	IV	1.5 mg/kg (S)	5	2.9	5.1 (±0.4)	0.5	2.9 (±0.3)	0.5–1	57	U, T, PD
62	Gentamicin	IV	1.5 mg/kg (S)	3	2.9	5.1 (±0.4)	0.5	0	0–8	0	I, T
187	Kanamycin	IM	0.5 (S)	3	2.0	9.3 (4–16)	2	0.8 (0–2.0)	2	9	
62	Netilmicin	IV	2.0 mg/kg (S)	4	3.2	5.4 (±0.5)	0.5	3.7 (±0.8)	1–2	69	U, PD, T
62	Netilmicin	IV	2.0 mg/kg (S)	3	3.2	5.4 (±0.5)	0.5	0	0–8	0	I, T
188	Sisomicin	IM	0.75 (S)	5	2.0	6.7 (±0.6)	1	1.9 (±0.66)	3	28	U
Cephalosporins and related β-lactams											
189	Aztreonam	IV	2 (S)	3	2	64 (±12 SE)	1–3	51 (±31 SE)	1–3	79	
44	Cefadroxil	Oral	0.5 (S)	7	1.3	2.15	8	2.46	8	114	U
190	Cefazolin	IV	1.0 (S)	9	2.0	72.5 (36–112)	0.5–2	21.3 (5–83)	0.5–2	30	U
191	Cefoperazone	IV	2.0 (S)	6	2.9	209 (108–270)	1	15.5 (7–25)	4–6	7	I, U, PD
192	Cefotaxime	IV	1.0 (S)	6	1.2	28	1.0	7.2 (±3.1 SD)	3.0	26	U
193	Cefotaxime	IM/IV	25 mg/kg (M/S)	6	1.2	19.9 (13–34)	0.5	4.8 (2.8–11.2)	3.0	24	I, P
194	Cefoxitin	IV	2.0 (S)	6	0.8	11.8 (4–18)	1–5	3.6 (1–6.4)	1–5	31	U
195	Cefpodoxime	Oral	0.2 (S)	6	1.9–3.2	2.72 (±0.32 SE)	6	1.84 (±0.33 SE)	6	67	U
196	Ceftazidime	IV	2.0 (S)	5	1.9	80 (±10)	1.0	17 (±3)	1	21	U, E
197	Ceftizoxime	IV	1.0 (S)	5	1.7	24.1 (±4.4 SD)	1.0	7.8 (±2.2 SD)	2–3	32	U

198	Ceftriaxone	IV	1.0 (S)	5	12.4	39.4 (34–50)	4	7.9 (7.0–8.7)	4	20	
178	Cefuroxime	IV	1.0 (S)	6	1.3	24 (14–40)	1.5–4.5	7.3 (5.6–9.1)	1.5–4.5	30	U
199	Cephalothin	IV	1.0 (M)	3	0.5	22.5 (14–34.5)	2.5–4.5	26.0 (21.5–28.5)	2.5–4.5	116	U
191	Moxalactam	IV	2.0 (S)	5	2.4	99 (43–122)	1	20 (9–35)	4–6	20	PD
Quinolones											
200	Ciprofloxacin	IV	0.2 (S)	7	3–5	3.8 (±2.4 SD)	0.1	1.0 (±0.6)	3.25	26	U, PD
200	Ciprofloxacin	Oral	0.75 BID (M)	3	3–5	4.3 (±0.6 SD)	3.5	2.3 (±0.4)	3.5	53	U, PD
200	Ciprofloxacin	Oral	0.75 BID (M)	3	3–5	2.3 (±2.2 SD)	0	2.9 (±1.5 SD)	2	126	I, PD
201	Lomefloxacin	Oral	0.2 (S)	7	7–8.5	2.16 (1.58–4.34)	1–6	1.36 (0.65–2.18)	6	63	U, PD
202	Ofloxacin	Oral	0.3 QD (M)	21	4–8	4.70 (±0.63 SD)	2	3.82 (±0.41 SD)	2	82	U
Penicillins											
203	Amoxicillin	Oral	0.75 (S)	9	2.4	4.5	4	1.6	5.3	36	U, T
204	Ampicillin	Oral	1.0 (S)	6	1.2	21.4 (±3.7)	1	10.5 (±1.5)	3	49	U
205	Ampicillin	IV	0.4 g/kg/day (M)	17	1.6 ± 1.1	11 ± 10.2	3	16.2 ± 7.9	4	147	I
206	Bacampicillin	Oral	0.8 (M)	9	2.2	7.0 (±4.3 SD)	1.5	2.9 (±1.9 SD)	3	41	U, T, PD
207	Mezlocillin	IV	10 (S)	6	1.1	778 (±270)	0.25	100 (±38)	1	13	U, T, PD
199	Penicillin	Oral	2–3 × 10^6 units (M)	4	0.5	33 (16–61)	1–3	28.5 (5–56)	1–3	86	I
199	Penicillin	Oral	1–2 × 10^6 units (M)	5	0.5	20.4 (11–25)	1–3	13.6 (3–26)	1–3	67	U
205	Penicillin	IV	200,000 IU/kg/day (M)	13	1.21 ± 1.1	3.9 ± 3.4	3	7.7 ± 3.4	4	197	I
208	Ticarcillin	IV	5.0 (S)	5	1.2	63 (56–70)	1	9 (6–11)	3	14	U, PD

(Continued)

Table 14.4 (Continued)

Antimicrobial Concentrations in Pleural Fluid

Reference	Antimicrobial	Administration Method[a]	Dose (g) (Multiple or Single)[b]	n	Serum Half-life (h)	Serum Concentration Mean (μg/mL) (Range)	Time Serum Obtained (h)	Site Concentration Mean (μg/mL) (Range)	Time Site Specimen Obtained (h)	Ratio of Site/ Serum (%)	Notes[c]
Tetracyclines											
209	Doxycycline	IV	0.2 (S)	16	20	5.0 (±0.4)	1	1.8 (±0.2)	10	36	
Others											
210	Clindamycin	Oral	0.15 (M)	3	2	10.1	1–2	9.3 (1.3–22)	1–2	92	U
211	Fosfomycin	IV	30 mg/kg (S)	6	2	195.2 (±49.2 SD)	0.25	42.6 (±16 SD)	3.7	22	U, PD
212	Rifampin	Oral	10 mg/kg (S)	8	3.0	6.5 (0.9–11.0)	8–9	2.6 (0.6–6.0)	8–9	40	U
213	Teicoplanin	IV	0.4 (M)	3	40–70	36.2 (±5.0 SE)	0.5	7.5 (±1.5)	5	21	PD
186	Vancomycin	IV	0.5 (S)	12	6	7.3 (2.9–10)	1.1–4.0	3.0 (0–8.1)	1.2–4.5	41	U
214	Vancomycin	IV (CI)	30 mg/kg/day	8	6.3 (±1.9 SD)	14.0[d] (±4.3 SD)	4	12.1 (±2.9 SD)	4	86	U, T
	Vancomycin	IV	15 mg/kg (M)	8	6.3 (±1.9 SD)	14.4[d] (±4.9 SD)	4	16 (±4.5 SD)	4	111	U, T

[a]IV, intravenously; IM, intramuscularly.
[b]S, single dose; M, multiple dose; BID, twice a day; QD, once a day; CI, continuous infusion.
[c]U, uninfected (causes other than empyema); T, tube drainage; PD, peak data; I, infected (empyema).
[d]Measured in the blood.

Table 14.5

Antimicrobial Concentrations in Joint Fluid

Reference	Antimicrobial	Administration Method[a]	Dose (g) (Multiple or Single)[b]	n	Serum Half-life (h)	Serum Concentration Mean (μg/mL) (Range)	Time Serum Obtained (h)	Site Concentration Mean (μg/mL) (Range)	Time Site Specimen Obtained (h)	Ratio of Site/Serum (%)	Notes[c]
Aminoglycosides											
215	Amikacin	IM	7.5–15.7 mg/kg/day (M)	4	2.0	15.3 (12.1–21.0)	4.0–7.0	17.0 (12.5–24.4)	4.0–7.0	111	I
216	Gentamicin	IM	1.0–1.5 mg/kg (S)	6	2.0	4.0 (2.4–6.5)	1.0–3.5	3.2 (2.4–4.4)	1.0–3.5	80	
217	Kanamycin	IM	15 mg/kg/day (M)	4	2.0	21.2 (11.0–28.0)	2.0	15.4 (8.7–21.0)	2.0	73	
216	Tobramycin	IM	1.0–1.5 mg/kg (S)	7	2.0	2.7 (1.0–5.6)	1.5–4.0	2.4 (1.3–4.6)	1.5–4.0	89	
Cephalosporins and related β-lactams											
218	Cefadroxil	Oral	0.5 (S)	5	1.3	7.30	2.0	7.14	2.0	98	
219	Cefamandole	IV	2 (S)	29	0.7	66.8	0.5	33.2	0.5	50	
220	Cefazolin	IV	1.0 (S)	15	1.8	81.4 (56–135)	0.25–0.5	26.2 (7.1–63)	0.25–0.5	32	
221	Cefotaxime	IV	2 (S)	22	1.2	25	2	29	2	116	E, I
222	Cephalexin	Oral	25 mg/kg (M)	5	0.8	17.1 (9.3–20)	2.0	11.3 (5.3–19)	2.0	66	I
Penicillins											
223	Ampicillin	IM	0.5 (M)	14	1.1	8.3 (2.1–19.0)	1.0	4.4 (1.1–12.0)	1.0	53	
217	Ampicillin	Oral	0.5 (M)	19	1.1	2.9 (0.03–10.0)	2.0	1.8 (0.03–5.4)	2.0	62	
219	Cloxacillin	IV	2.0 (S)	29	0.5	120.0	0.75	105.0	0.75	87	
222	Dicloxacillin	Oral	25 mg/kg (M)	6	0.5	13.6 (9.2–28)	2.0	9.5 (3.2–23)	2.0	70	I
224	Methicillin	IV	25–61 mg/kg (M)	6	0.5	23.2 (1.7–60.0)	0.5–4.0	27.8 (3.8–69)	0.5–4.0	120	
225	Nafcillin	IM	1.5 (S)	20	1.0	15.5 (7.9–26.0)	1.0	2.7 (0.5–7.0)	1.0	17	
226	Penicillin	IM	25–40 × 10³ units (M)	7	1.0	0.14 (0.06–0.25)	1.0	0.13 (0.09–0.19)	1.0	93	
224	Penicillin G	IV	25 mg/kg (M)	3	0.5	2.6 (0.16–5.1)	1.0–2.0	2.6 (0.08–5.1)	1.0–2.0	100	I
Other											
227	Linezolid	PO except for last dose which was IV	0.6 (M)	10	4.26–5.4	23 ± 6.5	1.5 h after last dose	20.1 ± 3.4	1.5 h after last dose	87.4	
228	Tigecycline	IV	0.1 (S)	5	42.4	0.196 ± 0.052	4	0.116 ± 0.059	4	58	
186	Vancomycin	IV	500 mg (M)	6	6.0	7.0 (5.2–8.7)	1.0–1.65	5.7 (4.0–6.4)	1.0–1.65	81	

[a]IM, intramuscularly; IV, intravenously; PO, by mouth.
[b]M, multiple dose; S, single dose; PO, by mouth.
[c]I, infected joint; E, extrapolated from graphical data.

Table 14.6

Antimicrobial Concentrations in Cutaneous Blisters, Disks, and Threads

Reference	Antimicrobial	Administration Method[a]	Dose (g) (Multiple or Single)[b]	n	Serum Half-life (h)	Serum Concentration Mean (μg/mL) (Range)	Time Serum Obtained (h)	Site Concentration Mean (μg/mL) (Range)	Time Site Specimen Obtained (h)	Ratio of Site/Serum (%)	Notes[c]
Aminoglycosides											
16	Amikacin	IM	7.5 mg/kg (S)	12	2.0	24.6 (±4.72)	2.0	4.2 (±2.1)	2.0	17	W
16	Gentamicin	IM	1.7 mg/kg (S)	12	2.0	5.9 (±2.7)	2.0	1.8 (±0.77)	2.0	31	W
229	Netilmicin	IM	200 mg (S)	3	2.3	5.8 (3.5–9)	2.0	5.6 (3.5–9)	2.0	97	SB
16	Tobramycin	IM	1.7 mg/kg (S)	12	2.0	6.4 (±3.5)	2.0	1.4 (±0.5)	2.0	22	W
Cephalosporins and related β-lactams											
21	Aztreonam	IV	1.0 (S)	6	1.93	24.1 (±3.5)	2.0	21.8 (±3.8)	2.0	90	CB
230	Cefaclor	Oral	0.5 (S)	8	1.0 (±0.3)	11.1 (±2.3)	2	9.5 (±2.4)	2	85.6	SB
20	Cefadroxil	Oral	1.0 (S)	10	1.5	28.4	1.5–3	20	1.5–3	70	CB
16	Cefamandole	IV	1.0 (S)	12	0.7	5.0 (±1.8)	2.0	1.4 (±0.4)	2.0	28	W
16	Cefazolin	IV	1.0 (S)	12	2.0	40.5 (±0.7)	2.0	4.2 (±1.3)	2.0	11	W
231	Cefepime	IV	2 (S)	6	2.1	58.8 (±9.3)	2	79.1 (±30.5)	2	134	CB
232	Cefixime	Oral	400 mg (S)	6	3.8	3.4 (±1.4)	4	2.3 (±1.5)	4	68	CB, E
233	Cefmenoxime	IM	1 (S)	5	1.4	36	2	21.5	2	60	SB, E
18	Cefmetazole	IV	2.0 (M)	12	1.1	12	1	17.8	1	148	W
234	Cefodizime	IV	1 (S)	6	2.4	34	3	8.4	3	25	SB, E
235	Cefodizime	IM	1 (S)	4	4.3 (±0.3)	54.2 (±20.6)	1	15.5 (±6.7)	1	28.4	PT
236	Cefonicid	IV	30 mg/kg (S)	6	4.1	140	4	31	4	22	SB, E
22	Cefoperazone	IV	2.0 (S)	14	2.4	47.1 (±8.5)	2.0	6.2 (±1.5)	2.0	13	T
22	Cefotaxime	IV	2.0 (S)	14	0.83	18.2 (±4.5)	2.0	6.3 (±2.4)	2.0	35	T

237	Cefotaxime	IM	1.0 (S)	4	1.2	7.0	2.0	2.0	2.0	29	W
238	Desacetyl-cefotaxime	IV		4	1.5	2.9 (1.2–5.2)	2.0	1.79 (1.06–2.78)	2.0	62	SB
239	Cefotetan	IV	2.0 (S)	4	3.9	65.1	2	57.7	2	87	SB
240	Cefotiam	IV	1 (S)	21	1.5	10.5 (±2.2)	2	11.6 (±2.2)	2	110	SB
22	Cefoxitin	IV	2.0 (S)	14	0.88	13.1 (±3.0)	2.0	5.9 (±1.8)	2.0	45	T
241	Cefpirome	IV	1.0 (S)	6	2.3	97.4 (70–147)	1.9	39.2 (31–49)	1.9	40	CB
242	Cefpodoxime	Oral	0.2	8	2.1	2.3	2.3	1.6	3.5	70	SB
			0.4	8	2.1	4.2	2.4	2.8	3.5	68	SB
243	Cefprozil	Oral	0.25 (M)	12	1.3	6.1	1.5	3.0	24	49	SB
244	Cefsulodin	IV	1.0 (S)	8	1.5	32	2.0	15.3	2.0	48	CB
245	Ceftazidime	IV	1.0 (M)	4	7.9		2.0		2.0		T, IR, PER
246	Ceftibuten	Oral	0.2 (M)	6	2.5	10	2.0	8.4	2	84	CB
247	Ceftizoxime	IV	30 mg/kg (S)	6	1.4	42	2	35	2	83	SB, E
247	Ceftizoxime	IV	30 mg/kg (S)	6	1.4	37	2	14	2	38	D, E
248	Ceftriaxone	IV	1 (M)	12	7.2	100	4	53	4	53	SB, E
22	Cefuroxime	IV	1.5 (S)	14	0.88	17.8 (±4.2)	2.0	6.7 (±2.1)	2.0	38	T
20	Cephalexin	Oral	1.0 (S)	10	1.0	23.3	1.5–2.0	13.7	1.5–2.0	59	CB
209	Cephalothin	IV	1.0 (S)	17	0.5		1.0		1.0	54	CB, PER
249	Cephalothin	IV	2.0 (M)	3	0.5	45.6	0.33	3.43	0.33	7.5	TC
17	Cephapirin	IV	1.0 (S)	12	0.5	1.2 (±0.4)	2.0	1.1 (±0.4)	2.0	91	W
249	Cephradine	IV	2.0 (M)	3	0.7	84.77	0.33	10.73	0.33	13	TC
12	CGP9000	Oral	1.0 (S)	6	1.0	24	2.0	16.6	2.0	69	D
250	FK-037	IV	2.0 (S)	6	2.0	143	0.5	63	1–2	44	CB
251	Meropenem	IV	30 mg/kg	8	1.0	6.3 (5.4–7.2)	4–12	5.5	4–12	87	SB
64	Imipenem	IV	0.5 (M)	4	0.9–1.3	32 (30–40)	1	2 (1–5)	1	30	MD, SP
			0.5 (S)	5	0.9–1.3	45	1	12	1	47	MD

(Continued)

Table 14.6 (Continued)

Antimicrobial Concentrations in Cutaneous Blisters, Disks, and Threads

Reference	Antimicrobial	Administration Method[a]	Dose (g) (Multiple or Single)[b]	n	Serum Half-life (h)	Serum Concentration Mean (µg/mL) (Range)	Time Serum Obtained (h)	Site Concentration Mean (µg/mL) (Range)	Time Site Specimen Obtained (h)	Ratio of Site/Serum (%)	Notes[c]
Penicillins											
252	Amoxicillin	IV	1.0 (S)	6	1.3	15.0	2.0	6.0	2.0	40	CB
253	Amoxicillin/clavulanic acid	Oral	500/250 mg (S)	6	1.2/1.0	4.36 (±1.5)/2.72 (±0.7)	2	3.3 (±3.6)/2.07 (±0.9)	2	76/76	CB
17	Ampicillin	Oral	2.0 (S)	12	1.1	7.5 (±3.6)	2.0	1.0 (±0.6)	2.0	13	W
254	Ampicillin	IV	2.0 (S)	6	0.83	24	1.5	10	1.5	42	T
17	Bacampicillin	Oral	1.6 (S)	12	1.1	13.0 (±5.4)	2.0	2.2 (±0.6)	2.0	17	W
255	Benzylpenicillin	IM	0.5 (S)	9	0.5	3.5 (2–5)	2.0	0.6 (0.4–1.0)	2.0	17	W
16	Carbenicillin	IV	3.0 (S)	12	1.5	48.8 (±15.4 SE)	2.0	10.8 (±5.9 SE)	2.0	22	W
256	Cloxacillin	IV	1.0 (S)	6	0.65	8.0	1.5	1.5	1.5	19	SB
252	Flucloxacillin	IV	1.0 (S)	6	1.1	9.0	2.0	5.0	2.0	56	CB
257	Flucloxacillin	IV	2.0 (S)	5	2.1	24	2.0	3.7	2.0	15	SB, E
15	Nafcillin	IM	0.5 (S)	11	1.0	3 (1.8–40)	2.0	0.1 (0.05–0.2)	2.0	3	W
15	Penicillin V	Oral	1.0 (S)	10	0.5	0.9 (0.4–2.0)	2.0	0.2 (0.1–0.4)	2.0	22	W
258	Piperacillin/tazobactam	IV	4.0 (S) / 0.5 (S)	6 / 6	1.0 / 1.1	224 (136–290) / 27 (17–36)	0.5 / 0.5	77 (43–126) / 113 (5.0–27)	0.5–3 / 0.5–3	35 / 42	CB / CB
259	Temocillin	IV	1 (S)	6	4.5	95 (±30)	2	40 (±16)	2	42	SB, E
16	Ticarcillin	IV	3.0 (S)	12	1.2	47.1 (±6.4)	2.0	10.9 (±4.6)	2.0	23	W
260	Timentin (ticarcillin/clavulanic acid)	IV	3.2 (S)	12	1.0/0.9	81 (±19)/1.5 (±0.3)	2	32 (±2.6)/2.6 (±0.8)	2	40/173	SB, E
260	Timentin (ticarcillin/clavulanic acid)	IV	3.2 (S)	12	1.0/0.9	81 (±19)/1.5 (±0.3)	2	71 (±23)/2.0 (±0.9)	2	88/133	T, E

Quinolones											
248	Ciprofloxacin	Oral	0.5 (S)	12	3.7	2.3 (±0.8)	1.3	1.8 (±0.8)	2.3	80	SB
	Ciprofloxacin	Oral	0.5 (M)	12	4.7	3.5 (±1.3)	1.0	1.9 (±0.7)	2.5	57	SB
261	Enoxacin	Oral	0.6 (S)	6	6.2	3.7 (±0.5)	1.9	2.9 (±0.5)	3.7	78	CB
	Enoxacin	IV	0.4 (S)	7	5.1	5.5 (±1.8)	Peak	2.2 (±0.5)	0.5	40	CB
262	Fleroxacin	Oral	0.4 (S)	6	12.0	6.1 (±2.2)	0.7	3.8 (±0.6)	4.0	62	CB
263	Gatifloxacin	Oral	0.4 (S)	9	6.8 (±0.72)	4.1 (±0.86) (2.9–5.4 range)	1.8 (± 0.94)	3.6 (±1.6) (2.2–7.6 range)	4.2 (±1.9)	87	CB
261	Ofloxacin	Oral	0.6 (S)	6	7.0	10.7 (±6.4)	1.2	5.2 (±6.9)	5.3	49	CB
261	Norfloxacin	Oral	0.4 (S)	6	3.25	1.5 (±0.1)	1.5	1.0 (±0.3)	2.3	67	CB
261	Pefloxacin	IV	0.4 (S)	8	10.5	5.1	Peak	3.3 (±0.7)	1.8	66	CB, E
Others											
264	Azithromycin	Oral	0.5 (S)	6	9.6	0.1 (0.06–15)	6	0.13 (0.1–0.15)	2–4	130	CB
265	Carumonam	IV	2 (S)	6	1.68	36.6 (±8.2)	2	48.1 (±11.4)	2	131	CB
266	CGP31608 (penem)	IV	1 (S)	6	0.5	2.8 (±0.2)	2	5.4 (±1.0)	2	193	CB
267	Clindamycin	Oral	0.5 (S)	4	2.0	3.75	1.5–2.5		1.5–2.5	9	W, PER
268	Dalbavancin	IV	1.0 (S)	9	168	46.5 ± 9.13	168	30.3 ± 4.43	168	65	CB
269	Daptomycin	4 mg/kg	7 (S)	7	7.74 (±0.63)	77.5 (±8.3)	0.5	14.5	2	18.7	CB
25	Dirithromycin	Oral	0.25 (S)	6	1.7	0.55 (±0.28)	3.3	0.20 (±0.08)	3.3	42	MD
270	Doxycycline	Oral	100 mg (M)	8	11.7	1.5	2	0.7	2	47	SB, E
271	Erythromycin base	Oral	0.5 (M)	8	1.5	2.92	4–6	1.33	4–6	46	SB, E
271	Erythromycin (EA)	Oral	0.5 (M)	8	1.5	1.24	4–6	0.68	4–6	55	SB, E
168	Erythromycin	Oral	0.5 (M)	4	1.5	1.9	3.0	0.12	3.0	6	SB
65	FCE22101 (penem)	IV	1 (S)	6	0.8	2.1 (±0.4)	2	5.0 (±1.9)	2	238	CB

(Continued)

Table 14.6 (Continued)

Antimicrobial Concentrations in Cutaneous Blisters, Disks, and Threads

Reference	Antimicrobial	Administration Method[a]	Dose (g) (Multiple or Single)[b]	n	Serum Half-life (h)	Serum Concentration Mean (μg/mL) (Range)	Time Serum Obtained (h)	Site Concentration Mean (μg/mL) (Range)	Time Site Specimen Obtained (h)	Ratio of Site/Serum (%)	Notes[c]
65	FCE22891 (penem)	Oral	1 (S)	5	0.6	2.0 (±1.5)	2	2.7 (±1.3)	2	135	CB
272	Fosfomycin	IV	8.0	6	5.7	395 (±46)	1	156 (±16)	1	53	MD, SE
273	Fusidic acid	Oral	0.25 (M)	8	16	39 (13.7–54.9)	3	21 (3.4–35)	6–12	53	SB
274	Linezolid	Oral	0.6 (M)	6	4.9	18.3 ± 0.6	0.7	16.4 ± 10.6	2–4	90	
275	Methioprim	Oral	320 mg (S)	5	9.3	2.6	4	0.9	4	35	SB, E
275	Methioprim	Oral	160 mg (S)	5	9.3	2.5	4	1.3	4	52	SB, E
276	Rifampin	Oral	450 mg (S)	3	2.5	13.2 (10.0–16.0)	3.0	2.7 (2.7–2.8)	6–9	20	SB
157	Sulfacarbamide	Oral	335 mg (M)	5	4–5	7 (±1)	2.0	4 (±1)	2.0	57	SB
157	Sulfadiazine	Oral	335 mg (M)	5	3–4	39 (±2)	2.0	15 (±2)	2.0	50	SB
157	Sulfadimidine	Oral	335 mg (M)	5	5–7	27 (±3)	2.0	6 (±2)	2.0	22	SB
157	Sulfamethoxazole	Oral	0.8 (M)	5	5–7	115 (±6)	2.0	43 (±4)	2.0	37	SB
277	Teicoplanin	IV	440 mg (S)	6	34.2	21.0 (±4.9)	2	13.2 (±2.1)	2	63	CB
278	Telithromycin	Oral	0.6 (S)	8	9.8 L[d]	0.83 (±0.35)	2.5 (±1.03)	0.44 (±0.23)	10.5 (±5.09)	53	CB
279	Tigecycline	IV	0.1, 0.05 (M)	10	44.9	0.82	0.5	0.27 ± 0.31	2.8		CB
157	Trimethoprim	Oral	320 mg (S)	5	8–10	2.8 (±0.4)	2.0	1.5 (±0.4)	2.0	54	SB
157	Trimethoprim	Oral	160 mg (M)	5	8–10	3.1 (±0.8)	2.0	1.7 (±0.3)	2.0	55	SB

[a]IM, intramuscularly; IV, intravenously.
[b]S, single dose; M, multiple dose.
[c]W, skin window; SB, suction blister; CB, cantharidin blister; E, values extrapolated from graph; PT, plastic template method of Kiistala and Mustakallio (18); T, threads; IR, impaired renal function; PER, actual levels not reported, only percentage penetration data; D, disk; TC, tissue cage; MD, microdialysis probe of interstitial fluid of muscle; SP, septic patients.
[d]Literature value.

Table 14.7

Antimicrobial Concentrations in Bile

Reference	Antimicrobial	Administration Method[a]	Dose (g) (Multiple or Single)[b]	n	Serum Half-life (h)	Serum Concentration Mean (μg/mL) (Range)	Time Serum Obtained (h)	Site Concentration Mean (μg/mL) (Range)	Time Site Specimen Obtained (h)	Ratio of Site/Serum (%)	Notes[c]
Aminoglycosides											
75	Amikacin	IV	0.5 (M)	10	2.0	13.4 (±5.4 SD)	2.0	7.2 (±3.9 SD)	2.0	54	U, T
280	Amikacin	IM	0.5 (S)	7	2.0	14.0 (6–17)	0.75–20	4.2 (<1–7.5)	0.75–2.0	30	U, GB
73	Gentamicin	IM	0.1 (S)	15	2.0	3.2 (2–4.9)	0.8–1.2	1.0 (0–3.9)	0.8–1.2	31	GB
73	Gentamicin	IM	0.12 (S, M)	11	2.0	4.4 (1.5–6.9)	1.0	2.8 (0–10)	1.0	64	T
280	Kanamycin	IM	0.5 (S)	5	2.0	15.4 (10–20)	1.5–2.25	4.6 (<1–12)	1.5–2.25	30	U, GB
281	Streptomycin	IV	0.5 (S)	11	2.5	7.7 (0.6–16)	~1.5–2.0	5.7 (0.5–32)	~1.5–2.0	74	GB
Cephalosporins and related β-lactams											
282	Aztreonam	IV	2.0 (S)	14	1.7	20.0 (±10 SD)	1–2	32.4 (±39.7 SD)	1–2	162	U, CD
282	Aztreonam	IV	2.0 (S)	14	1.7	20.0 (±10 SD)	1–2	9.3 (±3.0 SD)	1–2	47	U, GB
283	Cefaclor	Oral	1.0 (S)	6	0.7	8.3 (±3.7 SD)	2.5	522 (±342 SD)	2.2	6,289	U, E
284	Cefadroxil	Oral	1.0 (S)	4	1.3	20.4 (±6.7 SE)	3.0	4.5 (±2.0 SE)	3.0	22	U, T
285	Cefamandole	IV	1.0 (S)	8	0.7	93 (±5 SD)	0.5	352 (±64 SD)	0.5	378	U, T
78	Cefamandole	IV	2.0 (S)	6	0.7	37.5 (20–76)	1.0	6.1 (0.5–15)	1.0	16	CD, OD
286	Cefazolin	IV	1.0 (S)	8	2.0	65 (40–88)	0.5	51 (5–168)	1.0	78	U, T
287	Cefbuperazone	IV	1.0 (S)	13	1.7	96.7 (±12.3)	0.5	6.6 (±3.0)	0.5	7	U, GB
288	Cefepime	IV	2.0 (M)	20	2.0	7.6 (0.4–62)	8.6	15.5 (0.2–70)	8.6	204	A
289	Cefepime	IV	2.0 (S)	27	5.02	100 ± 85.5	4.73 ± 4.25	19.8 ± 12.9	4.73 ± 4.25	19.8	
290	Cefmenoxime	IV	1.0 (S)	6	1.1	22.4 (17–38)	0.9	117.9 (1.5–204)	0.9	526	U, GB
291	Cefoperazone	IV	1.0 (M)	10	1.9	45.1 (±7.9 SE)	2.9	19.2 (±9.6 SE)	2.9	43	I, GB
149	Ceforanide	IV	1.0 (S)	6	2.7	45 (±4 SD)	2.0	49 (±16 SD)	2.0	108	U, GB, PC

(Continued)

Table 14.7 (Continued)

Antimicrobial Concentrations in Bile

Reference	Antimicrobial	Administration Method[a]	Dose (g) (Multiple or Single)[b]	n	Serum Half-life (h)	Serum Concentration Mean (μg/mL) (Range)	Time Serum Obtained (h)	Site Concentration Mean (μg/mL) (Range)	Time Site Specimen Obtained (h)	Ratio of Site/Serum (%)	Notes[c]
149	Ceforanide	IV	1.0 (S)	5	2.7	45 (±4 SD)	2.0	149 (±59 SD)	2.0	331	U, CD, PD
148	Cefotaxime	IM	0.5 (M)	5	1.2	12.8 (7.4–17.5)	0.25	2.9 (0.8–7.8)	0–2	23	I, CD
148	Cefotaxime	IV	1.0 (M)	5	1.2	19.4 (8.6–48.2)	1.0	48.9 (34–82)	0.75	252	I, GB
292	Cefpiramide	IV	1.0 (S)	10		106 (±12)	2.0	116 (±392)	2.0	1095	CD, T
293	Ceftazidime	IV	1.0 (S)	20	1.7	24.9 (12.5–37)	1.75	18.5 (10.1–27)	1.75	74	GB
148	Ceftazidime	IV	1.0 (S)	13	1.7	36.1 (24–47)	1.0	31.8 (12.5–55)	1.0	88	CD
2	Ceftizoxime	IV	1.0 (S)	5	1.7	47.6 (±7.4 SD)	1.0	39.0 (±22.4 SD)	0–2	82	U, T
2	Ceftizoxime	IV	1.0 (S)	6	1.7	30.6 (±5.8 SD)	1.0	10.5 (±11.8 SD)	1–3	34	GB
291	Ceftriazone	IV	1.0 (M)	11	6.5	59.5 (±13 SE)	2.9	44.5 (±16 SE)	2.9	75	I, GB
294	Cefuroxime	IV	0.75 (S)	5	1.4	46 (36–69)	0–0.8	10.6 (1.4–19.6)	0.3–1.7	23	CD
79	Cephacetrile	IM	1.0 (S)	5	0.9	11.2 (8.5–17.5)	2.0	0.7 (0–2)	2.0	6	T
286	Cephaloridine	IM	1.0 (S)	7	1.5	32 (23–50)	0.5	17 (1–42)	1.0	53	U, T
74	Cephalothin	IV	1.0 (S)	11	0.5	12.7 (4–46)	0.8–1.2	2.8 (<0.1–10.5)	0.8–1.2	22	GB
74	Cephalothin	IV	1.0 (S)	13	0.5	11.4 (2.2–28)	1.0	5.7 (<0.1–13.1)	1.0	50	T
74	Cephalothin	IV	1.0 (M)	4	0.5	7.2 (3.2–10.3)	1.0	12.0 (0.4–25.7)	1.0	172	U, T
295	Imipenem	IV	1.0 (S)	12	1.2	36.2 (27–49)	0.5	17.5 (3.5–51.3)	0.5	48	T
69	Meropenem	IV	1.0 (S)	11	1.0	14.6 (2.6–44)	1–3.3	14.8 (3.9–20.2)	1–3.3	101	E, CD, PD
69	Meropenem	IV	1.0 (S)	13	1.0	20.0 (5.8–40)	1–3.3	8.1 (0.7–25.7)	1–3.3	41	E, CD, OD
296	Meropenem	IV	1.0 (S)	43	1.2	27.3 (1.9–87.0) / 4.8 (0.3–41.6)	0.5–1.5	4.9 (1.5–16.1) / 17.7 (1.3–18.9)	0.5–1.5 / 3–5	18 / 369	
Penicillins											
297	Amoxicillin	IM	1.0 (S)	5	1.1	10.4 (8.6–12)	1.2–1.5	11.6 (9–13.5)	1.2–1.5	110	CD
72	Ampicillin	Oral	0.5 (S)	10	1.1	3.4 (0.5–6.6)	2.0	3.5 (0.6–11)	2.0	103	T

72	Ampicillin	IV	0.5 (S)	5	1.1	16.5 (3.5–28)	1.0	15.7 (≤8.2–33)	1.0	95	GB
72	Ampicillin	IV	0.5 (S)	5	1.1	16.5 (3.5–28)	1.0	40.7 (13.5–72)	1.0	246	CD
298	Ampicillin/ sulbactam	IV	1.0 (S)	14	1.1	20.2 (611.3)	0.25–1.5	15.9 (612.9)	0.25–1.5	22	GB
		IV	0.5 (S)	14	0.8	19.9 (69.6)	0.25–1.5	4.3 (65.4)	0.25–1.5	22	GB
299	Apalcillin	IV	1.0 (S)	10	1.2	38.3 (±3.1 SEM)	3.0	2,093 (±859)	3.0	5,464	T
300	Methicillin	IM	1.0 (S)	5	0.5	5.7 (3–12.5)	0.75–2.0	5.5 (<0.8–0)	0.75–2.0	96	GB
82	Mezlocillin	IM	1.0 (S)	10	1.1	23.5 (14.5–38)	2.0	221 (13–680)	2.0	940	T
301	Nafcillin	IM	1.0 (S)	6	1.0	13.5 (9–18)	0.5–1.0	540 (173–1,030)	0.5–1.0	4,000	U, T
71	Penicillin G	IV	1×10^6 units (S)	10	0.5	9.9 (4.3–17.5)	1.0	45.7 (2.2–189)	1.0	461	GB
71	Penicillin G	IV	1×10^6 units (S)	10	0.5	9.9 (4.3–17.5)	1.0	93.5 (24–204)	1.0	944	CD
67	Piperacillin	IV	1.0 (S)	11	1.1	43.7 (2.1–120)	0.5	2.9 (0–18)	0.5	7	OD
68	Piperacillin	IV	2.0 (S)	10	1.1	81.7 (±20.5 SD)	1.0	382 (±110 SD)	1.0	468	CD
		IV	2.0 (S)	10	1.1	81.7 (±20.5 SD)	1.0	30.8 (±2.5 SD)	1.0	38	GB
		IV	2.0 (S)	10	1.1	187 (±62 SD)	1.0	170 (±47 SD)	1.0	91	T
302	Temocillin	IV	2.0 (M)	8	3.8	123 (56–168)	2.0	961 (24–2,303)	2.0	782	T
303	Ticarcillin/ clavulanic acid	IV	3.0 (S)	23	1.2	85 (35–210)	2.5	425 (225–700)	2.5	500	CD
		IV	0.2 (S)	23	1.1	2.8	2.5	1.2	2.5	43	CD
Quinolones											
304	Ciprofloxacin	IV	0.4 (S)	10	1.06	4.43 (1.88–6.24)	2.08 (1.58–2.5)	5.79 (0.76–12.47)	2.08 (1.58–2.5)	131	
304	Ciprofloxacin	Oral	0.5 (S)	10	3.74	0.81 (0.01–1.79)	1.92 (1.67–2.42)	9.2 (0.3–53.05)	1.92 (1.67–2.42)	1136	
281	Chlortetracycline	IV	0.5 (S)	7	9.0	12 (1.2–18)	~1.5–2.0	40 (2.4–72)	~1.5–2.0	333	GB
305	Demethylchlor- tetracycline	IV	0.5 (S)	4	14.0	6.8 (6.2–7.8)	2.0	197 (74–120)	2.0	1,426	U, T
76	Doxycycline	IV	0.2 (S)	5	20.0	3.9 (3.2–4.4)	2.0	12.4 (3.2–18.2)	2.0	318	U, GB
76	Doxycycline	IV	0.2/0.1 (M)	15	20.0	3.0 (0.1–5.0)	20	22.2 (0.1–3)	20	740	U, GB

(Continued)

Table 14.7 (Continued)

Antimicrobial Concentrations in Bile

Reference	Antimicrobial	Administration Method[a]	Dose (g) (Multiple or Single)[b]	n	Serum Half-life (h)	Serum Concentration Mean (μg/mL) (Range)	Time Serum Obtained (h)	Site Concentration Mean (μg/mL) (Range)	Time Site Specimen Obtained (h)	Ratio of Site/Serum (%)	Notes[c]
281	Oxytetracycline	IV	0.5 (S)	12	8.0	10.3 (0.6–18)	~1.5–2.0	45.6 (0.3–144)	~1.5–2.0	443	GB
281	Tetracycline	IV	0.5 (S)	9	10.0	80 (5–160)	~1.5–2.0	200 (40–320)	~1.5–2.0	250	GB
Others											
281	Bacitracin	IV	2.5×10^4 (S)	9		0.75 (0.04–1.3)	~1.5–2.0	1.6 (0.04–5.0)	~1.5–2.0	213	GB
281	Chloramphenicol	IV	0.5 (S)	8	2.5	1.4 (1.25–5)	~1.5–2.0	3.1 (1.3–10)	~1.5–2.0	221	GB
68	Clindamycin	IV	0.6 (S)	7	2.0	14.5 (9–26)	1.0	42 (14–168)	~1.0	290	CD, PD
68	Clindamycin	IV	0.6 (S)	7	2.0	11.3 (6–19)	1.0	0	~1.0	0	CD, OD
281	Erythromycin	Oral	0.4 (S)	5	1.5	1.6 (0.2–5.0)	~1.5–2.0	6.3 (0.1–20)	~1.5–2.0	394	GB
66	Metronidazole	IV	0.5 (S)	14	8.0	12.3 (8.3–16.1)	2.5	0	2.5	0	GB, OC
66	Metronidazole	IV	0.5 (S)	14	8.0	12.3 (8.3–16.1)	2.5	13.2 (10.7–15.1)	2.5	107	CD, PD
66	Metronidazole	IV	0.5 (S)	8	8.0	12.0 (7.7–16.2)	2.5	11.3 (9.8–14.8)	2.5	94	GB, PC
281	Polymyxin	IV	0.1 (S)	7	4.4	3.1 (0.6–8)	~1.5–2.0	2.0 (0.6–9.6)	~1.5–2.0	65	GB
77	Rifampin	Oral	0.15 (S)	4	2.5	1.4 (1.1–1.8)	3–5	258 (41–539)	3–5	18,400	GB
186	Vancomycin	IV	0.5 (S)	9	6.0	7.5 (5.2–10.0)	1.0	3.1 (2.0–3.6)	1.0	41	T

[a]IV, intravenously; IM, intramuscularly.
[b]M, multiple dose; S, single dose.
[c]U, uninfected; T, T-tube drain; GB, gallbladder; CD, common bile duct; A, acute cholecystitis; I, infected; PC, patent cystic duct; PD, patent common duct; OC, obstructed cystic duct; E, endoscopic retrograde duct cannulation; OD, obstructed common duct;

Although biliary penetration is often touted as advantageous in the therapy of biliary tract infection, it is not at all clear that this is an important treatment variable in view of the poor penetration in the presence of obstruction. Keighley et al. (83) have shown that biliary antibiotic concentrations have no influence on rates of bacteremia and wound infection associated with biliary tract surgery. Smith and LeFrock (84), Nagar and Berger (85), and Dooley et al. (86) have extensively reviewed biliary antibiotic penetration and clinical use in biliary infection.

Sputum

Both sputum and bronchial secretion specimens are included in Table 14.8. Bronchial secretions were obtained via bronchoscopy or by suction aspiration from patients with endotracheal tubes or tracheostomies. Some articles provide data on antimicrobial concentrations in epithelial lining fluid in the lung, which is indicated in Table 14.8 (87). Most subjects had chronic bronchitis, but some studies were done with children with cystic fibrosis, and occasionally patients had pneumonia. Nearly all studies were done with infected patients. Some studies suggest higher sputum antibiotic levels with the use of mucolytic agents (88–90). Ratios of sputum-to-serum concentrations are low for most drugs. Data on AUC ratios were limited but showed ratios of 2.7% and 4.5% for cefotaxime (91), 14% for cefuroxime (92), 106% for ciprofloxacin (93), and 19% for netilmicin by both intermittent and continuous intravenous infusions. Sputum concentrations of the cefotaxime metabolite desacetyl-cefotaxime are much higher than those of the parent drug (94).

Some studies have shown a relationship between clinical infection cure and antibiotic concentration in sputum (89,95) and have shown that the antibiotic concentration increases with the degree of sputum purulence for at least some antibiotics (96). Reviews of this topic have differed on the importance of sputum antibiotic concentrations to the cure of infection, with Lambert (97) taking a somewhat skeptical view, while Pennington (98) has taken a supportive stand with which Smith and LeFrock (99) have concurred. Readers are also directed to an excellent study by Wong et al. (100), which could not be included in Table 14.8 because of the graphical presentation of the data. Hitt and Gerding (43) have compiled ratios of sputum antimicrobial levels to the minimal inhibitory concentration for 90% of common bacterial pathogens that cause bronchitis and pneumonia. These ratios

may prove predictive of clinical outcome, but good clinical correlation is lacking.

Breast Milk

The studies of breast milk (Table 14.9) were performed in lactating mothers who were normal volunteers or were being treated for nonbreast infections. The results show that the secretion of most antibiotics into breast milk is insignificant. However, a few agents, notably metronidazole, chloramphenicol, tetracycline, and lincomycin, were found in milk at levels approaching the serum levels. Giamarellou et al. (101) reported a study showing that quinolones (ciprofloxacin, ofloxacin, and pefloxacin) also have excellent penetration into breast milk, posing a possible risk to newborn infants. In a single study addressing milk penetration during puerperal mastitis, concentrations of phenoxymethyl-penicillin were higher in the milk from the mastitic breasts than in the nonmastitic breasts, but serum concentrations were not determined for the patients with mastitis (102). Even though only small quantities of most antibiotics reach the breast milk, the potential still exists for allergy or toxicity in the infant.

Middle Ear Fluid

Antibiotic levels were assayed in middle ear fluid from patients categorized as infected (acute otitis media) or uninfected (serous otitis or otitis media with effusion) (Table 14.10). The middle ear fluid samples were usually removed by needle aspiration. Pediatric subjects were studied most often. Most antibiotics penetrated significantly into the middle ear fluid. In the few cases where direct comparison was possible, the presence of acute infection appeared to enhance antibiotic penetration into the middle ear fluid.

Sinus Secretions

The sinus secretion studies were done primarily in patients with either acute or chronic maxillary sinusitis. None of the studies corrected for blood contamination, but this was likely minimal. On the basis of the data presented in Table 14.11, tetracyclines, erythromycin, and trimethoprim seemed to achieve better penetration than the β-lactams. There may be an inverse correlation between degree of purulence and amount of antibiotic penetration (103,104). One clinical correlation showed that an antibiotic concentration higher than the minimal inhibitory concentration of the pathogen was associated with clearance of the bacteria (105).

(continued on page 716)

Table 14.8

Antimicrobial Concentrations in Sputum and Bronchial Secretions

Reference	Antimicrobial	Administration Method[a]	Dose (g) (Multiple or Single)[b]	n	Serum Half-life (h)	Serum Concentration Mean (μg/mL) (Range)	Time Serum Obtained (h)	Site Concentration Mean (μg/mL) (Range)	Time Site Specimen Obtained (h)	Ratio of Site/Serum (%)	Notes[c]
Aminoglycosides											
306	Amikacin	IM	7.5 mg/kg	13	2.8	23.7 (±2.9 SE)	1.5–2.0	5.2 (±1.5 SE)	1.5–2.0	21	U, B
307	Gentamicin	IM	0.08 (M)	8	2.0	6.3 (3–12)	1.0	<0.5	1.0	<8	I, B, P
308	Gentamicin	IV	0.24 (S)	24		4.7 ± 0.49	4	3.1 ± 0.39	4	66	I, ELF
309	Netilmicin	IV	0.45 (S)	5	2.7	12.0 (±0.7 SE)	2.0	2.0 (±0.3 SE)	2.0	17	I, B
310	Tobramycin	IV	7 mg/kg q24 (M)	12		22.4 ± 5.9	0.5	2.7 ± 0.7	0.5	11.9	I, ELF, PP
311	Sisomicin	IV	1.5 mg/kg (M)	20	2.0	1.0 (±0.25 SE)	1.0	0.5 (±0.1 SE)	1.0	50	I, SP
312	Tobramycin	IM/IV	1.7 mg/kg (M)	10	2.0	8.0 (5.6–12.0)	1–2.2	1.4 (0.5–2.8)	1–2.6	18	U, B
Cephalosporins and related β-lactams											
313	Aztreonam	IV	2.0 (S)	9	1.7	39 (12–69)	2	4.2 (0.04–14.1)	2	21	I, B
208	Cefazolin	IV	1.0 (S)	9	2.0	100 (±30 SD)	0.5	2.3 (±0.5 SD)	0–2	2	I, SP
230	Cefaclor	Oral	0.75 MR (M)	6	1.2	3.08 (±1.7 SD)	4	2.71 (±0.87 SD)	4	88	ELF
314	Cefdinir	Oral	0.3 (S)	9		2.00[d]	224[d] min	0.78[d]	224[d] min	41	U, BM
	Cefdinir	Oral	0.6 (S)	8		4.20[d]	223[d] min	1.14[d]	223[d] min	31	U, BM
	Cefdinir	Oral	0.3 (S)	9		2.00[d]	224[d] min	0.29[d]	224[d] min	15	U, ELF
	Cefdinir	Oral	0.6 (S)	8		4.20[d]	223[d] min	0.49[d]	223[d] min	12	U, ELF
315	Cefepime	IV	2.0 (S)	20		40.4 (±28.1 SD)	4.84	24.1[e] (±17.8 SD)	4.84	60	U, BM
316	Cefmenoxime	IV	1.0 (S)	3	1.4	3.4 (1.4–6.2)	2	0.3 (0.1–0.8)	2	9	I, SP
	Cefmenoxime	IV	1.0 (M)	5	1.4	3.5 (0.6–10)	2	0.3 (0.1–0.5)	2	8	
91	Cefotaxime	IM	1.0 (M)	30	1.2	37.5 (±2 SD)	1.0	0.6 (±0.1 SD)	3.0	2	I, SP, PP
317	Cefoxitin	IV	2.0 (S)	36	0.8	13.9	1.0	1.6	1.0	11	I, B
317	Cefoxitin	IV	2.0 (M)	21	0.8	19	1.0	3.0	1.0	16	I, B

318	Cefpirome	IV	1.0 (S)	8	2.0	20.1	0.5–7	7.2 (±1.1 SE)	0.5–7	36	U, ELF
319	Cefsulodin	IV	1.0 (S)	6	1.5	28	2	2.8	2	10	I, B
320	Cefazidime	IV	2.0 (S)	8	1.7	32 (±6.1 SD)	2	5.6 (±4.1 SD)	2	18	I, B
2	Ceftizoxime	IV	2.0 (S)	8	1.7	109 (±45 SD)	0.5	4.3 (±4.3 SD)	2.6	4	I, SP
321	Ceftriaxone	IV	2.0 (S)	22	6.5	43 (22–80)	3	1.9 (0–6.5)	3	2	I, B
		IV	2.0 (S)	22	6.5	11 (0–46)	24	3.4 (1.0–8.0)	24	33	I, B
		IV	2.0 (M)	12	6.5	34 (11–57)	6	4.5 (2.0–9.5)	6	14	I, B
92	Cefuroxime	IM	0.75 (M)	4	1.4	17.3 (14–25)	1.0	2.4 (1.4–4.8)	1.0	14	I, B
322	Cephalexin	Oral	0.5 (M)	20	0.8			0.3 (0.03–3.4)	0–12		I, P
323	Cephradine	Oral	1.0 (S)	8	0.7	7.8	2–3	1.3	2–3.3	20	I, B
94	Desacetyl cefotaxime	IV	2.0 (M)	7	1.5	9.3 (1.7–15.1)	1.3	5.8 (1.6–9.2)	1.3	62	U, B
324	Ertapenem	IV	1.0 (M)	15	8	4.8 (3.9–6.4)	12	2 (1.1–2.5)	12	41.7	I,ELF,P
325	Meropenem	IV	1.0 (S)	8	1.0	2.7 (±1.3 SD)	3	0.5 (±0.4 SD)	3	20	U, B
326	Meropenem	IV	1.0 (S)	6		14.98^f (±5.30 SD) 14.98^f (±5.30 SD)	1.0	7.07 (±2.87 SD)	1.0	47	U, ELF
	Meropenem	IV	1.0 (S)	6			1.0	0.086 (±0.033 SD)	1.0	0.6	U, L
327	Meropenem	IV	2.0 (M)	4	0.89	12.8 ± 2.7	3	2.8 ± 1.5	3	21.9	U, ELF
328	Moxalactam	IM	1.0 (M)	20	2.3	54.9	1.0	5.0	1.0	9	I, B
Penicillins											
90	Amoxicillin	Oral	0.5 (M)	12	1.0	30 (±5.0 SEM)	3	1.3 (±0.2 SEM)	3	4	I, B, E, MU
89	Amoxicillin	Oral	1.0 (M)	20	1.3	9.4	2	2.2	4	23	I, SP, PP, MU
329	Amoxicillin/ clavulanic acid	Oral	0.5 (S)	15	1.1	6.9 (8.6)	1–2	0.9 (3.5)	1–2	13	U, ELF
		Oral	0.25 (S)	15	1.1	5.3 (9.3)	1–2	1.0 (8.4)	1–2	14	U, ELF
95	Ampicillin	Oral	1.0 (M)	20	1.5	5.5 (3.5–9.8)	2.0	0.25 (0–0.5)	0–24	5	I, SP
330	Ampicillin/ sulbactam	IV	2.0 (S)	15	1.2	97 (±95 SE)	0.5	0.6 (±0.1 SE)	0.5	<1	U, B
		IV	1.0 (S)	15	1.1	38 (±3.8 SE)	0.5	0.3 (±0.1 SE)	0.5	<1	U, B

(Continued)

Table 14.8 (Continued)

Antimicrobial Concentrations in Sputum and Bronchial Secretions

Reference	Antimicrobial	Administration Method[a]	Dose (g) (Multiple or Single)[b]	n	Serum Half-life (h)	Serum Concentration Mean (μg/mL) (Range)	Time Serum Obtained (h)	Site Concentration Mean (μg/mL) (Range)	Time Site Specimen Obtained (h)	Ratio of Site/Serum (%)	Notes[c]
331	Apalcillin	IV	2.1 (S)	6	2.4	27.6	2.0	5.8	2.0	21	I, B, AUC
323	Bacampicillin	Oral	0.8 (S)	11	1.1	9.5	2–3	2.1	2–3.3	22	I, B
332	Benzylpenicillin	IM	10^6 units (M)	29	0.5	10.9 (1–>16)	2–3	0.2 (0–>0.5)	2–3	2	I, SP
208	Carbenicillin	IV	5.0 (S)	12	1.5	463 (±89 SD)	0.5	3.4 (±0.4 SD)	0–2	1	I, SP
333	Cloxacillin	Oral	0.25 (M)	12	0.5	5.6 (3.0–1)	1–2	0.6 (0.01–1.6)	1–2	11	I, C, CF
334	Piperacillin	IV	2.0 (M)	18	1.1	101	2	3.6	2	4	I, B
335	Talampicillin	Oral	0.75 (M)	8		6.8 (4.0–10.9)	1	0.5 (0.3–0.8)	2	7	I, B
208	Ticarcillin	IV	5.0 (S)	11	1.6	469 (±65 SD)	0.5	4.1 (±1.0 SD)	0–2	1	I, SP
Quinolones											
336	Ciprofloxacin	Oral	0.5 (M)	34	4.0	3.80 (2.0–7.5)	2	1.0	2	26	I, SP, AUC
		Oral	0.5 (M)	34	4.0	2.0	4	1.3 (0.7–3.6)	4	65	I, SP, AUC
		Oral	0.5 (M)	34	4.0	1.3	8	0.8	8	62	I, SP, AUC
337	Ciprofloxacin	Oral	0.5 (M)	4		2.11[f] (±0.35 SD)	4	1.87 (±0.91 SD)	4	89	U, ELF
93	Ciprofloxacin	IV	0.4 (M)	25	5.35 ± 2.21	47.41 ± 17.02		50.3 ± 20.27		106	I, BS, AUC
338	Enoxacin	Oral	0.6 (S)	15	5.5	1.8	1	1.1	1	58	U, I, E
		Oral	0.6 (S)	15	5.5	3.2	3	3.1	3	95	
		Oral	0.6 (S)	15	5.5	2.0	7	2.8	7	140	
339	Fleroxacin	Oral	0.4 (M)	6	15	8.7[f] (±1.3 SD)	1.4	10.0 (±5.3 SD)	2.2	115	I, SP
340	Garenoxacin	Oral	0.6 (S)	6		10.03[f] (±2.80 SD)	3.26	6.98[e] (±1.34 SD)	3.26	72	U, BM
	Garenoxacin	Oral	0.6 (S)	6		10.03[f] (±2.80 SD)	3.26	9.21 (±3.62 SD)	3.26	95	U, ELF
341	Gatifloxacin	Oral	0.4 (S)	5		3.96[f] (3.50–4.40)	2	6.24[e] (4.60–8.70)	2	157	U, BM
	Gatifloxacin	Oral	0.4 (S)	5		3.96[f] (3.50–4.40)	2	6.00 (3.90–8.50)	2	151	U, ELF

337	Levofloxacin	Oral	0.5 (M)	4		5.29^f (±1.23 SD)	4	9.94 (±2.74 SD)	4	188	U, ELF
	Levofloxacin	Oral	0.75 (M)	4		11.98^f (2.99 SD)	4	22.12 (±14.92 SD)	4	185	U, ELF
342	Lomefloxacin	Oral	0.4 (M)	4		3.2 (±1.4 SD)	2	2.5 (±1.2 SD)	2	78	I, B
	Lomefloxacin	Oral	0.4 (M)	4		3.2 (±1.4 SD)	2	5.9^g (±2.1 SD)	2	197	I, BM
	Lomefloxacin	Oral	0.4 (M)	4		3.2 (±1.4 SD)	2	6.9 (±2.8 SD)	2	216	I, ELF
343	Moxifloxacin	Oral	0.4 (S)	6		3.22^e (±1.25 SD)	2.2	5.36^e (±1.29 SD)	2.2	167	U, BM
	Moxifloxacin	Oral	0.4 (S)	6		3.22 (±1.25 SD)	2.2	20.7 (±1.92 SD)	2.2	678	U, ELF
344	Ofloxacin	Oral	0.4 (M)	18	7.0	4.7 (±2.5 SD)	2.0	2.8 (±1.5 SD)	2.0	60	I, C, F
345	Pefloxacin	IV	0.4 (S)	20	10.5	4.6	Peak	3.8	Peak	83	E, AUC
	Pefloxacin	Oral	0.4 (S)	30	10.5	5.1	Peak	4.6	Peak	89	I, E, AUC
Tetracyclines											
346	Doxycycline	Oral	0.1 (S)	10	20	2.3 (1.1–4.4)	2	<0.4 (0.4–0.6)	2–3	17	I, SP
346	Minocycline	Oral	0.1 (S)	11	14	4.5 (2.7–8.7)	2	<1.1 (0.4–2.6)	2–3	24	I, SP
347	Minocycline	Oral	0.1 (M)	13	14	0.8 (±0.5 SD)	13–20	1.5 (±1.1 SD)	13–20	188	U, B, PT
	Minocycline	Oral	0.1 (M)	10	14	0.8 (±0.4 SD)	13–20	4.5 (±3.2 SD)	13–20	563	U, B, DT
346	Tetracycline	Oral	0.25 (S)	12	10	4.0 (1.2–7.5)	4	<1.2 (<0.4–2.4)	4–5	30	I, SP
Others											
348	Azithromycin	Oral	0.5 (S)	20	30	0.13 (±0.05 SD)	12	2.2 (±0.9 SD)	48	1,692	U, ELF
349	Azithromycin ER	Oral	2 (S)	32		0.94 ± 0.54	4 (2–8)	3.2	48	340	PP, U, ELF
350	Clarithromycin	Oral	0.5 (M)	10	4.9	4.0 (±1.2 SE)	4.25	20.5 (±6.7 SE)	4.25	513	U, ELF
350	14-Hydroxy-clarithromycin	Oral		10	7.2	0.7 (±0.2 SE)	4.25	1.9 (±0.7 SE)	4.25	271	U, ELF
351	Clindamycin	Oral	0.3 (S)	24	2.0	2.7	2–4	1.6 (0.3–4.8)	2–4	60	B
352	Colistin	IV	0.174 (M)	13	5.9	2.21 ± 1.08	1	0	2	0	I, ELF, P, PP
353	Dirithromycin	Oral	0.5 (M)	13		0.17 (±0.03 SD)	24	1.26 (±0.30 SD)	24	741	I, B
	Dirithromycin	Oral	0.5 (M)	13/10		0.17 (±0.03 SD)	24	6.51^e (±1.44 SD)	24	3,829	I, BM

(Continued)

Table 14.8 (Continued)

Antimicrobial Concentrations in Sputum and Bronchial Secretions

Reference	Antimicrobial	Administration Method[a]	Dose (g) (Multiple or Single)[b]	n	Serum Half-life (h)	Serum Concentration Mean (μg/mL) (Range)	Time Serum Obtained (h)	Site Concentration Mean (μg/mL) (Range)	Time Site Specimen Obtained (h)	Ratio of Site/Serum (%)	Notes[c]
354	Erythromycin	Oral	1.0 (M)	8	1.5	4.4 (±1.6 SD)	2	1.1 (±0.5 SD)	2	25	I, B
355	Erythromycin ethylsuccinate	Oral	1.0 (M)	19	1.5	0.7 (0.4–1.4)	3	0.6 (0.1–2.5)	3	83	U, B
355	Erythromycin lactobionate	IV	0.5 (S)	11	1.5	1.5 (0.6–1.9)	3	1.3 (0.5–2.5)	3	89	U, B
356	Erythromycin proprionate	Oral	0.5 (M)	30	3.1	3.1 (±0.1 SD)	4	1.2 (±0.1 SD)	4	39	I, B, E
356	Erythromycin stearate	Oral	0.5 (M)	30	3.0	1.9 (±0.1 SD)	4	0.9 (±0.1 SD)	4	47	I, B, E
333	Fusidic acid	Oral	20 mg/kg/day	12	4–12	8.7 (4–14)	1–2	0.5 (0.1–1.6)	1–2	57	I, C, CF
357	Josamycin	Oral	1.0 (M)	10		0.6 (±0.5)	3	0.2 (±0.2)	3	33	U, L
358	Linezolid	Oral	0.6 (M)	5		15.5[f] (±4.9 SD)	4	64.3 (±33.1 SD)	4	414	U, ELF
359	Linezolid	IV	0.6 (M)	16	4.4	17.7 ± 4.4	0.3	14.4 ± 5.6	1	105 ± 34	PP, I, ELF, P
	Telithromycin	Oral	0.8 (M)	7		1.86[f] (±0.91 SD)	2.45	14.89 (±11.35 SD)	2.45	857	U, ELF

[a]M, intramuscularly; IV, intravenously.
[b]M, multiple dose; S, single dose; MR, modified release.
[c]U, uninfected; B, bronchial secretions; I, infected; P, pneumonia; ELF, epithelial lining fluid; SP, sputum; BM, bronchial mucosa; PP, peak-to-peak levels; L, lavage fluid; E, extrapolated from graphs; MU, mucolytic agent used; AUC, area under the curve; C, children; CF, cystic fibrosis; DT, distal to tumor; PT, proximal to tumor.
[d]Value reported as median.
[e]Milligrams per kilogram.
[f]Measured in plasma.
[g]Microgram per gram.

Table 14.9

Antimicrobial Concentrations in Breast Milk

Reference	Antimicrobial	Administration Method[a]	Dose (g) (Multiple or Single)[b]	n	Serum Half-life (h)	Serum Concentration Mean (µg/mL) (Range)	Time Serum Obtained (h)	Site Concentration Mean (µg/mL) (Range)	Time Site Specimen Obtained (h)	Ratio of Site/Serum (%)	Notes[c]
Aminoglycosides											
102	Amikacin	IM	0.10 (S)	23	2.0	3.0 (2.9–3.2)	2	0	2	0.0	
360	Kanamycin	IM	1.0 (S)	4	2.0	50	1	18.4	1	37.00	PD
361	Tobramycin	IM	0.08 (S)	5	2.0	2.63	2.5	<0.44 (trace–0.44)	3	<17.0	
Cephalosporins and related β-lactams											
362	Aztreonam	IM	1 (S)	6	1.7–2	40.0 (±1.8 SE)	1.5	0.34 (±0.08 SE)	6	1.0	PD
362	Aztreonam	IV	1 (S)	6	1.7–2	126.3 (±17.1 SE)	0.25	0.22 (±0.06 SE)	4	0.2	PD
363	Cefadroxil	Oral	1.0 (S)	6	1.3	21.6 (14.6–30.0)	3	1.64 (0.12–2.40)	6	8.0	PD
364	Cefamandole	IV	1.0 (S)	4	0.7	19.1	1	0.46	1	2.0	PD
365	Cefazolin	IV	2.0 (S)	20	2	54.33 (±15.9 SD)	2	1.51 (±0.16)	3	3.0	
366	Cefmenoxime	IV	1.0–2.0 (M)	5	0.8–1.2	1.1	12	1.75	12	159.0	
102	Cefmetazole	IV	1.0 (S)	23	1.1	19.2 (17.0–21.4)	2	0–trace	2		
367	Cefonicid	IM	1.0 (S)	10	4.4	67.4 (±15.8 SD)	1	0.16 (±0.09 SD)	1	0.2	
368	Cefoperazone	IV	1.0 (S)	4	2	54 (37–88)	0.2–0.6	0.41 (0–0.82)	2	1.0	
363	Cefotaxime	IV	1.0 (S)	12	1.2	9.4 (5.9–18.4)	1	0.32 (0.2–0.5)	2	3.0	PD
102	Cefotetan	IV	1.0 (S)	23	3–4.6	25.0 (21.6–28.5)	2	0.1 (0–0.3)	2	0.4	
102	Cefotiam	IM	0.5 (S)	23	0.7–1.0	5.9 (5.6–6.2)	2	0–trace	2		
369	Cefoxitin	IM	2.0 (S)	5	0.8	40.8 (15.3–77.6)	0.5–1	0.41 (0.31–0.65)	1–7	1.0	PD
370	Cefoxitin	IV	1.0 (S)	4	0.8	18.3 (5.6–25)	0.4–0.5	0.58 (0–1.5)	1	3.0	
371	Cefprozil[d]	Oral	1.0 (S)	9	1.69	14.8 (±3.2 SD)	2	3.4 (±2.3 SD)	6	23.0	PD
255	Cefsulodin	IV	1.0 (S)	5	1.2	56.8	1	0.8 (0.7–0.9)	2	1.0	
372	Ceftazidime	IV	2.0 (S)	12	1.8	71.8 (±47.7 SD)	1	5.2 (±3.0 SD)	1	7.0	

(Continued)

Table 14.9 (Continued)

Antimicrobial Concentrations in Breast Milk

Reference	Antimicrobial	Administration Method[a]	Dose (g) (Multiple or Single)[b]	n	Serum Half-life (h)	Serum Concentration Mean (μg/mL) (Range)	Time Serum Obtained (h)	Site Concentration Mean (μg/mL) (Range)	Time Site Specimen Obtained (h)	Ratio of Site/Serum (%)	Notes[c]
2	Ceftizoxime	IV	1.0 (S)	6	1.7	22.6 (±6.25 SD)	1	0.3 (±0.1 SD)	1	1.0	
373	Ceftriaxone	IV	1.0 (S)	10	5.3	30	4	0.5 (±0.1 SD)	4	2.0	
373	Ceftriaxone	IM	1.0 (S)	10	5.3	30	4	0.7 (±0.1 SD)	4	2.0	
363	Cephalexin	Oral	1.0 (S)	6	0.8	22.9 (16.9–32.1)	1	0.5 (0.24–0.85)	4	2.0	PD
102	Cephaloridine	IM	1.0 (S)	23	1–1.5	19.0 (18.0–20.0)	1	0.15 (0–0.3)	6	1.0	PD
363	Cephalothin	IV	1.0 (S)	6	0.5	5.9 (3.4–7.8)	1	0.47 (0.32–0.62)	2	8.0	PD
363	Cephapirin	IV	1.0 (S)	6	0.5	6.1 (3.1–8.0)	1	0.43 (0.28–0.64)	2	7.0	PD
374	Cephradine	Oral	0.5 (M)	6	0.7	4.44	2	0.62	2	14.0	
Penicillins											
363	Amoxicillin	Oral	1.0 (S)	6	1.0	14.6 (8.7–18.0)	2	0.81 (0.39–1.3)	5	6.0	PD
102	Ampicillin	Oral	0.5 (S)	23	0.5–1.0	3.3 (2.6–4.0)	2	0.1 (0–0.2)	2	3.0	
102	Bacampicillin	Oral	0.5 (S)	23	1	4.0 (3.2–4.8)	2	0	2	0.0	
102	Carbenicillin	IM	1.0 (S)	23	0.5–1.0	11.6 (7.6–17.0)	2	0.2 (0–0.4)	2	2.0	
102	Cloxacillin	IM	0.5 (S)	23	0.5	2.3 (1.7–2.7)	2	0.1 (0–0.2)	2	4.0	
102	Dicloxacillin	Oral	0.25 (S)	23	0.7	4.7 (4.6–4.8)	2	0.2 (0.2–0.3)	2	4.0	
128	Epicillin	Oral	0.5 (M)	5	1.0	1.1	4	0.16	4	15.0	PD
102	Methicillin	IM	1.0 (S)	23	0.5	5.5 (4.8–6.4)	2	0.26 (0.2–0.3)	2	5.0	
102	Mezlocillin	IM	1.0 (S)	23	1.1	6.8 (6.6–7.0)	2	0	2	0.0	
102	Oxacillin	IM	0.5 (S)	23	0.5	1.0 (0.7–1.3)	2	0.5 (0.23–0.7)	2	50.0	
375	Oxacillin	Oral	0.5 (M)	10	0.5	<1.31 (<0.3–5.6)	1–4	≤0.2	1–4	≤15.0	
376	Penicillin	IM	1 × 10⁵ units (M)	3	0.5	0.80 (0.49–0.96)	1–2	0.05 (0.03–0.06)	1–2	6.0	
377	Penicillin G	IM	3 × 10⁵ units 5 × 10⁵ units (S)	4	0.5	1.08 (0.72–1.92)	2	<0.11 (<0.03–0.24)	2	<10.0	

378	Penicillin V	Oral	1.32 (S)	4	1	4.7 (3.0–6.6)	1–3	0.3 (0.28–0.50)	4–8	6.0	
379	Piperacillin	IV	4.5 (M)	?	1.0	182	1	2	1	1.0	
380	Pivampicillin	Oral	0.35 (M)	9	0.5–1.0	2.13 (0.33–8.20)	1–4.3	0.1 (0.06–0.19)	1–4.5	5.0	
381	Sulbactam	IV	0.5 (S ± M)	6	1.0	2 (0.7–5)	2	0.52 (0–2.2)	0–8	26.0	
382	Ticarcillin	IV	1.0 (S)	5	1.2	52 (29–100)	0.2–1	Trace	2		
102	Ticarcillin	IM	1.0 (S)	23	1.2	8.9 (7.3–10.4)	2	0	2	0.0	
101	Ciprofloxacin	Oral	0.75 BID (M)	10	3–5	2.06 (±0.68 SD)	2	3.79 (±1.26 SD)	2	184.0	PD
383	Garenoxacin	Oral	0.6 (S)	6		8.9 (±2.7 SD)	3	3 (±0.6 SD)	0–6	36.0	
101	Ofloxacin	Oral	0.4 BID (M)	10	4–8	2.45 (±0.81 SD)	2	2.41 (±0.80 SD)	2	98.0	PD
101	Pefloxacin	Oral	0.4 BID (M)	10	8–12	4.75 (±1.57 SD)	2	3.54 (±1.25 SD)	2	75.0	PD
Tetracyclines											
384	Chlortetracycline	Oral	2.0–3.0 (M)	8	9	4.13 (1–8)	?	1.25 (1–2)	?	30.0	
385	Tetracycline	Oral	0.5 (M)	5	10	1.84 (0.65–3.2)	0–6	1.14 (0.43–2.58)	0–6	62.0	
386	Doxycline	Oral	0.1 (M)	15	20	2.42 (1.3–4.50)	3	0.77 (0.4–1.40)	3	32.0	PD
Others											
387	Chloramphenicol	Oral	0.5 (S)	4	1.9	5.33 (±0.39 SE)	2	3.24 (±0.88 SD)	2	61.0	PD
102	Clindamycin	Oral	0.15 (S)	23	2.4	2.4 (1.8–3.0)	2	0.7 (0.5–1.2)	2	29.0	
388	Clindamycin	Oral	0.15 (M)	5	2	<3.7 (<1–9.9)	6	<1.4 (<0.5–3.1)	6	38.0	
102	Erythromycin	Oral	0.5 (S)	23	1.4	4.3 (3.9–4.7)	1	1.2 (0.9–1.4)	4	28.0	PD
185	Lincomycin	Oral	0.5 (M)	9	4.5	1.4 (0.4–3.2)	6	1.3 (0.5–2.4)	6	93.0	
389	Metronidazole	Oral	0.2 (M)	11	6–14	5.0 (1.0–11.6)	0–4.5	5.7 (1.6–12.2)	0.3–4.5	99.0	
390	Nitrofurantoin	Oral	0.2 (M)	4	0.3	0.83 (0.2–1.6)	2	0.2 (0–0.5)	2	24.0	
391	Rosaramicin	Oral	0.25 (S)	10	4.4	0.28 (0.165–0.485)	2–4	0.03 (0.028–0.045)	2–4	11.0	PD
387	Thiamphenicol	Oral	0.5 (S)	7	2.0	3.64 (±1.76 SD)	2	2.16 (±1.04 SD)	4	59.0	
392	Tinidazole	IV	0.5 (S)	20	14.0	6.1 (±0.32 SE)	12	5.8 (±0.33 SE)	12	95.0	PD

[a]IM, intramuscularly; IV, intravenously.
[b]S, single dose; M, multiple dose; BID, twice a day.
[c]PD, peak data.
[d]Cis-isomer of cefprozil

Table 14.10

Antimicrobial Concentrations in Middle Ear Fluid

Reference	Antimicrobial	Administration Method[a]	Dose (g) (Multiple or Single)[b]	n[c]	Serum Half-life (h)	Serum Concentration Mean (μg/mL) (Range)	Time Serum Obtained (h)	Site Concentration Mean (μg/mL) (Range)	Time Site Specimen Obtained (h)	Ratio of Site/Serum (%)	Notes[d]
Cephalosporins and related β-lactams											
393	Cefaclor	Oral	20 mg/kg (S)	15	0.7	12.3 (±7.3 SD)	1.5–1.9	2.9 (±1.5 SD)	1.5–1.9	22.0	P, NS
394	Cefatrizine	Oral	0.5 (S)	3	1.7	6.2 (5.0–7.2)	3	9.5 (8.2–10.5)	3	153.0	I
395	Cefixime	Oral	8 mg/kg (S)	16	2.4–4	2.51 (1.2–4.12)	3–5	1.32 (0.35–2.86)	3–5	52.5	I
395	Cefixime	Oral	8 mg/kg (S)	9	2.4–4	4.21 (2.48–10.7)	3–5	1.51 (0.32–5.69)	3–5	32.5	U
396	Cefotaxime	IV	25 mg/kg (S)	5	1.2	2.1 (2–2.2)	1.0	2.6 (2.0–3.3)	1.0	123.0	P
397	Cefprozil	Oral	20 mg/kg (S)	40	0.9–1.5	9.56 (1.28–21.47)	0.4–6	1.69 (0.17–8.67)	0.4–6	18.0	P
398	Cefprozil	Oral	15 mg/kg (M)	22	0.98	9.18	1.5	2.4	3.5	26.1437	PD
399	Loracarbef	Oral	7.5 mg/kg (S)	12	1	4.2 (±2.0 SD)	1.3–3.3	2.0 (±2.6 SD)	1.3–3.3	48.0	P
Penicillins											
400	Amoxicillin	Oral	15 mg/kg (S)	12	1.0	4.0 (0.62–6.5)	0.5–3	1.8 (0.3–3.5)	0.5–3	45.0	I, P
401	Amoxicillin	Oral	15 mg/kg (S)	5	1.0	9.4 (±1.3 SD)	1.5–2	2.3 (±1.5 SD)	1.5–2	24.0	U, P
402	Ampicillin	Oral	10 mg/kg (S)	15	1.5	4.3 (1.0–9.0)	2	2.17 (0.85–8.0)	2	50.0	I, P
402	Ampicillin	Oral	10 mg/kg (S)	9	1.5	3.6 (1.1–6.6)	2	0.23 (0–0.39)	2	6.0	U, P
402	Azidocillin	Oral	15 mg/kg (S)	15	0.75	7.4 (1.7–27)	2	3.2 (0.58–14)	2	44.0	I, P
402	Azidocillin	Oral	15 mg/kg (S)	18	0.75	4.8 (1.2–12)	2	0.50 (0–1.60)	2	10.0	U, P
403	Penicillin G	IM	4 × 10^5 units (S)	83	0.5	3.6 (1.2–11.2)	1	1.3 (0–8.2)	1	35.0	I
403	Penicillin G	IM	4 × 10^5 units (S)	13	0.5	3.2 (1.6–7.1)	1	0–trace	1	0.0	U
404	Penicillin V	Oral	26 mg/kg (S)	6	0.5	13 (8–20)	1.0	6.0 (5–8)	1.0	46.0	I, PD

Tetracyclines

Ref	Drug	Route	Dose	n						
405	Doxycycline	Oral	0.2 (S)	10	18.5	2.4 (1.0–3.4)	2.3–4.3	1.0 (0–1.7)	2.3–4.3	42.0	
406	Oxytetracycline	IM	0.1 (S)	10	8	2.1 (0.6–7.0)	1–3	0.7 (0.125–1.8)	1–3	33.0	I, P
406	Oxytetracycline	IM	0.1 (S)	4	8	0.74 (0.35–1.3)	1.5–2.8	<0.1	1.5–2.8	<14.0	U
Others											
400	Erythromycin estolate	Oral	15 mg/kg (S)	13	1.5	3.54 (0.6–4.5)	0.5–2	1.66 (0.4–4.0)	0.5–2	47.0	I, P
400	Erythromycin ethylsuccinate	Oral	15 mg/kg (S)	6	1.5	1.55 (0.5–2.6)	1–2	0.6 (0.4–1.0)	1–2	39.0	I, P
407	Metronidazole	Oral	2.4 (S)	12	10	45.2 (±8.3 SD)	2–4	31.8 (±25.65 SD)	2–4	70.0	I
408	Sulfadiazine	Oral	5 mg/kg (M)	24	10–12	18.4 (9.0–30.0)	1.3–4.5	10.5 (0–25)	1.3–4.5	57.0	NS, C
401	Sulfamethoxazole	Oral	20 mg/kg (S)	5	10	62.4 (±15.5)	1.5–2	17.0 (±6.7)	1.5–2	27.0	U, P, C
401	Sulfisoxazole	Oral	37.5 mg/kg (S)	5	5–7	87.4 (±35.2)	1.5–2	3.7 (±0.7)	1.5–2	4.0	U, P, C
401	Trimethoprim	Oral	4 mg/kg (S)	5	10–12	1.6 (±1.1)	1.5–2	1.9 (±1.4)	1.5–2	119.0	U, P, C
400	Trisulfapyrimidine	Oral	80 mg/kg (S)	7	3–4	13.6 (5.5–24)	0.5–1.2	8.1 (4–12)	0.5–1.2	60.0	I, P

[a] IV, intravenously; IM, intramuscularly.
[b] S, single dose; M, multiple dose.
[c] Number of patients studied.
[d] P, pediatric cases; NS, number of site samples is different than number of serum samples; I, infected; U, uninfected; PD, peak data; C, given in combination with another antibiotic.

Table 14.11

Antimicrobial Concentrations in Sinus Secretions

Reference	Antimicrobial	Administration Method[a]	Dose (g) (Multiple or Single)[b]	n	Serum Half-life (h)	Serum Concentration Mean (μg/mL) (Range)	Time Serum Obtained (h)	Site Concentration Mean (μg/mL) (Range)	Time Site Specimen Obtained (h)	Ratio of Site/Serum (%)	Notes[c]
Cephalosporins and related β-lactams											
394	Cefatrizine	Oral	0.5 (S)	3	1.4	6.0 (5.8–6.2)	3	2.7 (2.1–3.1)	3	45	AC
409	Cefotiam nexetil	Oral	0.2 (M)	8		0.96 (0.5–1.65)	2	1.04 (0.1–1.45)	2	108	CH
410	Cephalexin	Oral	0.5 or 15 mg/kg	9	0.8	8.8 (1.9–19)	2.0	1.1 (<0.1–4.0)	2.0	10	
411	Loracarbef	Oral	0.4 (M)	20	0.7–1.2	7.9 (4.83–14.0)	2	1.75 (0–5.71)	2		AC
Penicillins											
412	Ampicillin	Oral	0.5 (M)	4	1.1	3.8 (1.8–8.0)	2–3	0.125 (0–0.3)	2–3	3	
413	Azidocillin	IM	0.75 (M)	15	0.75	4.0	2.5	0.70 (0.16–1.82)	2.5	17.5	CH
413	Azidocillin	IM	1.5 (M)	8	0.75	8.5	2.5	0.34 (0.16–0.8)	2.5	4	
103	Penicillin V	Oral	0.4 0.4 0.8	17	0.5	2.1 (0–2.4)	2.1	<0.6 (<0.2–1.2)	2.1	<29	AC
104	Penicillin V	Oral	0.4 0.4 0.8	7	0.5	1.0 (0.4–2.4)	2	<2 (0.2–0.5)	2	<20	P
104	Penicillin V	Oral	0.4 0.4 0.8	10	0.5	1.0 (<0.1–2.0)	2	0.5 (<0.2–1.2)	2.1	50	M
414	Sultamicillin	Oral	0.75 (S)	3		3.09 (0.67–5.2) (ampicillin)/3.12 (0.57–4.6) (sulbactam)	1.5–2 1.5–2	0.32 (0.1–0.65) (ampicillin)/0.26 (0.2–0.53) (sulbactam)	1.5–2 1.5–2	10 8	AC AC

Quinolones											
415	Enoxacin	Oral	0.4 (S)	5	5.5	1.3 (1.0–2.1)	5	1.4 (0.6–2.7)	5	108	AC
Tetracyclines											
416	Doxycycline	Oral	0.1 (M)	24	20	3.5 (1.2–6.0)	2–7	2.0 (0.5–7.5)	2–7	57	
417	Minocycline	Oral	1.0 (M)	8	14	2.5 (0.5–5.1)	2–7	1.06 (0.05–3)	2–7	34	AC, CH
104	Tetracycline HCl	Oral	0.25 (M)	21	10	2.4 (0.9–6.0)	2.1	1.9 (0.5–3.6)	2.1	79	P
104	Tetracycline HCl	Oral	0.25 (M)	14	10	2.9 (1.4–4.8)	2.0	3.0 (1.0–7.0)	2.0	103	M
Others											
418	Azithromycin	Oral	0.5 (M)	3		0.28 (±0.11)	2.5	1.87 (±1.08)	96	468	AC
419	Erythromycin stearate	Oral	0.5 (M)	10	1.5	2.2 (0.3–5.0)	4.7	1.3 (0.3–2.5)	4.7	59	AC
420	Erythromycin stearate	Oral	0.5 (M)	13	1.5	2.2 (0.2–5.0)	2–3	0.9 (0.1–3.0)	2–3	42	CH
421	Sulfadiazine	Oral	0.5 (M)	10	3.5	42 (24–66)	2–4	6.6 (2.3–15)	2–4	20	AC
421	Trimethoprim	Oral	0.16 (M)	10	9.0	3.0 (2.1–5.6)	2–4	3.9 (1.1–10.8)	2–4	133	AC

[a]IM, intramuscularly.
[b]S, single dose; M, multiple dose.
[c]AC, acute sinusitis; CH, chronic sinusitis; P, purulent; M, mucous.

Prostatic Secretions

There are only a limited number of human studies detailing antibiotic concentrations in human prostatic secretions (Table 14.12). Winningham et al. (106) have determined in a dog model, in which urinary contamination has been excluded, that the major factors controlling antibiotic penetration into the prostatic fluid are the degree of lipid solubility, the pK_a, and the amount of protein binding. Using the dog model, Madsen et al. (107), Meares (108,109), and Gasser et al. (110) have determined that only trimethoprim, erythromycin, rosamicin, oleandomycin, clindamycin, enoxacin, and fleroxacin concentrate into prostatic fluid. The dog model may not necessarily reflect the situation in humans, however, because prostatic secretions in humans with prostatitis are more alkaline than the secretion found in normal dogs (59,111). One study suggested that prostatic fluid concentrations of cephalosporins are increased in patients with acute prostatitis, compared with uninfected controls (112). The higher pH found in humans may favor the penetration of some quinolones that are zwitterions (110). The degree of antibiotic penetration into prostatic fluid may be more important than prostatic tissue concentration because bacteria that cause chronic bacterial prostatitis reside within the prostatic fluid, and the prostatic epithelium acts as a barrier to the passage of most antibiotics into the fluid (113). When prostatic fluid drug levels in normal patients were compared with levels in a patient with ureterosigmoidostomy, it was found that the drug concentrations of nitrofurantoin and ampicillin found in normal patients were almost entirely due to urinary contamination (114,115). One group measured iohexol in the prostatic fluid after intravenous injection to exclude urinary contamination (116–118). Clinical data have revealed that trimethoprim is only partially effective in the treatment of chronic bacterial prostatitis. Quinolones may be of some benefit in the treatment of chronic bacterial prostatitis, but long-term follow-up has often been inadequate (119).

Cerebrospinal Fluid

Table 14.13 lists antimicrobial studies investigating the penetration of various agents into human CSF. There have been several reviews on the same topic that also dealt with the kinetics of central nervous system handling of drugs (120,121). There was no correction for blood contamination in these studies, and the results demonstrated considerable variability in the ratios of antimicrobial concentrations in CSF and serum. Many studies, typified by that of Mullaney and John (122), provide useful information on CSF levels of drugs such as cefotaxime, but make evaluation of drug penetration impossible by not presenting data on concentrations in serum. Similarly, data for ampicillin (123), nafcillin (124), and rifampin (125) are available but include small numbers of patients or lack actual drug levels. The CSF-to-serum ratio ranged from 0% for rifampin in uninfected controls (126) and 0% for low-dose oxytetracycline (127) to 199% for amoxicillin when measured 4 hours after a single intravenous dose (128). In general, because samples were taken at longer time intervals following the systemic drug administration, serum levels were lower in relation to CSF concentrations and the CSF-to-serum ratios increased. Data for several antimicrobials are included in detail to illustrate changes in CSF concentrations with time after administration, duration of meningitis, and multiple dosing (128–130).

Aqueous Humor

In almost all studies, the antibiotic levels in aqueous humor were measured in uninfected patients undergoing cataract surgery (Table 14.14). Under those conditions, most antibiotics penetrated poorly into the aqueous humor when given systemically, resulting in levels that are inadequate for treating endophthalmitis. Data are limited on penetration of antibiotics into infected eyes. One study examined doxycycline levels in acutely inflamed eyes and found levels similar to those in uninflamed eyes (131). Animal studies of bacterial endopthalmitis have shown enhanced penetration into the aqueous and vitreous humors of infected eyes with some antibiotics (132,133).

Skeletal Muscle

The majority of studies measuring antibiotic concentrations in skeletal muscle were done on uninfected normal muscle obtained during surgical procedures (Table 14.15). One study measured drug concentrations in the muscle of a decubitus ulcer (134). The higher concentrations observed for clindamycin and ciprofloxacin (compared with β-lactams) probably reflect the higher intracellular concentrations of lincosamides and quinolones (135). Newer studies have used microdialysis techniques, which distinguishes whole tissue from interstitial fluid concentrations within muscle (136,137).

(continued on page 729)

Table 14.12

Antimicrobial Concentrations in Prostatic Secretions

Reference	Antimicrobial	Administration Method[a]	Dose (g) (Multiple or Single)[b]	n	Serum Half-life (h)	Serum Concentration Mean (μg/mL) (Range)	Time Serum Obtained (h)	Site Concentration Mean (μg/mL) (Range)	Time Site Specimen Obtained (h)	Ratio of Site/Serum (%)	Notes[c]
Aminoglycosides											
422	Amikacin	IM	0.20 (S)	10	2–3	12.44 (9.4–18.5)	2.5–3	3.18 (1.24–5.20)	2.5–3	25	U
423	Tobramycin	IM	0.080 (S)	3	2.5	4.0 (4.0–4.0)	1	<0.5	1	<12	U
Cephalosporins and related β-lactams											
112	Cefmenoxime	IV	2.0 (S)	11		39.5 ± 11.7	1	12.8 (2.6–30.8)	1	32	I
				18		52.8 ± 18.0	1	0.7 (0–2.3)	1	2	U
117	Cefpodoxime	Oral	0.2 (S)	3		1.39 (0.3–1.94)	3	0.15 (0–0.42)	3	11	U, UCE
112	Moxalactam	IV	2.0 (S)	11	2.3	84.6 ± 24.1	1	14.0 (1.3–529)	1	17	I
				12		100 ± 20.5	1	1.2 (0.4–2.2)	1	1	U
424	Moxalactam	IV	1.0 (S)	5	2.3	44.6 (26.3–57.9)	1	1.59 (0.33–4.52)	1	4	I
Penicillins											
115	Ampicillin	Oral	0.5 (M)	7	1.5	4.1 (2.9–5.9)	2	4.7 (0.5–10.6)	2	115	U
				9	1.5			17.6 (1.2–61.4)	2	429	I
422	Piperacillin	IV	1.0 (S)	9	1.3	5.7 (2.0–12.8)	2.5–3	0.30 (0.16–0.78)	2.5–3	5	U
Tetracyclines											
425	Minocycline	Oral	0.2 (S)	5	14	1.19 (±0.21)	3	2.95 (±1.29)	3	251	I
		IV	0.2 (S)	3	14	1.61 (±0.7)	3	2.6 (±1.66)	3	161	U
426	Tetracycline	IV	0.5 (S)	4	10	6.25 (5.0–10)	1	0.664 (0.156–1.25)	1	11	U

(Continued)

Table 14.12 (Continued)
Antimicrobial Concentrations in Prostatic Secretions

Reference	Antimicrobial	Administration Method[a]	Dose (g) (Multiple or Single)[b]	n	Serum Half-life (h)	Serum Concentration Mean (µg/mL) (Range)	Time Serum Obtained (h)	Site Concentration Mean (µg/mL) (Range)	Time Site Specimen Obtained (h)	Ratio of Site/Serum (%)	Notes[c]
Quinolones											
427	Ciprofloxacin	Oral	0.5 (S)	7	4.3	1.44 (0.27–2.48)	2.4	2.2 (0.02–5.5)	2–4.4	154	U
428	Ciprofloxacin	Oral	0.25 (S)	7	4.6	0.53	3	0.14 (0–0.40)	3	0.25	U
116	Enoxacin	IV	0.428 (S)	9	4.5	1.26 (1.1–1.71)	2–4	0.57 (0.29–0.96)	2–4	47	U, UCE
429	Fleroxacin	Oral	0.4 (S)	9	12	3.63 (0.44–5.54)	1–4	1.81 (0.53–4.15)	1–4	50	U
430	Gatifloxacin	Oral	0.4 (S)	7	7.2	1.92 (1.53–2.46)	4	2.35 (2.03–3.10)	4	110	U, UCE
428	Levofloxacin	Oral	0.25 (S)	8	5.6	1.7	3	0.84 (0.67–1.50)	3	51	U
116	Lomefloxacin	Oral	0.4 (S)	5	8	1.81 (1.39–3.0)	4	1.38 (0.6–3.06)	4	48	U, UCE
431	Moxifloxacin	Oral	0.4 (S)	8	3.5	2.38 (±0.30)	3.5	3.79 (±1.24)	3.5	160	U, UCE
116	Norfloxacin	Oral	0.8 (S)	8	3.5	1.4 (0.69–2.71)	1–4	0.14 (0.08–0.43)	1–4	12	U, UCE
118	Ofloxacin	IV	0.4 (S)	5	6	2.0 (1.93–2.01)	4	0.66 (0.11–1.31)	4	33	U, UCE
116	Temafloxacin	Oral	0.4 (S)	4	9	2.23 (1.7–2.65)	4	0.78 (0.56–0.92)	4	36	U, UCE
Others											
426	Bacitracin	IV	0.5 (S)	3		0.104 (0.078–1.56)	1	0.104 (<0.039–1.56)	1	100	U
432	Trimethoprim	Oral	0.005–0.0081/kg (M)	4	14.5	3.1 (2.5–3.7)	9–12	4.2 (2.4–5.6)	9–12	155	

[a]IM, intramuscularly; IV, intravenously.
[b]S, single dose; M, multiple dose.
[c]U, uninfected; I, infected; UCE, urine contamination excluded.

Table 14.13

Antimicrobial Concentrations in Cerebrospinal Fluid

Reference	Antimicrobial	Administration Method[a]	Dose (g) (Multiple or Single)[b]	n	Serum Half-life (h)	Serum Concentration Mean (µg/mL) (Range)	Time Serum Obtained (h)	Site Concentration Mean (µg/mL) (Range)	Time Site Specimen Obtained (h)	Ratio of Site/Serum (%)	Notes[c]
Aminoglycosides											
433	Amikacin	IV	7.5 mg/kg (M)	5	2.2 ± 1.1	15 (11–18)	2.0	52. (3.8–6.9)	2.0	34.7	I
434	Gentamicin	IM	1.5 mg/kg (S)	16	2.0	1.4 (0.8–3.0)	2.0	0.03 (0–0.10)	2.0	2.5	I
435	Kanamycin	IM	7.5 mg/kg (M)	4	2.0	13	2.0	3.2	2.0	25	I
Cephalosporins and related β-lactams											
436	Aztreonam	IV	2 (S)	6	1.9	44.7 (29.9–74.2)	2.0	2.98 (0.76–6.67)	2.0	6.7	I
437	Cefamandole	IV	125 mg/kg (M)	20	0.7	10–20	1.0–2.0	0.94 (0–3.4)	1.0–2.0	6.5 (0–19)	I
438	Cefazolin	IV	6.0/day (M)	4	2.0	29.1 (±5.2)	3.0	0	3.0	0	U
438	Cefazolin	IV	6.0/day (M)	4	2.0	52.6 (±6.5)	6	0	6	0	CI, U
439	Cefixime	IV	8 mg/kg (S)	10	2.6–5.6	2.9 (0.3–4.7)	1–8	0.2	1–5	12	I
129	Cefmenoxime	IV	6.0 (S)	5	1.4	25.09 (15.88–49.22)	1	2.10 (0.43–4.4)	1	8.4	I, CI
129	Cefmenoxime	IV	6.0 (S)	5	1.4	11.71 (7.94–15.88)	2	1.69 (0.65–4.5)	2	14.4	I, CI
129	Cefmenoxime	IV	6.0 (S)	5	1.4	9.08 (0.82–16.12)	4	4.99 (0.52–15)	4	55	I, CI
129	Cefmenoxime	IV	6.0 (S)	5	1.4	2.52 (1.84–4.37)	8	4.28 (0.8–7.7)	8	170	I, CI
440	Cefoperazone	IV	50 mg/kg (S)	6	1.9	85 (60–130)	1.25–3.25	1.53 (<0.8–5.2)	1.25–3.25	1.8	I
441	Cefotaxime	IV	0.15–3.0/day (M)	11	1.2	17 (2.2–42.8)	2.0	8.7 (8.2–27.2)	2.0	51	I

(Continued)

Table 14.13 (Continued)

Antimicrobial Concentrations in Cerebrospinal Fluid

Reference	Antimicrobial	Administration Method[a]	Dose (g) (Multiple or Single)[b]	n	Serum Half-life (h)	Serum Concentration Mean (μg/mL) (Range)	Time Serum Obtained (h)	Site Concentration Mean (μg/mL) (Range)	Time Site Specimen Obtained (h)	Ratio of Site/Serum (%)	Notes[c]
442	Cefotaxime	IV	40 mg/kg (M)	14	1.2	6.6 (1.7–13.6)	14	1.2 (0.63–3.1)	14	18	I, TD 14
129	Cefoxitin	IV	2.0 (M)	17	0.8	9	1.0–2.0	4.7 (±3.0)	1.0–2.0	52	I
443	Cefpirome	IV	2.0 (S)	9	2.0	20.5 (10.2–43)	4	4.2 (0.5–7.5)	4	20	I
444	Cefsulodin	IV	2.0 (M)	3	1.5	2.97 (1.5 4.4)	6.25–6.67	2.11 (1.31–3.1)	6.25–6.67	71	I
445	Ceftazidime	IV	2.0 (M)	5	1.85	28.2 (21–40)	3.0	7.2 (3–21)	2.0	23.5	I, TD 11–20
446	Ceftriaxone	IV	100 mg/kg/day (M)	15	4.0	128.2 (±44.2 SE)	2.0	11.0 (±3.1 SE)	2.0	8.6	I
447	Ceftizoxime	IV	30 mg/kg (S)	12	1.51	22.9 (8.3–60.8)	1.6–3.6	4.9 (0–17.0)	1.6–3.6	21	I
448	Ceftizoxime	IV	200 mg/kg/day (M)	4	1.7	26 (16–50)	3	7.25 (3.6–13)	3	27.9	I, TD 1–14
449	Cefuroxime	IV	3 (M)	9	1.4	5.2 (0.3–21.7)	6.0–8.5	5.6 (0.25–19.8)	6.0–8.5	108	I
450	Cephaloridine	IM	1.0 (S/M)	18	1.5	11.8 (5.9–19.6)	2.0–4.0	0.03 (0–0.26)	2.0–4.0	0.3	I
442	Cephalothin	IV	4.0 (S)	4	0.5	34.0	1.0	"Very low"	1.0	<0.1	U
442	Cephradine	IV	4.0 (S)	14	0.7	136.5	1.0	≤1.5	1.0	≤1	U
451	Imipenem	IV	1.0 (S)	4/10		20.0 (12–41)	1.0–2.0	1.7 (0.65–3.4)	2.0–6.0	8.5	I
451	Cilastatin	IV	1.0 (S)	4/10		19	1.0–2.0	0.9	2.0–6.0	4.7	I
452	Meropenem	IV	40 mg/kg (S)	6	1.0	13.3 (5.7–32)	2–3	2.8 (0.3–6.5)	1–4	21	I
Penicillins											
453	Amoxicillin	IV	1.0 (M)	7	1.1	20.0 (±10.0)	1.0	2.0 (±1.4)	1.0	10	1, TD 8–12
335	Ampicillin	IV	15 mg/kg (S)	11	1.1	8.8 (3.2–23.8)	1.0–2.0	0.3 (0–0.9)	1.0–2.0	3.4	I

#	Drug	Route	Dose								Notes
454	Methicillin	IM	2.0 (M)	3	0.5	50 (27.5–90)	1.0	3.6 (0.78–10.8)	1.0	7	I, P
455	Nafcillin	IV	50 mg/kg (M)	7	1.5–3.2	123.0	0.08–0.5	4.5	2.0–3.0	3.7	I
456	Nafcillin	IV	169–200 mg/kg/day (M)	3	1.0	229 (36–615)	1.0–2.0	33 (2.7–88)	1.0–2.0	14	I
457	Penicillin G	IV	2.5×10^5 units/day (M)	6	0.5	9.5	2.0	0.8	2.0	8	I, TD 5
458	Piperacillin	IV	324–436 mg/kg/day (M)	4	1.1	79 (21–121)	1–10 days	23 (4–35)	1–10	29	I, CI
459	Procaine penicillin	IM	0.6 (M)	10		1.04 (0.49–1.92)	2–3	0.002 (0–0.01)	2–3	0.19	I, TD 14–21
460	Sulbactam	IV	1.0 (S)	7	1	13.0 (5–29)	1.5–7	4.16 (0.65–12)	1.5	32	I
461	Temocillin	IV	2 (S)	4	4.5	86.2 (64.8–113.8)	2	10.15 (<0.5–21.9)	2	11.8	I, TD 1
Quinolones											
462	Ciprofloxacin	IV	0.2 (M)	7	4.0	1.59 (0.85–2.95)	1	0.39 (0.11–0.68)	1	25	I
				5	4.0	1.44 (0.83–2.60)	2	0.56 (0.23–1.20)	2	39	I
				6	4.0	0.24 (0.90–0.40)	8	0.35 (0.07–0.61)	8	146	I
462	Ciprofloxacin	Oral	0.5 (S)	8	4.0	2.41 (±0.8)	2	0.06 (±0.03)	2	3	U
				6	4.0	0.77 (±0.22)	4	0.14 (±0.07)	4	18	U
				7	4.0	0.45 (±0.24)	8	0.08 (±0.02)	8	18	U
463	Moxifloxacin	Oral	0.4 (S)	10	12.7	6.55 ± 3.61	2–4	3.00 ± 1.84	2–4	46	U
462	Ofloxacin	Oral	0.2 (M)	11	7.0	3.1 (0.5–7.75)	1.5	1.3 (0.32–3.60)	1.5	42	I, U, E
				6	7.0	1.16 (0.5–2.3)	12	0.83 (0.49–135)	12	72	I, U, E
462	Pefloxacin	IV	0.5 (M)	6	10.5	10.3 (6.2–16)	1	4.8 (2.40–9.00)	2	47	I
Others											
464	Chloramphenicol	IV	100 mg/kg/day (M)	11	2.5	15.2 (4.2–29.0)	3.0	5.7 (2.0–15.6)	3.0	38	I, TD 10
465	Daptomycin	IV	10 mg/kg (S)	11	8.6	43.3 ± 13.5	6	0.461 ± 0.51	6	1.5	

(Continued)

Table 14.13 (Continued)

Antimicrobial Concentrations in Cerebrospinal Fluid

Reference	Antimicrobial	Administration Method[a]	Dose (g) (Multiple or Single)[b]	n	Serum Half-life (h)	Serum Concentration Mean (μg/mL) (Range)	Time Serum Obtained (h)	Site Concentration Mean (μg/mL) (Range)	Time Site Specimen Obtained (h)	Ratio of Site/ Serum (%)	Notes[c]
466	Dimethylchlor-tetracycline	Oral	1.0 (S)	8	9	3.3 (1.7–7.5)	4.0	0.19 (0.17–0.21)	4.0	5.8	U
467	Doxycycline	Oral	400 mg/day (M)	5		5.8 (3.6–8.6)	4–6	1.3 (0.8–2.0)	4–6	22.4	I
468	Doxycycline	Oral	400 mg/day (M)	10	21	7.5 (4.3–12)	2–3	1.1 (0.6–1.9)	2–3	14.7	I, TD 5–8
469	Lincomycin	IM	20 mg/kg (S)	10	4.5	7.4 (2.3–23.8)	2.0	0.5 (0.14–1.6)	2.0	6.8	I
470	Linezolid	IV	0.6 (S)	9	5.0	6.83 ± 3.32	2	5.06 ± 3.53	2	74	U
471	Metronidazole	Oral	2.4 (S)	4	8.0	33.7	1.5	14.5 (6.0–22.7)	1.5	43	U
17	Oxytetracycline	IM	59–100 mg/kg/day (M)	7	8	34.3 (0–80)	24	2.3 (0–5)	24	6.7	I
126	Rifampin	Oral	25 mg/kg (S)	5	3.0	6.8 (4.4–9.3)	3.0	0.27 (0.23–0.33)	3.0	4	I
472	Sulfamethoxazole	IV	25 mg/kg (S)	4	1.0	82.5 (50–150)	1.75–3.0	33 (28–40)	1.75–3.0	40	U
228	Tigecycline	IV	0.1 (S)	6		0.062 ± 0.018	24	0.025 ± 0.005	24	11	U, AUC
471	Tinidazole	Oral	2.0 (S)	4		35.2	1.5	31 (17.0–39.0)	1.5	88	U
472	Trimethoprim	IV	5 mg/kg (S)	4	8–10	3.7 (3.0–4.1)	1.75–3.0	≤1.1 (≤0.5–1.5)	1.75–3.0	≤41	U
186	Vancomycin	IV	500 mg/kg (M)	9	6.0	6.3 (4.3–10.0)	1.0–2.5	0	1.0–2.5	0	U

[a]IV, intravenously; IM, intramuscularly.
[b]M, multiple dose; S, single dose.
[c]I, infected cerebrospinal fluid; U, uninfected; CI, continuous infusion; TD, treatment day; P, probenecid; E, extrapolated from graphs; AUC, area under the curve.

Table 14.14

Antimicrobial Concentrations in Aqueous Humor

Reference	Antimicrobial	Administration Method[a]	Dose (g) (Multiple or Single)[b]	n[c]	Serum Half-life (h)	Serum Concentration Mean (μg/mL) (Range)	Time Serum Obtained (h)	Site Concentration Mean (μg/mL) (Range)	Time Site Specimen Obtained (h)	Ratio of Site/Serum (%)	Notes[d]
Aminoglycosides											
313	Amikacin	IV	0.5 (S)	5	2	10.6 (±0.58 SE)	2.5	0	2.5	0.5	U
473	Amikacin	IM	7.5 mg/kg (S)	47	2.0	20.85 (5–40)	0.7–7.7	0.85 (0.04–3.1)	0.7–7.7	4.5	U
474	Gentamicin	IV	0.08 (S)	10	2	8.8 (±4.3 SD)	0.25	1.9 (±0.27 SD)	0.025	22.5	U
474	Gentamicin	IM	0.08 (S)	9	2	5.2 (±1.2 SD)	1	1.6 (±0.9 SD)	~1	27.5	U
475	Netilmicin	IM	1.5 mg/kg (S)	30	2	6.7	2	<1 (<1–1.4)	0–3.5	<15.5	U
476	Tobramycin	IV	0.08 (S)	6	2	4.9 (±0.5 SD)	1	1.6 (±0.5 SD)	1	32.5	U
477	Tobramycin	IM	0.08 (S)	9	2	4.07 (±2.28)	1	0.3 (±0.26)	1	7.4	U
Cephalosporins and related β-lactams											
478	Aztreonam	IV	2.0 (S)	5	1.3–2.2	90 (±28)	2	1.46 (±1.23)	2	2.5	U
479	Cefaclor	Oral	1.0 (S)	6	0.7	21.0 (7–34)	1–3	0.78 (0.09–1.56)	1–3	4.5	U
480	Cefadroxil	Oral	1.0 (S)	9	1.3	14.77	2	6.15	2	42.5	U
481	Cefamandole	IM	1.0 (S)	7	0.7	17.8 (7–34.4)	1–4.5	0	1–4.5	0.5	U
481	Cefamandole	IV	1.0 (S)	6	0.7	39.3 (31.5–64)	~1	0.59 (0–1.1)	~1	2.5	U
482	Cefazolin	IV	0.5 (S)	3	2.0	35 (32–39)	0.7	<0.6	0.7	<1.7	U
483	Cefepime	IV	1.0 (S) 2.0 (S)	3 3	2	41.67 (±7.93 SD) 78.34 (±8.66 SD)	1 1	4.87 (±0.06 SD) 5.70 (±1.30 SD)	1 1	11.7 7.3	U, HPC
484	Cefmenoxime	IV	2.0 (S)	4–5	1.1	67 (45–80)	2	3.19 (2.88–3.36)	2	5.5	U
485	Cefonicid	IV	1.0 (S)	7	4.4	89 (70–120)	1–2	0.23 (0.14–0.31)	1–2	0.3	U
486	Cefoperazone	IV	2.0 (M)	6	2	30.5 (16–55)	4–5	1.9 (0.4–3.4)	4–5	6.5	U
487	Cefotaxime	IV	1.0 (S)	17	1.2	58 (3–200)	1–2	0.95 (0.25–4.5)	1–2	2.5	U

(Continued)

Table 14.14 (Continued)

Antimicrobial Concentrations in Aqueous Humor

Reference	Antimicrobial	Administration Method[a]	Dose (g) (Multiple or Single)[b]	n[c]	Serum Half-life (h)	Serum Concentration Mean (µg/mL) (Range)	Time Serum Obtained (h)	Site Concentration Mean (µg/mL) (Range)	Time Site Specimen Obtained (h)	Ratio of Site/Serum (%)	Notes[d]
488	Cefoxitin	IV	2.0 (S)	5	0.8	48 (40–65)	~1	3.2 (3–3.4)	~1	7.5	U
488	Cefoxitin/probenecid	IV	2.0 (S)	4	?	79.4 (65–90)	~1	2.7 (2.2–3.2)	~1	3.5	U
489	Cefpirome	IV	2.0 (S)	7	?	57 (±23 SD)	2	2.25 (±0.75 SD)	2	3.9	U, E, HPC
490	Cefsulodin	IM	0.5 (S)	7	1.5	9.9 (±3.3)	1–1.5	0.36 (±0.38)	1–1.5	4.5	U
486	Cefsulodin	IV	2.0 (M)	6	1.5	31.8 (8–75)	3–5	5.0 (1.8–9.0)	3–5	16.5	U
491	Ceftazidime	IV	2.0 (S)	14	1.8	90.7 (53.2–137.5)	0.5–1	3.3 (2.0–4.5)	0.5–1	4.5	U
486	Ceftazidime	IM	1.0 (M)	5	1.8	21.8 (12–28)	3–5	2.6 (2.0–3.3)	3–5	12.5	U
492	Ceftizoxime	IV	2.0 (S)	6	1.7	48.9 (±21.5)	2	7.9 (±5.7)	2	16.5	U
493	Ceftriaxone	IV	2.0 (S)	10	5.8	198 (90–394)	1–8	1.16 (0.71–1.92)	1–8	1.5	
494	Cefuroxime	IV	2.0 (S)	5	1.3	14.6 (12.5–16.5)	1	1.46 (0.9–2.3)	1	10.5	U
494	Cefuroxime	IM	1.5 (S)	5	1.3	11.9 (8.0–15.5)	1	1.72 (1.0–2.2)	1	14.5	U
495	Cephalexin	Oral	0.5 (S)	10	0.8	17.8 (±3.4)	1	0.35 (±0.14)	1	2.5	U, S
495	Cephalexin/probenecid	Oral	1.0 (S)	13	?	50.0 (±4.7)	1	2.5 (±1.4)	1	5.5	U, NS
496	Cephaloridine	IM	1.0 (S)	6	1.5	28 (25–30)	2–4	1.9 (0.8–4.0)	2–4	7.5	U
497	Cephalothin	IV	1.0 (S)	18	0.5	12.9 (10–14)	0.5	0.48 (0–1.0)	0.5	4.5	U, S
498	Cephradine	Oral	0.5 (S)	8	0.7	9.13 (3.5–18)	0.5–3.4	0.45 (0–1.2)	0.5–3.4	5.5	U
499	Imipenem	IV	1.0 (S)	5	1	37.4 (13.5–56.5)	2	2.99 (2.40–3.90)	2	8.5	U
500	Meropenem	IV	2.0 (S)	5	1.2	46.11 (37.4–60.4)	0.5	13.39 (12.5–15.8)	0.5	29.0	U, V, HPC
486	Moxalactam	IV	2.0 (M)	5	2.3	26.1 (23–32)	3–5	4.1 (2.4–9.5)	3–5	16.5	U
501	Moxalactam	IV	2.0 (S)	15	2.3	105 (50–150)	0.5–2	1.26 (0.62–2.3)	0.5–2	1.5	U

Quinolones

462	Ciprofloxacin	Oral	1.0 (S)	12	4.0	5.7 (1.2–9.2)	1.4–3	0.44 (0.15–0.96)	2.0–3	8.5	U
462	Ciprofloxacin	Oral	0.75 (M)	6	4.0	3.6 (1.6–5.4)	1.4–1.6	0.61 (0.22–0.95)	1.4–1.6	17.5	U
462	Ciprofloxacin	IV	0.40 (S)	3	4.0	2.5 (0.9–3.8)	1.5–2.5	0.4 (0.28–0.59)	1.5–2.5	16.5	
502	Gatifloxacin	Oral	0.40 (M)	11	10.5	5.14 (±1.36 SD)	3.2 (±1.1 SD)	1.08 (±0.54 SD)	3.9 (±1.1 SD)	21.0	U, V, NS, HPC
503	Levofloxacin	i.v.	0.50 (S)	16	7	5.11 (±1.68 SD)	2.08–4.5	1.39 (±0.33 SD)	2.08–4.5	30	U, HPC
504	Moxifloxacin	Oral	0.40 (S)	25	12.4	1.34 (±0.98 SD)	2.02 ± 0.51	0.21 (±0.21 SD)	1.53 ± 0.45	15.6	U, V, HPC
505	Moxifloxacin	Oral	0.40 (M)	13	12.4	3.56 (±1.31 SD)	2.94 ± 0.81 SD	1.58 (±0.8 SD)	3.71 ± 0.89 SD	44.3	U, V, HPC
506	Ofloxacin	Oral	0.2 (S)	12	7.0	2.67 (±0.54 SD)	2	0.38 (±0.15 SD)	2	14.5	U
506	Ofloxacin	IV	0.2 (S)	6	7.0	2.49 (±1.31 SD)	2	0.33 (±0.19 SD)	2	13.5	U
462	Pefloxacin	IV	0.4 (S)	5	12.6	3.4 (2.9–3.5)	6	1.4 (1.20–1.75)	6	41.5	U, E, L
462	Pefloxacin	Oral	0.4 (S)	14	10.5	4.94	3.3	0.89	3.3	18.5	U, E

Penicillins

507	Azlocillin	IV	4.0 (S)	24	1	151 (±33)	<1	4.44 (±3.05)	<1	3.5	U, PD
508	Cloxacillin	IM	1–4 (S)	4	0.5	11.5	0.7–1.7	<1.0	1.2–1.6	<8.7	
491	Epicillin	IV	2.0 (S)	4	1.0	106 (80–136)	1–2	1.45 (1.09–1.75)	1–2	1.5	
509	Methicillin	IV	4.0 (C)	6	0.5	18.0	24	0	24	0.5	U
509	Methicillin/probenecid	IV	4.0 (C)	16	?	29.7	24	0	24	0.5	U
482	Methicillin	IV	2.0 (S)	5	0.5	76 (50–104)	0.4–1.2	<1.1 (<0.78–2.2)	0.4–1.2	<1.4	U
510	Mezlocillin	IV	4.0 (S)	4	1.1	180 (150–195)	1	4.4 (1.0–7.5)	1	2.5	U, E
482	Nafcillin	IV	2.0 (S)	5	1.0	97 (70–120)	0.5–0.8	<0.84 (<0.4–1.9)	0.5–0.8	<0.9	U
511	Oxacillin	IM	0.5 (M)	9	0.5	4.0	0–4	0	0–4	0.5	U
511	Oxacillin/probenecid	IM	0.5 (M)	10	0.5	5.70	0–4	0	0–4	0.5	U
493	Penicillin G	IV	10 × 10^6 units	4	0.5	121 (42–222)	2–5	2.94 (0.46–6.86)	2–5	2.5	
512	Piperacillin	IV	4.0 (S)	25	1.5	34	1–7	1.5	1–7	4.5	U, E

(Continued)

Table 14.14 (Continued)

Antimicrobial Concentrations in Aqueous Humor

Reference	Antimicrobial	Administration Method[a]	Dose (g) (Multiple or Single)[b]	n[c]	Serum Half-life (h)	Serum Concentration Mean (μg/mL) (Range)	Time Serum Obtained (h)	Site Concentration Mean (μg/mL) (Range)	Time Site Specimen Obtained (h)	Ratio of Site/Serum (%)	Notes[d]
Tetracyclines											
131	Doxycycline	Oral	0.1 (M)	10	21	3.56 (1.5–7.96)	4–4.5	0.34 (0.25–0.47)	4–4.5	10.5	U
131	Doxycycline	Oral	0.1 (M)	10	21	4.65 (2.07–7.90)	3.0–4.3	0.60 (0.23–1.45)	3–4.3	13.5	I
513	Minocycline	Oral	0.1 (M)	26	14	6.75 (±1.0)	1	1.15 (±0.05)	1	17.5	U
514	Tetracycline	Oral	3 (S)	3	10	26 (25–28)	3	2.9 (2.5–3.5)	3	11.5	U
514	Tetracycline	IV	7 mg/kg (M)	5	10	63 (34–98)	5	5.5 (3.4–8.6)	5	9.5	U
Macrolides											
515	Azithromycin	Oral	1.0 (S)	5	44	0.58 (±0.31 SD)	3	0.054 (±0.022 SD)	3	9.3	U, C, HPC
516	Clarithromycin	Oral	0.5 (S)	5	6	1.91 (±0.56 SD)	5.3	0.13 (±0.05 SD)	4.7	6.8	U, V, HPC
Others											
132	Fosfomycin	IV	4.0 (S)	8	2	75.2	2	18.8 (±3.4)	2	25.5	U
517	Lincomycin	IM	0.6 (M)	8	4.5	15.3 (10.2–23)	1–2	1.3 (1.0–2.0)	1–2	8.5	U
518	Linezolid	Oral	0.6 (S)	8	4–5	7.53 (± 2.7 SD)	3.57 ± 1.07 SD	3.85 (±1.1 SD)	3.65 ± 0.95 SD	51.1	U, V, HPC
518	Linezolid	Oral	0.6 (M)	7	4–5	10.3 (± 4.1 SD)	6.25 ± 3.70 SD	6.6 (±2.7 SD)	6.17 ± 3.67 SD	64.1	U, V, HPC
519	Metronidazole	IV	0.5 (S)	10	10	15.9 (±2.9 SE)	0.7–1.5	5.2 (±0.5 SE)	0.7–1.5	38.5	U
519	Tinidazole	IV	0.5 (S)	10	14	11.6 (±1.3 SE)	0.7–1.5	5.3 (±0.7 SE)	0.7–1.5	47.5	U
482	Vancomycin	IV	0.5 (S)	5	6	13.8 (11–17)	0.7–1.3	<0.78	0.7–1.3	<5.6	U
520	Vancomycin	IV	1.0 (M)	7	6	13.51 (±4.96 SD)	6	1.42 (±0.47 SD)	6	10.5	U

[a]IV, intravenously; IM, intramuscularly.

[b]S, single dose; M, multiple dose; C, continuous infusion.

[c]Number of subjects studied.

[d]U, uninfected; HPC, high-performance liquid chromatography; E, values extrapolated from graphs; S, secondary aqueous sampled; NS, number of site sample when different from number of serum samples; PD, peak data, I, infected; C, conjunctival concentrations measured also; L, lens concentration measured also; V, vitreous concentrations measured also.

Table 14.15

Antimicrobial Concentrations in Skeletal Muscle

Reference	Antimicrobial	Administration Method[a]	Dose (g) (Multiple or Single)[b]	n	Serum Half-life (h)	Serum Concentration Mean (µg/mL) (Range)	Time Serum Obtained (h)	Site Concentration Mean (µg/mL) (Range)	Time Site Specimen Obtained (h)	Ratio of Site/Serum (%)	Notes[c]
Aminoglycosides											
521	Amikacin	IM	7.5 mg/kg (S)	6	2.0	14.9 (7–19.3)	1.5	2.2 (0.8–4.5)	1.5	15	U, CH
134	Gentamicin	IM	0.08 (S)	~9	2.0	5.4 (3.6–7.3)	1.8–3.0	6.5 (<2.8)	1.8–3	111	U
188	Netilmicin	IV	0.0015/kg (S)	6	2.0	2.6 (±1.2)	2–3	0.8 (0–3.6)	2–3	31	U
Cephalosporins and related β-lactams											
189	Aztreonam	IV	2.0 (S)	6	1.7	108	0.25–0.68	16	0.25–0.68	20	U, C
522	Cefadroxil	Oral	1.0 (M)	12	1.3	20.7 (±2.9)	2	6.5 (±0.9)	2	31	U
134	Cefazolin	IM	1.0 (S)	~9	2.0	35 (7.3–82)	1.8–3.8	<6.0 (all)	1.8–3.8	<7–<82	U
523	Cefmenoxime	IV	2.0 (S)	41	1.0	52.4	1	12.96	0.75		U, MM
525	Cefotaxime	IV	2.0 (S)	11	1.0	81 (±10)	0–0.5	3.8 (±1.3)	0–0.5	5	U
255	Cefoxitin	IV	2.0 (S)	31	0.8	25	1.0	24	1.0	96	U, MM
525	Cefsulodin	IV	2.0 (S)	5	1.5	55.1 (50–90)	1.0	10.2 (5–40)	1.0	19	U
526	Ceftazidime	IV	2.0 (S)	35	1.8	36.5	2	9.4 (3–22)	2	25.8	U, C
527	Cetriaxone	IV	1.0 (S)	53	7.0	90.8	1.3	11.2	1.5		U, C
528	Cephradine	IM	2.0 (S)	10	0.7	119 (49–285)	0.41	21.5 (21–60)	1.5	18	U, P
528	Cephradine	IM	2.0 (S)	10	0.7	119 (49–285)	0.41	14.4 (0.5–26)	1.5	12	D
137	Ertapenem	IV	1.0 (S)S	3	3.77	103.3 (±26.3)	0.5	6.71 (±4.14)	1.5	13	U, MD, AUC
529	Imipenem	IV	1.0 (S)	10	0.9	47.2	0–1	2.5	0–1	5	U
Penicillins											
530	Dicloxacillin	IV	1 (S)	6	0.7	6	4	3 (2–4)	0.8	13	
531	Flucloxacillin	IV	2.0 (S)	20	0.7	125.2	0–1	14.2	0–1	11	U

(Continued)

TABLE 14.15 (Continued)

Antimicrobial Concentrations in Skeletal Muscle

Reference	Antimicrobial	Administration Method[a]	Dose (g) (Multiple or Single)[b]	n	Serum Half-life (h)	Serum Concentration Mean (µg/mL) (Range)	Time Serum Obtained (h)	Site Concentration Mean (µg/mL) (Range)	Time Site Specimen Obtained (h)	Ratio of Site/Serum (%)	Notes[c]
532	Mezlocillin	IV	5.0 (S)	10	0.99	100 (50–100)	1.5	26.4 (10–40)	1.5	26.4	U
533	Nafcillin	IV or IM	1.0 (S)	14	1.0	2.2 (0.3–10)	4.5	0.58	4.8	26	U
534	Oxacillin	IV	4.0 (S)	6	0.5	94.5 (44–117)	0.58	<2	0.58	<2	U, MM
535	Piperacillin	IV	5.0 (S)	14	1.1	95 (±25)	2.5	30 (±17)	2.5	32	I, C
536	Piperacillin	IV	2.0 (S)	30	1.1	16.4	1–2	8.1	1–2	49	U
537	Temocillin	IV	1.0	7	62.6	2.5–5.5	9.5 (<3.1–17.3)		2.5–5.5	27	U, C
538	Ticarcillin	IV	5.0 (S)	5	1.2	185 (118–242)	1.0–1.5	18 (9–44)	1.0–1.5	10	U
Tetracycline											
153	Tetracycline	Oral	0.5 (M)	5	10	3.7 (2.1–4.6)	3–4	1.9 (0–3.3)	3–4	50	U, C
Quinolones											
143	Ciprofloxacin	Oral	0.5 (S)	7	4.0	1.4 (0.4–2.0)	1.5–4.8	1.1 (0.5–1.9)	1.5–4.8	79	U, C
		Oral	0.75 (S)	7		2.6 (0.9–3.8)	1.5–4.8	1.3 (0.6–2.4)	1.5–4.8	50	U, C
Others											
539	Clindamycin	IV	5 mg/kg	11	2.0	4.9 (1.1–14)	0.8–1.9	6.1 (0–25)	0.5–2.6	124	U, CH
540	Linezolid	IV	0.6 (S)	12	4–5	15.8 (95% CI[d] 12.5–19.1)	0.33	13.4 (95% CI[d] 10.2–16.5)	0.33	94.3	U
541	Teicoplanin	IV	12 mg/kg	9		27.5 (±20.3)	1–2	6.7 (±8.8)	1–2	27	U
136	Telithromycin	Oral	0.8	10	8.6	1.73 (0.94–2.89)	2.8	0.13 (0.04–0.29)	4	27	U, AUC, MD
542	Vancomycin	IV	0.15 mg	5	6.0	14.2	1–2	3.2	1–2	23	U

[a]IM, intramuscularly; IV, intravenously.
[b]S, single dose; M, multiple dose.
[c]U, uninfected; CH, children; C, corrected; MM, blood contamination measured as minimal; P, proximal muscle; D, distal muscle; MD, microdialysis; AUC, area under curve data
[d]Confidence interval.

Bone

A multitude of studies on antibiotic penetration into bone have been published (Table 14.16). Most of the studies were performed on uninfected bone, following antibiotics given prophylactically to patients prior to orthopedic procedures. There is a wide variance in technique, making the results conflicting and difficult to interpret. The majority of studies reported techniques that cut or crushed the bone, suspended the material in a buffer for a variable amount of time, and then measured the antibiotic extracted into the buffer, using a microbiologic assay. Newer studies used microdialysis techniques measuring interstitial fluid concentrations within bone. Many investigators washed or rinsed the bone to remove blood after removing the sample. It is unknown whether this could also remove some of the antibiotic.

The buffer/bone mixture is usually shaken at 4°C to 6°C for 1 to 24 hours. An 8-hour shake/elution technique has resulted in 79.9% recovery of cefazolin and 77% recovery of cephradine, but only 10.8% recovery of cephalothin (138). Schurman et al. (139) found that when the extraction procedure was performed for more than 3 to 5 hours, the recovery of cephalothin, but not cefamandole, declined by 67% at 24 hours. Rosdahl et al. (140) added several antibiotics to cancellous and cortical bone specimens and then homogenized the specimens before microbiologic assay. Recovery of the antibiotic ranged from 4% to 100%. The fall in antibiotic concentration was primarily due to the instability of the antibiotics during the homogenization procedures and was not due to binding of the antibiotic to bone. Adam et al. (141) found that neither ticarcillin nor clavulanate was adsorbed to inorganic bone; however, Wittmann and Kotthaus (142) found that the hydroxyapatite portion of bone acts as a depot carrier for several quinolone antibiotics. Other investigators have found that the quinolones bind to bone samples (143) and require several extraction steps for full extraction of the antibiotic from the bone (142).

Numerous studies noted differences between cortical and cancellous bone antibiotic concentrations, with the cortical bone usually having lower drug levels. This may reflect the fact that many antibiotics do not bind to inorganic bone, or it may be due to a difference in the blood supply. Fitzgerald (144), using data compiled from animal models, concluded that there is no anatomic or physiologic barrier preventing antibiotic diffusion into bone. He concluded that, at least in the case of β-lactams and aminoglycosides, the osseous interstitial fluid concentration of an antibiotic was a reflection of the serum concentration. This agrees with the results of Williams et al. (145), who thought that, although the relationship was not clear-cut, antibiotics with high serum levels and long half-lives usually had higher bone concentrations. Hughes and Anderson (146) thought that the capillary blood supply to the bone was of critical importance in delivering the antibiotic to the bone. In one study in which necrotic bone was sampled, cefamandole concentration was usually not detectable (147). We are not aware of any conclusive studies that attempt to correlate clinical outcome with the degree of antibiotic bone penetration, either in treating osteomyelitis or in preventing postoperative infection.

Cardiac Tissue

Antibiotic levels in cardiac tissue were measured in atrial appendage, valve, or heart muscle (Table 14.17). Virtually all studies were done in uninfected hearts. Study patients received a dose of antibiotic prior to undergoing valve replacements, coronary artery bypass grafting, or repair of congenital heart abnormalities. The cephalosporins were most widely studied and showed moderate penetration into cardiac tissue, with cephalothin and cefonicid having the lowest site-to-serum ratios. Particularly high penetration into cardiac tissue was noted for clindamycin, teicoplanin, and the quinolones. Readers are cautioned to note that cardiac penetration may not correlate with the efficacy of an antibiotic in preventing infection in patients undergoing cardiac surgery.

Gallbladder

Studies of antibiotic concentration in gallbladder tissue (Table 14.18) are difficult to interpret because specimens may be contaminated by bile as well as blood. Only one study cited in Table 14.18 corrected assay results for blood contamination (148). One study failed to show any difference in gallbladder levels of ceforanide when the cystic duct was obstructed or unobstructed (149). Other studies, however, revealed higher gallbladder levels of clindamycin when the common duct was patent than when it was obstructed (68) and higher levels when the gallbladder functioned than when it did not (150).

(continued on page 740)

Table 14.16

Antimicrobial Concentrations in Bone

Reference	Antimicrobial	Administration Method[a]	Dose (g) (Multiple or Single)[b]	n	Serum Half-life (h)	Serum Concentration Mean (μg/mL) (Range)	Time Serum Obtained (h)	Site Concentration Mean (μg/mL) (Range)	Time Site Specimen Obtained (h)	Ratio of Site/Serum (%)	Notes[c]
Aminoglycosides											
543	Gentamicin	IM	1.7 mg/kg (M)	3	2.0	5.2 (3.7–7.1)	1–2	1.22 (<2.1–3.6)	1–2	~30.5	U
544	Isepamicin	IV	15 mg/kg (S)	12		43 (26–27)	1–2	6.3 (1.6–11.9) / 8.3 (2.4–20.9)	1–2 / 1–2	15 / 19	U, CO / U, CA
545	Tobramycin	IV	0.0015/kg	5	2.0	6 (2.4–8.3)	0.35	0.8 (0.6–1)	0.35	13.5	U
Cephalosporins and related β-lactams											
546	Aztreonam	IV	2.0 (S)	18	1.7	78 (42–129)	1.5	16 (0–49)	1.5	20.5	U, C, CA
547	Cefaclor	Oral	0.5 (S)	39	0.75	7.5	2	1.59 (0–3.2)	2	18.5	U
218	Cefadroxil	Oral	0.5 (S)	6	1.3	6.33	4	0.4 / 0.9	4	6.3 / 14.2	U, CO / U, CA
522	Cefadroxil	Oral	1.0 (M)	14	1.3	21.5 (±2.3)	2	5.0 (±0.9)	2	23.5	U
147	Cefamandole	IV	1.0–2.0 (S)	7	1.0	47.1 (22–67.5)	0.2–1.3	0.2 (0–1.5)	0.2–1.3		I
139	Cefamandole	IV	2.0 (S)	29	0.7	73.6 (±6.1)	0.85	9.4 (±1.1)	0.85	13.5	U
548	Cefazolin	IV	0.01/kg (S)	10	1.5	32.9 (±10.4)	1.2	3.03 (±1.78)	1.2	6.5	U, CA, C
543	Cefazolin	IM	1.0 (M)	3	2.0	42 (31–50)	0.5–2.0	~5 (<4.1–10)	0.5–2	~12.5	U
549	Cefazolin	IV or IM	50 mg/kg/day (M)	6	1.7	13 (±2)	2	3.8 (3–5)	2–6	29.5	I, CH
138	Cefazolin	IV	1.0 (S)	31	2.0	80	0.67	30	0.67	37.5	U, C
550	Cefazolin	IV	4.0 (S)	7	2.0	101 (74–138)	~1	14.4 (5.6–24.9) / 29 (3.3–48.9)	~1	14 / 29	U, CO / U, CA
145	Cefazolin	IV	1.0 (S)	17	2.0	51.7	1.15	5.9	1.15	11.4	U, CA
551	Cefepime	IV	2.0 (S)	10	2	72.9 (32–127)	0.8–1.9	35.6 (22–51) / 52.5 (35–68)	0.8–1.9 / 0.8–1.9	49 / 72	U, CO / U, CA

523	Cefmenoxime	IV	2.0	41		52.4	1.0	18.1 (±8.74)	0.83		U, MC, CA
		IV	2.0	41		52.4	1.0	16.5 (±6.23)	0.83	31.5	U, MC, CO
552	Cefodozime	IV	2.0 (S)	22	3–4	121	2.5	13.42	2.5	11	U, CO
								24.4	2.5	20	U, CA
553	Cefonicid	IV	0.03/kg (S)	12	2.6		1–3	18.7 (5.8–29.6)	1–3	12.5	U, C
554	Cefoperazone	IV	1.0 (M)	5	1.22	46	1.0	5	1.0	11.5	U, CA
		IV	1.0 (M)	5	1.22	46	1.0	4.2	1.0	9.5	U, CO
145	Ceforanide	IV	2.0 (S)	8	2.7	144.0	1.37	13.4	1.37	9.35	U, CA
555	Cefotaxime	IV	2.0 (S)	19	1.2	61	0.5–1	5.4	0.5–1	8.8	U, C
556	Cefotiam	IV	2.0 (S)	10	0.6–1.5	55.2 (±11.5)	1	14.7 (±4.4)	1	27	U
557	Cefoxitin	IV	45 mg/kg (S)	14	0.8	160 (±50)	2	8 (±3)	2	5	U, CO
								16 (±6)		10	U, CA
145	Cefoxitin	IV	2.0 (S)	20	0.8	39.0	1.15	6.3	1.15	16.2	U, CA
558	Ceftazidime	IV	1.0 (S)	12	1.9	49.1 (38.2–59.8)	0.5	14.8 (4.4–21.1)	0.5	30.5	U, C
2	Ceftizoxime	IV	1.0 (M)	5	1.7	33.7 (±6.9)	1	6.3 (±4.6)	1	19.5	U
527	Ceftriaxone	IV	1.0	53	7.0	67.3	1.8	32.4	1.56		U, C
559	Cefuroxime	IV	1.5 (S)	11	1.3	100 (±25)	0.75	5.5 (3–13)	0.75	5.5	U, CO
								12 (7–25)		12	U, CA
560	Cephalexin	Oral	0.5 (S)	36	0.9	11.7 ± 2.3	1.5	2.12 ± 0.33	2	19.5	U
549	Cephaloridine	IV or IM	100 mg/kg/day (M)	7	1.8	6.5	2	2.0 (0.7–6)	1–3	31.5	—
561	Cephalothin	IV	1.0 (S)	21	0.5	11.9 (6.6–20.8)	1	3.9 (0.9–17.5)	1	33.5	U
145	Cephalothin	IV	1.0 (S)	14	0.5	5.3	1.52	0.5	1.52	9.4	U, CA
63	Cephapirin	IV	1.0 (S)	10	0.28	70.8 (7.1–383)	0.25–1	9.1 (3.8–28.7)	0.25–1	45.5	U, C
562	Cephradine	IV	1.0 (S)	21	0.7	45	0.6	10	0.6	22.5	U, C
563	Cephradine	IM	1.0 (S)	24	0.7	11.7 (6.1–20.4)	1.7	1.79 (±0.98)	1.7	15	U, CA
								3.28 (±1.34)	1.7	28	U, CO

(Continued)

Table 14.16 (Continued)

Antimicrobial Concentrations in Bone

Reference	Antimicrobial	Administration Method[a]	Dose (g) (Multiple or Single)[b]	n	Serum Half-life (h)	Serum Concentration Mean (µg/mL) (Range)	Time Serum Obtained (h)	Site Concentration Mean (µg/mL) (Range)	Time Site Specimen Obtained (h)	Ratio of Site/Serum (%)	Notes[c]
548	Moxalactam	IV	0.01/kg (S)	10	3	33.3 (±7.7)	1.2	2.62 (±2.28)	1.2	7.5	U, CA, C
564	Ertapenem	IV	1.0 (S)	6		70.1 (47.7–76.0)	1	13.2 (8.9–18.1)	1	19	U, CA
564	Ertapenem	IV	1.0 (S)	6		70.1 (47.7–76.0)	1	8.0 (4.9–10.8)	1	13	U, CO
565	Imipenem	IV	1.0 (M)	10	1.4	35 (±4)	0.25	2.6 (0.4–5.4)	0.5–2.0		I
Penicillins											
566	Amoxicillin/ Clavulanic acid	IV	1.0 (M)	9	1.0	50.1	0.5	3.6	0.5	7.5	U
566	Clavulanic acid	IV	0.2 (M)	9	1.2	9.1	0.5	0.54	0.5	6.5	U
563	Ampicillin	IM	0.5 (S)	24	1.1	10.1 (1.1–34.8)	1.7	0.78 (±1.28) / 1.89 (±1.77)	1.7 / 1.7	8 / 19	U, CA / U, CO
556	Ampicillin/ sulbactam	IV	2.0 (S)	10	0.9	46.8 (±27.4)	1	20.7 (±9.6)	1	44	U
		IV	1.0 (S)	10	0.84	13.2 (±8.4)	1	7.7 (±4.1)	1	58	U
567	Azidocillin	Oral	0.75 (S)	6	0.75	12.2 (±5.0)	1	0.8 (±0.4)	1	65.5	U
568	Azlocillin	IV	5.0 (S)	8	1.0	14.3	1	24 (±1.35)	0.8–1.5	17.5	U
569	Carbenicillin	IV	5.0 (S)	15	1.5	281 (155–360)	0.5	32.3	0.5	11.6	U
570	Cloxacillin	Oral	0.5 (S)	10	0.5	3.2 (±0.5)	1	2.0 (±0.4)	1	62.5	U
		Oral	1.0 (S)	5	0.5	17.7 (±2.4)	2	2.9 (±1.3)	2	16	CA, MC, U
549	Dicloxacillin	IM	50 mg/kg/ day (M)	8	1.9	6 (±1)	2	6.4 (1.8–21)	2–6	106.5	I
570,571	Dicloxacillin	Oral	0.5 (S)	10	0.5	13 (±2.5)	1.5	2.0 (±0.5)	1.5	15.5	U
563	Flucloxacillin	IM	0.5 (S)	24		9.3 (2.7–17.8)	1.7	0.87 (±1.28) / 1.30 (±1.92)	1.7 / 1.7	9 / 13	U, CA / U, CO

572	Methicillin	IM	1.0 (M)	21	0.5	11.65 (±6.1)	~2	2.6 (0–7) 2.7 (0–10)	2	22 23	U, CO U, CA
549	Methicillin	IV	250 mg/kg/day (M)	10	0.8	18 (±8)	2	12.1 (1–46)	1–3	67.5	I
568	Mezlocillin	IV	5.0 (S)	10	1.3	135	1	21 (±2.75)	0.8–1.5	16.5	U
561	Oxacillin	IV	1.0 (S)	22	0.5	18.9 (5–33)	1	2.1 (0.3–14.5)	1	11.5	U
543	Penicillin G	IV	2 × 10⁶ units	3	0.5	5.0 (0.5–9.4)	0.5–1.0	<1	0.5–1.0	<20.5	U
555	Piperacillin	IV	50 mg/kg (S)	12	1.1	46.6	2	15.7	2	33.5	CO, U
573	Piperacillin/ tazobactam	IV	3.01	9	1	98.5 ± 19.1	1	21.3 ± 10.1	2	23	U, CA
			0.375			9.4 ± 2.2	1	18.7 ± 7.8 2.46 ± 0.96 2.29 ± 0.93		18 26 22	U, CO U, CA U, CO
574	Ticarcillin	IV	5.0 (S)	20	1.0	127 (28–214)	~1.1	32.4 (13.5–60.2) 30.5 (14–65.1)	~1.1 ~1.1	26 24	U, C, CO U, C, CA
574	Clavulanic acid	IV	0.2 (S)	20	1.2	8.4 (5–12.5)	~.1	14.8 (6.7–24.5) 9.6	~1.1 ~1.1	176 114	U, C, CO U, C, CA

Quinolones

143	Ciprofloxacin	Oral	0.5 (S)	7	4.0	1.4 (0.4–2.0)	1.5–4.8	0.4 (0.2–0.9)	1.5–4.8	28.5	U, C, CO
		Oral	0.75	7	4.0	2.6 (0.9–3.8)	1.5–4.8	0.7 (0.2–1.4)	1.5–4.8	27.5	U, C, CO
		Oral	0.5	6	4.0	2.0 (0.9–3.2)	2.0–4.5	0.7 (0.2–1.4)	2.0–4.5	35.5	I, C, CO
		Oral	0.75	4	4.0	2.9 (1.0–6.0)	2.0–4.5	1.4 (0.6–2.7)	2.0–4.5	48.5	I, C, CO
575	Enoxacin	Oral	0.4 (S)	5	5.5	2.0 (±0.4)	1.5–5.5	0.7 (±0.3)	1.5–5.5	35.5	U, C, CO
		Oral	0.4 (M)	6		2.1 (±0.3)	1.5–5.5	0.9 (±0.5)	1.5–5.5	45.5	U, C, CO
		Oral	0.4 (M)	6		2.8 (±1.6)	1.5–5.5	1.3 (±1.6)	1.5–5.5	39.5	I, C, CO
		IV	0.4 (S)	6		1.8 (±0.4)	1.5–5.5	0.9 (±0.5)	1.5–5.5	48.5	U, C, CO
		IV	0.4 (M)	6		3.1 (±0.9)	1.5–5.5	1.1 (±0.5)	1.5–5.5	35.5	U, C, CO
576	Levofloxacin	IV	0.5 (S)	146	6–7	8.57 (5.25–13.75)	1.5 1.5	6.61 (1.95–13.04) 3	1.5 1.5	77 35	CA CO
577	Lomefloxacin	Oral	0.2 (M)	5	8	1.65 ± 0.13	2.5	1.87 ± 0.66	2.5	103.5	U

(Continued)

Table 14.16 (Continued)

Antimicrobial Concentrations in Bone

Reference	Antimicrobial	Administration Method[a]	Dose (g) (Multiple or Single)[b]	n	Serum Half-life (h)	Serum Concentration Mean (μg/mL) (Range)	Time Serum Obtained (h)	Site Concentration Mean (μg/mL) (Range)	Time Site Specimen Obtained (h)	Ratio of Site/Serum (%)	Notes[c]
578	Moxifloxacin	Oral	0.4 (M)	10		6.26 (4.7–7.31)	2	2.97 (1.9–4.67)	2	48	U, CA
578	Moxifloxacin	Oral	0.4 (M)	10		6.26 (4.7–7.31)	2	2.54 (0.62–4.64)	2	40	U, CO
142	Ofloxacin	Oral	0.4 (S)	10	8.0	2.0 (±0.88)	4.0	1.22 (±1.54)	4.5	61.5	U
579	Pefloxacin	IV/Oral	0.4 (M)	15	10.5	9.2 (3.5–17.3)	2.0	4.1 (0.3–10.2)	2.0	44.5	U, C
567	Doxycycline	Oral	0.20 (S)	6	20	3.6 (±0.8)	3	2.6 (±2.0)	3	72.5	U
Others											
572	Clindamycin	IM	0.6 (M)	24	2.0	8.5 (±1.65)	~2	3.87 (1–9.6) 3.77 (0.7–7)	2	45 44	U, CO U, CA
567	Clindamycin	Oral	0.3 (M)	6	2.0	2.8 (±1.2)	1.5	0.6 (±0.4)	1.5	21.4	U
580	Daptomycin	IV	6 mg/kg (S)	8	10	72.9	0.5	4.7	0.5	9.7	U, AUC, CA, MD
567	Erythromycin	Oral	0.5 (S)	6	1.5	1.3 (0.1–2.1)	1	0.2 (±0.1)	1.5	18.5	U
581	Erythromycin	IV	1.0 (S)	4	1.5	9.8 (7.6–11)	0.25–2.5	3.8 (1.8–5.5)	0.25–2.5	39.5	U, CA
582	Fosfomycin	IV	100 mg/kg	9	3.6	377 (±73)	0.5	96.4 (±14.5)	3.9	43	U, CA, AUC, MD
583	Flurithromycin	Oral	0.5 (M)	8	9.9	1.5	1.5	1.5	1.5	100.5	U, C
584	Lincomycin	Oral	1.0 (M)	8	4.5	0.84 (0.25–1.5)	2–6	0.7 (0.25–1.3)	2–6	83.5	U
584	Lincomycin	IM	0.6 (M)	5	4.5	3.7 (2.6–5.0)	2–6	2.7 (1.0–5.2)	2–6	62.5	U
585	Lincomycin	Oral	1.0 (M)	10	4.5	5.8	~6	2.32	~6	40.5	I
540	Linezolid	IV	0.6 (S)	12	4–5	19.2 (10.7–38.2)	0.17	9.1 (4.3–13)	0.17	51	U
586	Linezolid	IV	0.6 (S)	11	4–5	17.1 (11.1–26.6)	0.9	3.9 (1.2–8.3)	0.9	22	I, CO

587	Linezolid	IV	0.6 (M)	3	9.3	22.4 (15.2–26.6)	0.5	17 (9.3–18.9)	2.5	92	U, AUC, CA, MD
588	Metronidazole	Rectal	1.0 (S)	13	8.0	9.82 (±4.05)	3	7.45 (±3.85)	3	75.5	U
589	Miokamycin	Oral	0.6 (S)	5		1.0 ±0.48	1	0.88 ±0.13	1	88.5	U
590	Rifampin	Oral	0.3 (M)	8	3.0	6.0 (±2.6)	3–4	0 / 1.2 (±0.5)	3–4	19 / 19	C, U, CO / C, U, CA
590	Rifampin	Oral	0.6 (M)	10	3.0	8.9 (±2.3)	3	1.7 (±1.0) / 3.6 (±0.7)	3	20 / 41	C, U, CO / C, U, CA
591	Rifampicin	IV	0.6 (S)	24	1.1	7.4 (3.2–12.8)	4	3.8 (1.9–8.2)	4	51.5	I, C
592	Roxithromycin	Oral	0.15 (M)	24	7.5	6.12	2.75	5.09	4.5	79.5	U, AU
545	Teicoplanin	IV	0.4	10	0.68	29.6 (18–74.4)	0.5	6.6 (2.6–18.4)	0.5	22.5	U
593	Telithromycin	Oral	0.8	6	9.8	0.73 (±0.32)	3.3	1.12 (±0.31)	3.3	150	U
228	Tigecycline	IV	0.1 (S)	6	42	0.098 (±0.013)	12	0.116 (±0.132)	12	41	U, AUC
594	Vancomycin	IV	0.015/kg	14 / 10	6.0	22.1 (10.5–52.9)	1.3	2.3 (0.5–16) / 0.81 (0–1.58)	1.3 / 1.3	13 / 4	U, CA, C / U, CO, C
	Variable (M)	5				17.5 (13.6–26.3)	2.5	2.4 (0–8.4)	2.5	14.5	I, CO, C

[a]IM, intramuscularly; IV, intravenously.
[b]M, multiple dose; S, single dose.
[c]U, uninfected; CO, cortical bone; CA, cancellous bone; C, corrected for blood; I, infected; MC, blood contamination was felt to be minimal; CH, children; AUC, ratios of areas under the curve; MD, use of microdialysis to determine interstitial fluid concentration.

Table 14.17

Antimicrobial Concentrations in Cardiac Tissue

Reference	Antimicrobial	Administration Method[a]	Dose (g) (Multiple or Single)[b]	n	Serum Half-life (h)	Serum Concentration Mean (μg/mL) (Range)	Time Serum Obtained (h)	Site Concentration Mean (μg/mL) (Range)	Time Site Specimen Obtained (h)	Ratio of Site/Serum (%)	Notes[c]
Aminoglycosides											
595	Amikacin	IM	0.5 (S)	9	2.0	17.4 (±2.5)	0.6–1.5	4.3 (±0.9)	0.6–1.5	25.5	A
	Gentamicin	IV	1.5 mg/kg (S)	33	2.0	2.7	1–2	0.5	1–2	19.5	V
Cephalosporins and related β-lactams											
189	Aztreonam	IV	2.0 (S)	12	1.7–2	76 (±5 SE)	0.9–1.6	22 (±2 SE)	0.9–1.6	29.5	A
596	Cefamandole	IV	2.0 (S)	23	0.6	78 (25–130)	0.3–2.0	34 (8–70)	0.3–2.0	44.5	A, C
597	Cefamandole	IM	20 mg/kg (S)	15	0.7	47 (22–70)	0.5–2	16 (6–35)	0.5–2	34.5	V
598	Cefazolin	IV	2.0 (S)	16	2	114.1 (50–200)	1	38.9 (25–60)	1	34.1	C
599	Cefazolin	IM	10 mg/kg (S)	9	2	34.0 (21–40)	0.5–1.4	10.1 (±3.2 SD)	0.5–1.4	30.5	A, C
600	Cefepime	IV	2 (S)	5	2	69.8 (±25.6 SD)	<1	21.5 (±8.9 SD)	<1	30.8	MS
601	Cefonicid	IM	1.0 (S)	7	3.5	85 (48–138)	2	7.5 (2.6–9.5)	2	8.8	
602	Ceforanide	IV	30 mg/kg (S)	11	2.3	127 (40–200)	0.3–1.7	52 (30–80)	0.3–1.7	41.5	A, C
603	Cefoxitin	IV	2.0 (S)	10	0.8	55.8 (29–78.1)	0.75–1	27.3 (18.2–43.2)	0.75–1	49.5	V
	Cefsulodin	IV	2.0 (S)	23	1.5	72.1	1–2	10.1	1–2	14.5	
604	Ceftizoxime	IV	2.0 (S)	22	1.7	80.9 (±7.3)	1	37.0 (±2.8)	1	46.5	A
604	Ceftizoxime	IV	2.0 (S)	7	1.7	56.5 (34.1–92.6)	2	16.9 (9.1–20.7)	2	30.5	MY
527	Ceftriaxone	IV	1.0 (S)	53	15.7	67.3	1.8	30.5	1.9	45.5	A
605	Cephalothin	IV	2.0 (S)	12	0.5	66 (10–140)	0.2–1.7	7.5 (0–17)	0.3–1.9	11.5	A, C
597	Cephalothin	IM	20 mg/kg (S)	15	0.5	30 (20–70)	0.5–1.5	<4 (<1–22)	0.5–1.5	<13.5	V
605	Cephapirin	IV	2.0 (S)	15	0.5	62 (10–140)	0.2–1.7	12 (0–32)	0.3–1.9	19.5	A, C
598	Cephradine	IV	2.0 (S)	17	0.7	40.9 (20–75)	1	18.1 (10–25)	1	44.3	A, C
599	Moxalactam	IV	10 mg/kg (S)	10	2.5	40.1 (±5.2 SD)	0.5–0.7	19.2 (±10.4 SD)	0.5–0.7	48.5	A, C

Quinolones

606	Ciprofloxacin	IV	0.4 (S)	6	3–5	6.19 (±1.73 SD)	0	31.6 (±25.0 SD)	0–1	510.5	MY, NS
606	Ciprofloxacin	IV	0.4 (S)	6	3–5	6.19 (±1.73 SD)	0	5.8 (±3.2 SD)	0–1	94.5	V, NS
606	Ciprofloxacin	Oral	0.75 (M)	6	3–5	11.59 (±3.95 SD)	0	21.8 (±13.0 SD)	0–1	188.5	MY, NS
606	Ciprofloxacin	Oral	0.75 (M)	8	3–5	11.59 (±3.95 SD)	0	8.3 (±3.1 SD)	0–1	72.5	V, NS
607	Ofloxacin	IV	0.4 (S)	3	4–8	15.9 (±2.5 SD)	0	8.89 (±2.16 SD)	0–1	56.5	MY, NS
607	Ofloxacin	IV	0.4 (S)	3	4–8	15.9 (±2.5 SD)	0	5.00 (±0.75 SD)	0–1	31.5	V, NS
608	Pefloxacin	IV	0.8 (S)	9	8–12	7.1 (±2.02)	4	6.90	4	97.5	V, NS
608	Pefloxacin	IV	0.8 (S)	3	8–12	7.1 (±2.02)	4	20.1 (±25.1)	4	284.5	MY, NS

Penicillins

531	Flucloxacillin	IV	2.0 (S)	9	2.1	125.2 (±11.7 SE)	0–1	16.5 (±2.6 SE)	1–2	13.5	V, NS, PD
609	Piperacillin	IV	100 mg/kg (S)	5	1.0	300 (240–400)	0.3–0.5	90 (85–100)	0.3–0.5	30.5	MY

Others

610	Clindamycin	IV	0.6 (M)	6	2	6.0 (5–8)	1	15.6 (12.5–18)	1	260.5	A
610	Doxycycline	IV	0.1 (M)	11	20	10.3 (8–13)	1	5.9 (5–6.3)	1	57.5	A
600	Fusidic acid	IV	1 (S)	5		117.9 (±42.2 SD)	<1	127.1 (±38.2 SD)	<1	107.8	MS
611	Lincomycin	IM	0.6 (M)	51	4.5	9.7	1	7.7	1	79.5	
612	Rifampin	Oral	0.6 (S)	10	2–5	15.9	2	3.8	2	24.5	V
613	Teicoplanin	IV	6 mg/kg (S)	32	40–70	22.2 (±0.7 SE)	1	70.6 (±1.7 SE)	1	318.5	A
614	Teicoplanin	IV	12 mg/kg (S)	8	40–70	16.2 (±10.5 SE)	2–3	5.5 (±5.1 SE)	2–3	34	V, NS
542	Vancomycin	IV	15 mg/kg (S)	7	4–6	14.2 (±2.0 SE)	1–2	4.2 (±1.0 SE)	1–2	30.5	V, NS

[a]IM, intramuscularly; IV, intravenously.
[b]S, single dose; M, multiple dose.
[c]A, atrial appendage; V, valve; C, corrected for blood; MY, myocardium; NS, number of site samples is different than number of serum samples; PD, peak data.

Table 14.18

Antimicrobial Concentrations in Gallbladder

Reference	Antimicrobial	Administration Method[a]	Dose (g) (Multiple or Single)[b]	n	Serum Half-life (h)	Serum Concentration Mean (µg/mL) (Range)	Time Serum Obtained (h)	Site Concentration Mean (µg/mL) (Range)	Time Site Specimen Obtained (h)	Ratio of Site/Serum (%)	Notes[c]
Aminoglycosides											
164	Amikacin	IM	0.5 (S)	8	2.0	31.3 (±8.4 SD)	1-2	2.7 (±2.0 SD)	1-2	9	
Cephalosporins and related β-lactams											
282	Aztreonam	IV	2.0 (S)	14	1.7	20.0 (±10 SD)	1-2	6.6 (±6.0 SD)	1-2	33	U
287	Cefbuperazone	IV	1.0 (S)	13	1.7	96.7 (52-168)	0.5	26.1 (3.2-99)	0.5	27	U
290	Cefmenoxime	IV	1.0 (S)	6	1.1	22.4 (17-38)	0.9	10.1 (2-29)	0.9	45	U
291	Cefoperazone	IV	1.0 (M)	10	1.9	45.1 (±7.9 SE)	2.9	21.7 (±3.25 SE)	2.9	49	A
149	Ceforanide	IV	1.0 (S)	5	2.7	45 (±4 SD)	2.0	20 (±2 SD)	2.0	44	U, OC
149	Ceforanide	IV	1.0 (S)	4	2.7	38 (±4 SD)	2.0	21 (±2 SD)	2.0	55	U
148	Cefotaxime	IM	1.0 (M)	5	1.2	19.4 (9-48)	1.0	2.0 (0.6-5.0)	1.0	10	U, C
79	Cefpiramide	IV	1.0 (S)	10		157 (±21)	1.0	22.6 (±4.2)	1.0	14	
293	Ceftazidime	IV	1.0 (S)	20	1.7	24.9 (12.5-37.3)	1.75	21.3 (8.6-46.5)	1.75	86	U, F
289	Cefepime	IV	2 (S)	27	2	100 (±85.5 SD)	4.73 ± 4.25	48.3 (±38.7 SD)	4.73 ± 4.25	38	F
288	Cefepime	IV	2.0 (M)	29	2.0	7.6 (0.4-62)	8.6	5.4 (0.4-28)	8.6	70	A
2	Ceftizoxime	IV	1.0 (S)	6	1.7	31 (±5.8 SD)	1.0	10.5 (±12 SD)	0.5-2.5	34	U
291	Ceftriaxone	IV	1.0 (M)	11	6.5	59.5 (±13 SE)	2.9	25.1 (±8.6 SE)	2.9	42	A
294	Cefuroxime	IV	0.75 (S)	5	1.3	46 (36-69)	0-0.8	12.1 (7.1-16.5)	0.3-1.7	26	F
296	Meropenem	IV	1.0 (S)	33	1.2	27.3 (1.9-87.0) / 4.8 (0.3-41.6)	0.5-1.5 / 3-5	3.2 (1.3-4.2) / 0.9 (0.8-1.4)	0.5-1.5 / 3-5	12 / 19	AD
Penicillins											
297	Amoxicillin	IM	1.0 (S)	5	1.0	10.4 (8.6-12)	1.2-1.5	4.2 (3-6)	1.2-1.5	40	
615	Ampicillin/ sulbactam	IV	2.0 (S)	8	0.8	18.8 (±4.5 SD)	2	8.7 (±8.3 SD)	2	46	
		IV	1.0 (S)	8	1.0	10.7 (±3.5 SD)	2	4.7 (±1.4 SD)	2	44	

		Route	Dose[a],[b]								[c]
70	Piperacillin	IV	2.0 (S)	10	1.1	81.7 (±20.5 SD)	1.0	10.5 (±2.6 SD)	1.0	13	
302	Temocillin	IV	2.0 (M)	10	3.9	87.5 (34–126)	4	52.5 (28–97)	4	60	U, F
303	Ticarcillin/ clavulanic acid	IV	3.0 (S)	11	1.2	82 (±30 SD)	1.0–3.8	26 (±12)	1.0–3.8	32	U, F, E
303		IV	0.2 (S)	11	1.1	2.0 (±1.0)	1.0–3.8	0.9 (±0.7)	1.0–3.8	45	
Quinolones											
616	Levofloxacin	IV	0.5 (S)	54	7	11.37	1.18 ± 0.35	15.61 (0.67–74.33)	1.18 ± 0.35	162	Medians
616	Levofloxacin	Oral	0.5 (S)	7	7	9.65 (8.01–40.56)	3.42 ± 1.05	17.93 (11.65–31.76)	3.42 ± 1.05	170	Medians
617	Moxifloxacin	IV	0.4 (S)	16	12.4	0.39–4.37	0.83– 21.17	1.73–17.08	0.83–21.17	300	AC, ranges
Tetracyclines											
76	Doxycycline	IV	0.2/0.1 (M)	15	20	3.0 (0.1–5.0)	20	5.4 (1.6–15.2)	20	180	U
618	Doxycycline	Oral	0.1 (M)	31	20	3.4	4–10	3.7 (1.4–8.7)	4–10	110	A
Others											
68	Clindamycin	IV	0.6 (S)	7	2.0	14.5 (9–26)	1.0	12 (5–44)	2.0	83	PD
68	Clindamycin	IV	0.6 (S)	5	2.0	11.3 (6–19)	1.0	6 (0–12)	2.0	53	OD
150	Clindamycin	Oral	0.3 (M)	6	2.0	1.6	2.0	1.7	2.0	106	F
150	Clindamycin	Oral	0.3 (M)	8	2.0	0.9	2.0	0.3	2.0	35	NF
77	Rifampin	Oral	0.15 (S)	4	2.5	1.4 (1.1–1.8)	3–5	1.8 (0.5–2.6)	3–5	129	
619	Trimethoprim	Oral	1.0 (S)	3	8–10	6.2 (3.0–8.2)	4	13.3 (7.1–19)	4	215	

[a] M, intramuscularly; IV, intravenously.
[b] S, single dose; M, multiple dose.
[c] U, uninfected; A, acute cholecystitis; OC, obstructed cystic duct; C, corrected for hemoglobin; E, extrapolated from graphical data; PD, patent duct; OD, obstructed duct; F, functioning gallbladder; NF, nonfunctioning gallbladder.

Lung Tissue

Antimicrobial concentrations in lung tissue (Table 14.19) have been measured almost exclusively following pulmonary resection of lung cancers. An exception involved a unique method of positron emission labeling of erythromycin followed by scanning of the lungs, while increasing numbers of samples of pulmonary tissue were obtained by transbronchial biopsy (151). Correction for blood contamination of specimens was done in only a few studies (151–155). The antimicrobial concentrations achieved in lung tissue were considerably higher than those in sputum (Table 14.8), but far fewer studies of lung tissue have been performed. Several drugs, such as ciprofloxacin (156), erythromycin (157), cefotaxime (158), and trimethoprim (159), showed much higher levels in lung than in blood. These studies were usually done 3 to 15 hours after the last doses of drug, at a time of relatively low serum levels, but nonetheless, they showed considerably more activity in lung tissue than in serum. Many of these agents (ciprofloxacin, erythromycin, and rifampin) are concentrated within cells, which may explain their high tissue levels. A few investigators have examined the concentrations of drug in infected or inflamed lung tissue (151,159–161). These levels were not substantially different from those in normal lung tissue from the same individuals. We are unaware of good correlation between lung antimicrobial concentrations and clinical therapeutic or prophylactic efficacy in humans. Therefore, clinical inferences from these data should be made with caution.

Prostatic Tissue

Numerous studies have measured antimicrobial concentrations in human prostatic tissue (Table 14.20). Most of the studies were performed with patients without infection, undergoing transurethral or suprapubic prostatectomy. Techniques for tissue preparation were variable. As is the case with prostatic secretions, the prostatic tissue concentrations observed in most of these studies may be due to urinary contamination and therefore must be interpreted with caution (107,162).

INTERPRETATION OF SERUM CONCENTRATIONS OF ANTIMICROBIALS

Interpretation of antimicrobial serum or plasma concentration data requires a basic understanding of the principles that govern pharmacokinetics: absorption, distribution, metabolism, and excretion of drug. In addition, method of administration, number of dosage administrations prior to sample collection, and timing of the sample collection with respect to the previous dose are equally important factors to consider when comparing data (163–165). Figure 14.2 depicts theoretical serum concentration data, using a two-compartment open simulation model, following a single 1-g dose of an antimicrobial by four different methods: intravenous bolus (1-minute infusion), 30-minute intravenous infusion, oral, and intramuscular administration. The apparent volume of distribution, bioavailability (100%), rate of elimination, and transfer rate constants between the central and peripheral compartments were all held constant in order to show just how different theoretical concentration-time curves may look when only one of these variables (administration) is altered.

Absorption

Absorption is the process by which antibiotic transfers from the site of administration (such as intravenous, intramuscular, oral, and topical) into the general circulation (central compartment) of the body, and it ranges from 0% to 100%. Percentage bioavailability (Table 14.21) is simply 100 times the ratio of the amount of active antibiotic (A) reaching the general circulation to the amount administered (dose).

$$\text{Percentage bioavailability} = 100 \times A/\text{dose}$$

For most antimicrobials administered intravenously or intramuscularly, percentage bioavailability is 100%. However, some, such as chloramphenicol succinate, are in an inactive form when given parenterally and the actual percentage bioavailability may be less than 100% because of partial conversion. Absorption from oral administration is less than 100% for most antimicrobials; therefore, the area under the serum concentration–time curve following oral administration is less than that following parenteral administration, with all other variables held constant. Percentage bioavailability refers only to the extent of absorption; it gives no indication of how rapidly the antimicrobial is absorbed and does not account for protein binding.

Rate of Administration

Difficulty in interpreting differences in concentration with various routes of administration is often attributed to the respective rates of antimicrobial

(continued on page 747)

Table 14.19

Antimicrobial Concentrations in Lung Tissue

Reference	Antimicrobial	Administration Method[a]	Dose (g) (Multiple or Single)[b]	n	Serum Half-life (h)	Serum Concentration Mean (μg/mL) (Range)	Time Serum Obtained (h)	Site Concentration Mean (μg/mL) (Range)	Time Site Specimen Obtained (h)	Ratio of Site/Serum (%)	Notes[c]
Aminoglycosides											
595	Amikacin	IM	0.5 (S)	10	2.0	20.7 (±1.5 SE)	0.8–1.5	8.3 (±1.0 SE)	0.8–1.5	40	SR
Cephalosporins and related β-lactams											
522	Cefadroxil	Oral	1.0 (S)	22	1.3	11.5 (±1.3 SD)	2–4	7.4 (±0.7 SD)	2–4	64	SR
620	Cefamandole	IV	2.0 (S)	6	0.7	23.1 (±9.4 SD)	1–2	18.1 (±9.7 SD)	1–2	78	SR, H
621	Cefepime	IV	2.0 (M)		2.96	127.85 (±27.51 SD)	0.5 (±0.05 SD)	119.29[d] (±4.89 SD)	0.5 (±0.05 SD)	94	SR
622	Cefonicid	IM	1.0 (S)	5	4.5	92 (±14 SD)	2.0	12 (±2.4 SD)	2.0	13	SR
155	Cefoperazone	IV	2.0 (S)	10	2.4	97 (44–149)	2	45 (21–68)	2	46	SR, C
158	Cefotaxime	IM	1.0 (M)	6	1.2	5.1 (2.6–7.5)	3	19.5 (16.1–20.5)	3	382	SR
623	Cefotetan	IM	2.0 (S)	4	3.2	70.3 (54–84)	3	6.6 (4.2–9.1)	3	9	SR
152	Cefoxitin	IV	1.0 (S)	11	0.8	38.5 (26–55)	1	13.2 (8.8–2.3)	1	35	SR, C
318	Cefpirome	IV	1.0 (S)	37	2.0	34.5 (±3.3 SE)	0.5–7	19.3 (±1.9 SE)	0.5–7	56	T
624	Ceftriaxone	IV	2.0 (S)	13	6.5	127 (±17.6 SD)	1–2	57.4 (±13.3 SD)	1–2	45	SR
625	Imipenem	IV	1.0 (S)	10	1.0	20 (±4)	1.0	12 (±9)	1.0	60	SR, E
		IV	1.0 (S)	10	1.0	5.5	2.25	0.3 (±0.1)	2.25	5	SR, E
Penicillins											
89	Amoxicillin	Oral	1.0 (S)	6	1.0	5.6 (4.9–6.9)	3	2.4 (1.9–2.9)	3	43	SR
355	Amoxicillin	Oral	0.5 (M)	10	1.0	3.3 (2.0–7.1)	3	3.1 (0.6–5.8)	3	94	SR
329	Amoxicillin/ clavulanic acid	Oral	0.5 (S)	15	1.1	6.9 (8.6)	1–2	3.0 (3.8)	1–2	32	T
		Oral	0.25 (S)	15	1.1	5.3 (9.3)	1–2	1.7 (3.7)	1–2	32	T

(Continued)

Table 14.19 (Continued)

Antimicrobial Concentrations in Lung Tissue

Reference	Antimicrobial	Administration Method[a]	Dose (g) (Multiple or Single)[b]	n	Serum Half-life (h)	Serum Concentration Mean (μg/mL) (Range)	Time Serum Obtained (h)	Site Concentration Mean (μg/mL) (Range)	Time Site Specimen Obtained (h)	Ratio of Site/Serum (%)	Notes[c]
330	Amoxicillin/sulbactam	IV	2.0 (S)	15	1.2	97 (±9.5 SE)	0.5	39 (±7.2 SE)	0.5	40	T
		IV	1.0 (S)	15	1.1	38 (±3.8 SE)	0.5	28 (±5.2 SE)	0.5	74	T
626	Flucloxacillin	IM	0.5 (S)	10	1.1	18.8 (13.2–22)	1.5–2.0	3.9 (3–5)	1.5–2.0	21	SR
626	Flucloxacillin	IM	0.5 (S)	4	1.1	16.2 (11.8–22)	2–2.2	2.4 (0.5–3.6)	2–2.2	15	SR, I
627	Piperacillin	IV	4.0 (M)	6	1.1	196.3 (119–296)	0.5–0.75	55.2 (17.1–98)	0.5–0.75	28	T
628	Piperacillin/tazobactam	IV	2.0 (S)	6	1.3	36.4	1–2	33.4	1–2	92	SR
629	Oxacillin	IV	0.5 (S)	6	0.9	10.2	1–2	7.9	1–2	78	SR
		IM	0.5 (S)	9	0.5	11.9 (6.6–16.2)	1	2.4 (0.5–4.4)	1	20	SR
Quinolones											
156	Ciprofloxacin	Oral	0.75 (S)	10	4.0	2.0	3.4	4.9 (±1.7 SD)	3.4	275	T
		IV	0.20 (S)	10	4.0	0.9	0.9	4.1 (±1.9 SD)	0.9	624	T
630	Levofloxacin	IV	0.5 (S)	4	5.68	3,375 (2,509–5,386)		2,267 (1,980–2,355)		67	SR, M, AUC
Tetracyclines											
154	Doxycycline	IV	0.1 (M)	12	20	9.3 (3.2–16)	1	6.8 (2.5–12)	1	73	SR, C
347	Minocycline	Oral	0.1 (M)	15	14	0.8 (±0.4 SD)	13–20	3.0 (±1.4 SD)	13–20	364	SR
153	Tetracycline phosphate	Oral	0.5 (M)	6	10	3.9 (1.9–7.6)	>3	2.1 (0–3.6)	>3	54	SR, C
Others											
348	Azithromycin	Oral	0.5 (S)	20	30	0.13 (±0.05 SD)	12	3.9 (±1.2 SD)	48	3,000	T
349	Azithromycin ER	Oral	2 (S)	32		0.94 (±0.54)	4(2–8)	37.9[d]	16	4,032	PP, I
350	Clarithromycin	Oral	0.5 (M)	10	4.9	4.0 (±1.2 SE)	4.25	16.8 (±5.0 SE)	4.25	420	T

	Drug	Route	Dose								
350	14-Hydroxy-clarithromycin	Oral		10	7.2	0.7 (±0.2 SE)	4.25	2.7 (±5.0 SE)	4.25	385	T
355	Erythromycin ethylsuccinate	Oral	1.0 (M)	19	1.5	0.7 (0.4–1.4)	3	4.2 (1.3–8.4)	3	547	SR
355	Erythromycin lactobionate	IV	0.5 (M)	11	1.5	1.5 (0.6–1.9)	3	6.5 (3.0–11.1)	3	462	SR
151	Erythromycin lactobionate	IV	0.27 (S)	5	0.7	7.3	0.3	5.5 (±2.2 SD)	02.–0.5	75	SR, I
631	Erythromycin stearate	Oral	0.5 (M)	14	1.5	3.1	2	4.7 (3.3–6.4)	3–4	152	SR
583	Flurithromycin	Oral	0.5 (M)	9	8.6	1.9	4	3.6	4	190	SR
160	Fosfomycin	IM	2.0 (S)	6	1.5	37.6 (±4.5 SE)	1.75–2.3	13.0 (±1.2 SE)	1.75–2.3	34	SR
160	Fosfomycin	IV	2.0 (S)	6	1.5	31.3 (±2.5 SE)	1.3–1.8	16.2 (±2.1 SE)	1.3–1.8	52	SR, I
161	Rifampin	Oral	0.6 (S)	8	3.0	6.4 (3–10)	2–3	2.1 (0.6–3.8)	2–3	33	SR
632	Roxithromycin	Oral	0.15 (M)	53	6.0	4.2 (±0.3 SD)	6	2.1 (±0.9 SD)	6	51	SR
633	Spiramycin	IV	0.5 (M)	6	5.5	0.31 (±0.03 SD)	3.0	1.2 (±0.14 SD)	3.0	371	SR
159	Trimethoprim	Oral	0.2 (M)	31	8–10	2.7 (0.7–11)	11–15	10.9 (2–34)	11–15	403	SR
159	Trimethoprim	Oral	0.2 (M)	14	8–10	3.0 (0.7–8.4)	11–15	16.4 (3.6–42)	11–15	547	SR, I

[a]IM, intramuscularly; IV, intravenously.
[b]S, single dose; M, multiple dose.
[c]SR, surgical resection; H, 2.5 g/100 mL hemoglobin contamination; C, corrected for hemoglobin contamination; T, transbronchial biopsy; E, extrapolated from graphical data; I, infected or inflamed lung tissue.
[d]Micrograms per gram.

Table 14.20

Antimicrobial Concentrations in Prostatic Tissue

Reference	Antimicrobial	Administration Method[a]	Dose (g) (Multiple or Single)[b]	n	Serum Half-life (h)	Serum Concentration Mean (μg/mL) (Range)	Time Serum Obtained (h)	Site Concentration Mean (μg/mL) (Range)	Time Site Specimen Obtained (h)	Ratio of Site/Serum (%)	Notes[c]
Aminoglycosides											
422	Amikacin	IM	0.2 (S)	10	2–3	12.44 (9.4–18.5)	2.5–3	6.09 (2.6–10.8)	2.5–3	49	U, UR
634	Sagamicin	IM	0.060 (S)	4	1.3	3.65 (2.9–4.4)	2.2–2.6	3.08 (2.7–3.3)	2.2–2.6	85	U
423	Tobramycin	IM	0.080 (S)	22	2.0	2.8 (1.5–4.4)	0.75–2	2.7 (0.9–6)	0.75–2	96	U, T, B, UR
Cephalosporins and related β-lactams											
635	Aztreonam	IV	1.0 (S)	8	1.7	31.4 (18–46.3)	0.8–3	8 (1.7–12.1)	0.8–3	25	U, UR
636	Cefaclor	Oral	0.5 (M)	5	0.7	1.87 (0.6–5.0)	2	0.74 (0.24–1.94)	2	39	U, T, O
637	Cefamandole	IV	2.0 (S)	21	0.7	51 (18–70)	1	17.1 (8–43)	1	34	U, T, A
638	Cefazolin	IV	2.0 (S)	14	1.0	139.07 (±39.68)	0.5	34.63 ± 9.75	0.5	25	I, T
639	Cefazolin	IV or IM	1.0 (M or S)	22	2	38 (±20)	~0.9	14 ± 14	~0.9	37	U, T, UR
640	Cefepime	IV	2.0 (S)	5	2.2	60	1	30 (21–38)	1	51	U
641	Cefminoxime	IV	1.0 (S)	15 / 21		72.3 ± 21.1 / 72.0 ± 55.8	1 / 1	7.4 ± 5.5 / 6.2 ± 3.5	1 / 1	11 / 9	I / U
642	Cefoperazone	IM	1.0 (M)	14	2.2	35.8 (4–67)	1.5	23.2 (4.7–44.7)	1.5	65	U
643	Cefotaxime	IV	2.0 (S)	25	1.2	45.2 (30–72)	1.5	22.9 (4–50)	1.5	51	U, T
644	Cefotaxime	IM	1.0 (M)	7	1.2	19.5 (11–30)	1–2	2.8 (1–4)	1–2	15	U, T, UR
645	Cefpirome	IV	1.0 (S)	6	3.0	50 ± 8	1–2	12 ± 5	1–2	28.5	U
646	Cefpodoxime	Oral	0.2 (S)	8	2.3	1.72 (0.72–2.77)	3	0.68 (0.41–1.23)	3	37	U
249	Cefsulodin	IV	2.0 (S)	10	1.5	55.3 (43–72)	0.5	30.25 (20–40)	0.5	55	U, T, A, UR
647	Ceftazidime	IV	2.0 (S)	4	1.9	73.3 (±12.3)	0.5–1.5	10.1 (±2.9)	0.5–1.5	14	U, UR
648	Ceftizoxime	IM	1.0 (S)	5	1.7	33.0 (29–43)	1–1.5	8.7 (5.7–15.1)	1–1.5	26	U
649	Ceftriaxone	IV	2.9 (S)	5	5.3	106.4 (73–158)	1.5	41.4 (11.7–75.4)	1.5	39	U, T, UR

141	Cefuroxime	IV	1.5 (S)	33	1.3	99.6 (40–210)	1	20.1 (6–35)	1	20	U, T, A
650	Cephacetrile	IV	2.0 (S)	19	0.9	65.8 (35.7–117.6)	1	8.5 (5.5–16.7)	1	13	U, T
651	Cephalexin	Oral	0.5 (S)	12	0.8	4.48 (0.17–16.55)	2–7	0.88 (0.09–3)	2–7	20	U, T
652	Cephalexin	Oral	0.5 (M)	17	0.8	~6–10 (0–715)	0.75–2	<5 (0.5–10)	0.75–2		U, I
650	Cephalothin	IV	2.0 (S)	13	0.5	19.3 (10.4–21.7)	1	4.9 (1.3–7.2)	1	25	U, T
653	Cephapirin	IV	2.0 (S)	13	0.5	50 (20–98)	0.5	20.8 (6.3–56)	0.5	42	U, T, A
654	Doripenem	IV	0.5 (S)	9	0.5	27.5 (20.4–33.5)	0.5	5.1 (2.8–8.3)	0.5	19	U, UR, T
655	Moxalactam	IM	0.5 (M)	5	2.3	13.5 (5.1–17.8)	<1	4.0 (2.3–7.3)	<1	30	U, T, O
Penicillins											
107	Ampicillin	Oral	0.5 (M)	12	1.5	8.9 (1.0–20.5)	2–3	4.0 (0.6–6.9)	2–3	75	U, T, B
107	Ampicillin	Oral	0.5 (M)	12	1.5	6.7 (3.0–10.2)	2–3	3.7 (1.0–9.3)	2–3	73	U, T, B, H
656	Ampicillin	IV	2.0 (S)	19	1.5	118 (±48.9)	0.5	47.18 (0.4–548)	0.5	40	U, UR
657	Azlocillin	IV	2.9 (M)	8	1.0	64.9 (39.8–97)	1.0–2.0	22.9 (13–37)	1.0–2.0	35	U
657	Mezlocillin	IV	2.0 (M)	8	1.0	36.3 (11.8–49)	1.3–2.5	9.4 (2.4–19)	1.3–3.0	25	U
422	Piperacillin	IV	1.0 (M)	9	1.3	5.70 (2.0–12.8)	2.5–3	1.28 (0.29–1.20)	2.5–3	21	U, UR
656	Sulbactam	IV	1.0 (S)	19	1–1.3	32.2 (±12.2)	0.5	19.7 (0.15–249)	0.5	61	U, UR
Quinolones											
658	Ciprofloxacin	IV	0.1 (S)	25	4.0	1.2 (0.9–1.8)	0.33–0.5	3.0 (1.1–4.6)	0.33	250	U
427	Ciprofloxacin	Oral	0.5 (S)	8	4.3	2.0 (1.1–2.3)	2–5	2.64 (1.1–5.5)	2–5	132	U
			0.5 (M)	8	4.3	1.5 (1.0–2.4)	2–6	3.6 (1.1–9.5)	6	240	U
462	Enoxacin	Oral	0.2 (M)	12	5.5	2.4 (±0.35)	3.9	4.1 (±1.18)	3.9	210	U
429	Fleroxacin	Oral	0.4 (S)	11	12.0	3.7 (0.4–5.5)	1.3–4	4.4 (0.6–6.8)	1.3–4	112	U, UR
659	Levofloxacin	Oral then IV	0.5 (M)	20	6–7	8	1	22	1	296	U, E
660	Lomefloxacin	Oral	0.4 (S)	20	8.0	2.4 (0.5–4.8)	3.5	5.4 (1.1–10.1)	3.5	225	U, T, UR
661	Norfloxacin	Oral	0.4 (M)	10	3.3	1.3 (<0.25–5.3)	1–2	1.6 (<0.25–4.65)	1–2	123	U, UR
462	Norfloxacin	Oral	0.4 (M)	9	3.3	1.45 (0.4–5.3)	1–2	1.74 (0.75–4.7)	1–2	120	
462	Ofloxacin	Oral	0.4 (S)	21	7.0	2.04 (±1.16)	8.5–13	3.47 (±1.35)	8.5–13	170	U, T, UR
662	Pefloxacin	IV	0.8 (S)	10	3.8–5.6	5.67 (±1.98)	6	3.36 (±1.26)	6	59	U, T, UR

(Continued)

Table 14.20 (Continued)

Antimicrobial Concentrations in Prostatic Tissue

Reference	Antimicrobial	Administration Method[a]	Dose (g) (Multiple or Single)[b]	n	Serum Half-life (h)	Serum Concentration Mean (µg/mL) (Range)	Time Serum Obtained (h)	Site Concentration Mean (µg/mL) (Range)	Time Site Specimen Obtained (h)	Ratio of Site/Serum (%)	Notes[c]
Tetracyclines											
425	Doxycycline	IV	0.200 (M)	5	20	1.1 (±0.27)	3	1.21 (±0.46)	3	110	U, T, B
618	Doxycycline	Oral	0.200 then 0.100	5	20	2.8	4–10	3.1 (1.8–8.2)	4–10	110	U, T
422	Minocycline	Oral	0.1 (S)	9	11–20	2.05 (1.56–2.55)	2.5–3	1.82 (0.99–1.43)	2.5–3	94	U, UR
Others											
663	Azithromycin	Oral	0.25 (M)	14	56	<0.1	14	2.54	11–18	>2,000	U
646	Carumonam	IV	1.0 (S)	4		29.0 (25–33.3)	1.3	5.7 (2.8–8.9)	1.3	20	U
664	Clarithromycin	Oral	0.75 (M)	45	3–5	1.51 (±0.57)	7	3.83 (±2.14)	7	253	U, O
665	Erythromycin gluceptate	Oral	0.250 (M)	9	1.5	0.42 (0.23–1.16)	2	0.58 (0.14–1.05)	2	138	U, T, B, UR
666	Myocamicin	Oral	0.6 (S)	5		2.6 (1.7–3.4)	1.0	3.8 (2.7–4.2)	1.0	146	U
665	Rosamicin	Oral	0.250 (M)	9	3.1	0.07 (0.06–0.14)	2	2.4 (0.5–3.8)	2	3,430	U, T, B, UR
667	Spiramycin	Oral	1.0 (M)	22	0.5	(0.3–0.7)	12–15	~9.0 (7–13)	12–15	1,800	U, T
668	Sulfamethoxazole	IM	0.400 (S)	6	11.0	17.8 (12.1–23.2)	4	5.19 (3.2–6.51)	4	29	U, T, O, B
668	Sulfamethoxazole	Oral	0.800 (S)	5	11.0	26.2 (2.3–32.9)	4	7.11 (0.45–13.4)	4	27	U, T, O, B
668	Sulfamethoxazole	Oral	0.800 (M)	8	11.0	65.9 (40–108)	4	34.9 (19–64)	4	53	U, T, O, B
669	Thiamphenicol	IV	1.0 (S)	11	1.5	20.7 (9.6–35)	0.8	32.1 (8.5–64.4)	0.8	191	U, T, O, A
668	Trimethoprim	IM	0.080 (S)	6	14.5	0.40 (0.22–0.51)	4	1.55 (0.81–2.5)	4	387	U, T, O, B
668	Trimethoprim	Oral	0.160 (S)	5	14.5	0.98 (0.4–1.3)	4	2.84 (0.47–5.0)	4	290	U, T, O, B
668	Trimethoprim	Oral	0.160 (S)	8	14.5	2.39 (0.7–3.0)	4	5.54 (4.1–27)	4	232	U, T, O, B

[a]IM, intramuscularly; IV, intravenously.
[b]S, single dose; M, multiple dose.
[c]U, uninfected; UR, transurethral resection of prostate; T, prostate tissue; B, benign; O, open prostatectomy; A, prostate adenoma; I, infected; H, hetacillin ester given to patients, ampicillin measured in serum and tissue; E, extrapolated from graphs.

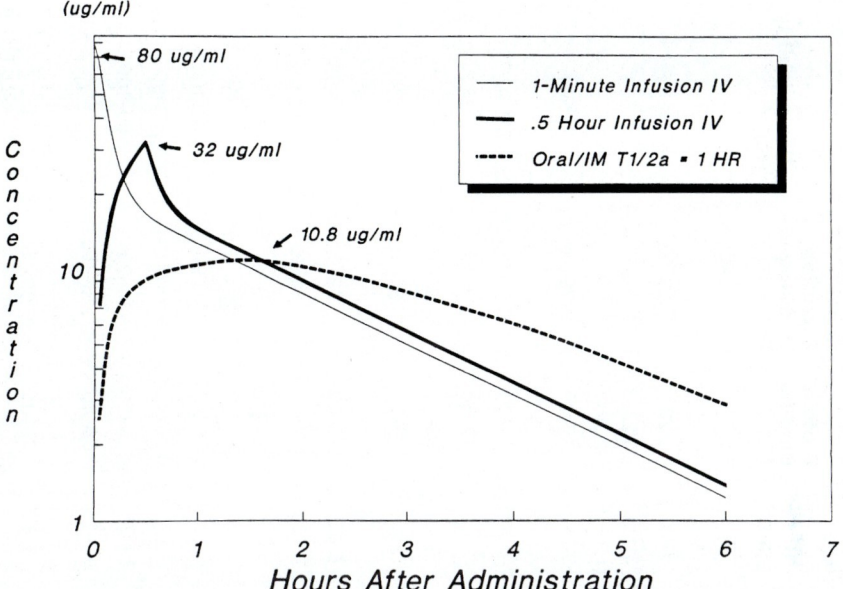

Figure 14.2 ■ **Serum kinetics of a single 1-g dose of an antimicrobial given by intravenous (*IV*) bolus infusion, 0.5-hour IV infusion, oral administration, or intramuscular (*IM*) injection.** An absorption half-life ($T_{1/2a}$) of 1 hour was assumed for the oral and intramuscular administrations.

administration. Generally, intravenous administration is achieved through a zero-order process (constant rate of administration over time) and intramuscular and oral administrations are thought to follow a first-order process (Fick's law of passive diffusion). Intramuscular and oral absorption rates are also influenced by a number of local factors, such as pH, gastrointestinal motility, dosage form, food, and muscle perfusion, to mention a few; each of which may be significant. As a result, peak serum concentration following intramuscular or oral administration tends to be lower and less predictable than that after intravenous administration. Again, the simulations in Figure 14.2, in which the oral and intramuscular half-life of drug absorption ($T_{1/2a}$) was held constant (1 hour) and the intravenous rates differ, show the effects observed by simply changing the rate of antibiotic administration.

Distribution

Once the antibiotic reaches the general circulation (central compartment), the antibiotic begins to diffuse into other body spaces and tissues (peripheral compartments) not at equilibrium with the central compartment (Fig. 14.1). This process is often referred to as *distribution*, and the time

period during which this is most evident on the serum concentration–time curve is often referred to as the *distribution phase* or α-phase. Although distribution takes place following all forms of antimicrobial administration, the distribution phase is most apparent immediately following intravenous bolus or short infusion, which makes timing of sample collection most critical for concentration comparisons. The distribution phase of the serum concentration–time curve is generally short-lived (less than 1 hour); however, minor differences in the time of serum sample collection during the distribution phase may result in major differences in antimicrobial concentrations and therefore interpretation. Because of the difficulty in timing and collecting samples in and around the distribution phase of the curve, peak serum concentration data reported in the literature are often conflicting and misleading. The distribution phase for most antibiotics is of brief duration and is difficult to characterize. In order to avoid confusion and subsequent misinterpretation, many authors choose not to sample during the distribution phase but rather report the time at which serum samples for determination of antibiotic concentration were obtained following antibiotic administration. Data on achievable serum

(continued on page 756)

TABLE 14.21

Serum Kinetics and Urinary Excretion of Antimicrobials in Humans

Antimicrobial	Dosage/Route[a]	Sampling Time[b]	Serum Concentration (μg/mL)[c]	Half-life (h) Normal	Half-life (h) ESRD[d]	Protein Binding (%)	Renal Excretion Unchanged (%)	Bioavailability (%)[e]
Amikacin	7.5 mg/kg IM 7.5 mg/kg IV	1 h 0.5 h	21 15–25	2–3	30	0–5	>90	T1
Amoxicillin	0.5 g orally	2 h	8	0.8–2	7–20	20	60–98	80 F
Amoxicillin/ clavulanic acid	0.5 g orally/ 0.5 g orally	1 h	7.6/2.3	0.8–2/0.8–1	7–20	20/22–30	60–98/28–47	80 F
Ampicillin	0.5 g orally 0.5 g IM	1 h 1 h	2 8	0.8–1.8	7–20	17–20	79–92	50 F
Ampicillin/sulbactam	0.5 g IV/0.5 g IV	1 h	14/20	0.8–1.8/1–1.3	7–20/21	17–20/21	17–20/38	79–92/75
Azithromycin	0.5 g orally	2–4 h	0.3–0.63	35–60		12–50	4–12	37 F
Azlocillin	2 g IV	5 min	142–363	0.8–1.5	5–6	30–46	50–75	
Aztreonam	1 g IV (0.5-h infusion) 1 g IM	125 1 h	1.6–1.7 46.5	1.6–1.7	8.4	56	65–94	
Bacampicillin	0.4 g orally	1 h	2.7	0.8–1.5	6–20	17–20	79–92	87–98
Carbenicillin	1 g IM 1 g IV	0.5–2 h 0.25 h	15–20 71–140	1.1	10–20	50	80–90	
(Indanyl salt)	0.382 g orally	0.5–1 h	5.1–6.5					30
Cefaclor	1 g orally	0.5–1 h	23	0.5–1	2.8	25	>90	70–100 F
Cefaclor MR	0.75 g orally	2.9 h	9.1 (±1.8 SD)	1.2		25	71	>90
Cefadroxil	1 g orally	1–2	28–35	1.2–1.7	20–25	20	>90	80–100 F
Cefamandole	1 g IM 1 g IV	0.5–2 h 10 min	25 140	0.5–1	7.9–18	56–80	75–100	
Cefazolin	1 g IM 1 g IV	1 h 5 min	60 190	1.4–2.5	18–36	70–85	90–96	
Cefdinir	0.3 g orally 0.6 g orally	224* min 223* min	2.00* 4.20*					

Cefepime	1 g IM 1 g IV	0.5–1.5 h	30–74 67	2	13.5	16–19	99	
Cefepime	2 g IV (M)	0.5 h (±0.05 SD)	127.85 (±27.51 SD)		2.96			
Cefetamet	1 g orally	3–5 h	5.5–6.5	2–2.5	11–30	22	90	30–50 F
Cefixime	0.2 g orally	2–6 h	1–4	3–9	11.5	65–69	20–50	50
Cefmenoxime	1 g IM 1 g IV	40 h 2 min	27 100	0.9–1.6	6–26	77–84	67–86	
Cefmetazole	30 mg/kg IM 30 mg/kg IV	0.5–0.75 h 1 h	80 97	0.8–1.8	15	68	71	
Cefodizime	1 g IM 1 g IV	1 h	75 177–215	2.5–3.7	7.7	81	69–95	88–100
Cefonicid	1 g IM 1 g IV	1 h 5 min	99 220	3.5–4.8	65	95–98	90–99	
Cefoperazone	1 g IM 1 g IV	1 h 5 min	63 200	1.6–2.4	2.1–2.5	82–93	75–99	
Ceforanide	1 g IM 1 g IV	1 h 0.25 h	70–80 140	2.2–3.5	25	80	85–95	
Cefotaxime	1 g IM 1 g IV (active metabolite)	0.5 h 5 min	21–25 100	1	2.6	35–51	40–60	
Cefotetan	1 g IM 1 g IV	1.5 h 2 min	75 140–240	3–4.6	10–20	78–91	66–100	
Cefotiam	1 g IV 1 g IM	0.25 h 0.75 h	77.6 13.5	0.6–1.5	5.3	62	50–67	
Cefoxitin	1 g IM 1 g IV	0.5 h 5 min	24–28 110	0.7–1	13–22	65–79	85–90	
Cefpirome	1 g IM 1 g IV	1.5 h 5 min	32 80–100	2	14.5	10	80–90	92–98
Cefpodoxime	0.2 g orally	2–3 h	2.5	2.5	9.8	18–23	80	41–50 FE
Cefprozil	1 g orally	1–2 h	18	1–2	6	35–45	89–95	

(Continued)

Table 14.21 (Continued)

Serum Kinetics and Urinary Excretion of Antimicrobials in Humans

Antimicrobial	Dosage/Route[a]	Sampling Time[b]	Serum Concentration (μg/mL)[c]	Half-life (h) Normal	Half-life (h) ESRD[d]	Protein Binding (%)	Renal Excretion Unchanged (%)	Bioavailability (%)[e]
Cefsulodin	1 g IM	1.5 h	20	1.7–2	10–13	15–30	50–70	
Ceftaroline	0.6 IV	0.92h	21.3	2.66	NA	20	88	
Ceftazidime	1 g IM / 1 g IV	1 h / 5 min	40 / 105	1.4–2	19–24	5–17	75–90	
Ceftibuten	0.2 g orally	2–3 h	11.6	1.5–2.5	18–29	65–77		80
Ceftizoxime	1 g IM / 1 g IV	1 h / 5 min	40 / 113	1.4–1.7	30–36	30–50	85–95	
Ceftriaxone	1 g IM / 1 g IV (0.5-h infusion)	1 h / 5 min	62–83 / 100–175	7.7–8.6	12–18	83–95	65–95	
Cefuroxime	1 g IM	1 h	40	1.1–2.2	15–22	33–50	95	
Cefuroxime	0.5 g IV	1 h	42–66					
Cefuroxime axetil	1 g orally	1.8 h	11					36–50 FE
Cephalexin	1 g orally	1 h	32	0.9	20–40	15	91–100	90–100 F
Cephaloridine	1 g IM	0.5–1 h	30	1–1.5	3–11	20	70–85	
Cephalothin	1 g IM / 1 g IV	0.5 h / 2 min	20 / 30	0.5–1	3–19	65–80	50–70	
Cephapirin	1 g IM / 1 g IV (also active metabolite)	0.5–1 h / 5 min	10–17 / 70	0.3–0.8	1.75–2.5	45–50	30–70	
Cephradine	0.5 g orally / 1 g IM / 1 g IV	1 h / 1 h / 5 min	11–16.6 / 4.4–14 / 60–86	0.6–0.7		8–17	80–100	90–100 F
Chloramphenicol base	1 g orally	0.5–4 h	10–13	1.6–4	3.2–7	50–60	5–15 (base)	76–93
Chloramphenicol succinate	1 g IV	0.5–1 h	4.9–12					70 IS

Chloramphenicol succinate	1 g IM	5–6						80
Chloramphenicol palmitate							F
Cinoxacin	0.5	2–4 h	10.8 ±5.7	1.1–2.7	8.5–12.1	63–73	60	
Ciprofloxacin	0.5 g orally 0.1 g IV	1–2 h	1.9–2.9	3–6	6–8.7	40	30–50	60–80 F
Clarithromycin	0.25 g orally	2	0.58–0.8	3–5[h]		42–50	20–30	50 F
Clindamycin	0.15 g orally 0.3 g IM 0.6 g IV	1 h 1–3 h	2–3 6 10	2–4	3–5	60–95		90
Cloxacillin	0.5 g orally	1–2 h	2–9	0.5	1–3	95	70–90	50–77 F
Colistin	2 mg/kg IM	1–2	5–13	2.7–4.8	48–72		>75	
Cyclacillin	0.5 g orally	1 h	11–12	0.5–0.6	8–10	18–25	65–85	95
Daptomycin	4 mg/kg IV	0.5 h	77.5** (±8.3 SD)**		7.74 (±0.63 SD)	90%	59.7 (±10.2 SD)	
Demeclocycline	0.3 g orally	4 h	1–2	10–15	1–2	41–90	38–56	F
Dicloxacillin	1 g orally 0.25 g IM	1 h 1 h	10–15 5	0.5	1–2	88–98	60–90	50
Dirithromycin[i]	0.5 g orally	4–4.5 h	01–0.5; E[j] 0.3	E[j] 20–50		E[j] 15–30	<5	6–14 FE
Dirithromycin	0.5 g orally (M)	24 h	0.17 (±0.03 SD)					
Doripenem	0.5 g IV	1 h	23	1	NA	8–9	70	
Doxycycline	1.2 g orally 0.2 g IV	2 h 0.25 h	2–3 6.4	12–22	16–24	80–95	35–40	90
Ertapenem	1.0 g IV	2 h	83	4	NA	85–95	80	
Erythromycin	0.5 g orally		0.3–1.9	1.2–2.6	4–6	75–90	2–15	F
Erythromycin estolate ester	0.5 g orally		4 (80% ester)					
Erythromycin ethylsuccinate ester	0.5 g orally		1.5 (66% ester)					

(Continued)

Table 14.21 (Continued)

Serum Kinetics and Urinary Excretion of Antimicrobials in Humans

Antimicrobial	Dosage/Route[a]	Sampling Time[b]	Serum Concentration (μg/mL)[c]	Half-life (h) Normal	Half-life (h) ESRD[d]	Protein Binding (%)	Renal Excretion Unchanged (%)	Bioavailability (%)[e]
Erythromycin stearate	0.5 g orally	3 h	0.13–1.3 (base)					F
Erythromycin lactobionate	1 g IV	1 h	10					
Erythromycin glucceptate	1 g IV	1 h	9.9					
Enoxacin	0.4 g orally	1–6 h	2.8–3.6	3.4–6.4	30	18–30	26–72	80–98
Fleroxacin	0.4 g orally	1–2 h	4.4–6.8	8–13		23–32	50–77	>95
Floxacillin	0.5 g orally	1 h	11–20	0.75–1.5		92–94	40–70	50–54 F
Garenoxacin	0.6 g orally	3.26 h	10.03** (2.80 SD)					
Gatifloxacin	0.4 g orally	1.8 h	4.1** (±0.86 SD)		6.8 (±0.72 SD)	20%	65 (±15 SD)	
Gemifloxacin	0.32 g orally	1.2 h	2.31** (±0.55 SD)		5.9 (+0.44 SD)		36.1 (±7.5 SD)	
Gentamicin	1 mg/kg IM 1.5 mg/kg IV	0.5 h	4 4–8	1–3	24–48	0–5	>90	TI
Imipenem/cilastitin	1 g IV (0.5-h infusion)		19–60	0.9–1.3	3	13–25	5–42	
Josamycin	0.5 g orally	1 h	0.65	0.9–2		15	<20	F
Kanamycin	7.5 mg/kg IM 7.5 mg/kg IV	1 h 0.5 h	22 20–25	2–3	27–30	0–5	>90	TI
Latamoxef	0.5 g IV 1 g IM	15 min 0.5–1 h	42 52	2–2.8	19.3	52	67–87	
Levofloxacin	0.1 g orally	1 h	1.4–1.8	6–7		50	61–86	>95 F
Levofloxacin	0.5 g orally (M) 0.75 g orally (M)	4 h 4 h	5.29** (±1.23 SD) 11.98** (±2.99 SD)					

Lincomycin	0.5 g orally 0.6 g IM 0.6 g IV	2–4 h 1–2 h	6–12 12–20					10–70	20–30 F
Linezolid	0.6 g orally (M)	4 h	15.5** (±4.9 SD)	6.9			31	30	100
Lomefloxacin	0.4 g orally	1–2 h	3.5–4.7	6.4–7.7	21–38	20	57–76	F
Loracarbef	0.2 g orally	1 h	8	0.7–1.2			59–66	90
Mecillinam (amdinocillin)	10 mg/kg IV 10 mg/kg IM	0 h 0.5 h	32–70 26	1	3–6	5–10	65	
Meropenem	1 g IV (S)	0.5 h	25.96** (±22.16 SD)	1	3.4–20	2	70	
Methicillin	1 g IM 1 g IV	0.5 h 60	10–15	0.5–1	4	28–49	62–80	
Metronidazole	0.5 g orally	1–2 h	12	6–12	8–15	<20	20	>80
Mezlocillin	1 g IM 1 g IV	0.75–1 h 5 min	15.4 64–142	0.7–1.1	2.5–5.5	45	61–72	
Minocycline	0.2 g IV (0.5–1-h infusion) 0.2 g orally	5 min 1 h	2.5–6.6 0.7–4.4	11–20	17–69	60–75	10–13	90 F
Moxalactam	1 g IM 1 g IV	1–2 h 0.25 h	27 101	1.7–2.3	18–23	35–50	67–90	
Moxifloxacin	0.4 g orally (S)	2.2 h	3.22 (±1.25 SD)					
Nafcillin	1 g IM	1 h	8	0.5–1	1.5	87–90	31–40	10–20
Nalidixic acid	1 g orally	1 h	15–50	6–7	21	0–5	0.5–30	F
Netilmicin	1 mg/kg IM 2 mg/kg IV	0.5 h	4 7	2.7	40	0–5	>90	TI
Nitrofurantoin	0.1 g orally		<2	0.3–1	1	90	27–56	80–95 D, FE
Norfloxacin	0.4 g orally	1–1.5 h	1.5	2–4	8.34	10–15	12–30	30–40
Ofloxacin	0.3 g orally	1–2 h	2.8–5.3	5–7.5	20	41	96	
Oritavancin	0.2 g orally (M) 0.8 g orally (S)	1.0 1.5	46.2** (±10.7 SD) 137** (±28.6 SD)	151 (±39 SD) 204 (±162)				

(Continued)

Table 14.21 (Continued)

Serum Kinetics and Urinary Excretion of Antimicrobials in Humans

Antimicrobial	Dosage/Route[a]	Sampling Time[b]	Serum Concentration (μg/mL)[c]	Half-life (h) Normal	Half-life (h) ESRD[d]	Protein Binding (%)	Renal Excretion Unchanged (%)	Bioavailability (%)[e]
Oxacillin	1 g orally 1 g IV 0.5 g IM	1 h 1 h 0.5 h	5–10 15.9 15	0.5	1	92–95	39–66	30–88 F
Oxytetracycline	0.5 g orally 0.25 g IM	3 h 2 h	0.5–2.3 1.4	8.5–9.6	50	20–40	60–70	75 F
Pefloxacin	0.4 g orally		3.8–5.6	8–14	16.4	20–30	8–9	80–98
Penicillin G	5 × 10⁶ units IV 1 × 10⁶ units IM	10 min 0.5 h	273 12	0.5	6–20	40–60	70–85	20–30
Penicillin V	0.5 g orally		3					60
Piperacillin	2 g IM 2 g IV	0.5 h 10 min	36 164–225	1.3	3–5	16–22	74–89	
Piperacillin/tazobactam	4 g IV/0.5 g IV		298/34	0.7–1.3/0.89	3–5	16–48/ 20–30	74–89	
Pivmecillin	0.4 g orally	1–2 h	2–5.1	1	3–6	5–10	65	F
Polymyxin B	50 mg IM	2 h	1–8	6	48–72	Low	60	
Rosoxacin	0.25 g orally	2–2.5 h	4.9	2–6			4	
Roxithromycin	0.3 g orally	2 h	10	12		85–95	10	F
Sparfloxacin	0.2 g orally	2.7–5.6 h	0.7–1.6	14–18			7–12	
Streptomycin	1 g IM	1 h	25–50	2.5	100	35	>90	TI
Sulfamethoxazole	2 g orally 0.8 g IV (1-h infusion)	2–4 h	50–120 46.3	9–12	20–50	62–70		95–100g
Sulfisoxazole	2 g IV 2 g IM	Mean concentration 1–4 h	16.7 16	4.6–8.3	11	85	40–60	96

Drug	Dose[a]	Time[b]						
Sultamicillin (prodrug of ampicillin/sulbactam)	0.5 g orally	1–2	Ampicillin, 5.6/ sulbactam, 4.0	0.8–1.8/1–1.3	7–20/21	17–20/38	79–92/75	80
Telithromycin	0.8 g orally (M)	2 h	1.14** (0.53–1.85)	9.8		60–70	13	57
Temocillin	1 g IV	5 min	161	4–6	26	63–88	70–85	
Tetracycline	0.5 g orally	2–3 h	3–4	8–10	15–100	25	65	75 F
Ticarcillin	1 g IM / 3 g IV	0.5–1 h / 0.25 h	21–31 / 190	1.2	13–16	45–65	80–99	
Ticarcillin/clavulanic acid	3 g IV/0.2 g IV	15 min	277/11.4	1.2/0.8–1	13–16	45–65/9	80–99	
Tigecycline	0.1 g IV	1 h	0.604	42.4		71–89	33	
Tobramycin	1 mg/kg IM / 1.5 mg/kg IV	0.5 h	4 / 4–8	2.5	56	0–5	>90	TI
Trimethoprim	0.16 g orally / 0.16 g IV (1-h infusion)	1–4 h	1–3 / 3.4	8–14	24–42	42–46		90 F
Vancomycin[k]	1 g IV (1-h infusion)	1–2 h	20–25	6–10	200–250	50–60	90–100	

[a] Single-dose studies, except for those denoted (M), which were multiple dose; IM, intramuscularly; intravenous (IV) doses were either bolus or infusions of less than 10-minute duration, except where noted.

[b] Time serum sample was taken after dose administration was completed; chosen to be near the peak level just following the distribution phase.

[c] Serum concentration data reported as a mean or range. *, values reported as median; **, concentrations measured in plasma.

[d] End-stage renal disease.

[e] IS, inactive succinate partially hydrolyzed to base, 30% excreted as inactive succinate by kidneys; TI, therapeutic index is low, serum concentrations are highly variable, recommend monitoring serum concentrations; F, food may alter bioavailability; FE, food may enhance bioavailability; D, bioavailability may be affected by dosage form.

[f] Protein binding is concentration-dependent.

[g] MR, modified release.

[h] Metabolism may be saturable.

[i] Rapidly metabolized tothromyclamine.

[j] E, erythromyclamine-active metabolites.

[k] Timing of samples is critical because of a significant α-phase; serum concentrations are highly variable.

concentrations in Table 14.21 are presented with the time at which samples were obtained. In general, intravenous administration results in serum concentrations that are greater than those following oral or intramuscular administration and are most vulnerable to misinterpretation due to the distribution phase.

Elimination

Elimination is the loss of active antibiotic from the body and is due to excretion and/or metabolism. Excretion is the loss of unchanged antibiotic, and metabolism is the loss due to conversion of the antibiotic to another chemical compound (metabolite). Metabolites may or may not have antimicrobial activity. For most antibiotics, elimination is a first-order process, which simply means that serum concentration declines exponentially with time:

$$C_t = C \times e^{-k_{el} \times t}$$

where C is serum concentration, C_t is the serum concentration at some time t after C was determined, and k_{ef} is an elimination rate constant. With first-order elimination, the time for the serum concentration to decline by one-half (half-life) is constant:

$$t_{1/2} = (\ln 2)/k_{el}$$

where $t_{1/2}$ is the serum half-life and k_{ef} is the elimination rate constant. Knowing the serum half-life, one can then estimate the fraction of the dose that remains in the body at any time after the dose was given:

$$\text{Fraction remaining} = e^{-0.693n}$$

where n is the number of half-lives that have elapsed since the dose was administered.

Renal Excretion

Most antimicrobials are eliminated in the urine, either unchanged or as metabolites. The data on achievable urinary concentration are often difficult to interpret. Urinary concentrations are constantly changing as a function of changing serum concentration and urine volume. The fraction of drug in general circulation that is excreted unchanged in the urine, fe, is a pharmacokinetic parameter that describes the contribution of urinary elimination to the overall elimination of antibiotic from the body.

fe = total drug excreted unchanged/total dose

The percentage of antibiotic excreted unchanged (fe 100) is high for antibiotics with renal excretion as the sole or primary route of elimination and low for antibiotics that are not readily excreted in the urine or that undergo significant metabolism. Determination of fe requires both an assay that is specific for the parent compound and a sampling time sufficiently long to ensure complete urinary excretion (at least five times the half-life).

Appendix 14.1 shows urinary excretion, metabolites, and reported urine levels for some selected antimicrobial agents.

Disease and Other Factors

A number of diseases are known to influence the absorption, distribution, and elimination of antimicrobials. Absorption may be enhanced or impaired by a number of factors. Gastrointestinal surgery, achlorhydria, malabsorption syndrome, stress, formulation differences, other drugs, and food are some of the more common conditions or factors that may alter drug absorption. Similarly, a number of conditions are associated with altered elimination. The two most readily identifiable conditions are decreased kidney function (renal excretion) and decreased hepatic function (metabolism). Each may be due to intrinsic loss of functional tissue alone or may be due to other causes such as decreased cardiac output, which may result in decreased blood flow to the kidney or liver (163–165). Severe peripheral vascular disease has been demonstrated to diminish the skeletal muscle concentration of gentamicin after a single intravenous dose (166). Data from human subjects with underlying conditions or disease states or from persons taking any other medications must be interpreted with caution.

Studies have used the microdialysis method to compare the tissue pharmacokinetics of antimicrobials in healthy individuals with those of critically ill with sepsis. Joukhadar et al. (167) found that the AUC in serum of piperacillin to be marginally reduced in critically ill patients with sepsis compared with healthy controls. However, the interstitial muscle and subcutaneous skin concentrations of piperacillin were markedly reduced in critically ill patients compared with that of healthy controls, with maximal antimicrobials in tissues in critically ill patients only about 10% of those in healthy controls. Tegeder et al. (63) found the AUC of imipenem in serum to be similar in critically ill patients compared with that of healthy controls, but the AUC in interstitial fluid of muscle and subcutaneous tissue of skin were markedly lower in critically ill patients than in healthy controls. Further, the C_{max} exceeded the usual minimum inhibitory concentration cutoff of 4 µg/mL in only one of four patients after administration of appropriate doses based on renal function. Studies performed with linezolid revealed a higher volume of distribution and increased clearance rates in septic patients, with a high degree of patient variability, and suggested that critically ill patients may need more frequent dosing (168).

The data in Table 14.21 have been extracted from published scientific literature and the respective manufacturer's published product information. All data are listed either as a mean value or as a range of values. The purpose of Table 14.21 is to serve as a general reference for the comparative evaluation of the basic pharmacokinetics of antimicrobials. Except where noted, listed serum concentrations and the sampling times, percentage renally excreted, and bioavailability are from single-dose studies. Elimination half-life data are broken into two categories: those from young healthy adults (normal) and those from persons with end-stage renal disease. As previously mentioned, most antimicrobials are eliminated to varying degrees by glomerular filtration or tubular secretion. Percentage renal excretion is that percentage of a single dose that has been reported to be recovered in the urine as the active parent compound. Some antimicrobials have metabolites with significant antimicrobial activity and are noted.

QUALITY CONTROL

The major considerations in quality control of antimicrobial determinations in extravascular sites are proper specimen processing and adequate controls for assay procedures. Blood and body fluid contamination (particularly urine and bile) are the most serious concerns in specimen processing, but care must also be given to possible drug inactivation due to prolonged vigorous specimen preparations such as are often used in assays of bone. These issues have been discussed earlier in the chapter and recommendations were made for optimal handling of specimens.

Problems in quality control of assays center primarily on the use of proper diluents in the preparation of standard curves for biologic assays. Again, these principles have been thoroughly discussed earlier in the chapter.

Finally, of major concern is the proper interpretation of extravascular antimicrobial concentrations with regard to any clinical application of this information. Clinical correlations of infection cure as a function of local antimicrobial concentration are still imperfect and probably will remain so until more definitive information becomes available.

ACKNOWLEDGMENTS

This chapter was based extensively on the work of Drs. Lance Peterson, Carolyn Hughes, Tom Larson, Darcie Bridwell, and Christopher Shain from previous editions of this text. Michelle Beattie and Susan Sanders have provided valued assistance in the literature search.

REFERENCES

1. Bamberger DM, Herndon BL, Suvarna PR. The effect of zinc on microbial growth and bacterial killing by cefazolin a Staphylococcus aureus abscess milieu. *J Infect Dis* 1993;168:893–896.
2. Gerding DN, Peterson LR. Comparative tissue and extravascular fluid concentrations of ceftizoxime. *J Antimicrob Chemother* 1982;10(Suppl C):105–116.
3. Gerding DN, Peterson LR, Legler DC, et al. Ascitic fluid cephalosporin concentrations: influence of protein binding and serum pharmacokinetics. *Antimicrob Agents Chemother* 1978;14:234–239.
4. Gerding DN, Peterson LR, Salomonson JK, et al. Prediction of the concentration of penicillins in ascitic fluid from serum kinetics and protein binding of the antibiotics in serum and ascitic fluid of dogs. *J Infect Dis* 1978;138:166–173.
5. Chisholm GD, Waterworth PM, Calnan JS, et al. Concentration of antibacterial agents in interstitial tissue fluid. *Br Med J* 1973;1:569–573.
6. Gerding DN, Hall WH, Schierl EA, et al. Cephalosporin and aminoglycoside concentrations in peritoneal capsular fluid in rabbits. *Antimicrob Agents Chemother* 1976;10:902–911.
7. Peterson LR, Gerding DN. Prediction of cefazolin penetration into high- and low-protein-containing extravascular fluid: new method for performing simultaneous studies. *Antimicrob Agents Chemother* 1978;14:533–538.
8. Dixon RL, Owens ES, Rall DP. Evidence of active transport of benzyl-^{14}C-penicillin from cerebrospinal fluid to blood. *J Pharm Sci* 1969;58:1106–1109.
9. Mouton JW, Theuretzbacher U, Craig WA, et al. Tissue concentrations: do we ever learn? *J Antimicrob Chemother* 2008;61:235–237.
10. Raeburn JA. A review of experimental models for studying the tissue penetration of antibiotics in man. *Scand J Infect Dis* 1978;14(Suppl):225–227.

11. Rebuck JW, Crowley JH. A method of studying leukocytic functions in vivo. *Ann NY Acad Sci* 1955;59:757–805.

12. Gillett AP, Wise R. Penetration of four cephalosporins into tissue fluid in man. *Lancet* 1978;1:962–964.

13. Peterson LR, Van Etta LL, Gerding DN. Interstitial concentration of antibiotics. *J Antimicrob Chemother* 1981;8:425.

14. Peterson LR, Schierl EA, Hall WH. Effect of protein concentration and binding on antibiotic assays. *Antimicrob Agents Chemother* 1975;7:540–542.

15. Tan JS, Trott A, Phair JP, et al. A method for measurement of antibiotics in human interstitial fluid. *J Infect Dis* 1972;126:492–497.

16. Tan JS, Salstrom SJ. Levels of carbenicillin, ticarcillin, cephalothin, cefazolin, cefamandole, gentamicin, tobramycin and amikacin in human serum and interstitial fluid. *Antimicrob Agents Chemother* 1977;11:698–700.

17. Tan JS, Salstrom SJ. Bacampicillin, ampicillin, cephalothin and cephapirin levels in human blood and interstitial fluid. *Antimicrob Agents Chemother* 1979;15:510–512.

18. Tan JS, Salstrom S, Signs SA, et al. Pharmacokinetics of intravenous cefmetazole with emphasis on comparison between predicted theoretical levels in tissue and actual skin window fluid levels. *Antimicrob Agents Chemother* 1989;33:924–927.

19. Kiistala V, Mustakallio KK. Dermo-epidermal separation with suction: electron microscopic and histochemical study of initial events of blistering of human skin. *J Invest Dermatol* 1967;48:466–467.

20. Simon VC, Malerczyk V. Serum and skin blister levels of cefadroxil in comparison to cephalexin. In: *Program and abstracts of the 18th Interscience Conference on Antimicrobial Agents and Chemotherapy*. Washington, DC: American Society for Microbiology; 1978. Abstract 225.

21. Wise R, Dyhs A, Hegarty A, et al. Pharmacokinetics and tissue penetration of aztreonam. *Antimicrob Agents Chemother* 1982;22:969–971.

22. Hoffstedt B, Walder M. Influence of serum protein binding and mode of administration on penetration of five cephalosporins into subcutaneous tissue fluid in humans. *Antimicrob Agents Chemother* 1981;20:783–786.

23. Hoffstedt B, Walder M. Penetration of ampicillin, doxycycline and gentamicin into interstitial fluid in rabbits and of penicillin V and pivampicillin in humans measured with subcutaneously implanted cotton threads. *Infection* 1981;9:7–11.

24. Howell A, Sutherland R, Rolinson GN. Effect of protein binding on levels of ampicillin and cloxacillin in synovial fluid. *Clin Pharmacol Ther* 1972;13:724–732.

25. Muller M, Haag O, Burgdorff T, et al. Characterization of peripheral-compartment kinetics of antibiotics by in vivo microdialysis in humans. *Antimicrob Agents Chemother* 1996;40:2703–2709.

26. Muller M, Rohde B, Kovar A, et al. Relationship between serum and free interstitial concentrations of cefodizime and cefpirome in muscle and subcutaneous adipose tissue of healthy volunteers measured by microdialysis. *J Clin Pharmacol* 1997;37:1108–1113.

27. Kaplan JM, McCracken GH, Snyder E. Influence of methodology upon apparent concentrations of antibiotics in tissues. *Antimicrob Agents Chemother* 1973;3:143–146.

28. Parker CW. Radioimmunoassay. *Annu Rev Pharmacol Toxicol* 1981;21:113–132.

29. Voller A, Bidwell DE, Bartlett A. Enzyme immunoassays in diagnostic medicine. *Bull World Health Organ* 1976;53:55–65.

30. Sabath LD. The assay of antimicrobial compounds. *Hum Pathol* 1976;7:287–295.

31. Yoshikawa TT, Maitra SK, Schotz MC, et al. High-pressure liquid chromatography for quantitation of antimicrobial agents. *Rev Infect Dis* 1980;2:169–181.

32. Fasching CE, Peterson LR. Anion-exchange extraction of cephapirin, cefotaxime, and cefoxitin from serum for liquid chromatography. *Antimicrob Agents Chemother* 1982;21:628–633.

33. Fasching CE, Peterson LR. High-pressure liquid chromatographic assay of azlocillin and mezlocillin with an anion-exchange extraction technique. *J Liq Chromatogr* 1983;6:2513–2520.

34. Fasching CE, Peterson LR, Bettin KM, et al. High-pressure liquid chromatographic assay of ceftizoxime with an anion-exchange extraction technique. *Antimicrob Agents Chemother* 1982;22:336–337.

35. Landersdorfer DB, Bulitta JB, Kinzig M, et al. Penetration of antibacterials into bone pharmacokinetic, pharmacodynamic and bioanalytical considerations. *Clin Pharmacokinet* 2009;48:89–124.

36. Rauws AG, Van Klingeren B. Estimation of antibiotic levels of interstitial fluid from whole tissue levels. *Scand J Infect Dis* 1978;14(Suppl):186–188.

37. Bergan T. Pharmacokinetics of tissue penetration of antibiotics. *Rev Infect Dis* 1981;3:45–66.

38. Plaue VR, Bethke RO, Fabricius K, et al. Kritische Untersuchungen zur Methodik von Antibiotikaspiegelbestimmungen in Menschlichen Geweben. *Arzneimittelforschung* 1980;30:1–5.

39. Kunin CM. Binding of antibiotics to tissue homogenates. *J Infect Dis* 1970;121:55–64.

40. Peterson LR, Gerding DN. Influence of protein binding of antibiotics on serum pharmacokinetics and extravascular penetration: clinically useful concepts. *Rev Infect Dis* 1980;2:340–348.

41. Peterson LR, Gerding DN, Zinneman HH, et al. Evaluation of three newer methods for investigating protein interactions of penicillin G. *Antimicrob Agents Chemother* 1977;11:993–998.

42. Peterson LR, Hall WH, Zinneman HH, et al. Standardization of a preparative ultracentrifuge method for quantitative determination of protein binding of seven antibiotics. *J Infect Dis* 1977;136:778–783.

43. Hitt JA, Gerding DN. Sputum antimicrobial levels and clinical outcome in bronchitis. *Semin Respir Infect* 1991;6:122–128.

44. Diaz Gomez ML, Rebora Guiterrez R, Galindo Hernandez E, et al. Cefadroxil, serum, and pleural fluid levels. In: *Program and abstracts of the 18th Interscience Conference on Antimicrobial Agents and Chemotherapy*. Washington, DC: American Society for Microbiology; 1978. Abstract 223.

45. Hall WH, Gerding DN, Schierl EA. Penetration of tobramycin into infected extravascular fluids and its therapeutic effectiveness. *J Infect Dis* 1977;135:957–961.

46. Kozak AJ, Gerding DN, Peterson LR, et al. Gentamicin intravenous infusion rate: effect on interstitial fluid concentration. *Antimicrob Agents Chemother* 1977;12:606–608.

47. Thys J, Klastersky J, Mombelli G. Peak or sustained antibiotic serum levels for optimal tissue penetration. *J Antimicrob Chemother* 1981;8(Suppl C):29–36.

48. Peterson LR, Gerding DN, Fasching CE. Effects of method of antibiotic administration on extravascular penetration: crossover study of cefazolin given by intermittent injection or constant infusion. *J Antimicrob Chemother* 1981;7:71–79.

49. Van Etta LL, Kravitz GR, Russ TE, et al. Effect of method of administration on extravascular penetration of four antibiotics. *Antimicrob Agents Chemother* 1982;21:873–880.

50. Cronberg S. A simple mathematical model of diffusion of drug into an infection site. *Scand J Infect Dis* 1978; 14(Suppl):100–104.

51. Gerding DN, Van Etta LL, Peterson LR. Role of serum protein binding and multiple antibiotic doses in the extravascular distribution of ceftizoxime and cefotaxime. *Antimicrob Agents Chemother* 1982;22:844–847.

52. Van Etta LL, Peterson LR, Fasching CE, et al. The effect of the ratio of surface area to volume on the penetration of antibiotics into extravascular spaces in an in vitro model. *J Infect Dis* 1982;146:423–428.

53. Gerding DN, Kromhout JP, Sullivan JJ, et al. Antibiotic penetrance of ascitic fluid in dogs. *Antimicrob Agents Chemother* 1976;10:850–855.

54. Gerding DN. Principles of antimicrobial therapy. In: Soule BM, ed. *The APIC curriculum for infection control practice.* Dubuque, IA: Kendall/Hunt Publishing Co, 1983: 508–509.

55. Benoni G, Arosio E, Raimondi MG, et al. Pharmacokinetics of ceftazidime and ceftriaxone and their penetration into the ascitic fluid. *J Antimicrob Chemother* 1985;16: 267–273.

56. el Touny M, el Guinaidy M, Abdel Bary M, et al. Pharmacokinetics of cefodizime in patients with liver cirrhosis and ascites. *Chemotherapy* 1992;38:201–205.

57. Grange JD, Gouyette A, Gutmann L, et al. Pharmacokinetics of amoxycillin/clavulanic acid in serum and ascitic fluid in cirrhotic patients. *J Antimicrob Chemother* 1989;23:605–611.

58. Hary L, Smail A, Ducroix JP, et al. Pharmacokinetics and ascitic fluid penetration of piperacillin in cirrhosis. *Fundam Clin Pharmacol* 1991;5:789–795.

59. Pfau A, Perlberg S, Shapira A. The pH of the prostatic fluid in health and disease: implications of treatment in chronic bacterial prostatitis. *J Urol* 1978;119:384–387.

60. Silvain C, Bouquet S, Breux JP, et al. Oral pharmacokinetics and ascitic fluid penetration of ofloxacin in cirrhosis. *Eur J Clin Pharmacol* 1989;37:261–265.

61. Van Gossum A, Quenon M, Van Gossum M, et al. Penetration of cefoperazone into ascites. *Eur J Clin Pharmacol* 1989;37:577–580.

62. Thys JP, Vanderhoeft P, Herchuelz A, et al. Penetration of aminoglycosides in uninfected pleural exudates and in pleural empyemas. *Chest* 1988;93:530–532.

63. Schurman OJ, Burton DS, Kajiyama G, et al. Sodium cephapirin disposition and distribution into human bone. *Curr Ther Res* 1976;20:194–203.

64. Tegeder I, Schmidtko A, Brautigam L, et al. Tissue distribution of imipenem in critically ill patients. *Clin Pharmacol Ther* 2002;71:325–333.

65. Webberly JM, Wise R, Andrews JM, et al. The pharmacokinetics and tissue penetration of FCE22101 following intravenous and oral administration. *J Antimicrob Chemother* 1988;21:445–450.

66. Nielson MW, Justesen T. Excretion of metronidazole in human bile. *Scand J Gastroenterol* 1977;12:1003–1008.

67. Blenkharn JI, Habib N, Mok D, et al. Decreased biliary excretion of piperacillin after percutaneous relief of extrahepatic obstructive jaundice. *Antimicrob Agents Chemother* 1985;28:778–780.

68. Brown RB, Martyak SN, Barza M, et al. Penetration of clindamycin phosphate into the abnormal human biliary tract. *Ann Intern Med* 1976;84:168–170.

69. Granai F, Smart HL, Triger DR. A study of the penetration of meropenem into bile using endoscopic retrograde cholangiography. *J Antimicrob Chemother* 1992;29:711–718.

70. Brogard JM, Blickle JF, Dorner M, et al. Biliary pharmacokinetic profile of piperacillin: experimental data and evaluation in man. *Int J Clin Pharmacol* 1990;28:462–470.

71. Brogard JM, Pinget M, Doffoel M, et al. Evaluation of the biliary excretion of penicillin G. *Chemotherapy* 1979; 25:129–139.

72. Brogard JM, Pinget M, Meyer C, et al. Biliary excretion of ampicillin: experimental and clinical study. *Chemotherapy* 1977;23:213–226.

73. Mendelson J, Portnoy J, Sigman H. Pharmacology of gentamicin in the biliary tract of humans. *Antimicrob Agents Chemother* 1973;4:538–541.

74. Mendelson J, Portnoy J, Sigman H, et al. Pharmacology of cephalothin in the biliary tract of humans. *Antimicrob Agents Chemother* 1974;6:659–665.

75. Bermudez RH, Lugo A, Ramirez-Ronda CH, et al. Amikacin sulfate levels in human serum and bile. *Antimicrob Agents Chemother* 1981;19:352–354.

76. Moorthi K, Wiederholt K. Is the administration of doxycycline still indicated in bacterial infections of the gallbladder and the bile ducts? *Eur J Clin Pharmacol* 1981;20: 35–38.

77. Binda GE, Domenichini E, Gottardi A, et al. Rifampicin, a general review. *Arzneimittelforschung* 1971;21:1942–1953.

78. Levi JU, Martinez OV, Malinin TI, et al. Decreased biliary excretion of cefamandole after percutaneous biliary decompression in patient with total common bile duct obstruction. *Antimicrob Agents Chemother* 1984;26:944–946.

79. Brogard JM, Haegele P, Dorner M, et al. Biliary excretion of a new semisynthetic cephalosporin, cephacetrile. *Antimicrob Agents Chemother* 1973;3:19–23.

80. Bouza E, Hellin T, Rodriquez-Creixems M, et al. Comparison of ceftazidime concentrations in bile and serum. *Antimicrob Agents Chemother* 1983;24:104–106.

81. Brogard JM, Kopferschmitt J, Pinget M, et al. Cefuroxime concentrations in serum, urine, and bile: pharmacokinetic profile. *Proc R Soc Med* 1977;70(Suppl 9):42–50.

82. Brogard JM, Kopferschmitt J, Arnaud JP, et al. Biliary elimination of mezlocillin: an experimental and clinical study. *Antimicrob Agents Chemother* 1980;18:69–76.

83. Keighley MRB, Drysdale RB, Quoraishi AH, et al. Antibiotics in biliary disease: the relative importance of antibiotic concentrations in bile and serum. *Gut* 1976;17: 495–500.

84. Smith BR, LeFrock J. Biliary tree penetration of parenteral antibiotics. *Infect Surg* 1983;2:110–121.

85. Nagar H, Berger SA. The excretion of antibiotics by the biliary tract. *Surg Gynecol Obstet* 1984;158:601–607.

86. Dooley JS, Hamilton-Miller JM, Brumfitt W, et al. Antibiotics in the treatment of biliary infection. *Gut* 1984; 25:988–998.

87. Honeybourne D, Baldwin DR. The site concentrations of antimicrobial agents in the lung. *J Antimicrob Chemother* 1992;30:249–260.

88. Bergogne-Berezin E, Berthelot G, Kafe H, et al. Influence of a fluidifying agent (bromhexine) on the penetration of antibiotics into respiratory secretions. *Int J Clin Pharmacol Res* 1985;5:341–344.

89. Braga PC, Scaglione F, Scarpazza G, et al. Comparison between penetration of amoxicillin combined with carbocysteine and amoxicillin alone in pathological bronchial secretions and pulmonary tissue. *Int J Clin Pharmacol Res* 1985;5:331–340.

90. Ricevuti G, Mazzone A, Vecilli E, et al. Influence of erdosteine, a mucolytic agent, on amoxycillin penetration into sputum in patients with an infective exacerbation of chronic bronchitis. *Thorax* 1988;43:585–590.

91. Maesen FPV, Davies BI, Drenth BMH, et al. Treatment of acute exacerbations of chronic bronchitis with cefotaxime: a controlled clinical trial. *J Antimicrob Chemother* 1980;6(Suppl A):187–192.

92. Bergogne-Berezin E, Even P, Berthelot G, et al. Cefuroxime: pharmacokinetic study in bronchial secretions. *Proc R Soc Med* 1977;70(Suppl 9):34–37.

93. Kontou P, Chatzika K, Pitsiou G, et al. Pharmacokinetics of ciprofloxacin and its penetration into bronchial secretions of mechanically ventilated patients with chronic pulmonary disease. *Antimicrob Agents Chemother* 2011;55(9):4149–4153.

94. Fick RB Jr, Alexander MR, Prince RA, et al. Penetration of cefotaxime into respiratory secretions. *Antimicrob Agents Chemother* 1987;31:815–817.

95. May JR, Delves DM. Treatment of chronic bronchitis with ampicillin: some pharmacological observations. *Lancet* 1965;1:929–933.

96. Klastersky J, Thys JP, Mombelli G. Comparative studies of intermittent and continuous administration of aminoglycosides in the treatment of bronchopulmonary infections due to Gram-negative bacteria. *Rev Infect Dis* 1981;3:74–83.

97. Lambert HP. Clinical significance of tissue penetration of antibiotics in the respiratory tract. *Scand J Infect Dis* 1978;14(Suppl):262–266.

98. Pennington JE. Penetration of antibiotics into respiratory secretions. *Rev Infect Dis* 1981;3:67–73.

99. Smith BR, LeFrock JL. Bronchial tree penetration of antibiotics. *Chest* 1983;83:904–908.

100. Wong GA, Pierce TH, Goldstein E, et al. Penetration of antimicrobial agents into bronchial secretions. *Am J Med* 1975;59:219–223.

101. Giamarellou H, Kolokythas E, Petrikkos G, et al. Pharmacokinetics of three newer quinolones in pregnant and lactating women. *Am J Med* 1989;87(Suppl 5A):49S–51S.

102. Matsuda S. Transfer of antibiotics into maternal milk. *Biol Res Pregnancy* 1984;2:57–60.

103. Gullers K, Lundberg C, Malmborg A-S. Penicillin in paranasal sinus secretions. *Chemotherapy* 1969;14:303–307.

104. Lundberg C, Malmborg A-S. Concentration of penicillin V and tetracycline in maxillary sinus secretion after repeated doses. *Scand J Infect Dis* 1973;5:123–133.

105. Eneroth C-M, Lundberg C. The antibacterial effect of antibiotics in treatment of maxillary sinusitis. *Acta Otolaryngol* 1976;81:475–483.

106. Winningham DG, Nemoy MJ, Stamey TA. Diffusion of antibiotics from plasma into prostatic fluid. *Nature* 1968;219:139–143.

107. Madsen PO, Kjaer TB, Baumueller A, et al. Antimicrobial agents in prostatic fluid and tissue. *Infection* 1976;4(Suppl 2):154–159.

108. Meares EM Jr. Long-term therapy of chronic bacterial prostatitis with trimethoprim-sulfamethoxazole. *Can Med Assoc J* 1975;112:22S–25S.

109. Meares EM Jr. Prostatitis: review of pharmacokinetics and therapy. *Rev Infect Dis* 1982;4:475–483.

110. Gasser TC, Graversen PH, Madsen PO. Fleroxacin (Ro 23–6240) distribution in canine prostatic tissue and fluids. *Antimicrob Agents Chemother* 1987;31:1010–1013.

111. Barza M, Cuchural G. The penetration of antibiotics into the prostate in chronic bacterial prostatitis. *Eur J Clin Microbiol* 1984;3:503–505.

112. Katoh N, Ono Y, Ohshima S, et al. Diffusion of cefmenoxime and latamoxef into prostatic fluid in the patients with acute bacterial prostatitis. *Urol Int* 1992;48:191–194.

113. Stamey TA, Meares EM Jr, Winningham DG. Chronic bacterial prostatitis and the diffusion of drugs into prostatic fluid. *J Urol* 1970;103:187–194.

114. Madsen PO, Wolf H, Barquin OP, Rhodes P. The nitrofurantoin concentration in prostatic fluid of humans and dogs. *J Urol* 1968;100:54–56.

115. Wolf H, Madsen PO, Rhodes P. The ampicillin concentration in prostatic tissue and prostatic fluid. *Urol Int* 1967;22:453–460.

116. Naber KG. The role of quinolones in the treatment of chronic bacterial prostatitis. *Infection* 1991;19(Suppl 3):S170–S177.

117. Naber KG, Kinzig M, Adam D, et al. Concentrations of cefpodoxime in plasma, ejaculate and in prostatic fluid and adenoma tissue. *Infection* 1991;19:30–35.

118. Naber KG, Kinzig M, Adam D, et al. Penetration of ofloxacin into prostatic fluid, ejaculate and seminal fluid. *Infection* 1993;21:98–100.

119. Naber KG. Use of quinolones in urinary tract infections and prostatitis. *Rev Infect Dis* 1989;11(Suppl 5):S1321–S1337.

120. Barling RWA, Selkon JB. The penetration of antibiotics into cerebrospinal fluid and brain tissue. *J Antimicrob Chemother* 1978;4:203–227.

121. Norrby R. A review of the penetration of antibiotics into CSF and its clinical significance. *Scand J Infect Dis* 1978;14(Suppl):296–309.

122. Mullaney DT, John JF. Cefotaxime therapy. *Arch Intern Med* 1983;143:1705–1708.

123. Thrupp LD, Leedom JM, Ivler D, et al. Ampicillin levels in the cerebrospinal fluid during treatment of bacterial meningitis. *Antimicrob Agents Chemother* 1965;5:206–213.

124. Ruiz DE, Warner JF. Nafcillin treatment of *Staphylococcus aureus* meningitis. *Antimicrob Agents Chemother* 1976;9:554–555.

125. Furesz S, Scotti R, Pallanza R, et al. Rifampicin: a new rifamyicin. *Arzneimittelforschung* 1967;17:534–537.

126. Sippel JE, Mikhail IA, Girgis NI, et al. Rifampin concentrations in cerebrospinal fluid of patients with tuberculous meningitis. *Am Rev Respir Dis* 1974;109:579–580.

127. Koch R. Blood and cerebrospinal fluid levels of intramuscular oxytetracycline. *J Pediatr* 1955;46:44–48.

128. Marmo E, Cuppola L, Pempinello R, et al. Levels of amoxycillin in the liquor during continuous intravenous administration. *Chemotherapy* 1982;28:171–175.

129. Humbert G, Leroy A, Rogez J, et al. Cefoxitin concentrations in the cerebrospinal fluids of patients with meningitis. *Antimicrob Agents Chemother* 1980;17:675–678.

130. Humbert G, Veyssier P, Fourtillan JB, et al. Penetration of cefmenoxime into cerebrospinal fluid of patients with bacterial meningitis. *J Antimicrob Chemother* 1986;18:503–506.

131. Tsacopoules M. The penetration of vibramycin (doxycycline) in human aqueous humor. *Ophthalmologica* 1969;159:418–429.

132. Adenis JP, Denis F, Frokco JL, et al. Etude de la penetration intraoculaire de la fosfomycine chez l'homme et chez lapin. *J Fr Ophthalmol* 1986;9:533–537.

133. Denis F, Adenis JP, Mounier M, et al. Intraocular passage (healthy eye and infected eye) of ceftriaxone in man and rabbit. *Chemioterapia* 1985;4(Suppl 2):338–339.

134. Berger SA, Barza M, Haher J, et al. Penetration of antibiotics into decubitus ulcers. *J Antimicrob Chemother* 1981;7:193–195.
135. Ryan DM, Cars O. A problem in the interpretation of beta-lactam antibiotic levels in tissue. *J Antimicrob Chemother* 1983;12:281–284.
136. Traunmuller F, Fille M, Thallinger C, et al. Multiple-dose pharmacokinetics of telithromycin in peripheral soft tissues. *Int J Antimicrob Agents* 2009;34:72–75.
137. Burkhard O, Brunner M, Schmidt S, et al. Penetration of ertapenem into skeletal muscle and subcutaneous adipose tissue in healthy volunteers measured by *in vivo* microdialysis. *J Antimicrob Chemother* 2006;58:632–636.
138. Cunha BA, Gossling HR, Pasteinak HS, et al. The penetration characteristics of cefazolin, cephalothin, and cephradine into bone in patients undergoing total hip replacement. *J Bone Joint Surg Am* 1977;59:856–859.
139. Schurman OJ, Hirshman HP, Burton DS. Cephalothin and cefamandole penetration into bone, synovial fluid, and wound drainage fluid. *J Bone Joint Surg Am* 1980;62:981–985.
140. Rosdahl VT, Sorensen TS, Colding H. Determination of antibiotic concentrations in bone. *J Antimicrob Chemother* 1979;5:275–280.
141. Adam D, Schalkhauser K, Boettger F. Zur Diffusion von Cefuroxim in das Prostataund andere Gewebe des urogenitalbereichs. *Med Klin* 1979;74:1867–1870.
142. Wittmann DH, Kotthaus E. Further methodological improvement in antibiotic bone concentration measurements: penetration of ofloxacin into bone and cartilage. *Infection* 1986;14(Suppl 4):270–273.
143. Fong IW, Ledbetter WH, Vandenbroucke AC, et al. Ciprofloxacin concentrations in bone and muscle after oral dosing. *Antimicrob Agents Chemother* 1986;29:405–408.
144. Fitzgerald RH. Antibiotic distribution in normal and osteomyelitic bone. *Orthop Clin North Am* 1984;15:537–546.
145. Williams DN, Gustilo RB, Bevesley R, et al. Bone and serum concentrations of five cephalosporin drugs: relevance to prophylaxis and treatment in orthopedic surgery. *Clin Orthop* 1983;179:254–265.
146. Hughes SPF, Anderson FM. Penetration of antibiotics into bone. *J Antimicrob Chemother* 1985;15:517–519.
147. Perry-Holly BA, Ritterbusch JK, Burdge RE, et al. Cefamandole levels in serum and necrotic bone. *Clin Orthop* 1985;1199:280–281.
148. Soussy CJ, Deforges LP, Le Van Thoi J, et al. Cefotaxime concentration in the bile and wall of the gallbladder. *J Antimicrob Chemother* 1980;6(Suppl A):125–130.
149. Kenady DE, Ram MB. Biliary levels of ceforanide. *Antimicrob Agents Chemother* 1983;23:706–709.
150. Sales JE, Sutcliffe M, O'Grady F. Excretion of clindamycin in the bile of patients with biliary tract disease. *Chemotherapy* 1973;19:11–15.
151. Wollmer P, Rhodes CG, Pike VW, et al. Measurement of pulmonary erythromycin concentration in patients with lobar pneumonia by means of positron tomography. *Lancet* 1982;2:1361–1363.
152. Perea EJ, Garcia-Iglesias MC, Ayarra J, et al. Comparative concentration of cefoxitin in human lungs and sera. *Antimicrob Agents Chemother* 1983;23:323–324.
153. Racz G. Tissue concentration of antibiotic following oral doses of tetracycline phosphate complex. *Curr Ther Res* 1971;13:553–557.
154. Thadepalli H, Mandal AK, Bach VT, et al. Tissue levels of doxycycline in the human lung and pleura. *Chest* 1980;78:304–305.
155. Warterberg K, Tohak J, Knapp W. Lung tissue concentrations of cefoperazone. *Infection* 1983;11:280–282.
156. Reid TMS, Gould IM, Goulder D, et al. Brief report: respiratory tract penetration of ciprofloxacin. *Am J Med* 1989;87(Suppl 5A):60S–61S.
157. Brun JN, Ostby N, Bredesen JE, et al. Sulfonamide and trimethoprim concentrations in human serum and skin blister fluid. *Antimicrob Agents Chemother* 1981;19:82–85.
158. Galy J, Mantel O. Concentrations of cefotaxime in tissue and body fluids. *Nouv Presse Med* 1981;10:565–579.
159. Hansen I, Lykkegaard Nielson M, Heerfordt L, et al. Trimethoprim in normal and pathological human lung tissue. *Chemotherapy* 1973;19:221–234.
160. Farago E, Kiss IJ, Nabradi Z. Serum and lung tissue levels of fosfomycin in humans. *Int J Clin Pharmacol Ther Toxicol* 1980;18:554–558.
161. Kiss IJ, Farago E, Juhasz I, et al. Investigation on the serum and lung tissue level of rifampicin in man. *Int J Clin Pharmacol Biopharm* 1976;13:42–47.
162. Borrero AJ. Doxycycline levels in serum and prostatic tissue. *Urology* 1973;1:490–491.
163. Evans WE, Schentag JJ, Jusko JJ. *Applied pharmacokinetics: principles of therapeutic drug monitoring.* 2nd ed. San Francisco: Applied Therapeutics, Inc, 1986.
164. Rowland M, Tozer TN. *Clinical pharmacokinetics: concepts and applications.* 2nd ed. Philadelphia: Lea & Febiger, 1989.
165. Wagner JG. *Fundamentals of clinical pharmacokinetics.* 2nd ed. Hamilton, IL: Drug Intelligence Publications, 1979.
166. Zammit MC, Fiorentino L, Cassar K, et al. Factors affecting gentamicin penetration in lower extremity ischemic tissues with ulcers. *Int J Lower Extrem Wounds* 2011;10:130–137.
167. Joukhadar C, Frossard M, Mayer BX, et al. Impaired target site penetration of beta-lactams may account for therapeutic failure in patients with septic shock. *Crit Care Med* 2001;29:385–391.
168. Buerger C, Plock N, Dehghanyar P, et al. Pharmacokinetics of unbound linezolid in plasma and tissue interstitium of critically ill patients after multiple dosing using microdialysis. *Antimicrob Agents Chemother* 2006;50:2455–2463.
169. Bergan T, Hellum KB, Schreiner A, et al. Passage of erythromycin into human suction skin blisters. *Curr Ther Res* 1982;32:597–603.
170. Lanao JM, Dominguez A, Mactas JG, et al. The influence of ascites on the pharmacokinetics of amikacin. *Int J Clin Pharmacol Ther Toxicol* 1980;18:57–61.
171. Gerding DN, Hall WH, Schierl EA. Antibiotic concentrations in ascitic fluid of patients with ascites and bacterial peritonitis. *Ann Intern Med* 1977;86:708–713.
172. Ariza J, Xiol X, Esteve M, et al. Aztreonam vs. cefotaxime in the treatment of Gram-negative spontaneous peritonitis in cirrhotic patients. *Hepatology* 1991;14:91–98.
173. Higuchi K, Ikawa K, Ikeda K, et al. Peritoneal pharmacokinetics of cefepime in laparotomy patients with inflammatory bowel disease, and dosage considerations for surgical intra-abdominal infections based on pharmacodynamic assessment. *J Infect Chemother* 2008;14:110–116.

174. Gomez-Jimenez J, Ribera E, Gasser I, et al. Randomized trial comparing ceftriaxone with cefonicid for treatment of spontaneous bacterial peritonitis in cirrhotic patients. *Antimicrob Agents Chemother* 1993;37:1587–1592.

175. Runyon BA, Akriviadis EA, Sattler FR, et al. Ascitic fluid and serum cefotaxime and desacetyl cefotaxime levels in patients treated for bacterial peritonitis. *Dig Dis Sci* 1991;36:1782–1786.

176. Moreau L, Durand H, Biclet P. Cefotaxime concentrations in ascites. *J Antimicrob Chemother* 1980;6(Suppl A): 121–122.

177. Garcia MJ, Dominguez-Gil A, Diaz Perez F. Disposition of cefoxitin in patients with ascites. *Eur J Clin Pharmacol* 1981;20:371–374.

178. Lechi A, Arosio E, Xerri L, et al. The kinetics of cefuroxime in ascitic and pleural fluid. *Int J Clin Pharmacol Ther Toxicol* 1982;20:493–496.

179. Wilson DE, Chalmers TC, Medoff MA. The passage of cephalothin into and out of ascitic fluid. *Am J Med Sci* 1967;253:449–452.

180. Arrigucci S, Garcea A, Fallani S, et al. Ertapenem peritoneal fluid concentrations in adult surgical patients. *Int J Antimicrob Agents* 2009;33:371–373.

181. Soga Y, Ohge H, Ikawa K, et al. Peritoneal pharmacokinetics and pharmacodynamic target attainment of meropenem in patients undergoing abdominal surgery. *J Chemother* 2010;22(2):98–102.

182. Rolando N, Wade JJ, Philpott-Howard JN, et al. The penetration of imipenem/cilastatin into ascitic fluid in patients with chronic liver disease. *J Antimicrob Chemother* 1994;33:163–167.

183. Martin WJ, Nichols DR, Heilman FR. Penicillin V: further observations. *Proc Staff Meet Mayo Clin* 1955;30: 521–526.

184. Stass H, Rink AD, Delesen H, et al. Pharmacokinetics and peritoneal penetration of moxifloxacin in peritonitis. *J Ant Chem* 2006;58:693–696.

185. Medina A, Fiske N, Hjelt-Harvey I, et al. Absorption, diffusion and excretion of a new antibiotic, lincomycin. *Antimicrob Agents Chemother* 1964;1963:189–196.

186. Geraci JE, Heilman FR, Nichols DR, et al. Some laboratory and clinical experiences with a new antibiotic, vancomycin. *Proc Staff Meet Mayo Clin* 1956;31: 564–582.

187. Pulaski EJ, Tubbs RS. Inhibitory effects of kanamycin and diffusion into various body fluids. *Antibiot Med Clin Ther* 1959;6:589–593.

188. Just HM, Eschenbruch E, Schmuziger M, et al. Penetration of netilmicin into heart valves, subcutaneous and muscular tissue of patients undergoing heart surgery. *Clin Cardiol* 1983;6:217–219.

189. Beam TR Jr, Galask RP, Friedhoff LT, et al. Aztreonam concentration in human tissues obtained during thoracic and gynecologic surgery. *Antimicrob Agents Chemother* 1986;30:505–507.

190. Cole DR, Pung J. Penetration of cefazolin into pleural fluid. *Antimicrob Agents Chemother* 1977;11:1033–1035.

191. Yamada H, Iwanaga T, Nakanishi H, et al. Penetration and clearance of cefoperazone and moxalactam in pleural fluid. *Antimicrob Agents Chemother* 1985;27:93–95.

192. Lode H, Kemmerich B, Gruhlke G, et al. Cefotaxime in bronchopulmonary infections: a clinical and pharmacological study. *J Antimicrob Chemother* 1980;6(Suppl A): 193–198.

193. Kafetzis DA. Penetration of cefotaximine into empyema fluid. *J Antimicrob Chemother* 1980;6(Suppl A):153.

194. Webb D, Thadepalli H, Bach V, et al. Clinical and experimental evaluation of cefoxitin therapy. *Chemotherapy* 1978;26(Suppl 1):306–312.

195. Dumont R, Guetat F, Andrews JM, et al. Concentrations of cefpodoxime in plasma and pleural fluid after a single oral dose of cefpodoxime proxetil. *J Antimicrob Chemother* 1990;26(Suppl E):41–46.

196. Walstad RA, Hellum KB, Blika S, et al. Pharmacokinetics and tissue penetration of ceftazidine: studies on lymph, aqueous humor, skin blister, cerebrospinal fluid and pleural fluid. *J Antimicrob Chemother* 1983; 12(Suppl A):275–282.

197. Takamoto M, Ishibashi T, Harada S, et al. Experience with ceftizoxime in respiratory tract infection and its transfer into pleural effusion. *Chemotherapy* 1980; 28(Suppl 5):394–404.

198. Benoni G, Arosio E, Cuzzolin L, et al. Penetration of ceftriaxone into human pleural fluid. *Antimicrob Agents Chemother* 1986;29:906–908.

199. Taryle DA, Good JT, Morgan EJ, et al. Antibiotic concentrations in human parapneumonic effusions. *J Antimicrob Chemother* 1981;7:171–177.

200. Joseph J, Vaughan LM, Basran GS. Penetration of intravenous and oral ciprofloxacin into sterile and empyemic human pleural fluid. *Ann Pharmacother* 1994;28: 313–315.

201. Kimura M, Matsushima T, Nakamura J, et al. Comparative study of penetration of lomefloxacin and ceftriaxone into transudative and exudative pleural effusion. *Antimicrob Agents Chemother* 1992;36:2774–2777.

202. Yew WW, Lee J, Chan CY, et al. Ofloxacin penetration into tuberculous pleural effusion. *Antimicrob Agents Chemother* 1991;35:2159–2160.

203. Daschner FD, Gier E, Lentzen H, et al. Penetration into the pleural fluid after bacampicillin and amoxicillin. *J Antimicrob Chemother* 1981;7:585–588.

204. Lode H, Dzwillo G. Investigation of the diffusion of antibiotics into the human pleural space. In: *Proceedings of the 10th International Congress of Chemotherapy.* Washington, DC: American Society for Microbiology, 1978;1:386–388.

205. Giachetto G, Catalina M, Nanni L, et al. Ampicillin and penicillin concentration in serum and pleural fluid of hospitalized children with community-acquired pneumonia. *Pediatr Infect Dis J* 2004;23(7):625–629.

206. Bronsveld W, Stam J, MacLaren DM. Concentrations of ampicillin in pleural fluid and serum after single and repetitive doses of bacampicillin. *Scand J Infect Dis* 1978;14(Suppl):274–278.

207. Knoller J, Schonfeld W, Mayer M, et al. Mezlocillin in pleural effusions: analysis by HPLC. *Zentralbl Bakteriol Hyg A* 1988;268:370–375.

208. Lode H, Gruhlke G, Hallermann W, et al. Significance of pleural and sputum concentrations for antibiotic therapy of bronchopulmonary infections. *Infection* 1980; 8(Suppl 1):S49–S53.

209. Simon C, Sommerwerck D, Friehoff J. Der Wert von Doxycyclin bei Atemwegsinfektionen (Serum, -Speichel, -Sputum-Lungen, und Pleuraexsudatspiegel). *Prax Klin Pneumol* 1978;32:266–270.

210. Panzer JD, Brown DC, Epstein WL, et al. Clindamycin levels in various body tissues and fluids. *J Clin Pharmacol* 1972;12:259–262.

211. Fernandez-Lastra C, Marino EL, Barrueco M, et al. Disposition of phosphomycin in patients with pleural effusion. *Antimicrob Agents Chemother* 1984;25:458–462.

212. Boman G, Malmberg AS. Rifampin in plasma and pleural fluid after single oral doses. *Eur J Clin Pharmacol* 1974; 7:51–58.

213. Jacobs F, Rocmans P, Motte S, et al. Penetration and bactericidal activity of teichoplanin in post-thoracotomy pleural fluids. In: *Program and abstracts of the 26th Interscience Conference on Antimicrobial Agents and Chemotherapy.* Washington, DC: American Society for Microbiology; 1986. Abstract 1251.

214. Byl B, Jacobs F, Wallemacq P, et al. Vancomycin penetration of uninfected pleural fluid exudates after continuous or intermittent infusion. *Antimicrob Agents Chemother* 2003;47:2015–2017.

215. Honda DH, Adams HG, Barriere SL. Amikacin penetration into synovial fluid during treatment of septic arthritis. *Drug Intell Clin Pharm* 1981;15:284–286.

216. Dee TH, Kozin F. Gentamicin and tobramycin penetration into synovial fluid. *Antimicrob Agents Chemother* 1977;12:548–549.

217. Baciocco EA, Iles RL. Ampicillin and kanamycin concentrations in joint fluid. *Clin Pharmacol Ther* 1971;12: 858–863.

218. Valencia-Chinas A, Galindo-Hernandez F, Reyes-Sanchez J, et al. Concentrations of cefadroxil in osteoarticular tissues. In: *Program and abstracts of the 11th International Congress of Chemotherapy and 19th Interscience Conference on Antimicrobial Agents and Chemotherapy.* Washington, DC: American Society for Microbiology; 1979. Abstract 338.

219. Vainiopaa S, Wilppula E, Lalla M, et al. Cefamandole and isoxazolyl penicillins in antibiotic prophylaxis of patients undergoing total hip or knee-joint arthroplasty. *Arch Orthop Trauma Surg* 1988;107:228–230.

220. Schurman OJ, Hirshman HP, Kajiyama G, et al. Cefazolin concentrations in bone and synovial fluid. *J Bone Joint Surg Am* 1978;60:359–362.

221. Harle A, Ritzerfeld W, Kluppelberg FH. Cefotaxime levels in synovial fluid following intravenous administration. *Z Orthop* 1988;126:425–430.

222. Nelson JD, Howard JB, Shelton S. Oral antibiotic therapy for skeletal infections of children. *Pediatrics* 1978; 92:131–134.

223. Parker RH, Birbara C, Schmid FR. Passage of nafcillin and ampicillin into synovial fluid. *Zentralbl Bakteriol* 1976;(Suppl 5):1115–1123.

224. Nelson JD. Antibiotic concentrations in septic joint effusions. *N Engl J Med* 1971;284:349–353.

225. Viek P. Concentration of sodium nafcillin in pathological synovial fluid. *Antimicrob Agents Chemother* 1962; 1961:379–383.

226. Balboni VG, Shapiro IM, Kydd DM. The penetration of penicillin into joint fluid following intramuscular administration. *Am J Med Sci* 1945;210:588–591.

227. Rana B, Butcher I, Grigoris P, et al. Linezolid penetration into osteo-articular tissues. *J Antimicrob Chemother* 2002; 50:747–750.

228. Rodvold KA, Gotfried MH, Cwik M, et al. Serum, tissue and body fluid concentrations of tigecycline after a singled 100 mg dose. *J Antimicrob Chemother* 2006;58: 1221–1229.

229. Solberg CO, Madsen ST, Digranes A, et al. High dose netilmicin therapy: efficacy, tolerance and tissue penetration. *J Antimicrob Chemother* 1980;6:133–141.

230. Mazzei T, Novelli A, Esposito S, et al. New insight into the clinical pharmacokinetics of cefaclor: tissue penetration. *J Chemother* 2000;12:53–62.

231. Nye KJ, Shi YG, Andrews JM, et al. Pharmacokinetics and tissue penetration of cefepime. *J Antimicrob Chemother* 1989;24:23–28.

232. Stone JW, Linong G, Andrews JM, et al. Cefixime in-vitro activity, pharmacokinetics and tissue penetration. *J Antimicrob Chemother* 1989;23:221–228.

233. Korting HC. Plasma and skin blister fluid levels of cefotriam and cefmenoxime after single intramuscular application of 1 gm in gonorrhea. *Chemotherapy* 1984; 30:277–282.

234. Korting HC, Schafer-Korting M, Maass L, et al. Cefodizime in serum and skin blister fluid after single intravenous and intramuscular doses in healthy volunteers. *Antimicrob Agents Chemother* 1987;31:1822–1825.

235. Mazzei T, Novelli A, Esposito S, et al. Cefodizime in skin suction blister fluid and serum following a single intravenous or intramuscular dose in adult patients. *J Chemother* 2000;12:306–313.

236. Shyu WC, Quintiliani R, Nightingale CH, et al. Effect of protein binding on drug penetration into blister fluid. *Antimicrob Agents Chemother* 1988;32:128–130.

237. Frossard M, Joukhadar C, Erovic BM, et al. Distribution and antimicrobial activity of fosfomycin in the interstitial fluid of human soft tissues. *Antimicrob Agents Chemother* 2000;44:2728–2732.

238. Bergan T, Kalager T, Hellum KB, et al. Penetration of cefotaxime and desacetylcefoxamine into skin blister fluid. *J Antimicrob Chemother* 1982;10:193–196.

239. Mazzei T, Tonelli F, Novelli A, et al. Penetration of cefotetan into suction skin blister fluid and tissue homogenates in patients undergoing abdominal surgery. *Antimicrob Agents Chemother* 1994;38:2221–2223.

240. Bryskier A, Elbaz P, Fourtillan JB, et al. Evaluation of the extravascular distribution of cefotiam (SLE 963) by the skin blister technic. *Pathol Biol* 1984;32:506–508.

241. Kavi J, Andrews JM, Ashby JP, et al. Pharmacokinetics and tissue penetration of cefpirome, a new cephalosporin. *J Antimicrob Chemother* 1988;22:911–916.

242. Borin MT, Hughes GS, Spillers CR, et al. Pharmacokinetics of cefpodoxime in plasma and skin blister fluid following oral dosing of cefpodoxime proxetil. *Antimicrob Agents Chemother* 1990;34:1094–1099.

243. Barbhaiya RH, Shukla UA, Gleason CR, et al. Comparison of cefprozil and cefaclor pharmacokinetics and tissue penetration. *Antimicrob Agents Chemother* 1990; 34:1204–1209.

244. Findlay CD, Wise R, Allcock JE, et al. The tissue penetration, as measured by a blister technique, and pharmacokinetics of cefsulodin compared with carbenicillin and ticarcillin. *J Antimicrob Chemother* 1981;7:637–642.

245. Hoffstedt B, Walder M. Penetration of ceftaxidime into extracellular fluid in patients. *J Antimicrob Chemother* 1981;8(Suppl B):289–292.

246. Wise R, Nye K, O'Neill P, et al. Pharmacokinetics and tissue penetration of ceftibuten. *Antimicrob Agents Chemother* 1990;34:1053–1055.

247. Shyu WC, Quintiliani R, Nightingale CH. An improved method to determine interstitial fluid pharmacokinetics. *J Infect Dis* 1985;152:1328–1331.

248. LeBel M, Gregoire S, Caron M, et al. Difference in blister fluid penetration after single and multiple doses of ceftriaxone. *Antimicrob Agents Chemother* 1985;28: 123–127.

249. Adam D, Reichart B, Beyer J, et al. Diffusion of cephradine and cephalothin into interstitial fluid of human volunteers with tissue cages. *Infection* 1978;6:578–581.

250. Wise R, Andrews JM, O'Neill P, et al. Pharmacokinetics and distribution in tissue of FK-037, a new parenteral cephalosporin. *Antimicrob Agents Chemother* 1994; 38:2369–2372.

251. Mouton JW, Michel MF. Pharmacokinetics of meropenem in serum and suction blister fluid during continuous and intermittent infusion. *J Antimicrob Chemother* 1991;28:911–918.

252. Wise R, Gillett AP, Cadge B, et al. The influence of protein binding upon tissue fluid levels of six-lactam antibiotics. *J Infect Dis* 1980;42:77–82.

253. Wise R, Bennett SA, Dent J. The pharmocokinetics of orally absorbed cefuroxime compared with amoxycillin/clavulanic acid. *J Antimicrob Chemother* 1984;13:603–610.

254. Herlitz V, Langmaack H, Metzger M, et al. Serum and tissue levels of cefoxitin in perioperative prophylaxis. *J Antimicrob Chemother* 1980;6:717–722.

255. Takase Z; Obstetrics and Gynecology Research Group. Basic and clinical research on cefsulodin in the field of obstetrics and gynecology. *Jpn J Antibiot* 1982;35: 2861–2877.

256. Hoffstedt B, Walder M, Forsgren A. Comparison of skin blisters and implanted cotton threads for the evaluation of antibiotic tissue concentrations. *Eur J Clin Microbiol* 1982;1:33–37.

257. Bergan T, Engeset A, Olszewski W, et al. Extravascular penetration of highly protein-bound flucloxacillin. *Antimicrob Agents Chemother* 1986;30:729–732.

258. Wise R, Logan M, Cooper M, et al. Pharmacokinetics and tissue penetration of tazobactam administered alone and with piperacillin. *Antimicrob Agents Chemother* 1991;35:1081–1084.

259. Lockley MR, Brown RM, Wise R. Pharmacokinetics and tissue penetration of temocillin. *Drugs* 1985;29(Suppl 5): 106–108.

260. Walstad RA, Hellum KB, Thurmann-Nielsen E, et al. Pharmacokinetics and tissue penetration of timentin: a simultaneous study of serum, urine, lymph, suction blister and subcutaneous thread fluid. *J Antimicrob Chemother* 1986;17(Suppl C):71–80.

261. Wise R, Lister D, McNulty CAM, et al. The comparative pharmacokinetics of five quinolones. *J Antimicrob Chemother* 1986;18(Suppl D):71–81.

262. Wise R, Kirkpatrick B, Ashby J, et al. Pharmacokinetics and tissue penetration of Ro 23–6240, a new trifluoroquinolone. *Antimicrob Agents Chemother* 1987;31: 161–163.

263. Wise R, Andrews JM, Ashby JP, et al. A study to determine the pharmacokinetics and inflammatory fluid penetration of gatifloxacin following a single oral dose. *J Antimicrob Chemother* 1999;44:701–704.

264. Cooper MA, Nye K, Andrews JM, et al. The pharmacokinetics and inflammatory fluid penetration of orally administered azithromycin. *J Antimicrob Chemother* 1990; 26:533–538.

265. McNulty CA, Garden GM, Ashby J, et al. Pharmacokinetics and tissue penetration of carumonam, a new synthetic monobactam. *Antimicrob Agents Chemother* 1985; 28:425–427.

266. Wise R, Webberly JM, Andrews JM, et al. The pharmacokinetics and tissue penetration of intravenously administered CGP31608. *J Antimicrob Chemother* 1988; 21:85–91.

267. Raeburn JAA. A method for studying antibiotic concentrations in inflammatory exudate. *J Clin Pathol* 1971;24: 633–635.

268. Nicolau D, Sun HK, Seltzer E, et al. Pharmacokinetics of dalbavancin in plasma and skin blister fluid. *J Antimicrob Chemother* 2007;60:681–684.

269. Wise R, Gee T, Andrews JM, et al. Pharmacokinetics and inflammatory fluid penetration of intravenous daptomycin in volunteers. *Antimicrob Agents Chemother* 2002;46:31–33.

270. Schreiner A, Digranes A. Pharmocokinetics of lymecycline and doxycycline in serum and suction blister fluid. *Chemotherapy* 1985;31:261–265.

271. Tuominen RK, Mannisto PT, Solkinen A, et al. Antibiotic concentration in suction skin blister fluid and saliva after repeated dosage of erythromycin acistrate and erythromycin base. *J Antimicrob Chemother* 1988; 21(Suppl D):57–65.

272. Frossard M, Joukhadar C, Erovic BM, et al. Distribution and antimicrobial activity of fosfomycin in the interstitial fluid of human soft tissues. *Antimicrob Agents Chemother* 2000;44:2728–2732.

273. Vaillant L, Machet L, Taburet AM, et al. Levels of fusidic acid in skin blister fluid and serum after repeated administration of two dosages (250 and 500 mg). *Br J Dermatol* 1992;126:591–595.

274. Gee T, Ellis R, Marshall G, et al. Pharmacokinetics and tissue penetration of linezolid following multiple oral doses. *J Antimicrob Chemother* 2001;45:1843–1846.

275. Bergan T, Bruun JN, Ostby N, et al. Human pharmacokinetics and skin blister levels of sulfonamides and dihydrofolate reductase inhibitors. *Chemotherapy* 1986; 32:319–328.

276. Solberg CO, Halstensen A, Digranes A, et al. Penetration of antibiotics into human leukocytes and dermal suction blisters. *Rev Infect Dis* 1983;5:S468–S473.

277. McNulty CA, Garden GM, Wiser R, et al. The pharmacokinetics and tissue penetration of teicoplanin. *J Antimicrob Chemother* 1985;16:743–749.

278. Namour F, Sultan E, Pascual MH, et al. Penetration of telithromycin (HMR 3647) a new ketolide antimicrobial, into inflammatory blister fluid following oral administration. *J Antimicrob Chemother* 2002;49:1035–1038.

279. Sun HK, Ong CT, Umer A, et al. Pharmacokinetic profile of tigecycline in serum and skin blister fluid of healthy subjects after multiple intravenous administrations. *Antimicrob Agents Chemother* 2005;49:1629–1932.

280. Hansbrough SF, Clark JE, Reimer LG. Concentrations of kanamycin and amikacin in human gallbladder bile and wall. *Antimicrob Agents Chemother* 1981;20: 515–517.

281. Pulaski EJ, Fusillo MH. Gallbladder bile concentrations of the major antibiotics following intravenous administration. *Surg Gynecol Obstet* 1955;100:571–574.

282. Moseley JG, Chaudhuri AK, Desai AL, et al. The distribution of aztreonam in serum, bile, skin and subcutaneous tissues in patients undergoing cholecystectomy. *J Hosp Infect* 1990;15:389–392.

283. Ohnhaus EE, Halter F, Lebek G. Estimation of the biliary excretion of different cephalosporins utilizing retrograde cholongiopancreatography (ERCP). *Endoscopy* 1981;13: 13–32.

284. Palmu A, Jarvinen H, Hallynck T, et al. Cefadroxil levels in bile in biliary infection. In: Nelson JD, Grassi C, eds. *Current chemotherapy and infectious disease: proceedings of the 11th International Congress of Chemotherapy and 19th Interscience Conference on Antimicrobial Agents and Chemotherapy.* Washington, DC: American Society for Microbiology, 1979:643–644.

285. Ratzan KR, Baker HB, Lauredo I. Excretion of cefa-mandole, cefazolin and cephalothin into T-tube bile. *Antimicrob Agents Chemother* 1978;13:985–987.

286. Ratzan KR, Ruiz C, Irvin GL III. Biliary tract excretion of cefazolin, cephalothin, and cephaloridine in the presence of biliary tract disease. *Antimicrob Agents Chemother* 1974;6:426–431.

287. Tanaka H, Nishino H, Sawada T, et al. Biliary penetration of cefbuperazone in the presence and absence of obstructive jaundice. *J Antimicrob Chemother* 1987; 20:417–420.

288. Okamoto MP, Gill MA, Nakahiro RK, et al. Tissue concentrations of cefepime in acute cholecystitis patients. *Ther Drug Monit* 1992;14:220–225.

289. Petrikkos G, Kastanakis M, Markogiannakis A, et al. Pharmacokinetics of cefepime in bile and gall bladder tissue after prophylactic administration in patients with extrahepatic biliary diseases. *Int J Antimicrob Agents* 2006;27:331–334.

290. Smith BR, LeFrock J, Carr BB. Cefmenoxime penetration into gallbladder bile and tissue. *Antimicrob Agents Chemother* 1983;23:941–943.

291. Orda R, Berger SA, Levy Y, et al. Penetration of ceftriaxone and cefoperazone into bile and gallbladder tissue in patients with acute cholecystitis. *Dig Dis Sci* 1992; 37:1691–1693.

292. Brogard JM, Jehl F, Blickle JF, et al. Experimental and clinical evaluation of the biliary phamacokinetic profile of cefpiramide, a new cephalosporin with high hepatic elimination. *Drugs Exp Clin Res* 1988;14:519–527.

293. Walstad RA, Wiig JN, Thurmann-Nielsen E, et al. Pharmacokinetics of ceftazidime in patients with biliary tract disease. *Eur J Clin Pharmacol* 1986;31:327–331.

294. Severn M, Powis SJA. Biliary excretion and tissue levels of cefuroxime: a study in eleven patients undergoing cholecystectomy. *J Antimicrob Chemother* 1979;5: 183–188.

295. Mayer M, Tophof C, Opferkuch W. Bile levels of imipenem in patients with T-drain following the administration of imipenem/cilastatin. *Infection* 1988;16: 225–228.

296. Condon RE, Walker AP, Hanna CB, et al. Penetration of meropenem in plasma and abdominal tissues from patients undergoing intraabdominal surgery. *Clin Infect Dis* 1997;24(Suppl 2):S181–S183.

297. Kiss IJ, Farago E, Schnitzler J, et al. Amoxycillin levels in human serum, bile, gallbladder, lung and liver tissue. *Int J Clin Pharmacol Ther Toxicol* 1981;19:69–74.

298. Morris DL, Ubhi CS, Robertson CS, et al. Biliary pharmacokinetics of sulbactam plus ampicillin in humans. *Rev Infect Dis* 1986;8(Suppl 5):S589–S592.

299. Brogard JM, Arnaud JP, Blickle JF, et al. Biliary elimination of apalcillin. *Antimicrob Agents Chemother* 1984;26:428–430.

300. Henegar GC, Silverman M, Gardner RJ, et al. Excretion of methicillin in human bile. *Antimicrob Agents Chemother* 1962;1961:348–351.

301. Green GR, Geraci JE. A note on the concentration of nafcillin in human bile. *Mayo Clin Proc* 1965;40: 700–704.

302. Wittke RR, Adam D, Klein HE. Therapeutic results and tissue concentrations of temocillin in surgical patients. *Drugs* 1985;29(Suppl 5):221–226.

303. Owen AWMC, Faragher EB. Biliary pharmacokinetics of ticarcillin and clauvulanic acid. *J Antimicrob Chemother* 1986;17(Suppl C):65–70.

304. Zurbuchen U, Ritz JP, Lehmann KS, et al. Oral vs intravenous antibiotic prophylaxis in elective laparoscopic cholecystectomy—an exploratory trial. *Langenbecks Arch Surg* 2008;393:479–485.

305. Kunin CM, Finland M. Excretion of demethylchlortetracycline into the bile. *N Engl J Med* 1959;261: 1069–1071.

306. Dull WL, Alexander MR, Kasik JE. Bronchial secretion levels of amikacin. *Antimicrob Agents Chemother* 1979; 16:767–771.

307. Klastersky J, Greening C, Mouawad E, et al. Endotracheal gentamicin in bronchial infections in patients with tracheostomy. *Chest* 1971;61:117–120.

308. Panidis D, Markantonis SL, Boutzouka E, et al. Penetration of gentamicin into the alveolar lining fluid of critically ill patients with ventilator-associated pneumonia. *Chest* 2005;128(2):545–552.

309. Valcke YJ, Vogelaers DP, Colardyn FA, et al. Penetration of netilmicin in the lower respiratory tract after once-daily dosing. *Chest* 1992;101:1028–1032.

310. Boselli E, Breilh D, Djabarouti S, et al. Reliability of mini-bronchioalveolar lavage for the measurement of epithelial lining fluid concentrations of tobramycin in critically ill patients. *Intensive Care Med* 2007;33: 1519–1523.

311. Klastersky J, Carpentier-Meunier F, Kahan-Coppens L, et al. Endotracheally administered antibiotics for Gram-negative bronchopneumonia. *Chest* 1979;75:586–591.

312. Alexander M, Schoell S, Hicklin G, et al. Bronchial secretion concentrations of tobramycin. *Am Rev Respir Dis* 1982;125:208–209.

313. Barrera V, Sinues B, Martinez P, et al. Penetration de l'amikacine daus la chambre anterieure de l'oell humain. *J Fr Ophthalmol* 1984;7:539–543.

314. Cook PJ, Andrews JM, Wise R, et al. Distribution of cefdinir, a third generation cephalosporin antibiotic, in serum and pulmonary compartments. *J Antimicrob Chemother* 1996;37:331–339.

315. Chadha D, Wise R, Baldwin DR, et al. Cefepime concentrations in bronchial mucosa and serum following a single 2 gram intravenous dose. *J Antimicrob Chemother* 1990;25:959–963.

316. Serieys C, Bergogne-Berezin E, Kafe H, et al. Study of the diffusion of cefmenoxine into the bronchial secretions. *Chemotherapy* 1986;32:1–6.

317. Bergogne Berezin E, Kafe H, Berthelot G, et al. Pharmacokinetic study of cefoxitin in bronchial secretions. In: Siegenthaler W, Luethy R, eds. *Current chemotherapy: proceedings.* Washington, DC: American Society for Microbiology, 1978:758–760.

318. Baldwin DR, Maxwell SRJ, Honeybourne D, et al. The penetration of cefpirome into the potential sites of pulmonary infection. *J Antimicrob Chemother* 1991;28: 79–86.

319. Bergogne-Berezin E, Berthelot G, Safran D, et al. Penetration of cefsulodin into bronchial secretions. *Chemotherapy* 1984;30:205–210.

320. Bergogne-Berezin E, Pierre J, Berthelot G, et al. Diffusion bronchique des nouvelles beta-lactimes anti-pseudomonas. *Pathol Biol* 1984;32:421–425.

321. Husson MO, Debout J, Krivosic-Horber R. Etude de la diffusion bronchique de la ceftriaxone. *Pathol Biol* 1986; 34:325–327.

322. Halprin GM, McMahon SM. Cephalexin concentrations in sputum during acute respiratory infections. *Antimicrob Agents Chemother* 1973;3:703–707.

323. Bergogne-Berezin E, Morel C, Benard Y, et al. Pharmacokinetic study of beta-lactam antibiotics in bronchial secretions. *Scand J Infect Dis* 1978;14(Suppl):267–272.

324. Boselli E, Breilh D, Saux MC, et al. Pharmacokinetics and lung concentrations of ertapenem in patients with ventilator-associated pneumonia. *Intensive Care Med* 2006; 32:2059–2062.

325. Bergogne-Berezin E, Muller-Serieys C, Aubier M, et al. Concentration of meropenem in serum and in bronchial secretions in patients undergoing fiberoptic bronchoscopy. *Eur J Clin Pharmacol* 1994;46:87–88.

326. Allegranzi B, Cazzadori A, Di Perri G, et al. Concentrations of single-dose meropenem (1 g IV) in bronchoalveolar lavage and epithelial lining fluid. *J Antimicrob Chemother* 2000;46:319–322.

327. Conte JE Jr, Golden JA, Kelley MG, et al. Intrapulmonary pharmacokinetics and pharmacodynamics of meropenem. *Int J Antimicrob Agents* 2005;26:449–456.

328. Mouton Y, Caillaux M, Beaucaire G, et al. Penetration of moxalactam in bronchial secretions and clinical evaluation in intensive care patients. In: *Program and abstracts of the 21st Interscience Conference on Antimicrobial Agents and Chemotherapy*. Washington, DC: American Society for Microbiology; 1981. Abstract 732.

329. Cook PJ, Andrews JM, Woodcock J, et al. Concentrations of amoxycillin and clavulante in lung compartments in adults without pulmonary infection. *Thorax* 1994; 49:1134–1138.

330. Wildfeuer A, Rühle KH, Balk PL, et al. Concentrations of ampicillin and sulbactam in serum and in various compartments of the respiratory tract of patients. *Infection* 1994;22:149–151.

331. Bergogne-Berezin E, Pierre J, Chastre J, et al. Pharmacokinetics of apalcillin in intensive-care patients: study of penetration into the respiratory tract. *J Antimicrob Chemother* 1984;14:67–73.

332. Hafez FF, Stewart SM, Burnet ME. Penicillin levels in sputum. *Thorax* 1965;20:219–225.

333. Saggers BA, Lawson D. In vivo penetration of antibiotics into sputum in cystic fibrosis. *Arch Dis Child* 1968; 43:404–409.

334. Mouton Y, Caillaux M, Deboscker Y, et al. Etude de la diffusion bronchique de la piperacilline chez dix-huit patients de reanimation. *Pathol Biol* 1985;33:359–362.

335. Vacek V, Hejzlar M, Skalova M. Penetration of antibiotics into the cerebrospinal fluid in inflammatory conditions. I. Preface and comparative study of ampicillin with hetacillin. *Int J Clin Pharmacol* 1968;1:87–90.

336. Hoogkamp-Korstanje JAA, Klein SJ. Ciprofloxacin in acute exacerbations of chronic bronchitis. *J Antimicrob Chemother* 1986;18:407–413.

337. Gotfried MH, Danziger LH, Rodvold KA. Steady-state plasma and intrapulmonary concentrations of levofloxacin and ciprofloxacin in healthy adult subjects. *Chest* 2001;119:1114–1122.

338. Davies BI, Maesen FPV, Teengs JP. Serum and sputum concentrations of enoxacin after single oral dosing in a clinical and bacteriological study. *J Antimicrob Chemother* 1984;14(Suppl C):83–89.

339. Begg EJ, Robson RA, Saunders DA, et al. The pharmacokinetics of oral fleroxacin and ciprofloxacin in plasma and sputum during acute and chronic dosing. *J Clin Pharmacol* 1999;49:32–38.

340. Andrews J, Honeybourne D, Jevons G, et al. Concentrations of garenoxacin in plasma, bronchial mucosa, alveolar macrophages and epithelial lining fluid following a single oral 600 mg dose in healthy adult subjects. *J Antimicrob Chemother* 2003;51:727–730.

341. Honeybourne D, Banerjee D, Andrews J, et al. Concentrations of gatifloxacin in plasma and pulmonary compartments following a single 400 mg oral dose in patients undergoing fibre-optic bronchoscopy. *J Antimicrob Chemother* 2001;48:63–66.

342. Cazzola M, Matera MG, Tufano MA, et al. Pulmonary disposition of lomefloxacin in patients with acute exacerbation of chronic obstructive pulmonary disease. A multiple-dose study. *J Chemother* 2001;13:407–412.

343. Soman A, Honeybourne D, Andrews J, et al. Concentrations of moxifloxacin in serum and pulmonary compartments following a single 400 mg oral dose in patients undergoing fibre-optic bronchoscopy. *J Antimicrob Chemother* 1999;44:835–838.

344. Pedersen SS, Jensen T, Hvidberg EF. Comparative pharmacokinetics of ciprofloxacin and ofloxacin in cystic fibrosis patients. *J Antimicrob Chemother* 1987;20: 575–583.

345. Davies BI, Maesen FPV, Teengs JP, et al. The quinolones in chronic bronchitis. *Pharm Weekbl Sci* 1986;8:53–59.

346. Ruhen RW, Tandon MK. Minocycline, doxycycline and tetracycline levels in serum and bronchial secretions of patients with chronic bronchitis. *Pathology* 1975; 7:193–197.

347. Naline E, Sanceaume M, Taty L, et al. Penetration of minocycline into lung tissues. *Br J Clin Pharmacol* 1991; 32:402–404.

348. Baldwin DR, Wise R, Andrews JM, et al. Azithromycin concentrations at the sites of pulmonary infection. *Eur Respir J* 1990;3:886–890.

349. Lucchi M, Damle B, Fang A, et al. Pharmacokinetics of azithromycin in serum, bronchial washings, alveolar macrophages and lung tissue following a single oral dose of extended or immediate release formulations of azithromycin. *J Antimicrob Chemother* 2008;61:884–891.

350. Honeybourne D, Kees F, Andrews JM, et al. The levels of clarithromycin and its 14-hydroxy metabolite in the lung. *Eur Respir J* 1994;7:1275–1280.

351. Bergogne-Berezin E, Morel C, Even P, et al. Pharmacocinetique des antibiotiques dans les voies respiratoires. *Nouv Presse Med* 1978;7:2831–2836.

352. Imberti R, Cusato M, Villani P, et al. Steady-state pharmacokinetics and BAL concentration of colistin in critically ill patients after IV colistin methanesulfonate administration. *Chest* 2010;138(6):1333–1339.

353. Leroyer C, Muller-Serieys C, Quiot JJ, et al. Dirithromycin concentrations in bronchial mucosa and secretions. *Respiration* 1998;65:381–385.

354. Pierre J, Bergogne-Berezin E, Kafe H, et al. The penetration of macrolides into bronchial secretions. *J Antimicrob Chemother* 1985;16(Suppl A):217–220.

355. Brun Y, Forey F, Gamondes JP, et al. Levels of erythromycin in pulmonary tissue and bronchial mucus compared to those of amoxicillin. *J Antimicrob Chemother* 1981;8:459–466.

356. Ricevuti G, Pasotti D, Mazzone A, et al. Serum, sputum and bronchial concentrations of erythromycin in chronic bronchitis after single and multiple treatments with either propionate-17-acetylcysteinate or stearate erythromycin. *Chemotherapy* 1988;34:374–379.

357. Panteix G, Harf R, deMontclos H, et al. Josamycin pulmonary penetration determined by bronchoalveolar lavage in man. *J Antimicrob Chemother* 1988;22: 917–921.

358. Conte JE Jr, Golden JA, Kipps J, et al. Intrapulmonary pharmacokinetics of linezolid. *Antimicrob Agents Chemother* 2002;46:1475–1480.

359. Boselli E, Breilh D, Rimmele T, et al. Pharmacokinetics and intrapulmonary concentrations of linezolid administered to critically ill patients with ventilator-associated pneumonia. *Crit Care Med* 2005;33(7):1529–1533.

360. Chyo N, Sunada H, Nohara S. Clinical studies of kanamycin applied in the field of obstetrics and gynecology. *Asian Med J* 1962;5:293–297.

361. Takase Z. Laboratory and clinical studies of tobramycin in the field of obstetrics and gynecology. *Chemotherapy* 1975;23:1390–1403.

362. Fleiss PM, Richward GA, Gordon J, et al. Aztreonam in human serum and breast milk. *Br J Clin Pharmacol* 1985; 19:509–511.

363. Kafetzis DA, Siafas CA, Georgakopoulos PA, et al. Passage of cephalosporins and amoxicillin into the breast milk. *Acta Paediatr Scand* 1981;70:285–288.

364. Lily and Co. Mandol in lactating mothers. Data on file. Indianapolis, IN: Elilily and Co.

365. Yoshioka H, Cho K, Takimoto M, et al. Transfer of cefazolin into human milk. *J Pediatr* 1979;94:151–152.

366. Weissenbacher ER, Adams D, Gutschow K, et al. Clinical results and concentrations of cefmenoxime in serum, amniotic fluid, mother's milk, and placenta. *Am J Med* 1984;77(Suppl 6A):11–12.

367. Lou MA, Wu YH, Jacob LS, et al. Penetration of cefonicid into human breast milk and various body fluids and tissues. *Rev Infect Dis* 1984;6(Suppl 4): 5816–5820.

368. Takase Z, Shirafuji H, Uchida M. Fundamental and clinical studies of cefoperazone in the field of obstetrics and gynecology. *Chemotherapy* 1980;28(Suppl 6): 825–836.

369. Dresse A, Lambotte R, Dubois M, et al. Transmammary passage of cefoxitin: additional results. *J Clin Pharmacol* 1983;23:438–440.

370. Takase Z, Shirafuji H, Uchida M. Clinical and laboratory studies on cefoxitin in the field of obstetrics and gynecology. *Chemotherapy* 1978;26:502–505.

371. Shyu WC, Shah VR, Campbell DA, et al. Excretion of cefprozil into human breast milk. *Antimicrob Agents Chemother* 1992;36:938–941.

372. Blanco JD, Jorgensen JH, Castaneda YS, et al. Ceftazidime levels in human breast milk. *Antimicrob Agents Chemother* 1983;23:479–480.

373. Kafetzis DA, Brater DC, Fanourgakis JE, et al. Ceftriaxone distribution between maternal blood and fetal blood and tissues at parturition and between blood and milk postpartum. *Antimicrob Agents Chemother* 1983;23: 870–873.

374. Mischler TW, Corson SL, Larranaga A, et al. Cephradine and epicillin in body fluids of lactating and pregnant women. *J Reprod Med* 1973;26:130–136.

375. Prigot A, Froix KJ, Rubin E. Absorption, diffusion and excretion of a new penicillin, oxacillin. *Antimicrob Agents Chemother* 1962;1962:402–409.

376. Greene HJ, Burkhart B, Hobby GL. Excretion of penicillin in human milk following parturition. *Am J Obstet Gynecol* 1946;51:732–733.

377. Rosansky R, Brzczinsky A. The excretion of penicillin in human milk. *J Lab Clin Med* 1949;34:497–500.

378. Matheson I, Samseth M, Loberg R, et al. Milk transfer of phenoxymethyl-penicillin during puerperal mastitis. *Br J Clin Pharmacol* 1988;25:33–40.

379. Lederle Laboratories. Piperacil [package insert]. Data on file. Lederle Laboratories, 1982.

380. Braneberg PE, Heisterberg L. Blood and milk concentrations of ampicillin in mothers treated with pivampicillin and in their infants. *J Perinatal Med* 1987;15:555–558.

381. Foulds G, Miller RD, Knirsch AK, et al. Sulbactam kinetics and excretion into breast milk in postpartum women. *Clin Pharmacol Ther* 1985;38:692–696.

382. Cho N, Nakayama T, Uehara K, et al. Laboratory and clinical evaluation of ticarcillin in the field of obstetrics and gynecology. *Chemotherapy* 1977;25:2911–2923.

383. Amsden GW, Nicolau DP, Whitaker AM, et al. Characterization of the penetration of garenoxacin into the breast milk of lactating women. *J Clin Pharmacol* 2004; 44:188–192.

384. Guilbeau JA, Schoenbach EB, Schaub IG, et al. Aureomycin in obstetrics. *JAMA* 1950;143:520–526.

385. Posner AC, Prigot A, Konicoff NG. Further observations on the use of tetracycline hydrochloride in prophylaxis and treatment of obstetric infections. *Antibiot Annu* 1954;5:594–598.

386. Morgan G, Ceccarelli G, Ciaffi G. Comparative concentrations of a tetracycline antibiotic in serum and maternal milk. *Antibiotica* 1968;6:216–222.

387. Plomp TA, Thiery M, Maes RAA. The passage of thiamphenicol and chloramphenicol into human milk after single and repeated oral administration. *Vet Hum Toxicol* 1983;25:167–172.

388. Steen B, Rane A. Clindamycin passage into milk. *Br J Clin Pharmacol* 1982;13:661–664.

389. Heisterberg L, Branebjerg PE. Blood and milk concentrations of metronidazole in mothers and infants. *J Perinat Med* 1983;11:114–120.

390. Varsano J, Fischl J, Shochet SB. The excretion of orally ingested nitrofurantoin in human milk. *J Pediatr* 1973;82:886–887.

391. Stoehr GP, Juhl RP, Veals J, et al. The excretion of rosaramicin into breast milk. *J Clin Pharmacol* 1985; 25:89–94.

392. Mannisto PT, Karhunen M, Koskela O, et al. Concentrations of tinidazole in breast milk. *Acta Pharmacol Toxicol* 1983;53:254–256.

393. Ernstson S, Anari M, Eden T, et al. Penetration of cefaclor to adenoid tissue and middle ear effusion in chronic OME. *Acta Otolaryngol* 1985;424(Suppl):7–12.

394. Santacroce F, Dainelli B, Mignini F, et al. Determination of cefatrizine levels in blood, tonsils, paranasal sinuses and middle ear. *Drugs Exp Clin Res* 1985;11:453–456.

395. Harrison CJ, Chartrand SA, Rodriguez W, et al. Middle ear fluid concentrations of cefixime in acute otitis media and otitis media with effusion. In: *Program and abstracts of the 34th Interscience Conference on Antimicrobial Agents and Chemotherapy.* Washington, DC: American Society for Microbiology, 1994. Abstract A67.

396. Danon J. Cefotaxime concentrations in otitis media effusions. *J Antimicrob Chemother* 1980;6(Suppl A): 131–132.

397. Shyu WC, Haddad J, Reilly J, et al. Penetration of cefprozil into middle ear fluid of patients with otitis media. *Antimicrob Agents Chemother* 1994;38:2210–2212.

398. Nicolau DP, Sutherland CA, Arguedas A, et al. Pharmacokinetics of cefprozil in plasma and middle ear fluid. *Pediatr Drugs* 2007;9:119–123.

399. Kusmiesz H, Shelton S, Brown O, et al. Loracarbef concentrations in middle ear fluid. *Antimicrob Agents Chemother* 1990;34:2030–2031.

400. Ginsburg CM, McCracken GH, Nelson JD. Pharmacology of oral antibiotics used for treatment of otitis media and tonsillopharyngitis in infants and children. *Ann Otol Rhinol Laryngol* 1981;90(Suppl 84):37–43.

401. Krause PJ, Owens NJ, Nightingale CH, et al. Penetration of amoxicillin, cefaclor, erythromycin-sulfisoxazole, and trimethoprim-sulfamethoxazole into the middle ear fluid of patients with chronic serous otitis media. *J Infect Dis* 1982;145:815–821.

402. Lahikainen EA, Vuori M, Virtanen S. Azidocillin and ampicillin concentrations in middle ear effusion. *Acta Otolaryngol* 1977;84:227–232.

403. Lahikainen EA. Penicillin concentration in middle ear secretion in otitis. *Acta Otolaryngol* 1970;70: 358–362.

404. Kamme C, Lundgren K, Rundcrantz H. The concentration of penicillin V in serum and middle ear exudate in acute otitis media in children. *Scand J Infect Dis* 1969; 1:77–83.

405. Sundberg L, Eden T, Ernstson S. Penetration of doxycycline in respiratory mucosa. *Acta Otolaryngol* 1983; 96:501–508.

406. Silverstein H, Bernstein JM, Lerner PI. Antibiotic concentrations in middle ear effusions. *Pediatrics* 1966;38: 33–39.

407. Jokipii AM, Jokipii L. Metronidazole, tinidazole, ornidazole and anaerobic infections of the middle ear, maxillary sinus and central nervous system. *Scand J Infect Dis* 1981;26(Suppl):123–129.

408. Kohonen A, Palmgren O, Renkonen O. Penetration of trimethoprim-sulfadiazine into middle ear fluid in secretory otitis media. *Int J Pediatr Otorhinolaryngol* 1983; 6:89–94.

409. Cherrier P, Tod M, Le Gros V, et al. Cefotiam concentrations in the sinus fluid of patients with chronic sinusitis after administration of cefotiam hexetil. *Eur J Clin Microbiol Infect Dis* 1993;12:211–215.

410. Kohonen A, Paavolainen M, Renkonen OV. Concentration of cephalexin in maxillary sinus mucosa and secretion. *Ann Clin Res* 1975;7:50–53.

411. Stenquist M, Olen L, Jannert M, et al. Penetration of loracarbef into the maxillary sinus: a pharmacokinetic assessment. *Clin Ther* 1996;18:273–284.

412. Gnarpe H, Lundberg C. L-phase organisms in maxillary sinus secretions. *Scand J Infect Dis* 1971;3:257–259.

413. Jokinen K, Raunto V. Penetration of azidocillin into the secretion and tissues in chronic maxillary sinusitis and tonsilitis. *Acta Otolaryngol* 1975;79:460–465.

414. Jones S, Yu VL, Johnson JT, et al. Pharmacokinetic and therapeutic trial of sultamicillin in acute sinusitis. *Antimicrob Agents Chemother* 1985;28:832–833.

415. Malmborg AS, Kumlien J, Samuelsson A, et al. Concentrations of enoxacin in sinus secretions. *Rev Infect Dis* 1989;11(Suppl 5):S1205–S1206.

416. Eneroth C-M, Lundberg C, Wretlind B. Antibiotic concentrations in maxillary sinus secretions and in the sinus mucosa. *Chemotherapy* 1975;21(Suppl 1):1–7.

417. Worgan D, Daniel RJE. The penetration of minocycline into human sinus secretions. *Scott Med J* 1976;21: 197–199.

418. Ehnhage A, Rautiainen M, Fang AF, et al. Pharmacokinetics of azithromycin in serum and sinus fluid after administration of extended-release and immediate-release formulations in patients with acute bacterial sinusitis. *Int J Antimicrob Agents* 2008;31:561–566.

419. Kalm O, Kamme C, Bergstrom B, et al. Erythromycin stearate in acute maxillary sinusitis. *Scand J Infect Dis* 1973;7:209–217.

420. Paavolainen M, Kohonen A, Palva T, et al. Penetration of erythromycin stearate into maxillary sinus mucosa and secretion in chronic maxillary sinusitis. *Acta Otolaryngol* 1977;84:292–295.

421. Mattila J, Mannisto PT, Luodeslampi M. Penetration of trimethoprim and sulfadiazine into sinus secretion in acute maxillary sinusitis. *Chemotherapy* 1983;29: 174–177.

422. Goto T, Makinose S, Ohi Y, et al. Diffusion of piperacillin, cefotiam, minocycline, amikacin and ofloxacin into the prostate. *Int J Urol* 1998;5:243–246.

423. Williams CB, Litvak AS, McRoberts JW. Comparison of serum and prostatic levels of tobramycin. *Urology* 1979;13:589–591.

424. Shimada J, Ueda Y. Moxalactam: absorption, excretion, distribution, and metabolism. *Rev Infect Dis* 1982; 4(Suppl):S569–S580.

425. Frongillo RF, Galuppo L, Moretti A. Suction skin blisters, skin window, and skin chamber techniques to determine extravascular passage of cefotaxime in humans. *Antimicrob Agents Chemother* 1981;19:22–28.

426. Borski AA, Pulaski EJ, Kimbrough JC, et al. Prostatic fluid, semen, and prostatic tissue concentrations of the major antibiotics following intravenous administration. *Antibiot Chemother* 1954;4:905–910.

427. Boerma JBJ, Dalhoff A, Debruyne FMY. Ciprofloxacin distribution in prostatic tissue and fluid following oral administration. *Chemotherapy* 1985;31:13–18.

428. Bulitta JB, Kinzig M, Naber CK, et al. Population pharmacokinetics and penetration into prostatic, seminal and vaginal fluid for ciprofloxacin, levofloxacin and their combination. *Chemotherapy* 2011;57:402–416.

429. Kees F, Naber KG, Schumacher H, et al. Penetration of fleroxacin into prostatic secretion and prostatic adenoma tissue. *Chemotherapy* 1988;34:437–443.

430. Naber CK, Steghafner M, Kinzig-Schippers M, et al. Concentrations of gatifloxacin in plasma and urine and penetration into prostatic and seminal fluid, ejaculate, and sperm cells after single oral administrations of 400 milligrams to volunteers. *Antimicrob Agents Chemother* 2001;45:293–297.

431. Wagenlehner FME, Kees F, Weidner W, et al. Concentrations of moxifloxacin in plasma and urine, and penetration into prostatic fluid and ejaculate, following single oral administration of 400 mg to healthy volunteers. *Int J Antimicrob Agents* 2008;31:21–26.

432. Nielson ML, Hansen IT. Trimethoprim in human prostatic tissue and prostatic fluid. *Scand J Urol Nephrol* 1972; 6:244–248.

433. Yogev R, Kolling WM. Intraventricular levels of amikacin after intravenous administration. *Antimicrob Agents Chemother* 1981;20:583–586.

434. Vacek V, Hejzlar M, Skalova M. Penetration of antibiotics into the cerebrospinal fluid in inflammatory conditions. III. Gentamicin. *Int J Clin Pharmacol* 1969;2:277–279.

435. Howard JB, McCracken GH. Reappraisal of kanamycin usage in neonates. *J Pediatr* 1975;86:949–956.

436. Greenman RL, Arcey SM, Dickenson GM, et al. Penetration of aztreonam into human cerebrospinal fluid in the presence of meningeal inflammation. *J Antimicrob Chemother* 1985;15:637–640.

437. Korzeniowski OM, Carvalho EM Jr, Rocha H, et al. Evaluation of cefamandole therapy in patients with bacterial meningitis. *J Infect Dis* 1978;137:S169–S179.

438. Thys JP, Vanderkelen B, Klastersky J. Pharmacological study of cefazolin during intermittent and continuous infusion: a crossover investigation in humans. *Antimicrob Agents Chemother* 1976;10:395–398.

439. Nahata MC, Kohlbrenner VM, Barson WJ. Pharmacokinetics and cerebrospinal fluid concentrations of cefixime in infants and young children. *Chemotherapy* 1993; 39:1–5.

440. Cable D, Overturf G, Edralin G. Concentrations of cefoperazone in cerebrospinal fluid during bacterial meningitis. *Antimicrob Agents Chemother* 1983;23:688–691.

441. Belohradsky BH, Geiss D, Marget W, et al. Intravenous cefotaxime in children with bacterial meningitis. *Lancet* 1980;1:61–63.

442. Asmar BI, Thirumoorthi MC, Buckley JA, et al. Cefotaxime diffusion into cerebrospinal fluid of children with meningitis. *Antimicrob Agents Chemother* 1985;28: 138–140.

443. Wolff M, Chavanet P, Kazmierczak A, et al. Diffusion of cefpirome into the cerebrospinal fluid of patients with purulent meningitis. *J Antimicrob Chemother* 1992; 29(Suppl A):59–62.

444. Bruckner O, Friess D, Schaaf D, et al. Cure of pseudomonal meningitis dependent on levels of cefsulodin in cerebrospinal fluid. *Drugs Exp Clin Res* 1983;9: 291–297.

445. Modai J, Decazes JM, Wolff M, et al. Penetration of ceftazidime into cerebrospinal fluid of patients with bacterial meningitis. *Antimicrob Agents Chemother* 1983; 24:126–128.

446. Steele RW, Bradsher RW. Comparison of ceftriaxone with standard therapy for bacterial meningitis. *J Pediatr* 1983;103:138–141.

447. Cable D, Edralin G, Overturf GP. Human cerebrospinal fluid pharmacokinetics and treatment of bacterial meningitis with ceftizoxime. *J Antimicrob Chemother* 1982;10(Suppl C):121–127.

448. Overturf GD, Cable DC, Forthal DN, et al. Treatment of bacterial meningitis with ceftizoxime. *Antimicrob Agents Chemother* 1984;25:258–262.

449. Swedish Study Group. Cefuroxime versus ampicillin and chloramphenicol for the treatment of bacterial meningitis. *Lancet* 1982;1:295–298.

450. Lerner PI. Penetration of cephaloridine into cerebrospinal fluid. *Am J Med Sci* 1971;262:321–326.

451. Dealy DH, Duma RJ, Tarktaglione TA, et al. Penetration of primaxin (*N*-formimidoyl thienamicin and cilastatin) into human cerebrospinal fluid. In: *Proceedings of the 14th International Congress of Chemotherapy*. Kyoto, Japan: International Society of Chemotherapy, 1985. Abstract S-78–4.

452. Dagan R, Velghe L, Rodda JL, et al. Penetration of meropenem into the cerebrospinal fluid of patients with inflamed meninges. *J Antimicrob Chemother* 1994; 34:175–179.

453. Lacut JY, Humbert G, Aubertin J, et al. Treatment of purulent meningitis in adults with injectable amoxycillin: clinical and pharmacokinetic results. *Curr Ther Res* 1981;29:36–46.

454. Combined Clinical Staff Conference of the National Institutes of Health. A new penicillin derivative resistant to penicillinase, dimethoxyphenyl penicillin. *Antibiot Chemother* 1961;11:537.

455. Yogev R, Schultz WE, Rosenman SB. Penetrance of nafcillin into human ventricular fluid: correlation with ventricular pleocytosis and glucose levels. *Antimicrob Agents Chemother* 1981;19:545–548.

456. Kane JG, Parker RH, Jordan GW, et al. Nafcillin concentration in cerebrospinal fluid during treatment of staphylococcal infections. *Ann Intern Med* 1977;87: 309–311.

457. Hieber JP, Nelson JD. A pharmacologic evaluation of penicillin in children with purulent meningitis. *N Engl J Med* 1977;197:410–413.

458. Dickinson GM, Droller DG, Greeman RL, et al. Clinical evaluation of piperacillin with observations on penetrability into cerebrospinal fluid. *Antimicrob Agents Chemother* 1981;20:481–486.

459. Goh BT, Smith GW, Samarasinghe L, et al. Penicillin concentrations in serum and cerebrospinal fluid after intramuscular injection of aqueous procaine penicillin 0.6 MU with and without probenecid. *Br J Vener Dis* 1984;60:371–373.

460. Stahl JP, Bru JP, Fredji G, et al. Penetration of sulbactam into the cerebrospinal fluid of patients with bacterial meningitis receiving ampicillin therapy. *Rev Infect Dis* 1986;8(Suppl 5):S612–S616.

461. Bruckner O, Trautmann M, Borner K. A study of the penetration of temocillin in the cerebrospinal fluid. *Drugs* 1985;29(Suppl 5):162–166.

462. Gerding DN, Hitt JA. Tissue penetration of new quinolones in humans. *Rev Infect Dis* 1989;11(Suppl 5): S1046–S1057.

463. Kanellakopoulou K, Pagoulatou A, Stroumpoulis K, et al. Pharmacokinetics of moxifloxacin in non-inflamed cerebrospinal fluid of humans: implication for a bactericidal effect. *J Antimicrob Chemother* 2008;61:1328–1331.

464. Van Niekerk CH, Steyn DL, Davis WG, et al. Chloramphenicol levels in cerebrospinal fluid in meningitis. *S Afr Med J* 1980;58:159–160.

465. Kullar R, Chin JN, Edwards DJ, et al. Pharmacokinetics of single-dose daptomycin in patients with suspected or confirmed neurological infections. *Antimicrob Agents Chemother* 2011;55:3505–3509.

466. Boger WP, Gavin JJ. Demethylchlortetracycline: serum concentration studies and cerebrospinal fluid diffusion. *Antibiot Annu* 1960;1959:393–400.

467. Yim CW, Flyan NM, Fitzgerald FT. Penetration of oral doxycycline into the cerebrospinal fluid of patients with latent neurosyphilis. *Antimicrob Agents Chemother* 1985;28:347–348.

468. Dotevall L, Hagberg L. Penetration of doxycycline into cerebrospinal fluid in patients treated for suspected Lyme neuroborreliosis. *Antimicrob Agents Chemother* 1989;33: 1078–1080.

469. Vacek V, Hejzlar M, Skalova M. Penetration of antibiotics into the cerebrospinal fluid in inflammatory conditions. II. Lincomycin. *Int J Clin Pharmacol* 1968;1:501–503.

470. Tsona A, Metallidis S, Foroglou N, et al. Linezolid penetration into cerebrospinal fluid and brain tissue. *J Chemother* 2010;22:17–19.

471. Jokipii AMM, Myllvia VV, Hokkanen E, et al. Penetration of the blood brain barrier by metronidazole and tinidazole. *J Antimicrob Chemother* 1977;3:239–245.

472. Wang EEL, Prober CG. Ventricular cerebrospinal fluid concentrations of trimethoprim-sulphamethoxazole. *J Antimicrob Chemother* 1983;11:385–389.

473. Wingfield DL, McDougal RL, Roy FH, et al. Ocular penetration of amikacin following intramuscular injection. *Arch Ophthalmol* 1983;101:117–120.

474. Sinues B, Martinez P, Palomar A, et al. Niveles de gentamicina en humor acuoso y plasma segun la via de administracion. *Ard Farmacol Toxicol* 1982;8:219–226.

475. Orr W, Jackson WB, Colden K. Intraocular penetration of netilmicin. *Can J Ophthalmol* 1985;20:171–175.

476. Sinues B, Martinez P, Barrera V, et al. Taux de la tobramycine dans l'humeur aqueuse et le plasma humains apres administration par voie intraveineuse et sous-conjonctivale. *Therapie* 1983;38:345–353.

477. Petounis A, Papapanos G, Karageorgiou-Makromihelaki C. Penetration of tobryamycin sulfate into the human eye. *Br J Ophthalmol* 1978;62:660–662.

478. Haroche G, Salvanet A, Lafaix C, et al. Pharmacokinetics of aztreonam in the aqueous humor. *J Antimicrob Chemother* 1986;18:195–198.

479. Axelrod JL, Damask LJ, Kochman RS. Cefaclor levels in human aqueous humor. In: *Program and abstracts of the 17th Interscience Conference on Antimicrobial Agents and Chemotherapy.* Washington, DC: American Society for Microbiology, 1977. Abstract 311.

480. Bidart B, Galindo Hernandez E, Flores Mercado F. Cefadroxil levels in human aqueous humors. In: *Program and abstracts of the 11th International Congress of Chemotherapy and 19th Interscience Conference on Antimicrobial Agents and Chemotherapy.* Washington, DC: American Society for Microbiology, 1979. Abstract 339.

481. Axelrod JL, Kochman RS. Cefamandole levels in primary aqueous humor in man. *Am J Ophthalmol* 1978;85: 342–348.

482. MacIlwaine WA, Sande MA, Mandell GL. Penetration of antistaphylococcal antibiotics into the human eye. *Am J Ophthalmol* 1974;77:589–592.

483. Ozdamar A, Aras C, Ozturk R, et al. Ocular penetration of cefepime following systemic administration in humans. *Ophthalmic Surg Lasers* 2001;32:25–29.

484. Axelrod JL, Kochman RS, Horowitz MA, et al. Comparison of ceftizoxime and cefmenoxime levels in human aqueous humor. In: *Program and abstracts of the 23rd Interscience Conference on Antimicrobial Agents and Chemotherapy.* Washington, DC: American Society for Microbiology, 1983. Abstract 644.

485. Axelrod JL, Kochman RS. Cefonicid concentrations in human aqueous humor. *Arch Ophthalmol* 1984;102: 433–434.

486. Giamarellou H, Kavouklis E, Grammatikou M, et al. Penetration of four-lactam antibiotics with antipseudomonal activity into human aqueous humor. In: Periti P, Grassi G, eds. *Current chemotherapy and immunotherapy: proceedings.* Washington, DC: American Society for Microbiology, 1982:153–155.

487. Quentin CD, Ansorg R. Penetration of cefotaxime into the aqueous humour after intravenous application. *Graefes Arch Clin Exp Ophthalmol* 1983;220:245–247.

488. Axelrod JL, Kochman RS. Cefoxitin levels in human aqueous humor. *Am J Ophthalmol* 1980;90:388–393.

489. Egger SF, Alzner E, Georgopoulos M, et al. Penetration of cefpirome into the anterior chamber of the human eye after intravenous application. *J Antimicrob Chemother* 2000;45:213–216.

490. Rubinstein E, Avni I, Tuizer H, et al. Cefsulodin levels in the human aqueous humor. *Arch Ophthalmol* 1985; 103:426–427.

491. Axelrod JL, Kochman RS, Horowitz MA, et al. Ceftazidime concentrations in human aqueous humor. *Arch Ophthalmol* 1984;102:923–925.

492. Martinelli D, Mazzei T, Fallani S, et al. Ceftizoxime concentrations in human aqueous humor following intravenous administration. *Chemioterapia* 1988;7:317–319.

493. Ziak E, Schuhmann G, Konstantinou D, et al. Levels in aqueous humour of eight relevant antibiotics in humans. In: *Recent advances in chemotherapy: proceedings of the 14th International Congress of Chemotherapy.* Kyoto, Japan: University of Tokyo Press, 1985.

494. Guerra R, Casu L, Giola K, et al. Penetration of parenteral cefuroxime into the human aqueous humor. *Arzneimittelforschung* 1981;31:861–863.

495. Records RE. The human intraocular penetration of a new orally effective cephalosporin antibiotic, cephalexin. *Ann Ophthalmol* 1971;3:309–313.

496. Riley FC, Boyle GL, Leopold IH. Intraocular penetration of cephaloridine in humans. *Am J Ophthalmol* 1968;66:1042–1049.

497. Records RE. Intraocular penetration of cephalothin. *Am J Ophthalmol* 1968;66:441–443.

498. Axelrod JL, Kochman RS. Cephradine levels in human aqueous humor. *Arch Ophthalmol* 1981;99:2034–2036.

499. Axelrod JL, Newton JC, Klein RM, et al. Penetration of imipenem into human aqueous and vitreous humor. *Am J Ophthalmol* 1987;104:649–653.

500. Schauersberger J, Amon M, Wedrich A, et al. Penetration and decay of meropenem into the human aqueous humor and vitreous. *J Ocul Pharmacol Ther* 1999;15:439–445.

501. Axelrod JL, Kochman RS. Moxalactam concentration in human aqueous humor after intravenous administration. *Arch Ophthalmol* 1982;100:1334–1336.

502. Hariprasad SM, Mieler WF, Holz ER. Vitreous and aqueous penetrations of orally administered gatifloxacin in humans. *Arch Ophthalmol* 2003;121:345–350.

503. Garcia-Vazquez E, Mensa J, Sarasa M, et al. Penetration of levofloxacin into the anterior chamber (aqueous humor) of the human eye after intravenous administration. *Eur J Clin Microbiol Infect Dis* 2007;26:137–140.

504. Vedantham V, Lalitha P, Velpandian T, et al. Vitreous and aqueous penetration of orally administered moxifloxacin in humans. *Eye* 2006;20:1273–1278.

505. Hariprasad SM, Shah GK, Mieler WF, et al. Vitreous and aqueous penetration of orally administered moxifloxacin in humans. *Arch Ophthalmol* 2006;124:178–182.

506. Von Gunten S, Lew D, Paccolat F, et al. Aqueous humor penetration of ofloxacin given by various routes. *Am J Ophthalmol* 1994;117:87–89.

507. Johnson AP, Scoper SV, Woo FL, et al. Azlocillin levels in human tears and aqueous humor. *Am J Ophthalmol* 1985;99:469–472.

508. Uwaydah MM, Faris BM, Samara IN, et al. Cloxacillin penetration. *Am J Ophthalmol* 1976;82:114–116.

509. Records RE. The human intraocular penetration of methicillin. *Arch Ophthalmol* 1966;76:720–722.

510. Behrens-Baumann W, Ansorg R. Mezlocillin concentrations in human aqueous humor after intravenous and subconjunctival administration. *Chemotherapy* 1985;31: 169–172.

511. Records RE. Human intraocular penetration of sodium oxacillin. *Arch Ophthalmol* 1967;77:693–695.

512. Woo FL, Johnson AP, Caldwell DR, et al. Piperacillin levels in human tears and aqueous humor. *Am J Ophthalmol* 1984;98:17–20.

513. Poirier RH, Ellison AC. Ocular penetration of orally administered minocycline. *Ann Ophthalmol* 1979;11: 1859–1861.

514. Abraham RK, Burnett HH. Tetracycline and chloramphenicol studies on rabbit and human eyes. *Arch Ophthalmol* 1955;54:641–659.

515. Tabbara KF, Al-Kharashi SA, Al-Mansouri SM, et al. Ocular levels of azithromycin. *Arch Ophthalmol* 1998; 116:1625–1628.

516. Al-Sibai MB, Al-Kaff AS, Raines D, et al. Ocular penetration of oral clarithromycin in humans. *J Ocul Pharmacol Ther* 1998;14:575–583.

517. Becker EF. The intraocular penetration of lincomycin. *Am J Ophthalmol* 1969;67:963–965.

518. Fiscella RG, Lai WW, Buerk B, et al. Aqueous and vitreous penetration of linezolid (Zyvox) after oral administration. *Ophthalmology* 2004;111:1191–1195.

519. Mattila J, Nerdrum K, Rouhiainen H, et al. Penetration of metronidazole and tinidazole into the aqueous humor in man. *Chemotherapy* 1983;29:188–191.

520. Souli M, Kopsinis G, Kavouklis E, et al. Vancomycin levels in human aqueous humour after intravenous and subconjunctival administration. *Int J Antimicrob Agents* 2001;18:239–243.

521. Daschner F, Reiss E, Engert J. Distribution of amikacin in serum, muscle, and fat in children after a single intramuscular injection. *Antimicrob Agents Chemother* 1977; 11:1081–1083.

522. Quintiliani R. A review of the penetration of cefadroxil into human tissue. *J Antimicrob Chemother* 1982;19(Suppl B):33–38.

523. Robens W. Concentrations of cefmenoxime in human tissues. *Am J Med* 1984;77(Suppl 6A):32–33.

524. Just HM, Bassler M, Frank U, et al. Penetration of cefotaxime into heart valves, subcutaneous and muscle tissue of patients undergoing open-heart surgery. *J Antimicrob Chemother* 1984;14:431–434.

525. Adam D, Wittke RR, Eisenberger F. Tissue penetration of cefsulodin, a new antipseudomonas-cephalosporin antibiotic. *Drugs Exp Clin Res* 1981;7:227–231.

526. Adam D, Reichart B, Williams KJ. Penetration of ceftazidime into human tissue in patients undergoing cardiac surgery. *J Antimicrob Chemother* 1983;12(Suppl A): 269–273.

527. Beam TR, Raab TA, Spooner JA, et al. Comparison of ceftriaxone and cefazolin prophylaxis against infection in open heart surgery. *Am J Surg* 1984;148(Suppl 4A): 8–14.

528. Bullen BR, Ramsden CT, Kester RC. Tissue levels of cephradine in ischemic limbs, following a single intravenous injection. *Curr Med Res Opin* 1980;6:585–588.

529. Kummel A, Scholsser V, Petersen E, et al. Pharmacokinetics of imipenem-cilastatin in serum and tissue. *Eur J Clin Microbiol* 1985;4:609–610.

530. Jorgensen LN, Andreasen JJ, Nielsen PT, et al. Dicloxacillin concentrations in amputation. *Acta Orthop Scand* 1989;60:617–620.

531. Fraschini F, Braga PC, Copponi V, et al. Tropism of erythromycin for the respiratory system. In: Nelson JD, Grassi C, eds. *Current chemotherapy and infectious disease: proceedings*. Washington, DC: American Society for Microbiology, 1979:659–662.

532. Helwing E, Lux M, Duben W, et al. Mezlocillin: Zur Gewebekonzentration und Wirksamkeit. *Med Klin* 1979; 74:112–116.

533. Nunes HL, Pecora CC, Judy K. Turnover and distribution of nafcillin in tissues and body fluids of surgical patients. *Antimicrob Agents Chemother* 1965;1964: 237–249.

534. Adam D, Wilhelm K, Chysky V. Antibiotic concentrations in blood and tissue. *Arzneimittelforschung* 1981;31:1972–1976.

535. Russo J, Thompson MIB, Russo ME. Piperacillin distribution into bile, gallbladder wall, abdominal skeletal muscle, and adipose tissue in surgical patients. *Antimicrob Agents Chemother* 1982;22:488–492.

536. Silbermann M, Niederdellmann H, Kluge D, et al. Concentration of piperacillin and cefotaxime in human muscle and fat tissue. In: *Program and abstracts of the 20th Interscience Conference on Antimicrobial Agents and Chemotherapy*. Washington, DC: American Society for Microbiology, 1980. Abstract 755.

537. Gould JG, Meikle G, Cooper DL, et al. Temocillin concentrations in human tissues. *Drugs* 1985;29(Suppl 5): 167–169.

538. Daschner FD, Thema G, Langmaack H, et al. Ticarcillin concentrations in serum, muscle, and fat after a single intravenous injection. *Antimicrob Agents Chemother* 1980;17:738–739.

539. Bell MJ, Shackelford PG, Schroeder KF. Penetration of clindamycin into peritoneal fluid, intestine and muscle in neonates and infants. *Curr Ther Res* 1983;33: 751–757.

540. Lovering AM, Zhang J, Bannister GC, et al. Penetration of linezolid into bone, fat, muscle and haematoma of patients undergoing routine hip replacement. *J Antimicrob Chemother* 2002;50:73–77.

541. Frank UK, Schmidt-Eisenlohr E, Mlangeni D, et al. Penetration of teicoplanin into heart valves and subcutaneous and muscle tissues of patients undergoing open-heart surgery. *Antimicrob Agents Chemother* 1997;41:2559–2561.

542. Daschner FD, Frank U, Kummel A, et al. Pharmacokinetics of vancomycin in serum and tissue of patients undergoing open heart surgery. *J Antimicrob Chemother* 1987;19:359–362.

543. Smilak JD, Flittie WH, Williams TW. Bone concentrations of antimicrobial agents after parenteral administration. *Antimicrob Agents Chemother* 1976;9: 169–171.

544. Boselli E, Breilh D, Bel JC, et al. Diffusion of isepamicin into cancellous and cortical bone tissue. *Chemother* 2002;14(4):361–365.

545. Wilson APR, Taylor B, Treasure T, et al. Antibiotic prophylaxis in cardiac surgery: serum and tissue levels of teicoplanin, flucloxacillin and tobramycin. *J Antimicrob Chemother* 1988;21:210–212.

546. MacLeod CM, Bartley EA, Galante JO, et al. Aztreonam penetration into synovial fluid and bone. *Antimicrob Agents Chemother* 1986;29:710–712.

547. Akimoto Y, Mochizuki Y, Uda A, et al. Cefaclor concentrations in human serum, gingiva, mandibular bone, and dental follicle following a single oral administration. *Gen Pharmacol* 1992;23:639–642.

548. Hume AL, Polk R, Kline B, et al. Comparative penetration of latamoxef (moxalactam) and cefazolin into human knee following simultaneous administration. *J Antimicrob Chemother* 1983;12:623–627.

549. Tetzlaff TR, Howard JB, McCracken GH, et al. Antibiotic concentrations in pus and bone of children with osteomyelitis. *J Pediatr* 1978;92:135–140.

550. Parsens RL, Beavis JP, David JA, et al. Plasma, bone, hip capsule, and drain fluid concentrations of cephazolin during total hip replacement. *Br J Clin Pharmacol* 1978; 5:331–336.

551. Breilh D, Boselli E, Bel JC, et al. Diffusion of cefepime into cancellous and cortical bone tissue. *J Chemother* 2003;15(2):134–138.

552. Scaglione F, De Martini G, Peretto L, et al. Pharmacokinetic study of cefodizime and ceftriaxone in sera and bones of patients undergoing hip arthroplasty. *Antimicrob Agents Chemother* 1997;41:2292–2294.

553. Nightingale CH, Quintiliani R, Dudley MN, et al. Tissue penetration and half-life of cefonicid. *Rev Infect Dis* 1984;6(Suppl 4):821–828.

554. Braga PC, Scaglione F, Villa S, et al. Cefoperazone pharmacokinetics and sputum levels after single/multiple I.M. injections in bronchopneumopathic patients and bone, pulmonary and prostatic tissue penetration. *Int J Clin Pharmacol Res* 1983;5:349–355.

555. Wittmann DH, Schassan HH. Bone levels, tissue fluid and peritoneal fluid measurements following piperacillin administration. In: *Program and abstracts of the 20th Interscience Conference on Antimicrobial Agents and Chemotherapy.* Washington, DC: American Society of Microbiology; 1980. Abstract 757.

556. Dehne MG, Muhling J, Sablotzki A, et al. Pharmacokinetics of antibiotic prophylaxis in major orthopedic surgery and blood-saving techniques. *Orthopedics* 2001;24(7):665–669.

557. Plaue R, Muller O, Fabricius K, et al. Verlaufiger Bericht uber Cefoxitinspiegel-Bestimmungen in menschlichen geweben. *Infection* 1979;7(Suppl 1):S80–S84.

558. Leigh DA, Griggs J, Tighe CM, et al. Pharmacokinetic study of ceftazidime in bone and serum of patients undergoing hip and knee arthroplasty. *J Antimicrob Chemother* 1985;16:637–642.

559. Wittmann DH, Schassan HH, Seidel H. Untersuchungen uber die Bioverfugbarkeit von Cefuroxim im Knochen und im Wiundsekret. *Med Welt* 1979;30:227–232.

560. Akimoto Y, Uda A, Omata H, et al. Cephalexin concentrations in human serum, gingiva, and mandibular bone following a single oral administration. *Clin Pharmacol* 1990;21:621–623.

561. Fitzgerald RH, Kelly PJ, Snyder RJ, et al. Penetration of methicillin, oxacillin, and cephalothin into bone and synovial tissues. *Antimicrob Agents Chemother* 1978;14:723–726.

562. Davies AJ, Lockley RM, Jones A, et al. Comparative pharmacokinetics of cefamandole, cefuroxime and cephradine during total hip replacement. *J Antimicrob Chemother* 1986;17:637–640.

563. Brooks S, Dent AR. Comparison of bone levels after intramuscular administration of cephradine (Velosef) or flucloxacillin/ampicillin in hip replacement. *Pharmatherapeutica* 1984;3:642–649.

564. Boselli E, Breilh D, Djabarouti S, et al. Diffusion of ertapenem into bone and synovial tissues. *J Antimicrob Chemother* 2007,60:893–896.

565. MacGregor RR, Gibson GA, Bland JA. Imipenem pharmacokinetics and body fluid concentrations in patients receiving high-dose treatment for serious infections. *Antimicrob Agents Chemother* 1986;29:188–192.

566. Grimer RJ, Karpinski MRK, Andrews JM, et al. Penetration of amoxycillin and clavulanic acid into bone. *Chemotherapy* 1986;32:185–191.

567. Bystedt H, Dahlback A, Dornbusch K, et al. Concentration of azidocillin, erythromycin, doxycycline plus clindamycin in human mandibular bone. *Int J Oral Surg* 1978;7:442–449.

568. Wittmann DH, Schassan HH, Seidel H. Pharmakokinetische Untersuchungen zur Penetration von Azlocillin und Mezlocillin in den Knochen und in die Gewebsflussigkeit. *Arzneimittelforschung* 1981;31:1157–1162.

569. Kramer J, Weuta H. Utersuchungen uber Serumund Knocheuspiegel nach Injektion von Oxacillin und Carbenicillin. *Z Orthop* 1972;110:216–233.

570. Kondell PA, Nord CE, Nordeniam A. Concentrations of cloxacillin, dicloxacillin, and flucloxacillin in dental alveolar serum and mandibular bone. *Int J Oral Surg* 1982;11:40–43.

571. Sirot J, Lopitaux R, Sirot J, et al. Diffusion de la cloxacilline dans le tissue osseux human apies administration par voie orale. *Pathol Biol* 1982;30:332–335.

572. Schurman DJ, Johnson BL, Finerman G, et al. Antibiotic bone penetration concentration of methicillin and clindamycin phosphate in human bone taken during total hip replacement. *Clin Orthop* 1975;111:142–146.

573. Incavo SJ, Ronchetti PJ, Choi JH, et al. Penetration of piperacillin-tazobactam into cancellous and cortical bone tissues. *Antimicrob Agents Chemother* 1994;38:905–907.

574. Adam D, Heilmann HD, Weismeier K. Concentrations of ticarcillin and clavulanic acid in human bone after prophylactic administration of 5.2 g of Timentin. *Antimicrob Agents Chemother* 1987;31:935–939.

575. Fong IW, Rittenhouse BR, Simbul M, et al. Bone penetration of enoxacin in patients with and without osteomyelitis. *Antimicrob Agents Chemother* 1988;32:834–837.

576. von Baum H, Bottcher S, Abel R, et al. Tissue and serum concentrations of levofloxacin in orthopaedic patients. *Int J Antimicrob Agents* 2001;18:335–340.

577. Akimoto Y, Mochizuki Y, Uda A, et al. Concentrations of lomefloxacin in radicular cyst and oral tissues following single or multiple oral administration. *Univ Sch Dent* 1993;35:267–275.

578. Malincarne L, Ghebregzabher M, Moretti MV, et al. Penetration of moxifloxacin into bone in patients undergoing total knee arthroplasty. *J Antimicrob Chemother* 2006;57:950–954.

579. Dellamonica P, Bernard E, Etesse H, et al. The diffusion of pefloxacin into bone and the treatment of osteomyelitis. *J Antimicrob Chemother* 1986;17(Suppl B):93–102.

580. Traunmüller F, Schintler MV, Metzler J, et al. Soft tissue and bone penetration abilities of daptomycin in diabetic patients with bacterial foot infections. *J Antimicrob Chemother* 2010;65:1252–1257.

581. Sorensen TS, Colding H, Schroeder E, et al. The penetration of cefazolin, erythromycin and methicillin into human bone tissue. *Acta Orthop Scand* 1978;49:549–553.

582. Schintler MV, Traunmüller F, Metzler J et al. High fosfomycin concentrations in bone and peripheral soft tissue in diabetic patients resenting with bacterial foot infection. *J Antimicrob Chemother* 2009;64:574–578.

583. Benoni G, Cuzzolin L, Leone R, et al. Pharmacokinetics and human tissue penetration of flurithromycin. *Antimicrob Agents Chemother* 1988;32:1875–1878.

584. Vacek V, Hejzlar M, Pavlansky R. Certain problems of rational lincomycin therapy of staphylococcal osteomyelitis. *Rev Czech Med* 1969;15:92–102.

585. Linzenmeier G, Schafer P, Volk H, et al. Determination of lincomycin concentration in chronically inflamed bone and soft tissue of man. *Arzneimittelforschung* 1968;18:204–207.

586. Kutscha-Lissberg F, Hebler U, Muhr G, et al. Linezolid penetration into bone and joint tissues infected with methicillin-resistant staphylococci. *Antimicrob Agents Chemother* 2003;47:3964–3966.

587. Traunmüller F, Schintler MV, Spendel S, et al. Linezolid concentrations in infected soft tissue and bone following repetitive doses in diabetic patients with bacterial foot infections. *Int J Antimicrob Agents* 2010;36:84–86.

588. Rood JP, Collier J. Metronidazole levels in alveolar bone. In: *Metronidazole. Royal Society of Medicine International Congress and Symposium, series 18.* London: Royal Society of Medicine and Academic Press, 1979:45–47.

589. Fraschini F, Scaglione F, Mezzetti M, et al. Pharmacokinetic profile of cefotetan in different clinical conditions. *Drugs Exp Clin Res* 1988;14:547–553.

590. Sirot J, Prive L, Lopitaux R, et al. Etude de la diffusion de la rifampicine dans le tissu osseux spong ieux et compact au cours de protheses totales de hanches. *Pathol Biol* 1983;31:438–441.

591. Roth B. Penetration of parenterally administered rifampicin into bone tissue. *Chemotherapy* 1984;30:358–365.

592. Del Tacca M, Danesi R, Bernardini N, et al. Roxithromycin penetration into gingiva and alveolar bone of odontoiatric patients. *Chemotherapy* 1990;36:332–336.

593. Kuehnel TS, Schurr C, Lotter K, et al. Penetration of telithromycin into the nasal mucosa and ethmoid bone of patients undergoing rhinosurgery for chronic sinusitis. *J Antimicrob Chemother* 2005;55:591–594.

594. Graziani AL, Lawson LA, Gibson GA, et al. Vancomycin concentrations in infected and noninfected human bone. *Antimicrob Agents Chemother* 1988;32:1320–1322.

595. Farago E, Kiss J, Gomory A, et al. Amikacin: in vitro bacteriologic studies, levels in human serum, lung, and heart tissue, and clinical results. *Int J Clin Pharmacol Biopharm* 1979;17:421–428.

596. Olson NH, Nightingale CH, Quintiliani R. Penetration characteristics of cefamandole into the right atrial appendage and pericardial fluid in patients undergoing open heart surgery. *Ann Thorac Surg* 1979;29:104–108.

597. Archer GL, Polk RE, Dumg RJ, et al. Comparison of cephalothin and cefamandole prophylaxis during insertion of prosthetic heart valves. *Antimicrob Agents Chemother* 1978;13:924–929.

598. Nightingale CH, Klimek JJ, Quintiliani R. Effect of protein binding on the penetration of nonmetabolized cephalosporins into atrial appendage and pericardial fluids in open heart surgical patients. *Antimicrob Agents Chemother* 1980;17:595–598.

599. Polk RE, Smith JE, Ducey K, et al. Penetration of moxalactam and cefazolin into atrial appendage after simultaneous intramuscular or intravenous administration. *Antimicrob Agents Chemother* 1982;22:201–203.

600. Kanellakopoulou K, Tselikos D, Giannitsioti E, et al. Pharmacokinetics of fusidic acid and cefepime in heart tissues: implications for a role in surgical prophylaxis. *J Chemother* 2008;20:468–471.

601. Sterling RP, Connor DJ, Norman JC, et al. Cefonicid concentration in serum and atrial tissue during open heart surgery. *Antimicrob Agents Chemother* 1983;23:790–792.

602. Mullany LD, French MA, Nightingale CH, et al. Penetration of ceforanide and cefamandole into the right atrial appendage, pericardial fluid, sternum, and intercostal muscle of patients undergoing open heart surgery. *Antimicrob Agents Chemother* 1982;21:416–420.

603. Martin CM. *Tissue levels and body fluid levels of cefoxitin in man after therapeutic doses of the antibiotic.* Data on file. Rahway, NJ: Merck Sharp & Dohme, 1979.

604. Kobayashi M, Washio M, Eishin H, et al. Ceftizoxime level in the myocardium (right atrial muscle and mitral papillary muscle) during open heart surgery. *Jpn J Surg* 1988;18:136–141.

605. Quintiliani R, Klimek J, Nightingale CH. Penetration of cephapirin and cephalothin into the right atrial appendage and pericardial fluid of patients undergoing open heart surgery. *J Infect Dis* 1979;139:348–352.

606. Mertes PM, Voiriot P, Dopff C, et al. Penetration of ciprofloxacin into heart valves, myocardium, mediastinal fat, and sternal bone marrow in humans. *Antimicrob Agents Chemother* 1990;34:398–401.

607. Mertes PM, Jehl F, Burtin P, et al. Penetration of ofloxacin into heart valves, myocardium, mediastinal fat, and sternal bone marrow in humans. *Antimicrob Agents Chemother* 1992;36:2493–2496.

608. Brion N, Lessana A, Mosset F, et al. Penetration of pefloxacin in human heart valves. *J Antimicrob Chemother* 1986;17(Suppl B):89–92.

609. Adam D, Reichart B, Rothenfusser B. Diffusion of piperacillin into human heart muscle. In: Nelson JD, Grassi C, eds. *Current chemotherapy and infectious disease: proceedings.* Washington, DC: American Society for Microbiology, 1980:307–308.

610. Mandal AK, Thadepalli H, Bach VT, et al. Antibiotic concentration in the human right atrial appendage. *Curr Ther Res* 1980;28:504–510.

611. Vitt TG, Panzer JD. *Lincomycin at the tissue level following intramuscular lincocin.* Kalamazoo, MI: The Upjohn Co, 1973. Lincocin Study C5 034. Data on file.

612. Archer GL, Armstrong BC, Kline BJ. Rifampin blood and tissue levels in patients undergoing cardiac valve surgery. *Antimicrob Agents Chemother* 1982;21:800–803.

613. Foucault P, Desauliniers D, Saginur R, et al. Concentration of teicoplanin in human heart tissue. In: *Program and abstracts of the 28th Interscience Conference on Antimicrobial Agents and Chemotherapy.* Washington, DC: American Society for Microbiology, 1988. Abstract 937.

614. Frank UK, Schmidt-Eisenlohr E, Mlangeni D, et al. Penetration of teicoplanin into heart valves and subcutaneous and muscle tissues of patients undergoing open-heart surgery. *Antimicrob Agents Chemother* 1997;41:2559–2561.

615. Wildfeuer A, Laufen H, Muller-Wening D, et al. The effect of antibiotics on the intracellular survival of bacteria in human phagocytic cells. *Arzneimittelforschung* 1987;37:1367–1370.

616. Swoboda S, Oberdorfer K, Klee F, et al. Tissue and serum concentrations of levofloxacin 500 mg administered intravenously or orally for antibiotic prophylaxis in biliary surgery. *J Antimicrob Chemother* 2003;51:459–462.

617. Ober MC, Hoppe-Tichy T, Koninger J, et al. Tissue penetration of moxifloxacin into human gallbladder wall in patients with biliary tract infections. *J Antimicrob Chemother* 2009;64:1091–1095.

618. Fabre J, Milek E, Kalfopoulos P, et al. The kinetics of tetracyclines in man. II. Excretion, penetration in normal and inflammatory tissues, behavior in renal insufficiency and hemodialysis. *Schweiz Med Wochenschr* 1971;101:625–633.

619. Burroughs Wellcome Company. *Septra: a monograph.* Research Triangle Park, NC: Burroughs Wellcome Company, 1973;73.

620. Daschner F, Blume E, Langmaack H, et al. Cefamandole concentrations in pulmonary and subcutaneous tissue. *J Antimicrob Chemother* 1979;5:474–475.

621. Breilh D, Saux MC, Delaisement C, et al. Pharmacokinetic population study to describe cefepime lung concentrations. *Pulm Pharmacol Ther* 2001;14:69–74.

622. Cozzola M, Polverino M, Guidetti E, et al. Penetration of cefonicid into human lung tissue and lymph nodes. *Chemotherapy* 1990;36:325–331.

623. Fraschini F, Scaglione F, Pintucci G, et al. The diffusion of clarithromycin and roxithromycin into nasal mucosa, tonsil and lung in humans. *J Antimicrob Chemother* 1991;27(Suppl A):61–65.

624. Just HM, Frank U, Simon A, et al. Concentrations of ceftriaxone in serum and lung tissue. *Chemotherapy* 1984;30:81–83.

625. Benoni G, Cuzzolin L, Bertrand C, et al. Imipenem kinetics in serum, lung tissue and pericardial fluid in patients undergoing thoracotomy. *J Antimicrob Chemother* 1987;20:725–728.

626. Kiss IJ, Farago E, Gomory A, et al. Investigations on the flucloxacillin levels in human serum, lung tissue, pericardial fluid and heart tissue. *Int J Clin Pharmacol Ther Toxicol* 1980;18:405–411.

627. Marlin GE, Burgess KR, Burgoyne J, et al. Penetration of piperacillin into bronchial mucosa and sputum. *Thorax* 1981;36:774–780.

628. Kinzig M, Sorgel F, Naber KG, et al. Tissue penetration of piperacillin/tazobactam. In: *Proceedings of the 31st Interscience Conference on Antimicrobial Agents and Chemotherapy*. Washington, DC: American Society for Microbiology, 1991. Abstract 862.

629. Kiss IJ, Farago E, Fabian E. Study of oxacillin levels in human serum and lung tissue. *Ther Hung* 1974;22:55–59.

630. Zeitlinger MA, Traunmuller F, Abrahim A, et al. A pilot study testing whether concentrations of levofloxacin in interstitial space fluid of soft tissues may serve as a surrogate for predicting its pharmacokinetics in lung. *Int J Antimicrob Agents* 2007;29:44–50.

631. Fraschini F, Braga PC, Scaglione F, et al. Study on pulmonary, prostatic and renal (medulla and cortex) distribution of sagamicin at different time intervals. *Int J Clin Pharmacol Res* 1987;7:51–58.

632. Friesen VA, Streifinger W, Hofstetter A, et al. Minocyclin- und Doxycyclin-Konzentrationen in Serum, Urin, Prostataexprimat und -gewebe. *Fortschr Med* 1982;100:605–608.

633. Kitzis M, Desnottes JF, Brunel D, et al. Spiramycin concentrations in lung tissue. *J Antimicrob Chemother* 1988;22(Suppl B):123–126.

634. Fraschini F, Scaglione F, Cicchetti F, et al. Prostatic tissue concentrations and serum levels of myocamicin in human subjects. *Drugs Exp Clin Res* 1988;24:253–255.

635. Madsen PO, Dhruv R, Friedhoff LT. Aztreonam concentrations in human prostatic tissue. *Antimicrob Agents Chemother* 1984;26:20–21.

636. Smith RP, Schmid GP, Baltch AL, et al. Concentration of cefaclor in human prostatic tissue. *Am J Med Sci* 1981;281:19–24.

637. Adam D, Hofstetter AG, Eisenberger F. Zur Diffusion von Cefamandol in das Prostatagewebe. *Med Klin* 1979;74:235–238.

638. Adam D, Hofstetter AG, Reichart B, et al. Zur Diffusion von Cefazedon in das Herzmuskel-, Prostataund Hautgewebe sowie in die Gallenflussigkeit. *Arzneimittelforschung* 1979;29:1901–1906.

639. Iversen P, Madsen PO. Short-term cephalosporin prophylaxis in transurethral surgery. *Clin Ther* 1982;5 (Suppl A):58–66.

640. Arkell D, Ashrap M, Andrews JM, et al. An evaluation of the penetration of cefepime into prostate tissue in patients undergoing elective prostatectomy. *J Antimicrob Chemother* 1992;29:473–474.

641. Sasagawa I, Yamaguchi O, Shiraiwa Y. Cefminox sodium penetration into prostatic tissue with and without inflammation. *Int Urol Nephrol* 1991;23:569–572.

642. Melloni D, Ammatuna P, Formica P, et al. Pharmacokinetic study on adenomatous prostate tissue concentration of cefoperazone. *Chemotherapy* 1989;35:410–415.

643. Schalkhauser K, Adam D. Zur diffusion von Cefotaxim in verschiedene Gewebe des urologischen Bereichs. *Infection* 1980;8(Suppl 3):S327–S329.

644. Grabe M, Andersson K-E, Forsgren A, et al. Concentrations of cefotaxime in serum, urine and tissues of urological patients. *Infection* 1981;9:154–158.

645. Saxby MF, Arkell DG, Andrews JM, et al. Penetration of cefpirome into prostatic tissue. *J Antimicrob Chemother* 1990;25:488–490.

646. Whitby M, Hempenstall J, Gilpin C, et al. Penetration of monobactam antibiotics (aztreonam, carumonam) into human prostatic tissue. *Chemotherapy* 1989;35:7–11.

647. Abbas AMA, Taylor MC, DaSilva C, et al. Penetration of ceftazidime into the human prostate gland following intravenous injection. *J Antimicrob Chemother* 1985;15:119–121.

648. Smith Kline & French Laboratories. Data on file. Philadelphia, PA.

649. Adam D, Naber KG. Concentrations of ceftriaxone in prostate adenoma tissue. *Chemotherapy* 1984;30:16.

650. Adam D, Hofstetter AG, Eisenberger F, et al. Zur Diffusion von Cefacetril in das Prostatagewebe. *Med Welt* 1978;29:1216–1217.

651. Symes JM, Jarvic JD, Tresidder GC. An appraisal of cephalexin monohydrate levels in semen and prostatic tissue. *Chemotherapy* 1975;20:257–262.

652. Litvak AS, Franks CD, Vaught SK, et al. Cefazolin and cephalexin levels in prostatic tissue and sera. *Urology* 1976;7:497–498.

653. Adam D, Hofstetter AG, Staehler G. Studies on diffusion of cephapirin into prostatic tissue. *Fortschr Med* 1977;95:2107–2109.

654. Yamada Y, Ikawa K, Nakamura K, et al. Penetration of doripenem into prostatic tissue following intravenous administration in prostatectomy patients. *Int J Antimicrob Agents* 2010;35:504–506.

655. Smith RP, Wilbur H, Sutphen NT, et al. Moxalactam concentrations in human prostatic tissue. *Antimicrob Agents Chemother* 1983;24:15–17.

656. Klotz T, Braun M, Bin Saleh A, et al. Penetration of a single infusion of ampicillin and sulbactam into prostatic tissue during transurethral prostatectomy. *Int Urol Nephrol* 1999;31:203–209.

657. Smith R, Wilbur H, Bassey C, et al. Azlocillin and mezolocillin concentration in human prostatic tissue. *Chemotherapy* 1988;34:267–271.

658. Hoogkamp-Korstanje JAA, van Oort HJ, Schipper JJ, et al. Intraprostatic concentration of ciprofloxacin and its activity against urinary pathogens. *J Antimicrob Chemother* 1984;14:641–645.

659. Drusano GL, Preston SL, Van Guilder M, et al. A population pharmacokinetic analysis of the penetration of the prostate by levofloxacin. *Antimicrab Agents Chemother* 2000;44(8):2046–2051.

660. Kovarik JM, De Hond JAPM, Hoepelman IM, et al. Intraprostatic distribution of lomefloxacin following multiple-dose administration. *Antimicrob Agents Chemother* 1990;34:2398–2401.

661. Bergeron MG, Thabet M, Toy R, et al. Norfloxacin penetration into human renal and prostatic tissues. *Antimicrob Agents Chemother* 1985;28:349–350.

662. Giannopoulos A, Koratzanis G, Giamarellos-Bourboulis EJ. Pharmacokinetics of intravenously administered pefloxacin in the prostate; perspectives for its application in surgical prophylaxis. *Int J Antimicrob Agents* 2001;17:221–224.

663. Foulds G, Madsen P, Cox C, et al. Concentration of azithromycin in human prostatic tissue. *Eur J Clin Microbiol Infect Dis* 1991;10:868–871.

664. Giannopoulos A, Koratzanis G, Giamarellos-Bourboulis EJ, et al. Pharmacokinetics of clarithromycin in the prostate: implications for the treatment of chronic abacterial prostatitis. *J Urol* 2001;165:97–99.

665. Baumueller A, Hoyme U, Madsen PO. Rosamicin: a new drug for the treatment of bacterial prostatitis. *Antimicrob Agents Chemother* 1977;12:240–242.

666. Fraschini F, Scaglione F, Falchi M, et al. Miokamycin penetration into oral cavity tissues and crevicular fluid. *Int J Clin Pharmacol Res* 1989;9:293–296.

667. Macfarlane JA, Walsh JM, Mitchell AAB, et al. Spiramycin in the prevention of postoperative staphylococcal infection. *Lancet* 1968;1:1–4.

668. Oosterlinck W, Defoort R, Renders G. The concentration of sulphamethoxazole and trimethoprim in human prostate gland. *Br J Urol* 1975;47:301–304.

669. Plomp TA, Mattelaer JJ, Maes RAA. The concentration of thiamphenicol in seminal fluid and prostatic tissue. *J Antimicrob Chemother* 1978;4:65–71.

APPENDIX 14.1

Urinary Excretion, Metabolites, and Reported Urine Levels (with Normal Renal Function) of Selected Antimicrobials

Drug	Excretion[a]	Metabolites	Urine Levels (µg/mL); Dose[b]
Penicillins			
Natural penicillins			
Penicillin G	TS, GF, some TR	Predominantly parent compound, small amount of inactive penicil-loic acid (169)	Mean, 597 in 3 h; 500 mg
Phenoxymethyl-penicillin	TS, GF, some TR	34% penicilloic acid	400–600 units/mL; 500 mg
Aminopenicillins			
Ampicillin	TS, GF	11% penicilloic acid	160–700 in 6 h; 500 mg p.o. 1,000–2,250 in 6 h; 1 g/i.m.
Amoxicillin	TS, GF	20% penicilloic acid	300–1,300 over 6 h; 250–500 mg p.o.
Penicillinase-resistant penicillins			
Cloxacillin, oxacillin, dicloxacillin, flucloxacillin	TS, GF	90% parent compound, <10% bioactive metabolites	>1,000; 1 g i.v.
Methicillin	GF, TS	Parent compound	
Nafcillin	GF, TS	30% parent compound	285–1,188 for 0–6 h; 500 mg i.m.
Carboxypenicillins			
Carbenicillin	TS, GF	>95% parent compound	5,000–10,000; 5 g i.v. >1,000 for 0–3 h; 1 g p.o.
Ticarcillin	TS, GF	Predominantly parent compound, 10%–15% inactive penicilloic acid	600–2,500; 3 g i.v.
Ureidopenicillins			
Piperacillin	TS, GF	Parent compound	Mean, 13,000 over 8 h; 2 g i.v.
Azlocillin	TS, GF	Parent compound	2,240–5,000 in 2 h; 2–4 g i.v.
Mezlocillin	TS, GF	Parent compound	Mean, 3,400 over 6 h; 3 g i.v.
Amdinocillin (mecillinam)	GF, TS	Four metabolites, three bioactive	92–365 for 0–6 h; 400 mg pivmecillinam p.o.
β-Lactamase inhibitors			
Clavulanic acid	GF	Several metabolities	Mean, 403 for 0–4 h; 125 mg
Sulbactam	TS, GF	75% parent compound	
Tazobactam	GF, TS	25% open-ring metabolite	
Cephalosporins			
Cephalothin	GF, TS	33% desacetyl derivative (less active)	707 at 6 h; 500 mg i.m.
Cephalexin	GF, TS	Parent compound	Mean, 2,300 at 1–2 h; 500 mg q.i.d. 5,000–10,000 at 1–2 h; 1.0 g q.i.d.
Cefazolin	GF, TS	Parent compound	700–2,000 in 4–6 h; 1 g i.v.
Cephapirin	GF, TS	40% desacetyl derivatives (active)	300–2,500 over 6 h; 1 g i.v.
Cephradine	GF, TS	Parent compound	Mean, 1.1–3.2 mg/mL first 2 h; 500 mg p.o.
Cefonicid	GF, TR	Parent compound	162–1,017 for 0–2 h; 7.5 mg/kg i.v.
Cephaloridine	GF, some TS	Parent compound	400–1,200 over 6 h; 500 mg i.m.
Cefamandole	GF, TS	Parent compound	1,500–3,100 for 0–2 h; 1 g i.v.
Cefoxitin	GF, TS	About 1% descarbamyl derivative	450–7,200; 1 g i.v. 300–3,600; 500 mg every 6 h over 6 h

APPENDIX 14.1 *(Continued)*

Urinary Excretion, Metabolites, and Reported Urine Levels (with Normal Renal Function) of Selected Antimicrobials

Drug	Excretion[a]	Metabolites	Urine Levels (μg/mL); Dose[b]
Cefotetan	GF, little TS	Parent compound, some bioactive tautomer	1,000 at 1 h; 0.5 g i.m. 2,000 at 1 h; 1 g i.m.
Cefotiam	GF, TS	Insufficient data	>25 at 8–10 h; 2 g i.v.
Ceforanide	GF, TS	Parent compound	
Cefuroxime	GF, TS	Parent compound	1,000–7,000 at 1–2 h; 750 mg to 1 g i.v.
Cefmenoxime	GF, TS	Parent compound	Mean, 3,000; 1 g i.v.
Cefaclor	GF, TS	Some metabolites	1,017 for 0–2 h; 250 mg p.o.
Cefadroxil	GF, TS	Parent compound	1,200; 0.5 p.o.
Cefetamet	GF, some TS	Unchanged	832–1,120 at 2–4 h; 1.5 g p.o.
Cefpodoxime proxetil	24%–36% of dose in 24 h	Little metabolism	19.8 for 8–12 h; 200 mg p.o. for 4 h; 0.25–1 g
Ceprozil	GF, TS	Unchanged	175–658 for 4 h; 0.25–1 g
Cefepime	70%–99%	Unchanged	292–3,120 for 4 h; 0.5–2.0 g
Cefotaxime	GF, TS	30% parent compound, substantial active desacetyl cefotaxime	250–1,500 for 0–6 h; 500 mg i.m. 1,900–4,000, 0–6 h; 2 g i.v.
Cefoperazone	15%–37% excreted by GF, little TS	Parent compound	1,000–2,000 for 0–6 h; 2 g i.v. 120–600 for 0–6 h; 500 mg i.m.
Cefixime	20% excreted	Insufficient data	21–139 at 2–4 h; 400 mg p.o.
Ceftizoxime	GF, TS	Parent compound	≤95 over 18 h; 2–4 g i.v. Mean, 6,150 over 2 h; 1 g i.v.
Ceftazidime	GF	Parent compound	Mean, 526 for 0–2 h; 1 g i.v.
Ceftriaxone	CF	Parent compound	Mean, 855; 1 g i.v.
Cefsulodin	GF, little TS, possible TR	Insufficient data	Mean, 1,400 for 0–2 h; 1 g i.v.
Cefpiramide	23% excreted by GF, little TS	No active metabolities	377–1,087 for 0–2 h; 500–1,000 mg i.v.
Other β-lactams			
Doripenem	GF, TS	70% unchanged, 15% inactive metabolite	601 in 4 h, 500 mg i.v.
Ertapenem		80%, 38% unchanged, 37% inactive metabolite	
Loracabef	GF, TS	Unchanged	12 at 6–12 h; 200 mg
Moxalactam	GF, some TS	Parent compound	565–1,700 for 0–6 h; 500 mg i.m. 1,900–7,500 for 0–6 h; 2 g i.v.
Imipenem/cilastatin	GF, 30% TS	Imipenem: 6%–30% parent without cilastatin, 70% with cilastatin; cilastatin: 76% parent, 14% N-acetyl derivative	500 at 2 h; for 500 mg i.v.
Meropenem	GF, TS	80% unchanged, 20% open-ring metabolite	
Monobactams			
Aztreonam	GF, some TS	Some hydrolysis	1,000–5,000 for 0–2.5 h; 1 g i.v.
Carumonam	GF	10%–15% inactive opening form	26–792; 2 g i.v.

(Continued)

APPENDIX 14.1 *(Continued)*

Urinary Excretion, Metabolites, and Reported Urine Levels (with Normal Renal Function) of Selected Antimicrobials

Drug	Excretion[a]	Metabolites	Urine Levels (μg/mL); Dose[b]
Aminoglycosides			
Amikacin	GF, some TR	Parent compound	170–1,720; 300 mg/m^2 i.v.
Gentamicin	GF	Parent compound	400–500 at 2–4 h;1.6 mg/kg i.m.
Kanamycin	GF, some TR	Parent compound	250–3,100; 300 mg/m^2 i.v.
Netilmicin	GF (?), some TR	Parent compound	Mean, 110 for 0–8 h; 2 mg/kg i.v.
Tobramycin	GF	Parent compound	94–443 in 1 h; 1 mg/kg i.m.
Macrolides and lincosamides			
Erythromycin	TS (?), TR (?)	5%–10% unchanged, N-demethyl metabolite	Mean, 30 for 0–6 h; 1 g every 8 h
Lincomycin	5%–25% excreted	Insufficient data	2–255 for 0–4 h; 500 mg p.o.
Clindamycin	≤6% excreted	N-demethyl and sulfoxide metabolites (both bioactive)	8–20 over 24 h; 150 mg p.o.
Roxithromycin	7%–8% excreted	Three major metabolites	
Clarithromycin	40% in 24 h	32% parent compound or 14-OH metabolite (active), several other metabolites	
Azithromycin	6% in 24 h	Parent compound	
Tetracyclines			
Tetracycline	GF	Parent compound	Mean, 273 for 0–8 h; 500 mg
Doxycycline	GF, some TR	Parent compound	Mean, 134 over 4 h; 100 mg p.o.
Minocycline	<10% in urine GF	Uncharacterized metabolites	Mean, 9.4; 150 mg 8.1–19.4 over 12 h; 200 mg
Sulfonamides and trimethoprim			
Sulfadiazine	GF, TS	Substantial inactive acetyl derivative, some glucuronide	13–150 at 8 h; 3 g p.o.
Sulfisoxazole	GF, TS	30%–50% acetyl derivative	65% of 500 mg over 24 h; 4 g i. v. 67% of 2,377 mg over 24 h; 3 g p.o.
Sulfamethoxazole	GF, TS, TR	20%–40% parent compound, glucuronide, hydroxymethyl, and acetyl metabolites	100–600; 500 mg p.o. b.i.d.
Trimethoprim	GF, TS	25%–60% parent compound, several metabolites	70–100 for 0–4 h; 100 mg
Trimethoprim/ sulfamethoxazole			31–165/10–133; 160/800 b.i.d.
Quinolones			
Nalidixic acid	Insufficient data	85% inactive glucuronide, some active hydroxynalidixic acid	63–1,000; 1 or 2 g p.o. q.i.d.
Cinoxacin	GF	50%–60% parent compound, four inactive metabolites	Mean, 390 for 0–2 h; 500 mg p.o.
Norfloxacin	GF, TS	25%–40% parent compound, 15%–20% as six metabolites (some active)	168–417 for 0–3 h; 400 mg
Ciprofloxacin	GF, TS	25%–50% parent compound, 10%–15% as four metabolites	>2 at 12–24 h; 500 mg

APPENDIX 14.1 *(Continued)*

Urinary Excretion, Metabolites, and Reported Urine Levels (with Normal Renal Function) of Selected Antimicrobials

Drug	Excretion[a]	Metabolites	Urine Levels (μg/mL); Dose[b]
Enoxacin	GF, TS	40%–60% parent compound, 10%–15% metabolites	>8 at 24–48 h; 600 mg p.o.
Moxifloxacin	20% unchanged	Primarily glucuronide conjugate	
Ofloxacin	GF, TS	70%–90% parent compound, 5%–15% as two metabolites	126–438 for 0–3 h; 100 mg i.v.
Pefloxacin	8%–9% excreted unchanged	24%–50% metabolites, major norfloxacin (active), four others	Mean, 42 for 0–24 h; 800 mg p.o.
Fleroxacin	GF	60% unchanged, 7% N-demethyl (active), 4.5% N-oxide (inactive)	100–200 for 8 h; 200–800 mg p.o.
Lomefloxacin	GF, TS	Small amount of unidentified metabolites	100–250 for 12 h; 200 mg
Levofloxacin	GF	Mainly unchanged	286 at 2–4 h; 200 mg
Other antimicrobials			
Chloramphenicol	GF	<10% parent compound, inactive glucuronide (TS, GF), unhydrolyzed succinate ester	15–200 at 2 h; 1 g p.o.
Colistimethate	Insufficient data	Sulfomethyl derivative	2.6–3.6 for 0–6 h; 30 mg i.m.
Daptomycin	78%	Unchanged	
Fusidic acid	Not excreted	Insufficient data	<0.8 μg; 500 p.o. t.i.d.
Linezolid	30% unchanged	10%–40% as hydroxyethyl glycine metabolite and aminoethoxyacetic acid metabolite	
Methenamine mandelate	GF, some TR	Insufficient data	300–3,000 formaldehyde; 1 g q.i.d. p.o.
Metronidazole	GF, TR (?)	15% parent compound, oxidative metabolites (some bioactive) glucuronic acid conjugates	Mean, 15–67 for 4–8 h; 0.25 mg p.o. 76–115 for 4–8 h; 0.50 mg
Nitrofurantoin	GF, TS, TR	30% parent compound	25–300; 100 mg p.o. q.i.d.
Polymyxin B	Insufficient data	60% parent compound	20–100; 2.5–3.0 mg/kg/day
Rifabutin	50% recovered	8% unchanged, >20 metabolites (some bioactive)	
Rifampin	6%–30% excreted GF	Desacetyl derivative (active)	Mean, 34–50 at 12 h; 300 mg p.o. even, 12 h
Tigecycline	33%	22% unchanged	
Spectinomycin	GF	Parent compound	Mean, 1,600 for 0–6 h; 2 g/day
Teicoplanin	GF	<5% metabolites in rats	Mean, 43 for 0–4 h; 440 mg i.v.
Vancomycin	GF	Parent compound	800; 1 g i.v.
Antifungals			
Amphotercin B	GF, <10% excreted		0.51–4.61 mg/24 h; 5–105 mg
5-Fluorocytocine	GF	99% parent	>2,000 for 0–6 h; 3–5 g
Fluconazole	GF, TR	80% parent compound, 11% metabolites	118 for 0–24 h
Itraconazole	<1%	10 urinary metabolites	

[a]TS, tubular secretion; GF, glomerular filtration; TR, tubular resorption.
[b]p.o., orally; i.m., intramuscularly; i.v., intravenously; b.i.d., twice per day; t.i.d., three times per day; q.i.d., four times per day.
From Nicolle LE. Measurement and significance of antibiotic activity in the urine. In: Lorian V, ed. *Antibiotics in laboratory medicine.* 4th ed. Baltimore: Lippincott Williams & Wilkins, 1996:794–798, with permission.

Antiinfective Resistance Resource Guide

Daniel Amsterdam

Antimicrobial resistance is recognized as a significant worldwide public health concern. Several key health care quality indicators focus on infection prevention and treatment, including selective use of antimicrobial agents, length of hospital stay, ventilator-associated pneumonia, catheter-associated infections, surgical site infections, and readmission rates. These indicators are clearly influenced by resistance to antimicrobial agents (1).

The recognition that resistance to therapeutic agents has increased in recent decades has been reported by laboratories identifying clinical isolates exhibiting resistance to many antimicrobial agents (2,3). Resistance is relevant to all microbiologic species, encompassing viruses, bacteria, mycobacteria, fungi, protozoa, and parasites. Commonly identified bacteria exhibiting resistance to antibiotics have broad implications in our hospitals and clinics (1). Such organisms include *Staphylococcus aureus*, *Streptococcus pneumoniae*, *Enterococcus* species, *Acinetobacter* species, *Pseudomonas* species, and *Klebsiella* (2–4). Antibiotic stewardship programs and antibiograms are approaches used by experts in clinical microbiology and pharmacology to inform clinicians about the state and extent of antimicrobial resistance in their institutions to ensure appropriate use of antimicrobial agents (1). These practitioners also evaluate and compare changes in resistance patterns at their institutions with those reported elsewhere. The data repositories documenting these changes are demonstrated by the Web sites provided in the attached tables.

Given the rapid changes in resistance of microbes in recent decades, clinical microbiologists, pharmacologists, and clinicians, including infectious disease experts, must be able to quickly retrieve this information. Such data resources will also assist those caring for individuals harboring resistant organisms from other areas of the world, and may prevent the spread of antibiotic-resistant microorganisms. These resources can also provide materials to educate the community about issues of resistance.

Web sites that contained information on antimicrobial resistance have been previously published (2–4). Provided in this Appendix are updated representative Web sites, links, and international networks relevant to the problem of antimicrobial resistance to facilitate the work of clinicians, laboratorians, and pharmacologists involved with prevention, research, education, and care of individuals infected by potentially resistant microorganisms.

Table 1

General Resources			
Title/Subject	**Web Address**	**Source**	**Comments**
Antimicrobial Resistance in Canada	www.can-r.com	CARA	Online research portal for Canadian health care providers on antimicrobial resistance in Canada
Antibiotic resistance threats in the United States	http://www.cdc.gov /drugresistance/threat-report-2013/	CDC	Site and links regarding antibiotic-resistant organisms with greatest risk to human health
Common resistant organisms	http://www.cdc.gov /drugresistance /diseasesconnectedar.html	CDC	Excellent updated overview of the most common resistant organisms
Antibiotic/antimicrobial resistance	http://www.cdc.gov /drugresistance/index.html	CDC National Center for Emerging and Zoonotic Infectious Diseases	Several links to updated reports from CDC
Antibiotic awareness European health initiative	http://www.ecdc.europa.eu/en /activities/surveillance/EARS-Net /Pages/index.aspx	ECDC	Excellent maps showing changes in resistance patterns and links to other useful sites
Antimicrobial resistance	http://www.idsociety.org/Topic _Antimicrobial_Resistance/	IDSA	Updated site on IDSA policies, initiatives, and advocacy efforts to address resistance concerns
Antibiotic resistance policy newsletter	http://www.idsociety .org/uploadedFiles/IDSA /Policy_and_Advocacy /Current_Topics_and_Issues /Antimicrobial_Resistance /Strengthening_US_Efforts /STAAR_Act/	IDSA	Excellent links to policies and information on resistance
Joint program initiative on antimicrobial resistance	http://www.jpiamr.eu/	JPIAMR	Resource from the European Union to coordinate research on antimicrobial resistance
"Bugs & Drugs on the Web" Web site	http://www.antibioticresistance .org.uk/	National Electronic Library of Infection	Provides information for the public on appropriate use of antimicrobials
Antimicrobial resistance	http://www.niaid.nih.gov/Pages	NIAID	Updates and links to reports from NIH and NIAID
Antimicrobial (drug) resistance	http://www.niaid.nih.gov /topics/antimicrobialResistance /Understanding/Pages/causes .aspx	NIAID	Public site with information and updates on resistance and drug use
UK 5-year antimicrobial resistance strategy 2013 to 2018	https://www.gov.uk /government/publications /uk-5-year-antimicrobial-resistance-strategy-2013-to-2018	UK DOH site	Site covering cross-government UK strategy to decrease antimicrobial resistance
Drug resistance	http://www.who.int /drugresistance/en/	WHO	Global health emergency data exemplified by resistance to virtually all antimicrobials

Table 2

Antibacterial Resources			
Title/Subject	**Web Address**	**Source**	**Comments**
Antibiotic resistance threats	http://www.cdc.gov/drugresistance/index.html	CDC	Resource covering a broad range of topics with links to policies, educational materials, and research
CRE	http://www.cdc.gov/hai/organisms/cre/	CDC	Updated Web page about CRE in health care settings
Health care–associated infections with VISA/VRSA	http://www.cdc.gov/HAI/organisms/visa_vrsa/visa_vrsa.html	CDC	Updated information on VISA/VRSA organisms and links to other sites
MRSA resource	http://www.cdc.gov/mrsa/	CDC	Resources focused on research, updates, and education regarding MRSA infections
NARMS	http://www.cdc.gov/narms	CDC	Site to provide updates in tracking of resistant bacteria
VRE	http://www.cdc.gov/hai/organisms/vre/vre.html	CDC	Updated Web page about VRE in health care settings
VRE and other resistant organisms	http://www.cddep.org/ResistanceMap/bug-drug/VRE	CDDEP	Links and networks about health policy surrounding resistance in VRE and other organisms
VRE, *Clostridium difficile*, CRE	http://www.ipac-canada.org/links_aro.php	IPAC	Site with lots of excellent links for public awareness and policy about resistance
Antibiotics and antibiotic resistance	http://www.fda.gov/Drugs/ResourcesForYou/Consumers/BuyingUsingMedicineSafely/AntibioticsandAntibioticResistance/default.htm	FDA	Site with resources, links, and information for consumers
Antibiotic resistance Web page	http://www.harfordcountyhealth.com/wp-content/uploads/2011/02/Antibiotic-Resistance-Web-Page	Harford County Health Department	Resource and links: summary for consumers and professionals
Antibiotic resistance in Australia	http://www.nps.org.au/about-us/what-we-do/campaigns-events/antibiotic-resistance-fighter	National Prescribing Service; Australian DOH and Ageing	Resources and links on efforts to address antibiotic resistance in Australia
Clinical research network on antibacterial resistance	http://www.niaid.nih.gov/topics/antimicrobialresistance/Pages/default.aspx	NIAID, Division of Microbiology and Infectious Diseases	Resource for clinical research opportunities to address antibacterial resistance
ESBLs as a source of resistance	http://www.hpa.org.uk/Topics/InfectiousDiseases/InfectionsAZ/ESBLs/	Public Health England	Updated information and links to other sites/networks in England and Europe

(Continued)

Table 2 (continued)

Antibacterial Resources			
Title/Subject	**Web Address**	**Source**	**Comments**
VISA/VRSA and CRE	http://www.dshs.state .tx.us/idcu/health /antibiotic_resistance/	Texas Department of State Health Services	Networks and links on VISA/ VRSA and CRE
Bacterial Epidemiology and Antimicrobial Resistance Research Unit	http://www.ars.usda .gov/main/site_main .htm?modecode=66-12-05	USDA Agricultural Research Service	Resource focused on antimi- crobial resistance in zoonotic foodborne pathogens and commensal bacteria
VISA/VRSA	http://www.dhhr.wv.gov /oeps/disease/IBD_VPD /IBD/Pages/MRSA.aspx	West Virginia Department of Health and Human Resources	Updated information on VISA/VRSA organisms and links to other sites

Table 3

Antimycobacterial Resources			
Title/Subject	**Web Address**	**Source**	**Comments**
Extensively drug-resistant TB	http://www.cdc.gov/tb/topic /laboratory/BiosafetyGuidance _xdrtb.htm	CDC	Information on laboratory safety for XDR *Mycobacterium* TB; multiple links to other resources
MDR-TB	http://www.eurosurveillance .org/ViewArticle.aspx ?ArticleId=20742	ECDC	Eurosurveillance article on MDR-TB and links to many other resistance data and scholarly articles
MDR-TB	http://www.european-lung- foundation.org/16166 -multidrug-resistant -tuberculosis-mdr-tb.htm	European Lung Foundation	Updated information about TB for public health education; documents in multiple languages; links to additional resources
TB	http://www.tbfacts.org /drug-resistant-tb.html	GHE of the United Kingdom	Great information on TB and other coinfections from a nonprofit whose focus is TB
Drug-resistant TB	http://www.who.int/tb /challenges/mdr/tdrfaqs/en/	WHO	FAQs with multiple links to other resources

Table 4

Antifungal Resources			
Title/Subject	**Web Address**	**Source**	**Comments**
Fungal resistance	http://ec.europa.eu/research /health/infectious-diseases /antimicrobial-drug-resistance /projects/041_en.html	EURESFUN network	Fungal drug resistance Web site for funding information for research
Antifungal susceptibility testing	http://mycology.adelaide.edu .au/Laboratory_Methods /Antifungal_Susceptibility _Testing/methods.html	University of Adelaide, Australia	Methods to identify resistance to antimycotics with links to detailed information

Table 5

Antiviral Resources

Title/Subject	Web Address	Source	Comments
Influenza viral resistance	http://www.cdc.gov/flu/professionals/antivirals/antiviral-drug-resistance.htm	CDC	Updated information on influenza virus resistance
Resistance by HIV, hepatitis C, and other viral infections	https://www.iasusa.org/	IAS-USA	Up-to-date information and resource for those caring for patients with resistant viral infections
Hepatitis and HIV coinfection and resistance	http://www.hivandhepatitis.com/2009icr/icaac/docs/091509_f.html	ICAAC	HIV and hepatitis B coinfection may cause resistance; links to other resources on hepatitis B and hepatitis C as well
HIV resistance	http://home.ncifcrf.gov/hivdrp/related_sites.html	National Cancer Institute	Excellent site on HIV viral resistance with multiple links to other sites and networks
HIV resistance	http://hivdb.stanford.edu/pages/links.html	Stanford University HIV drug resistance database	HIV treatment and resistance Web site with multiple links

Table 6

Antiinfective Agents: Guidelines for Use

Title/Subject	Web Address	Source	Comments
Influenza	http://www.cdc.gov/flu/PROFESSIONALS/ANTIVIRALS/index.htm http://www.ammi.ca/guidelines	CDC Association of Medical Microbiology and Infectious Disease Canada	
Hepatitis B and C	http://www.hepatitis.va.gov/provider/guidelines/	U.S. Department of Veterans Affairs	
Hepatitis C	http://www.hcvguidelines.org	IDSA	Up-to-date summary of Hepatitis C and its treatment.
HIV/ARV	http://aidsinfo.nih.gov/guidelines	NIH	
Tuberculosis	http://www.cdc.gov/tb/publications/guidelines/treatment.htm	CDC	
Pneumococcus	http://www.cdc.gov/pneumococcal/clinicians/diagnosis-medical-mgmt.html	CDC	
Organism by organism	http://www.idsociety.org/organism/	IDSA	Up-to-date references for bacteria, fungi, parasites, mycobacteria, and viruses/HIV

Abbreviations and Acronyms

CARA	Canadian Antimicrobial Resistance Alliance	ICAAC	Interscience Conference on Antimicrobial Agents and Chemotherapy
CDC	Centers for Disease Control and Prevention	IDSA	Infectious Disease Society of America
CDDEP	The Center for Disease Dynamics, Economics & Policy	IPAC	Infection Prevention and Control Canada
CRE	Carbapenem-resistant Enterobacteriaceae	JPIAMR	Joint Programming Initiative on Antimicrobial Resistance
DOH	Department of Health	MRSA	Methicillin-resistant *Staphylococcus aureus*
EARS-Net EU	European Antimicrobial Resistance Surveillance Network	NARMS	National Antimicrobial Resistance Monitoring System for Enteric Bacteria
ECDC	European Centre for Disease Prevention and Control	NCI	National Cancer Institute, USA
ESBL	Extended-spectrum β-lactamase	NIAID	National Institute of Allergy and Infectious Diseases
EURESFUN	European Resistance Fungal Network consortium	NIH	National Institutes of Health
FDA	U.S. Food and Drug Administration	TB; MDR-TB; XDR	*Mycobacterium* tuberculosis; multidrug-resistant TB; Extensively drug-resistant
GHE of the United Kingdom	Global Health Education	USDA	U.S. Department of Agriculture
HIV	Human Immunodeficiency Virus	VISA/VRSA	Vancomycin-intermediate *Staphylococcus aureus* /vancomycin-resistant *Staphylococcus aureus*
HR	Human Resources	VRE	Vancomycin-resistant Enterococcus
IAS-USA	International Antiviral Society-USA	WHO	World Health Organization

REFERENCES

1 Davey P, Brown E, Charani E, et al. Interventions to improve antibiotic prescribing practices for hospital inpatients. *Cochrane Database Syst Rev* 2013;(4):CD003543.

2 Harbarth S, Emonet S. Navigating the World Wide Web in search of resources on antimicrobial resistance. *Clin Infect Dis* 2006;43:72–78.

3 Falagas ME, Karveli EA. World Wide Web resources on antimicrobial resistance. *Clin Infect Dis* 2006;43:630–633.

4 Zhanel GG, Low DE. Launching of the CAN-R Web site—the official Web site of the Canadian Antimicrobial Resistance Alliance. *Can J Infect Dis Med Microbiol* 2007;18:151–152.

NOTE: Page numbers in *italics* indicate figures; page numbers followed by t indicate tables.

Cefsulodin
  in aqueous humor, 724t
  in breast milk, 709t
  in cerebrospinal fluid, 720t
  concentration in cutaneous blisters,
      disks, threads, 695t
  concentrations in cardiac tissue, 736t
  concentrations in prostatic tissue,
      744t
  serum kinetics and urinary
      excretion, 750t
  in skeletal muscle, 727t
  in sputum, 705t
  susceptibility of *C. trachomatis* and
      C. pneumoniae, 293t
Ceftaroline
  serum kinetics and urinary
      excretion, 750t
  solvents and diluents for
      preparation, 65t
Ceftazidime
  in aqueous humor, 724t
  in breast milk, 709t
  in cerebrospinal fluid, 720t
  concentration in ascites, 687t
  concentration in bile, 700t
  concentration in cutaneous blisters,
      disks, threads, 695t
  concentration in pleural fluid, 690t
  concentrations in bone, 731t
  concentrations in gallbladder, 738t
  concentrations in prostatic tissue,
      744t
  pH effects, 70t
  QC ranges of MIC, 87t
  screening and confirmatory tests,
      127t
  serum kinetics and urinary
      excretion, 750t
  in skeletal muscle, 727t
  solvents and diluents for
      preparation, 65t
Ceftibiprole, solvents and diluents for
      preparation, 65t
Ceftibuten
  concentration in cutaneous blisters,
      disks, threads, 695t
  QC ranges of MIC, 87t
  serum kinetics and urinary
      excretion, 750t
  solvents and diluents for
      preparation, 65t
Ceftizoxime
  in aqueous humor, 724t
  in breast milk, 710t
  in cerebrospinal fluid, 720t
  concentration in bile, 700t
  concentration in cutaneous blisters,
      disks, threads, 695t
  concentration in pleural fluid, 690t
  concentrations in bone, 731t
  concentrations in cardiac tissue,
      736t
  concentrations in gallbladder, 738t
  concentrations in prostatic tissue,
      744t

QC ranges of MIC, 87t
  serum kinetics and urinary
      excretion, 750t
  in sputum, 705t
Ceftriaxone
  against *A. phagocytophilum*, *E. canis*,
      and *E. chaffeensis*, 305t
  in aqueous humor, 724t
  in breast milk, 710t
  in cerebrospinal fluid, 720t
  concentration in ascites, 687t
  concentration in bile, 700t
  concentration in cutaneous blisters,
      disks, threads, 695t
  concentration in pleural fluid, 691t
  concentrations in bone, 731t
  concentrations in cardiac tissue,
      736t
  concentrations in gallbladder, 738t
  concentrations in lung tissue, 741t
  concentrations in prostatic tissue,
      744t
  pH effects, 70t
  QC ranges of MIC, 87t
  screening and confirmatory tests,
      127t
  serum kinetics and urinary
      excretion, 750t
  in skeletal muscle, 727t
  in sputum, 705t
  standard buffer for, 330t
  standard curve concentrations for,
      333t
  susceptibility of *B. burgdorferi*, 310t
  susceptibility of *C. trachomatis* and
      C. pneumoniae, 293t
  susceptibility of *T. pallidum*, 311t
Ceftrizine, in sinus secretions, 714t
Cefuroxime
  in aqueous humor, 724t
  in cerebrospinal fluid, 720t
  concentration in ascites, 687t
  concentration in bile, 700t
  concentration in cutaneous blisters,
      disks, threads, 695t
  concentration in pleural fluid, 691t
  concentrations in bone, 731t
  concentrations in gallbladder, 738t
  concentrations in prostatic tissue,
      745t
  QC ranges of MIC, 87t
  serum kinetics and urinary
      excretion, 750t
  solvents and diluents for
      preparation, 65t
  in sputum, 705t
Cell wall/biofilm structures, gram-
      positive and gram-negative
      microorganisms, 454–457,
      455
Cellular reservoirs, in resistance testing,
      508
Cephacetrile
  concentration in bile, 700t
  concentrations in prostatic tissue,
      745t

Cephalexin
  in aqueous humor, 724t
  in breast milk, 710t
  concentration in cutaneous blisters,
      disks, threads, 695t
  concentration in joint fluid, 693t
  concentrations in bone, 731t
  concentrations in prostatic tissue,
      745t
  HPLC performance data, 382t
  pH effects, 70t
  serum kinetics and urinary
      excretion, 750t
  in sinus secretions, 714t
  solvents and diluents for
      preparation, 65t
  in sputum, 705t
Cephaloridine
  in aqueous humor, 724t
  in breast milk, 710t
  in cerebrospinal fluid, 720t
  concentration in bile, 700t
  concentrations in bone, 731t
  serum kinetics and urinary
      excretion, 750t
  standard buffer for, 330t
  standard curve concentrations for,
      333t
Cephalosporins
  gene transfer factors and antibiotic
      resistance, 153t
  HPLC, 376, 382
  increasing inoculum concentrations,
      79t
  inoculum effect, 78t
  mechanisms of action, 466
  pH effects, 69t
  susceptibility of *B. burgdorferi*, 310t
  susceptibility of *C. trachomatis* and
      C. pneumoniae, 293t
Cephalothin
  in aqueous humor, 724t
  in breast milk, 710t
  in cerebrospinal fluid, 720t
  concentration in ascites, 687t
  concentration in bile, 700t
  concentration in cutaneous blisters,
      disks, threads, 695t
  concentration in pleural fluid, 691t
  concentrations in bone, 731t
  concentrations in cardiac tissue,
      736t
  concentrations in prostatic tissue,
      745t
  conditions for plate diffusion assay,
      332t
  filtration effects, 67t
  growth media effects, 69t
  increase of MIC, 73t
  inoculum concentration *E. coli*, 79t
  microdilution and macrodilution
      results, 83t
  pH effects, 70t
  QC ranges of MIC, 87t
  serum kinetics and urinary
      excretion, 750t